# Mosby's Textbook for
# NURSING
# ASSISTANTS

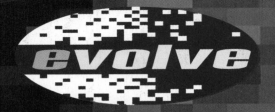

# The Latest *Evolution* in Learning.

Evolve provides online access to free learning resources and activities designed specifically for the textbook you are using in your class. The resources will provide you with information that enhances the material covered in the book and much more.

Visit the Web address listed below to start your learning evolution today!

## Think outside the book... *evolve.*

# Mosby's Textbook for NURSING ASSISTANTS

**6th Edition**

*With 983 Illustrations*

## Sheila A. Sorrentino

### RN, MSN, PhD

**Curriculum and Health Care Consultant**
Normal, Illinois

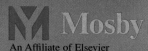
Mosby
An Affiliate of Elsevier

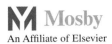
Mosby
An Affiliate of Elsevier

11830 Westline Industrial Drive
St. Louis, Missouri 63146

---

**Notice**

Nursing is an ever-changing field. Standard safety precautions must be followed, but as new research and clinical experience broaden our knowledge, changes in treatment may become necessary or appropriate. Readers are advised to check the most current product information provided by the manufacturer. It is the responsibility of the licensed health care provider, relying on experience and knowledge of the patient or resident, to determine the best treatment for each individual patient or resident. Neither the publisher nor the author assumes any liability for any injury and/or damage to persons or property arising from this publication.

---

Previous editions copyrighted 2000, 1996, 1992, 1987, 1984

International Standard Book Code Number 0-323-02580-3 (SC) 0-323-02579-X (HC)

*Executive Editor:* Suzi Epstein
*Senior Developmental Editor:* Maria Broeker
*Publishing Services Manager:* John Rogers
*Project Manager:* Helen Hudlin, Kathy Teal
*Senior Designer:* Kathi Gosche

Printed in the United States of America

Last digit is the print number:  9  8  7  6  5  4  3  2  1

*To my cousin, Kristine—who studied from a previous edition of this book
and then continued her higher education,*

*and*

*To her husband, Michael, for loving Kristine and for having kissed her hand.*

*Wishing them a lifetime of happiness and joy.*

*Sheila A. Sorrentino*

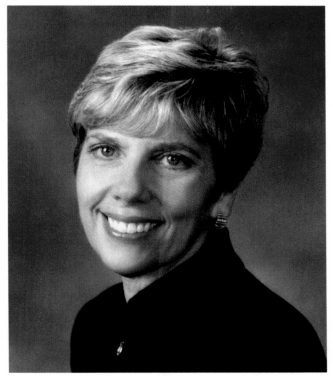

Sheila A. Sorrentino

Sheila A. Sorrentino is currently a curriculum and health care consultant focusing on career ladder nursing programs and effective delegation and partnering with assistive personnel in hospitals, long-term care centers, and home care agencies.

Dr. Sorrentino was instrumental in the development and approval of CNA-PN-ADN programs in the Illinois Community College System and has taught in nursing assistant, practical nursing, associate degree, and baccalaureate and higher degree programs. Her career includes experiences as a nursing assistant, staff nurse, charge nurse, head nurse, nursing educator, assistant dean, dean, and consultant.

A Mosby author since 1982, Dr. Sorrentino has written several textbooks for nursing assistants and other assistive personnel. She was also involved in the development of *Mosby's Nursing Assistant Skills Videos* and *Mosby's Nursing Skills Videos.* An earlier version of

nursing assistant skills videos won the 1992 International Medical Films Award on caregiving.

Dr. Sorrentino has a bachelor of science degree in nursing, a master of arts in education, a master of science degree in community nursing, and a PhD in higher education administration. She is a member of Sigma Theta Tau and Lewis University's Nursing and Health Professions Advisory Committee and a former member and chair of the Central Illinois Higher Education Health Care Task Force. She has also served on the Iowa-Illinois Safety Council Board of Directors and the Board of Directors of Our Lady of Victory Nursing Center in Bourbonnais, Illinois. In 1998 she received an alumni achievement award from Lewis University for outstanding leadership and dedication in nursing education. Her presentations at national conferences focus on delegation and other issues relating to assistive personnel.

# ■ REVIEWERS ■

**Sharon Dillion Alba,** RN, BSN
Associate Professor of Nursing
Western New Mexico University
Silver City, New Mexico

**Lena L. Deter,** MPH, RN
Health Educator & Consultant
DELHEC Educational Services & Consulting
Webster, Massachusetts

**Catherine M. Homard,** RN, MSN
Nurse Aide Instructor
Central Campus Career & Technical Programs
Des Moines, Iowa

**Catherine R. Van Son,** RN, MSN
Older Adult Focus Project Faculty
School of Nursing
Oregon Health & Science University
Portland, Oregon

# ■ ACKNOWLEDGMENTS ■

As with previous editions of *Mosby's Textbook for Nursing Assistants*, many individuals and agencies have contributed to this new, sixth edition by providing information, insights, and resources. I am especially grateful and appreciative of the efforts by:

- Mary Beth Sorrentino-Herron of Illinois Valley Community Hospital in Peru, Illinois, for providing human resource information and forms.
- Linda Sorrentino-Ferrari of Dr. Thomas Curry's office in Peru, Illinois, for providing policy information.
- Deborah Smith of OSF St. Joseph's Medical Center in Bloomington, Illinois, for graciously inviting Mosby to conduct a photo shoot at the hospital.
- Jane DeBlois of OSF St. Joseph's Medical Center in Bloomington, Illinois, for her coordination efforts before and during the photo shoot, which surpassed all expectations and truly defied description. An "angel on earth," Jane made this photo shoot the smoothest and most efficient that I have experienced. Plus, she made it fun for all involved. To her, many more thanks than I can express.
- The OSF St. Joseph's Medical Center staff and volunteers for participating in the photo shoot, especially Joni Schenkel and Staci Sutton. You are gracious, kind, photogenic, and a wonderful group to work with.
- Bernie Gorek, my co-author on *Mosby's Textbook for Long-Term Care Assistants*, edition 4, and *Mosby's Essentials for Nursing Assistants*, edition 2; Pam Randolph of the Arizona State Board of Nursing in Phoenix, Arizona; Tammy Taylor of Heartland Community College in Normal, Illinois; and Julie White of Wilbur Wright College in Chicago, Illinois, for providing valuable insights and information and for serving as informal consultants.
- Photographer Michael DeFilippo of St. Louis, Missouri, for the great photos. It was a pleasure working with him.
- The artists at Graphic World in St. Louis, Missouri, for their talented work.
- Sharon Alba, Lena Deter, Catherine Homard, and Catherine Van Son for reviewing the manuscript and for their candor and suggestions. They have contributed to the thoroughness and accuracy of this book.
- Betty Hazelwood, copy editor, for her attention to detail, questions, and humor. Once again, she made the copyediting process painless, efficient, and pleasant.
- And, finally, to the talented and dedicated Elsevier staff, especially Suzi Epstein, Maria Broeker, Marken Gannon, and the members of John Rogers' production team—Helen Hudlin, Jeanne Genz, Kathi Gosche, and Kathy Teal. In her role as editor, Suzi once again gave guidance and support and kept the project on track. She also stressed the importance of taking care of self. Maria Broeker handled numerous details and manuscript needs. As always, what would I do without Maria? And Marken provided clerical and secretarial assistance. In Kathy Teal's absence (Kathy, I know you were there in spirit), Helen and Jeanne made the production process easy and pleasant. They produced a book that is user friendly and pleasing to the student. And Kathi Gosche created another unique and colorful book and cover design. As always, she made the book distinctive from the rest.
- And to all those who contributed to this effort in any way, I am sincerely grateful.

*Sheila A. Sorrentino*

# ■ INSTRUCTOR PREFACE ■

As with previous editions of *Mosby's Textbook for Nursing Assistants*, this sixth edition serves to prepare students to function as nursing assistants in hospitals, nursing centers, and home care settings. This textbook serves the needs of students and instructors in community colleges, technical schools, high schools, hospitals, nursing centers, and other agencies. As students complete their education, the book is a valuable resource for competency test review. As part of one's personal library, the book is a reference for the nursing assistant who seeks to review or learn additional information for safe care.

The book emphasizes the needs of individuals across the life span, from infancy through old age. Patients and residents are presented as persons with dignity and value who have a past, a present, and a future. Caring, understanding, ensuring the person's rights, and respecting patients and residents as persons with dignity and value are attitudes conveyed throughout the book.

The nursing assistants of today and tomorrow must have a firm understanding of the legal principles affecting their role. Both federal and state laws directly and indirectly define their roles and limitations. Nursing assistant roles and functions also vary among agencies. Therefore emphasis is given to nursing assistant responsibilities and limitations, specifically in Chapter 2, which focuses on the legal and ethical aspects of the nursing assistant role. It includes the reporting of elder, child, and domestic abuse.

Nursing assistant functions and role limits also depend on effective delegation. Building on the delegation principles presented in Chapter 2, *Delegation Guidelines* are presented as they relate to procedures. They empower the student to seek information from the nurse and from the care plan about critical aspects of the procedure and the observations to report and record.

Safety has always been a core value of *Mosby's Textbook for Nursing Assistants.* Because safety issues in health care agencies receive local, state, and national attention, the safety content of this edition has been strengthened and expanded (Chapter 10). A new feature, *Safety Alert,* is integrated throughout the book, but is mainly related to the procedures. The intent is to focus the student's attention on the need to be safe and cautious when giving care.

In addition to legal aspects, delegation, and safety issues, work ethics also affect how nursing assistants function. To foster a positive work ethic, Chapter 3 focuses on workplace behaviors and practices. The goal is for the nursing assistant to be a proud, professional member of the nursing and health teams.

## ORGANIZATIONAL STRATEGIES

These concepts and principles—treating the patient or resident as a person, ethical and legal aspects, delegation, safety, and work ethics—serve as the guiding framework for this book. Other organizational strategies and values include:

- Awareness and understanding of the work setting and the individuals in that setting
- Respect for the patient or resident as a physical, social, psychological, and spiritual being who has basic needs and protected rights
- Respect for personal choice and dignity of person
- Appreciating the role of cultural heritage and religion in health and illness practices
- Understanding body structure and function to give safe care and to safely perform psychomotor skills
- That learning proceeds from the simple to the complex
- That certain concepts and functions are foundational and central to other procedures—safety, body mechanics, and preventing infection
- That the nursing process is the basis for planning and delivering nursing care and that nursing assistants must follow the person's care plan

## CONTENT ISSUES

With every edition, revision and content decisions are made. When changes are made in laws or in guidelines and standards issued by government or accrediting agencies, the decisions are simple. The content is revised or added as needed. Other content issues are more difficult. The learning needs and abilities of the student, instructor desires, and book length are among the factors considered. With such issues in mind, new and expanded content includes:

### Chapter 1: Introduction to Health Care Agencies
- Assisted living *(new)*
- Skilled nursing facilities *(new)*
- Meeting standards (licensure, certification, and accreditation) *(new)*

## CHAPTER 3: WORK ETHICS
- New employee orientation *(new)*
- Managing stress *(new)*

## CHAPTER 4: COMMUNICATING WITH THE HEALTH TEAM
- Problem solving *(new)*
- Medical terminology *(moved)*
- Using computers *(enhanced)*

## CHAPTER 5: ASSISTING WITH THE NURSING PROCESS *(NEW)*
- Assignment sheets *(new)*

## CHAPTER 6: UNDERSTANDING THE PERSON
- FOCUS ON LONG-TERM CARE: SAFETY AND SECURITY NEEDS *(new)*
- FOCUS ON LONG-TERM CARE: PERSONS YOU WILL CARE FOR *(new)*
- FOCUS ON CHILDREN: TOUCH *(new)*
- Disability etiquette *(new)*
- The person who is comatose *(new)*
- Behavior issues *(new)*

## CHAPTER 9: CARE OF THE OLDER PERSON
- Homesharing *(new)*
- Board and care homes *(new)*
- Foster care *(new)*
- Ombudsman program *(new)*

## CHAPTER 10: SAFETY (MOST AREAS EXPANDED)
- Bed rail entrapment *(new)*
- Bed rail 4-inch rule *(new)*
- FOCUS ON CHILDREN: BED RAILS *(enhanced)*
- Household poisons *(new)*
- Electrical shock *(enhanced)*
- Wheelchair and stretcher safety *(new)*
- Bomb threats *(new)*

## CHAPTER 11: RESTRAINT ALTERNATIVES AND SAFE RESTRAINT USE *(NEW)*

## CHAPTER 12: PREVENTING INFECTION
- Preventing foodborne illnesses *(new)*
- FOCUS ON OLDER PERSONS: INFECTION *(new)*
- FOCUS ON OLDER PERSONS: ASEPTIC PRACTICES *(new)*
- Drug-resistant organisms *(new)*

## CHAPTER 13: BODY MECHANICS
- Ergonomics *(new)*
- PROCEDURE: TRANSFERRING THE PERSON FROM THE CHAIR OR WHEELCHAIR TO BED *(new)*
- Transferring a person to and from a toilet *(new)*
- PROCEDURE: TRANSFERRING THE PERSON TO AND FROM THE TOILET *(new)*
- Repositioning in a chair or wheelchair *(new)*

## CHAPTER 15: BEDMAKING
- Alternate method of putting a pillowcase on the pillow *(new)*
- Toe pleat *(new)*

## CHAPTER 16: PERSONAL HYGIENE
- FOCUS ON CHILDREN: ORAL HYGIENE (for infants) *(new)*
- Towel baths *(new)*
- FOCUS ON OLDER PERSONS: TOWEL BATHS *(new)*

## CHAPTER 17: GROOMING
- FOCUS ON OLDER PERSONS: SHAVING *(new)*

## CHAPTER 18: URINARY ELIMINATION
- FOCUS ON CHILDREN: NORMAL URINATION *(new)*

## CHAPTER 19: BOWEL ELIMINATION
- FOCUS ON CHILDREN: NORMAL BOWEL MOVEMENTS *(new)*

## CHAPTER 20: NUTRITION AND FLUIDS
- PROCEDURE: PREPARING THE PERSON FOR MEALS *(new)*
- The dysphagia diet *(new)*
- Box 20-6 Dysphagia Diet *(new)*
- Box 20-7 Signs and Symptoms of Dysphagia *(new)*
- Box 20-8 Aspiration Precautions *(new)*

## CHAPTER 26: COLLECTING AND TESTING SPECIMENS (NEW)

## CHAPTER 27: THE PERSON HAVING SURGERY
- Marking the surgical site *(new)*

## CHAPTER 28: WOUND CARE
- Box 28-1 Types of Wounds *(new)*
- Risk factors for stasis ulcers *(new)*
- Prevention of stasis ulcers *(new)*
- Box 28-4 Measures to Prevent Circulatory Ulcers *(new)*

## CHAPTER 30: OXYGEN NEEDS
- FOCUS ON CHILDREN: COUGHING AND DEEP BREATHING *(new)*

## CHAPTER 31: REHABILITATION AND RESTORATIVE CARE
- Restorative nursing *(new)*
- Restorative aides *(new)*

## CHAPTER 32: HEARING AND VISION PROBLEMS
- FOCUS ON CHILDREN: OTITIS MEDIA *(new)*

## CHAPTER 33: COMMON HEALTH PROBLEMS
- Hormone therapy (cancer) *(new)*
- Biological therapy (cancer) *(new)*
- Multiple sclerosis *(expanded)*
- Diverticular disease *(new)*

## CHAPTER 34: MENTAL HEALTH PROBLEMS
- Box 34-3 Signs and Symptoms of Bipolar Disorder *(new)*
- FOCUS ON OLDER PERSONS: DEPRESSION *(new)*

## CHAPTER 35: CONFUSION AND DEMENTIA
- Box 35-4 Other Signs and Symptoms of Alzheimer's Disease (AD) *(new)*
- Box 35-6 Care of Persons With AD and Other Dementias *(expanded)*
- Validation therapy *(new)*

## CHAPTER 39: ASSISTED LIVING (NEW)

## FEATURES AND DESIGN

Besides content issues, attention is also given to improving the book's features and designs. To make the book more readable and user friendly, new features and design elements were added while others were retained (see Student Preface, p. xvii).

- *ILLUSTRATIONS*—the book contains numerous full-color photographs and line art.
- *KEY TERMS WITH DEFINITIONS*—are at the beginning of each chapter.
- *KEY TERMS IN BOLD PRINT*—are throughout the text. The definition is presented in narrative in the text. Unlike other books, students do not have to turn to the margin for the definition, return to the text, and then try to understand the context of the term.
- *BOXES AND TABLES*—list principles, guidelines, signs and symptoms, nursing measures, and other information. They are an efficient way for instructors to highlight content. They are also useful study guides for students.
- *ICONS*—in section headings alert the reader to an associated procedure. Procedure boxes contain the same icon.
- *DELEGATION GUIDELINES*—are associated with procedures. As stated earlier, they focus on the information needed from the nurse and the care plan about critical aspects of the procedure and which observations to report and record. Step 1 of most procedures refers the student to the appropriate *Delegation Guidelines*. **New!**
- *SAFETY ALERTS*—focus the student's attention on the need to be safe and cautious when giving care. Step 1 of most procedures refers the student to the appropriate *Safety Alerts*. **New!**
- *CHARTING SAMPLES*—are provided for many content areas and procedures. Incorporating documentation principles, they show how to correctly record care and observations. **New!**
- *PROCEDURE BOXES DIVIDED INTO PRE-PROCEDURE, PROCEDURE, AND POST-PROCEDURE STEPS*—labeling and color gradients also differentiate the sections. Including the *Pre-Procedure* and *Post-Procedure* steps, rather than simply referring the student to them as is done in other texts, serves to show the procedure as a whole and reinforces learning.
- *QUALITY OF LIFE*—this section in the procedure boxes reminds the student of fundamental courtesies—knock before entering the room, address the person by name, and introduce one's self by name and title.
- *NNAAP*™—appears in the procedure box title bar for skills included in the National Nurse Aide Assessment Program (NNAAP™).

- *CARING ABOUT CULTURE BOXES*—serve to sensitize the student to cultural diversity and how culture influences health and illness practices.
- *FOCUS ON CHILDREN BOXES*—provide age-specific information about needs, considerations, and special circumstances of children. This feature is useful in meeting age-specific training requirements of the Joint Commission on Accreditation of Healthcare Organizations.
- *FOCUS ON OLDER PERSONS BOXES*—provide age-specific information about the needs, considerations, and special circumstances of older persons. This feature is useful in meeting age-specific training requirements of the Joint Commission on Accreditation of Healthcare Organizations.

- *FOCUS ON HOME CARE BOXES*—highlight information necessary for safe functioning in the home setting.
- *FOCUS ON LONG-TERM CARE BOXES*—highlight information unique to the long-term care setting. Such information includes requirements of the Omnibus Budget Reconciliation Act of 1987 (OBRA).
- *REVIEW QUESTIONS*—are found at the end of each chapter. A page number for the answer section is given.

May this book serve you and your students well. My intent is to provide you and your students with the information needed to teach and learn safe and effective care during this time of dynamic change in health care.

*Sheila A. Sorrentino, RN, BSN, MA, MSN, PhD*

# ■ STUDENT PREFACE ■

This book was designed for you. It was designed to help you learn. The book is a useful resource as you gain experience and expand your knowledge.

This preface gives some study guidelines and helps you use the book. When given a reading assignment, do you read from the first page to the last page without stopping? How much do you remember? You will learn more if you use a study system. A useful study system has these steps:

- Survey or preview
- Question
- Read and record
- Recite and review

## SURVEY OR PREVIEW

Before you start a reading assignment, survey or preview the assignment. This gives you an idea of what the assignment covers. It also helps you recall what you already know about the subject. Carefully look over the assignment. Preview the chapter title, headings, subheadings, and terms or ideas in bold print or italics. Also survey the objectives, key terms, boxes, and the review questions at the end of the chapter. Previewing only takes a few minutes. Remember, previewing helps you become familiar with the material.

## QUESTION

After previewing, you need to form questions to answer while you read. Questions should relate to what might be asked on a test or how the information applies to giving care. Use the title, main headings, and subheadings to form questions. Avoid questions that have one word answers. Questions that begin with what, how, or why are helpful. While reading, you may find that a question does not help you study. If so, just change the question. Remember, questioning sets a purpose for reading. So changing a question only makes this step more useful.

## READ AND RECORD

Reading is the next step. Reading is more productive after you determine what you already know and what you need to learn. Read to find answers to your questions. The purpose of reading is to:

- Gain new information
- Connect new information to what you know already

Break the assignment into smaller parts. Then answer your questions as you read each part. Also, mark important information—underline, highlight, or make notes. Underlining and highlighting remind you what you need to learn. Go back and review the marked parts later. Making notes results in more immediate learning. To make notes, write down important information in the margins or in a notebook. Use words and statements to jog your memory about the material.

You need to remember what you read. To do so, work with the information. Organize information into a study guide. Study guides have many forms. Diagrams or charts show relationships or steps in a process. Note taking in outline format is also very useful. The following is a sample outline.

I. Main heading
  a. Second level
  b. Second level
    1. Third level
    2. Third level
II. Main heading

## RECITE AND REVIEW

Finally, recite and review. Use your notes and study guides. Answer the questions you formed earlier. Also answer other questions that came up when reading and answering the *Review Questions* at the end of a chapter. Answer all questions out loud (recite).

Reviewing is more about *when* to study rather than *what* to study. You already determined what to study during the preview, question, and reading steps. The best times to review are right after the first study session, one week later, and before a quiz or test.

This book was also designed to help you study. Special design features are described on the next pages.

I hope you enjoy learning and your work. You and your work are important. You and the care you give may be bright spots in a person's day!

## OBJECTIVES

- Define the key terms listed in this chapter
- Explain why grooming is important
- Identify the factors that affect hair care
- Explain how to care for matted and tangled hair
- Describe how to shampoo hair
- Describe the measures practiced when shaving a person
- Describe the measures practiced when shaving a person
- Describe why nail and foot care are important
- Explain why nail and foot care are important
- Describe the rules for changing gowns and clothing
- Perform the procedures described in this chapter

## KEY TERMS

**alopecia** Hair loss
**dandruff** Excessive amount of dry, white flakes from the scalp
**hirsutism** Excessive body hair in women and children
**pediculosis (lice)** Infestation with lice

**pediculosis capitis** Infestation of the scalp (capitis) with lice
**pediculosis corporis** Infestation of the body (corporis) with lice
**pediculosis pubis** Infestation of the pubic (pubis) hair with lice

Hair care, shaving, and nail and foot care are important to many people. Like hygiene, these grooming measures prevent infection and promote comfort. They also affect love, belonging, and self-esteem needs.

People differ in their [...] clean hair. Othe [...] want only clean hair [...] and polished nails [...] beards. Likewise [...] underarms. Som [...] shave or use oth [...]

## HAIR C[...]

How the [...]
Some pe[...]
hair car[...]
Care: H[...]

Th[...]
perso[...]
tory [...]
car[...]

women with aging. Cancer treatments (radiation therapy to the head and chemotherapy) often cause alopecia in males and females. Skin disease is another cause. Stress, poor nutrition, pregnancy, some drugs, and hormone changes are other causes. Except for hair loss from aging, hair usually grows back.

- **Hirsutism** is excessive body hair in women and children. It results from heredity and abnormal amounts of male hormones.

[...]**ff** is the excessive amount of dry, white flakes [...]. Itching often occurs. Sometimes eye-[...] are involved. Medicated sham-[...] tion with lice. [...] are par-

### Objectives tell what is presented in the chapter.

### Key terms are the important words and phrases in the chapter. Definitions are given for each term. The key terms introduce you to the chapter content. They are also a useful study guide.

### Bolded type is used to highlight the key terms in the text. You again see the key term and read its definition. This helps reinforce your learning.

---

## BRUSHING AND COMBING HAIR

Brushing and combing hair are part of early morning care, morning care, and afternoon care. They also are done whenever needed. Many people want hair care done before visitors arrive. Encourage patients and residents to do their own hair care. Assist as needed. Perform hair care for those who cannot do so. The person chooses how to brush, comb, and style hair.

Brushing increases blood flow to the scalp. It also brings scalp oils along the hair shaft. Scalp oils help keep hair soft and shiny. Brushing and combing prevent tangled and matted hair. When brushing and combing hair, start at the scalp. Then brush or comb to the hair ends.

Long hair easily mats and tangles. Daily brushing and combing prevent the problem. So does braiding. Do not braid hair without the person's consent. *Never cut matted or tangled hair.* Tell the nurse if the person has matted or tangled hair. The nurse may have you comb or brush through the matting and tangling. To do this:

- Take a small section of hair near the ends.
- Comb or brush through to the hair ends.
- Working up to the scalp, add small sections of hair.
- Comb or brush through each longer section to the hair ends.
- Brush or comb from the scalp to the hair ends.

Special measures are needed for curly, coarse, and dry hair. Use a wide-tooth comb for curly hair. Start at the neckline. Working upward, lift and fluff hair outward. Continue to the forehead. Wet hair or apply a conditioner or petroleum jelly as directed. This makes combing easier. The person may have certain practices or hair care products. They are part of the care plan. Also, the person can guide you when giving hair care. *See Caring About Culture: Braiding Hair.*

When giving hair care, place a towel across the shoulders to protect the person's garments. If the person is in bed, give hair care before changing the pillowcase. If done after a linen change, place a towel across the pillow to collect falling hair. *See Focus on Children: Brushing and Combing Hair.*

### DELEGATION GUIDELINES: Brushing and Combing Hair

You need this information from the nurse and care plan before brushing and combing hair:

- How much help the person needs
- What to do if hair is matted and tangled
- What measures are needed for curly, coarse, or dry hair
- What hair care products to use
- The person's preferences and routine hair care measures
- What observations to report and record:
  —Scalp sores
  —Flaking
  —Presence of lice
  —Patches of hair loss
  —Very dry or very oily hair

### SAFETY ALERT: Brushing and Combing Hair

Sharp brush bristles can injure the scalp. So can a comb with sharp or broken teeth. Tell the nurse if you have concerns about the person's brush or comb.

### CARING ABOUT CULTURE
#### BRAIDING HAIR

Styling hair in small braids is a common practice of some cultural groups. The braids are left intact for shampooing. To undo these braids, the nurse obtains the person's consent.

### Delegation Guidelines describe what information you need from the nurse and care plan before performing a procedure. They also tell you what information to report and record.

### Safety Alerts focus your attention on the need to be safe and cautious when giving care.

### Caring About Culture boxes contain information to help you learn about the various practices of other cultures.

354  CHAPTER 17  Grooming

### FOCUS ON OLDER PERSONS
SHAMPOOING

Oil gland secretion decreases with aging. Therefore older persons have dry hair. They may shampoo less often than younger adults.

When shampooing during the tub bath or shower, the person tips his or her head back to keep shampoo and water out of the eyes. Support the back of the head with one hand as you shampoo with the other. Some older people cannot tip their heads back. They lean forward and hold a washcloth over the eyes. Support the forehead with one hand as you shampoo with the other. Make sure the person can breathe easily.

Many older people have limited range of motion in their necks. They cannot tolerate shampooing at the sink or on a stretcher.

### FOCUS ON CHILDREN
SHAMPOOING

Oil gland secretion increases during puberty. Therefore adolescents tend to have oily hair. Frequent shampooing is often necessary.

### FOCUS ON HOME CARE
SHAMPOOING

You can make a trough from a plastic shower curtain or tablecloth. Or use a plastic drop cloth for painting. (Avoid plastic trash bags. They slip and slide easily and are not sturdy.) Place the plastic under the person's head. Make a raised edge around the plastic to prevent water from spilling over the sides. Direct the ends of the plastic into the basin. Water flows into the basin.

### FOCUS ON LONG-TERM CARE
SHAMPOOING

Shampooing is usually done weekly on the person's bath or shower day. If a woman's hair is done in the beauty shop, do not shampoo her hair. She wears a shower cap during the tub bath or shower.

Focus on Older Persons boxes provide age-specific information about the needs, considerations, and special circumstances of older persons.

Focus on Children boxes provide age-specific information about the needs, considerations, and special circumstances of children.

Focus on Home Care boxes highlight information necessary for safe functioning in the home setting.

Focus on Long-Term Care boxes highlight information unique to the long-term care setting. Such information includes requirements of the Omnibus Budget Reconciliation Act of 1987 (OBRA).

Color illustrations and photographs visually present key ideas, concepts, or procedure steps. They help you apply and remember the written material.

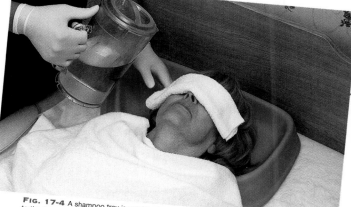

FIG. 17-4 A shampoo tray is used to shampoo a person in bed. The tray is directed to the side of the bed so water drains into a collecting basin.

### SHAMPOOING

Most people shampoo at least once a week. Some shampoo two or three times a week. Others shampoo every day. Many factors affect frequency. They include the condition of the hair and scalp, hairstyle, and personal choice.

Some persons use certain shampoos and conditioners. Others use medicated shampoo ordered by the doctor.

The person may need help shampooing. After shampooing, dry and style hair as quickly as possible. Women may want hair curled or rolled up before drying. Check with the nurse before doing so.

Tell the nurse if a shampoo is requested. Do not wash a person's hair unless a nurse asks you to do so. The shampooing method used depends on the person's condition, safety factors, and personal choice. The nurse tells you what method to use:

* *Shampoo* ... *the shower or tub bath.* The person ... A hand-held nozzle is used ...

353

* *Shampoo on a stretcher.* The stretcher is front of the sink. A towel is placed under the neck. The head is tilted over the edge of the sink (Fig. 17-3). A water pitcher or hand-held nozzle is used to wet and rinse the hair. Remember to lock the stretcher wheels and use the safety straps and side rails.
* *Shampoo in bed.* The person's head and shoulders are moved to the edge of the bed if possible. A shampoo tray is placed under the head to protect the linens and mattress from water. The tray also drains water into a basin placed on a chair by the bed (Fig. 17-4, p. 354). Use a water pitcher to wet and rinse the hair. See *Focus on Children: Shampooing.* See *Focus on Older Persons: Shampooing,* p. 354. See *Focus on Home Care: Shampooing,* p. 354. See *Focus on Long-Term Care: Shampooing.*

Heading icons alert you to associated procedures. Procedure boxes contain the same icon.

355

MOSBY'S TEXTBOOK FOR NURSING ASSISTANTS

SHAMPOOING THE PERSON'S HAIR

NNAAP™

### QUALITY OF LIFE

Remember to:
- Knock before entering the person's room
- Address the person by name
- Introduce yourself by name and title

### PRE-PROCEDURE

1 Follow *Delegation Guidelines: Shampooing*, p. 353.
   See *Safety Alert: Shampooing*, p. 353.
2 Explain the procedure to the person.
3 Practice hand hygiene.
4 Collect the following:
   - Two bath towels
   - Hand towel or washcloth
   - Shampoo
   - Hair conditioner (if requested)
   - Bath thermometer
   - Pitcher or nozzle (if needed)
   - Shampoo tray (if needed)

   - Basin or pan (if needed)
   - Waterproof pad (if needed)
   - Gloves (if needed)
   - Comb and brush
   - Hair dryer
5 Arrange items nearby.
6 Identify the person. Check the ID bracelet against the assignment sheet. Call the person by name.
7 Provide for privacy.
8 Raise the bed for body mechanics for a shampoo in bed. The far bed rail is up if bed rails are used.

### PROCEDURE

9 Position the person for the method you will use. Place the waterproof pad and shampoo tray under the head and shoulders if needed.
10 Place a bath towel across the shoulders or across the pillow.
11 Brush and comb the hair to remove snarls and tangles.
12 Raise the bed rail if used.
13 Obtain water. Water temperature should be about 105° F (40.5° C). Test temperature according to agency policy.
14 Lower the bed rail (if used).
15 Put on gloves (if needed).
16 Ask the person to hold a dampened hand towel or washcloth over the eyes. It should not cover the nose and mouth. (A damp towel or washcloth is easier to hold. It will not slip.)
17 Use the pitcher or nozzle to wet the hair.

18 Apply a small amount of shampoo.
19 Work up a lather with both hands. Start at the hairline. Work toward the back of the head.
20 Massage the scalp with your fingertips. Do not scratch the scalp.
21 Rinse the hair.
22 Repeat steps 18 through 21.
23 Apply conditioner. Follow directions on the container.
24 Squeeze water from the person's hair.
25 Cover hair with a bath towel.
26 Dry the person's face with a towel.
27 Help the person raise the head if appropriate.
28 Rub the hair and scalp with the towel. Use the second towel if the first is wet.
29 Comb the hair to remove snarls and tangles as quickly as possible.
30 Dry and style hair as quickly as possible.

### POST-PROCEDURE

31 Remove and discard the gloves (if used). Decontaminate your hands.
32 Provide for comfort.
33 Lower the bed to its lowest position.
34 Raise or lower bed rails. Follow the care plan.
35 Place the signal light within reach.
36 Unscreen the person.
37 Clean and return equipment to its proper place. Discard disposable items.
38 Follow agency policy for dirty linen.
39 Decontaminate your hands.

---

**Procedure icons** in the title bar of the procedure alert you to associated content areas. Heading icons and procedure icons are the same.

**Procedures** are written in a step-by-step format. They are divided into *Pre-procedure, Procedure,* and *Post-procedure* sections for easy studying.

**Boxes and tables** contain important rules, principles, guidelines, signs and symptoms, nursing measures, and other information in a list format. They identify important information and are useful study guides.

**NNAAP™** in the procedure title bar alerts you to those skills that are part of the National Nurse Aide Assessment Program (NNAAP™). *Note: All states do not participate in NNAAP™. Ask your instructor for a list of the skills tested in your state.*

**Quality of Life** in the procedure boxes reminds you to knock before entering the room, to call the person by name, and to introduce yourself by name and title. These simple courtesies show respect for the patient or resident as a person.

---

**BOX 17-1    RULES FOR SHAVING**

- Use electric shavers for persons taking anticoagulant drugs. Never use safety razors.
- Protect bed linens. Place a towel under the part being shaved. Or place a towel across the shoulders to protect clothing.
- Soften the skin before shaving.
- Encourage the person to do as much as safely possible.
- Hold the skin taut as needed.
- Shave in the direction of hair growth when shaving the face and underarms.
- Shave up from the ankles when shaving legs. This is against hair growth.
- Do not cut, nick, or irritate the skin.
- Rinse the body part thoroughly.
- Apply direct pressure to nicks or cuts.
- Report nicks, cuts, or irritation to the nurse at once.

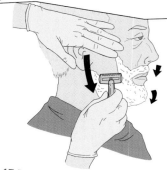

**FIG. 17-5** Shave in the direction of hair growth. Use longer strokes on the larger areas of the face. Use short strokes around the chin and lips.

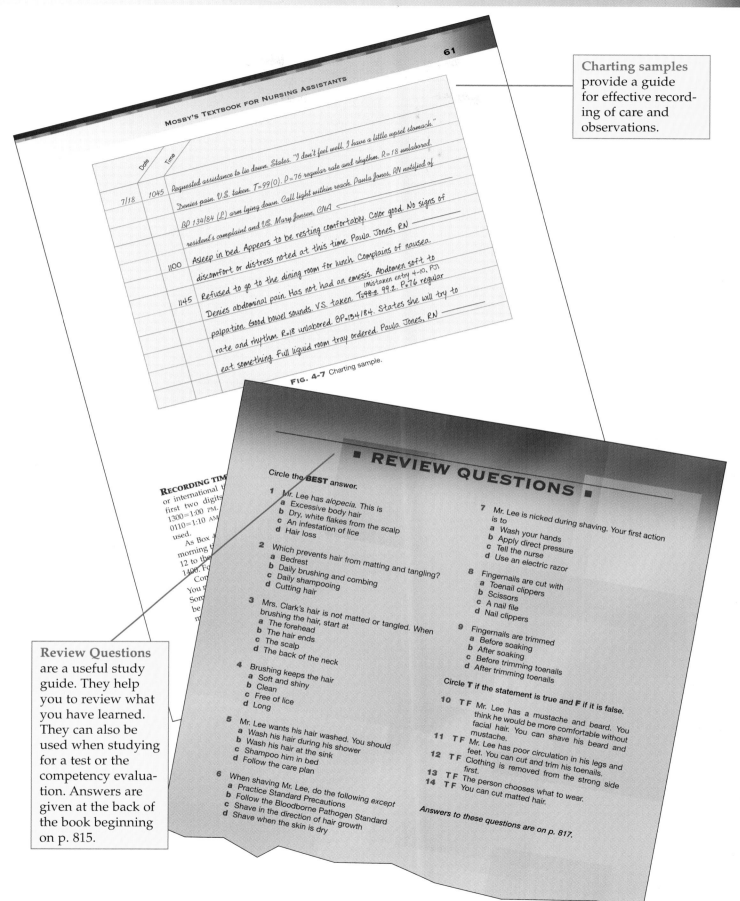

**Charting samples** provide a guide for effective recording of care and observations.

61

MOSBY'S TEXTBOOK FOR NURSING ASSISTANTS

| Date | Time | |
|------|------|---|
| 7/18 | 1045 | Requested assistance to lie down. States: "I don't feel well. I have a little upset stomach." Denies pain. V.S. taken. T=99(0). P=76 regular rate and rhythm. R=18 unlabored. BP 134/84 (L) arm lying down. Call light within reach. Mary Jensen, CNA Paula Jones, RN notified of resident's complaint and V.S. |
| | 1100 | Asleep in bed. Appears to be resting comfortably. Color good. No signs of discomfort or distress noted at this time. Paula Jones, RN |
| | 1145 | Refused to go to the dining room for lunch. Complains of nausea. Denies abdominal pain. Has not had an emesis. Abdomen soft to palpation. Good bowel sounds. V.S. taken. T=98.2 99.2. P=76 regular (Mistaken entry 4-10, PJ) rate and rhythm. R=18 unlabored. BP=134/84. States she will try to eat something. Full liquid room tray ordered. Paula Jones, RN |

**FIG. 4-7** Charting sample.

**RECORDING TIM**
or international t
first two digits
1300=1:00 PM.
0110=1:10 AM
used.
As Box
morning
12 to the
1400. F
Co
You
Som
be
m

**Review Questions** are a useful study guide. They help you to review what you have learned. They can also be used when studying for a test or the competency evaluation. Answers are given at the back of the book beginning on p. 815.

## ■ REVIEW QUESTIONS ■

Circle the **BEST** answer.

1  Mr. Lee has *alopecia*. This is
   a  Excessive body hair
   b  Dry, white flakes from the scalp
   c  An infestation of lice
   d  Hair loss

2  Which prevents hair from matting and tangling?
   a  Bedrest
   b  Daily brushing and combing
   c  Daily shampooing
   d  Cutting hair

3  Mrs. Clark's hair is not matted or tangled. When brushing the hair, start at
   a  The forehead
   b  The hair ends
   c  The scalp
   d  The back of the neck

4  Brushing keeps the hair
   a  Soft and shiny
   b  Clean
   c  Free of lice
   d  Long

5  Mr. Lee wants his hair washed. You should
   a  Wash his hair during his shower
   b  Wash his hair at the sink
   c  Shampoo him in bed
   d  Follow the care plan

6  When shaving Mr. Lee, do the following except
   a  Practice Standard Precautions
   b  Follow the Bloodborne Pathogen Standard
   c  Shave in the direction of hair growth
   d  Shave when the skin is dry

7  Mr. Lee is nicked during shaving. Your first action is to
   a  Wash your hands
   b  Apply direct pressure
   c  Tell the nurse
   d  Use an electric razor

8  Fingernails are cut with
   a  Toenail clippers
   b  Scissors
   c  A nail file
   d  Nail clippers

9  Fingernails are trimmed
   a  Before soaking
   b  After soaking
   c  Before trimming toenails
   d  After trimming toenails

Circle **T** if the statement is true and **F** if it is false.

10  T F  Mr. Lee has a mustache and beard. You think he would be more comfortable without facial hair. You can shave his beard and mustache.

11  T F  Mr. Lee has poor circulation in his legs and feet. You can cut and trim his toenails.

12  T F  Clothing is removed from the strong side first.

13  T F  The person chooses what to wear.

14  T F  You can cut matted hair.

Answers to these questions are on p. 817.

# ■ CONTENTS ■

# Mosby's Textbook for
# NURSING
# ASSISTANTS

# Introduction to Health Care Agencies

## OBJECTIVES

- Define the key terms listed in this chapter
- Explain the purposes and services of health care agencies
- Identify members of the health team and the nursing team
- Describe the nursing service department
- Describe the nursing team members
- Describe four nursing care patterns
- Describe programs that pay for health care
- Explain why standards are met

## KEY TERMS

**acute illness** A sudden illness from which a person is expected to recover

**assisted living facility** Provides housing, personal care, support services, health care, and social activities in a homelike setting

**case management** A nursing care pattern; a case manager (an RN) coordinates a person's care from admission through discharge and into the home setting

**chronic illness** An ongoing illness, slow or gradual in onset, for which there is no known cure; the illness can be controlled and complications prevented

**functional nursing** A nursing care pattern focusing on tasks and jobs; each nursing team member has certain tasks and jobs to do

**health team** Staff members who work together to provide health care

**hospice** A health care agency or program for persons who are dying

**licensed practical nurse (LPN)** A nurse who has completed a 1-year nursing program and has passed a licensing test; called *licensed vocational nurse* (*LVN*) in some states

**licensed vocational nurse (LVN)** Licensed practical nurse

**nursing assistant** A person who gives basic nursing care under the supervision of an RN or LPN/LVN

**nursing team** The individuals who provide nursing care—RNs, LPNs/LVNs, and nursing assistants

**patient-focused care** A nursing care pattern; services are moved from departments to the bedside

**primary nursing** A nursing care pattern; an RN is responsible for the person's total care

**registered nurse (RN)** A nurse who has completed a 2-, 3-, or 4-year nursing program and has passed a licensing test

**team nursing** A nursing care pattern; a team of nursing staff is led by an RN who decides the amount and kind of care each person needs

**terminal illness** An illness or injury for which there is no reasonable expectation of recovery

Health care agencies offer services to persons needing health care (Box 1-1). Staff members have special talents, knowledge, and skills. All work to meet the person's needs. The *person* is the focus of care.

### BOX 1-1 TYPES OF HEALTH CARE AGENCIES

- Hospitals
- Long-term care centers (nursing homes, nursing centers)
- Home care agencies
- Adult day-care centers
- Assisted living facilities
- Board and care homes
- Rehabilitation and subacute care facilities
- Hospices
- Doctors' offices
- Clinics
- Centers for persons with mental illnesses
- Centers for persons with developmental disabilities
- Drug and alcohol treatment centers
- Crisis centers for rape, abuse, suicide, and other mental health emergencies

## AGENCY PURPOSES AND TYPES

Services range from simple to complex. Some agencies have one purpose and offer one service. Others have many purposes. They offer many services.

### PURPOSES OF AGENCIES

The purposes of health care are:

- *Health promotion.* This includes physical and mental health. The goal is to reduce the risk of illness. People receive teaching and counseling about healthy living. Diet, exercise, and changing unhealthy habits are discussed. They learn the warning signs and symptoms of illness. Ill persons learn how to manage and cope with their diseases.
- *Disease prevention.* Risk factors and early warning signs of disease are identified. Measures are taken to reduce risk factors and prevent disease. Simple lifestyle changes can prevent health problems. For example, high blood pressure can lead to heart attacks and strokes. Diet and exercise can help lower blood pressure. Immunizations prevent some infectious diseases. Polio, measles, mumps, smallpox, and hepatitis are examples.
- *Detection and treatment of disease.* This involves diagnostic tests, physical exams, surgery, emergency care, and drugs. Often respiratory, physical, and occupational

therapies are needed. The nursing team observes signs and symptoms, gives care, and carries out the doctor's orders.
- *Rehabilitation and restorative care.* The goal is to return persons to their highest possible level of physical and psychological functioning. It starts when the person first seeks health care. The person learns or relearns skills needed to live, work, and enjoy life. Maintaining function is important. Help is given with making needed changes at home.

These purposes are all related. For example, Mr. Parsons has severe chest pain and problems breathing. He goes to the emergency room. After an exam and laboratory tests, the doctor diagnoses a heart attack. Mr. Parsons is admitted to the hospital for treatment. He also receives teaching and counseling about heart attack risk factors and changing habits. This includes no smoking, a low-fat diet, and exercise. The goals are to promote health and prevent another heart attack. He has fears about dying and about not being able to lead an active life. A rehabilitation program is planned. It starts activity slowly. Activity may progress to walking, jogging, or swimming. More teaching and counseling focus on diet, drugs, life-style, and activity. Mr. Parsons and his family are encouraged to talk about fears and concerns. They are given help in learning to cope. Successful rehabilitation helps promote health and may prevent another heart attack.

**STUDENT LEARNING.** Many agencies are learning sites for students. They study to become nurses, doctors, x-ray and laboratory technicians, dietitians, or nursing assistants. These students also assist in the purposes of health care. They are involved in patient and resident care.

### TYPES OF AGENCIES

Nursing assistants work in many settings. Some work in doctors' offices and clinics. Most work in the following agencies.

**HOSPITALS.** Hospital services include emergency care, surgery, nursing care, x-ray procedures and treatments, and laboratory testing. Services also include respiratory, physical, occupational, and speech therapies.

People of all ages need hospital care. They go to have babies, for physical and mental health problems, to have surgery, to heal broken bones, or to die. They have acute, chronic, or terminal illnesses:
- **Acute illness** is a sudden illness from which the person is expected to recover.
- **Chronic illness** is an ongoing illness that is slow or gradual in onset. There is no known cure. The illness can be controlled and complications prevented.
- **Terminal illness** is an illness or injury for which there is no reasonable expectation of recovery. The person will die (Chapter 41).

Some hospital stays are less than 24 hours. The person needs hospital services but does not stay 24 hours. Some surgeries, diagnostic procedures, and therapies do not require 24-hour stays. Outpatient services are common.

Others persons need to stay days, weeks, or months. The length of stay depends on the person's condition and illness.

**REHABILITATION AND SUBACUTE CARE AGENCIES.** Hospital stays are usually short. This is because of insurance coverage. A person does not need hospital care but is too sick to go home. The person's condition is stable. However, medical care, nursing care, or rehabilitation is still needed. Care needs fall between hospital care and long-term care. Complex equipment and care measures are needed. Common programs include:

- *Ventilator weaning.* A person needs a mechanical ventilator to breathe (Chapter 30). The goal is to breathe without the ventilator.
- *Pulmonary rehabilitation.* For example, a person has a tracheostomy (Chapter 30). If it is temporary, the goal is for the person to breathe without it. If it is permanent, the person learns tracheostomy care and management.
- *Wound management.* The person has a chronic wound from surgery or trauma (Chapter 28). Wound healing is the goal.
- *Neurological rehabilitation.* The person had a stroke or has a nervous system disease or injury (Chapter 33).

- *Orthopedic rehabilitation.* The person had joint replacement surgery. Or the person has a bone, joint, or muscle injury or disease (Chapter 33).
- *Complex medical care.* The person has a complex heart, kidney, digestive, or other disorder. Persons with cancer or AIDS may need complex medical care (Chapter 33).

Some hospitals and long-term care centers have rehabilitation and subacute care units. Some are separate agencies. Many persons fully recover. Others may need long-term care.

**ASSISTED LIVING FACILITIES.** An **assisted living facility** provides housing, personal care, support services, health care, and social activities in a homelike setting (Chapter 39). Some are part of retirement communities or nursing centers (Chapter 9).

The person has a room or an apartment. Three meals a day are provided. So are housekeeping, laundry, and transportation services. Help is given with personal care and drugs. Social and recreational activities are provided. There is access to health and medical care.

**LONG-TERM CARE CENTERS.** Some persons cannot care for themselves at home. But they do not need hospital care. Long-term care centers (nursing homes, nursing facilities, nursing centers) can help them.

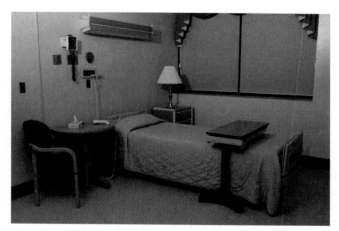

**FIG. 1-1** Room in a long-term care center.

Medical, nursing, dietary, recreational, rehabilitative, and social services are provided.

Persons in long-term care centers are called *residents*. They are not *patients*. This is because the center is their temporary or permanent home.

Most residents are older. They have chronic diseases, poor nutrition, or poor health. Long-term care centers are designed to meet their needs (Fig. 1-1).

Not all residents are old. Some are disabled from birth defects, accidents, or diseases. People are often discharged from hospitals while still sick or still recovering from surgery. Home care is an option for some. Others need long-term care. Some recover and return home. Others need nursing care until death.

**Skilled nursing facilities.** Skilled nursing facilities (SNFs) provide more complex care than do nursing centers. They are part of hospitals or nursing centers. SNFs are for persons with health problems that do not require hospital care. They need rehabilitation or time to recover from illness or surgery. Often they return home after a short stay. Others become permanent nursing center residents.

**MENTAL HEALTH CENTERS.** Mental health centers are for persons with mental illnesses. Some persons have problems dealing with life events. Others present dangers to themselves or others because of how they think and behave. Outpatient care is common. Some need short-term or life-long inpatient care.

**HOME CARE AGENCIES.** Care is given in the person's home. Public health departments, private businesses, and hospitals provide home care services. Services range from health teaching and supervision to bedside nursing care. Physical therapy, rehabilitation, and food services are common. Some older persons need home care. So do some persons who are dying.

**HOSPICES.** A **hospice** is a health care agency or program for persons who are dying. The physical, emotional, social, and spiritual needs of the person and family are met in a setting that allows much freedom. The person and family have much control over the person's quality of life. Children and pets usually can visit at any time. Family and friends can assist with care. Hospitals, nursing centers, and home care agencies provide hospice care.

**HEALTH CARE SYSTEMS.** Agencies join together as one provider of care. A system usually has hospitals, nursing centers, home care agencies, hospice settings, and doctors' offices (Fig. 1-2). An ambulance service and medical supply store for home care are common. The system may serve a community or a large region.

The goal is to serve all health care needs. A person uses other system providers as needed (Box 1-2).

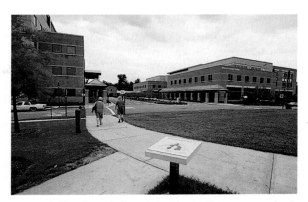

**FIG. 1-2** The hospital and doctors' offices are part of a health care system. (Courtesy Anne Arundel Health System, Inc., Annapolis, Md.)

| BOX 1-2 | USING A HEALTH CARE SYSTEM |
| --- | --- |

A health care system owns Mercy Hospital. Dr. Moore and Dr. Gills work there. The hospital has a rehabilitation unit and a home care service. LifeCare Ambulance Service and a medical supply store are part of the system. So is Lakeside Nursing Center.

June Adams is 78 years old. She sees Dr. Moore in his office. She complains of tightness in her chest, dizziness, and a "pounding heart beat." Dr. Moore admits her to the hospital. He asks Dr. Gills, a heart specialist, to take over her care. While in the hospital, she has a heart attack. A few days later she has a stroke. She cannot move her left side. She is given needed medical care. When her condition is stable, she is transferred to the rehabilitation unit.

Mrs. Adams spends 2 weeks on the rehabilitation unit. She needs home care if she returns home. Or she can go to a nursing center. She wants to go home. Her family wants to help care for her. They need a hospital bed, commode, bedpan, wheelchair, and other items. They rent some items and buy others at the medical supply store.

Mrs. Adams is transported home by LifeCare Ambulance Service. Mercy Hospital's home care agency provides home care services. A nursing assistant visits every day. Mrs. Adams is assisted with hygiene and grooming needs. A nurse visits three times a week.

A month later Mrs. Adams has another stroke. She returns to Mercy Hospital by LifeCare Ambulance Service. After 8 days, she is transferred to the rehabilitation unit. The second stroke has caused more disabilities. Dr. Gills suggests nursing home care. Mrs. Adams and her family agree with him.

The nurse arranges for Mrs. Adams to be admitted to Lakeside Nursing Center. She is transferred there by LifeCare Ambulance Service.

## ORGANIZATION

An agency has a governing body called the *board of trustees.* The board makes policies. It makes sure that good, safe care is given at the lowest possible cost. Local, state, and federal standards are followed.

An administrator manages the agency. He or she reports directly to the board. Directors or department heads manage certain areas (Fig. 1-3).

## THE HEALTH TEAM

The **health team** involves staff members who work together to provide health care. (It also is called the *interdisciplinary health care team.*) Their skills and knowledge focus on the person's total care (Table 1-1). The goal is to provide quality care. The person is the focus of their care (Fig. 1-4, p. 9).

Many staff members are involved in the care of one person. Coordinated care is important. A registered nurse (RN) usually coordinates the person's care (p. 8).

## NURSING SERVICE

Nursing service is a large department. The director of nursing (DON) is an RN. (*Vice president of nursing* and *vice president of patient services* are other titles.) Usually a bachelor's or master's degree is required. The DON is responsible for the entire nursing staff and the care given. Nurse managers (RNs) assist the DON. They manage and carry out nursing department functions.

Nurse managers are responsible for a work shift or nursing area. Hospital nursing areas include surgical and medical nursing units, intensive care units, maternity departments, and pediatric units. They also include operating and recovery rooms, an emergency department, and mental health units. Nurse managers are responsible for all nursing care and the actions of nursing staff in their areas.

In nursing centers, nurse managers may coordinate resident care for a certain shift. Or they are responsible for a certain function. Examples include staff development, restorative nursing, infection control, or continuous quality improvement.

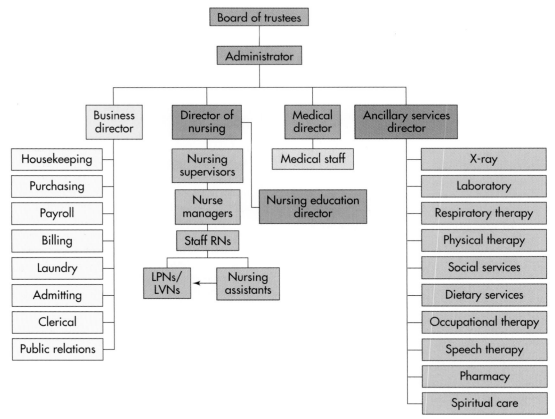

**FIG. 1-3** The organizational chart of a health care agency.

| TABLE 1-1 HEALTH TEAM MEMBERS | | |
|---|---|---|
| **Title** | **Description** | **Credentials** |
| Activities director | Assesses, plans, and implements recreational needs | Required training varies with state and/or employer; ranges from no training to bachelor's degree |
| Assistive personnel | Assist nurses in giving bedside nursing care; supervised by a nurse (see "Nursing assistant") | Completion of state-approved training and competency evaluation program to work in long-term care and home care agencies receiving Medicare funds |
| Audiologist | Tests hearing; prescribes hearing aids; works with hearing-impaired persons | Master's degree; 1 year of supervised employment; national examination; license in some states |
| Cleric (clergyman; clergywoman) | Assists with spiritual needs | Priest, minister, rabbi, sister (nun), deacon, or other pastoral training |
| Dental hygienist | Focuses on preventing dental disorders; supervised by a licensed dentist | Completion of an accredited dental hygiene program; state license |
| Dentist | Prevents and treats disorders and diseases of the teeth, gums, and oral structures | Doctor of dental science (DDS); state license |
| Dietitian | Assesses and plans for nutritional needs; teaches good nutrition, food selection, and preparation | Bachelor's degree; registered dietitian (RD) must pass a national registration examination; license or certification in some states |
| Licensed practical/ vocational nurse (LPN/LVN) | Provides direct nursing care, including the administration of drugs, under the direction of an RN | Certificate or diploma (usually 1 year in length); state license |
| Medical laboratory technician (MLT) | Collects samples and performs laboratory tests on blood, urine, and other body fluids, secretions, and excretions | Associate's degree; national certifying examination; license in some states |
| Medical records and health information technician | Maintains medical records; transcribes medical reports, files records, completes required reports | Associate's degree; national examination |
| Medical technologist (MT) | Performs complicated laboratory tests on blood, urine, and other body fluids, secretions, and excretions; organizes, supervises, and performs diagnostic analyses; supervises MLTs | Bachelor's degree; national certification examination; license in some states |
| Nurse practitioner | Works with other health care providers to plan and provide care; does physical examinations, health assessments, and health education | RN with master's degree and clinical experience in an area of nursing; certification examination may be required |
| Nursing assistant | Assists nurses and gives nursing care; supervised by a licensed nurse | Completion of a state-approved training and competency evaluation program to work in long-term care or in home care agencies receiving Medicare funds; state registry |
| Occupational therapist (OT) | Assists persons to learn or retain skills needed to perform activities of daily living; designs adaptive equipment for activities of daily living | Bachelor's degree; national certification; state license |
| Occupational therapy assistant | Performs tasks and services supervised by an OT | Associate's degree; national certification; license in some states |
| Pharmacist | Fills drug orders written by doctors; monitors and evaluates drug interactions; consults with doctors and nurses about drug actions and interactions | Degree from a college of pharmacy; state license |

| TABLE 1-1 | HEALTH TEAM MEMBERS—CONT'D | |
|---|---|---|
| Title | Description | Credentials |
| Physical therapist (PT) | Assists persons with musculoskeletal problems; focuses on restoring function and preventing disability | Bachelor's degree; state license |
| Physical therapy assistant | Performs selected physical therapy tasks and functions; supervised by a PT | Associate's degree; national certification or license in many states |
| Physician (doctor) | Diagnoses and treats diseases and injuries | Medical school graduation, residency, and national board examination; state license |
| Physician assistant | Assists doctors in diagnosis and treatment; performs many medical tasks; supervised by a doctor | Associate's, bachelor's, or master's degree; national certification or state license |
| Podiatrist | Prevents, diagnoses, and treats foot disorders | Doctor of podiatric medicine (DPM); state license |
| Radiographer/ radiologic technologist | Takes x-rays and processes film for viewing | Certificate, associate's, or bachelor's degree; national registry examination; license in some states |
| Registered nurse (RN) | Assesses, makes nursing diagnoses, plans, implements, and evaluates nursing care; supervises LPNs/LVNs and nursing assistants | Associate's, diploma, or bachelor's degree; state license |
| Respiratory therapist | Assists in treatment of lung and heart disorders; gives respiratory treatments and therapies | Associate's or bachelor's degree; national certification examination; license in some states |
| Social worker | Helps patients, residents, and families with social, emotional, and environmental issues affecting illness and recovery; coordinates community agencies to assist patients, residents, and families | Bachelor's or master's degree in social work; license, certification, or registration |
| Speech-language pathologist | Evaluates speech and language and treats persons with speech, voice, hearing, communication, and swallowing disorders | Master's degree; 1 year supervised work experience; national examination; license in some states |

Each nursing area has RNs. They provide nursing care and supervise LPNs/LVNs and nursing assistants. Staff RNs report to the nurse manager. LPNs/LVNs report to staff RNs or to the nurse manager. You report to the RN or LPN/LVN supervising your work.

Nursing education is part of nursing service. Nursing education staff:
- Plan and present educational programs
- Provide the nursing team with new and changing information
- Instruct the nursing team on the use of new equipment
- Educate and train nursing assistants
- Conduct orientation programs for new employees

## THE NURSING TEAM

The **nursing team** involves the individuals who provide nursing care—RNs, LPNs/LVNs, and nursing assistants. Each has different roles and responsibilities. All are concerned with the physical, social, emotional, and spiritual needs of the person and family.

### REGISTERED NURSES

A **registered nurse (RN)** has completed a 2-, 3-, or 4-year nursing program and has passed a licensing test:
- Community college programs—2 years
- Hospital-based diploma programs—2 or 3 years
- College or university programs—4 years

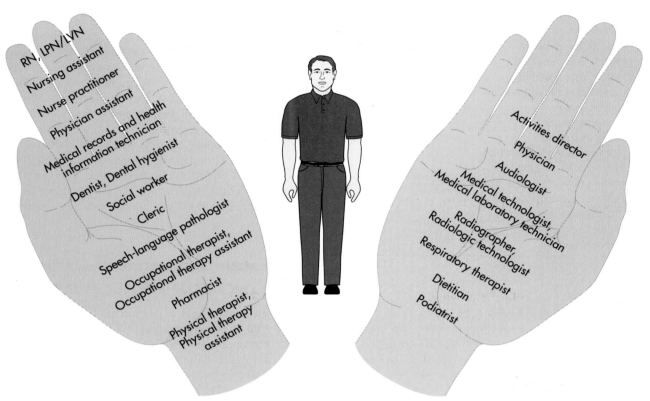

**FIG. 1-4** Members of the health team. The person is the focus of care.

Nursing and the biological, social, and physical sciences are studied. The graduate nurse takes a licensing test offered by a state board of nursing. The nurse receives a license and becomes *registered* when the test is passed. RNs must have a license recognized by the state in which they work.

RNs assess, make nursing diagnoses, plan, implement, and evaluate nursing care (Chapter 5). They develop care plans for each person and provide care. They also delegate nursing care and tasks to the nursing team. They make sure that the nursing team follows the care plans. They evaluate how the care plans and nursing care affect each person. RNs teach persons how to improve health and independence. They also teach the family.

RNs carry out the doctor's orders. They may delegate them to LPNs/LVNs or nursing assistants. RNs do not diagnose diseases or illnesses. They do not prescribe treatments or drugs. However, RNs can study to become clinical nurse specialists or nurse practitioners. A master's degree or special certification is required. These RNs have diagnosing and prescribing functions.

RNs work as staff nurses, nurse managers, directors of nursing, and instructors. Job options depend on education, abilities, and experience.

## LICENSED PRACTICAL NURSES AND LICENSED VOCATIONAL NURSES

A **licensed practical nurse** (**LPN**) has completed a 1-year nursing program and has passed a licensing test. Hospitals, community colleges, vocational schools, and technical schools offer programs. Some programs are 10 months long; others take 18 months. Some high schools offer 2-year programs.

Students study nursing, body structure and function, psychology, mathematics, and communication. Graduates take a licensing test for practical nursing. When the graduate nurse passes the test, he or she receives a license and the title of *licensed practical nurse*. Some states use the term **licensed vocational nurse** (**LVN**). Like RNs, practical or vocational nurses must have a license to work.

LPNs/LVNs are supervised by RNs, licensed doctors, and licensed dentists. They have fewer responsibilities and functions than RNs do. LPNs/LVNs have less education than RNs. They need little supervision when the person's condition is stable and care is simple. They assist RNs in caring for acutely ill persons and with complex procedures.

| BOX 1-3 | TITLES FOR NURSING ASSISTANTS |

**BOX 1-3 TITLES FOR NURSING ASSISTANTS**

- Certified nursing assistant
- Clinical technician
- Health care assistant
- Health care technician
- Licensed nursing assistant
- Nurse's aide
- Nurse extender
- Nurse technician
- Nursing support technician
- Patient care assistant
- Patient care attendant
- Patient care monitor
- Patient care technician
- Patient care worker
- Support partner

## NURSING ASSISTANTS

**Nursing assistants** give basic nursing care under the supervision of an RN or LPN/LVN. There are many titles for nursing assistants (Box 1-3). The title depends on the setting, roles, and functions.

Hospitals, nursing centers, community colleges, technical schools, and high schools offer nursing assistant courses. Nursing assistants are discussed in Chapter 2.

## NURSING CARE PATTERNS

Nursing care is given in many ways. The nursing care pattern depends on how many persons need care, the staff, and the cost.

- **Functional nursing** focuses on tasks and jobs. Each nursing team member has certain tasks and jobs to do. For example, one nurse gives all drugs. Another nurse gives all treatments. Nursing assistants give baths, make beds, and serve meals.
- **Team nursing** involves a team of nursing staff led by an RN. The RN decides the amount and kind of care each person needs. The team leader delegates the care of certain persons to other nurses. Nursing tasks and procedures are delegated to nursing assistants. Delegation is based on the person's needs and team members' abilities. Team members report to the team leader about observations made and the care given.
- **Primary nursing** involves total care. An RN is responsible for the person's total care. The nursing team assists as needed. The RN (called a *primary nurse*) gives care and plans the person's discharge. If needed, home care or long-term care is arranged. The RN teaches and counsels the person and family.

- **Case management** is like primary nursing. A case manager (an RN) coordinates a person's care from admission through discharge and into the home setting. He or she communicates with the doctor and other health team members. There also is communication with the insurance company and community agencies involved in the person's care. Some case managers work with certain doctors. Others deal only with certain health problems. Heart diseases and cancer are examples.
- **Patient-focused care** is when services are moved from departments to the bedside. The nursing team performs basic skills performed by other health team members (Chapter 2). The number of people caring for each person is reduced. This reduces care costs.

## PAYING FOR HEALTH CARE

Health care is costly. Even after a person leaves the hospital or nursing center, bills often continue for doctor visits, drugs, medical supplies, and home care. Most people cannot afford these bills. Some avoid medical care because they cannot pay. Others pay doctor bills even if it means going without food or drugs. Health care bills cause worry, fear, and emotional upset. If the person has insurance, some care costs are covered.

Health care is a major focus of society. The goals are to provide health care to everyone and to reduce care costs. Cost-cutting efforts include managed care and prospective payment systems. More changes are likely.

You need to know the following:
- *Private insurance* is bought by individuals and families. The insurance company pays for some or all health care costs.
- *Group insurance* is bought by groups for individuals. Many employers provide health insurance for employees under group coverage.
- *Medicare* is a federal health insurance program for persons 65 years of age or older. Some younger people with certain disabilities are covered. Medicare has two parts. Part A pays for some hospital, SNF, hospice, and home care costs. Part B helps pay for doctors' services, outpatient hospital care, physical and occupational therapists, some home care, and many other services. Part B is voluntary. The person pays a monthly premium.
- *Medicaid* is a health care payment program. It is sponsored by federal and state governments. Benefits, rules, and eligibility requirements vary from state to state. Older, blind, and disabled people are usually eligible. So are families with low incomes. There is no insurance premium. The amount paid for each covered service is limited.

## PROSPECTIVE PAYMENT SYSTEMS

Prospective payment systems limit the amounts paid by insurers, Medicare, and Medicaid. Prospective means *before* care. The amount paid for services is determined before the person enters the hospital, SNF, or rehabilitation center.

*Diagnosis-related groups (DRGs)* help reduce Medicare and Medicaid costs. So do *resource utilization groups (RUGs)*. Payment is determined *before* the person receives care. RUGs are for SNF payments. *Case mix groups (CMGs)* are used to decide payments to rehabilitation centers. If treatment costs are less than the amount paid, the agency keeps the extra money. If costs are greater, the agency takes the loss.

## MANAGED CARE

Managed care deals with health care delivery and payment (Box 1-4). Insurers contract with doctors and hospitals for reduced rates or discounts. The insured person uses doctors and agencies providing the lower rates. If others are used, care is covered in part or not at all. The person pays for costs not covered by insurance.

Managed care limits the choice of where to go for health care. It also limits the care that doctors provide. Many states require managed care for Medicaid and Medicare coverage.

**MANAGED CARE AS PRE-APPROVAL FOR SERVICES.** Many insurers must approve the need for health care services. If the need is approved, the insurer pays for the services. If the need is not approved, the person pays for the costs. The pre-approval process depends on the insurance company.

This pre-approval process is also called *managed care*. It includes monitoring care. The purpose is to reduce unneeded services and procedures. The insurer decides what to pay. With health maintenance organization (HMO) or preferred provider organization (PPO) contracts, the insurer may decide where the person goes for the services.

## MEETING STANDARDS

Health care agencies must meet certain standards. Standards are set by the federal and state governments. They also are set by accrediting agencies. Standards relate to agency policies and procedures, budget and finances, and quality of care. An agency must meet standards for:

- *Licensure.* A license is issued by the state. An agency must have a license to operate and provide care.
- *Certification.* This is required to receive Medicare and Medicaid funds.
- *Accreditation.* This is voluntary. It signals quality and excellence.

### THE SURVEY PROCESS

Surveys are done to see if the agency meets set standards. A survey team will:

- Review policies and procedures
- Review medical records
- Interview staff, patients and residents, and families
- Observe how care is given
- Check for cleanliness and safety
- Review budgets and finances
- Make sure the staff meets state requirements (Are doctors and nurses licensed? Are nursing assistants on the state registry?)

The survey team decides if the agency meets the standards. If standards are met, the agency receives a license, certification, or accreditation.

Sometimes problems are found. A problem is called a *deficiency*. The agency is given time to correct it. Usually 60 days is given. The agency can be fined for uncorrected or serious deficiencies. Or it can lose its license, certification, or accreditation.

### YOUR ROLE

You have an important role in meeting standards and in the survey process. You must:

- Provide quality care
- Protect the person's rights
- Provide for the person's and your own safety
- Help keep the agency clean and safe
- Conduct yourself in a professional manner
- Have good work ethics
- Follow agency policies and procedures
- Answer surveyor questions honestly and completely

---

**BOX 1-4   TYPES OF MANAGED CARE**

**Health Maintenance Organization (HMO)**—provides health care services for a prepaid fee. For the fee, persons receive needed services offered by the HMO. Some need just an annual physical exam. Others require hospital care. Whatever services are used, the cost is covered by the prepaid fee. HMOs focus on preventing disease and maintaining health. Keeping someone healthy costs far less than treating illness.

**Preferred Provider Organization (PPO)**—is a group of doctors and hospitals. They provide health care at reduced rates. Usually the arrangement is made between the PPO and an employer or an insurance company. Employees or those insured are given reduced rates for the services used. The person can choose any doctor or hospital in the PPO.

# ■ REVIEW QUESTIONS ■

Circle the **BEST** answer.

**1** Helping persons return to their highest physical and mental functioning is called
   a Detection and treatment of disease
   b Promotion of health
   c Rehabilitation
   d Disease prevention

**2** Rehabilitation starts when the
   a Person is ready for discharge
   b Person first seeks health care
   c Doctor writes the order
   d Health team thinks the person is ready

**3** A health care program for persons who are dying is called a
   a Hospice
   b Nursing center
   c Skilled nursing facility
   d Hospital

**4** Who controls policy in a health care agency?
   a The survey team
   b The health team
   c The board of trustees
   d The administrator

**5** Who is responsible for the entire nursing staff and safe nursing care?
   a The case manager
   b The director of nursing
   c The nursing supervisor
   d An RN

**6** You are a member of
   a The health team and the nursing team
   b The health team and the medical team
   c The nursing team and the medical team
   d An HMO and a PPO

**7** The nursing team includes the following *except*
   a RNs
   b Doctors
   c Nursing assistants
   d LVNs/LPNs

**8** Who does *not* supervise LPNs/LVNs?
   a Doctors
   b RNs
   c Dentists
   d Therapists

**9** Nursing tasks are delegated according to the person's needs and staff member abilities. This nursing care pattern is called
   a Functional nursing
   b Primary nursing
   c Team nursing
   d Case management

**10** These statements are about insurance programs. Which is *false?*
   a PPOs provide health care at reduced rates.
   b HMOs provide health care for a prepaid fee.
   c Medicare and Medicaid are for anyone in need.
   d DRGs and RUGs affect Medicare payments.

**11** Which is required for an agency to operate and provide care?
   a A license
   b Certification
   c Accreditation
   d A survey

**12** Which process is voluntary for health care agencies?
   a Licensure
   b Certification
   c Accreditation
   d Surveys

*Answers to these questions are on p. 815.*

# The Nursing Assistant

## OBJECTIVES

- Define the key terms listed in this chapter
- Explain the history and current trends affecting nursing assistants
- Explain the laws that affect nursing assistants
- Explain what nursing assistants can do and their role limits
- Explain why you need a job description
- Describe the educational requirements for nursing assistants
- Describe the delegation process
- Explain how to accept or refuse a delegated task
- Explain how to prevent negligent acts
- Give examples of false imprisonment, defamation, assault, battery, and fraud
- Describe how to protect the right to privacy
- Explain the purpose of informed consent
- Explain your role in relation to wills
- Describe child, elder, and domestic abuse

## KEY TERMS

**abuse** The intentional mistreatment or harm of another person

**accountable** Being responsible for one's actions and the actions of others who perform delegated tasks; answering questions about and explaining one's actions and the actions of others

**assault** Intentionally attempting or threatening to touch a person's body without the person's consent

**battery** Touching a person's body without his or her consent

**civil law** Laws concerned with relationships between people

**crime** An act that violates a criminal law

**criminal law** Laws concerned with offenses against the public and society in general

**defamation** Injuring a person's name and reputation by making false statements to a third person

**delegate** To authorize another person to perform a task

**ethics** Knowledge of what is right conduct and wrong conduct

**false imprisonment** Unlawful restraint or restriction of a person's freedom of movement

**fraud** Saying or doing something to trick, fool, or deceive a person

**invasion of privacy** Violating a person's right not to have his or her name, picture, or private affairs exposed or made public without giving consent

**job description** A list of responsibilities and functions the agency expects you to perform

**law** A rule of conduct made by a government body

**libel** Making false statements in print, writing, or through pictures or drawings

**malpractice** Negligence by a professional person

**negligence** An unintentional wrong in which a person fails to act in a reasonable and careful manner and causes harm to a person or to the person's property

**responsibility** The duty or obligation to perform some act or function

**slander** Making false statements orally

**standard of care** The skills, care, and judgment required by the health team member under similar conditions

**task** A function, procedure, activity, or work that does not require an RN's professional knowledge or judgment

**tort** A wrong committed against a person or the person's property

**will** A legal statement of how a person wants property distributed after death

Federal and state laws and agency polices combine to define the roles and functions of each health team member. Everyone must protect patients and residents from harm. To do so, you need to know:

- What you can and cannot do
- What is right conduct and wrong conduct
- Your legal limits

Laws, job descriptions, and the person's condition shape your work. So does the amount of supervision you need.

Protecting persons from harm also involves a complex set of rules and standards of conduct. They form the legal and ethical aspects of care.

## HISTORY AND CURRENT TRENDS

For decades, nursing assistants have helped nurses with basic nursing care. Often called *nurse's aides,* they gave baths and made beds. They helped with grooming, elimination, and other needs. Their work was similar in hospitals and nursing homes. Until the 1980s, training was not required by law. RNs gave on-the-job training. Some hospitals, nursing homes, and schools offered nursing assistant courses.

Before the 1980s, team nursing was common. An RN was the team leader. The RN assigned care to nurses and nursing assistants. Care was assigned according to each person's needs and condition. It also depended on the staff member's education and experiences.

Primary nursing was common in the 1980s. RNs planned and gave care. Many hospitals did not hire LPNs/LVNs and nursing assistants. Meanwhile, nursing homes relied on nursing assistants for resident care.

Home care increased during the 1980s. Prospective payment systems limit health care payments (Chapter 1). To reduce care costs, hospital stays also are limited. Therefore patients are discharged earlier than in the past. Often they are still quite ill and need home care.

Health care is a major political issue. The goals are to reduce costs and provide all persons with health care. Efforts to reduce health care costs include:

- *Hospital closings.* Many do not make enough money to stay open.
- *Hospital mergers.* Hospitals merge to share resources and to avoid the same costly services. For example, one hospital offers heart surgery. The other serves women and children.
- *Health care systems.* Agencies join together as one provider of care (Chapter 1). For example, the person transfers from the hospital to a system nursing center.

The person is transported by the system's ambulance service. After rehabilitation, the person returns home. The system's home care agency provides needed home care. The person's care is kept within the system from the hospital to the home setting.

- *Managed care.* Insurers have contracts with doctors, hospitals, and health care systems for reduced rates or discounts (Chapter 1). The insured person uses the services with the lower rates. If others are used, the care is covered in part or not at all. The person pays for costs not covered by insurance.
- *Staffing mix.* Hospitals hire RNs, LPNs/LVNs, and nursing assistants. Most hospitals require a state-approved nursing assistant training and competency evaluation program for employment. More training is given for tasks not in the training program.
- *Patient-focused care and cross-training.* Services are moved from departments to the bedside. Staff members are cross-trained to perform basic skills performed by other health team members. For example, a blood test was ordered for Ms. Tyler. The nurse tells the unit secretary, who then calls the laboratory. The laboratory secretary tells a medical laboratory technician. The technician sends a staff member to Ms. Tyler's room to draw the blood sample. Five people are involved so far. With patient-focused care and cross-training, Ms. Tyler's blood is drawn by a nursing team member when the order is given. Ms. Tyler does not wait for laboratory staff to arrive. She is served faster and with fewer staff members. Fewer staff members reduce costs.

## STATE AND FEDERAL LAWS

The tasks performed by nursing assistants vary from state to state. They also can vary among and within agencies. For example, emergency room tasks may differ from those on a surgical nursing unit. You might do other tasks in home care.

State nurse practice acts and the Omnibus Budget Reconciliation Act of 1987 (OBRA) provide direction for what you can do.

### NURSE PRACTICE ACTS

Each state has a nurse practice act. It regulates nursing practice in that state. It does so to protect the public's welfare and safety. A nurse practice act:

- Defines RN and LPN/LVN.
- Describes the scope of practice for RNs and LPNs/LVNs.
- Describes education and licensing requirements for RNs and LPNs/LVNs .
- Protects the public from persons practicing nursing without a license. Persons who do not meet the state's requirements cannot perform nursing functions.

The law allows for revoking or suspending a nurse's license. Reasons include:
- Being convicted of a crime in any state
- Selling or distributing drugs
- Using the person's drugs for oneself
- Placing a person in danger from the overuse of alcohol or drugs
- Demonstrating grossly negligent nursing practice
- Being convicted of abusing or neglecting children or older persons
- Violating a nurse practice act and its rules and regulations
- Demonstrating incompetent behaviors
- Aiding or assisting another person to violate a nurse practice act and its rules and regulations
- Making medical diagnoses
- Prescribing drugs and treatments

A state's nurse practice act is used to decide what nursing assistants can do. Legal and advisory opinions about nursing assistants are based on the act. So are any state laws about their roles and functions. If you perform a task beyond the legal limits of your role, you could be practicing nursing without a license. This creates serious legal problems for you and the nurse supervising your work.

## THE OMNIBUS BUDGET RECONCILIATION ACT OF 1987

The Omnibus Budget Reconciliation Act of 1987 (OBRA) applies to all 50 states. Its purpose is to improve the quality of life of nursing center residents.

This law sets minimum training and competency evaluation requirements for nursing assistants. The law requires each state to have a nursing assistant training and competency evaluation program. It must be completed by nursing assistants working in nursing centers and hospital long-term care units. *See Focus on Home Care: The Omnibus Budget Reconciliation Act of 1987.*

**THE TRAINING PROGRAM.** OBRA requires at least 75 hours of instruction. Some states require more hours. Sixteen hours is supervised practical training. It occurs in a laboratory or clinical setting (Fig. 2-1). The student performs nursing care and procedures on another person. A nurse supervises this practical training (clinical practicum or clinical experience).

The training program includes the knowledge and skills needed to give basic nursing care. Areas of study include:
- Communication
- Infection control
- Safety and emergency procedures
- Residents' rights
- Basic nursing skills
- Personal care skills
- Feeding methods
- Elimination procedures
- Skin care
- Transferring, positioning, and turning methods
- Dressing
- Ambulating the person
- Range-of-motion exercises
- Signs and symptoms of common diseases
- How to care for cognitively impaired persons (those who have problems with thinking and memory)

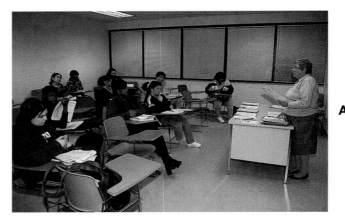

A

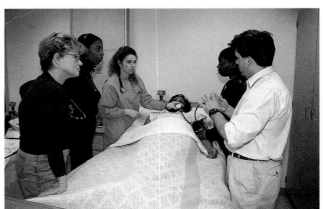

B

**FIG. 2-1** Nursing assistant training program. **A,** Students study in a classroom setting. **B,** Students practice nursing skills in a laboratory setting.

---

### FOCUS ON HOME CARE
#### THE OMNIBUS BUDGET RECONCILIATION ACT OF 1987

Many states have training and competency requirements for home health care assistants (home health aides). If a home care agency receives Medicare funds, such workers must meet OBRA's training and competency evaluation requirements.

**COMPETENCY EVALUATION.** The competency evaluation has a written test and a skills test (see Appendix A, p. 821). The written test has multiple-choice questions. Each has four choices. Only one answer is correct. The number of questions varies from state to state.

The skills test involves performing nursing skills. You will perform certain skills learned in your training program.

You take the competency evaluation after your training program. Your instructor tells you where the tests are given. He or she helps you complete the application. There is a fee for the evaluation. Send the fee with your application. If you work in a nursing center, the employer pays this fee. You are told the place and time of the tests after your application is processed. Some states give you a choice of test dates.

Your training prepares you for the competency evaluation. If you listen, study hard, and practice safe care, you should do well. If the first attempt was not successful, you can retest. OBRA allows at least three attempts to successfully complete the evaluation.

**NURSING ASSISTANT REGISTRY.** OBRA requires a nursing assistant registry in each state. It is an official record or listing of persons who have successfully completed a state-approved nursing assistant training and competency evaluation program. The registry has information about each nursing assistant:

- Full name, including maiden name and any married names.
- Last known home address.
- Registration number and its expiration date.
- Date of birth.
- Last known employer, date hired, and date employment ended.
- Date the competency evaluation was passed.
- Information about findings of abuse, neglect, or dishonest use of property. It includes the nature of the offense and supporting evidence. If a hearing was held, the date and its outcome are included. The person has the right to include a statement disputing the finding. All information stays in the registry for at least 5 years.

Any agency can access registry information. You also receive a copy of your registry information. The copy is provided when the first entry is made and when information is changed or added. You can correct wrong information.

**OTHER OBRA REQUIREMENTS.** Retraining and a new competency evaluation program are required for nursing assistants who have not worked for 2 consecutive years (24 months). It does not matter how long someone worked as a nursing assistant. What matters is how long that person did *not* work. States can require:

- A new competency evaluation
- Both retraining and a new competency evaluation

Regular in-service education and performance reviews also are required. Nursing centers must provide educational programs to nursing assistants. Their work is evaluated. These requirements help ensure that nursing assistants have current knowledge and skills to give safe, effective care.

## ROLES AND RESPONSIBILITIES

Nurse practice acts, OBRA, state laws, and legal and advisory opinions direct what you can do. To protect persons from harm, you must understand what you can do, what you cannot do, and the legal limits of your role. In some states this is called *scope of practice.*

RNs supervise your work. In some states, LPNs/LVNs can do so. You assist nurses in giving care. You also perform nursing procedures and tasks involved in the person's care. Often you function without a nurse in the room. At other times you help nurses give care. In some agencies, you assist doctors with procedures. The rules in Box 2-1 will help you understand your role.

Nursing assistant functions and responsibilities vary among states and agencies. Before you perform a procedure make sure that:

- Your state allows nursing assistants to perform the procedure
- The procedure is in your job description
- You have the necessary training and education
- A nurse is available to answer questions and to supervise you

---

**BOX 2-1 RULES FOR NURSING ASSISTANTS**

- You are an assistant to the nurse.
- A nurse assigns and supervises your work.
- You report observations about the person's physical or mental status to the nurse. Report changes at once.
- The nurse decides what should be done for a person. The nurse decides what should not be done for a person. You do not make these decisions.
- Review directions with the nurse before going to the person.
- Perform no function or task that you are not trained to do.
- Perform no function or task that you are not comfortable doing without a nurse's supervision.
- Perform only those functions and tasks that your state and job description allow.

You perform tasks and procedures that meet hygiene, safety, comfort, nutrition, exercise, and elimination needs. You lift and move persons and collect specimens. You observe the person. This includes measuring temperatures, pulses, respirations, and blood pressures. You assist with admitting and discharging patients and residents. Promoting psychological comfort also is part of your role. *See Focus on Home Care: Roles and Responsibilities.*

Box 2-2 describes the limits of your role. These are the procedures and tasks that you never perform. You must know what you can do in the state in which you are working. For example, you move from New York to New Hampshire. You must learn the laws and rules in New Hampshire. Some nursing assistants work in two states. For example, you work at nursing centers in Illinois and Iowa. Your functions in Illinois may differ from those in Iowa. You must know the laws and rules of both states.

Some nursing assistants are also emergency medical technicians (EMTs). EMTs give emergency care outside of health care settings. These settings are called "in the field." EMTs work under the direction of doctors in hospital emergency rooms. State laws and rules for EMTs differ from those for nursing assistants. For example, Joan Woods is an EMT for a fire department. When off duty, she is a nursing assistant at St. John's Hospital. Her state allows EMTs to start intravenous infusions (IVs) in the field. However, nursing assistants do not start IVs. Joan cannot start IVs when working at the hospital as a nursing assistant.

The situation is similar for persons who were medics or corpsmen in military service. They can suture wounds. Nursing assistants cannot do so. When working as a nursing assistant, medics and corpsmen must follow their state's laws and rules for nursing assistants. As with EMTs, the ability to perform a task does not give the right to do so in all settings.

State laws and rules limit nursing assistant functions. Nursing assistant job descriptions reflect those laws and rules.

## JOB DESCRIPTION

The **job description** is a list of responsibilities and functions the agency expects you to perform (Fig. 2-2). Always request a written job description when you apply for a job. Ask questions about it during your job

*Text continued on p. 23.*

---

### BOX 2-2 ROLE LIMITS FOR NURSING ASSISTANTS

- *Never give medications.* This includes drugs given orally, rectally, vaginally, by injection, by application to the skin, or directly into the bloodstream through an intravenous (IV) line. Licensed nurses give drugs. Some states allow nursing assistants to give drugs under certain conditions. To do so, you must complete a state-required medication training program. The function must be in your job description. You must have the necessary supervision.

- *Never insert tubes or objects into body openings. Do not remove them from the body.* You must not insert tubes into a person's bladder, esophagus, trachea, nose, ears, bloodstream, or surgically created body openings. Exceptions to this rule are those procedures in this textbook (giving enemas, inserting rectal tubes). You may study and practice these procedures during your training. To perform them, they must be in your job description. And you must have the necessary supervision.

- *Never take oral or telephone orders from doctors.* Politely give your name and title, and ask the doctor to wait. Promptly find a nurse to speak with the doctor.

- *Never perform procedures that require sterile technique.* With sterile technique, all objects in contact with the person's body are free of microorganisms. Sterile technique and procedures require skills, knowledge, and judgment beyond your training. You can assist a nurse with a sterile procedure. However, you will not perform the procedure yourself.

- *Never tell the person or family the person's diagnosis or medical or surgical treatment plans.* This is the doctor's responsibility. Nurses may clarify what the doctor has said.

- *Never diagnose or prescribe treatments or drugs for anyone.* Only doctors can diagnose and prescribe.

- *Never supervise other nursing assistants or assistive personnel.* This is a nurse's responsibility. You will not be trained to supervise others. Supervising others can have serious legal consequences.

- *Never ignore an order or request to do something that you cannot do or that is beyond your legal limits.* Promptly explain to the nurse why you cannot carry out the order or request. The nurse assumes you are doing what you were told to do unless you explain otherwise. You cannot neglect the person's care.

---

### FOCUS ON HOME CARE
#### ROLES AND RESPONSIBILITIES

You provide personal care and home services. Home services depend on the needs of the person and family. They may include:

- Laundry. Clothing and linens are washed, ironed, and mended. (This may include family laundry.)
- Shopping for groceries and household items.
- Preparing and serving meals. You plan menus, follow special diets, and feed the person if necessary.
- Light housekeeping. You do not do heavy housekeeping. This includes moving heavy furniture, waxing floors, shampooing carpets, washing windows, and cleaning rugs or drapes. You do not carry firewood, coal, or ash containers.

**JOB DESCRIPTION**

**Illinois Valley Community Hospital**
925 West Street, Peru, Illinois 61354
815-223-3300

Caring Professionals

CRITERIA: NURSE ASSISTANT          NAME: _____          UNIT: _____

The following criteria are to be considered as an integral part of this job description and are used in the evaluation process.

| ASSISTING WITH NURSING CARE | Met | Not Met |
|---|---|---|
| **ASSISTS WITH ASSESSING**<br>Recognizes abnormal vital signs and reports them to the nurse in charge immediately. | | |
| Observes patients and reports problems (e.g., bleeding, drainage, voiding, machine functions, IV drip, safety situations) immediately and/or current status to the nurse in charge. | | |
| Checks on patients regularly, making frequent rounds. | | |
| **ASSISTS WITH PLANNING/ORGANIZING**<br>Consistently organizes and appropriately executes personal work assignments in an effort to achieve maximum productivity and efficiency during the assigned shift. | | |
| Demonstrates a time-conscious awareness and consistently strives to use time effectively, completing assigned procedures during scheduled shift. | | |
| Responds to changes in the unit workload, patient census, and staffing levels; plans patient care accordingly. | | |
| Demonstrates an ability to recognize and deal with priorities promptly. | | |
| **ASSISTS WITH IMPLEMENTING**<br>Administers patient care based on the plan of care. | | |
| Effectively implements nursing orders after consulting appropriate sources regarding unfamiliar or questionable orders. | | |
| Responds to patient's condition/needs and acts in a timely and appropriate manner. | | |
| Demonstrates a reliable and dependable ability to follow through with designated responsibilities in collecting, labeling, and transporting specimens to the proper area at the appropriate time: always correctly labels type of specimen collected, including patient's name and room number. | | |
| Assists the nurse with complicated treatment procedures. | | |
| Completes work left from previous shifts and reports all incomplete assignments to ensure continuity of care. | | |
| As required, provides for patient comfort (by positioning, extra bathing, straightening linens, putting personal articles within reach) with courtesy and responsiveness. | | |
| Routinely assists patients with elimination (bedpan, bathroom) as required. | | |
| Regularly ambulates patients as assigned; demonstrates proper techniques. | | |

**FIG. 2-2** Nursing assistant job description. Note that the job description is also a performance evaluation tool. (Modified from Illinois Valley Community Hospital, Peru, Ill.)
*Continued.*

| ASSISTING WITH NURSING CARE (CONT'D) | Met | Not Met |
|---|---|---|
| Consistently demonstrates competence in providing morning, evening, and general care routines in accordance with established nursing care procedures to ensure patients' comfort and safety. | | |
| Regularly prepares patients for meals, sets up each patient and patient's tray, assists in feeding patients (if necessary), positions patients to avoid choking and for ease in eating, and distributes water and other nourishments according to patients' needs; regularly provides patients with fresh water. | | |
| Always follows the nursing care plan; observes established policies and procedures for proper patient treatment and care. | | |
| Promptly answers patient signal lights, whether that of assigned patient or not. | | |
| ASSISTS WITH EVALUATING<br>Checks physical environment of unit to determine what needs to be done in terms of smooth operation. | | |
| Evaluates need for linen changes. | | |
| Reviews basic care provided to patients and reports if changes are needed. | | |
| ASSISTS WITH TEACHING/LEARNING<br>Regularly provides patient information on admission in regard to: correct storage of patients' valuables, eyeglasses, and dentures; use of equipment, bed controls, nurse/patient communication system; location of bathroom and emergency call signals; and specimen collection. | | |
| Serves as a resource person for new employees during orientation. | | |
| Demonstrates the knowledge and skills necessary to provide care appropriate to pediatric, adolescent, adult, and geriatric patients. (Attends two age-specific in-services.) | | |
| Demonstrates the knowledge of the principles of growth and development over the life span. (Score at least 80% on post-test.) | | |
| Recognizes own inadequacies, and seeks assistance appropriately. | | |
| COMMUNICATING | | |
| Communicates to appropriate members of the health care team specific observations or changes in patient's condition. | | |
| Explains information to patients, visitors, and co-workers in a clear and thorough manner; leaves no questions unanswered and follows up on information not readily available. | | |
| Consistently communicates appropriately with patients: speaks respectfully, addresses patients by name, responds to patients' needs or requests for assistance. | | |
| JUDGMENT/LEADERSHIP | | |
| Promotes teamwork among staff. | | |
| Reports all patient care or management problems as appropriate, using chain of command. | | |
| Functions in a calm manner during emergency and crisis situations. | | |

**FIG. 2-2, CONT'D** Nursing assistant job description. Note that the job description is also a performance evaluation tool.

| | Met | Not Met |
|---|---|---|
| **MAINTAINING SAFETY/INFECTION CONTROL/PATIENT RIGHTS** | | |
| Always demonstrates knowledge of and rationale for safe use of equipment; reports any equipment malfunctions and orders service, as necessary. | | |
| Ensures patient safety by maintaining bed in a low position and signal light within reach at all times. Identifies patients before performing procedures. Follows the care plan for bed rail use. | | |
| Uses proper techniques of body mechanics. | | |
| Assists in maintaining a clean, safe, and attractive environment in all areas of the patient unit. | | |
| Practices hand hygiene before and after each patient contact; uses aseptic technique during procedures and treatments. | | |
| Uses principles of Standard, Airborne, Droplet, and Contact Precautions. Follows the Bloodborne Pathogen Standard. | | |
| Adheres to The Patient Care Partnership: Understanding Expectations, Rights, and Responsibilities, and respects the patient's right to privacy, dignity, and confidentiality. | | |
| Handles all patients' clothing, dentures, glasses, and other valuables with care. | | |
| **RELATIONSHIP WITH OTHERS** | | |
| Demonstrates a high level of mental and emotional tolerance and even temperament when dealing with ill people; uses tact, sensitivity, sound judgment, and a professional attitude when relating with patients, families, co-workers, and physicians. | | |
| Greets all patients in a courteous manner by introducing self and calling the patient by name. | | |
| Displays an unhurried, caring manner in all personal contact; demonstrates the ability to remain friendly and cooperative during all work situations. | | |
| Consistently responds to others in a helpful manner, especially in times of increased patient activities or short staffing situations. | | |
| Promotes an atmosphere of acceptance for new staff members on the unit. | | |
| **ATTENDANCE AND RELIABILITY** | | |
| Consistently is on time and ready to work at the start of the shift; requires no start-up time. | | |
| Willingly accepts reassignments to other units when necessary. | | |
| Consistently returns promptly from errands, coffee breaks, and meals. | | |
| Complies with Absenteeism Policy. | | |
| **COOPERATION/SUPPORT** | | |
| Attends and actively participates in unit meetings. (75% of the time) | | |
| Accepts additional assignments willingly. | | |

**FIG. 2-2, CONT'D** Nursing assistant job description. Note that the job description is also a performance evaluation tool.

*Continued.*

| | Met | Not Met |
|---|---|---|
| COOPERATION/SUPPORT (CONT'D) | | |
| Consistently promotes good public relations for the unit, nursing department, and hospital. | | |
| Supports hospital philosophy, policies and procedures, and management decisions. | | |
| INITIATIVE | | |
| Takes initiative in recognition and resolution of problems. | | |
| Reports to the nurse manager or appropriate supervisor any suggestions or recommendations for positive changes within the departmental policies and procedures. | | |
| Ensures that supplies are maintained according to established guidelines, and notifies appropriate person to restock. | | |
| PROFESSIONAL GROWTH/APPEARANCE | | |
| Always appears well-groomed and observes the hospital dress code; wears identification badge while on duty; maintains a professional appearance at all times; is clean and well-groomed. | | |
| Maintains professional code of ethics. | | |
| Attends all mandatory programs including those on safety, infection control, and CPR. | | |
| Attends a minimum of 5 other programs throughout the year. | | |
| Identifies own self-development needs, and writes goals for same. Strives to achieve those goals. | | |
| Demonstrates ability to perform unit-specific competencies. | | |
| PARTICIPATES IN PROFESSIONAL/COMMUNITY ORGANIZATIONS/ACTIVITIES OR HOSPITAL-RELATED COMMUNITY ACTIVITIES.  LIST:                                                                                  **BONUS** | | |
| DEMONSTRATES PROFESSIONAL GROWTH BY ACQUIRING COLLEGIATE CREDIT, CBU'S, OR CERTIFICATION.                                                                            **BONUS** | | |
| REGULARLY CONTRIBUTES TO NURSING AND HOSPITAL FUNCTIONS THROUGH ACTIVE PARTICIPATION ON COMMITTEES.                                                                  **BONUS** | | |
| WORKS EXTRA WEEKENDS/HOLIDAYS TO ASSIST IN PROVIDING ADEQUATE STAFFING.    **BONUS** | | |
| ROTATES SHIFTS AND WORKS EXTRA HOURS TO ASSIST IN PROVIDING ADEQUATE STAFFING.   **BONUS** | | |

**FIG. 2-2, CONT'D** Nursing assistant job description. Note that the job description is also a performance evaluation tool.

interview. Before accepting a job, tell the employer about any functions you did not learn. Also advise the employer of functions you cannot do for moral or religious reasons. Clearly understand what is expected before taking a job. Do not take a job that requires you to:
- Act beyond the legal limits of your role
- Function beyond your training limits
- Perform acts that are against your morals or religion

No one can force you to do something beyond the legal limits of your role. Jobs may be threatened for refusing to follow a nurse's orders. Often staff members obey out of fear. That is why you must understand your roles and responsibilities. You also need to know the functions you can safely perform, the things you should never do, and your job description. Understanding the ethical and legal aspects of your role is equally important (p. 25).

## EDUCATIONAL REQUIREMENTS

Each agency has educational requirements for nursing assistants. They are based on state laws and guidelines that limit what nursing assistants can do.

## DELEGATION

Nurse practice acts give nurses certain responsibilities. They also give them the legal authority to perform nursing tasks. A **responsibility** is the duty or obligation to perform some act or function. For example, RNs are responsible for supervising LPNs/LVNs and nursing assistants. Only RNs can carry out this responsibility.

In nursing, a **task** is a function, procedure, activity, or work that does not require an RN's professional knowledge or judgment. **Delegate** means to authorize another person to perform a task. The person must be competent to perform the task in a given situation. For example, you know how to give a bed bath. However, Mr. Jones is a new resident. The RN wants to spend time with him and assess his nursing needs. The RN gives the bath.

## WHO CAN DELEGATE

RNs can delegate tasks to LPNs/LVNs and nursing assistants. In some states, LPNs/LVNs can delegate tasks to nursing assistants. *See Focus on Long-Term Care: Who Can Delegate.*

### FOCUS ON LONG-TERM CARE
#### WHO CAN DELEGATE
Some states allow LPNs/LVNs to have supervisory roles in long-term care settings. The LPN/LVN delegates tasks to nursing assistants. The LPN/LVN follows the delegation process and the "five rights of delegation" (p. 24).

Delegation decisions must protect the person's health and safety. The delegating nurse is legally accountable for the task. To be **accountable** means to be responsible for one's actions and the actions of others who perform delegated tasks. It also involves answering questions about and explaining one's actions and the actions of others.

The delegating nurse must make sure that the task was completed safely and correctly. If the RN delegates, the RN is responsible for the delegated task. If the LPN/LVN delegates, the LPN/LVN is responsible for the delegated task. The RN also supervises LPNs/LVNs. Therefore the RN also is legally accountable for the tasks that LPNs/LVNs delegate to nursing assistants. The RN is accountable for all nursing care.

*Nursing assistants cannot delegate.* You cannot delegate any task to other nursing assistants. You can ask someone to help you. But you cannot ask or tell someone to do your work.

## DELEGATION PROCESS

Delegated tasks must be within the legal limits of what you can do. The nurse must know:
- What tasks your state allows nursing assistants to perform
- The tasks in your job description
- What you were taught in your education program
- What skills you learned
- How your skills were evaluated
- About your work experiences

The nurse discusses these areas with you. The nurse needs to learn about you, your abilities, and your concerns. You may be a new employee or new to the nursing unit. Or the nurse may be new. In any case, the nurse needs to know about you. You need to know about the nurse.

Agency policies, guidelines, and your job description state what tasks nurses can delegate to you. These documents must follow state laws, rules, and legal opinions about nursing assistants.

To make delegation decisions, the nurse reviews the questions in Box 2-3, p. 24. The person's needs, the task, and the staff member doing the task must fit. The nurse can decide to delegate the task to you. Or the nurse can decide not to delegate the task. The person's needs and the task may require a nurse's knowledge, judgment, and skill. You may be asked to assist.

Do not get offended or angry if you are not asked to perform a task that is usually delegated to you. The nurse decides what is best for the person at the time. That decision is also best for you at that time. You should not do something that requires a nurse's judgment and critical thinking skills. For example, you often care for Mrs. Mills. She has bruises on her face and arms after her son visits. She reports falling in the bathroom. The RN suspects abuse. Instead of asking you to assist Mrs. Mills with bathing, the RN does so.

- What is the person's condition? Is it stable or likely to change?
- What are the person's basic needs at this time?
- What is the person's mental function at this time?
- What are the person's emotional and spiritual needs at this time?
- Can the person assist with his or her care? Does the person depend on others for care?
- Is the task something the nurse can delegate?
- For this person, does the task require the knowledge, judgment, and skill of an RN or LPN/LVN?
- How often will the nurse have to assess the person?
- Can the task harm the person? If yes, how?
- What effect will the task have on the person?
- Is it safe for the person if the task is delegated to you?
- Do you have the training and experience to perform the task, given the person's current status? Is your training documented? How were your training and skills evaluated?
- How often have you performed the task?
- What other tasks were delegated to you?
- Do you have the time to perform the task safely?
- Is a nurse available to supervise you?
- How much supervision will you need?
- Will you need more directions as you perform the task?
- Is a nurse available to help or take over if the person's condition changes or problems arise?

The RN wants to assess Mrs. Mills for other signs of abuse and to talk with her. At this time Mrs. Mills needs the RN's knowledge and judgment.

The person's circumstances are central factors in making delegation decisions. They must result in the best care for the person. A nurse risks a person's health and safety with poor delegation decisions. Also, the nurse may face serious legal problems. If you perform a task that places the person at risk, you can also face serious legal problems.

**THE FIVE RIGHTS OF DELEGATION.** The National Council of State Boards of Nursing's five rights of delegation sum up the delegation process:

- *The right task.* Can the task be delegated? Is the nurse allowed to delegate the task? Is the task in your job description?
- *The right circumstances.* What are the person's physical, mental, emotional, and spiritual needs at this time?
- *The right person.* Do you have the training and experience to safely perform the task for this person?
- *The right directions and communication.* The nurse must give clear directions. The nurse tells you what to do

and when to do it. The nurse tells you what observations to make and when to report back. The nurse allows questions and helps you set priorities.
- *The right supervision.* The nurse guides, directs, and evaluates the care you give. The nurse demonstrates tasks as necessary and is available to answer questions. The less experience you have with a task, the more supervision you need. Complex tasks require more supervision than do basic tasks. Also, the person's circumstances affect how much supervision you need. The nurse assesses how the task affected the person and how well you performed the task. The nurse tells you what you did well and what you can do to improve your work. This is to help you learn and give better care.

## YOUR ROLE IN DELEGATION

You perform delegated tasks for or on *a person*. You must perform the task safely. This protects the person from harm. You have two choices when a task is delegated to you. You either *agree* or *refuse* to do the task. Use the "five rights of delegation" to decide. Answer the questions in Box 2-4.

**ACCEPTING A TASK.** When you agree to perform a task, you are responsible for your own actions. What you do or fail to do can harm the person. *You must complete the task safely.* Ask for help when you are unsure or have questions about a task. Report to the nurse what you did and the observations you made.

**REFUSING A TASK.** You have the right to say "no." Sometimes refusing to follow the nurse's directions is your right and duty. You should refuse to perform a task when:
- The task is beyond the legal limits of your role
- The task is not in your job description
- You were not prepared to perform the task
- The task could harm the person
- The person's condition has changed
- You do not know how to use the supplies or equipment
- Directions are unethical, illegal, or against agency policies
- Directions are unclear or incomplete
- A nurse is not available for supervision

Use common sense. This protects you and the person. Ask yourself if what you are doing is safe for the person.

Never ignore an order or a request to do something. Tell the nurse about your concerns. If the task is within the legal limits of your role and in your job description, the nurse can help increase your comfort with the task. The nurse can:
- Answer your questions
- Demonstrate the task
- Show you how to use supplies and equipment
- Help you as needed

**THE FIVE RIGHTS OF DELEGATION FOR NURSING ASSISTANTS**

**THE RIGHT TASK**

- Does your state allow you to perform the task?
- Were you trained to do the task?
- Do you have experience performing the task?
- Is the task in your job description?

**THE RIGHT CIRCUMSTANCES**

- Do you have experience performing the task given the person's condition and needs?
- Do you understand the purpose of the task for the person?
- Can you perform the task safely under the current circumstances?
- Do you have the equipment and supplies to safely complete the task?
- Do you know how to use the equipment and supplies?

**THE RIGHT PERSON**

- Are you comfortable performing the task?
- Do you have concerns about performing the task?

**THE RIGHT DIRECTIONS AND COMMUNICATION**

- Did the nurse give clear directions and instructions?
- Did you review the task with the nurse?
- Do you understand what the nurse expects?

**THE RIGHT SUPERVISION**

- Is a nurse available to answer questions?
- Is a nurse available if the person's condition changes or if problems occur?

Modified from the National Council of State Boards of Nursing, Inc., Chicago.

- Observe you performing the task
- Check on you often
- Arrange for needed training

You must not refuse a task because you do not like it or do not want to do it. You must have sound reasons. Otherwise, you place the person at risk for harm. You also risk losing your job.

## ETHICAL ASPECTS

**Ethics** is knowledge of what is right conduct and wrong conduct. Morals are involved. It also deals with choices or judgments about what should or should not be done. An ethical person behaves and acts in the right way. He or she does not cause a person harm.

Ethical behavior also involves not being *prejudiced* or *biased*. To be prejudiced or biased means to make judgments and have views before knowing the facts.

**BOX 2-5** **RULES OF CONDUCT FOR NURSING ASSISTANTS**

- Respect each person as an individual.
- Perform no act that is not within the legal limits of your role.
- Perform only those acts that you have been prepared to do.
- Take no drug without the prescription and supervision of a doctor.
- Carry out the directions and instructions of the nurse to your best possible ability.
- Complete each task safely.
- Be loyal to your employer and co-workers.
- Act as a responsible citizen at all times.
- Know the limits of your role and knowledge.
- Keep the person's information confidential.
- Protect the person's privacy.
- Consider the person's needs to be more important than your own.
- Perform no action that will cause the person harm.

Judgments and views usually are based on one's values and standards. They are based in the person's culture, religion, education, and experiences. The person's situation may be very different from your own. For example:

- Children want their mother to have nursing home care. In your culture, children care for older parents at home.
- A person has many tattoos and body piercings. You do not like tattoos or body piercings.
- An 80-year-old man does not want lifesaving measures. You believe that everything should be done to save life.

Do not judge the person by your values or standards. Do not avoid persons whose standards and values differ from your own.

Ethical problems involve making choices. You must decide what is the right thing to do. For example:

- A co-worker is often late for work. You find her in an empty room drinking from a cup. You also smell alcohol on her breath. She asks you not to tell anyone.
- An older person has bruises all over her body. She told the RN that she fell. She tells you that her son is very mean to her. She asks you not to tell the nurse.

Professional groups have codes of ethics. The code has rules, or standards of conduct, for group members to follow. The American Nurses Association (ANA) has a code of ethics for RNs. The National Federation of Licensed Practical Nurses (NFLPN) has one for LPNs/LVNs. The rules of conduct in Box 2-5 can guide your thinking and behavior. See Chapter 3 for ethics in the workplace.

## LEGAL ASPECTS

Ethics is concerned with what you *should or should not do*. Laws tell you what you *can and cannot do*. A **law** is a rule of conduct made by a government body. The U.S. Congress and state legislatures make laws. Enforced by the government, laws protect the public welfare.

**Criminal laws** are concerned with offenses against the public and against society in general. An act that violates a criminal law is called a **crime**. A person found guilty of a crime is fined or sent to prison. Murder, robbery, rape, and kidnapping are some crimes.

**Civil laws** are concerned with relationships between people. Examples of civil laws are those that involve contracts and nursing practice. A person found guilty of breaking a civil law usually has to pay a sum of money to the injured person.

### TORTS

*Tort* comes from a French word meaning wrong. Torts are part of civil law. A **tort** is a wrong committed against a person or the person's property. Torts may be intentional or unintentional.

**UNINTENTIONAL TORTS.** **Negligence** is an unintentional wrong. The negligent person failed to act in a reasonable and careful manner. As a result, harm was caused to the person or property of another. The person did not mean or intend to cause harm. The person failed to do what a reasonable and careful person would have done. Or he or she did what a reasonable and careful person would not have done. The negligent person may have to pay damages (a sum of money) to the one injured.

**Malpractice** is negligence by a professional person. A person has professional status because of training, education, and the service provided. Nurses, doctors, dentists, lawyers, and pharmacists are examples.

What you do or do not do can lead to a lawsuit if harm results to the person or property of another. **Standard of care** refers to the skills, care, and judgment required by the health team under similar conditions. Standards of care come from:
- Laws, including nurse practice acts
- Textbooks
- Agency policies and procedures (Fig. 2-3)
- Manufacturer instructions for equipment
- Job descriptions
- Approval and accrediting agency standards

Negligent actions are likely to occur when:
- A nurse asks you to apply a hot soak. You fail to test water temperature. The water is too hot. The person is burned.
- Mrs. Parks needs help getting to the bathroom. You do not answer the signal light promptly. She gets up without help. She falls and breaks a hip.

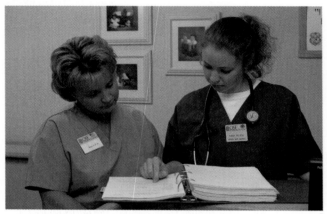

**FIG. 2-3** Nurse and nursing assistant review the policy and procedure manual. It is kept at the nurses' station.

- A mechanical lift is used to transfer Mr. Brown from his bed to a chair. You do not follow the manufacturer's instructions for using the lift. Mr. Brown slips out of the lift and falls to the floor. He breaks a hip.
- Mrs. Clark complains of chest pain. You do not tell the nurse. Mrs. Clark has a heart attack and dies.
- Two residents have the same last name. You do not identify the person before a procedure. You perform the procedure on the wrong person. Both residents are harmed. One had a procedure that was not ordered. The other did not have a needed procedure.

You are legally responsible *(liable)* for your own actions. The nurse is liable as your supervisor. However, you are not relieved of personal liability. Remember, sometimes refusing to follow the nurse's directions is your right and duty (p. 24).

**INTENTIONAL TORTS.** Intentional torts are acts meant to be harmful. Defamation (libel and slander), false imprisonment, invasion of privacy, fraud, and assault and battery are intentional torts.

**Defamation** is injuring a person's name and reputation by making false statements to a third person. **Libel** is making false statements in print, writing, or through pictures or drawings. **Slander** is making false statements orally. Never make false statements about a patient, resident, co-worker, or any other person. Examples of defamation include:
- Implying or suggesting that a person abuses drugs
- Saying that a person is insane or mentally ill
- Implying or suggesting that a person steals money from the staff

**False imprisonment** is the unlawful restraint or restriction of a person's freedom of movement. It involves:
- Threatening to restrain a person
- Restraining a person
- Preventing a person from leaving the agency

| BOX 2-6 | PROTECTING THE RIGHT TO PRIVACY |
| --- | --- |

- Keep all information about the person confidential.
- Cover the person when he or she is being moved in hallways.
- Screen the person as in Figure 2-4. Close the door when giving care. Also close drapes and window shades.
- Expose only the body part involved in a treatment or procedure.
- Do not discuss the person or the person's treatment with anyone except the nurse supervising your work. "Shop talk" is a common cause of invasion of privacy.
- Ask visitors to leave the room when care is given.
- Do not open the person's mail.
- Allow the person to visit with others in private.
- Allow the person to use the telephone in private.

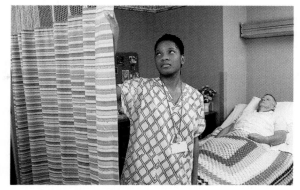

**FIG. 2-4** Pulling the curtain around the bed helps protect the person's privacy.

**Invasion of privacy** is violating a person's right not to have his or her name, picture, or private affairs exposed or made public without giving consent. You must treat the person with respect and ensure privacy. Only staff involved in the person's care should see, handle, or examine his or her body. See Box 2-6 for measures to protect privacy.

The Health Insurance Portability and Accountability Act of 1996 (HIPAA) protects the privacy and security of a patient's health information. *Protected health information* refers to identifying information and information about the person's health care. Failure to comply with HIPAA rules can result in fines, penalties, and criminal action including jail time. You must follow agency policies and procedures. Direct any questions about the person or the person's care to the nurse. Also follow the rules for computer use (Chapter 4).

**Fraud** is saying or doing something to trick, fool, or deceive a person. The act is fraud if it does or could cause harm to a person or the person's property. Telling a person or family that you are a nurse is fraud. So is giving wrong or incomplete information on a job application.

Assault and battery may result in both civil and criminal charges. **Assault** is intentionally attempting or threatening to touch a person's body without the person's consent. The person fears bodily harm. Threatening to "tie down" a person is an example of assault. **Battery** is touching a person's body without his or her consent. Consent is the important factor in assault and battery. The person must consent to any procedure, treatment, or other act that involves touching the body. The person has the right to withdraw consent at any time.

Protect yourself from being accused of assault and battery. Explain to the person what is to be done and get the person's consent. Consent may be verbal— "yes" or "okay." Or it can be a gesture—a nod, turning over for a back rub, or holding out an arm so you can take a pulse.

## INFORMED CONSENT

A person has the right to decide what will be done to his or her body and who can touch his or her body. The doctor is responsible for informing the person about all aspects of treatment. Consent is informed when the person clearly understands:

- The reason for a treatment
- What will be done
- How it will be done
- Who will do it
- The expected outcomes
- Other treatment options
- The effects of not having the treatment

Persons under legal age (usually 18 years of age) cannot give consent. Nor can mentally incompetent persons. Such persons are unconscious, sedated, or confused or have certain mental health problems. Informed consent is given by a responsible party—a husband, wife, daughter, son, or a legal representative.

Consent is given when the person enters the agency. A form is signed giving general consent to treatment. Special consent forms are required for surgery and other complex and invasive measures. The doctor informs the person about all aspects of the procedure. The RN may be given this responsibility.

*You are never responsible for obtaining written consent.* However, you can witness the signing of a consent. To be a witness, you must be present when the person signs the consent.

## WILLS

A **will** is a legal statement of how a person wants property distributed after death. You can ethically and legally witness the signing of a will. You can also refuse to do so without fear of legal action.

A person may ask you to help prepare a will. You must politely refuse. Explain that you do not have the legal knowledge or ability to prepare a will. Ask a nurse to speak to the person or family member about contacting a lawyer.

Do not witness a person's will if you are named in the will. To do so prevents you from receiving what was left to you. If you are a witness, be prepared to testify that:

- The person was of sound mind when the will was signed
- The person stated that the document being signed was his or her last will

Many agencies do not let employees witness wills. Know your agency's policy before you agree to witness a will. If you have questions, ask the nurse. If you witness a will, tell the nurse.

## REPORTING ABUSE

**Abuse** is the intentional mistreatment or harm of another person. Abuse is a crime. It can occur at home or in a health care agency. Abuse has one or more of these elements:

- Willful causing of injury
- Unreasonable confinement
- Intimidation (to make afraid with threats of force or violence)
- Punishment
- Depriving the person of goods or services needed for physical, mental, or psychosocial well-being

Abuse causes physical harm, pain, or mental anguish. Protection against abuse extends to persons in a coma. With child and elder abuse, the abuser is usually a family member or a caregiver. The abuser can be a friend, neighbor, landlord, or other person.

### ELDER ABUSE

Elder abuse can take these forms:

- *Physical abuse.* Grabbing, hitting, slapping, kicking, pinching, hair-pulling, or beating. It also includes corporal punishment—punishment inflicted directly on the body. Beatings, lashings, or whippings are examples. Neglect is also physical abuse. The person is deprived of needed health care or treatment. Neglect is also failure to provide food, clothing, hygiene, and other needs. In health care, neglect includes but is not limited to:
  —Leaving persons lying or sitting in urine or feces
  —Isolating persons in their rooms or other areas
  —Failing to answer signal lights
- *Verbal abuse.* Using oral or written words or statements that speak badly of, sneer at, criticize, or condemn the person. It includes unkind gestures.
- *Involuntary seclusion.* Confining the person to a cer-

tain area. People have been locked in closets, basements, attics, and other spaces.

- *Financial abuse.* The person's money is stolen or used by another person. It is also misusing a person's property. For example, a daughter sells her father's house without his consent.
- *Mental abuse.* Humiliation, harassment, ridicule, and threats of punishment. It includes being deprived of needs such as food, clothing, care, a home, or a place to sleep.
- *Sexual abuse.* The person is harassed about sex or is attacked sexually. The person may be forced to perform sexual acts out of fear of punishment or physical harm.

There are many signs of elder abuse. The abused person may show only some of the signs in Box 2-7.

Federal and state laws require the reporting of elder abuse. If abuse is suspected, it must be reported. Where and how to report suspected abuse vary among

---

**BOX 2-7 SIGNS OF ELDER ABUSE**

- Living conditions are unsafe, unclean, or inadequate.
- Personal hygiene is lacking. The person is unclean. Clothes are dirty.
- Weight loss—there are signs of poor nutrition and inadequate fluid intake.
- Assistive devices are missing or broken—glasses, hearing aids, dentures, cane, walker.
- Frequent injuries—conditions behind the injuries are strange or seem impossible.
- Old and new injuries—bruises, welts, scars, and punctures.
- Complaints of pain or itching in the genital area.
- Bleeding and bruising in the genital area.
- Burns on the feet, hands, or buttocks. Cigarettes and cigars cause small circle-like burns.
- Pressure ulcers (Chapter 28) or contractures (Chapter 22).
- The person seems very quiet or withdrawn.
- The person seems fearful, anxious, or agitated.
- The person does not seem to want to talk or answer questions.
- The person is restrained. Or the person is locked in a certain area for long periods.
- The person cannot reach toilet facilities, food, water, and other necessary items.
- Private conversations are not allowed. The caregiver is present during all conversations.
- The person seems anxious to please the caregiver.
- Drugs are not taken properly. Drugs are not purchased. Or too much or too little of the drug is taken.
- Visits to the emergency room may be frequent.
- The person may change doctors often. Some people do not have a doctor.

states. You may suspect that a person is being abused. If so, discuss the matter and your observations with the RN. Give as much information as possible. The RN contacts health team members as needed.

The RN also contacts community agencies that investigate elder abuse. They act at once if the problem is life-threatening. Sometimes the help of police or the courts is necessary.

*See Focus on Long-Term Care: Elder Abuse.*

Helping abused older persons is not always easy or possible. The abuse may never be reported or recognized. Or the investigating agency cannot gain access to the person. Sometimes older persons are abused by their children. A victim may want to protect the child. Some victims are embarrassed or believe they deserve abuse. A victim may fear what will happen. He or she may think that the present situation is better than no care at all. Some people fear not being believed if they report the abuse themselves.

## CHILD ABUSE

Child abuse occurs at every social level. It occurs in low-, middle-, and high-income families. The abuser may have little education or be highly educated. The abuser is usually a household member (parent, a parent's partner, brother or sister, nanny). The abuser is

someone the family knows. Risk factors for child abuse include:

- Stress
- Family crisis (divorce, unemployment, moving, poverty, crowded living conditions)
- Drug or alcohol abuse
- Abuser history of being abused as a child
- Discipline beliefs that include physical punishment
- Lack of emotional attachment to the child
- A child with birth defects or chronic illness
- A child with a personality or behaviors that the abuser considers "different" or unacceptable
- Unrealistic expectations for the child's behavior or performance
- Families that move often and do not have family or friends nearby

**TYPES OF CHILD ABUSE.** Abuse differs from neglect. *Physical neglect* means to deprive the child of food, clothing, shelter, and medical care. *Emotional neglect* is not meeting the child's need for affection and attention.

*Physical abuse* is injuring the child on purpose. It can cause death. *Sexual abuse* is using, persuading, or forcing a child to engage in sexual conduct. It may take many forms:

- *Rape*—forced sexual intercourse with a person who is not of legal age to give consent.
- *Molestation*—sexual advances toward a child. It includes kissing, touching, or fondling sexual areas. The abuser may kiss, touch, or fondle the child. Or the child is forced to kiss, touch, or fondle the abuser.
- *Incest*—sexual activity between family members. The abuser may be a parent, stepparent, brother or sister, stepbrother or stepsister, aunt or uncle, cousin, or grandparent.
- *Child pornography*—taking pictures or videotaping a child involved in sexual acts.
- *Child prostitution*—forcing a child to engage in sexual activity for money. Usually the child is forced to have many sexual partners.

Box 2-8, p. 30, lists the signs of child abuse. Child and parent behaviors may signal that something is wrong. The child may be quiet and withdrawn. He or she may fear adults. Sometimes children are afraid to go home. Sudden behavior changes are common in sexual abuse. Bedwetting, thumb-sucking, loss of appetite, poor grades, and running away from home are examples.

Parents give different stories about what happened. Injuries are blamed on play accidents or other children. Frequent emergency room visits are common.

Child abuse is complex. Many more behaviors, signs, and symptoms are present than discussed here. The health team must be alert for signs and symptoms of child abuse. State laws require the reporting of suspected child abuse. However, someone should not be falsely accused.

---

### FOCUS ON LONG-TERM CARE
#### ELDER ABUSE

OBRA does not allow nursing centers to employ persons who were convicted of abuse, neglect, or mistreatment of persons in any health care agency. Before hiring a person, the center must thoroughly check the applicant's work history. All references must be checked. Efforts must be made to find out about any criminal prosecutions.

The employer also checks the nursing assistant registry for any findings about abuse, neglect, or mistreatment of residents. It also is checked for misusing or stealing a resident's property. For nurses or other staff, the licensing authority is contacted.

The center must take certain actions if abuse is suspected within the center.

- The incident is reported at once to the administrator and to other officials as required by federal and state laws.
- All claims of abuse are thoroughly investigated.
- The center must prevent further potential for abuse while the investigation is in progress.
- Investigation results are reported to the center administrator and to other officials as required by federal and state laws within 5 days of the incident.
- Corrective actions are taken if the claim is found to be true.

<table>
<tr><td>

**BOX 2-8   SIGNS AND SYMPTOMS OF CHILD ABUSE**

**PHYSICAL ABUSE**

- Bruises on the face (lips, mouth, cheeks), back, buttocks, abdomen, chest, and inner thighs
- Welts on the face (lips, mouth, cheeks), back, buttocks, abdomen, chest, and inner thighs
  —The shape of the object causing the welt may be seen. The shape may be of a belt, belt buckle, wooden spoon, chain, clothes hanger, rope, or other object.
- Burns and scalds on the feet, hands, back, or buttocks
  —Intentional burns leave a pattern from the item causing the burn: cigarettes, irons, curling irons, ropes, stove burners, and radiators.
  —In scalds, the area immersed in the hot liquid is clearly marked. For example, a scald to the hand looks like a glove. A scald to a foot looks like a sock.
- Fractures of the nose, skull, arms, or legs
- Bite marks

**SEXUAL ABUSE**

- Bleeding, cuts, and bruises of the genitalia, anus, or mouth
- Stains or blood on underclothing
- Painful urination
- Vaginal discharge
- Genital odor
- Difficulty walking or sitting
- Pregnancy

</td></tr>
</table>

If you suspect child abuse, share your concerns with the RN. Give as much information as you can. The RN contacts health team members and child protection agencies as needed.

## DOMESTIC ABUSE

Domestic abuse occurs in relationships. One partner has power and control over the other. Such power and control occur through abuse. Fear and harm occur. Abuse may be physical, sexual, verbal, economic, or social. Usually more than one type of abuse is present:

- *Physical abuse*—unwanted punching, slapping, grabbing, choking, poking, biting, pulling hair, twisting arms, or kicking. It may involve burns and the use of weapons. Physical injuries occur. Death is a constant threat.
- *Sexual abuse*—unwanted sexual contact.
- *Verbal abuse*—unkind and hurtful remarks. They make the person feel unwhole, unattractive, and without value.
- *Economic abuse*—controlling money. Having or not having a job is controlled by the abuser. So are paychecks, money gifts from family and friends, and money for household expenses (food, clothing).
- *Social abuse*—controlling friendships and other relationships. The abuser controls phone calls, car use, leaving the home, and visits with family and friends.

Like child and elder abuse, domestic abuse is complex. The victim often hides the abuse. He or she may protect the abusive partner. State laws vary about reporting domestic abuse. However, the health team has an ethical duty to provide emotional support. They also have the duty to give information about safety and community resources. If you suspect domestic abuse, share your concerns with the RN. The RN gathers information as needed to help the person.

Circle the **BEST** answer.

1   Which trend moves services from departments to the bedside?
   a   Managed care
   b   Health care systems
   c   Staffing mix
   ✓ d   Patient-focused care

2   Nursing practice is regulated by
   a   OBRA
   b   Medicare and Medicaid
   ✓ c   Nurse practice acts
   d   Codes of ethics

3   What state law affects what you can do?
   a   The state's nurse practice act
   b   OBRA
   c   Medicare
   d   Medicaid

4   You perform a task not allowed by your state. Which is *true?*
   a   If an RN delegated the task, there is no legal problem.
   ✓ b   You could be found guilty of practicing nursing without a license.
   c   Performing the task is allowed if it is in your job description.
   d   If you complete the task safely, there is no legal problem.

5   An RN asks you to start an IV. Which is *true?*
   a   Nursing assistants do not start IVs.
   b   The RN must supervise your work.
   c   You must be trained to start IVs.
   d   You must know why the person needs the IV.

6   These statements are about delegation. Which is *false?*
   a   RNs can delegate their responsibilities to you.
   b   A delegated task must be safe for the person.
   c   The delegated task must be in your job description.
   d   The delegating nurse is responsible for the safe completion of the task.

7   A task is in your job description. Which is *false?*
   a   The RN must always delegate the task to you.
   b   The RN delegates the task to you if the person's circumstances are right.
   c   The RN must make sure you have the necessary education and training.
   d   You must have clear directions before you perform the task.

8   A nurse delegates a task to you. You must
   a   Complete the task
   b   Decide to accept or refuse the task
   c   Delegate the task if you are busy
   d   Ignore the request if you do not know what to do

9   You are responsible for
   a   Completing tasks safely
   b   Delegation
   c   The "five rights of delegation"
   d   Delegating tasks to nursing assistants

10  You can refuse to perform a task for these reasons *except*
   a   The task is beyond the legal limits of your role
   b   The task is not in your job description
   ✓ c   You do not like the task
   d   A nurse is not available to supervise you

11  You decide to refuse a task. What should you do?
   a   Delegate the task to someone else.
   b   Communicate your concerns to the nurse.
   c   Ignore the request.
   d   Talk to the nurse's supervisor.

12  Ethical standards
   a   Are federal laws
   b   State laws
   c   Are about right conduct and wrong conduct
   d   Are rules stating what you can and cannot do

13  Mr. Jones wants to know the reason for an x-ray. Who is responsible for telling him?
   a   The doctor
   b   You are
   c   The RN
   d   Any health team member

14  Which is *not* a crime?
   a  Negligence
   b  Murder
   c  Robbery
   d  Rape

15  These statements are about negligence. Which is *false*?
   a  It is an unintentional tort.
   b  The negligent person did not act in a reasonable manner.
   c  Harm was caused to a person or a person's property.
   d  A prison term is likely.

16  The intentional attempt or threat to touch a person's body without the person's consent is
   a  Assault
   b  Battery
   c  Defamation
   d  False imprisonment

17  The illegal restraint of a person's freedom of movement is
   a  Assault
   b  Battery
   c  Defamation
   d  False imprisonment

18  Mr. Blue's picture is made public without his consent. This is
   a  Battery
   b  Fraud
   c  Invasion of privacy
   d  Malpractice

19  Which will *not* protect the person's right to privacy?
   a  Informed consent
   b  Screening the person when giving care
   c  Exposing only the body part involved in the treatment or procedure
   d  Asking visitors to leave the room when care is given

20  A person asks if you are a nurse. You answer "yes." This is
   a  Negligence
   b  Fraud
   c  Libel
   d  Slander

21  Who obtains the person's informed consent?
   a  The doctor
   b  The RN
   c  The LPN
   d  The nursing assistant

22  Which is *not* a sign of elder abuse?
   a  Stiff joints and joint pain
   b  Old and new bruises
   c  Poor personal hygiene
   d  Frequent injuries

23  A child is deprived of food and clothing. This is
   a  Physical neglect
   b  Physical abuse
   c  Emotional neglect
   d  Sexual abuse

24  These statements are about domestic abuse. Which is *true*?
   a  Domestic abuse involves physical harm.
   b  Domestic abuse always involves violence.
   c  One partner has control over the other partner.
   d  Only one type of abuse is usually present.

25  You suspect a person was abused. What should you do?
   a  Tell the family.
   b  Call a state agency.
   c  Tell an RN.
   d  Ask the person if he or she was abused.

*Answers to these questions are on p. 815.*

# Work Ethics

## OBJECTIVES

- Define the key terms listed in this chapter
- Identify good health and personal hygiene practices
- Describe how to look professional
- Describe the qualities and traits of a successful nursing assistant
- Explain how to get a job
- Explain how to plan for childcare and transportation
- Describe ethical behavior on the job
- Explain how to manage stress
- Explain the aspects of harassment
- Explain how to resign from a job
- Identify the common reasons for losing a job

## KEY TERMS

**confidentiality** Trusting others with personal and private information

**courtesy** A polite, considerate, or helpful comment or act

**gossip** To spread rumors or talk about the private matters of others

**harassment** To trouble, torment, offend, or worry a person by one's behavior or comments

**preceptor** A staff member who guides another staff member

**stress** The response or change in the body caused by any emotional, physical, social, or economic factor

**stressor** The event or factor that causes stress

**work ethics** Behavior in the workplace

Ethics deals with right conduct and wrong conduct. It involves choices and judgments about what to do or what not to do. An ethical person does the right thing. In the workplace, certain behaviors (conduct), choices, and judgments are expected. **Work ethics** deals with behavior in the workplace. Your conduct reflects your choices and judgments. Work ethics involves:

- How you look
- What you say
- How you behave
- How you treat others
- How you work with others

To get and keep a job, you must conduct yourself in the right way.

## PERSONAL HEALTH, HYGIENE, AND APPEARANCE

Patients, residents, and families expect the health team to look and act healthy. For example, a person is told to stop smoking. Yet he or she sees health team members smoking. If you are not clean, people wonder if you give good care. You are a member of the health team. Your personal health, appearance, and hygiene need careful attention.

## YOUR HEALTH

You must give careful and effective care. To do so, you must be physically and mentally healthy. Otherwise you cannot function at your best.

- *Diet.* You need a balanced diet from the Food Guide Pyramid (Chapter 20). Start your day with a good breakfast. To maintain your weight, balance the calories you take in with your energy needs. To lose weight, take in fewer calories than your energy needs. Avoid foods from the fats, oils, and sweets group. Also avoid salty foods and crash diets.
- *Sleep and rest.* Sleep and rest are needed for health and to do your job well. Most adults need about 7 hours of sleep daily. Fatigue, lack of energy, and irritability mean you need more rest and sleep.
- *Body mechanics.* You will bend, carry heavy objects, and lift, move, and turn persons. These tasks place stress and strain on your body. You need to use your muscles correctly (Chapter 13).
- *Exercise.* Exercise is needed for muscle tone, circulation, and weight control. Walking, running, swimming, and biking are good forms of exercise. You will feel better physically and mentally with regular exercise. Consult your doctor before starting a vigorous exercise program.
- *Your eyes.* You will read instructions and take measurements. Wrong readings can cause the person harm. Have your eyes checked. Wear needed glasses or contact lenses. Provide enough light when reading or doing fine work.
- *Smoking.* Smoking causes lung, heart, and circulatory disorders. Smoke odors stay on your breath, hands, clothing, and hair. Hand hygiene and good personal hygiene are needed.
- *Drugs.* Some drugs affect thinking, feeling, behavior, and function. Working under the influence of drugs affects patient and resident safety. Take only those drugs ordered by a doctor. Take them in the prescribed way.
- *Alcohol.* Alcohol is a drug that depresses the brain. It affects thinking, balance, coordination, and mental alertness. Never report to work under the influence of alcohol. Do not drink alcohol while working. Like other drugs, alcohol affects the person's safety.

## YOUR HYGIENE

Personal hygiene needs careful attention. Bathe daily. Use a deodorant or antiperspirant to prevent body odors. Brush your teeth after meals. Use a mouthwash to prevent breath odors. Shampoo often. Style hair in an attractive and simple way. Keep fingernails clean, short, and neatly shaped.

Menstrual hygiene is important. Change tampons or sanitary napkins often, especially if flow is heavy. Wash your genital area with soap and water at least twice a day. Also practice good hand washing.

Foot care prevents odors and infection. Bathe your feet daily. Dry thoroughly between the toes. Cut toenails straight across after bathing or soaking them.

## YOUR APPEARANCE

Good health and personal hygiene practices help you look and feel well. Follow the practices in Box 3-1. They help you look neat, clean, and professional (Fig. 3-1, p. 36).

---

**BOX 3-1   PRACTICES FOR A PROFESSIONAL APPEARANCE**

- Practice good hygiene.
- Wear uniforms that fit well. They are modest in length and style. Follow the agency's dress code.
- Keep uniforms clean, pressed, and mended. Sew on buttons. Repair zippers, tears, and hems.
- Wear a clean uniform daily.
- Wear your name badge or photo ID at all times when on duty.
- Wear underclothes that are clean and fit properly. Change them daily. Do not wear colored undergarments. They can be seen through white and light-colored uniforms.
- Cover tattoos. They may offend others.
- Do not wear jewelry. Wedding and engagement rings may be allowed. Rings and bracelets can scratch a person. Confused or combative persons can easily pull on jewelry. So can young children.
- Do not wear jewelry in pierced eyebrows, nose, lips, or tongue while on duty.
- Follow the agency's dress code for earrings. Usually small, simple earrings are allowed. For multiple ear piercings, usually only one set of earrings is allowed.
- Wear a wristwatch with a second hand.
- Wear clean stockings and socks that fit well. Change them daily.
- Wear shoes that fit properly, are comfortable, and give needed support. Do not wear sandals or open-toed shoes.
- Clean and polish shoes often. Wash and replace laces as needed.
- Keep fingernails clean, short, and neatly shaped. Long nails can scratch a person.
- Do not wear nail polish. Chipped nail polish may provide a place for microorganisms to grow.
- Have a simple, attractive hairstyle. Hair is off your collar and away from your face. Use simple pins, combs, barrettes, and bands to keep long hair up and in place.
- Keep beards and mustaches clean and trimmed.
- Use makeup that is modest in amount and moderate in color. Avoid a painted and severe look.
- Do not wear perfume, cologne, or after-shave lotion. They may offend, nauseate, or cause breathing problems in patients and residents.

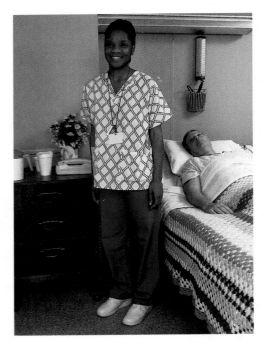

**FIG. 3-1** This nursing assistant is well-groomed. Her uniform and shoes are clean. Her hair has a simple style. It is away from her face and off of her collar. She does not wear jewelry.

## GETTING A JOB

There are easy ways to find out about jobs:
- Newspaper classified ads
- Local state employment service
- Agencies you would like to work at
- Phone book yellow pages
- People you know—your instructor, family, and friends
- The Internet
- Your school's or college's job placement counselors
- Your clinical experience site

Your clinical experience site is an important source. The staff always looks at students as future employees. They look for good work ethics. They watch how students treat patients, residents, and co-workers. They look for the qualities and traits described in Box 3-2. If that agency is not hiring, the staff may advise you about where to apply.

### WHAT EMPLOYERS LOOK FOR

If you had your own business, who would you want to hire? Your answer helps you better understand the employer's point of view. Employers want employees who:
- Are dependable
- Are well-groomed
- Have the needed job skills and training
- Have values and attitudes that fit with the agency

---

| BOX 3-2 | QUALITIES AND TRAITS FOR GOOD WORK ETHICS |
|---|---|

- **Caring.** Have concern for the person. Help make the person's life happier, easier, or less painful.
- **Dependable.** Report to work on time and when scheduled. Perform delegated tasks. Keep obligations and promises.
- **Considerate.** Respect the person's physical and emotional feelings. Be gentle and kind toward patients, residents, families, and co-workers.
- **Cheerful.** Greet and talk to people in a pleasant manner. Do not be moody, bad-tempered, or unhappy while at work.
- **Empathetic.** Empathy is seeing things from the person's point of view—putting yourself in the person's position. How would you feel if you had the person's problem?
- **Trustworthy.** Patients, residents, and staff members have confidence in you. They believe you will keep information confidential. They trust you not to gossip about patients, residents, or the health team.
- **Respectful.** Patients and residents have rights, values, beliefs, and feelings. They may differ from yours. Do not judge or condemn the person. Treat the person with respect and dignity at all times. Also show respect for the health team.
- **Courteous.** Be polite and courteous to patients, residents, families, visitors, and co-workers. See p. 46 for common courtesies in the workplace.
- **Conscientious.** Be careful, alert, and exact in following instructions. Give thorough care. Do not lose or damage the person's property.
- **Honest.** Accurately report the care given, your observations, and any errors.
- **Cooperative.** Willingly help and work with others. Also take that "extra step" during busy and stressful times.
- **Enthusiastic.** Be eager, interested, and excited about your work. Your work is important.
- **Self-aware.** Know your feelings, strengths, and weaknesses. You need to understand yourself before you can understand patients and residents.

You need to care about others. You must care enough to want to make a person's life happier, easier, or less painful. Good work ethics involves certain traits, attitudes, and manners (see Box 3-2). They are necessary for you to function well (Fig. 3-2). *See Focus on Home Care: What Employers Look For.*

Being dependable is important. You must be at work on time and when scheduled. Undependable people cause everyone problems. Other staff members take on extra work. Fewer people give care. Quality of care suffers. Supervisors spend time trying to find out if the person is coming to work. They also have to find someone to cover for the absent employee. You want co-workers to work when scheduled. Otherwise, you

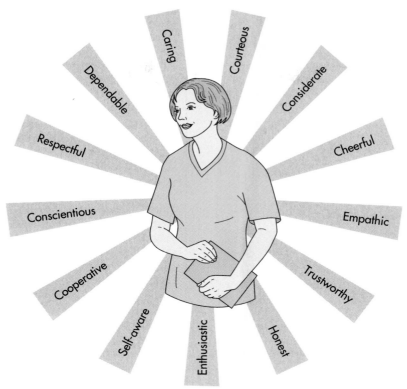

**FIG. 3-2** Good work ethics involves these qualities and traits.

have extra work. You have less time to spend with patients and residents. Likewise, co-workers also expect you to work when scheduled.

Applicants who look good communicate many things to the employer. You have only one chance to make a good first impression. A well-groomed person is likely to get the job. A sloppy person, with wrinkled or dirty clothes and body or breath odors, is not likely to get the job. Proper dress for an interview is discussed on p. 42.

**JOB SKILLS AND TRAINING.** Employers need to know that you can do required job skills. The employer requests proof of required training. Proof of training includes:
- A certificate of course completion
- A high school, college, or technical school transcript
- An official grade report (report card)

Give the employer only a *copy* of your certificate, transcript, or grade report. Never give the original to the employer. Keep it for future use. The employer may want a transcript sent directly from the school or college. *See Focus on Long-Term Care: Job Skills and Training*, p. 38. *See Focus on Home Care: Job Skills and Training*, p. 38.

---

## FOCUS ON HOME CARE
### WHAT EMPLOYERS LOOK FOR

- You must *be able to work alone.* The RN makes some home visits. However, an RN is not right there to help you at the bedside if problems occur. You can reach an RN by phone. You must provide care skillfully and safely.
- *Self-discipline* is essential. You must arrive at homes on time. Plan activities so personal care needs and housekeeping tasks get done. Avoid temptations. This includes watching TV, talking on the phone, visiting, and stopping for a cup of coffee.
- *Honesty* is very important. You might need to shop. Be honest and thrifty with the person's money. Accurately report to the person or family the items purchased, their cost with receipts, amount spent, and amount of money returned.
- *Respect* the person's property. You will handle valuables and personal property in health care settings. However, access to the person's property is greater in the home. Home furnishings, appliances, linens, and household items are used for personal care and housekeeping. Treat personal and family property with respect. Prevent damage. Read the manufacturer's instructions before using any appliance. Clean the appliance after use.

## FOCUS ON LONG-TERM CARE
### JOB SKILLS AND TRAINING

To work in long-term care, you must complete a state-approved training and competency evaluation program. This is an OBRA requirement. The employer requests proof of training. Your record in the state nursing assistant registry is checked. Nursing centers cannot hire persons who were convicted of abusing, neglecting, or mistreating a person. This also is an OBRA requirement.

## FOCUS ON HOME CARE
### JOB SKILLS AND TRAINING

Home care agencies receiving Medicare funds must meet OBRA requirements. You must meet the training and competency evaluation requirements outlined in OBRA. Some states have additional training requirements if you want to work in home care.

## JOB APPLICATIONS

You get a job application from the *personnel office* or *human resources office* (Fig. 3-3). You can complete the application there. Or you can complete it at home, and return it by mail or in person. You must be well-groomed and behave pleasantly when seeking or returning a job application. It may be your first chance to make a good impression.

To complete a job application, follow the guidelines in Box 3-3. How you fill it out may mean getting or not getting the job. Often the application is your first chance to impress the employer. A neat, readable, and complete application gives a good image. A sloppy or incomplete one does not.

Some agencies provide job applications on-line. Follow the agency's instructions for completing and sending an on-line application.

*Text continued on p. 42.*

### BOX 3-3 GUIDELINES FOR COMPLETING A JOB APPLICATION

- Read and follow the directions. They may ask you to use black ink and to print. Following directions is needed on the job. Employers look at job applications to see if you can follow directions.
- Write neatly. Your writing must be readable. A messy application gives a bad image. Readable writing gives the correct information. The agency cannot contact you if unable to read your phone number. You may miss getting the job.
- Complete the entire form. Something may not apply to you. If so, write "N/A" for nonapplicable. Or draw a line through the space. This tells the employer that you read the section. It also shows that you did not skip the item on purpose.
- Report any felony arrests or convictions as directed. Write "no" or "none" as appropriate. Some states require criminal background checks.
- Give information about employment gaps. If you did not work for a time, the employer wonders why. Provide this information to give a good impression about your honesty. Some reasons are going to school, raising children, caring for an ill or older family member, or your own illness.
- Tell why you left a job, if asked. Be brief, but honest. People leave jobs for one that pays better. Some leave for career advancement. Other reasons include those given for employment gaps. If you were fired from a job, give an honest but positive response. Do not talk badly about a former employer.
- Provide references. Be prepared to give the names, titles, addresses, and telephone numbers of at least three references who are not relatives. You should have this information written down before completing an application. (Always ask references if an employer can contact them.) You may get the job faster or over another applicant if the employer can quickly check references. If they are missing or incomplete, the employer waits for all of the information. This wastes your time and the employer's time. Also, the employer wonders if you are hiding something with incomplete reference information.
- Be prepared to provide the following:
  —Social security number
  —Proof of citizenship or legal residency
  —Proof of required training and competency evaluation
  —Identification—driver's license or government-issued ID card
- Give honest responses. Lying on an application is fraud. It is grounds for being fired.

## (Please Print in Ink)

In considering your application for employment, the facility may conduct a detailed and thorough investigation which may include but is not limited to a criminal record check, interviews or inquiries of prior employers, coworkers, acquaintances, relatives or friends.

**PERSONAL**

| LAST NAME | FIRST | MIDDLE | SOCIAL SECURITY NO. |

| PRESENT ADDRESS | CITY | STATE | ZIP CODE | HOME TELEPHONE NO. |

| PERMANENT ADDRESS | CITY | STATE | ZIP CODE | CONTACT TELEPHONE NO. |

ANY PREVIOUS NAME(S)? YES ☐ NO ☐ IF YES, IDENTIFY ALL OTHER NAMES INCLUDING MAIDEN NAME:

BEST TIME TO CONTACT YOU: | DATE AVAILABLE FOR WORK:

ARE YOU APPLYING FOR:
FULL TIME ☐ PART TIME ☐
REGULAR ☐ TEMPORARY ☐

POSITION APPLIED FOR: | SALARY DESIRED:

HOW WERE YOU REFERRED TO THIS FACILITY?

WOULD YOU CONSIDER WORKING:
WEEKENDS & HOLIDAYS YES ☐ NO ☐
ROTATING SHIFTS YES ☐ NO ☐
ON CALL YES ☐ NO ☐
ANY SHIFT YES ☐ NO ☐

RELATIVES OR FRIENDS EMPLOYED IN THIS FACILITY? YES ☐ NO ☐
NAME: DEPT: RELATIONSHIP:

SHIFT PREFERENCE:
DAYS ☐ EVENINGS ☐ NIGHTS ☐

HAVE YOU EVER BEEN EMPLOYED BY THIS FACILITY?
YES ☐ NO ☐ WHEN? | ARE YOU 18 YRS OF AGE OR OLDER? YES ☐ NO ☐

LONG RANGE OCCUPATIONAL GOALS:

ARE YOU A U.S. CITIZEN OR AN ALIEN LEGALLY AUTHORIZED TO WORK IN THE UNITED STATES? YES ☐ NO ☐

HAVE YOU EVER BEEN CONVICTED OF, OR PLEAD GUILTY TO, A CRIME OTHER THAN MISDEMEANOR TRAFFIC VIOLATIONS? YES ☐ NO ☐ IF YES, EXPLAIN:

HAVE YOU EVER BEEN INVOLVED IN THE SUBSTANTIATED ABUSE OR NEGLECT OF CHILDREN OR ADULTS UNDER THE LAWS OF THIS OR ANY OTHER STATE OF THE UNITED STATES? YES ☐ NO ☐ IF YES, EXPLAIN:

If your answer is "yes" to either of the above, you will not be automatically disqualified from employment consideration, except as required by state or federal law.

**EDUCATION / SKILLS**

| SCHOOL | NAME AND ADDRESS OF SCHOOL | COURSE OF STUDY | CHECK LAST YEAR COMPLETED | | | | DID YOU GRADUATE? | LIST DIPLOMA OR DEGREE |
|---|---|---|---|---|---|---|---|---|
| HIGH | | | 1 | 2 | 3 | 4 | ☐ YES ☐ NO | |
| COLLEGE | | | 1 | 2 | 3 | 4 | ☐ YES ☐ NO | |
| COLLEGE | | | 1 | 2 | 3 | 4 | ☐ YES ☐ NO | |

OTHER Business College or Special Courses: (Include Special Military Training, Post Graduate and Nursing)

AREA(S) OF SPECIALIZATION OR MAJOR INTEREST: | LIST OFFICE SKILLS INCLUDING COMPUTER/SOFTWARE EXPERIENCE:

LIST HEALTH CARE, BUSINESS, OR INDUSTRIAL EQUIPMENT OPERATED: | WORD PROCESSING: APPROX. WPM

**PROFESSIONAL LICENSES**
☐ CURRENTLY LICENSED ☐ ELIGIBLE FOR LICENSE
☐ CURRENTLY REGISTERED ☐ ELIGIBLE FOR REGISTRATION
LICENSE OR REGISTRATION **EVER** SUSPENDED, REVOKED OR ON PROBATION?
☐ YES ☐ NO IF YES, EXPLAIN
TYPE: STATE:
NO: DATE:

**PROFESSIONAL CERTIFICATIONS**
☐ CURRENTLY CERTIFIED
☐ ELIGIBLE FOR CERTIFICATION
TYPE:
STATE: DATE:

☐ CURRENTLY LICENSED ☐ ELIGIBLE FOR LICENSE
☐ CURRENTLY REGISTERED ☐ ELIGIBLE FOR REGISTRATION
LICENSE OR REGISTRATION **EVER** SUSPENDED, REVOKED OR ON PROBATION?
☐ YES ☐ NO IF YES, EXPLAIN
TYPE: STATE:
NO: DATE:

☐ CURRENTLY CERTIFIED
☐ ELIGIBLE FOR CERTIFICATION
TYPE:
STATE: DATE:

**FIG. 3-3** A sample job application. (Courtesy Association Management Resources, Naperville, Ill. Copyright © 2002.) *Continued.*

Read job description

**Briefly describe duties and skills acquired through military or volunteer service: (include dates)**

_____
_____
_____

## PREVIOUS EXPERIENCE

**PROVIDE INFORMATION REGARDING PREVIOUS EMPLOYMENT BEGINNING WITH MOST RECENT EMPLOYER.**

| | FROM: (MO/YR) | TO: (MO/YR) | SUPERVISOR'S NAME: | SALARY(Hr/ Mo/Yr): |
|---|---|---|---|---|

JOB TITLE: _____

EMPLOYER: _____ PHONE: _____

ADDRESS: _____

DUTIES:_____
_____

REASON FOR LEAVING: _____

MAY WE CONTACT YOUR CURRENT EMPLOYER?    YES ☐    NO ☐

| | FROM: (MO/YR) | TO: (MO/YR) | SUPERVISOR'S NAME: | SALARY(Hr/ Mo/Yr): |
|---|---|---|---|---|

JOB TITLE: _____

EMPLOYER NAME:_____ PHONE: _____

ADDRESS: _____

DUTIES:_____
_____

REASON FOR LEAVING: _____

| | FROM: (MO/YR) | TO: (MO/YR) | SUPERVISOR'S NAME: | SALARY(Hr/ Mo/Yr): |
|---|---|---|---|---|

JOB TITLE: _____

EMPLOYER NAME:_____ PHONE: _____

ADDRESS: _____

DUTIES:_____
_____

REASON FOR LEAVING: _____

| | FROM: (MO/YR) | TO: (MO/YR) | SUPERVISOR'S NAME: | SALARY(Hr/ Mo/Yr): |
|---|---|---|---|---|

JOB TITLE: _____

EMPLOYER NAME:_____ PHONE: _____

ADDRESS: _____

DUTIES:_____
_____

REASON FOR LEAVING: _____

**PLEASE IDENTIFY AND EXPLAIN ANY GAPS IN EMPLOYMENT LONGER THAN THREE (3) MONTHS:**

_____
_____

**FIG. 3-3, CONT'D** A sample job application. (Courtesy Association Management Resources, Naperville, Ill. Copyright © 2002.)

**LANGUAGE**

**LANGUAGE SKILLS - DO NOT COMPLETE UNLESS REQUESTED**

| LANGUAGE | DO YOU? | ☐ SPEAK | ☐ FAIR ☐ GOOD ☐ FLUENT | ☐ READ | ☐ FAIR ☐ GOOD ☐ FLUENT | ☐ WRITE | ☐ FAIR ☐ GOOD ☐ FLUENT |
|---|---|---|---|---|---|---|---|
| LANGUAGE | DO YOU? | ☐ SPEAK | ☐ FAIR ☐ GOOD ☐ FLUENT | ☐ READ | ☐ FAIR ☐ GOOD ☐ FLUENT | ☐ WRITE | ☐ FAIR ☐ GOOD ☐ FLUENT |

**REFERENCES**

**LIST AT LEAST THREE (3) REFERENCES WHO ARE NOT RELATIVES:**

| NAME AND RELATIONSHIP | TITLE | COMPANY NAME AND ADDRESS | TELEPHONE |
|---|---|---|---|
| | | | |
| | | | |
| | | | |

**SIGNATURE**

**CAREFULLY READ THIS SECTION PRIOR TO PROVIDING SIGNATURE BELOW**

I hereby affirm that the information provided on this application (and accompanying resume, if any) is true and complete. I understand that any false or misleading representations or omissions made on the application or during the hiring process may disqualify me from further consideration for employment and may result in discharge even if discovered at a later date.

I understand that employment may be conditioned upon successfully passing a medical examination and that I may be required to satisfactorily complete a drug screening as a condition of employment.

I hereby authorize persons, schools, my current employer (if applicable) and previous employers and other organizations to provide this facility and its affiliates with any requested information regarding my application or suitability for employment, and I completely release all such persons or entities from any and all liability related to the providing or use of such information.

I understand that my employment is at-will which means that I may terminate the employment relationship at any time and for any reason with or without notice, and that the facility has the same right. I understand that no one has the authority to enter into any agreement contrary to the preceding sentence, except for a written agreement signed by an administrative representative of this facility and notarized.

Date _____ Signature _____

**FOR OFFICE USE ONLY**

**TO BE COMPLETED AFTER EMPLOYED** HIRED? YES ☐ NO ☐ SEE COMMENTS BELOW

REFERENCES CHECKED AND BY WHOM: REFERENCE #1 DATE REFERENCE #2 DATE REFERENCE #3 DATE

PERSONNEL NOTES (these notes are open to inspection -- keep information factual)_____

IF APPLICANT IS 18 YRS. OLD OR LESS, IS PROOF OF AGE ON FILE? YES ☐ NO ☐

INTERVIEWER'S SIGNATURE

STARTING DATE | ☐ EXEMPT ☐ NON-EXEMPT | COMPLETION OF EVALUATION PERIOD APPROVED BY DATE

DEPARTMENT | COST CENTER | SIGNATURE

POSITION/JOB SITE | ☐ FULL TIME ☐ PART TIME ☐ ON CALL STATUS ☐ ROTATION

STARTING SALARY/GRADE | DIFFERENTIAL | SHIFT | EMPLOYEE NUMBER

NOTIFY IN CASE OF EMERGENCY NAME RELATIONSHIP ADDRESS TELEPHONE

Reorder #HOS-001 ● Association Management Resources ● 1151 East Warrenville Road ● P.O. Box 3015 ● Naperville, IL 60566 ● 630/505-7777

**FIG. 3-3, CONT'D** A sample job application. (Courtesy Association Management Resources, Naperville, Ill. Copyright © 2002.)

## THE JOB INTERVIEW

A job interview is the employer's chance to get to know and evaluate you. You also find out more about the agency. Remember, employers hire well-groomed, dependable, and skilled people.

The interview may be at the time you ask for and complete the job application. Some agencies review the application first to see if you are qualified. If yes, an interview is scheduled. Write down the interviewer's name and the date and time of the appointment. If you need directions to the agency, ask for them at this time.

Box 3-4 lists common interview questions. Prepare your answers before the interview. Also type a list of your skills to give to the interviewer.

You must present a good image. You need to be neat, clean, and well-groomed (Fig. 3-4). How you dress is important. Follow the guidelines in Box 3-5.

You must be on time. It shows you are dependable. Go to the agency some day before your interview. Note how long it takes to get there and where to park. Also find the personnel office. A *dry run* (practice run) gives an idea of how long it takes to get from your home to the personnel office.

When you arrive for the interview, tell the receptionist your name and why you are there. Also give the interviewer's name. Then sit quietly in the waiting room. Do not smoke or chew gum. Use the time to review your answers to the common interview questions. Waiting may be part of the interview. The interviewer may ask the receptionist about how you acted while waiting. Smile, and be polite and friendly.

Greet the interviewer in a polite manner. A firm handshake is correct for men and women. Address the interviewer as Mr., Mrs., Ms., Miss, or Doctor. Stand until asked to take a seat. When sitting, use good posture. Sit in a professional manner. If offered a beverage, it is correct to accept. Be sure to thank the person.

Good eye contact is needed. Look directly at the interviewer when answering or asking questions. Poor eye contact sends negative information—being shy, insecure, or dishonest or lacking interest. Also watch your body language (Chapter 6). Body language involves facial expressions, gestures, posture, and body movements. What you say is important. However, how you use and move your body also tells a great deal. Avoid distracting habits—biting nails, playing with jewelry or clothing, crossing your arms, and swinging legs back and forth. Keep your mind on the interview. Do not touch or read things on the person's desk.

The interview lasts 15 to 45 minutes. Give complete and honest answers. Speak clearly and with confidence. Avoid short and long answers. "Yes" and "no" answers give little information. Briefly explain "yes" and "no" responses.

The interviewer will ask about your skills. Share your skills list. He or she may ask about a skill not on

| BOX 3-4 | COMMON INTERVIEW QUESTIONS |
| --- | --- |

- Tell me about yourself.
- Tell me about your career goals.
- What are you doing to reach these goals?
- Describe your idea of *professional* behavior.
- Tell me about your last job. Why did you leave?
- What did you like the most about your last job? What did you like the least?
- What would your supervisor and co-workers tell me about you? Your dependability? Your skills? Your flexibility?
- Which functions were the hardest for you? How did you handle this difficulty?
- How do you set priorities?
- How have your past experiences prepared you for this job?
- What would you like to change about your last job?
- How do you handle problems with patients, residents, and co-workers?
- Why do you want to work here?
- Why should this agency hire you?

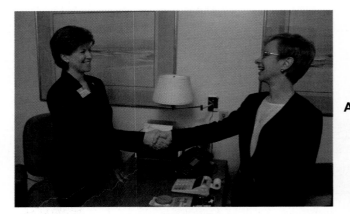

**A**

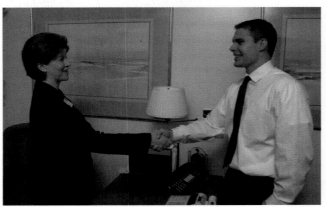

**B**

**FIG. 3-4 A,** A simple suit is worn for a job interview. **B,** This man wears slacks and a shirt and tie for his interview.

**GROOMING AND DRESSING FOR AN INTERVIEW**

- Bathe, brush your teeth, and wash your hair.
- Use a deodorant or antiperspirant.
- Make sure your hands and fingernails are clean.
- Apply makeup in a simple, attractive manner.
- Style your hair so that it is neat and attractive. Wear it as you would for work.
- Do not wear jeans, shorts, tank tops, halter tops, or other casual clothing.
- Iron clothing. Sew on loose buttons and mend garments as needed.
- Wear a simple dress, skirt and blouse, or suit (women). Men should wear a suit or dark slacks and a shirt and tie. A jacket is optional. A long-sleeved white or light blue shirt is best.
- Wear socks (men and women) or hose (women). Hose should be free of runs and snags.
- Make sure shoes are clean and in good repair.
- Avoid heavy perfumes, colognes, and after-shave lotions. A lightly scented fragrance is okay.
- Wear only simple jewelry that complements your clothes. Avoid adornments in body piercings. If you have multiple ear piercings, wear only one set of earrings.
- Stop in the restroom when you arrive for the interview. Check your hair, makeup, and clothes.

**BOX 3-6** **QUESTIONS TO ASK THE INTERVIEWER**

- Which job functions do you think are the most important?
- What employee qualities and traits are most important to you?
- What nursing care pattern is used here (Chapter 1)?
- Who will I work with?
- When are performance evaluations done? Who does them? How are they done?
- What performance factors are evaluated?
- How does the supervisor handle problems?
- What are the most common reasons that nursing assistants quit their jobs here?
- What are the most common reasons that nursing assistants lose their jobs here?
- How do you see this job in the next year? In the next 5 years?
- What is the greatest reward from this job?
- What is the greatest challenge of this job?
- What do you like the most about nursing assistants who work here?
- What do you like the least about nursing assistants who work here?
- Why should I work here rather than in another agency?
- Why are you interested in hiring me?
- May I have a tour of the agency and the unit I will work on? Will you introduce me to the nurse manager and unit staff?
- Can I have a few minutes to talk to the nurse manager?

your list. Explain that you are willing to learn the skill if your state allows nursing assistants to perform the task.

You want to find the right job for you. A right match is important. You want to enjoy your job and the agency. The agency wants to hire someone who will be happy in the job or at the agency. You can ask questions at the end of the interview. Box 3-6 lists some questions to ask. The person's answers will help you decide if the job is right for you.

Review the job description with the interviewer. If you have questions, ask them at this time. Advise him or her of those functions you cannot perform because of training, legal, ethical, or religious reasons. Honesty now prevents problems later.

Ask questions about pay rate, work hours, and uniform requirements. Also ask about the new-employee orientation program. Remember to ask about benefits—health and disability insurance, vacation, and continuing education. *See Focus on Home Care: The Job Interview.*

The interviewer signals when the interview is over. You may be offered a job at this time. Or you are told when to expect a call or letter. Follow-up is acceptable. Ask when you can check on your application. Before leaving, thank the interviewer. Say that you look forward to hearing from him or her. Shake the person's hand before you leave.

A thank-you note is advised (Fig. 3-5, p. 44). Write it within 24 hours of the interview. Your writing must be neat and readable. Use a computer or typewriter if your writing is hard to read. The thank-you note should include:
- The date
- The interviewer's formal name using Mr., Mrs., Ms., Miss, or Dr.
- A statement thanking the person for the interview
- Comments about the interview, the agency, and your eagerness to hear about the job
- Your signature using your first and last names

**FOCUS ON HOME CARE**
THE JOB INTERVIEW

You need to ask more questions when interviewing with a home care agency:
- What part of the community does the agency serve?
- What neighborhoods will you go to?
- How far will you travel between homes?
- Do you use your own car or is an agency car provided?
- If you use your own car, how are you reimbursed for mileage?
- Will you use public transportation? If yes, who pays for bus or train fares? If the agency pays, are you given fare money beforehand or reimbursed later?

> *December 12*
>
> *Dear Ms. Miller,*
>
> *Thank you for the interview yesterday. I enjoyed meeting you and learning more about the nursing center. I was impressed by the friendliness of the staff and would enjoy working in that environment.*
>
> *Again, thank you. I look forward to hearing from you soon.*
>
> *Sincerely,*
> *Jane M. Doe*

**FIG. 3-5** Sample thank-you note written after a job interview.

## ACCEPTING A JOB

Accept the job that is best for you. You can apply several places and have many interviews. Think about offers before accepting one. You might have more questions about the agency. Ask them before accepting the job. It might help to discuss the offer with a relative, friend, co-worker, or your instructor. Then you can decide what to do.

When you accept a job, agree on a starting date, pay rate, and work hours. Find out where to report on your first day. Ask for such information in writing. That way you and the employer have the same understanding of the job offer. You can use the written offer later if questions arise. Also ask for the employee handbook and other agency information. Read everything before you start working.

## NEW EMPLOYEE ORIENTATION

Agencies have orientation programs for new employees. The policy and procedure manual is reviewed. Your skills are checked. That is, the agency has you perform procedures in your job description. This is to make sure you do them safely and correctly. Also, you are shown how to use the agency's supplies and equipment.

Some agencies have preceptor programs. A **preceptor** is a staff member who guides another staff member. In a preceptor program, a nurse or nursing assistant:

- Helps you learn the agency's layout so you can find what you need
- Introduces you to patients, residents, and staff
- Helps you organize your work
- Helps you feel comfortable as part of the nursing team
- Answers questions about the policy and procedure manual

A nursing assistant preceptor is not your supervisor. Only nurses can supervise. A preceptor program usually lasts 2 to 4 weeks. Its purpose is to help you succeed in your new role. It also helps ensure quality care. When the preceptor program ends, you should feel comfortable with the setting and your role. If not, ask for more orientation time.

## PREPARING FOR WORK

Having a job is a privilege. It is not a right. It is not something owed to you. You obtained the necessary education and training. You succeeded in a job interview. To keep your job, you must function well and work well with others. You must:

- Work when scheduled
- Get to work on time
- Stay the entire shift

Absences and tardiness (being late) are common reasons for losing a job. Childcare and transportation issues often interfere with getting to work. You must plan for them in advance.

## CHILDCARE

Someone needs to care for your children when you leave for work, while you are at work, and before you get home from work. Also plan for emergencies:

- Your childcare provider is ill or cannot care for your children that day.
- A child becomes ill while you are at work.
- You will be late getting home from work.

## TRANSPORTATION

Plan for how you get to and from work. If you drive, keep your car in good working order. Keep plenty of gas in the car. Or leave early enough to get gas.

Carpooling is an option. Carpool members depend on each other. If the driver is late leaving, everyone is late for work. If one person is not ready when the driver arrives, everyone is late for work. Carpool with persons you trust to be ready and on time. When you drive, leave and pick up others on time. As a passenger, be ready to be picked up.

Know your bus or train schedule. Know what other bus or train to take if delays occur. Always carry enough money for fares to and from work.

Always have a back-up plan for getting to work. Your car may not start, the carpool driver may not go to work, or public transportation may not operate.

# ON THE JOB

How you look, how you behave, and what you say affect everyone in the agency. Practice good work ethics:

- Work when scheduled
- Be cheerful and friendly
- Perform delegated tasks
- Help others
- Be kind to others

The *Employee Handbook* of OSF Saint Francis Medical Center (Peoria, Ill.) says it best:

> You are what people see when they arrive here; yours are the eyes they look into when they're frightened and lonely. Yours are the voices people hear when they ride the elevators, when they try to sleep, and when they try to forget their problems. You are what they hear on their way to appointments which could affect their destinies, and what they hear after they leave those appointments. Yours are the comments people hear when you think they can't.
>
> Yours is the intelligence and caring that people hope they'll find here. If you're noisy, so is the medical center. If you're rude, so is the medical center. And if you're wonderful, so is the medical center.

You are an important member of the health team. Quality care is affected by how you work with others and how you feel about your job.

## ATTENDANCE

Report to work when scheduled and on time. The entire unit is affected when just one person is late. Call the agency if you will be late or cannot go to work. Follow the agency's attendance policies. They are explained in the employee handbook. Poor attendance can cause you to lose your job.

Be *ready to work* when your shift starts. Store your coat, purse, backpack, and other items before your shift starts. Use the restroom when you arrive at the agency. Arrive on your nursing unit a few minutes early. This gives you time to greet others and settle yourself.

Attendance also means staying the entire shift. You must prepare for childcare emergencies. Watching the clock for when your shift ends gives a bad image. You may need to work overtime. You need to prepare to stay longer if necessary. When it is time to leave, report off-duty to the nurse. *See Focus on Home Care: Attendance.*

## YOUR ATTITUDE

A good attitude is needed. Show that you enjoy your work. Listen to others. Be willing to learn. Stay busy, and use your time well.

Your work is very important. Nurses, patients, residents, and families rely on you to give good care. They expect you to be pleasant and respectful. You must believe that you and your work have value.

Always think before you speak. These statements signal a bad attitude:

- "That's not my patient (resident)."
- "I can't. I'm too busy."
- "I didn't do it."
- "I don't feel like it."
- "It's not my fault."
- "Don't blame me."
- "It's not my turn. I did it yesterday."
- "Nobody told me."
- "I can't come to work today. I have a headache."
- "That's not my job."
- "You didn't tell me that you needed it right away."
- "I work harder than anyone else."
- "No one appreciates what I do."
- "Is it time to leave yet?"

### FOCUS ON HOME CARE
#### ATTENDANCE

You must complete home care assignments. Never leave in the middle of an assignment. Nor should you leave before someone from the next shift arrives. Sometimes conflicts or problems occur. Make every effort to finish the assignment. Explain the problem to your supervisor. The supervisor tries to make needed changes. Do not walk out on the person. That would leave the person in an unsafe situation. Walking out is a very unethical behavior.

## GOSSIP

To **gossip** means to spread rumors or talk about the private matters of others. Gossiping is unprofessional and hurtful. To avoid being a part of gossip:

- Remove yourself from a group or situation where gossip is occurring.
- Do not make or repeat any comment that can hurt a person, family member, co-worker, or the agency.
- Do not make or repeat any comment that you do not know to be true. Making or writing false statements about another person is defamation (Chapter 2).
- Do not talk about patients, residents, visitors, families, co-workers, or the agency at home or in social settings.

## CONFIDENTIALITY

The person's information is private and personal. **Confidentiality** means to trust others with personal and private information. The person's information is shared only among health team members involved in his or her care. The person has the right to privacy and confidentiality. Agency and co-worker information also is confidential.

Avoid talking about patients, residents, the agency, or co-workers when others are present. Share information only with the nurse. Do not talk about patients, residents, the agency, or co-workers in hallways, elevators, dining areas, or outside the agency. Others may overhear you. Patients, residents, and visitors are very alert to comments. They think you are talking about them or their loved ones. This leads to misinformation and wrong impressions about the person's condition. You can easily upset the person or family. Be very careful about what, how, when, and where you say things.

Avoid eavesdropping. To eavesdrop means to listen in or overhear what others are saying. It invades a person's privacy.

Many agencies have intercom systems. They allow for communication between the bedside and the nurses' station (Chapter 14). The person uses the intercom to signal when help is needed. Someone at the nurses' station answers the intercom. The nursing team also uses the intercom to communicate with each other. Be careful what you say over the intercom. It is like a loud speaker. Others nearby can hear what you are saying.

## PERSONAL HYGIENE AND APPEARANCE

How you look affects the way people think about you and the agency. If staff members are clean and neat, people think the agency is clean and neat. They think the agency is unclean if staff members are messy and unkempt. People also wonder about the quality of care given.

Home and social attire are often improper at work. You cannot wear jeans, halter tops, tank tops, or short skirts. Clothing must not be tight, revealing, or sexual. Females cannot show cleavage, the tops of breasts, or upper thighs. Males must avoid tight pants and exposing their chests. Only the top shirt button is open. Follow the practices in Box 3-1.

## SPEECH AND LANGUAGE

Your speech and language must be professional. Speech and language used in home and social settings may be improper at work. Words used with family and friends may offend patients, residents, visitors, and co-workers. Remember the following:

- Do not swear or use foul, vulgar, or abusive language.
- Do not use slang.
- Control the volume and tone of your voice. Speak softly and gently.
- Speak clearly. The person may have a hearing problem (Chapter 32).
- Do not shout or yell.
- Do not fight or argue with the person, family, or co-workers.

## COURTESIES

A **courtesy** is a polite, considerate, or helpful comment or act. Courtesies are easy. They require little time or energy. And they mean so much to people. Even the smallest kind act can brighten someone's day:

- Address others by Miss, Mrs., Ms., Mr., or Doctor. Use a first name only if the person asks you to do so.
- Say "please." Begin or end each request with "please."
- Say "thank you" whenever someone does something for you.
- Apologize. Say "I'm sorry" when you make a mistake or hurt someone. Even little things—like bumping into someone in the hallway—need an apology.
- Be thoughtful. Compliment others. Wish others a happy birthday, a happy day or weekend off, or a happy holiday.
- Wish the person and family well when they leave the agency. "Stay well" or "stay healthy" are good phrases to use.
- Hold doors open for others. If you are at the door first, open the door and let others pass through. In business, men and women hold doors open for each other.
- Hold elevator doors open for others coming down the hallway.
- Let patients, residents, families, and visitors enter elevators first.
- Help others willingly when asked.
- Give praise. If you see a co-worker do or say something that impresses you, tell that person. Also tell your co-workers.
- Do not take credit for another person's deed. Give the person credit for the action.

## PERSONAL MATTERS

You were hired to do a job. Personal matters cannot interfere with the job. Otherwise care is neglected. You could lose your job for tending to personal matters while at work. To keep personal matters out of the workplace:

- Make personal phone calls only during meals and breaks. Use pay phones or your wireless phone.
- Do not let family and friends visit you on the unit. If they must see you, arrange for them to meet you during a meal or break.
- Make appointments (doctor, dentist, lawyer, beauty, and others) for your days off.
- Do not use agency computers, printers, fax machines, photocopiers, or other equipment for your personal use.
- Do not take agency supplies (pens, paper, and others) for your personal use.
- Do not discuss personal problems at work.
- Control your emotions. If you need to cry or express anger, do so in a private place. Get yourself together quickly and return to your work.
- Do not borrow money from or lend it to co-workers. This includes meal money and bus or train fares. Borrowing and lending can lead to problems with co-workers.
- Do not sell things or engage in fund-raising at work. Do not sell your child's candy or raffle tickets to co-workers.
- Do not have personal pagers or wireless phones turned on while at work.

## MEALS AND BREAKS

Meal breaks are usually for 30 minutes. Other breaks are usually for 15 minutes. Meals and breaks are scheduled so that some staff are always on the unit. Staff remaining on the unit cover for the staff on break.

Staff members depend on each other. Leave for and return from breaks on time. That way other staff can have their turn. Do not take longer than allowed. Tell the nurse when you leave and return to the unit.

## JOB SAFETY

You must protect patients, residents, visitors, co-workers, and yourself from harm. Everyone is responsible for safety. Negligent behavior affects the safety of others (Chapter 2). Safety practices are presented throughout this book. These guidelines apply to everything you do:

- Understand the roles, functions, and responsibilities in your job description.
- Know the contents and policies in personnel and procedure manuals.
- Know what is right and wrong.
- Know what you can and cannot do.
- Develop the desired qualities and traits of nursing assistants.
- Follow the nurse's directions and instructions.
- Question unclear instructions and things you do not understand.
- Help others willingly when asked.
- Follow agency rules and regulations.
- Ask for any training that you might need.
- Report measurements, observations, the care given, the person's complaints, and any errors accurately. (See Chapter 4.)
- Accept responsibility for your actions. Admit when you are wrong or make mistakes. Do not blame others. Do not make excuses for your actions. Learn what you did wrong and why. Always try to learn from your mistakes.
- Handle the person's property carefully and prevent damage.

## PLANNING YOUR WORK

You will give care and perform routine tasks on the nursing unit. You must complete some things by a certain time. Others are done by the end of the shift. Plan your work to give safe, thorough care and to make good use of your time (Box 3-7).

---

**BOX 3-7 PLANNING YOUR WORK**

- Discuss priorities with the nurse.
- Know the routine of your shift and nursing unit.
- List care or procedures that are on a schedule. Some persons are turned or offered the bedpan every 2 hours.
- Judge how much time you need for each person, procedure, and task.
- Identify which tasks and procedures can be done while patients or residents are eating, visiting, or involved in activities or therapies.
- Plan care around meal times, visiting hours, and therapies. If working in a nursing center, also consider daily recreation and social activities.
- Identify when you will need help from a co-worker. Ask a co-worker to help you. Give the time when you will need help.
- Schedule equipment or rooms for the person's use. Some agencies have only one shower or bathtub to a nursing unit.
- Review delegated procedures. Gather needed supplies beforehand.
- Do not waste time. Stay focused on your work.
- Do not leave a messy work area. Make sure rooms are neat and orderly. Also clean utility areas.
- Be a self-starter. Have initiative. Ask others if they need help, follow unit routines, stock supply areas, and clean utility rooms. Stay busy.

## MANAGING STRESS

**Stress** is the response or change in the body caused by any emotional, physical, social, or economic factor. Stress is normal. It occurs every minute of every day. It occurs in everything you do. A **stressor** is the event or factor that causes stress. Many stressors are pleasant—watching a child play, planning a party, laughing with family and friends, enjoying a nice day. Some are not pleasant—illness, injury, family problems, death of loved ones, divorce, money concerns. Many parts of your job are stressful.

No matter the cause, stress affects the whole person:

- *Physically*—sweating, increased heart rate, faster and deeper breathing, increased blood pressure, dry mouth, and so on
- *Psychologically*—anxiety, fear, anger, dread, depression, and using defense mechanisms (Chapter 34)
- *Socially*—changes in relationships, avoiding others, needing others, blaming others, and so on
- *Spiritually*—changes in beliefs and values and strengthening or questioning one's beliefs in God or a higher power

Prolonged or frequent stress can threaten your health. Physical and mental problems can occur. Some problems are minor (headaches, sleep problems, muscle tension, and so on). Others are life-threatening (high blood pressure, heart attack, stroke, ulcers, and so on).

Dealing with stress is important. If your job causes stress, it affects your family and friends. If you have stress in your personal life, it affects your work. Stress affects you, the care you give, the person's quality of life, and how you relate to co-workers. These guidelines can help you reduce or cope with stress:

- Exercise regularly. It has physical and mental benefits—cardiovascular health, weight control, tension release, emotional well-being, and relaxation.
- Get enough rest and sleep (p. 35).
- Eat healthy (p. 35).
- Plan personal and quiet time for you. Read, take a hot bath, go for a walk, meditate, or listen to music. Do what makes you feel good.
- Use common sense about what you can do. Do not try to do everything that family and friends ask you to do. Consider the amount of time and energy that you have.
- Do one thing at a time. The demands on you may seem overwhelming. List each thing that you have to do. Set priorities.
- Do not judge yourself harshly. Do not try to be perfect or expect too much from yourself.
- Give yourself praise. You do good and wonderful things every day.
- Have a sense of humor. Laugh at yourself. Laugh with others. Spend time with those who make you laugh.
- Talk to the nurse if your work or a person is causing you too much stress. The nurse can help you deal with the matter.

## HARASSMENT

**Harassment** means to trouble, torment, offend, or worry a person by one's behavior or comments. Harassment can be sexual. Or it can involve age, race, ethnic background, religion, or disability. You must respect others. Do not offend others by your gestures, remarks, or use of touch. Do not offend others with jokes or pictures. Harassment is not legal in the workplace.

### SEXUAL HARASSMENT

Sexual harassment involves unwanted sexual behaviors by another. The behavior may be a sexual advance. Or it may be a request for a sexual favor. Some comments or touching are sexual. The behavior affects the person's work and comfort. In extreme cases, the person's job is threatened if sexual favors are not granted.

Victims of sexual harassment may be men or women. Men harass women or men. Women harass men or women. You might feel that you are being harassed. If so, report the matter to your supervisor and the human resource officer.

Be careful about what you say or do. Even innocent remarks and behaviors can be viewed as harassment. Employee orientation programs address harassment. You might not be sure about your own or another person's remarks or behaviors. If so, discuss the matter with the nurse. You cannot be too careful.

## RESIGNING FROM A JOB

A job closer to home, better pay, or new opportunities may prompt you to leave your job. School, childcare, and illness are other reasons. Whatever the reason, you need to tell your employer. Give a written notice. Write a resignation letter or complete a form in the human resource office. Giving 2-weeks' notice is a good practice. Do not leave a job without notice. Doing so can affect patient and resident care. Include the following in your written notice:

- Reason for leaving
- The last date you will work
- Comments thanking the employer for the opportunity to work in the agency

An exit interview is common practice. You and the employer talk before you leave the agency. Usually the employer asks what you liked about the agency and your job. Often employees are asked how the agency can improve.

## LOSING A JOB

A job is a privilege. You must perform your job well and protect patients and residents from harm. No pay raise or losing your job results from poor performance. Failure to follow an agency policy is often grounds for termination. So is failure to get along with others. Box 3-8 lists the many reasons why you can lose your job. To protect your job, function at your best. Always practice good work ethics.

---

| BOX 3-8 | COMMON REASONS FOR LOSING A JOB |
|---|---|

- Poor attendance—not showing up for work or excessive tardiness (being late)
- Abandonment—leaving the job during your shift
- Falsifying a record—job application or a person's record
- Violent behavior in the workplace
- Having weapons in the work setting—guns, knives, explosives, or other dangerous items
- Having, using, or distributing alcohol in the work setting
- Having, using, or distributing drugs in the work setting (this excludes taking drugs ordered by a doctor)
- Taking a person's drug for your own use or giving it to others
- Harassment
- Using offensive speech and language
- Stealing the agency's or a person's property
- Destroying the agency's or a person's property
- Showing disrespect to patients, residents, visitors, co-workers, or supervisors
- Abusing or neglecting a person
- Invading a person's privacy
- Failing to maintain patient, resident, agency, or co-worker confidentiality (includes access to computer information)
- Using the agency's supplies and equipment for your own use
- Defamation—see Chapter 2 and Gossip, p. 46
- Abusing meal breaks and break periods
- Sleeping on the job
- Violating agency dress code
- Violating any agency policy
- Failing to follow agency procedures for providing care
- Tending to personal matters while on duty

# ■ REVIEW QUESTIONS ■

Circle the **BEST** answer.

**1** To perform your job well you need the following *except*
   a Adequate sleep and rest
   b Regular exercise
   c To use drugs and alcohol
   d Good nutrition

**2** Good hygiene for work involves the following *except*
   a Bathing daily
   b Using a deodorant or antiperspirant
   c Brushing teeth after meals
   d Keeping fingernails long and polished

**3** You are getting ready for work. You should do the following *except*
   a Press and mend your uniform
   b Wear your name badge or photo ID
   c Wear jewelry
   d Style hair so it is up and off the collar

**4** When should you ask questions about your job description?
   a After completing the application
   b Before completing the application
   c When your interview is scheduled
   d During the interview

**5** Lying on an employment application is
   a Negligence
   b Fraud
   c Libel
   d Slander

**6** When completing a job application you should do the following *except*
   a Write neatly and clearly
   b Provide references
   c Give information about employment gaps
   d Leave spaces blank that do not apply to you

**7** Which of these qualities and traits do employers look for the *most?*
   a Cooperation
   b Courtesy
   c Dependability
   d Empathy

**8** Empathy is
   a Feeling sorry for a person
   b Seeing things from the other person's point of view
   c Being polite to others
   d Saying kind things

**9** What should you wear to a job interview?
   a A uniform
   b Party clothes
   c A simple dress or suit
   d What is most comfortable

**10** Which behavior is poor during a job interview?
   a Good eye contact with the interviewer
   b Shaking hands with the interviewer
   c Asking the interviewer questions
   d Crossing your arms and legs

**11** Which response to an interview question is best?
   a "Yes" or "no"
   b Long answers
   c Brief explanations
   d A written response

**12** Which statement reflects a good work attitude?
   a "It's not my fault."
   b "Please show me how this works."
   c "That's not my job."
   d "I did it yesterday. It's her turn."

**13** A co-worker tells you that a doctor and nurse are dating. This is
   a Gossip
   b Eavesdropping
   c Confidential information
   d Sexual harassment

**14** Which is professional speech and language?
   a Speaking clearly
   b Using vulgar and abusive words
   c Shouting
   d Arguing

**15** Which is *not* a courteous act?
   a Saying "please" and "thank you"
   b Expecting others to open doors for you
   c Saying "I'm sorry"
   d Complimenting others

# ■ REVIEW QUESTIONS ■

**16** You are on your meal break. Which is *false?*
 a You can make personal phone calls.
 b Family members can meet you.
 c You can take a few extra minutes if necessary.
 d The nurse needs to know that you are off the unit.

**17** You are planning your work. You should do the following *except*
 a Discuss priorities with the nurse
 b Ask others if they need help
 c Stay busy
 d Plan care so that you can watch the person's TV

**18** These statements are about stress. Which is *false?*
 a Stress affects the whole person.
 b A stressor is an event that cause stress.
 c All stress is unpleasant.
 d Stress is normal.

**19** Which does *not* help reduce stress?
 a Exercise, rest, and sleep
 b Blaming yourself for things you did not do
 c Planning quiet time
 d Having a sense of humor

**20** Which is *not* harassment?
 a Using touch to comfort a person
 b Joking about a person's religion
 c Asking for a sexual favor
 d Imitating a person's disability

**21** A letter of resignation should include the following *except*
 a Your reason for leaving
 b The last day you will work
 c A thank-you to the employer
 d What problems you had during your work

**22** You can lose your job for the following reasons *except*
 a Sharing the person's information with others
 b Arriving at the agency after your shift begins
 c Following the agency's dress code
 d Using the agency's computer for your own use

*Answers to these questions are on p. 815.*

# Communicating With the Health Team

4

## OBJECTIVES

- Define the key terms listed in this chapter
- Explain why health team members need to communicate
- Describe the rules for good communication
- Explain the purpose, parts, and information found in the medical record
- Describe the legal and ethical aspects of medical records
- Describe the purpose of the Kardex
- List the information you need to report to the nurse
- List the basic rules for recording
- Use the 24-hour clock, medical terminology, and abbreviations
- Explain how computers are used in health care
- Explain how to protect the right to privacy when using computers
- Describe the rules for answering phones
- Explain how to deal with conflict

## KEY TERMS

**abbreviation** A shortened form of a word or phrase

**anterior** At or toward the front of the body or body part; ventral

**chart** The medical record

**combining vowel** A vowel added between two roots or between a root and a suffix to make pronunciation easier

**communication** The exchange of information—a message sent is received and interpreted by the intended person

**conflict** A clash between opposing interests or ideas

**distal** The part farthest from the center or from the point of attachment

**dorsal** At or toward the back of the body or body part; posterior

**Kardex** A type of card file that summarizes information found in the medical record—drugs, treatments, diagnosis, routine care measures, equipment, and special needs

**lateral** At the side of the body or body part

**medial** At or near the middle or midline of the body or body part

**medical record** A written account of a person's condition and response to treatment and care; chart

**posterior** Dorsal

**prefix** A word element placed before a root; it changes the meaning of the word

**proximal** The part nearest to the center or to the point of origin

**recording** The written account of care and observations

**reporting** The oral account of care and observations

**root** A word element containing the basic meaning of the word

**suffix** A word element placed after a root; it changes the meaning of the word

**ventral** Anterior

**word element** A part of a word

Health team members communicate with each other to give coordinated and effective care. They share information about:

- What was done for the person
- What needs to be done for the person
- The person's response to treatment

For example: Dr. Hart orders a blood test for Mr. Barr. Food affects the test results. Mr. Barr must fast from midnight until the blood is drawn. He cannot have breakfast at the usual time. A nurse tells the dietary department that Mr. Barr's meal will be served later. A technician tells the nurse that the blood sample was drawn. The nurse orders the meal. A dietary worker brings the tray to the nursing unit. You serve Mr. Barr's tray. After he is done eating, you remove the tray and observe what he ate. You report your observations to the nurse. The nurse records the information in Mr. Barr's record.

Team members communicated with one another. Mr. Barr had coordinated and effective care.

You need to understand the basic aspects and rules of communication. Then you can learn how to communicate information to the nursing and health teams.

## COMMUNICATION

**Communication** is the exchange of information—a message sent is received and interpreted by the intended person. For good communication:

- Use words that mean the same thing to the sender and the receiver of the message. "Small," "moderate," and "large" mean different things to different people. Is small the size of a dime? Or is it the size of a quarter? In health care, different meanings can cause serious problems. Avoid words with more than one meaning.
- Use familiar words. You will learn medical terminology. If someone uses an unknown term, ask what it means. You must understand the message. Otherwise communication does not occur. Likewise, do not use terms unfamiliar to the person and family.
- Be brief and concise. Do not add unrelated or unneeded information. Stay on the subject. Avoid wandering in thought. Do not get wordy. Being brief and concise reduces the chance of omitting important details.
- Give information in a logical and orderly manner. Organize your thoughts. Present them step by step.
- Give facts, and be specific. The receiver should have a clear picture of what you are saying. You report a pulse rate of 110. It is more specific and factual than saying the "pulse is fast."

## THE MEDICAL RECORD

The **medical record (chart)** is a written account of a person's condition and response to treatment and care. It is a way for the health team to share information about the person. The record is permanent. It can be used years later if the person's health history is needed. The record is a legal document. It can be used as evidence in a court of law of the person's problems, treatment, and care.

The record has many forms. They are organized into sections for easy use. Each page is stamped with the person's name, room number, and other identifying information. This helps prevent errors and improper placement of records. The record includes the person's:

- Admission sheet
- Nursing history
- Physical exam results
- Doctor's orders
- Progress notes
- Graphic sheet
- Flow sheets
- Laboratory results
- X-ray reports
- IV therapy record
- Respiratory therapy record
- Consultation reports
- Surgery and anesthesia reports
- Other reports (for example: physical, occupational, and speech therapies)
- Special consents

Health team members record information on forms for their department. Other health team members read the information. It tells the care provided and the person's response (Fig. 4-1).

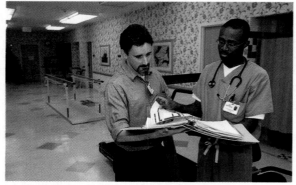

**FIG. 4-1** The nurse and physical therapist review a person's chart.

Each agency has policies about medical records and who can see them. Policies address:
- Who records
- When to record
- Abbreviations
- Correcting errors
- Ink color
- Signing entries

Some agencies allow nursing assistants to record. Others do not. You must know your agency's policies.

Professional staff involved in a person's care can look at the chart. Cooks, laundry and housekeeping staff, and office clerks have no need to read charts. Some agencies let nursing assistants read charts. If not, the nurse shares information as needed.

You have an ethical and legal duty to keep the person's information confidential. You may know someone in the agency. If you are not involved in that person's care, you have no right to review that person's chart. To do so is an invasion of privacy.

Many agencies let patients and residents see their records if they ask to do so. A person's legal representative may ask too. A person may ask you for the chart. If so, report the request to the nurse. The nurse will deal with the request.

The following parts of the medical record relate to your work.

## THE ADMISSION SHEET

The admission sheet is completed when the person is admitted to the agency. It has identifying information about the person—legal name, birth date, age, gender (male or female), current address, and marital status. It also has the person's Medicare or Social Security number. Other information includes diagnosis, known allergies, date and time of admission, and doctor's name. Religion, church, occupation, and employer are also found in this record. So is the name of the person's nearest relative or legal representative.

An identification (ID) number is given to each person. It is recorded on the admission sheet. So is information about advance directives. An advance directive is a document about a person's wishes about life support measures (Chapter 41).

The admission sheet is used to fill out other forms that require the same information. That way the person does not have to answer the same question many times.

## NURSING HISTORY

The nursing history is completed when the person is admitted. The nurse interviews the person. You can use the form to learn about the person's background and health history. It contains information about:
- The person's chief complaint—why the person sought health care
- History of the current illness—sudden or gradual in onset, when it started, signs and symptoms, and so on
- Childhood illnesses
- Past health problems, surgeries, and injuries
- Current drugs
- Allergies
- Family health history
- Life-style—habits, diet, sleep, hobbies, and so on
- Problems with activities of daily living
- Education and occupation

## THE GRAPHIC SHEET

The graphic sheet is used to record measurements and observations made daily, every shift, or 3 to 4 times a day (Fig. 4-2, p. 56). Information includes blood pressure, temperature, pulse, respirations, and weight. Intake and output, bowel movements, and doctor visits also are recorded on the graphic sheet.

*Med-Forms, Inc.*
FORM #MF37079 (Rev 9/95)

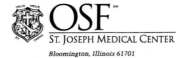

**OSF**
ST. JOSEPH MEDICAL CENTER
*Bloomington, Illinois 61701*

**DAILY SUMMARY AND GRAPHIC**

**TEMPERATURE**
Write in 105$^1$ or over

| DATE | | | | | | | | | | | | | | | | | | | | | | | | |
|---|---|---|---|---|---|---|---|---|---|---|---|---|---|---|---|---|---|---|---|---|---|---|---|---|
| HOSPITAL DAY | | | | | | | | | | | | | | | | | | | | | | | | |
| POST OP DAY | | | | | | | | | | | | | | | | | | | | | | | | |
| HOUR | 2400 | 0400 | 0800 | 1200 | 1600 | 2000 | 2400 | 0400 | 0800 | 1200 | 1600 | 2000 | 2400 | 0400 | 0800 | 1200 | 1600 | 2000 | 2400 | 0400 | 0800 | 1200 | 1600 | 2000 |
| B/P | | | | | | | | | | | | | | | | | | | | | | | | |

TEMPERATURE

104 40
102.2 39
100.4 38
98.6 37
96.6 36

| PULSE | | | | | | | | | | | | | | | | | | | | | | | | |
|---|---|---|---|---|---|---|---|---|---|---|---|---|---|---|---|---|---|---|---|---|---|---|---|---|
| RESPIRATION | | | | | | | | | | | | | | | | | | | | | | | | |
| WEIGHT | | | | | | | | | | | | | | | | | | | | | | | | |
| DR. VISIT | | | | | | | | | | | | | | | | | | | | | | | | |

| INTAKE | 2300-0700 | 0700-1500 | 1500-2300 | TOTAL | 2300-0700 | 0700-1500 | 1500-2300 | TOTAL | 2300-0700 | 0700-1500 | 1500-2300 | TOTAL | 2300-0700 | 0700-1500 | 1500-2300 | TOTAL |
|---|---|---|---|---|---|---|---|---|---|---|---|---|---|---|---|---|
| Oral | | | | | | | | | | | | | | | | |
| IV | | | | | | | | | | | | | | | | |
| Tube Feedings | | | | | | | | | | | | | | | | |
| PPN/TPN/Lipids | | | | | | | | | | | | | | | | |
| Blood/Blood Products | | | | | | | | | | | | | | | | |
| IV Meds | | | | | | | | | | | | | | | | |
| Chemotherapy | | | | | | | | | | | | | | | | |
| Unreturned irr. sol. | | | | | | | | | | | | | | | | |
| TOTAL INTAKE | | | | | | | | | | | | | | | | |
| OUTPUT | 2300-0700 | 0700-1500 | 1500-2300 | TOTAL | 2300-0700 | 0700-1500 | 1500-2300 | TOTAL | 2300-0700 | 0700-1500 | 1500-2300 | TOTAL | 2300-0700 | 0700-1500 | 1500-2300 | TOTAL |
| Urine | | | | | | | | | | | | | | | | |
| GI | | | | | | | | | | | | | | | | |
| Emesis | | | | | | | | | | | | | | | | |
| Drains | | | | | | | | | | | | | | | | |
| | | | | | | | | | | | | | | | | |
| | | | | | | | | | | | | | | | | |
| TOTAL OUTPUT | | | | | | | | | | | | | | | | |
| Feces | | | | | | | | | | | | | | | | |

**FIG. 4-2** Graphic sheet. (Courtesy OSF St. Joseph Medical Center, Bloomington, Ill.)

## PROGRESS NOTES

Progress notes describe the care given and the person's response (Fig. 4-3). The nurse records:

- The person's signs and symptoms
- Information about special treatments and drugs
- Information about patient or resident teaching and counseling
- Procedures performed by the doctor
- Visits by other health team members

*See Focus on Long-Term Care: Progress Notes.*

## FLOW SHEETS

A flow sheet is used to record frequent measurements or observations. For example, vital signs are measured every 15 minutes. The graphic sheet does not have room for frequent measurements. A flow sheet designed for this purpose does. The bedside intake and output record is another flow sheet (Chapter 20).

*See Focus on Long-Term Care: Flow Sheets. See Focus on Home Care: Flow Sheets.*

---

**FOCUS ON LONG-TERM CARE**
**PROGRESS NOTES**

Interdisciplinary progress notes are used in long-term care. Nurses chart about a change in the person's condition, unusual events, or problems. Summaries of care are written about the person's progress toward goals and response to care.

Daily recordings are not necessary. Center policies state how often recordings are made. However, OBRA requires a written summary every 3 months.

---

**FOCUS ON LONG-TERM CARE**
**FLOW SHEETS**

An activities of daily living (ADL) flow sheet is common in long-term care (Fig. 4-4, p. 58). It has information about hygiene, food and fluids, elimination, rest and sleep, activity, and social interactions.

---

**FOCUS ON HOME CARE**
**FLOW SHEETS**

A weekly care record has boxes for each day of the week and for care activities. There are boxes for temperature, pulse, respirations, blood pressure, and weight. You check the box for the day care was given or record the measurement on the day it was done.

---

| Date | Time | Nursing Margin | Other Depts Margin |
|------|------|----------------|--------------------|
| 3-19 | 1700 | Out with family for dinner. Jane Doe, LPN | ——————— |
|      | 1930 | Returned from outing accompanied by her son. States she had a pleasant time. Mary Smith, CNA ——————— | |
| 3-20 | 0900 | In bed. Complains of headache. T. 98.4 orally, radial pulse 72 and regular, respiration 18 and unlabored. BP 134/84 left arm lying down. Alice Jones, RN notified of resident complaint and vital signs. Ann Adams, CNA ——————— | |
|      | 0910 | In bed resting. States she has had a headache for about 1/2 hour. Denies nausea and dizziness. No other complaints. PRN Tylenol given. Instructed resident to use signal light if headache worsens or other symptoms occur. Alice Jones, RN ——————— | |
|      | 0945 | Resting quietly. Denies headache at this time. T. 98.4 orally, radial pulse 70 and regular, respirations 18 and unlabored. BP 132/84 left arm lying down. Alice Jones, RN ——————— | |

**FIG. 4-3** Progress notes. Note that other members of the health team also record on this form. (Modified from The Evangelical Lutheran Good Samaritan Society, Sioux Falls, SD.)

## Activities of Daily Living Flow Sheet

JAN   FEB   (MAR)   APR   MAY   JUN   JUL   AUG   SEP   OCT   NOV   DEC

| ORDER/INSTRUCTION | TIME | 1 | 2 | 3 | 4 | 5 | 6 | 7 | 8 | 9 | 10 | 11 | 12 | 13 | 14 | 15 | 16 | 17 | 18 | 19 | 20 | 21 | 22 | 23 | 24 | 25 | 26 | 27 | 28 | 29 | 30 | 31 |
|---|---|---|---|---|---|---|---|---|---|---|---|---|---|---|---|---|---|---|---|---|---|---|---|---|---|---|---|---|---|---|---|---|---|
| Bowel Movements<br>L = Large  M = Medium<br>S = Small  IC = Incontinent | 11-7 | M | | | | | | | | | | | | | | | | | | | | | | | | | | | | | | |
| | 7-3 | | | L | | | | | | | | | | | | | | | | | | | | | | | | | | | | |
| | 3-11 | | | | | | | | | | | | | | | | | | | | | | | | | | | | | | | |
| Bladder Elimination<br>I = Independent<br>IC = Incontinent<br>FC = Foley Catheter | 11-7 | / | / | / | / | | | | | | | | | | | | | | | | | | | | | | | | | | | |
| | 7-3 | / | / | / | / | | | | | | | | | | | | | | | | | | | | | | | | | | | |
| | 3-11 | / | IC | / | / | | | | | | | | | | | | | | | | | | | | | | | | | | | |
| Weight Bearing Status<br>TT = Toe Touch  AT = As tol.<br>P = Partial  F = Full<br>NWB = No wt. Bearing | 11-7 | AT | AT | AT | AT | | | | | | | | | | | | | | | | | | | | | | | | | | | |
| | 7-3 | AT | AT | AT | AT | | | | | | | | | | | | | | | | | | | | | | | | | | | |
| | 3-11 | AT | AT | AT | AT | | | | | | | | | | | | | | | | | | | | | | | | | | | |
| Transfer Status<br>ML = Medilift  SBA = Stand<br>By Assist;<br>Assist of 1 or 2 | 11-7 | SBA | SBA | SBA | SBA | | | | | | | | | | | | | | | | | | | | | | | | | | | |
| | 7-3 | SBA | SBA | SBA | SBA | | | | | | | | | | | | | | | | | | | | | | | | | | | |
| | 3-11 | SBA | SBA | SBA | A-1 | | | | | | | | | | | | | | | | | | | | | | | | | | | |
| Activity<br>A = Ambulate  GC = Gerichair<br>T = Turn every 2 hrs.<br>W/C = Wheelchair | 11-7 | T | T | T | T | | | | | | | | | | | | | | | | | | | | | | | | | | | |
| | 7-3 | A | A | A | A | | | | | | | | | | | | | | | | | | | | | | | | | | | |
| | 3-11 | A | A | A | A | | | | | | | | | | | | | | | | | | | | | | | | | | | |
| Safety<br>LT = Lap Tray  BR = Bed rails<br>BA = Bed Alarm<br>SB = Seat Belt | 11-7 | | | | | | | | | | | | | | | | | | | | | | | | | | | | | | | |
| | 7-3 | | | | | | | | | | | | | | | | | | | | | | | | | | | | | | | |
| | 3-11 | | | | | | | | | | | | | | | | | | | | | | | | | | | | | | | |
| Feeding Status<br>I = Independent  S = Set up<br>F = Staff feed  SP = Swallow<br>precautions  TL = Thickened<br>Liquids | Breakfast | S | S | S | S | | | | | | | | | | | | | | | | | | | | | | | | | | | |
| | Lunch | S | S | S | S | | | | | | | | | | | | | | | | | | | | | | | | | | | |
| | Supper | S | S | S | S | | | | | | | | | | | | | | | | | | | | | | | | | | | |
| Amount of food taken in % | Breakfast | 75 | 100 | 100 | 75 | | | | | | | | | | | | | | | | | | | | | | | | | | | |
| | Lunch | 75 | 75 | 100 | 75 | | | | | | | | | | | | | | | | | | | | | | | | | | | |
| | Supper | 50 | 50 | 50 | 75 | | | | | | | | | | | | | | | | | | | | | | | | | | | |
| Bath and Shampoo every<br>_Monday_ & _Thursday_ on<br>_7-3_ shift<br>T = Tub  S = Shower<br>B = Bedbath | 11-7 | | | | | | | | | | | | | | | | | | | | | | | | | | | | | | | |
| | 7-3 | | T | | | | | | | | | | | | | | | | | | | | | | | | | | | | | |
| | 3-11 | | | | | | | | | | | | | | | | | | | | | | | | | | | | | | | |
| Oral Care<br>Own/Dentures/None<br>I = Independent  S = Set up<br>A = Assist | 11-7 | S | S | S | S | | | | | | | | | | | | | | | | | | | | | | | | | | | |
| | 7-3 | S | S | S | S | | | | | | | | | | | | | | | | | | | | | | | | | | | |
| | 3-11 | S | S | S | S | | | | | | | | | | | | | | | | | | | | | | | | | | | |
| Dressing<br>I = Independent  S = Set up<br>A = Assist  T = Total Care | 11-7 | A | A | S | S | | | | | | | | | | | | | | | | | | | | | | | | | | | |
| | 7-3 | | | | | | | | | | | | | | | | | | | | | | | | | | | | | | | |
| | 3-11 | A | A | A | A | | | | | | | | | | | | | | | | | | | | | | | | | | | |
| Grooming: Washing Face and<br>Hands<br>Combing Hair<br>I = Independent  S = Set up<br>A = Assist  T = Total Care | 11-7 | A | A | A | A | | | | | | | | | | | | | | | | | | | | | | | | | | | |
| | 7-3 | A | A | A | A | | | | | | | | | | | | | | | | | | | | | | | | | | | |
| | 3-11 | A | A | A | A | | | | | | | | | | | | | | | | | | | | | | | | | | | |
| Trim Nails Weekly | 11-7 | | | | | | | | | | | | | | | | | | | | | | | | | | | | | | | |
| | 7-3 | | ✓ | | | | | | | | | | | | | | | | | | | | | | | | | | | | | |
| | 3-11 | | | | | | | | | | | | | | | | | | | | | | | | | | | | | | | |
| Lotion Arms and Legs twice<br>daily | 11-7 | | | | | | | | | | | | | | | | | | | | | | | | | | | | | | | |
| | 7-3 | ✓ | ✓ | ✓ | ✓ | | | | | | | | | | | | | | | | | | | | | | | | | | | |
| | 3-11 | ✓ | ✓ | ✓ | ✓ | | | | | | | | | | | | | | | | | | | | | | | | | | | |
| Shave Men Daily | 11-7 | | | | | | | | | | | | | | | | | | | | | | | | | | | | | | | |
| Shave Women every _3_<br>days | 7-3 | ✓ | | | ✓ | | | | | | | | | | | | | | | | | | | | | | | | | | | |
| | 3-11 | | | | | | | | | | | | | | | | | | | | | | | | | | | | | | | |
| Amount snacks taken in % | AM | 100 | 75 | 100 | 50 | | | | | | | | | | | | | | | | | | | | | | | | | | | |
| | PM | 100 | 100 | 75 | 75 | | | | | | | | | | | | | | | | | | | | | | | | | | | |
| | HS | 50 | 75 | 75 | 75 | | | | | | | | | | | | | | | | | | | | | | | | | | | |
| Intake and Output | 11-7 | | | | | | | | | | | | | | | | | | | | | | | | | | | | | | | |
| | 7-3 | | | | | | | | | | | | | | | | | | | | | | | | | | | | | | | |
| | 3-11 | | | | | | | | | | | | | | | | | | | | | | | | | | | | | | | |
| Vital Signs<br>Every _Week_ | 11-7 | | | | | | | | | | | | | | | | | | | | | | | | | | | | | | | |
| | 7-3 | | ✓ | | | | | | | | | | | | | | | | | | | | | | | | | | | | | |
| | 3-11 | | | | | | | | | | | | | | | | | | | | | | | | | | | | | | | |
| Weight<br>Every _Week_ | 11-7 | | ✓ | | | | | | | | | | | | | | | | | | | | | | | | | | | | | |
| | 7-3 | | | | | | | | | | | | | | | | | | | | | | | | | | | | | | | |
| | 3-11 | | | | | | | | | | | | | | | | | | | | | | | | | | | | | | | |

**FIG. 4-4** Some items on an activities of daily living flow sheet.

## THE KARDEX

The **Kardex** is a type of card file. It summarizes information found in the medical record—drugs, treatments, diagnosis, routine care measures, equipment, and special needs. The Kardex is a quick, easy source of information about the person (Fig. 4-5, p. 60).

## REPORTING AND RECORDING

The health team communicates by reporting and recording. Both are accounts of what was done for and observed about the person. **Reporting** is the oral account of care and observations. **Recording** (*charting*) is the written account of care and observations.

### REPORTING

You report care and observations to the nurse. Follow these rules:
- Be prompt, thorough, and accurate.
- Give the person's name and room and bed number.
- Give the time your observations were made or the care was given.
- Report only what you observed or did yourself.
- Give reports as often as the person's condition requires. Or give them as often as the nurse asks you to.
- Report any changes from normal or changes in the person's condition. Report these changes at once.
- Use your written notes to give a specific, concise, and clear report (Fig. 4-6).

**END-OF-SHIFT REPORT.** The nurse gives a report at the end of the shift. This is called the *end-of-shift report.* It is given to the nursing team of the oncoming shift. Information is shared about the care given and the care that must be given. Information about the person's condition is included.

Some agencies have all nursing team members hear the end-of-shift report as they come on duty. Others have nursing assistants perform routine tasks while nurses hear the report. After report, nurses share important information with the nursing assistants.

### RECORDING
When recording on the person's chart, you must communicate clearly and thoroughly. Follow the rules in Box 4-1. The charting sample in Figure 4-7, p. 61 shows how the rules apply. Anyone who reads your charting should know:
- What you observed
- What you did
- The person's response

> **BOX 4-1** **RULES FOR RECORDING**
>
> - Always use ink. Use the ink color required by the agency.
> - Include the date and the time for every recording. Use conventional time (AM or PM) or 24-hour clock time according to agency policy (p. 61).
> - Make sure writing is readable and neat.
> - Use only agency-approved abbreviations (p. 65).
> - Use correct spelling, grammar, and punctuation.
> - Never erase errors or use correction fluid. Cross out the incorrect part and write "error" or "mistaken entry" over it. Sign your initials to the error or mistaken entry. Then rewrite the part. Follow agency policy for correcting errors.
> - Sign all entries with your name and title as required by agency policy.
> - Do not skip lines. Draw a line through the blank space of a partially completed line or to the end of a page. This prevents others from recording in a space with your signature.
> - Make sure each form is stamped with the person's name and other identifying information.
> - Record only what you observed and did yourself.
> - Never chart a procedure or treatment until after it is completed.
> - Be accurate, concise, and factual. Do not record judgments or interpretations.
> - Record in a logical and sequential manner.
> - Be descriptive. Avoid terms with more than one meaning.
> - Use the person's exact words whenever possible. Use quotation marks to show that the statement is a direct quote.
> - Chart any changes from normal or changes in the person's condition. Also chart that you informed the nurse (include the nurse's name), what you told the nurse, and the time you made the report.
> - Do not omit information.
> - Record safety measures such as placing the signal light within reach or reminding someone not to get out of bed. This helps protect you if the person falls.

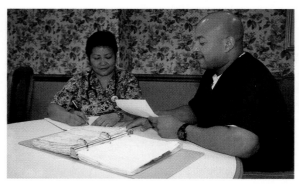

**FIG. 4-6** The nursing assistant uses notes when reporting to the nurse.

**DIET** Regular c̄ ground meat

Hold:

**NOURISHMENT/SPECIAL FEEDING** Health shake at HS

**INTAKE/OUTPUT**

Encourage/(Restrict) Fluids ___2000___ cc/24 Hr.

7-3 ___1000___  3-11 ___800___  11-7 ___200___

## FUNCTIONAL STATUS

| | SELF | ASSIST | TOTAL | OTHER | SPECIFY |
|---|---|---|---|---|---|
| Feeding | ☐ | ☒ | ☐ | ☐ | |
| Bathing | ☐ | ☒ | ☐ | ☐ | |
| Toileting | ☐ | ☒ | ☐ | ☐ | |
| Oral Care | ☐ | ☒ | ☐ | ☐ | |
| Positioning | ☒ | ☐ | ☐ | ☐ | |
| Transferring | ☒ | ☐ | ☐ | ☐ | |
| Wheeling | ☐ | ☐ | ☐ | ☐ | NA |
| Walking | ☒ | ☐ | ☐ | ☐ | |
| | ☐ | ☐ | ☐ | ☐ | |

## ACTIVITIES

Bedrest & BRP ___
Bedside Commode ___
Up ad Lib ___X___
Chair ___
Ambulatory ___X___
Ambulate & Assist Q ___
Turn Q ___
Dangle Q ___
Mode of Travel ___

## ELIMINATION

Bladder - Cont. (Incont)
Catheter ___
Date Changed ___
Irrigations ___

Bowel - (Cont.)/ Incont.
Ostomy ___
Irrigations ___ ___

## VITALS

Temp. ___QID___
Pulse ___QID___
Resp. ___QID___
BP ___QID___
Weight ___daily___
Other:
  Pulse OX
  QD

## COMMUNICATION DEFICITS ☐ None

Hearing ___Impaired___
Vision ___Impaired___
Speech ___
Language ___Impaired___

## SPECIAL CONDITIONS (Paralysis, Pressure Ulcers, Etc.)

NA

## SAFETY/SUPPORTIVE MEASURES

Bed rails: ☐ Nights Only ☐ Constant ☐ No Need
Restraints: ☐ PRN ☐ Constant    NA
Support Devices: ☐ PRN ☐ Constant    NA

## RESPIRATORY THERAPY

Aerosol
IPPB
Ultrasonic    NA
Rx Med ___

## OXYGEN

___2___ Liter/Minute
☒ PRN ☐ Constant
___ Tent ___ Catheter
___ Mask ___X___ Cannula

## PROSTHESIS ☐ None

Glasses ___X___  Dentures ___X___
Contacts ___  Limb ___
Hearing Aid ___(L) ear___

| DATE | TREATMENTS/MISCELLANEOUS |
|---|---|
| | |

## SPECIAL EQUIPMENT/PROCEDURES/ANCILLARY SERVICES/ETC.

Speech therapy 3 times/wk.

| ORDERED | SCHEDULED | COMPLETED | X-RAY AND SPECIAL DIAGNOSTIC EXAMS |
|---|---|---|---|
| 10-20 | 10-20 | 10-20 | Chest x-ray |
| | | | |
| | | | |
| | | | |
| | | | |
| | | | |

| START DATE | SCHEDULED MEDICATIONS | STOP DATE | RENEW | START DATE | STOP OR RENEW | SITE | IV FLUID & RATE | DATE & TIME CHANGED TUBING | DRESS. | SITE |
|---|---|---|---|---|---|---|---|---|---|---|
| 10-19 | Lasix 40 mgm QD | | | | | | | | | |
| 10-19 | Lanoxin .25 mgm QD | | | | | | | | | |

| DATE | ONE TIME ORDERS |
|---|---|
| | |

| DATE | DAILY/REPEATING ORDERS |
|---|---|
| 10-20 | Serum potassium daily |

| DATE | TIME | PRN MEDICATIONS |
|---|---|---|
| 10-19 | HS | Ativan .25 mgm QHS |

**MISCELLANEOUS**

**ALLERGIES:**
☒ None Known

**ISOLATION PRECAUTIONS/NURSING ALERTS:**
NA

**EMERGENCY CONTACT:**
Telephone No.
Name: Parker, Marie  Home: 555-1212
Relationship: Wife  Bus: NA

| ROOM | NAME | PHYSICIAN | ADMITTING DIAGNOSIS/PROBLEM | HOSP. NO. |
|---|---|---|---|---|
| 310 | Parker, Edwin | Dr. S Epstein | 1. CHF  2. Dementia | 1035B |

**FIG. 4-5** A sample Kardex. (Courtesy Briggs Corporation, Des Moines, Iowa.)

| Date | Time | |
|------|------|---|
| 7/18 | 1045 | Requested assistance to lie down. States: "I don't feel well. I have a little upset stomach." Denies pain. V.S. taken. T=99(O). P=76 regular rate and rhythm. R=18 unlabored. BP 134/84 (L) arm lying down. Call light within reach. Paula Jones, RN notified of resident's complaint and VS. Mary Jensen, CNA |
| | 1100 | Asleep in bed. Appears to be resting comfortably. Color good. No signs of discomfort or distress noted at this time. Paula Jones, RN |
| | 1145 | Refused to go to the dining room for lunch. Complains of nausea. Denies abdominal pain. Has not had an emesis. Abdomen soft to palpation. Good bowel sounds. VS. taken. T=98.2 (Mistaken entry 4-10, PJ) 99.2. P=76 regular rate and rhythm. R=18 unlabored. BP=134/84. States she will try to eat something. Full liquid room tray ordered. Paula Jones, RN |

**FIG. 4-7** Charting sample.

**RECORDING TIME.** The 24-hour clock (military time or international time) has four digits (Fig. 4-8). The first two digits are for the hour: 0100=1:00 AM; 1300=1:00 PM. The last two digits are for minutes: 0110=1:10 AM. The AM and PM abbreviations are not used.

As Box 4-2, p. 62, shows, the hour is the same for morning times, but AM is not used. For PM times, add 12 to the clock time. If it is 2:00 PM, add 12 and 2 for 1400. For 8:35 PM, add 12 and 835 for 2035.

Communication is better with the 24-hour clock. You must use AM and PM with conventional clock time. Someone may forget to use AM or PM. Or writing may be unclear. This means that the correct time is not communicated. Harm to the person could result.

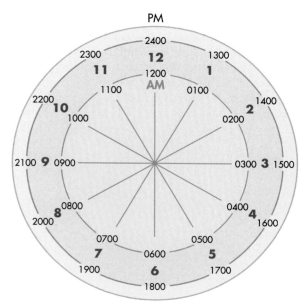

**FIG. 4-8** The 24-hour clock.

## BOX 4-2  24-HOUR CLOCK

| Conventional Time | 24-Hour Clock |
|---|---|
| 1:00 AM | 0100 |
| 2:00 AM | 0200 |
| 3:00 AM | 0300 |
| 4:00 AM | 0400 |
| 5:00 AM | 0500 |
| 6:00 AM | 0600 |
| 7:00 AM | 0700 |
| 8:00 AM | 0800 |
| 9:00 AM | 0900 |
| 10:00 AM | 1000 |
| 11:00 AM | 1100 |
| 12:00 NOON | 1200 |
| 1:00 PM | 1300 |
| 2:00 PM | 1400 |
| 3:00 PM | 1500 |
| 4:00 PM | 1600 |
| 5:00 PM | 1700 |
| 6:00 PM | 1800 |
| 7:00 PM | 1900 |
| 8:00 PM | 2000 |
| 9:00 PM | 2100 |
| 10:00 PM | 2200 |
| 11:00 PM | 2300 |
| 12:00 MIDNIGHT | 2400 or 0000 |

## MEDICAL TERMINOLOGY AND ABBREVIATIONS

Medical terminology and abbreviations are used in health care. You will learn many of them as you study to become a nursing assistant. You may want to buy a medical dictionary so you can learn new words.

Like all words, medical terms are made up of parts or **word elements.** They are combined to form medical terms. A term is translated by separating the word into its elements. Word elements are prefixes, roots, and suffixes (Box 4-3). Most are from Greek or Latin.

## PREFIXES, ROOTS, AND SUFFIXES

A **prefix** is a word element placed before a root. It changes the meaning of the word. The prefix *olig* (scant, small amount) is placed before the root *uria* (urine) to make *oliguria.* It means a scant amount of urine. Prefixes are always combined with other word elements. They are never used alone.

The **root** is a word element containing the basic meaning of the word. It is combined with another root, with prefixes, and with suffixes. Often a **combining vowel** is needed. It is a vowel (an *o* or an *i*) added between two roots or between a root and a suffix. The vowel makes pronunciation easier.

A **suffix** is a word element placed after a root. It changes the meaning of a word. Suffixes are not used alone. When translating medical terms, begin with the suffix. For example, *nephritis* means inflammation of the kidney. It was formed by combining *nephro* (kidney) and *itis* (inflammation).

Medical terms are formed by combining word elements. Remember, prefixes always come before roots. Suffixes always come after roots. A root can be combined with prefixes, roots, or suffixes. The prefix *dys* (difficult) can be combined with the root *pnea* (breathing). This forms *dyspnea.* It means difficulty breathing.

Roots can be combined with suffixes. The root *mast* (breast) combined with the suffix *ectomy* (excision or removal) forms *mastectomy.* It means the removal of a breast.

Combining a prefix, root, and suffix is another way to form medical terms. *Endocarditis* has the prefix *endo* (inner), the root *card* (heart), and the suffix *itis* (inflammation). *Endocarditis* means inflammation of the inner part of the heart.

## BOX 4-3  MEDICAL TERMINOLOGY

| PREFIX | MEANING |
|---|---|
| a-, an- | without, not, lack of |
| ab- | away from |
| ad- | to, toward, near |
| ante- | before, forward, in front of |
| anti- | against |
| auto- | self |
| bi- | double, two, twice |
| brady- | slow |
| circum- | around |
| contra- | against, opposite |
| de- | down, from |
| dia- | across, through, apart |
| dis- | apart, free from |
| dys- | bad, difficult, abnormal |
| ecto- | outer, outside |
| en- | in, into, within |
| endo- | inner, inside |
| epi- | over, on, upon |
| eryth- | red |
| eu- | normal, good, well, healthy |
| ex- | out, out of, from, away from |
| hemi- | half |
| hyper- | excessive, too much, high |
| hypo- | under, decreased, less than normal |
| in- | in, into, within, not |
| infra- | within |
| inter- | between |
| intro- | into, within |
| leuk- | white |
| macro- | large |
| mal- | bad, illness, disease |
| meg- | large |
| micro- | small |
| mono- | one, single |
| neo- | new |
| non- | not |
| olig- | small, scant |
| para- | beside, beyond, after |
| per- | by, through |
| peri- | around |
| poly- | many, much |
| post- | after, behind |
| pre- | before, in front of, prior to |
| pro- | before, in front of |
| re- | again, backward |
| retro- | backward, behind |

| PREFIX—CONT'D | MEANING |
|---|---|
| semi- | half |
| sub- | under, beneath |
| super- | above, over, excess |
| supra- | above, over |
| tachy- | fast, rapid |
| trans- | across |
| uni- | one |

| ROOT (COMBINING VOWEL) | MEANING |
|---|---|
| abdomin (o) | abdomen |
| aden (o) | gland |
| adren (o) | adrenal gland |
| angi (o) | vessel |
| arterio | artery |
| arthr (o) | joint |
| broncho | bronchus, bronchi |
| card, cardi (o) | heart |
| cephal (o) | head |
| chole, chol (o) | bile |
| chondr (o) | cartilage |
| colo | colon, large intestine |
| cost (o) | rib |
| crani (o) | skull |
| cyan (o) | blue |
| cyst (o) | bladder, cyst |
| cyt (o) | cell |
| dent (o) | tooth |
| derma | skin |
| duoden (o) | duodenum |
| encephal (o) | brain |
| enter (o) | intestines |
| fibr (o) | fiber, fibrous |
| gastr (o) | stomach |
| gloss (o) | tongue |
| gluc (o) | sweetness, glucose |
| glyc (o) | sugar |
| gyn, gyne, gyneco | woman |
| hem, hema, hemo, hemat (o) | blood |
| hepat (o) | liver |
| hydr (o) | water |
| hyster (o) | uterus |
| ile (o), ili (o) | ileum |
| laparo | abdomen, loin, or flank |

*Continued*

| ROOT (COMBINING VOWEL)—CONT'D | MEANING | SUFFIX | MEANING |
|---|---|---|---|
| laryng (o) | larynx | -algia | pain |
| lith (o) | stone | -asis | condition, usually abnormal |
| mamm (o) | breast, mammary gland | -cele | hernia, herniation, pouching |
| mast (o) | mammary gland, breast | -centesis | puncture and aspiration of |
| meno | menstruation | -cyte | cell |
| my (o) | muscle | -ectasis | dilation, stretching |
| myel (o) | spinal cord, bone marrow | -ectomy | excision, removal of |
| necro | death | -emia | blood condition |
| nephr (o) | kidney | -genesis | development, production, creation |
| neur (o) | nerve | -genic | producing, causing |
| ocul (o) | eye | -gram | record |
| oophor (o) | ovary | -graph | a diagram, a recording instrument |
| ophthalm (o) | eye | -graphy | making a recording |
| orth (o) | straight, normal, correct | -iasis | condition of |
| oste (o) | bone | -ism | a condition |
| ot (o) | ear | -itis | inflammation |
| ped (o) | child, foot | -logy | the study of |
| pharyng (o) | pharynx | -lysis | destruction of, decomposition |
| phleb (o) | vein | -megaly | enlargement |
| pnea | breathing, respiration | -meter | measuring instrument |
| pneum (o) | lung, air, gas | -metry | measurement |
| proct (o) | rectum | -oma | tumor |
| psych (o) | mind | -osis | condition |
| pulmo | lung | -pathy | disease |
| py (o) | pus | -penia | lack, deficiency |
| rect (o) | rectum | -phagia | to eat or consume; swallowing |
| rhin (o) | nose | -phasia | speaking |
| salping (o) | eustachian tube, uterine tube | -phobia | an exaggerated fear |
| splen (o) | spleen | -plasty | surgical repair or reshaping |
| sten (o) | narrow, constriction | -plegia | paralysis |
| stern (o) | sternum | -ptosis | falling, sagging, dropping, down |
| stomat (o) | mouth | -rrhage, -rrhagia | excessive flow |
| therm (o) | heat | -rrhaphy | stitching, suturing |
| thoraco | chest | -rrhea | profuse flow, discharge |
| thromb (o) | clot, thrombus | -scope | examination instrument |
| thyr (o) | thyroid | -scopy | examination using a scope |
| toxic (o) | poison, poisonous | -stasis | maintenance, maintaining a constant level |
| toxo | poison | -stomy, -ostomy | creation of an opening |
| trache (o) | trachea | -tomy, -otomy | incision, cutting into |
| urethr (o) | urethra | -uria | condition of the urine |
| urin (o) | urine | | |
| uro | urine, urinary tract, urination | | |
| uter (o) | uterus | | |
| vas (o) | blood vessel, vas deferens | | |
| ven (o) | vein | | |
| vertebr (o) | spine, vertebrae | | |

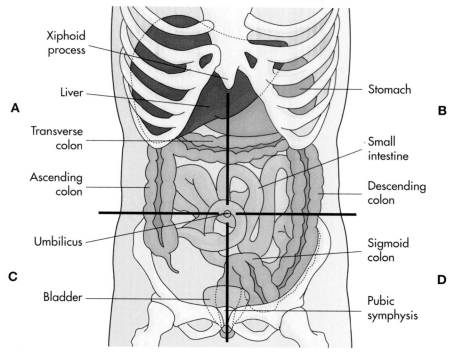

**FIG. 4-9** The four abdominal regions. **A,** Right upper quadrant. **B,** Left upper quadrant. **C,** Right lower quadrant. **D,** Left lower quadrant.

## ABDOMINAL REGIONS

The abdomen is divided into regions (Fig. 4-9). They are used to describe the location of body structures, pain, or discomfort. The regions are the:
- Right upper quadrant (RUQ)
- Left upper quadrant (LUQ)
- Right lower quadrant (RLQ)
- Left lower quadrant (LLQ)

## DIRECTIONAL TERMS

Certain terms describe the position of one body part in relation to another. These terms give the direction of the body part when a person is standing and facing forward (Fig. 4-10, p. 66):
- **Anterior (ventral)**—at or toward the front of the body or body part
- **Distal**—the part farthest from the center or from the point of attachment
- **Lateral**—at the side of the body or body part
- **Medial**—at or near the middle or midline of the body or body part
- **Posterior (dorsal)**—at or toward the back of the body or body part
- **Proximal**—the part nearest to the center or to the point of origin

## ABBREVIATIONS

**Abbreviations** are shortened forms of words or phrases. They save time and space when recording. Each agency has a list of accepted abbreviations. Obtain the list when you are hired. Use only those accepted by the agency. If you are unsure if an abbreviation is acceptable, write the term out in full. This ensures accurate communication.

Common abbreviations are on the inside of this book's back cover for easy use.

## USING COMPUTERS

Computer systems collect, send, record, and store information. It is retrieved when needed. Many agencies store charts and care plans (Chapter 5) on computers. Entering information on a computer is easier and faster than charting.

The health team uses computers to send messages and reports to the nursing unit. This reduces clerical work and phone calls. And information is sent with greater speed and accuracy.

Computers also are used for measurements such as blood pressures, temperatures, heart rates, and heart

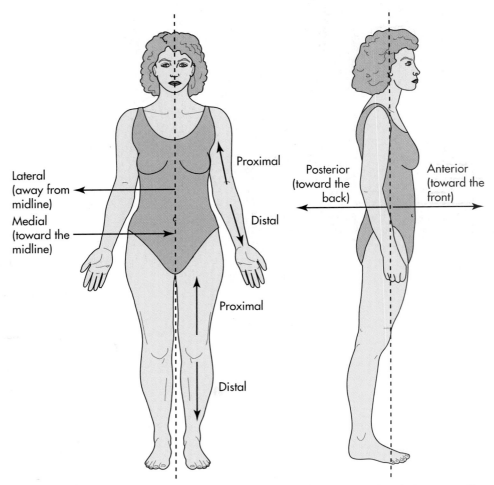

**FIG. 4-10** Directional terms describe the position of one body part in relation to another.

function. The computer senses normal and abnormal measurements. When the abnormal is sensed, an alarm alerts the nursing staff. Life-threatening events are detected early with computer monitoring.

Doctors can use computers when diagnosing. Signs and symptoms are entered into the computer. The computer asks questions, and the doctor responds. The computer offers possible diagnoses. Doctors also can use computers to prescribe drugs. The diagnosis is entered along with any requested information. The computer analyzes the information and suggests drugs and dosages.

Computers save time. Quality care and safety increase. Fewer recording errors are made. Records are more complete. Staff is more efficient.

Computers are easy to use. They contain vast amounts of information. Therefore the right to privacy must be protected. Only certain staff members use the computer. Each member has a code (password) to access computer files. If allowed access, you will learn how to use the agency's system. You must follow the agency's policy. Also follow the rules in Box 4-4 and the ethical and legal rules about privacy, confidentiality, and defamation.

## PHONE COMMUNICATIONS

You may have to answer phones at the nurses' station or in the person's room. Good communication skills are needed. The caller cannot see you. But you give much information by your tone of voice, how clearly you speak, and your attitude. Behave as if you are speaking to someone face-to-face. Be professional and courteous. Also practice good work ethics. Follow the agency's policy and the guidelines in Box 4-5. *See Focus on Home Care: Phone Communications.*

## BOX 4-4  USING THE AGENCY'S COMPUTER

- Do not tell anyone your password. If someone has your password, he or she can access the computer under your name. It will be hard to prove that someone else made the entries.
- Change your password often.
- Do not use another person's password.
- Follow the rules for recording (see Box 4-1).
- Enter information carefully. Double-check your entries.
- Prevent others from seeing what is on the screen. Do not leave the computer unattended.
- Log off after making an entry.
- Position equipment so the screen cannot be seen in the hallway.
- Do not leave printouts where others can read them or pick them up.
- Destroy or shred computer-printed worksheets.
- Send e-mail and messages only to those needing the information.
- Do not use e-mail for information or messages that require immediate reporting. Give the report in person. (The person may not read e-mail in a timely manner.)
- Do not use e-mail or messages to report confidential information. This includes addresses, phone numbers, and Social Security numbers. The computer system may not be secure.
- Do not use the agency's computer to:
  —Send personal e-mail or messages
  —Send or receive e-mail or messages that are offensive, illegal, or sexual
  —Send or receive e-mail or messages for illegal activities, jokes, politics, gambling (including football and other pools), chain letters, advertising, or other non-work activities
  —Post information, opinions, or comments on Internet message boards
  —Take part in Internet discussion groups
  —Upload, download, or transmit materials containing a copyright, trademark, or patent
- Remember that any communication may be read or heard by someone other than the intended person.
- Remember that deleted communications can be retrieved by authorized personnel.
- Remember that the agency has the right to monitor your computer use. This includes Internet use.
- Do not open another person's e-mail or messages.

## BOX 4-5  GUIDELINES FOR ANSWERING PHONES

- Answer the call after the first ring if possible. Be sure to answer by the fourth ring.
- Do not answer the phone in a rushed or hasty manner.
- Give a courteous greeting. Give your name, title, and department. For example: "Good morning. Three center. Jack Parks, nursing assistant."
- Write the following information when taking a message:
  —The caller's name and telephone number (include area code and extension number)
  —The date and time
  —The message
- Repeat the message and phone number back to the caller.
- Ask the caller to "Please hold" if necessary. First find out who is calling. Then ask if the caller can hold. Do not put callers with an emergency on hold.
- Do not lay the phone down or cover the receiver with your hand when not speaking to the caller. The caller may overhear confidential conversations.
- Return to a caller on hold within 30 seconds. Ask if the caller can wait longer or if the call can be returned.
- Do not give confidential information to any caller. Information about patients, residents, and employees is confidential. Refer such calls to an RN.
- Transfer the call if appropriate:
  —Tell the caller that you are going to transfer the call.
  —Give the name of the department if appropriate.
  —Give the caller the phone number in case the call gets disconnected or the line is busy.
- End the conversation politely. Thank the person for calling, and say good-bye.
- Give the message to the appropriate person.

## FOCUS ON HOME CARE
### PHONE COMMUNICATIONS

When answering phones in patients' homes, simply answer with "hello." This is for everyone's safety—the person, family, and you. The caller has too much information when you give the person's name ("Price residence") or your name and title.

People call homes for many reasons. Some make sales calls or to obtain donations. Others have criminal intent. They want to know who is there. Saying that you are a home health assistant tells that an ill, older, or disabled person is in the home. These people have difficulty defending themselves. They are easy prey for criminals. Do not give your name or the person's name until you know who is calling and why. Make sure that it is someone you want to talk to—the person's family or friend, your supervisor, or a caller expected by the person.

# DEALING WITH CONFLICT

People bring their values, attitudes, opinions, experiences, and expectations to the work setting. Differences often lead to conflict. **Conflict** is a clash between opposing interests or ideas. People disagree and argue. There are misunderstandings and unrest.

Conflicts arise over issues or events. Work schedules, absences, and the amount and quality of work performed are examples. The problems must be worked out. Otherwise, unkind words or actions may occur. The work setting becomes unpleasant. Care is affected.

To resolve a conflict, you need to identify the real problem. This is part of *problem solving*. The problem solving process involves these steps:

- Step 1: Define the problem. *A nurse ignores me.*
- Step 2: Collect information. The information must be about the problem. Do not include unrelated information. *The nurse does not look at me. The nurse does not talk to me. The nurse does not respond when I call her by name. The nurse does not ask me to help with tasks that require two people. The nurse talks to other staff members.*
- Step 3: Identify possible solutions. *Ignore the nurse. Talk to my supervisor. Talk to co-workers about the problem. Change jobs.*
- Step 4: Select the best solution. *Talk to my supervisor.*
- Step 5: Carry out the solution. *See below.*
- Step 6: Evaluate the results. *See below.*

Communication and good work ethics help prevent and resolve conflicts. Identify and solve problems before they become major issues. These guidelines can help you deal with conflict:

- Ask your supervisor for some time to talk privately. Explain the problem. Give facts and specific examples. Ask for advice in solving the problem.
- Approach the person with whom you have a conflict. Ask to talk privately. Be polite and professional.
- Agree on a time and place to talk.
- Talk in a private setting. No one should see or hear you and the other person.
- Explain the problem and what is bothering you. Give facts and specific behaviors. Focus on the problem. Do not focus on the person.
- Listen to the person. Do not interrupt.
- Identify ways to solve the problem. Offer your thoughts. Ask for the co-worker's ideas.
- Set a date and time to review the matter.
- Thank the person for meeting with you.
- Carry out the solutions.
- Review the matter as scheduled.

# CROSS-TRAINING OPPORTUNITIES

Receptionists and unit secretaries (ward clerks) use what you learned in this chapter. A receptionist answers the telephone and greets visitors. Information is also given about where to find patient or resident rooms and agency departments.

A unit secretary or ward clerk works on a nursing unit. The person maintains the medical record and Kardex, orders supplies, and communicates with the health team. Answering phones, taking messages, and computer work are other duties.

You may be asked to cross-train for one or both of these roles. If so, you will have greater job options. You will learn more about what these workers do. That will help you better understand and appreciate their roles and functions.

# ■ REVIEW QUESTIONS ■

Circle the **BEST** answer.

1 To communicate, you should do the following *except*
   a Use terms with many meanings
   b Be brief and concise
   c Present information logically and in sequence
   d Give facts and be specific

2 Mr. Barr is discharged from the agency. His medical record is
   a Destroyed to protect privacy
   b Sent home with him
   c Permanent
   d On computer

3 These statements are about medical records. Which is *false?*
   a The record is used to communicate information about the person.
   b The record is a written account of the person's illness and response to treatment.
   c The record can be used as evidence of the care given.
   d Anyone working in the agency can read the medical record.

4 A person is weighed daily. The measurement is recorded on the
   a Admission sheet
   b Graphic sheet
   c Flow sheet
   d Progress notes

5 Where does the nurse describe the nursing care given?
   a Admission sheet
   b Nursing history
   c Graphic sheet
   d Progress notes

6 When recording, you do the following *except*
   a Use ink
   b Include the date and time
   c Erase errors
   d Sign all entries with your name and title

7 These statements are about recording. Which action is *false?*
   a Use the person's exact words when possible.
   b Record only what you did and observed.
   c Sign your initials to a mistaken entry.
   d Chart a procedure before completing it.

8 In the evening the clock shows 9:26. In 24-hour clock time this is
   a 9:26 PM
   b 926
   c 0926
   d 2126

9 These statements are about computers in health care. Which is *false?*
   a Computers are used to collect, send, record, and store information.
   b The person's privacy must be protected.
   c All employees have the same password.
   d Computers link one department to another.

10 You answer a person's phone in the hospital. How should you answer?
   a "Good morning. Mr. Barr's room."
   b "Good morning. Third floor."
   c "Hello."
   d "Good morning. Mr. Barr's room. Joan Bates, nursing assistant, speaking."

11 A co-worker is often late for work. This means extra work for you. To resolve the conflict you should do the following *except*
   a Explain the problem to your supervisor
   b Discuss the matter during the end-of-shift report
   c Give facts and specific behaviors
   d Suggest ways to solve the problem

**Fill in the blanks**

12 Word elements used in medical terminology are
   a Prefixes
   b roots
   c suffixes

13 A _____ is placed at the beginning of a word to change the meaning of the word.

14 A _____ is placed at the end of a word to change the meaning of the word.

**15** The four regions of the abdomen are
a _Right upper quadrant (RUQ)_
b _Left upper quadrant (LUQ)_
c _Right lower quadrant (RLQ)_
d _Left lower quadrant (LLQ)_

Match the item in column A with the item in column B.

| Column A | | Column B |
|---|---|---|
| **16** Distal | d | **a** The part nearest to the center or point of origin |
| **17** Proximal | a | **b** Relating to or located at the side of the body or body part |
| **18** Anterior (ventral) | c | **c** Located at or toward the front part of the body or body part |
| **19** Medial | f | **d** The part farthest from the center or point of attachment |
| **20** Posterior (dorsal) | e | **e** Located at or toward the back of the body or body part |
| **21** Lateral | b | **f** Relating to or located at or near the middle or the midline of the body or body part |

Write the definition of the following prefixes.

**22** a- _w/o, lack of_

**23** dys- _bad, abnormal_

**24** bi- _two, double_

**25** ab- _away from_

**26** trans- _across_

**27** post- _after / behind_

**28** olig- _small_

**29** hyper- _excessive, too much, high_

**30** per- _by, through_

**31** hemi- _half_

**32** hypo- _under, less than normal_

**33** ad- _to, toward, near_

Write the definition of the following suffixes.

**34** -algia _____

**35** -itis _____

**36** -ostomy _____

**37** -ectomy _____

**38** -emia _____

**39** -osis _____

**40** -rrhage _____

**41** -penia _____

**42** -pathy _____

**43** -otomy _____

**44** -rrhea _____

**45** -plasty _____

Write the definition of the following roots.

**46** cranio _____

**47** cardio _____

**48** mammo _____

**49** veno _____

**50** urino _____

**51** pnea _____

**52** cyano _____

**53** arterio _____

**54** colo _____

**55** arthro _____

**56** litho _____

**57** gastro _____

# ■ REVIEW QUESTIONS ■

58  encephalo _____

59  gluco _____

60  hemo _____

61  hystero _____

62  hepato _____

63  myo _____

64  nephro _____

65  phlebo _____

66  oculo _____

67  osteo _____

68  neuro _____

69  pneumo _____

70  toxico _____

71  psycho _____

72  thoraco _____

**Write the abbreviation for the following terms.**

83  Bathroom privileges _BRP_

84  As desired _ad lib_

85  Complains of _c/o_

86  Twice a day _bid_

87  Hour of sleep _HS_

88  Intake and output _I & O_

89  Nothing by mouth _npo_

90  When necessary _prn_

91  Postoperative _____

92  Every _____

93  Wheelchair _____

94  At once, immediately _____

*Answers to these questions are on p. 815.*

**Match the item in column A with the item in column B.**

**Column A**
73  Intravenous ___
74  Apnea ___
75  Hemiplegia ___
76  Thoracotomy ___
77  Arthritis ___
78  Bronchitis ___
79  Anuria ___
80  Hematuria ___
81  Hysterectomy ___
82  Hemorrhage ___

**Column B**
a  Inflammation of a joint
b  Blood in the urine
c  Excessive flow of blood
d  Paralysis on one side
e  Surgical removal of the uterus
f  No breathing
g  Inflammation of the bronchi
h  Incision into the chest
i  No urine
j  Within a vein

# Assisting With the Nursing Process

5

## OBJECTIVES

- Define the key terms listed in this chapter
- Explain the purpose of the nursing process
- Describe the steps of the nursing process
- Explain your role in each step of the nursing process
- Explain the difference between objective data and subjective data
- Identify the observations that you need to report to the nurse
- Explain the purpose of care conferences

## KEY TERMS

**assessment** Collecting information about the person; a step in the nursing process

**evaluation** To measure if goals in the planning step were met; a step in the nursing process

**goal** That which is desired in or by the person as a result of nursing care

**implementation** To perform or carry out measures in the care plan; a step in the nursing process

**medical diagnosis** The identification of a disease or condition by a doctor

**nursing care plan** A written guide about the person's care

**nursing diagnosis** Describes a health problem that can be treated by nursing measures; a step in the nursing process

**nursing intervention** An action or measure taken by the nursing team to help the person reach a goal

**nursing process** The method RNs use to plan and deliver nursing care; its five steps are assessment, nursing diagnosis, planning, implementation, and evaluation

**objective data** Information that is seen, heard, felt, or smelled; signs

**observation** Using the senses of sight, hearing, touch, and smell to collect information

**planning** Setting priorities and goals; a step in the nursing process

**signs** Objective data

**subjective data** Things a person tells you about that you cannot observe through your senses; symptoms

**symptoms** Subjective data

---

Nurses communicate with each other about the person's strengths, problems, needs, and care. This information is shared through the nursing process. The **nursing process** is the method RNs use to plan and deliver nursing care. It has five steps:

- Assessment
- Nursing diagnosis
- Planning
- Implementation
- Evaluation

The nursing process focuses on the person's nursing needs. Good communication is needed between the person and the nursing team.

Each step is important. If done in order with good communication, nursing care is organized and has purpose. All nursing team members do the same things for the person. They have the same goals. The person feels safe and secure with consistent care.

The nursing process is used in all health care settings. It is used for all age-groups. The nursing process is ongoing. It changes as new information is gathered and as the person's needs change. You will see the continuous nature of the nursing process as each step is explained.

## ASSESSMENT

**Assessment** involves collecting information about the person. Nurses use many sources. A nursing history is taken (Chapter 4). This tells about current and past health problems. The family's health history also is important. Many diseases are genetic. That is, the risk for certain diseases is inherited from parents. For example, a mother had breast cancer. Her daughters are at risk. Information from the doctor is reviewed. So are test results and past medical records.

The RN assesses the person's body systems and mental status. You play a key role in assessment. You make many observations as you give care and talk to the person.

**Observation** is using the senses of sight, hearing, touch, and smell to collect information:

- You *see* how the person lies, sits, or walks. You see flushed or pale skin. You see red and swollen body areas.
- You *listen* to the person breathe, talk, and cough. You use a stethoscope to listen to the heartbeat and to measure blood pressure.
- Through *touch,* you feel if the skin is hot or cold, or moist or dry. You use touch to take the person's pulse.
- *Smell* is used to detect body, wound, and breath odors. You also smell odors from urine and bowel movements.

**Objective data** (signs) are information that is seen, heard, felt, or smelled. You can feel a pulse. You can see urine. You cannot feel or see the person's pain, fear, or nausea. **Subjective data (symptoms)** are things a person tells you about that you cannot observe through your senses.

Box 5-1 lists the basic observations you need to make and report to the nurse. Make notes of your observations. Use them when reporting and recording observations. Carry a note pad and pen in your pocket. That way you can note observations as you make them. Your agency may provide electronic hand-held devices for this purpose (Fig. 5-1).

The assessment step never ends. New information is collected with every patient or resident contact. New observations are made. The person shares more information. The family often adds more information. *See Focus on Long-Term Care: Assessment. See Focus on Home Care: Assessment*

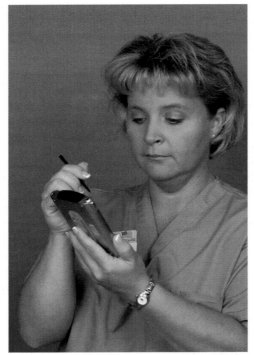

**FIG. 5-1** The nursing assistant uses an electronic, hand-held device to note observations.

**FOCUS ON LONG-TERM CARE**

ASSESSMENT

OBRA requires the *minimum data set (MDS)* for nursing center residents (Appendix B, p. 822). The MDS is an assessment and screening tool. The form is completed when the person is admitted to the center. It provides extensive information about the person. Examples are memory, communication, hearing and vision, physical function, and activities. The form is updated before each care conference. A new MDS is completed once a year and whenever the person's condition changes.

**FOCUS ON HOME CARE**

ASSESSMENT

Medicare-certified home health care agencies use the Outcome and Assessment Information Set (OASIS). It is used for adult home care patients. Besides assessment, OASIS is used for planning care.

BOX
5-1    BASIC OBSERVATIONS

### ABILITY TO RESPOND

- Is the person easy or hard to arouse?
- Can the person give his or her name, the time, and location when asked?
- Does the person identify others correctly?
- Does the person answer questions correctly?
- Does the person speak clearly?
- Are instructions followed correctly?
- Is the person calm, restless, or excited?
- Is the person conversing, quiet, or talking a lot?

### MOVEMENT

- Can the person squeeze your fingers with each hand?
- Can the person move arms and legs?
- Are the person's movements shaky or jerky?
- Does the person complain of stiff or painful joints?

### PAIN OR DISCOMFORT

- Where is the pain located? (Ask the person to point to the pain.)
- Does the pain go anywhere else?
- When did the pain begin?
- What was the person doing when the pain began?
- How long does the pain last?
- How does the person describe the pain?
  —Sharp
  —Severe
  —Knifelike
  —Dull
  —Burning
  —Aching
  —Comes and goes
  —Depends on position
- Was medication given?
- Did medication help relieve the pain? Is pain still present?
- Is the person able to sleep and rest?
- What is the position of comfort?

### SKIN

- Is the skin pale or flushed?
- Is the skin cool, warm, or hot?
- Is the skin moist or dry?
- What color are the lips and nails?
- Is the skin intact? Are there broken areas? If so, where?
- Are sores or reddened areas present?
- Are bruises present? Where are they located?
- Does the person complain of itching?

### EYES, EARS, NOSE, AND MOUTH

- Is there drainage from the eyes? What color is the drainage?
- Are the eyelids closed?
- Are the eyes reddened?
- Does the person complain of spots, flashes, or blurring?
- Is the person sensitive to bright lights?
- Is there drainage from the ears? What color is the drainage?
- Can the person hear? Is repeating necessary? Are questions answered appropriately?
- Is there drainage from the nose? What color is the drainage?
- Can the person breathe through the nose?
- Is there breath odor?
- Does the person complain of a bad taste in the mouth?
- Does the person complain of painful gums or teeth?

### RESPIRATIONS

- Do both sides of the person's chest rise and fall with respirations?
- Is breathing noisy?
- Does the person complain of difficulty breathing?
- What is the amount and color of sputum?
- What is the frequency of the person's cough? Is it dry or productive?

### BOWELS AND BLADDER

- Is the abdomen firm or soft?
- Does the person complain of gas?
- What are the amount, color, and consistency of bowel movements?
- What is the frequency of bowel movements?
- Can the person control bowel movements?
- Does the person have pain or difficulty urinating?
- What is the amount of urine?
- What is the color of urine?
- Is urine clear? Are there particles in the urine?
- Does urine have a foul smell?
- Can the person control the passage of urine?
- What is the frequency of urination?

### APPETITE

- Does the person like the diet?
- How much of the meal is eaten?
- What are the person's food preferences?
- Can the person chew food?
- How much liquid was taken?
- What are the person's liquid preferences?
- How often does the person drink liquids?
- Can the person swallow food and fluids?
- Does the person complain of nausea?
- What is the amount and color of material vomited?
- Does the person have hiccups?
- Is the person belching?
- Does the person cough when swallowing?

### ACTIVITIES OF DAILY LIVING

- Can the person perform personal care without help?
  —Bathing?
  —Brushing teeth?
  —Combing and brushing hair?
  —Shaving?
- Which does the person use: toilet, commode, bedpan, or urinal?
- Does the person feed himself or herself?
- Can the person walk?
- What amount and kind of help is needed?

# NURSING DIAGNOSIS

The RN uses assessment information to make a nursing diagnosis. A **nursing diagnosis** describes a health problem that can be treated by nursing measures. The problem may exist or may develop. Nursing diagnoses and medical diagnoses are not the same. A **medical diagnosis** is the identification of a disease or condition by a doctor. Cancer, pneumonia, chickenpox, stroke, heart attack, infection, AIDS, and diabetes are examples. Doctors use drugs, therapies, and surgery to cure or heal.

A person can have many nursing diagnoses. Nursing deals with the total person. Nursing diagnoses involve the person's physical, emotional, social, and spiritual needs (Box 5-2).

---

| BOX 5-2 | NURSING DIAGNOSES APPROVED BY THE NORTH AMERICAN NURSING DIAGNOSIS ASSOCIATION (NANDA) |
|---|---|

- Activity Intolerance
- Activity Intolerance, Risk for
- Adjustment, Impaired
- Airway Clearance, Ineffective
- Anxiety
- Aspiration, Risk for
- Bathing/Hygiene Self-Care Deficit
- Body Image, Disturbed
- Breastfeeding, Effective
- Breastfeeding, Ineffective
- Breastfeeding, Interrupted
- Breathing Pattern, Ineffective
- Cardiac Output, Decreased
- Caregiver Role Strain
- Caregiver Role Strain, Risk for
- Communication, Impaired Verbal
- Communication, Readiness for Enhanced
- Community Coping, Readiness for Enhanced
- Confusion, Acute
- Confusion, Chronic
- Constipation
- Constipation, Perceived
- Constipation, Risk for
- Coping, Defensive
- Coping, Ineffective
- Coping, Readiness for Enhanced
- Death Anxiety
- Decisional Conflict (Specify)
- Denial, Ineffective
- Dentition, Impaired
- Development, Risk for Delayed
- Diarrhea
- Disuse Syndrome, Risk for
- Diversional Activity, Deficient

- Dressing/Grooming Self-Care Deficit
- Dysreflexia, Autonomic
- Dysreflexia, Autonomic, Risk for
- Energy Field, Disturbed
- Environmental Interpretation Syndrome, Impaired
- Failure to Thrive, Adult
- Falls, Risk for
- Family Coping, Compromised
- Family Coping, Disabled
- Family Coping, Readiness for Enhanced
- Family Processes, Dysfunctional: Alcoholism
- Family Processes, Interrupted
- Family Processes, Readiness for Enhanced
- Fatigue
- Fear
- Feeding Self-Care Deficit
- Fluid Balance, Readiness for Enhanced
- Fluid Volume, Deficient
- Fluid Volume, Excess
- Fluid Volume, Risk for Deficient
- Fluid Volume, Risk for Imbalanced
- Gas Exchange, Impaired
- Grieving, Anticipatory
- Grieving, Dysfunctional
- Growth, Risk for Disproportionate
- Growth and Development, Delayed
- Health Maintenance, Ineffective
- Health-Seeking Behaviors (Specify)
- Home Maintenance, Impaired
- Hopelessness
- Hyperthermia
- Hypothermia
- Incontinence, Bowel
- Incontinence, Urinary, Functional

**BOX 5-2** | **NURSING DIAGNOSES APPROVED BY THE NORTH AMERICAN NURSING DIAGNOSIS ASSOCIATION (NANDA)—CONT'D**

- Incontinence, Urinary, Reflex
- Incontinence, Urinary, Stress
- Incontinence, Urinary, Total
- Incontinence, Urinary, Urge
- Incontinence, Urinary, Urge, Risk for
- Infant Behavior, Disorganized
- Infant Behavior, Risk for Disorganized
- Infant Behavior, Organized, Readiness for Enhanced
- Infant Feeding Pattern, Ineffective
- Infection, Risk for
- Injury, Risk for
- Intracranial Adaptive Capacity, Decreased
- Knowledge Deficient (Specify)
- Knowledge, Readiness for Enhanced (Specify)
- Latex Allergy Response
- Latex Allergy Response, Risk for
- Loneliness, Risk for
- Memory, Impaired
- Mobility, Impaired Bed
- Mobility, Impaired Wheelchair
- Nausea
- Noncompliance (Specify)
- Neglect, Unilateral
- Neurovascular Dysfunction, Risk for Peripheral
- Nutrition, Imbalanced: Less Than Body Requirements
- Nutrition, Imbalanced: More Than Body Requirements
- Nutrition, Imbalanced: More Than Body Requirements, Risk for
- Nutrition, Readiness for Enhanced
- Oral Mucous Membrane, Impaired
- Pain, Acute
- Pain, Chronic
- Parent/Infant/Child Attachment, Risk for Impaired
- Parental Role Conflict
- Parenting, Impaired
- Parenting, Readiness for Enhanced
- Parenting, Risk for Impaired
- Perioperative-Positioning Injury, Risk for
- Personal Identity, Disturbed
- Physical Mobility, Impaired
- Poisoning, Risk for
- Post-Trauma Syndrome
- Post-Trauma Syndrome, Risk for
- Powerlessness
- Powerlessness, Risk for
- Protection, Ineffective
- Rape-Trauma Syndrome
- Rape-Trauma Syndrome: Compound Reaction
- Rape-Trauma Syndrome: Silent Reaction
- Relocation Stress Syndrome
- Relocation Stress Syndrome: Risk for
- Role Performance, Ineffective
- Self-Concept, Readiness for Enhanced
- Self-Esteem, Chronic Low
- Self-Esteem, Situational Low
- Self-Esteem, Situational Low, Risk for
- Self-Mutilation
- Self-Mutilation, Risk for
- Sensory Perception, Disturbed (Specify type: visual, auditory, kinesthetic, gustatory, tactile, olfactory)
- Sexual Dysfunction
- Sexuality Patterns, Ineffective
- Skin Integrity, Impaired
- Skin Integrity, Risk for Impaired
- Sleep Deprivation
- Sleep Pattern, Disturbed
- Sleep, Readiness for Enhanced
- Social Interaction, Impaired
- Social Isolation
- Sorrow, Chronic
- Spiritual Distress
- Spiritual Distress, Risk for
- Spiritual Well-Being, Readiness for Enhanced
- Sudden Infant Death Syndrome, Risk for
- Suffocation, Risk for
- Suicide, Risk for
- Surgical Recovery, Delayed
- Swallowing, Impaired
- Therapeutic Regimen Management, Effective
- Therapeutic Regimen Management, Ineffective
- Therapeutic Regimen Management, Ineffective Community
- Therapeutic Regimen Management, Ineffective Family
- Therapeutic Regimen Management, Readiness for Enhanced
- Thermoregulation, Ineffective
- Thought Processes, Disturbed
- Tissue Integrity, Impaired
- Tissue Perfusion, Ineffective (Specify type: renal, cerebral, cardiopulmonary, gastrointestinal, peripheral)
- Toileting Self-Care Deficit
- Transfer Ability, Impaired
- Trauma, Risk for
- Urinary Elimination, Impaired
- Urinary Elimination, Readiness for Enhanced
- Urinary Retention
- Ventilation, Impaired Spontaneous
- Ventilatory Weaning Response, Dysfunctional (DVWR)
- Violence, Risk for Other-Directed
- Violence, Risk for Self-Directed
- Walking, Impaired
- Wandering

Modified from NANDA International 2002: *NANDA Nursing diagnoses: definitions and classification 2003-2004,* Philadelphia, NANDA.

# PLANNING

**Planning** involves setting priorities and goals. Nursing measures or actions are chosen to help the person meet the goals (Fig. 5-2). The person, family, and health team help the RN plan care.

Priorities relate to what is most important for the person. Maslow's theory of basic needs is useful for setting priorities (Chapter 6). The needs are arranged in order of importance. Some needs are required for life and survival (oxygen, water, and food). They must be met before all other needs. They have priority and must be done first.

Goals are then set. A **goal** is that which is desired in or by a person as a result of nursing care. Goals are aimed at the person's highest level of well-being and functioning: physical, emotional, social, spiritual. Goals promote health and prevent health problems. They also promote rehabilitation.

Nursing interventions are chosen after goals are set. An intervention is an action or measure. A **nursing intervention** is an action or measure taken by the nursing team to help the person reach a goal. Nursing intervention, nursing action, and nursing measure mean the same thing. A nursing intervention does not need a doctor's order. However, some nursing measures come from a doctor's order. For example, a doctor orders that Mrs. Kemp walk 50 yards two times a day. The RN includes this order in the care plan.

The **nursing care plan** is a written guide about the person's care. It has the person's nursing diagnoses and goals. It also has the measures or actions for each goal. The care plan is a communication tool. Nursing staff use it to see what care to give. The care plan helps ensure that the nursing team give the same care. It is found in the medical record, on the Kardex, or on computer (see Fig. 5-2).

The RN may conduct a care conference to share information and ideas about the person's care. The purpose is to develop or revise a person's nursing care plan. Effective care is the goal. Nursing assistants usually take part in the conference. You should share your suggestions and observations.

The plan is carried out. It may change if the person's nursing diagnoses change. Remember, nursing diagnoses may change as new information is gained during assessment.

*See Focus on Long-Term Care: Planning.*

---

## FOCUS ON LONG-TERM CARE
### PLANNING

OBRA requires two types of resident care conferences:
- The *interdisciplinary care planning (IDCP) conference* is held regularly to develop, review, and update care plans. The RN, doctor, and other health team members attend. The person and a family member also attend.
- *Problem-focused conferences* are held when one problem affects a person's care. Only staff directly involved in the problem attend. The person and family may be asked to attend.

OBRA requires the use of *resident assessment protocols (RAPs)*. They are guidelines used to develop the person's care plan (Appendix B, p. 822). The problems identified on the minimum data set (MDS) give *triggers* (clues) for the RAPs. Triggers direct the health team to the appropriate RAP. For example, Mrs. Reece is weak from illness and lack of exercise. She cannot do her activities of daily living (ADL). This triggers the RAPs. They provide guidelines to solve the problem. The goal is for Mrs. Reece to perform her ADL. The actions to help her reach the goal are:
- Occupational therapy to work with Mrs. Reece on ADL daily
- Physical therapy to work with Mrs. Reece on exercises daily
- Nursing staff to walk Mrs. Reece 50 feet twice daily

---

# IMPLEMENTATION

Implementation means to perform or carry out. The **implementation** step is performing or carrying out nursing measures in the care plan. Care is given in this step.

Nursing measures range from simple to complex. The nurse delegates measures and tasks that are within your legal limits and job description. The nurse may ask you to assist with complex measures.

You report the care given to the nurse. Some agencies allow you to record the care given. Reporting and recording are done *after* giving care, not before. Also report or record your observations. Observing is part of assessment. New observations may change the nursing diagnoses. If so, care plan changes are made. To give correct care, you need to know about any changes in the care plan.

## ASSIGNMENT SHEETS

The nurse communicates delegated measures and tasks to you. An assignment sheet is used for this purpose (Fig. 5-3, p. 80). The assignment sheet tells you about:
- Each person's care
- What measures and tasks need to be done
- When to take meal and lunch breaks
- Which nursing unit tasks to do

Talk to the nurse about any assignment that is unclear. You can also check the care plan and Kardex if you need more information.

| Nursing diagnosis | Goal | Intervention |
|---|---|---|
| Constipation related to lack of privacy. | Patient will have regular bowel movements by 6/30. | Ask patient to use signal light when urge to have bowel movement is felt. |
| | | Answer call light promptly. |
| | | Assist patient to bathroom. |
| | | Close bathroom door for privacy. |
| | | Leave the room if the patient can be alone; tell the patient you are leaving and that you will return when he turns on the signal light. |
| Disturbed Sleep Pattern related to noisy environment. | Patient will report a restful sleep by 6/29. | Perform any necessary care measures before bedtime. |
| | | Close the door to the patient's room. |
| | | Turn off television or radio or keep volume low if patient prefers. |
| | | Ask staff to avoid unnecessary talking outside the patient's room. |
| | | Ask staff to speak in low voices. |
| | | Turn off unneeded equipment. |

**FIG. 5-2** Nursing care plan. Each nursing diagnosis has a goal. There are nursing measures for each goal.

## EVALUATION

Evaluation means to measure. The **evaluation** step involves measuring if the goals in the planning step were met. Progress is evaluated. Goals may be met totally, in part, or not at all. Assessment information is used for this step. Changes in nursing diagnoses, goals, and the care plan may result.

The nursing process never ends. Nurses constantly collect information about the person. Nursing diagnoses, goals, and the care plan may change as the person's needs change.

## YOUR ROLE

You have a key role in the nursing process. The RN uses your observations for nursing diagnoses and planning. You may help develop the care plan. In the implementation step, you perform nursing actions and measures in the care plan. Your assignment sheet tells you what to do. Your observations are used for the evaluation step.

**Daily Assignment Sheet**

Group _____
Date _____

| Room _____ | Room _____ |
|---|---|
| Name _____ | Name _____ |
| BM _____ Shower | BM _____ Shower |
| VD _____ Sponge | VD _____ Sponge |
| Intake _____ | Intake _____ |
| Foley _____ | Foley _____ |
| Up in w/c _____ | Up in w/c _____ |
| Bed rest _____ | Bed rest _____ |
| Position _____ | Position _____ |
| Ambulate _____ | Ambulate _____ |
| Circle one: Appetite – Good  Fair  Poor | Circle one: Appetite – Good  Fair  Poor |
| Room _____ | Room _____ |
| Name _____ | Name _____ |
| BM _____ Shower | BM _____ Shower |
| VD _____ Sponge | VD _____ Sponge |
| Intake _____ | Intake _____ |
| Foley _____ | Foley _____ |
| Up in w/c _____ | Up in w/c _____ |
| Bed rest _____ | Bed rest _____ |
| Position _____ | Position _____ |
| Ambulate _____ | Ambulate _____ |
| Circle one: Appetite – Good  Fair  Poor | Circle one: Appetite – Good  Fair  Poor |
| Room _____ | Room _____ |
| Name _____ | Name _____ |
| BM _____ Shower | BM _____ Shower |
| VD _____ Sponge | VD _____ Sponge |
| Intake _____ | Intake _____ |
| Foley _____ | Foley _____ |
| Up in w/c _____ | Up in w/c _____ |
| Bed rest _____ | Bed rest _____ |
| Position _____ | Position _____ |
| Ambulate _____ | Ambulate _____ |
| Circle one: Appetite – Good  Fair  Poor | Circle one: Appetite – Good  Fair  Poor |

**FIG. 5-3** Sample assignment sheet.

Circle the **BEST** answer.

1   Which is *not* a step in the nursing process?
    a   Observation
    b   Assessment
    c   Planning
    d   Implementation

2   The nursing process
    a   Involves guidelines for care plans
    b   Is a care conference
    c   Involves triggers
    d   Is the method nurses use to plan and deliver nursing care

3   What happens during assessment?
    a   Goals are set.
    b   Information is collected.
    c   Nursing measures are carried out.
    d   Progress is evaluated.

4   Which is a symptom?
    a   Redness
    b   Vomiting
    c   Pain
    d   Pulse rate of 78

5   Which is a sign?
    a   Nausea
    b   Headache
    c   Dizziness
    d   Dry skin

6   Measures in the nursing care plan are carried out. This is
    a   A nursing diagnosis
    b   Planning
    c   Implementation
    d   Evaluation

7   Which statement is *true?*
    a   The nursing process is done without the person's input.
    b   You are responsible for the nursing process.
    c   The nursing process is used to communicate the person's care.
    d   Nursing process steps can be done in any order.

8   The nursing care plan
    a   Is written by the doctor
    b   Has actions the nursing team takes to help a person
    c   Is the same for all persons
    d   Is also called the Kardex

9   What is used to communicate the tasks and measures delegated to you?
    a   The care plan
    b   The Kardex
    c   An assignment sheet
    d   Care conferences

10   Which is a nursing diagnosis?
    a   Cancer
    b   Heart attack
    c   Kidney failure
    d   Pain

*Answers to these questions are on p. 816.*

# Understanding the Person

6

## OBJECTIVES

- Define the key terms listed in this chapter
- Identify the parts that make up the whole person
- Explain Abraham Maslow's theory of basic needs
- Explain how culture and religion influence health and illness
- Identify the emotional and social effects of illness
- Describe the persons cared for in health care agencies
- Explain the American Hospital Association's *The Patient Care Partnership: Understanding Expectations, Rights, and Responsibilities*
- Identify the elements needed to communicate
- Describe how to use verbal and nonverbal communication
- Explain the methods and barriers to good communication
- Explain why family and visitors are important to the person
- Identify the courtesies given to the person and visitors
- Explain how to deal with behavior issues

## KEY TERMS

**body language** Messages sent through facial expressions, gestures, posture, hand and body movements, gait, eye contact, and appearance

**culture** The characteristics of a group of people—language, values, beliefs, habits, likes, dislikes, customs—passed from one generation to the next

**disability** A lost, absent, or impaired physical or mental function

**esteem** The worth, value, or opinion one has of a person

**geriatrics** The branch of medicine concerned with the problems and diseases of old age and older persons

**holism** A concept that considers the whole person; the whole person has physical, social, psychological, and spiritual parts that are woven together and cannot be separated

**need** Something necessary or desired for maintaining life and mental well-being

**nonverbal communication** Communication that does not use words

**obstetrics** The branch of medicine concerned with the care of women during pregnancy, labor, and childbirth and for the 6 to 8 weeks after birth

**paraphrasing** Restating the person's message in your own words

**pediatrics** The branch of medicine concerned with the growth, development, and care of children; they range in age from the newborn to teenagers

**psychiatry** The branch of medicine concerned with mental health problems

**religion** Spiritual beliefs, needs, and practices

**self-actualization** Experiencing one's potential

**self-esteem** Thinking well of oneself and seeing oneself as useful and having value

**verbal communication** Communication that uses written or spoken words

The patient or resident is the most important person in the agency. Age, religion, and nationality make each person unique. So does culture, education, occupation, and life-style. Each person is important and special. Each has value. Each has fears, needs, and rights. You must treat the person as someone who can think, act, and make decisions.

## HOLISM

The person lives, works, loves, and has fun. When ill or disabled, things are done to and for the person. He or she is told when to eat, sleep, bathe, visit, sit in a chair, walk, and use the bathroom. Patients and residents often complain that they are treated as things, not as people.

Often they are treated as physical diseases or problems. For example: "The heart attack in 310," not "John Porter in 310." To provide good care, you must consider the whole person.

Holism means *whole*. **Holism** is a concept that considers the whole person. The whole person has physical, social, psychological, and spiritual parts. The parts are woven together and cannot be separated (Fig. 6-1).

Each part relates to and depends on the others. As a social being, a person speaks and communicates with others. Physically, the brain, mouth, tongue, lips, and throat structures must function for speech. Communication is also psychological. It involves thinking and reasoning.

To consider only the physical part is to ignore the person's ability to think, make decisions, and interact with others. It also ignores the person's experiences, life-style, culture, joys, sorrows, and needs.

## BASIC NEEDS

A **need** is something necessary or desired for maintaining life and mental well-being. According to Abraham Maslow, a famous psychologist, basic needs must be met for a person to survive and function. According to this theory, the needs are arranged in order of importance (Fig. 6-2). Lower-level needs must be met before the higher-level needs. Basic needs, from the lowest level to the highest level, are:

- Physiological or physical needs
- Safety and security needs
- Love and belonging needs
- Self-esteem needs
- The need for self-actualization

People normally meet their own needs. When they cannot, it is usually because of illness, injury, or advanced age. When people cannot meet their own needs, they usually seek health care.

## PHYSICAL NEEDS

Oxygen, food, water, elimination, rest, and shelter are needed for life. They are needed to survive. A person dies within minutes without oxygen. Without food or water, a person feels weak and ill within a few hours. The kidneys and intestines must function. Otherwise poisonous wastes build up in the blood. This can cause death. Without enough rest and sleep, a person becomes very tired. Without shelter, the person is exposed to extremes of heat and cold.

## SAFETY AND SECURITY NEEDS

Safety and security needs relate to feeling safe from harm, danger, and fear. Many people are afraid of health care agencies. Some care involves strange equipment or entering the body. Some care causes pain or discomfort. People feel safer and more secure if they know what will happen. For every procedure, they should know:
- Why it is needed
- Who will do it
- How it will be done
- What sensations or feelings to expect

*See Focus on Long-Term Care: Safety and Security Needs.*

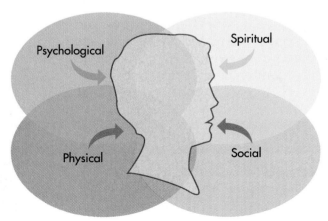

**FIG. 6-1** A person is a physical, psychological, social, and spiritual being. The parts overlap and cannot be separated.

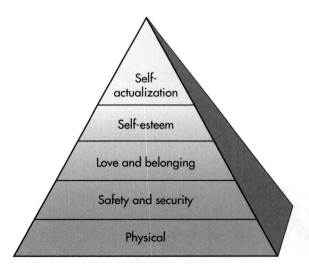

**FIG. 6-2** Basic needs for life as described by Maslow. (From Maslow, Abraham H: *Motivation and personality,* ed 3. Reprinted by permission of Pearson Education, Inc., Upper Saddle River, NJ.)

## LOVE AND BELONGING NEEDS

Love and belonging needs relate to love, closeness, and affection. They also involve meaningful relationships with others. Some people become weaker or die from the lack of love and belonging. This is seen in children and older persons. Family, friends, and the health team can meet love and belonging needs.

## SELF-ESTEEM NEEDS

**Esteem** is the worth, value, or opinion one has of a person. **Self-esteem** means to think well of oneself and to see oneself as useful and having value. People often lack self-esteem when ill, injured, older, or disabled. For example:

- A man is ill. How might he feel about not being able to work and support his family?
- A woman had a breast removed. Will she feel whole and pretty?
- A man had a leg amputated. Will he feel whole and manly?

## THE NEED FOR SELF-ACTUALIZATION

**Self-actualization** means experiencing one's potential. It involves learning, understanding, and creating to the limit of a person's capacity. This is the highest need. Rarely, if ever, is it totally met. Most people constantly try to learn and understand more. This need can be postponed, and life will continue.

## CULTURE AND RELIGION

**Culture** is the characteristics of a group of people—language, values, beliefs, habits, likes, dislikes, and customs. They are passed from one generation to the next. The person's culture influences health beliefs and practices. Culture also affects behavior during illness.

People come from many cultures, races, and nationalities. Their family practices and food choices may differ from yours. So might their hygiene habits and clothing styles. Some speak a foreign language. Some cultures have beliefs about what causes and cures illness. *See Caring About Culture: Health Care Beliefs.* They may perform rituals to rid the body of disease. *See Caring About Culture: Sick Care Practices.* Many have beliefs and rituals about dying and death (Chapter 41). Culture also is a factor in communication.

---

### CARING ABOUT CULTURE
#### HEALTH CARE BELIEFS

Some cultures believe that health is a balance between hot and cold. In *Mexico* and the *Dominican Republic*, hot and cold imbalances are thought to cause disease. "Hot" conditions include fever, infections, diarrhea, constipation, and ulcers. "Cold" conditions include cancer, earaches, menstrual periods, headaches, colds, and paralysis.

In *Vietnam*, foods and medicine are given to restore the hot-cold balance. Hot foods and medicines are for "cold" illnesses. Cold foods and medicines are for "hot" illnesses.

From Giger JN, Davidhizar RE: *Transcultural nursing: assessment and interventions*, ed 3, St Louis, 1999, Mosby.

---

### FOCUS ON LONG-TERM CARE
#### SAFETY AND SECURITY NEEDS

Many persons do not feel safe and secure when admitted to a nursing center. They are not in their usual, secure home setting. They are in a strange place with strange routines. Strangers care for them. Some become scared and confused.

Be kind and understanding. Show them the new setting. Listen to their concerns. Explain all routines and procedure. You may have to repeat information many times. Sometimes the information may need to be repeated for many days or weeks until they feel safe and secure. Be patient.

---

### CARING ABOUT CULTURE
#### SICK CARE PRACTICES

Folk practices are common in *Vietnam.* They include *cao gio*—rubbing the skin with a coin to treat the common cold. Skin pinching *(bat gio)* is used for headaches and sore throats. Herbal teas and soups are used for many signs and symptoms.

*Russian* folk practices also include herbs. Herbs are taken through drinks or enemas. For headaches, an ointment is placed behind the ears and temples and at the back of the neck. There are treatments for backaches. One involves making a dough of dark rye flour and honey. The dough is placed on the spinal column.

Folk healers are seen in *Mexico* and among some *Mexican Americans.* Folk healers may be family members skilled in healing practices. Some folk healers are from outside the family. A *yerbero* uses herbs and spices to prevent or cure disease. A *curandero (curandera* if female) deals with serious physical and mental illnesses. Witches use magic. A male witch is a called a *brujos.* A female witch is called a *brujas.*

From Giger JN, Davidhizar RE: *Transcultural nursing: assessment and interventions*, ed 3, St Louis, 1999, Mosby.

**Religion** relates to spiritual beliefs, needs, and practices. A person's religion influences health and illness practices. Religions may have beliefs and practices about daily living, behaviors, relationships with others, diet, healing, days of worship, birth and birth control, medicine, and death.

Many people find comfort and strength from religion during illness. They may want to pray and observe religious practices. Hospitals and nursing centers have chapels for prayer and religious services. Some broadcast the services through closed-circuit TV. Assist the person to attend services as needed (Fig. 6-3).

A person may want to see a spiritual leader or advisor. Report this to the nurse. Make sure the room is neat and orderly. Have a chair near the bed. Provide privacy during the visit.

The nursing process reflects the person's culture and religion. The care plan includes the person's cultural and religious practices.

You must respect and accept the person's culture and religion. You will meet people from other cultures and religions. Learn about their beliefs and practices. This helps you understand the person and give better care.

*A person may not follow all beliefs and practices of his or her culture or religion. Some people do not practice a religion. Each person is unique. Do not judge the person by your standards.*

*See Focus on Home Care: Culture and Religion.*

### FOCUS ON HOME CARE
#### CULTURE AND RELIGION

Culture is reflected in the home. Homes vary in size, cleanliness, and furnishings. Some are expensive. Others reflect poverty. Whether rich or poor, treat each person and family with respect, kindness, and dignity. Do not judge the person's life-style, habits, religion, or culture.

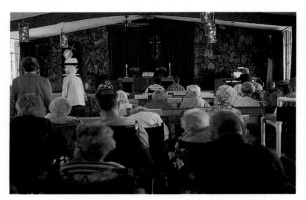

**FIG. 6-3** Residents attend a religious service in the nursing center.

## BEING SICK

People do not choose sickness or injury. However, they do occur. They have physical, psychological, and social effects. Some result in disabilities. A **disability** is a lost, absent, or impaired physical or mental function. It may be temporary or permanent.

Normal activities—work, going to school, fixing meals, driving, yard work, sports, or hobbies—may be hard or impossible. Daily activities bring pleasure, worth, and contact with others. People often feel angry, upset, and useless when unable to perform them. These feelings may increase if others must help with routine functions.

Sick people fear death, disability, chronic illness, and loss of function. Some explain why they are afraid. Others do not share feelings. They fear being laughed at for being afraid. A person with a broken leg may fear having a limp or not walking again. Persons having surgery often fear cancer. These feelings are normal and expected. You need to understand the effects of illness. How would you feel and react if you had the person's illness and problems?

Sick people are expected to behave in a certain way. They need to see a doctor, rest, and have others provide care and comfort. Sometimes recovery is delayed or does not occur. Then the psychological and social effects of illness become greater.

Culture and religion affect how people think and behave when ill. *See Caring About Culture: Sick Care Practices*, p. 85.

## PERSONS YOU WILL CARE FOR

People are grouped in health care agencies by their problems, needs, and age. Doctors and nurses have special knowledge and skills to care for these groups.

- *Mothers and newborns.* **Obstetrics** is the branch of medicine concerned with the care of women during pregnancy, labor, and childbirth and for the 6 to 8 weeks after birth. They are seen in clinics or doctors' offices during pregnancy. When labor begins, mothers usually go to a hospital's obstetric (maternity) department. Pregnancy, labor, and childbirth are normal and natural events. However, problems can occur during pregnancy and the 6 to 8 weeks after childbirth.
- *Children.* **Pediatrics** is the branch of medicine concerned with the growth, development, and care of children. They range in age from the newborn to teenagers. Pediatric units are designed and equipped to meet the needs of children and parents. The nursing staff meets the child's physical, safety, and emotional needs (Fig. 6-4).

- *Adults with medical problems.* Medical problems are illnesses, diseases, or injuries that do not need surgery. There are acute, chronic, and terminal illnesses. Examples are infections, strokes, and heart attacks.
- *Persons having surgery.* Surgical patients need care before and after surgery. Surgeries range from simple to very complex. Removal of the appendix (appendectomy) is a simple surgery. Open-heart and brain surgeries are complex. Before surgery, the person is prepared for the surgery and for what happens after surgery. The person's fears and concerns are dealt with. Needs after surgery relate to relieving pain, preventing complications, and adjusting to body changes.
- *Persons with mental health problems.* **Psychiatry** is the branch of medicine concerned with mental health problems. Problems vary from mild to severe mental and emotional disorders (Chapter 34). Some persons need help making decisions or coping with life stresses. Others are severely disturbed. They cannot do simple things—eat, bathe, or get dressed. Some persons are dangerous to themselves or others. They need special care and treatment.
- *Persons in special care units.* Some people are seriously ill or injured. Special care units are designed and equipped to treat and prevent life-threatening problems. They include intensive care units, coronary care units, kidney dialysis units, burn units, and emergency rooms (Fig. 6-5).
- *Persons needing subacute care or rehabilitation.* Some persons need more time to recover than hospital care allows. Others need rehabilitation (Chapter 31). They need to regain functions lost from surgery, illness, or accidents. Persons with birth defects learn skills using existing abilities.
- *Older persons.* **Geriatrics** is the branch of medicine concerned with the problems and diseases of old age and older persons. Aging is a normal process (Chapter 9). It is not an illness or disease. Many older people enjoy good health. Others have acute or chronic illnesses. Some have diseases common in older persons. Body changes normally occur with aging. Social and psychological changes also occur. *See Focus on Long-Term Care: Persons You Will Care For.*

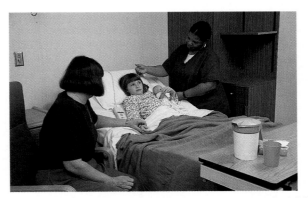

**FIG. 6-4** The nursing assistant gives care to a sick child.

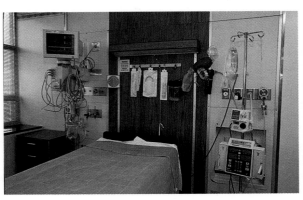

**FIG. 6-5** A room in an intensive care unit.

> ### FOCUS ON LONG-TERM CARE
> PERSONS YOU WILL CARE FOR
>
> Some older persons need long-term care. Their problems and needed care vary:
> - *Alert and oriented persons.* They know who and where they are. They have physical problems. The amount and care required depend on the disability.
> - *Confused and disoriented persons.* These persons are mildly to severely confused and disoriented. Some have Alzheimer's disease or other dementias (Chapter 35).
> - *Persons needing complete care.* They are severely disabled, confused, or disoriented. They cannot meet their own needs. Nor can they say what they need or want.
> - *Short-term residents.* These persons need to recover from fractures, acute illness, or surgery. They usually return home after subacute care or rehabilitation.
> - *Lifelong residents.* Some disabilities occur before age 22 years (Chapter 36). They are caused by birth defects and childhood diseases and injuries. Impairments may be physical, intellectual, or both. The person needs lifelong assistance, support, and special services.
> - *Mentally ill persons.* Mental illness affects behavior and function. In severe cases, self-care and independent living are impaired.
> - *Terminally ill persons.* The person with a terminal illness is dying. The goal is a peaceful, dignified death.

### BOX 6-1  THE PATIENT CARE PARTNERSHIP: UNDERSTANDING EXPECTATIONS, RIGHTS, AND RESPONSIBILITIES

When you need hospital care, your doctor and the nurses and other professionals at our hospital are committed to working with you and your family to meet your health care needs. Our dedicated doctors and staff serve the community in all its ethnic, religious, and economic diversity. Our goal is for you and your family to have the same care and attention we would want for our families and ourselves.

The sections below explain some of the basics about how you can expect to be treated during your hospital stay. They also cover what we will need from you to care for you better. If you have questions at any time, please ask them. Unasked or unanswered questions can add to the stress of being in the hospital. Your comfort and confidence in your care are very important to us.

#### WHAT TO EXPECT DURING YOUR HOSPITAL STAY

- **High quality hospital care.** Our first priority is to provide you the care you need, when you need it, with skill, compassion, and respect. Tell your caregivers if you have concerns about your care or if you have pain. You have the right to know the identity of doctors, nurses and others involved in your care, and you have the right to know when they are students, residents or other trainees.
- **A clean and safe environment.** Our hospital works hard to keep you safe. We use special policies and procedures to avoid mistakes in your care and keep you free from abuse or neglect. If anything unexpected and significant happens during your hospital stay, you will be told what happened, and any resulting changes in your care will be discussed with you.
- **Involvement in your care.** You and your doctor often make decisions about your care before you go to the hospital. Other times, especially in emergencies, those decisions are made during your hospital stay. When decision-making takes place, it should include:
  - *Discussing your medical condition and information about medically appropriate treatment choices.* To make informed decisions with your doctor, you need to understand:
    —The benefits and risks of each treatment.
    —Whether your treatment is experimental or part of a research study.
    —What you can reasonably expect from your treatment and any long-term effects it might have on your quality of life.
    —What you and your family will need to do after you leave the hospital.
    —The financial consequences of using uncovered services or out of network providers.
    Please tell your caregivers if you need more information about treatment choices.
  - *Discussing your treatment plan.* When you enter the hospital, you sign a general consent to treatment. In some cases, such as surgery or experimental treatment, you may be asked to confirm in writing that you understand what is planned and agree to it. This process protects your right to consent to or refuse a treatment. Your doctor will explain the medical consequences of refusing recommended treatment. It also protects your right to decide if you want to participate in a research study.
  - *Getting information from you.* Your caregivers need complete and correct information about your health and coverage so that they can make good decisions about your care. That includes:
    —Past illnesses, surgeries, or hospital stays.
    —Past allergic reactions.
    —Any medicines or dietary supplements (such as vitamins and herbs) that you are taking.
    —Any network or admission requirements under your health plan.
  - *Understanding your health care goals and values.* You may have health care goals and values or spiritual beliefs that are important to your well-being. They will be taken into account as much as possible throughout your hospital stay. Make sure your doctor, your family, and your care team know your wishes.
  - *Understanding who should make decisions when you cannot.* If you have signed a health care power of attorney stating who should speak for you if you become unable to make health care decisions for yourself, or a "living will" or "advance directive" that states your wishes about end-of-life care, give copies to your doctor, your family, and your care team. If you or your family need help making difficult decisions, counselors, chaplains and others are available to help.
- **Protection of your privacy.** We respect the confidentiality of your relationship with your doctor and other caregivers and the sensitive information about your health and health care that are part of that relationship. State and federal laws and hospital operating policies protect the privacy of your medical information. You will receive a Notice of Privacy Practices that describes the ways that we use, disclose, and safeguard patient information and that explains how you can obtain a copy of information from our records about your care.
- **Preparing you and your family for when you leave the hospital.** Your doctor works with hospital staff and professionals in your community. You and your family also play an important role in your care. The success of your treatment often depends on your efforts to follow medication, diet and therapy plans. Your family may need to help care for you at home.

  You can expect us to help you identify sources of follow-up care and let you know if our hospital has a financial interest in any referrals. As long as you agree we can share information about your care with them, we will coordinate our activities with your caregivers outside the hospital. You can also expect to receive information and, where possible, training about the self-care you will need when you go home.
- **Help with your bill and filing insurance claims.** Our staff will file claims for you with health care insurers or other programs such as Medicare and Medicaid. They also will help your doctor with needed documentation. Hospital bills and insurance coverage are often confusing. If you have questions about your bill, contact our business office. If you need help understanding your insurance coverage or health plan, start with your insurance company or health benefits manager. If you do not have health coverage, we will try to help you and your family find financial help or make other arrangements. We need your help with collecting needed information and other requirements to obtain coverage or assistance.

While you are here, you will receive more detailed notices about some of the rights you have as a hospital patient and how to exercise them. We are always interested in improving. If you have questions, comments, or concerns, please contact _____.

Courtesy American Hospital Association. Copyright 2003.

## THE PERSON'S RIGHTS

People want information about their health problems and treatment. They also want better care at lower costs. They want to be involved in treatment decisions. They are not willing to accept the doctor's advice without question.

In April, 2003, The American Hospital Association (AHA) adopted *The Patient Care Partnership: Understanding Expectations, Rights, and Responsibilities* (Box 6-1). The document explains the person's rights and expectations during hospital stays. The relationship between the doctor, the health team, and the patient is stressed. *See Focus on Long-Term Care: The Person's Rights.*

## COMMUNICATING WITH THE PERSON

For effective communication between you and the person, you must:
- Follow the rules of communication (Chapter 4):
  —Use words that have the same meaning for you and the person.
  —Avoid medical terms and words unfamiliar to the person.
  —Communicate in a logical and orderly manner. Do not wander in thought.
  —Give facts and be specific.
  —Be brief and concise.
- Understand and respect the patient or resident as a person.
- View the person as a physical, psychological, social, and spiritual human being.
- Appreciate the person's problems and frustrations.
- Respect the person's rights.
- Respect the person's religion and culture.
- Give the person time to process (understand) information.

**FOCUS ON LONG-TERM CARE**
### THE PERSON'S RIGHTS

Residents have rights as United States citizens. They also have rights under OBRA (Chapter 9). They relate to everyday life and care in nursing centers. Centers must protect and promote residents' rights. Residents must be free to exercise their rights without interference. Some residents are incompetent (not able). They cannot exercise their rights. Legal representatives do so for them.

Residents are informed of their rights orally and in writing. This occurs before or during admission to the center. It is given in the language the person uses and understands.

- Repeat information as often as needed. Repeat exactly what you said. Do not give the person a new message to process.
- Ask questions to see if the person understood you.
- Be patient. People with memory problems may ask the same question many times. Do not say that you are repeating information. Accept the memory loss as a disability.

You send messages by what you say and do. You use verbal and nonverbal communication. You must use both methods well.

## VERBAL COMMUNICATION

Words are used in **verbal communication.** Words are spoken or written. You find out how the person is feeling and share information. Most verbal communication involves the spoken word. Follow these rules:
- Face the person.
- Control the loudness and tone of your voice.
- Speak clearly, slowly, and distinctly.
- Do not use slang or vulgar words.
- Repeat information as needed.
- Ask one question at a time. Wait for the answer.
- Do not shout, whisper, or mumble.
- Be kind, courteous, and friendly.

The written word is used when a person cannot speak or hear. The nurse and care plan tell you how to communicate with the person. The devices shown in Figure 6-6, p. 90 are often used. The person also may have poor vision. When writing messages:
- Keep them brief and concise.
- Use a black felt pen on white paper.
- Print in large letters.

Some persons can hear but cannot speak or read. Ask questions that have "yes" or "no" answers. The person can nod, blink, or use other gestures for "yes" and "no." Follow the care plan. A picture board may be helpful (Fig. 6-7, p. 90).

Persons who are deaf may use sign language (Chapter 32).

## NONVERBAL COMMUNICATION

**Nonverbal communication** does not use words. Messages are sent with gestures, facial expressions, posture, body movements, touch, and smell. Nonverbal messages more accurately reflect a person's feelings than words do. They are usually involuntary and hard to control. A person may say one thing but act another way. Watch the person's eyes, hand movements, gestures, posture, and other actions. Sometimes they can tell you more than words.

**TOUCH.** Touch is a very important form of nonverbal communication. It conveys comfort, caring, love, affection, interest, trust, concern, and reassurance. Touch means different things to different people. The

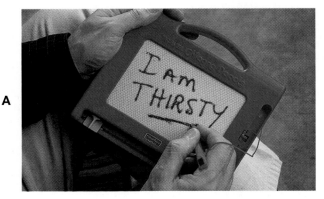

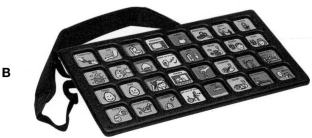

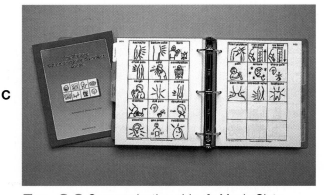

**FIG. 6-6** Communication aids. **A,** Magic Slate. **B,** Electronic talking aid. **C,** Communication binder. (**B,** Courtesy Mayer-Johnson Co., Solana Beach, Calif.)

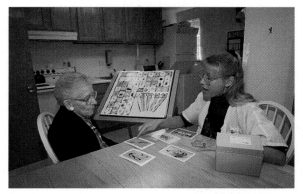

**FIG. 6-7** A person uses a picture board and picture cards to communicate.

meaning depends on age, gender (male or female), experiences, and culture.

Cultural groups have rules or practices about touch. They relate to who can touch, when it can occur, and where to touch the body. *See Caring About Culture: Touch Practices.*

Some people do not like to be touched. However, touch can show caring and warmth. Stroking or holding a hand can comfort a person. Touch should be gentle. It should not be hurried, rough, or sexual. To use touch, follow the person's care plan.

*See Focus on Children: Touch.*

**BODY LANGUAGE.** People send messages through their **body language:**

- Facial expressions *See Caring About Culture: Facial Expressions in Americans. Also see Caring About Culture: Facial Expressions in Other Cultures.*
- Gestures
- Posture
- Hand and body movements
- Gait
- Eye contact
- Appearance (dress, hygiene, jewelry, perfume, cosmetics, tattoos, and so on)

## CARING ABOUT CULTURE
### TOUCH PRACTICES

Touch practices vary among cultural groups. Touch is used often in *Mexico*. Some people believe that using touch while complimenting a person is important. It is thought to neutralize the power of the evil eye *(mal de ojo)*. Touch also is important in the *Philippine* culture.

Persons from the *United Kingdom* tend not to use touch. Touch is socially acceptable in *Poland*.

In *India*, men shake hands with other men. Men do not shake hands with women. Similar practices occur in *Vietnam*.

People from *China* do not like being touched by strangers. A nod or slight bow is given during introductions.

From D'Avanzo CE, Geissler EM: *Pocket guide to cultural health assessment*, ed 3, St Louis, 2003, Mosby.

## FOCUS ON CHILDREN
### TOUCH

Infants and young children respond to touch. It soothes and comforts them. They like to be held, stroked, rocked, and patted. They also like cuddling.

Older children and teenagers like to give and receive hugs. Contact must be professional, casual, and with consent. It should not be sexual or involve sexual areas.

Slumped posture may mean the person is not happy or feeling well. A person may deny pain. However, he or she protects the affected body part by standing, lying, or sitting in a certain way. Many messages are sent through body language.

Your actions, movements, and facial expressions send messages. So does how you stand, sit, walk, and look at a person. Your body language should show interest and enthusiasm. It should show caring and respect for the person. Often you will need to control your body language. Control reactions to odors from fluids, excretions, or the person's body. Many odors are beyond the person's control. Embarrassment and humiliation increase if you react to odors.

## CARING ABOUT CULTURE
### FACIAL EXPRESSIONS IN AMERICANS
- Coldness—there is a constant stare. Face muscles do not move.
- Fear—eyes are wide open. Eyebrows are raised. The mouth is tense with the lips drawn back.
- Anger—eyes are fixed in a hard stare. Upper lids are lowered. Eyebrows are drawn down. Lips are tightly compressed.
- Tiredness—eyes are rolled upward.
- Disapproval—eyes are rolled upward.
- Disgust—narrowed eyes. The upper lip is curled. There are nose movements.
- Embarrassment—eyes are turned away or down. The face is flushed. The person pretends to smile. He or she rubs the eyes, nose, or face. He or she twitches hair, beard, or mustache.
- Surprise—direct gaze with raised eyebrows.

From Giger JN, Davidhizar RE: *Transcultural nursing: assessment and intervention,* ed 3, St Louis, 1999, Mosby.

## CARING ABOUT CULTURE
### FACIAL EXPRESSIONS IN OTHER CULTURES
*Italian, Jewish, African-American,* and *Spanish-speaking persons* smile readily. They use many facial expressions and gestures for happiness, pain, or displeasure. Irish, English, and Northern European persons tend to have less facial expression.

In some cultures, facial expressions mean the opposite of what the person is feeling. For example, Asians may conceal negative emotions with a smile.

From Giger JN, Davidhizar RE: *Transcultural nursing: assessment and intervention,* ed 3, St Louis, 1999, Mosby.

## COMMUNICATION METHODS
Certain methods help you communicate with others. They result in better relationships. More information is gained for the nursing process.

**LISTENING.** Listening means to focus on verbal and nonverbal communication. You use sight, hearing, touch, and smell. You focus on what the person is saying. You observe nonverbal clues. They can support what the person says. Or they can show other feelings. For example, Mr. Kerr says, "I want to go to a nursing home. That way my daughter won't have to care for me." You see tears, and he looks away from you. His verbal says *happy.* His nonverbal shows *sadness.*

Listening requires that you care and have interest. Follow these guidelines:
- Face the person.
- Have good eye contact with the person. *See Caring About Culture: Eye Contact Practices.*
- Lean toward the person (Fig. 6-8, p. 92). Do not sit back with your arms crossed.
- Respond to the person. Nod your head. Say "uh huh," "mmm," and "I see." Repeat what the person says. Ask questions.
- Avoid the communication barriers (p. 92).

## CARING ABOUT CULTURE
### EYE CONTACT PRACTICES
In the *American* culture, eye contact signals a good self-concept. It also shows openness, interest in others, attention, honesty, and warmth. Lack of eye contact can mean:
- Shyness
- Lack of interest
- Humility
- Guilt
- Embarrassment
- Low self-esteem
- Rudeness
- Dishonesty

For some *Asian* and *Native American* cultures, eye contact is impolite. It is an invasion of privacy. In certain *Indian* cultures, eye contact is avoided with persons of higher or lower socioeconomic class. It is also given a special sexual meaning.

Direct eye contact is practiced in *Poland* and *Russia.* However, direct eye contact is rude in *Mexican* and *Vietnamese* cultures. In the *United Kingdom,* staring is a part of good listening.

Blinking has meaning. In *Vietnam,* it means that a message is received. It shows understanding in the *United Kingdom.*

From Giger JN, Davidhizar RE: *Transcultural nursing: assessment and intervention,* ed 3, St Louis, 1999, Mosby; D'Avanzo CE, Geissler EM: *Pocket guide to cultural health assessment,* ed 3, St Louis, 2003, Mosby.

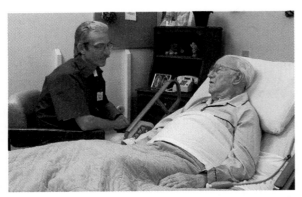

FIG. 6-8 Listen by facing the person. Have good eye contact. Lean toward the person.

**CARING ABOUT CULTURE**
THE MEANING OF SILENCE

In the *English* and *Arabic* cultures, silence is used for privacy. Among *Russian, French,* and *Spanish* cultures, silence means agreement between parties. In some *Asian* cultures, silence is a sign of respect, particularly to an older person.

From Giger JN, Davidhizar RE: *Transcultural nursing: assessment and interventions,* ed 3, St Louis, 1999, Mosby.

**PARAPHRASING.** **Paraphrasing** is restating the person's message in your own words. You use fewer words than the person did. Paraphrasing:
- Shows you are listening
- Lets the person see if you understand the message sent
- Promotes further communication

The person usually responds to your statement. For example:

*Mr. Kerr:* My wife was crying after talking to the doctor. I don't know what they talked about.

*You:* You don't know why your wife was crying.

*Mr. Kerr:* He must have told her that I have a tumor.

**DIRECT QUESTIONS.** Direct questions focus on certain information. You ask the person something you need to know. Some direct questions have "yes" or "no" answers. Others require that the person give more information. For example:

*You:* Mr. Kerr, do you want to shave this morning?

*Mr. Kerr:* Yes.

*You:* Mr. Kerr, when would you like to do that?

*Mr. Kerr:* Could we start in 15 minutes? I want to call my son first.

*You:* Yes, we can start in 15 minutes. Did you have a bowel movement today?

*Mr. Kerr:* No.

*You:* You said you didn't eat well this morning. Can you tell me what you ate?

*Mr. Kerr:* I had toast and coffee. I just don't feel like eating.

**OPEN-ENDED QUESTIONS.** Open-ended questions lead or invite the person to share thoughts, feelings, or ideas. The person chooses what to talk about. He or she controls the topic and the information given. Answers require more than a "yes" or "no." For example:
- "What do you like about living with your daughter?"
- "Tell me about your grandson."
- "What was your wife like?"
- "What do you like about being retired?"

The person chooses how to answer. Responses to open-ended questions are longer. They give more information than do responses to direct questions.

**CLARIFYING.** Clarifying lets you make sure that you understand the message. You can ask the person to repeat the message, say you do not understand, or restate the message. For example:
- "Could you say that again?"
- "I'm sorry, Mr. Kerr. I don't understand what you mean."
- "Are you saying that you want to go home?"

**FOCUSING.** Focusing is dealing with a certain topic. It is useful when a person rambles or wanders in thought. For example, Mr. Kerr talks at length about food and places to eat. You need to know why he did not eat much breakfast. To focus on breakfast you say: "Let's talk about breakfast. You said you don't feel like eating."

**SILENCE.** Silence is a very powerful way to communicate. Sometimes you do not need to say anything. This is true during sad times. Just being there shows you care. At other times, silence gives time to think, organize thoughts, or choose words. Silence is useful when making decisions. It also helps when the person is upset and needs to regain control. Silence on your part shows caring and respect for the person's situation and feelings.

Sometimes pauses or long silences are uncomfortable. You do not need to talk when the person is silent. The person may need silence. Dealing with silence gets easier as you gain experience in your role. *See Caring About Culture: The Meaning of Silence.*

## COMMUNICATION BARRIERS

Communication barriers prevent sending and receiving messages. Communication fails. You must avoid these barriers:
- *Using unfamiliar language.* You and the person must use and understand the same language. If not, messages are not accurately interpreted. See Appendix C, p. 833, for useful Spanish words and phrases.

- *Cultural differences.* The person may attach different meanings to verbal and nonverbal communication. *See Caring About Culture: Communicating With Persons From Other Cultures.*
- *Changing the subject.* Someone changes the subject when the topic is uncomfortable. Avoid changing the subject whenever possible.
- *Giving your opinion.* Opinions involve judging values, behavior, or feelings. Let others express feelings and concerns without adding your opinion. Do not make judgments or jump to conclusions.
- *Talking a lot when others are silent.* Talking too much is usually because of nervousness and discomfort with silence. Silences have meaning. They show acceptance, rejection, and fear. They also show the need for quiet and time to think.
- *Failure to listen.* Do not pretend to listen. It shows lack of interest and caring. This causes poor responses. You can miss complaints of pain, discomfort, or other symptoms that you must report to the nurse.
- *Pat answers.* "Don't worry." "Everything will be okay." "Your doctor knows best." These make the person feel that you do not care about his or her concerns, feelings, and fears.

- *Illness and disability.* Some illnesses, injuries, and birth defects affect speech, hearing, vision, cognitive function, and body movements. Verbal and nonverbal communication are affected. See Box 6-2 for disability etiquette.

## THE PERSON WHO IS COMATOSE

The person who is comatose is unconscious. The person cannot respond to others. Often the person can hear and can feel touch and pain. Assume that the person hears and understands you. Use touch and give care gently. Practice these measures:

- Knock before entering the person's room.
- Tell the person your name, the time, and the place every time you enter the room.
- Give care on the same schedule every day.
- Explain what you are going to do. Explain care measures step by step as you do them.
- Tell the person when you are finishing care.
- Use touch to communicate care, concern, and comfort (p. 89).
- Tell the person what time you will be back to check on him or her.
- Tell the person when you are leaving the room.

### CARING ABOUT CULTURE

#### COMMUNICATING WITH PERSONS FROM OTHER CULTURES

- Ask the nurse about the beliefs and values of the person's culture. Learn as much as you can about the person's culture.
- Do not judge the person by your own attitudes, values, beliefs, and ideas.
- Follow the person's care plan. It includes the person's cultural beliefs and customs.
- Do the following when communicating with foreign speaking persons:
  —Convey comfort by your tone of voice and body language.
  —Do not speak loudly or shout. It will not help the person understand English.
  —Speak slowly and distinctly.
  —Keep messages short and simple.
  —Be alert for words the person seems to understand.
  —Use gestures and pictures.
  —Repeat the message in other ways.
  —Avoid using medical terms and abbreviations.
  —Be alert for signs that the person is pretending to understand. Nodding and answering "yes" to all questions are signs that the person does not understand what you are saying.

Modified from Geissler EM: *Pocket guide to cultural assessment,* ed 2, St Louis, 1998, Mosby.

### BOX 6-2  DISABILITY ETIQUETTE

- Extend the same courtesies to the person as you would to anyone else.
- Allow the person privacy.
- Do not hang or lean on a person's wheelchair.
- Treat adults as adults. Do not use the person's first name unless he or she asks you to do so.
- Do not pat an adult in a wheelchair on the head.
- Speak directly to the person. Do not address questions intended for the person to his or her companion.
- Do not be embarrassed if you use words that relate to the disability. For example, you say "Did you see that?" to a person with a vision problem.
- Sit or squat to talk to a person in a wheelchair. This puts you and the person at eye level.
- Ask the person if he or she needs help before acting. If the person says "no," respect the person's wishes. If the person wants help, ask the person what to do and how to do it.
- Think before giving directions to a person in a wheelchair. Think about distance, weather conditions, stairs, curbs, steep hills, and other obstacles.
- Allow the person extra time to say or do things. Let the person set the pace in walking, talking, or other activities.

Modified from *Disability Etiquette,* Easter Seals, 2003.

# THE FAMILY AND VISITORS

Family and friends help meet safety and security, love and belonging, and self-esteem needs. They offer support and comfort. They lessen loneliness. Some also help with the person's care. *See Caring About Culture: Family Roles in Sick Care.* The presence or absence of family or friends can affect recovery and quality of life.

The person has the right to visit with family and friends in private and without unnecessary interruptions (Fig. 6-9). You may need to give care when visitors are there. Do not expose the person's body in front of them. Politely ask them to leave the room. Show them where to wait. Promptly tell them when they can return.

Treat family and visitors with courtesy and respect. They have concerns about the person's condition and care. They need support and understanding. However, do not discuss the person's condition with them. Refer their questions to the nurse.

Visiting rules depend on agency policy and the person's age and condition. Parents can visit children as often and as long as they want. Only short visits are allowed in special care units. Dying persons usually can have family present all the time. Know your agency's policies and each person's needs.

Visitors may have questions about the chapel, gift shop, business office, lounge, or dining room. Know the location, special rules, and hours of these areas.

A visitor may upset or tire a person. Report your observations to the nurse. The nurse will speak with the visitor about the person's needs. *See Focus on Older Persons: Family and Visitors. See Focus on Home Care: Families and Visitors.*

---

### CARING ABOUT CULTURE
#### FAMILY ROLES IN SICK CARE

In *Vietnam,* all family members are involved in the person's care. A similar practice is common in *China.* Family members bathe, feed, and comfort the person. However, women in *Mexico* cannot give care at home if it involves touching the genitals of adult men.

From D'Avanzo CE, Geissler EM: *Pocket guide to cultural health assessment,* ed 3, St Louis, 2003, Mosby.

---

### FOCUS ON OLDER PERSONS
#### FAMILY AND VISITORS

Sometimes older brothers, sisters, and cousins live together. They provide companionship and share living expenses. They care for each other during illness or disability.

Some older people live with their children. The older parent may be healthy, need some supervision, or be ill or disabled. The older parent moves in with the child. Or the child moves into the parent's home. Living with a child can help the older person feel safe and secure. Often the adult child gives care to an ill or disabled parent.

Adult children often need to work even though the parent cannot be left alone. Adult day care centers provide meals, supervision, and supervised activities for older persons. Cards, board games, movies, crafts, dancing, walks, and lectures are common. Some provide bowling and swimming. Help is given as needed. Some provide transportation from home to the center.

Living with an adult child is a social change. The parent, child, and the child's family need to adjust. The child's family needs time alone. Other family members may help give care. Respite care provides a break for the family. The parent enters a nursing center for a few days or weeks. Caregivers can rest, go on vacation, or take a break from care-giving stresses. Church and community groups may have volunteers who help give care.

---

### FOCUS ON HOME CARE
#### FAMILY AND VISITORS

Family personalities and attitudes affect the mood in the home. Many families are happy and supportive. Others have poor relationships. Mental or physical illness, drug or alcohol abuse, unemployment, and delinquency may affect the family. Some families have problems coping with or accepting the person's illness or disability.

Your supervisor explains family problems to you. Do not get involved. Be professional and have empathy. Do not give advice, take sides, or make judgments about family conflicts.

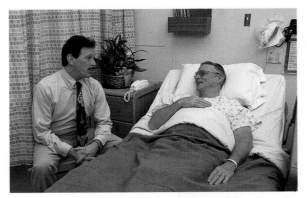

**FIG. 6-9** This man has a private visit with his son.

## BEHAVIOR ISSUES

Some patients, residents, and families have a hard time with illness, injury, or disability. They may have some of the following behaviors. These behaviors are new for some people. For others, they are lifelong. They are part of one's personality.

- *Anger.* Anger is a common emotion. Causes include fear, pain, and dying and death. Loss of function and loss of control over health and life are causes. So are long waits for care or to see the doctor. Anger is a symptom of diseases that affect thinking and behavior. Some people are generally angry. Few things please or make them happy. Anger is shown verbally and nonverbally. Verbal outbursts, shouting, raised voices, and rapid speech are common. Some people are silent. Others are uncooperative. They may refuse to answer questions. Nonverbal signs include rapid movements, pacing, clenched fists, and a red face. Glaring and getting close to you when speaking are other signs. Violent behaviors can occur.
- *Demanding behavior.* Nothing seems to please the person. The person is critical of others. He or she wants care given at a certain time and in a certain way. Causes include loss of independence, loss of health, loss of control of life, and unmet needs.
- *Self-centered behavior.* The person cares only about his or her own needs. The needs of others are ignored. The person demands the time and attention of others.
- *Aggressive behavior.* The person may swear, bite, hit, pinch, scratch, or kick. Fear, anger, pain, and dementia (Chapter 35) are causes. Protect the person, others, and yourself from harm (Chapter 10).
- *Withdrawal.* The person has little or no contact with others. He or she spends time alone and does not take part in social or group events. This may signal physical illness or depression.
- *Inappropriate sexual behavior.* Some people make inappropriate sexual remarks. Or they touch others. Some disrobe or masturbate in public. These behaviors may be on purpose. Or they are caused by disease, confusion, dementia, or drug side effects.

A person's behavior may be unpleasant. You cannot avoid the person or lose control. Good communication is needed. Follow the guidelines in Box 6-3.

---

**BOX 6-3  DEALING WITH BEHAVIOR ISSUES**

- Recognize frustrating and frightening situations. Put yourself in the person's situation. How would you feel? How would you want to be treated?
- Treat the person with dignity and respect.
- Answer questions clearly and thoroughly. Ask the nurse to answer questions you cannot answer.
- Keep the person informed. Tell the person what you are going to do and when.
- Do not keep the person waiting. Answer signal lights promptly. If you tell the person that you will do something for him or her, do it promptly.
- Explain the reason for long waits. Ask if you can get or do something to increase the person's comfort.
- Stay calm and professional if the person is angry or hostile. Often the person is not angry at you. He or she is angry at another person or situation.
- Do not argue with the person.
- Listen and use silence. The person may feel better if able to express feelings.
- Protect yourself from violent behaviors (Chapter 10).
- Report the person's behavior to the nurse. Discuss how you should deal with the person.

# ■ REVIEW QUESTIONS ■

Circle the **BEST** answer.

**1** Sally Jones had surgery. You focus on her
    **a** Care plan
    **b** Physical, safety and security, and self-esteem needs
    **c** As a physical, psychological, social, and spiritual person
    **d** Cultural and religious needs

**2** Which basic need is the most essential?
    **a** Self-actualization
    **b** Self-esteem
    **c** Love and belonging
    **d** Safety and security

**3** Using Maslow's theory of basic needs, which person's needs must be met first?
    **a** Mr. Kerr, who wants another blanket
    **b** Ms. Parks, who wants her mail opened
    **c** Ms. Street, who asks for more water
    **d** Mr. Hill, who is crying

**4** Sally Jones says "What are they doing to me?" What basic needs are not being met?
    **a** Physical needs
    **b** Safety and security needs
    **c** Love and belonging needs
    **d** Self-esteem needs

**5** Mr. Kerr has a garden behind the nursing center's garage. This relates to
    **a** Self-actualization
    **b** Self-esteem
    **c** Love and belonging
    **d** Safety and security

**6** Which is *false*?
    **a** Culture influences health and illness practices.
    **b** Culture and religion influence food practices.
    **c** Religious and cultural practices are allowed in health care agencies.
    **d** A person must follow all beliefs and practices of his or her religion or culture.

**7** Which is *true*?
    **a** Psychiatry is concerned with mental health problems.
    **b** Pediatrics focuses only on sick children.
    **c** Geriatric persons suffer from the disease of aging.
    **d** Nursing center residents need complete care.

**8** Sally Jones has the right to the following *except*
    **a** Compassionate and respectful care
    **b** Information about her treatment
    **c** Refuse treatment
    **d** Free care

**9** Which is *false*?
    **a** Verbal communication uses the written or spoken word.
    **b** Verbal communication is the truest reflection of a person's feelings.
    **c** Messages are sent by facial expressions, gestures, posture, and body movements.
    **d** Touch means different things to different people.

**10** To communicate with Sam Long, you should
    **a** Use medical words and phrases
    **b** Change the subject often
    **c** Give your opinions
    **d** Be quiet when he is silent

**11** Which might mean that you are *not* listening?
    **a** You sit facing the person.
    **b** You have good eye contact with the person.
    **c** You sit with your arms crossed.
    **d** You ask questions.

**12** Which is a direct question?
    **a** "Do you feel better now?"
    **b** "What are your plans for home."
    **c** "What will you do when you get home?"
    **d** "You said that you can't work."

**13** Sally Jones wants to take a shower. You say "You would like a shower." This is
    **a** Focusing
    **b** Clarifying
    **c** Paraphrasing
    **d** An open-ended question

**14** Focusing is useful when
    **a** A person is rambling
    **b** You want to make sure you understand the message
    **c** You want the person to share thoughts and feelings
    **d** You need certain information

# ■ REVIEW QUESTIONS ■

**15** Which promotes communication?
   a "Don't worry."
   b "Everything will be just fine."
   c "This is a good hospital."
   d "Why are you crying?"

**16** Miss Smith uses a wheelchair. To communicate with her, you should
   a Lean on her wheelchair
   b Pat her on the head
   c Speak to her companion
   d Sit or squat next to her

**17** Ms. Parker is comatose. Which action is *false*?
   a Assume that she can hear and can feel touch.
   b Explain what you are going to do.
   c Use listening and silence to communicate.
   d Tell her when you are leaving the room.

**18** A person is angry. Which is *true*?
   a The person has a disease that affects thinking and behavior.
   b Drug or alcohol abuse is likely.
   c You can tell the person to calm down.
   d Listening and silence are important.

**19** Sally Jones has many visitors. Which is *false*?
   a They can help meet her basic needs.
   b Privacy should be allowed.
   c Politely ask them to leave the room when you need to give care.
   d Direct questions about the gift shop and chapel to the nurse.

**20** A visitor seems to tire a person. What should you do?
   a Ask the person to leave
   b Tell the nurse
   c Stay in the room to observe the person and visitor
   d Find out the visitor's relationship to the person

**21** Nothing seems to please Mr. Kerr. He is critical of others. His behavior is described as
   a Angry
   b Demanding
   c Self-centered
   d Aggressive

*Answers to these questions are on p. 816.*

# Body Structure and Function

# OBJECTIVES

- Define the key terms listed in this chapter
- Identify the basic structures of the cell
- Explain how cells divide
- Describe four types of tissue
- Identify the structures of each body system
- Describe the functions of each body system

# KEY TERMS

**artery** A blood vessel that carries blood away from the heart

**capillary** A tiny blood vessel; food, oxygen, and other substances pass from the capillaries to the cells

**cell** The basic unit of body structure

**digestion** The process of physically and chemically breaking down food so that it can be absorbed for use by the cells

**hemoglobin** The substance in red blood cells that carries oxygen and gives blood its color

**hormone** A chemical substance secreted by the glands into the bloodstream

**immunity** Protection against a disease or condition; the person will not get or be affected by the disease

**menstruation** The process in which the lining of the uterus breaks up and is discharged from the body through the vagina

**metabolism** The burning of food for heat and energy by the cells

**organ** Groups of tissues with the same function

**peristalsis** Involuntary muscle contractions in the digestive system that move food through the alimentary canal

**respiration** The process of supplying the cells with oxygen and removing carbon dioxide from them

**system** Organs that work together to perform special functions

**tissue** A group of cells with similar functions

**vein** A blood vessel that carries blood back to the heart

---

You help patients and residents meet basic needs. Their bodies do not work at peak levels because of illness, disease, or injury. Your care promotes comfort, healing, and recovery. You need to know the body's normal structure and function. It will help you understand signs, symptoms, and the reasons for care and procedures. You will give safer and more efficient care.

## CELLS, TISSUES, AND ORGANS

The basic unit of body structure is the **cell.** Cells have the same basic structure. Function, size, and shape may differ. Cells are very small. You will need a microscope to see them. Cells need food, water, and oxygen to live and function.

Figure 7-1, p. 100 shows the cell and its structures. The *cell membrane* is the outer covering. It encloses the cell and helps it hold its shape. The *nucleus* is the control center of the cell. It directs the cell activities. The nucleus is in the center of the cell. The *cytoplasm* surrounds the nucleus. Cytoplasm contains smaller structures that perform cell functions. *Protoplasm* means "living substance." It refers to all structures, substances, and water within the cell. Protoplasm is a semiliquid substance much like an egg white.

*Chromosomes* are threadlike structures in the nucleus. Each cell has 46 chromosomes. Chromosomes contain *genes.* Genes control the traits children inherit from their parents. Height, eye color, and skin color are examples.

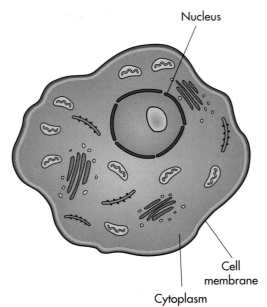

FIG. 7-1 Parts of a cell.

Nucleus

Cell membrane

Cytoplasm

The nucleus controls cell reproduction. Cells reproduce by dividing in half. The process of cell division is called *mitosis.* It is needed for tissue growth and repair. During mitosis, the 46 chromosomes arrange themselves in 23 pairs. As the cell divides, the 23 pairs are pulled in half. The two new cells are identical. Each has 46 chromosomes (Fig. 7-2).

Cells are the body's building blocks. Groups of cells with similar functions combine to form **tissues:**

- *Epithelial tissue* covers internal and external body surfaces. Tissue lining the nose, mouth, respiratory tract, stomach, and intestines is epithelial tissue. So are the skin, hair, nails, and glands.
- *Connective tissue* anchors, connects, and supports other tissues. It is in every part of the body. Bones, tendons, ligaments, and cartilage are connective tissue. Blood is a form of connective tissue.
- *Muscle tissue* stretches and contracts to let the body move (p. 103).
- *Nerve tissue* receives and carries impulses to the brain and back to body parts.

Groups of tissues with the same function form **organs.** An organ has one or more functions. Examples of organs are the heart, brain, liver, lungs, and kidneys. **Systems** are formed by organs that work together to perform special functions (Fig. 7-3).

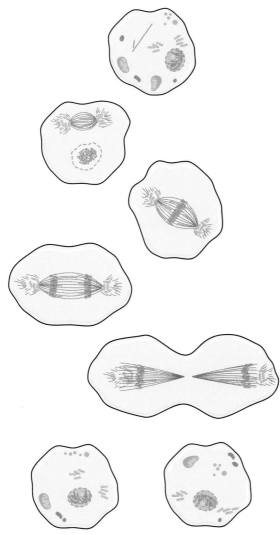

FIG. 7-2 Cell division.

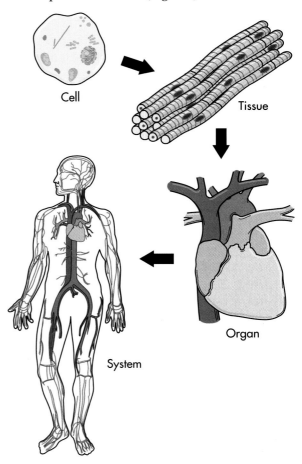

Cell

Tissue

Organ

System

FIG. 7-3 Organization of the body.

# THE INTEGUMENTARY SYSTEM

The *integumentary system,* or skin, is the largest system. *Integument* means covering. The skin covers the body. It has epithelial, connective, and nerve tissue. It also has oil glands and sweat glands. There are two skin layers (Fig. 7-4):

- The *epidermis* is the outer layer. It has living cells and dead cells. The dead cells were once deeper in the epidermis. They were pushed upward as cells divided. Dead cells constantly flake off. They are replaced by living cells. Living cells also die and flake off. Living cells of the epidermis contain *pigment.* Pigment gives skin its color. The epidermis has no blood vessels and few nerve endings.
- The *dermis* is the inner layer. It is made up of connective tissue. Blood vessels, nerves, sweat glands and oil glands, and hair roots are found in the dermis.

*Oil glands* and *sweat glands, hair,* and *nails* are skin appendages. The entire body, except the palms of the hands and soles of the feet, is covered with hair. Hair in the nose and ears and around the eyes protects these organs from dust, insects, and other foreign objects. Nails protect the tips of fingers and toes. Nails help fingers pick up and handle small objects. Sweat glands help the body regulate temperature. Sweat consists of water, salt, and a small amount of wastes. Sweat is secreted through pores in the skin. The body is cooled as sweat evaporates. Oil glands lie near hair shafts. They secrete an oily substance into the space near the hair shaft. Oil travels to the skin surface. This helps keep the hair and skin soft and shiny.

The skin has many functions:

- It is the body's protective covering.
- It prevents bacteria and other substances from entering the body.
- It prevents excess amounts of water from leaving the body.
- It protects organs from injury.
- Nerve endings in the skin sense both pleasant and unpleasant stimulation. Nerve endings are over the entire body. They sense cold, pain, touch, and pressure to protect the body from injury.
- It helps regulate body temperature. Blood vessels dilate (widen) when temperature outside the body is high. More blood is brought to the body surface for cooling during evaporation. When blood vessels constrict (narrow), the body retains heat. This is because less blood reaches the skin.

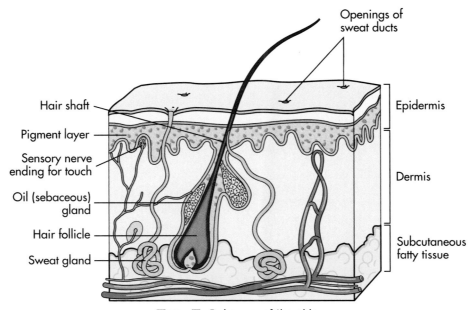

FIG. 7-4 Layers of the skin.

## THE MUSCULOSKELETAL SYSTEM

The musculoskeletal system provides the framework for the body. It lets the body move. This system also protects and gives the body shape.

### BONES

The human body has 206 bones (Fig. 7-5). There are four types of bones:

- *Long bones* bear the body's weight. Leg bones are long bones.
- *Short bones* allow skill and ease in movement. Bones in the wrists, fingers, ankles, and toes are short bones.
- *Flat bones* protect the organs. They include the ribs, skull, pelvic bones, and shoulder blades.
- *Irregular bones* are the vertebrae in the spinal column. They allow various degrees of movement and flexibility.

Bones are hard, rigid structures. They are made up of living cells. They are covered by a membrane called *periosteum.* Periosteum contains blood vessels that supply bone cells with oxygen and food. Inside the hollow centers of the bones is a substance called *bone marrow.* Blood cells are manufactured in the bone marrow.

### JOINTS

A *joint* is the point at which two or more bones meet. Joints allow movement (Chapter 22). *Cartilage* is the connective tissue at the end of long bones. It cushions the joint so that bone ends do not rub together. The *synovial membrane* lines the joints. It secretes *synovial fluid.* Synovial fluid acts as a lubricant so the joint can move smoothly. Bones are held together at the joint by strong bands of connective tissue called *ligaments.*

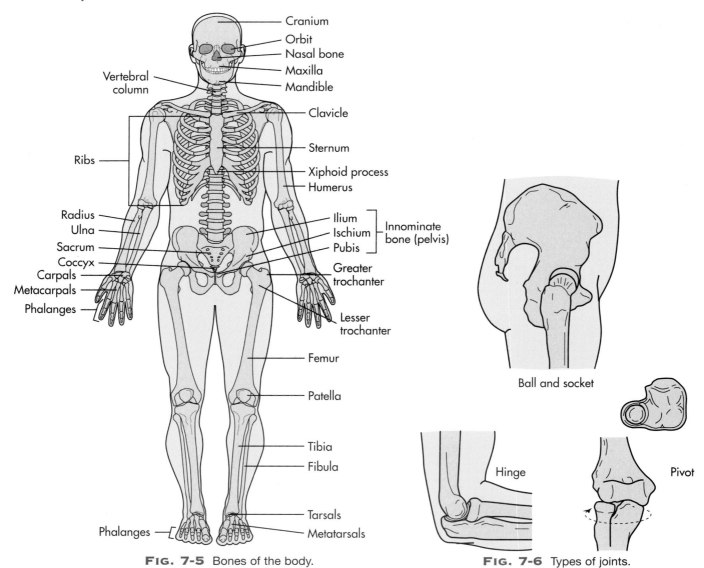

**FIG. 7-5** Bones of the body.

**FIG. 7-6** Types of joints.

There are three types of joints (Fig. 7-6):

- *Ball-and-socket joint* allows movement in all directions. It is made up of the rounded end of one bone and the hollow end of another bone. The rounded end of one fits into the hollow end of the other. The joints of the hips and shoulders are ball-and-socket joints.
- *Hinge joint* allows movement in one direction. The elbow is a hinge joint.
- *Pivot joint* allows turning from side to side. A pivot joint connects the skull to the spine.

## MUSCLES

The human body has more than 500 muscles (Figs. 7-7 and 7-8). Some are voluntary. Others are involuntary.

- *Voluntary* muscles can be consciously controlled. Muscles attached to bones *(skeletal muscles)* are voluntary. Arm muscles do not work unless you move your arm; likewise for leg muscles. Skeletal muscles are *striated*. That is, they look striped or streaked.
- *Involuntary muscles* work automatically. You cannot control them. They control the action of the stomach, intestines, blood vessels, and other body organs. Involuntary muscles are also called *smooth muscles*. They look smooth, not streaked or striped.
- *Cardiac muscle* is in the heart. It is an involuntary muscle. However, it appears striated like skeletal muscle.

Muscles have three functions:

- Movement of body parts
- Maintenance of posture
- Production of body heat

Strong, tough connective tissues called *tendons* connect muscles to bones. When muscles contract (shorten), tendons at each end of the muscle cause the

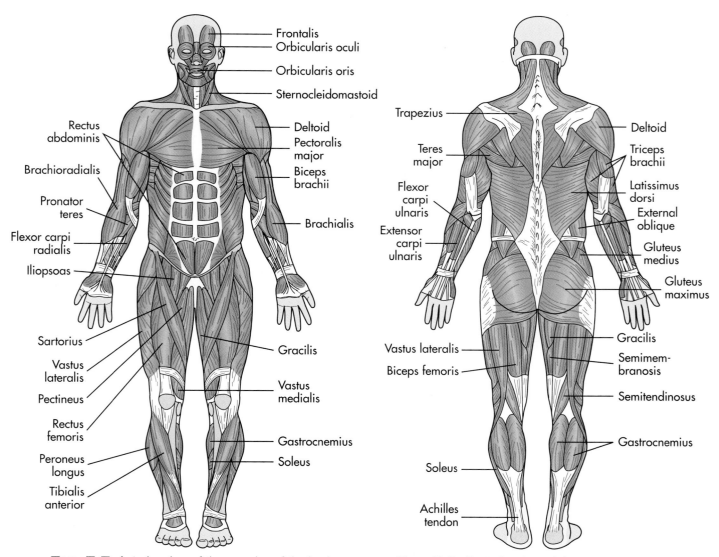

**FIG. 7-7** Anterior view of the muscles of the body.

**FIG. 7-8** Posterior view of the muscles of the body.

bone to move. The body has many tendons. See the Achilles tendon in Figure 7-8. Some muscles constantly contract to maintain the body's posture. When muscles contract, they burn food for energy. Heat is produced. The more muscle activity, the greater the amount of heat produced. Shivering is how the body produces heat when exposed to cold. Shivering is from rapid, general muscle contractions.

## THE NERVOUS SYSTEM

The nervous system controls, directs, and coordinates body functions. Its two main divisions are:
- The *central nervous system* (CNS). It consists of the *brain* and *spinal cord* (Fig. 7-9).
- The *peripheral nervous system*. It involves the *nerves* throughout the body (Fig. 7-10).

Nerves carry messages or impulses to and from the brain. Nerves connect to the spinal cord. They are easily damaged and take a long time to heal. Some nerve fibers have a protective covering called a *myelin sheath.* The myelin sheath also insulates the nerve fiber. Nerve fibers covered with myelin conduct impulses faster than those fibers without it.

### THE CENTRAL NERVOUS SYSTEM

The brain and spinal cord make up the central nervous system. The brain is covered by the skull. The three main parts of the brain are the *cerebrum,* the *cerebellum,* and the *brainstem* (see Fig. 7-9).

The cerebrum is the largest part of the brain. It is the center of thought and intelligence. The cerebrum is divided into two halves called the right and left *hemispheres.* The right hemisphere controls movement and activities on the body's left side. The left hemisphere controls the right side.

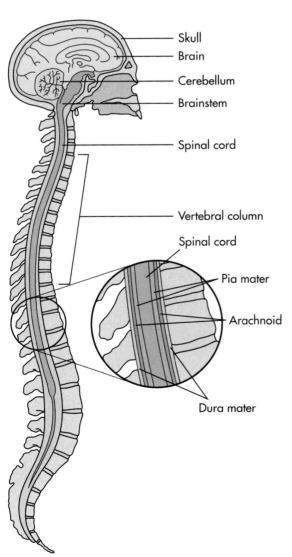

**FIG. 7-9**  Central nervous system.

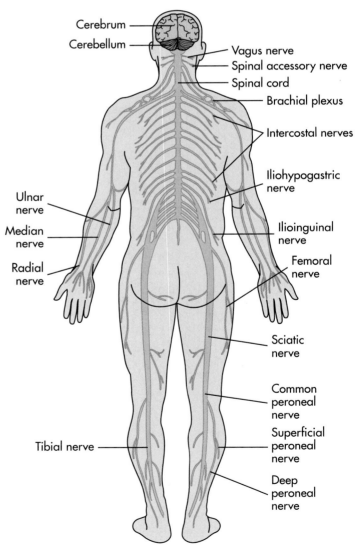

**FIG. 7-10**  Peripheral nervous system.

The outside of the cerebrum is called the *cerebral cortex* (Fig. 7-11). It controls the highest functions of the brain. These include reasoning, memory, consciousness, speech, voluntary muscle movement, vision, hearing, sensation, and other activities.

The cerebellum regulates and coordinates body movements. It controls balance and the smooth movements of voluntary muscles. Injury to the cerebellum results in jerky movements, loss of coordination, and muscle weakness.

The brainstem connects the cerebrum to the spinal cord. The brainstem contains the *midbrain, pons,* and *medulla.* The midbrain and pons relay messages between the medulla and the cerebrum. The medulla is below the pons. The medulla controls heart rate, breathing, blood vessel size, swallowing, coughing, and vomiting. The brain connects to the spinal cord at the lower end of the medulla.

The spinal cord lies within the spinal column. The cord is about 18 inches long. It contains pathways that conduct messages to and from the brain.

The brain and spinal cord are covered and protected by three layers of connective tissue called *meninges.* The outer layer lies next to the skull. It is a tough covering called the *dura mater.* The middle layer is the *arachnoid.* The inner layer is the *pia mater.* The space between the middle and inner layers is the *arachnoid space.* The space is filled with *cerebrospinal fluid.* It circulates around the brain and spinal cord. Cerebrospinal fluid protects the central nervous system. It cushions shocks that could easily injure brain and spinal cord structures.

## THE PERIPHERAL NERVOUS SYSTEM

The peripheral nervous system has 12 pairs of *cranial nerves* and 31 pairs of *spinal nerves.* Cranial nerves conduct impulses between the brain and the head, neck, chest, and abdomen. They conduct impulses for smell, vision, hearing, pain, touch, temperature, and pressure. They also conduct impulses for voluntary and involuntary muscles. Spinal nerves carry impulses from the skin, extremities, and the internal structures not supplied by cranial nerves.

Some peripheral nerves form the *autonomic nervous system.* This system controls involuntary muscles and certain body functions. The functions include the heartbeat, blood pressure, intestinal contractions, and glandular secretions. These functions occur automatically.

The autonomic nervous system is divided into the *sympathetic nervous system* and the *parasympathetic nervous system.* They balance each other. The sympathetic nervous system speeds up functions. The parasympathetic nervous system slows functions. When you are angry, scared, excited, or exercising, the sympathetic nervous system is stimulated. The parasympathetic system is activated when you relax or when the sympathetic system is stimulated for too long.

## THE SENSE ORGANS

The five senses are sight, hearing, taste, smell, and touch. Receptors for taste are in the tongue. They are called *taste buds.* Receptors for smell are in the nose. Touch receptors are in the dermis, especially in the toes and fingertips.

**THE EYE.** Receptors for vision are in the eyes (Fig. 7-12, p. 106). The eye is easily injured. Bones of the skull, eyelids and eyelashes, and tears protect the eyes from injury. The eye has three layers:
- The s*clera,* the white of the eye, is the outer layer. It is made of tough connective tissue.
- The *choroid* is the second layer. Blood vessels, the *ciliary muscle,* and the *iris* make up the choroid. The iris gives the eye its color. The opening in the middle of the iris is the *pupil.* Pupil size varies with the amount of light entering the eye. The pupil constricts (narrows) in bright light. It dilates (widens) in dim or dark places.
- The *retina* is the inner layer. It has receptors for vision and the nerve fibers of the optic nerve.

Light enters the eye through the *cornea.* It is the transparent part of the outer layer that lies over the eye. Light rays pass to the *lens,* which lies behind the pupil. The light is then reflected to the retina. Light is carried to the brain by the optic nerve.

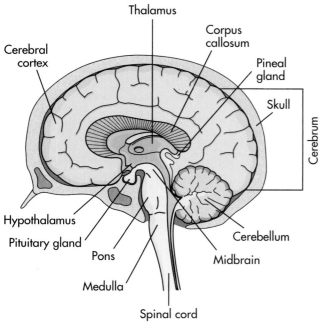

**FIG. 7-11** The brain.

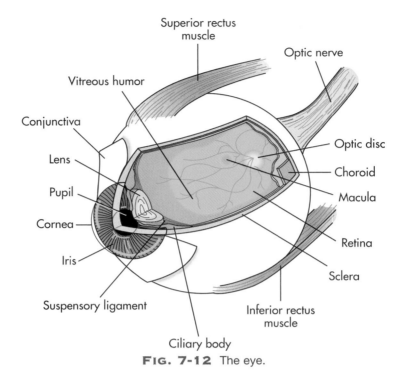

**FIG. 7-12** The eye.

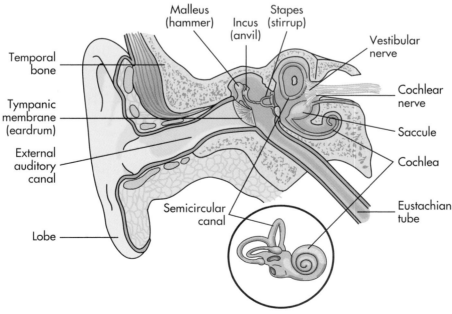

**FIG. 7-13** The ear.

The *aqueous chamber* separates the cornea from the lens. The chamber is filled with a fluid called *aqueous humor.* The fluid helps the cornea keep its shape and position. The *vitreous body* is behind the lens. It is a gelatin-like substance that supports the retina and maintains the eye's shape.

**THE EAR.** The ear is a sense organ (Fig. 7-13). It functions in hearing and balance. It has three parts: the *external ear, middle ear,* and *inner ear.*

The external ear (outer part) is called the *pinna* or *auricle.* Sound waves are guided through the external ear into the *auditory canal.* Glands in the auditory canal secrete a waxy substance called *cerumen.* The auditory canal extends about 1 inch to the *eardrum.* The eardrum *(tympanic membrane)* separates the external and middle ear.

The middle ear is a small space. It contains the *eustachian tube* and three small bones called *ossicles.* The eustachian tube connects the middle ear and the throat. Air enters the eustachian tube so that there is equal pressure on both sides of the eardrum. The ossicles amplify sound received from the eardrum and transmit the sound to the inner ear. The three ossicles are:
- The *malleus.* It looks like a hammer.
- The *incus.* It looks like an anvil.
- The *stapes.* It is shaped like a stirrup.

The inner ear consists of the *semicircular canals* and the *cochlea.* The cochlea looks like a snail shell. It contains fluid. The fluid carries sound waves from the middle ear to the *auditory nerve.* The auditory nerve then carries the message to the brain.

The three semicircular canals are involved with balance. They sense the head's position and changes in position. They send messages to the brain.

# THE CIRCULATORY SYSTEM

The circulatory system is made up of the blood, heart, and blood vessels. The heart pumps blood through the blood vessels. The circulatory system has many functions:
- Blood carries food, oxygen, and other substances to the cells.
- Blood removes waste products from cells.
- Blood and blood vessels help regulate body temperature. The blood carries heat from muscle activity to other body parts. Blood vessels in the skin dilate to cool the body. They constrict to retain heat.
- The system produces and carries cells that defend the body from microbes that cause disease.

## THE BLOOD

The blood consists of blood cells and *plasma.* Plasma is mostly water. It carries blood cells to other body cells. Plasma also carries substances that cells need to function. This includes food (proteins, fats, and carbohydrates), hormones (p. 116), and chemicals.

*Red blood cells (RBCs)* are called *erythrocytes.* They give the blood its red color because of a substance in the cell called **hemoglobin.** As *RBCs* circulate through the lungs, hemoglobin picks up oxygen. Hemoglobin carries oxygen to the cells. When blood is bright red, hemoglobin in the RBCs is saturated (filled) with oxygen. As blood circulates through the body, oxygen is given to the cells. Cells release carbon dioxide (a waste product). It is picked up by the hemoglobin. RBCs saturated with carbon dioxide make the blood look dark red.

The body has about 25 trillion (25,000,000,000,000) RBCs. About 4½ to 5 million cells are in a cubic millimeter of blood (the size of a tiny drop). RBCs live for 3 or 4 months. They are destroyed by the liver and spleen as they wear out. Bone marrow produces new RBCs. About 1 million RBCs are produced every second.

*White blood cells (WBCs)* are called *leukocytes.* They have no color. They protect the body against infection. There are 5,000 to 10,000 WBCs in a cubic millimeter of blood. At the first sign of infection, WBCs rush to the infection site. There they multiply rapidly. The number of WBCs increases when there is an infection. WBCs are produced by the bone marrow. They live about 9 days.

*Platelets (thrombocytes)* are needed for blood clotting. They are produced by the bone marrow. There are about 200,000 to 400,000 platelets in a cubic millimeter of blood. A platelet lives about 4 days.

## THE HEART

The heart is a muscle. It pumps blood through the blood vessels to the tissues and cells. The heart lies in the middle to lower part of the chest cavity toward the left side (Fig. 7-14, p. 108). The heart is hollow and has three layers (Fig. 7-15, p. 108):
- The *pericardium* is the outer layer. It is a thin sac covering the heart.
- The *myocardium* is the second layer. It is the thick, muscular part of the heart.
- The *endocardium* is the inner layer. A membrane, it lines the inner surface of the heart.

The heart has four chambers (see Fig. 7-15). Upper chambers receive blood and are called the *atria.* The *right atrium* receives blood from body tissues. The *left atrium* receives blood from the lungs. Lower chambers are called *ventricles.* Ventricles pump blood. The *right ventricle* pumps blood to the lungs for oxygen. The *left ventricle* pumps blood to all parts of the body.

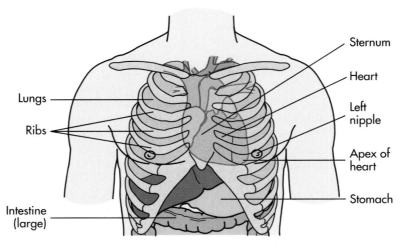

**FIG. 7-14** Location of the heart in the chest cavity.

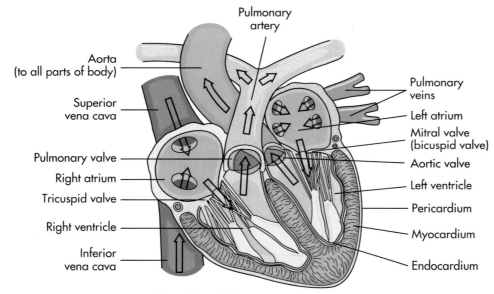

**FIG. 7-15** Structures of the heart.

*Valves* are between the atria and ventricles. The valves allow blood flow in one direction. They prevent blood from flowing back into the atria from the ventricles. The *tricuspid valve* is between the right atrium and right ventricle. The *mitral valve (bicuspid valve)* is between the left atrium and left ventricle.

Heart action has two phases:

- *Diastole.* It is the resting phase. Heart chambers fill with blood.
- *Systole.* It is the working phase. The heart contracts. Blood is pumped through the blood vessels when the heart contracts.

## THE BLOOD VESSELS

Blood flows to body tissues and cells through the blood vessels. There are three groups of blood vessels: arteries, capillaries, and veins.

**Arteries** carry blood away from the heart. Arterial blood is rich in oxygen. The *aorta* is the largest artery. It receives blood directly from the left ventricle. The aorta branches into other arteries that carry blood to all parts of the body (Fig. 7-16). These arteries branch into smaller parts within the tissues. The smallest branch of an artery is an *arteriole.*

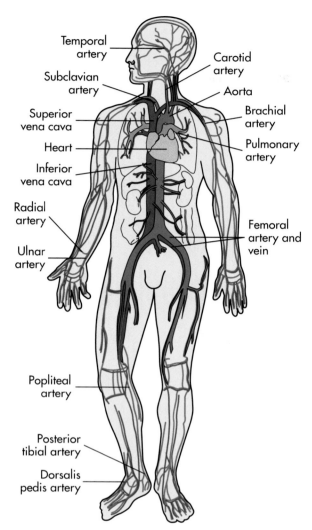

**FIG. 7-16** Arterial and venous systems.

Arterioles connect to **capillaries.** Capillaries are very tiny blood vessels. Food, oxygen, and other substances pass from capillaries into the cells. The capillaries pick up waste products (including carbon dioxide) from the cells. Veins carry waste products back to the heart.

**Veins** return blood to the heart. They connect to the capillaries by *venules.* Venules are small veins. Venules branch together to form veins. The many veins also branch together as they near the heart to form two main veins (see Fig. 7-16). The two main veins are the *inferior vena cava* and the *superior vena cava.* Both empty into the right atrium. The inferior vena cava carries blood from the legs and trunk. The superior vena cava carries blood from the head and arms. Venous blood is dark red. It has little oxygen and a lot of carbon dioxide.

Blood flow through the circulatory system is shown in Figure 7-15.

- Venous blood, poor in oxygen, empties into the right atrium.
- Blood flows through the tricuspid valve into the right ventricle.
- The right ventricle pumps blood into the lungs to pick up oxygen.
- Oxygen-rich blood from the lungs enters the left atrium.
- Blood from the left atrium passes through the mitral valve into the left ventricle.
- The left ventricle pumps the blood to the aorta. It branches off to form other arteries.
- The arterial blood is carried to the tissues by arterioles and to the cells by capillaries.
- Cells and capillaries exchange oxygen and nutrients for carbon dioxide and waste products.
- Capillaries connect with venules.
- Venules carry blood that has carbon dioxide and waste products.
- Venules form veins.
- Veins return blood to the heart.

## THE RESPIRATORY SYSTEM

Oxygen is needed to live. Every cell needs oxygen. Air contains about 21% oxygen. This meets the body's needs under normal conditions. The respiratory system (Fig. 7-17, p. 110) brings oxygen into the lungs and removes carbon dioxide. **Respiration** is the process of supplying the cells with oxygen and removing carbon dioxide from them. Respiration involves *inhalation* (breathing in) and *exhalation* (breathing out). The terms *inspiration* (breathing in) and *expiration* (breathing out) are also used.

Air enters the body through the *nose.* The air then passes into the *pharynx* (throat). It is a tube-shaped passageway for air and food. Air passes from the pharynx into the *larynx* (the voice box). A piece of cartilage, the *epiglottis,* acts like a lid over the larynx. The epiglottis prevents food from entering the airway during swallowing. During inhalation the epiglottis lifts up to let air pass over the larynx. Air passes from the larynx into the *trachea* (the windpipe).

The trachea divides at its lower end into the *right bronchus* and *left bronchus.* Each bronchus enters a lung. Upon entering the lungs, the bronchi divide many times into smaller branches. The smaller branches are called *bronchioles.* Eventually the bronchioles subdivide. They end up in tiny one-celled air sacs called *alveoli.*

Alveoli look like small clusters of grapes. They are supplied by capillaries. Oxygen and carbon dioxide are exchanged between the alveoli and capillaries. Blood in the capillaries picks up oxygen from the alveoli. Then the blood is returned to the left side of the

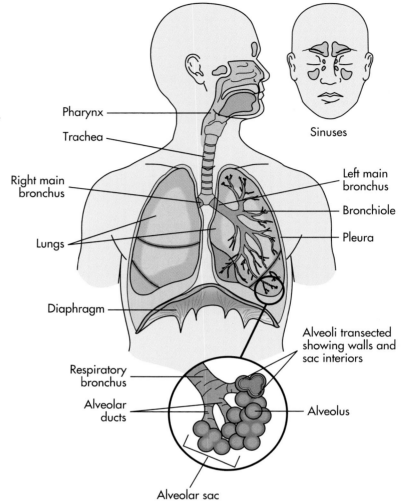

**FIG. 7-17** Respiratory system.

heart and pumped to the rest of the body. Alveoli pick up carbon dioxide from the capillaries for exhalation.

The lungs are spongy tissues. They are filled with alveoli, blood vessels, and nerves. Each lung is divided into lobes. The right lung has three lobes; the left lung has two. The lungs are separated from the abdominal cavity by a muscle called the *diaphragm.*

Each lung is covered by a two-layered sac called the *pleura.* One layer is attached to the lung and the other to the chest wall. The pleura secretes a very thin fluid that fills the space between the layers. The fluid prevents the layers from rubbing together during inhalation and exhalation. A bony framework made up of the ribs, sternum, and vertebrae protects the lungs.

## THE DIGESTIVE SYSTEM

The digestive system breaks down food physically and chemically so it can be absorbed for use by the cells. This process is called **digestion.** The digestive system is also called the *gastrointestinal system (GI system).* The system also removes solid wastes from the body.

The digestive system involves the *alimentary canal (GI tract)* and the accessory organs of digestion (Fig. 7-18). The alimentary canal is a long tube. It extends from the mouth to the anus. Its major parts are the mouth, pharynx, esophagus, stomach, small intestine, and large intestine. Accessory organs are the teeth, tongue, salivary glands, liver, gallbladder, and pancreas.

Digestion begins in the *mouth.* The mouth is also called the *oral cavity.* It receives food and prepares it for digestion. Using chewing motions, the *teeth* cut, chop, and grind food into small particles for digestion and swallowing. The *tongue* aids in chewing and swallowing. *Taste buds* on the tongue's surface contain nerve endings. Taste buds allow sweet, sour, bitter, and salty tastes to be sensed. *Salivary glands* in the mouth secrete *saliva.* Saliva moistens food particles to ease swallowing and begin digestion. During swallowing, the tongue pushes food into the pharynx.

The *pharynx* (throat) is a muscular tube. Swallowing continues as the pharynx contracts. Contraction of the

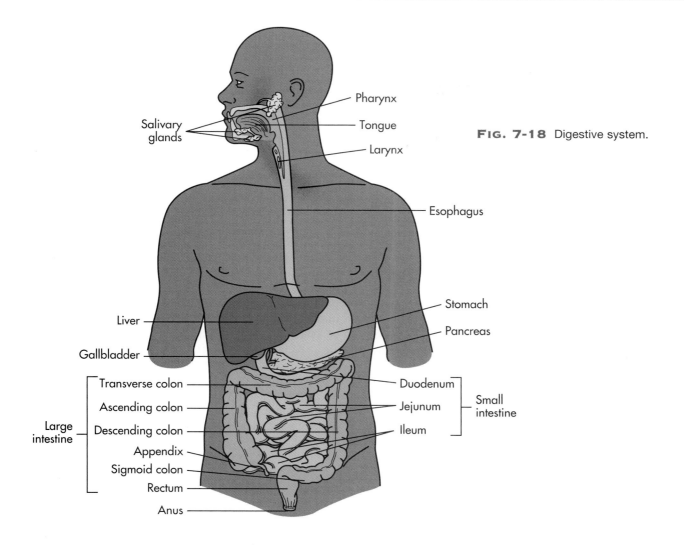

**FIG. 7-18** Digestive system.

Salivary glands
Pharynx
Tongue
Larynx
Esophagus
Liver
Gallbladder
Stomach
Pancreas
Transverse colon
Ascending colon
Descending colon
Appendix
Sigmoid colon
Rectum
Anus
Large intestine
Duodenum
Jejunum
Ileum
Small intestine

pharynx pushes food into the *esophagus*. The esophagus is a muscular tube about 10 inches long. It extends from the pharynx to the stomach. Involuntary muscle contractions called **peristalsis** move food down the esophagus into the stomach.

The *stomach* is a muscular, pouchlike sac. It is in the upper left part of the abdominal cavity. Strong stomach muscles stir and churn food to break it up into even smaller particles. A mucous membrane lines the stomach. It contains glands that secrete *gastric juices*. Food is mixed and churned with the gastric juices to form a semiliquid substance called *chyme*. Through peristalsis, the chyme is pushed from the stomach into the small intestine.

The *small intestine* is about 20 feet long. It has three parts. The first part is the *duodenum*. There more digestive juices are added to the chyme. One is called *bile*. Bile is a greenish liquid made in the *liver*. Bile is stored in the *gallbladder*. Juices from the *pancreas* and small

intestine are added to the chyme. Digestive juices chemically break down food so it can be absorbed.

Peristalsis moves the chyme through the two other parts of the small intestine: the *jejunum* and the *ileum*. Tiny projections called *villi* line the small intestine. Villi absorb the digested food into the capillaries. Most food absorption takes place in the jejunum and ileum.

Some chyme is not digested. Undigested chyme passes from the small intestine into the *large intestine* (*large bowel* or *colon*). The colon absorbs most of the water from the chyme. The remaining semisolid material is called *feces*. Feces contain a small amount of water, solid wastes, and some mucus and germs. These are the waste products of digestion. Feces pass through the colon into the *rectum* by peristalsis. Feces pass out of the body through the *anus*.

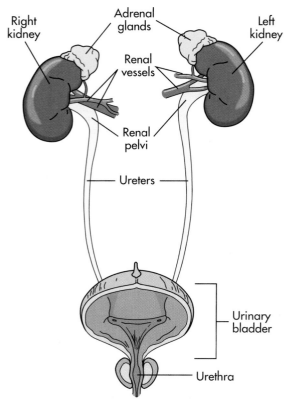

FIG. 7-19 Urinary system.

## THE URINARY SYSTEM

The digestive system rids the body of solid wastes. The lungs rid the body of carbon dioxide. Water and other substances are in sweat. There are other waste products in the blood from cells burning food for energy. The urinary system (Fig. 7-19):

- Removes waste products from the blood
- Maintains water balance within the body

The *kidneys* are two bean-shaped organs in the upper abdomen. They lie against the back muscles on each side of the spine. They are protected by the lower edge of the rib cage.

Each kidney has over a million tiny *nephrons* (Fig. 7-20). The nephron is the basic working unit of the kidney. Each nephron has a *convoluted tubule,* which is a tiny coiled tubule. Each convoluted tubule has a *Bowman's capsule* at one end. The capsule partly surrounds a cluster of capillaries called a *glomerulus.* Blood passes through the glomerulus and is filtered by the capillaries. The fluid part of the blood is squeezed into the Bowman's capsule. The fluid then passes into the tubule. Most of the water and other needed substances are reabsorbed by the blood. The rest of the fluid and the waste products form *urine* in the tubule. Urine flows through the tubule to a *collecting tubule.*

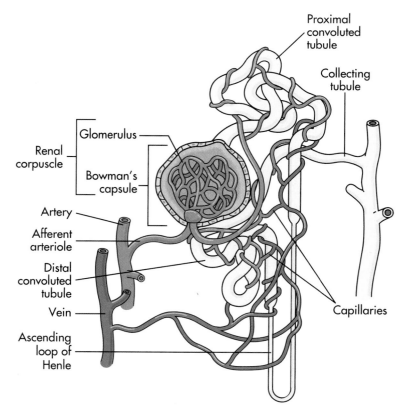

FIG. 7-20 A nephron.

All collecting tubules drain into the *renal pelvis* in the kidney.

A tube, called the *ureter*, is attached to the renal pelvis of the kidney. Each ureter is about 10 to 12 inches long. The ureters carry urine from the kidneys to the *bladder*. The bladder is a hollow, muscular sac. It lies toward the front in the lower part of the abdominal cavity.

Urine is stored in the bladder until the need to urinate is felt. This usually occurs when there is about half a pint (250 ml) of urine in the bladder. Urine passes from the bladder through the *urethra*. The opening at the end of the urethra is the *meatus*. Urine passes from the body through the meatus. Urine is a clear, yellowish fluid.

# THE REPRODUCTIVE SYSTEM

Human reproduction results from the union of a female sex cell and a male sex cell. The male and female reproductive systems are different. This allows for the process of reproduction.

## THE MALE REPRODUCTIVE SYSTEM

The male reproductive system is shown in Figure 7-21. The *testes (testicles)* are the male sex glands. Sex glands are also called *gonads*. The two testes are oval or almond-shaped glands. Male sex cells are produced in the testes. Male sex cells are called *sperm* cells.

*Testosterone*, the male hormone, is produced in the testes. This hormone is needed for reproductive organ function. It also is needed for the development of the male secondary sex characteristics. There is facial hair; pubic and axillary (underarm) hair; and hair on the arms, chest, and legs. Neck and shoulder sizes increase.

The testes are suspended between the thighs in a sac called the *scrotum*. The scrotum is made of skin and muscle.

Sperm travel from the testis to the *epididymis*. The epididymis is a coiled tube on top and to the side of the testis. From the epididymis, sperm travel through a tube called the *vas deferens*. Each vas deferens joins a *seminal vesicle*. The two seminal vesicles store sperm and produce *semen*. Semen is a fluid that carries sperm from the male reproductive tract. The ducts of the seminal vesicles unite to form the *ejaculatory duct*. It passes through the prostate gland.

The *prostate gland* lies just below the bladder. It is shaped like a donut. The gland secretes fluid into the semen. As the ejaculatory ducts leave the prostate, they join the *urethra*. The urethra runs through the prostate. The urethra is the outlet for urine and semen. The urethra is contained within the penis.

The *penis* is outside of the body and has *erectile* tissue. When a man is sexually excited, blood fills the erectile tissue. The penis enlarges and becomes hard and erect. The erect penis can enter a female's vagina. The semen, which contains sperm, is released into the vagina.

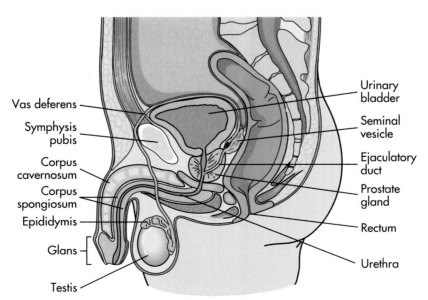

**FIG. 7-21** Male reproductive system.

# THE FEMALE REPRODUCTIVE SYSTEM

Figure 7-22 shows the female reproductive system. The female gonads are two almond-shaped glands called *ovaries.* An ovary is on each side of the uterus in the abdominal cavity.

The ovaries secrete the female hormones *estrogen* and *progesterone.* These hormones are needed for reproductive system function. They also are needed for the development of secondary sex characteristics in the female. These include increased breast size, pubic and axillary (underarm) hair, slight deepening of the voice, and widening and rounding of the hips.

When an ovum is released from an ovary, it travels through a *fallopian tube.* There are two fallopian tubes, one on each side. The tubes are attached at one end to the uterus. The ovum travels through the fallopian tube to the uterus.

The *uterus* is a hollow, muscular organ shaped like a pear. It is in the center of the pelvic cavity behind the bladder and in front of the rectum. The main part of the uterus is the *fundus.* The neck or narrow section of the uterus is the *cervix.* Tissue lining the uterus is called the *endometrium.* The endometrium has many blood vessels. If sex cells from the male and female unite into one cell, that cell implants into the endometrium, where it grows into a baby. The uterus serves as a place for the unborn baby to grow and receive nourishment.

The cervix of the uterus projects into a muscular canal called the *vagina.* The vagina opens to the outside of the body. It is just behind the urethra. The vagina receives the penis during intercourse. It also is part of the birth canal. Glands in the vaginal wall keep it moistened with secretions. In young girls, the external vaginal opening is partially closed by a membrane called the *hymen.* The hymen ruptures when the female has intercourse for the first time.

The external genitalia of the female are referred to as the *vulva* (Fig. 7-23):

- The *mons pubis* is a rounded, fatty pad over a bone called the *symphysis pubis.* The mons pubis is covered with hair in the adult female.
- The *labia majora* and *labia minora* are two folds of tissue on each side of the vaginal opening.
- The *clitoris* is a small organ composed of erectile tissue. It becomes hard when sexually stimulated.

The *mammary glands (breasts)* secrete milk after childbirth. The glands are on the outside of the chest. They are made up of glandular tissue and fat (Fig. 7-24). The milk drains into ducts that open onto the nipple.

**MENSTRUATION.** The endometrium is rich in blood to nourish the cell that grows into an unborn baby (*fetus*). If pregnancy does not occur, the endometrium breaks up. It is discharged through the vagina to the outside of the body. This process is called **menstruation.** Menstruation occurs about every 28 days. Therefore it is also called the *menstrual cycle.*

The first day of the cycle begins with menstruation. Blood flows from the uterus through the vaginal opening. Menstrual flow usually lasts 3 to 7 days. Ovulation occurs during the next phase. An ovum matures in an ovary and is released. Ovulation usually occurs on or about day 14 of the cycle.

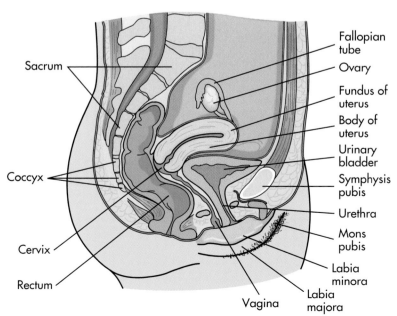

**FIG. 7-22** Female reproductive system.

Meanwhile, estrogen and progesterone (the female hormones) are secreted by the ovaries. These hormones cause the endometrium to thicken for pregnancy. If pregnancy does not occur, the hormones decrease in amount. This causes blood supply to the endometrium to decrease. The endometrium breaks up. It is discharged through the vagina. Another menstrual cycle begins.

## FERTILIZATION

To reproduce, a male sex cell (sperm) must unite with a female sex cell (ovum). The uniting of the sperm and ovum into one cell is called *fertilization*. A sperm has 23 chromosomes. An ovum has 23 chromosomes. When the two cells unite, the fertilized cell has 46 chromosomes.

During intercourse, millions of sperm are deposited into the vagina. Sperm travel up the cervix, through the uterus, and into the fallopian tubes. If a sperm and an ovum unite in a fallopian tube, fertilization results. Pregnancy occurs. The fertilized cell travels down the fallopian tube to the uterus. After a short time, the fertilized cell implants in the thick endometrium and grows during pregnancy.

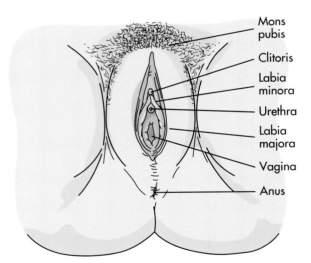

FIG. 7-23 External female genitalia.

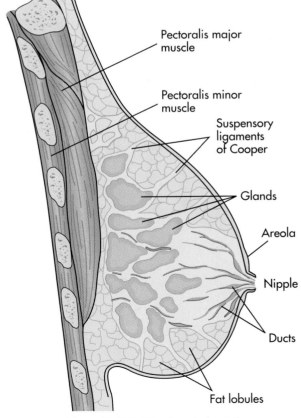

FIG. 7-24 The female breast.

# THE ENDOCRINE SYSTEM

The endocrine system is made up of glands called the *endocrine glands* (Fig. 7-25). The endocrine glands secrete chemical substances called **hormones** into the bloodstream. Hormones regulate the activities of other organs and glands in the body.

The *pituitary gland* is called the *master gland.* About the size of a cherry, it is at the base of the brain behind the eyes. The pituitary gland is divided into the anterior pituitary lobe and the posterior pituitary lobe. The *anterior pituitary lobe* secretes:
- *Growth hormone*—needed for the growth of muscles, bones, and other organs. It is needed throughout life to maintain normal-size bones and muscles. Growth is stunted if a baby is born with deficient amounts of the growth hormone. Too much of the hormone causes excessive growth.
- *Thyroid-stimulating hormone* (TSH)—needed for thyroid gland function.
- *Adrenocorticotropic hormone* (ACTH)—stimulates the adrenal gland.

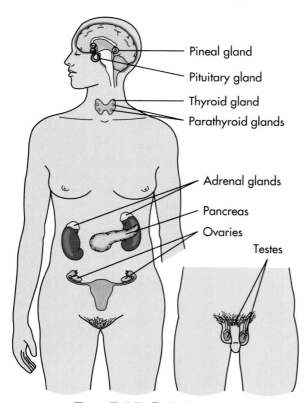

Pineal gland

Pituitary gland

Thyroid gland

Parathyroid glands

Adrenal glands

Pancreas

Ovaries

Testes

**FIG. 7-25** Endocrine system.

The anterior lobe also secretes hormones that regulate the growth, development, and function of the male and female reproductive systems.

The *posterior pituitary lobe* secretes *antidiuretic hormone* (ADH) and *oxytocin.* ADH prevents the kidneys from excreting excessive amounts of water. Oxytocin causes uterine muscles to contract during childbirth.

The *thyroid gland,* shaped like a butterfly, is in the neck in front of the larynx. *Thyroid hormone* (TH, thyroxine) is secreted by the thyroid gland. It regulates **metabolism.** Metabolism is the burning of food for heat and energy by the cells. Too little TH results in slowed body processes, slowed movements, and weight gain. Too much TH causes increased metabolism, excess energy, and weight loss. Some babies are born with deficient amounts of TH. Their physical growth and mental growth are stunted.

The four *parathyroid glands* secrete *parathormone.* Two lie on each side of the thyroid gland. Parathormone regulates calcium use. Calcium is needed for nerve and muscle function. Insufficient amounts of calcium cause *tetany.* Tetany is a state of severe muscle contraction and spasm. If untreated, tetany can cause death.

There are two *adrenal glands.* An adrenal gland is on the top of each kidney. The adrenal gland has two parts: the *adrenal medulla* and the *adrenal cortex.* The adrenal medulla secretes *epinephrine* and *norepinephrine.* These hormones stimulate the body to quickly produce energy during emergencies. Heart rate, blood pressure, muscle power, and energy all increase.

The adrenal cortex secretes three groups of hormones that are needed for life:
- *Glucocorticoids*—regulate metabolism of carbohydrates. They also control the body's response to stress and inflammation.
- *Mineralocorticoids*—regulate the amount of salt and water that is absorbed and lost by the kidneys.
- Small amounts of male and female sex hormones—see p. 113.

The *pancreas* secretes *insulin.* Insulin regulates the amount of sugar in the blood available for use by the cells. Insulin is needed for sugar to enter the cells. If there is too little insulin, sugar cannot enter the cells. If sugar cannot enter the cells, excess amounts of sugar build up in the blood. This condition is called *diabetes.*

The *gonads* are the glands of human reproduction. Male sex glands (testes) secrete *testosterone.* Female sex glands (ovaries) secrete *estrogen* and *progesterone.*

# THE IMMUNE SYSTEM

The immune system protects the body from disease and infection. Abnormal body cells can grow into tumors. Sometimes the body produces substances that cause the body to attack itself. Microorganisms (bacteria, viruses, and other germs) can cause an infection. The immune system defends against threats inside and outside the body.

The immune system gives the body immunity. **Immunity** means that a person has protection against a disease or condition. The person will not get or be affected by the disease:

- *Specific immunity* is the body's reaction to a certain threat.
- *Nonspecific immunity* is the body's reaction to anything it does not recognize as a normal body substance.

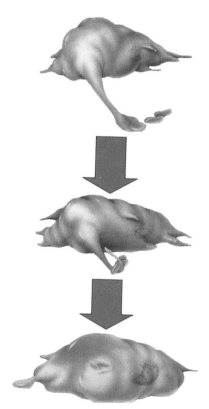

**FIG. 7-26** A phagocyte digests and destroys a microorganism. (From Thibodeau GA, Patton KT: *Structure and function of the body*, ed 11, St Louis, 2000, Mosby.)

Special cells and substances function to produce immunity:

- *Antibodies*—normal body substances that recognize abnormal or unwanted substances. They attack and destroy such substances.
- *Antigens*—abnormal or unwanted substances. An antigen causes the body to produce antibodies. The antibodies attack and destroy the antigens.
- *Phagocytes*—white blood cells that digest and destroy microorganisms and other unwanted substances (Fig. 7-26).
- *Lymphocytes*—white blood cells that produce antibodies. Lymphocyte production increases as the body responds to an infection.
- *B lymphocytes (B cells)*—cause the production of antibodies that circulate in the plasma. The antibodies react to specific antigens.
- *T lymphocytes (T cells)*—cells that destroy invading cells. *Killer T cells* produce poisonous substances near the invading cells. Some T cells attract other cells. These other cells destroy the invaders.

When the body senses an antigen (an unwanted substance), the immune system acts. Phagocyte and lymphocyte production increases. Phagocytes destroy the invaders through digestion. The lymphocytes produce antibodies that attack and destroy the unwanted substances.

# ■ REVIEW QUESTIONS ■

Circle the **BEST** answer.

1 The basic unit of body structure is the
   a Cell
   b Neuron
   c Nephron
   d Ovum

2 The outer layer of the skin is called the
   a Dermis
   b Epidermis
   c Integument
   d Myelin

3 Which is *not* a function of the skin?
   a Provides the protective covering for the body
   b Regulates body temperature
   c Senses cold, pain, touch, and pressure
   d Provides the shape and framework for the body

4 Which allows movement?
   a Bone marrow
   b Synovial membrane
   c Joints
   d Ligaments

5 Skeletal muscles
   a Are under involuntary control
   b Appear smooth
   c Are under voluntary control
   d Appear striped and smooth

6 The highest functions of the brain take place in the
   a Cerebral cortex
   b Medulla
   c Brainstem
   d Spinal nerves

7 The ear is involved with
   a Regulating body movements
   b Balance
   c Smoothness of body movements
   d Controlling involuntary muscles

8 The liquid part of the blood is the
   a Hemoglobin
   b Red blood cell
   c Plasma
   d White blood cell

9 Which part of the heart pumps blood to the body?
   a Right atrium
   b Right ventricle
   c Left atrium
   d Left ventricle

10 Which carry blood away from the heart?
   a Capillaries
   b Veins
   c Venules
   d Arteries

11 Oxygen and carbon dioxide are exchanged
   a In the bronchi
   b Between the alveoli and capillaries
   c Between the lungs and the pleura
   d In the trachea

12 Digestion begins in the
   a Mouth
   b Stomach
   c Small intestine
   d Colon

13 Most food absorption takes place in the
   a Stomach
   b Small intestine
   c Colon
   d Large intestine

14 Urine is formed by the
   a Jejunum
   b Kidneys
   c Bladder
   d Liver

15 Urine passes from the body through
   a The ureters
   b The urethra
   c The anus
   d Nephrons

16 The male sex gland is called the
   a Penis
   b Semen
   c Testis
   d Scrotum

**17** The male sex cell is the
a Semen
b Ovum
c Gonad
d Sperm

**18** The female sex gland is the
a Ovary
b Cervix
c Uterus
d Vagina

**19** The discharge of the lining of the uterus is called
a The endometrium
b Ovulation
c Fertilization
d Menstruation

**20** The endocrine glands secrete
a Hormones
b Mucus
c Semen
d Insulin

**21** The immune system protects the body from
a Low blood sugar
b Disease and infection
c Falling and loss of balance
d Stunted growth and loss of fluid

*Answers to these questions are on p. 816.*

# Growth and Development

# OBJECTIVES

- Define the key terms listed in this chapter
- Explain the principles of growth and development
- Identify the stages of growth and development
- Identify the developmental tasks for each age-group
- Describe the normal growth and development for each age-group

# KEY TERMS

**adolescence** The time between puberty and adulthood; a time of rapid growth and physical and social maturity

**development** Changes in mental, emotional, and social function

**developmental task** A skill that must be completed during a stage of development

**ejaculation** The release of semen

**growth** The physical changes that are measured and that occur in a steady, orderly manner

**infancy** The first year of life

**menarche** The first menstruation and the start of menstrual cycles

**menopause** The time when menstruation stops and menstrual cycles end

**primary caregiver** The person mainly responsible for providing or assisting with the child's basic needs

**puberty** The period when reproductive organs begin to function and secondary sex characteristics appear

**reflex** An involuntary movement

You care for people of all ages. They are in different stages of growth and development. An understanding of growth and development helps you give better care. The person's needs are easier to understand. This chapter presents the basic changes that occur in normal, healthy persons from birth through old age.

Growth and development are presented in stages. Age ranges and normal characteristics are given for each stage. The stages overlap. It is hard to see the start and end of each stage. Also, the rate of growth and development varies with each person.

Growth and development theories usually involve the two-parent family. However, single-parent households are common. A relative may care for children while the parent works or is in school. In this chapter, *primary caregiver* is used in place of *mother* or *father*. The **primary caregiver** is the person mainly responsible for providing or assisting with the child's basic needs. A mother, father, grandparent, aunt, uncle, or court-appointed guardian may have this role. *Parent* and *parents* are sometimes used here. However, another primary caregiver may have the parent role.

# PRINCIPLES

**Growth** is the physical changes that are measured and that occur in a steady and orderly manner. Growth is measured in height and weight. Changes in appearance and body functions also measure growth.

**Development** relates to changes in mental, emotional, and social function. A person behaves and thinks in certain ways in each stage of development. A 2-year-old thinks in simple terms. A primary caregiver is needed for basic needs. A 40-year-old thinks in complex ways. Most basic needs are met without help.

The entire person is affected. Although they differ, growth and development:
- Overlap
- Depend on each other
- Occur at the same time

For example, an infant cannot coo or babble (development) until the physical structures needed for speech are strong enough (growth). Basic principles of growth and development are:

- The process starts at fertilization and continues until death.
- The process proceeds from the simple to the complex. A baby sits before standing, stands before walking, and walks before running.
- The process occurs in certain directions:
  —From head to the foot: babies hold up their heads before they sit; they sit before they stand.
  —From the center of the body outward: babies control shoulder movements before they control hand movements.
- The process occurs in a sequence, order, and pattern. Certain skills must be completed during each stage. A **developmental task** is a skill that must be completed during a stage of development. A stage cannot be skipped. Each stage is the basis for the next stage.
- The rate of the process is uneven. It is not at a set pace. Growth is rapid during infancy. Children have growth spurts. Some children develop fast. Others develop slowly.
- Each stage has its own characteristics and developmental tasks.

## INFANCY (BIRTH TO 1 YEAR)

**Infancy** is the first year of life. Growth and development are rapid during this time. The developmental tasks of infancy are:

- Learning to walk
- Learning to eat solid foods
- Beginning to talk and communicate with others
- Beginning to have emotional relationships with parents, brothers, and sisters
- Developing stable sleep and feeding patterns

### THE NEWBORN (BIRTH TO 1 MONTH)

The *neonatal period* of infancy is from birth to 1 month. A baby is called a *neonate* or a *newborn* during this time.

The average newborn is about 20 inches long and weighs 7 to 8 pounds. Birth weight doubles by 6 months of age. It triples by 1 year of age. Babies are about 30 inches long by 1 year of age.

The newborn's head is large compared with the rest of the body. Skin is pink and wrinkled. The skin turns red when the baby cries. The trunk is long. The abdomen is large, round, and soft. Eyes are a deep blue in light-skinned babies. Dark-skinned babies have brown eyes. The newborn has fat, pudgy cheeks, a flat nose, and a receding chin (Fig. 8-1).

The central nervous system is not well developed in newborns. Movements are uncoordinated and lack purpose. Newborns can see clearly up to about 8 inches. They see in color. They prefer primary colors (red, green, blue, and so on) as they develop. Babies hear well. Loud sounds startle them. Soft sounds soothe them. Babies prefer female voices. They react to touch and feel pain. They can taste and smell.

Newborns have certain **reflexes** (involuntary movements). These reflexes decline and then disappear as the central nervous system develops:

- *Moro reflex (startle reflex)*— occurs when a baby is startled by a loud noise, a sudden movement, or the head falling back. The arms are thrown apart. The legs extend and then flex. A brief cry is common.
- *Rooting reflex*—occurs when the cheek is touched near the mouth. The mouth opens, and the head turns toward the touch. The rooting reflex is necessary for feeding. It guides the baby's mouth to the nipple.
- *Sucking reflex*—occurs when the lips are touched.
- *Grasp (palmar) reflex*—occurs when the palm is stroked. The fingers close firmly around the object (Fig. 8-2).
- *Step reflex*—occurs when the baby is held upright and the feet touch a surface. The feet move up and down as in stepping motions.

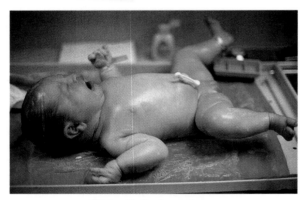

**FIG. 8-1** A newborn.

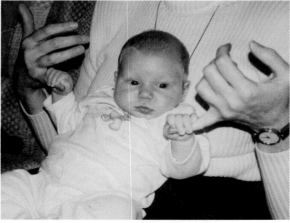

**FIG. 8-2** The grasp reflex.

Newborns sleep 20 hours a day. They awaken when hungry and fall asleep right after a feeding. Bottle-fed infants eat every 2½ to 4 hours. Breast-fed infants eat more often. The time between feedings lengthens as infants grow and develop. They also stay awake more and sleep less.

Movements are uncoordinated and lack purpose. They are mainly involuntary. Specific, voluntary, and coordinated movements occur as the nervous and muscular systems develop. Newborns cannot hold their heads up. They turn their heads from side to side.

## INFANTS (1 MONTH TO 1 YEAR)

When lying on their stomachs, 1-month-old infants can lift their heads up briefly (Fig. 8-3). They also can turn their heads. They smile.

Two-month-old infants can hold their heads up when held upright. When on their stomachs, they can turn their heads from side to side. They need support to sit in an angled position. They have tears and can follow objects with their eyes (Fig. 8-4). They can smile when responding to others. At 2 to 3 months, they laugh, squeal, and coo.

Infants 3 to 4 months of age can hold their heads up (Fig. 8-5). They reach for objects. They babble, coo, and make sounds. At 4 months, they can belly-laugh. The Moro, rooting, and grasp reflexes disappear.

By 4 to 5 months, infants can roll from front to back. They roll from back to front by 5 to 6 months. They also can sit by leaning forward on their hands (Fig. 8-6). Teething may begin with the bottom front teeth. They may sleep all night. They can play "peek-a-boo."

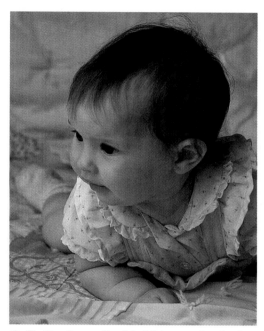

**FIG. 8-5** The 3-month-old child can raise the head and shoulders.

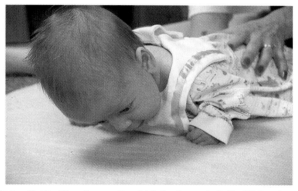

**FIG. 8-3** The 1-month-old infant can briefly lift her head when lying on her stomach.

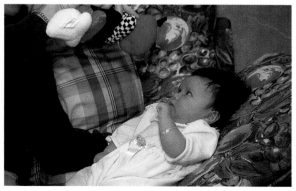

**FIG. 8-4** A 2-month-old child follows an object with her eyes.

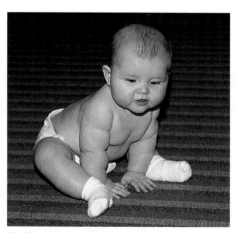

**FIG. 8-6** A 6-month-old sits forward, leaning on the hands. (From James SR, Ashwill JW, Droske SC: *Nursing care of children: principles and practice,* ed 2, Philadelphia, 2002, WB Saunders.)

Solid foods are given at 4 to 6 months. Rice cereal mixed with milk is given first. It is given with an infant spoon. Fruits, vegetables, and meats are introduced slowly. These foods are thin in consistency at first. Thicker and chunkier foods are given as more teeth erupt and chewing and swallowing skills increase.

Infants have more skills at 6 months. They can bear weight when pulled into a standing position. They sit with support and move around by rolling. Some start to drink from a cup. They smile at themselves in a mirror. They respond to their names.

Some infants start to crawl at 7 months. They can stand while holding on for support. They make sounds in response to caregivers.

Eight-month-old infants can sit for long periods. They also can change from lying to sitting and from sitting to lying positions. The pincer grasp develops. This means that they can hold small objects with the thumb and index finger. They can pick up small finger foods. They learn to drink from a cup with handles. Language skills increase. They can say "mama" and "dada." They respond to their names. Eye color is permanent.

When holding onto something, 9-month-olds can pull up into a standing position. They can hold a bottle, play "pat-a-cake," and drink from a cup or glass. They understand their names and "no." They point and use gestures to communicate.

Ten-month-old infants can stand alone. They may walk with help or while holding onto something (Fig. 8-7). They also may climb up and down stairs. At 11 months, they may walk alone and use push toys.

At 12 months, walking skills increase. They can climb onto furniture. They can turn book pages and put objects into a container. They can say a few words. Bottle weaning may begin.

## TODDLERHOOD (1 TO 3 YEARS)

Growth rate is slower than during infancy. Developmental tasks during this period are:

- Tolerating separation from the primary caregiver
- Gaining control of bowel and bladder function
- Using words to communicate
- Becoming less dependent on the primary caregiver

Toddlers need to assert independence. Therefore this time is called the "terrible twos." They learn to walk well. They are curious. Toddlers get into anything and everything. They touch, smell, and taste everything within reach. They climb on tables, chairs, counters, and other high areas. With these new skills, toddlers can explore their environment. They venture farther away from primary caregivers. Toddlers learn to do some things without a primary caregiver. By the age of 3, they can run, jump, climb, ride a tricycle, and walk up and down stairs.

Hand coordination increases. They learn to feed themselves. They progress from eating with fingers to using a spoon (Fig. 8-8). Toddlers can drink from cups. They can scribble, build towers with blocks, string beads, and turn book pages. Right- or left-handedness is seen during the second year.

Toilet training is a major task for toddlers. Bowel and bladder control is related to central nervous system development. Children must be mentally and physically ready for toilet training. Some children are ready at age 2 years. Others are ready at 2½ to 3 years of age. The process starts with bowel control. Bladder control during the day occurs before bladder control at night.

Speech and language skills increase. Speech is clearer. Toddlers learn words by imitating others. They understand more words than they use. An 18-month-old knows 6 to 18 words. By age 2 years, the child knows about 300 words. "Me" and "mine" are used often.

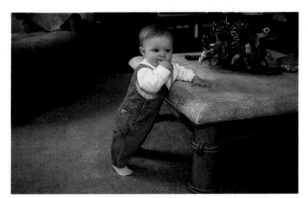

**FIG. 8-7** A 10-month-old infant can walk while holding onto furniture.

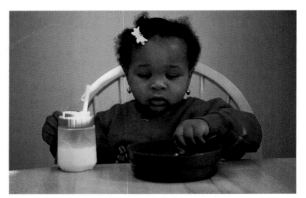

**FIG. 8-8** A toddler uses a spoon.

Play skills increase. The child plays alongside other children but not with them. Toddlers do not share toys. They are very possessive and do not understand sharing.

Temper tantrums and saying "no" are common during this stage. Toddlers express anger and frustration by kicking and screaming. This is how they object to having independence challenged. Using "no" can frustrate primary caregivers. Almost every request may be answered "no," even if the child is following the request.

Another task is tolerating separation from the primary caregiver. As toddlers start to explore, they move away from primary caregivers. With discomfort, frustration, or injury, they quickly return to primary caregivers or cry for their attention. If primary caregivers are consistently present when needed, children learn to feel secure. They learn to tolerate brief periods of separation.

# PRESCHOOL (3 TO 6 YEARS)

The preschool years are from the ages of 3 to 6 years. Children grow 2 to 3 inches per year. They gain about 5 pounds per year. Preschoolers are thinner, more coordinated, and more graceful than toddlers.

Developmental tasks of the preschool years include:
- Increasing the ability to communicate and understand others
- Performing self-care
- Learning the gender differences and developing sexual modesty
- Learning right from wrong and good from bad
- Learning to play with others
- Developing family relationships

## THE 3-YEAR-OLD

Three-year-olds become more coordinated. They can walk on tiptoe, balance on one foot for a few seconds, and run, jump, kick a ball, and climb with ease.

Personal care skills increase. They can put on shoes and clothes, manage buttons, wash their hands, and brush their teeth (Fig. 8-9). They can feed themselves, pour from a bottle, and help set the table without breaking dishes. Hand skills also include drawing circles and crosses.

Language skills increase. They know about 900 words. They talk and ask questions ("how" and "why") constantly. Three-year-olds can name body parts, family members, and friends. They like talking dolls and musical toys.

Play is important. They play with two or three other children and can share. They play simple games and learn simple rules. Imaginary friends and imitating adults are common. They enjoy crayons, cutting, pasting, painting, and playing "house" and "dress-up" (Fig. 8-10). They also like wagons, tricycles, and other riding toys.

Three-year-olds know that there are two sexes. They know that male and female bodies differ. They also know their own sex. Little girls may wonder how the penis works and why they do not have one. Little boys may wonder how girls can urinate without a penis.

The concept of time develops. Three-year-olds may speak of the past, present, and future. "Yesterday" and "tomorrow" are confusing. Children may fear the dark and need night-lights in bedrooms. Nightmares are common.

Three-year-olds are less fearful of strangers. They can be away from primary caregivers for short periods. They are less jealous than toddlers of a new baby. They try to please primary caregivers.

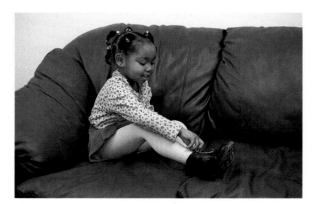

**FIG. 8-9** A 3-year-old has increased coordination.

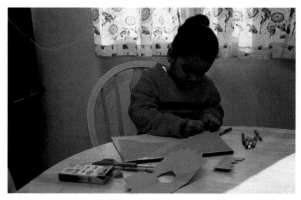

**FIG. 8-10** This 3-year-old enjoys cutting paper.

## THE 4-YEAR-OLD

Four-year-olds can hop, skip, and throw and catch a ball. They can lace shoes, draw faces, and copy a square. They try to print letters. With help, they can bathe and tend to toileting needs.

They know about 1500 words. They continue to ask many questions and tend to exaggerate stories. They can sing simple songs, repeat four numbers, count to five, and name a few colors.

Four-year-olds tend to tease, tattle, and tell fibs. When bad, they may blame an imaginary friend. Bragging, telling tales about family members, and showing off are common. They can play with other children. They are proud of accomplishments but have mood swings.

These children enjoy playing "dress-up," wearing costumes, and telling and hearing stories. They like to draw and make things. Imagination, drama, and imitating adults are part of play (Fig. 8-11). They play in groups of two or three and tend to be bossy. Playing "doctor and nurse" is common as curiosity about the other sex continues.

Four-year-olds prefer the primary caregiver of the other sex. Rivalries with brothers and sisters are seen, especially when a younger child takes the 4-year-old's things. Rivalries also occur when older children have more and different privileges. The family is often the focus of the child's frustrations and aggressive behavior. A 4-year-old may try to run away from home.

## THE 5-YEAR-OLD

Coordination increases. Five-year-olds can jump rope, skate, tie shoelaces, dress, and bathe. They can use a pencil well and copy diamond and triangle shapes. They can print a few letters, numbers, and their first names. Drawings of people include body parts.

Communication skills increase. They speak in full sentences. Questions are fewer than before but have more meaning. They want words defined and take part in conversations. They can name colors, coins, days, and the months. They specify and describe drawings.

Five-year-olds are more responsible and truthful. They quarrel less than before. They are more aware of rules and are eager to do things correctly. They have manners, are independent, and can be trusted within limits. Fears are fewer, but nightmares and dreams are common. They are proud of accomplishments.

These children like books about animals and other children. They like board games and try to follow rules. They imitate adults during play and are interested in TV. They also enjoy doing things with the primary caregiver of the same sex (Fig. 8-12). These include cooking, housecleaning, shopping, yard work, and sports.

Younger children are considered a nuisance. However, 5-year-olds usually protect them. They tolerate brothers and sisters well.

## SCHOOL AGE (6 TO 9 OR 10 YEARS)

School-age children enter the world of peer groups, games, and learning. They grow 2 to 3 inches a year. They gain 2 to 5 pounds a year. Their developmental tasks are:

- Developing the social and physical skills needed for playing games
- Learning to get along with children of the same age and background (peers)
- Learning gender-appropriate behaviors and attitudes
- Learning basic reading, writing, and arithmetic skills
- Developing a conscience and morals
- Developing a good feeling and attitude about oneself

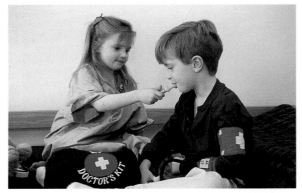

**FIG. 8-11** Four-year-olds play "dress-up" and imitate adults.

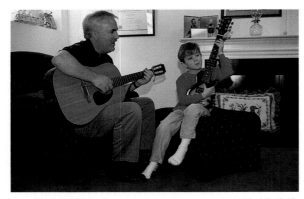

**FIG. 8-12** This 5-year-old enjoys music with his father.

Baby teeth are lost. This starts at around age 6 years. Permanent teeth erupt.

Children are very active. They can run, jump, skip, hop, and ride a two-wheeled bike. They can swim, skate, dance, and jump rope. These children can take part in team sports. Soccer, T-ball, baseball, and football are examples (Fig. 8-13). Children learn to play in groups. They learn teamwork and sportsmanship. Quiet play involves collections, board games, computer and electronic games, and crafts.

Language skills increase rapidly. Reading, writing, grammar, and math skills develop. They learn to print first. Printing is followed by cursive writing. Sentences are longer and more complex. As reading skills increase, so do language skills. Children like to read and to be read to. Older girls prefer romantic stories. They also like adventure stories about female heroines. Older boys like science fiction, horror, sports, and adventure stories. Both boys and girls like mysteries.

Pretend and imaginary play is seen in preschoolers. In school-age children, such play is replaced with activities that have purpose and involve "work." They like household tasks (cleaning, cooking, yard work). They also like crafts, building things, and scout groups. Rewards are important—good grades, trophies, pay for chores, scouting badges.

School-age children are concerned about being well liked. Being part of a peer group is important for love, belonging, and self-esteem needs. These children get along with and need adults. However, they prefer peer group fads, opinions, and activities (Fig. 8-14).

## LATE CHILDHOOD (9 OR 10 TO 12 YEARS)

Late childhood (preadolescence) is the time between childhood and adolescence. Developmental tasks are like those for school-age children. Preadolescents are expected to show more refinement and maturity in achieving these tasks:

- Becoming independent of adults and learning to depend on oneself
- Developing and keeping friendships with peers
- Understanding the physical, psychological, and social roles of one's sex
- Developing moral and ethical behavior
- Developing greater muscular strength, coordination, and balance
- Learning how to study

Many permanent teeth erupt. Girls have a growth spurt. By age 12 years, they are taller and heavier than boys. The body movements of both boys and girls are more graceful and coordinated (Fig. 8-15). Muscle strength and physical skills increase. Skill in team sports is important.

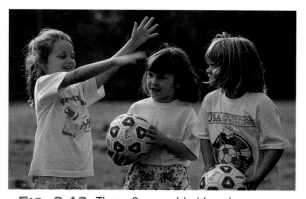

**FIG. 8-13** These 6-year-old girls enjoy soccer.

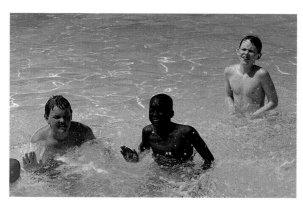

**FIG. 8-14** Belonging to a peer group is important to school-age children.

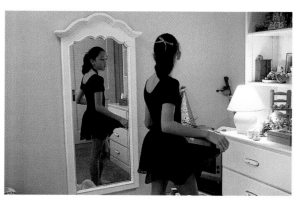

**FIG. 8-15** Movements are smooth and graceful in late childhood.

The onset of puberty nears. In girls, the hips widen and breast buds appear. Some 9-, 10-, and 11-year-old girls begin puberty. Boys show fewer signs of maturing sexually. Genital organs begin to grow.

These children need factual sex education. Friends share information about sex. It is often incomplete and inaccurate. Parents and children may be uncomfortable discussing sex with each other. They may avoid the subject. When children ask questions, answers must be honest and complete. They must be given in terms that children understand.

Peer groups are the center of activities. The group affects the child's attitudes and behavior. Children prefer friends of the same sex. Friends are loyal and share problems. Boys need to show their strength and toughness. They may have nicknames. Boys often tease girls. Girls may become "boy crazy."

These children are aware of the mistakes and faults of adults. They do not accept adult standards and rules without question. It is common to rebel against adults and test limits. Parents and children disagree. However, parents are needed for the child's development.

Math and language skills increase. These children read newspapers and enjoy comic books. They also like romantic, mystery, adventure, horror, and science fiction books and stories.

# ADOLESCENCE (12 TO 18 YEARS)

**Adolescence** is the time between puberty and adulthood. It is a time of rapid growth and physical and social maturity. The stage begins with puberty. **Puberty** is the period when reproductive organs begin to function and the secondary sex characteristics appear. Girls reach puberty between the ages of 9 and 15 years. Boys reach puberty between the ages of 12 and 16 years.

The developmental tasks of adolescence include:
- Accepting changes in the body and appearance
- Developing appropriate relationships with males and females of the same age
- Accepting the male or female role appropriate for one's age
- Becoming independent from parents and adults
- Developing morals, attitudes, and values needed to function in society

**Menarche** is the first menstruation and the start of menstrual cycles (Chapter 7). It marks the onset of puberty in girls. Secondary sex characteristics appear. These include:
- Increase in breast size
- Pubic and axillary (underarm) hair
- Slight deepening of the voice
- Widening and rounding of the hips

During late childhood, male sex organs begin to increase in size. This growth continues during adolescence. **Ejaculation** (the release of semen) signals the onset of puberty in boys. *Nocturnal emissions* ("wet dreams") occur. During sleep *(nocturnal)*, the penis becomes erect. Semen is released *(emission)*. Other secondary sex characteristics include:
- Facial hair
- Pubic and axillary (underarm) hair
- Hair on the arms, chest, and legs
- Deepening of the voice
- Increases in neck and shoulder sizes

A growth spurt occurs. Boys grow about 4 to 16 inches and gain 15 to 60 pounds. They usually stop growing between the ages of 18 and 21 years. Girls grow about 2 to 9 inches and gain between 15 and 50 pounds. They usually stop growing between the ages of 17 and 18 years. Some boys and girls continue to grow for a few more years.

Movements often seem awkward and clumsy. Growth of muscles and bones is uneven. Coordination and graceful movements develop as muscle and bone growth even out.

Changes in appearance are often hard to accept. Breast development can embarrass girls, especially if breasts are very large or small. Some do not like or want to wear a bra. Others wear clothes that will show off the breasts. Boys may worry about genital size. Height is a problem for both genders. Being small limits play in some sports. Boys do not like being shorter than their peers. Tall girls may feel embarrassed about being different and taller than other girls and boys.

Emotional reactions vary from high to low. Teenagers can be happy one moment and sad the next. It is hard to predict their reaction to a comment or event. They control emotions better later in this stage. Fifteen- to 18-year-olds can still become sad and depressed. However, they have more control over the time and place of emotional reactions.

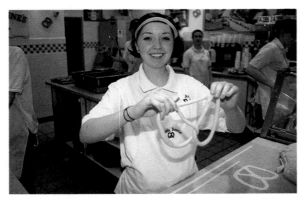

**FIG. 8-16** This teenager has a part-time job.

Adolescents need to become independent of adults, especially parents. They must learn to function, make decisions, and act responsibly without adult supervision. Many teenagers have part-time jobs or baby-sit (Fig. 8-16). They go to dances and parties, shop without an adult, and stay home alone. Many take part in school clubs and organizations.

Judgment and reasoning are not always sound. They still need guidance, discipline, and emotional and financial support from parents. The child and parents often disagree about behavior and activity restrictions and limits. Teenagers prefer being with peers than doing things with their family. They tend to confide in and seek advice from adults other than their parents.

Interests and activities reflect the need to become independent. They also reflect the need to develop relationships with the other sex and to act like males or females. Around age 15 to 17 years, a child may express homosexual feelings. Both sexes like parties, dances, and other social events. Clothing, makeup, and hairstyles are important. Baby-sitting or a part-time job may pay for clothes, makeup, and hair-care and skin-care products. Parents and teens rarely agree about clothing styles. Teenagers spend time experimenting with makeup and hairstyles. They spend time talking to friends on the phone, listening to music, and reading teen magazines.

Dating begins during adolescence. The age when dating begins varies. At first, dating is related to school events, such as a dance or football game. Group dating is common. The same group of girls just happens to be with the same group of boys. Pairing off and dating as a couple replaces group dating. Couples may be sexual partners.

Many difficult choices and conflicts result as teens mature physically, mentally, and emotionally. Parents and teens often disagree about dating. Parents worry about sexual activities, pregnancy, and sexually transmitted diseases. Teens usually do not understand or appreciate these concerns. "Going steady" helps meet security, love and belonging, and self-esteem needs. Teens may have problems controlling sexual urges and considering the consequences of sexual activity.

Adolescents begin to think about careers and what to do after high school. Interests, skills, and talents are some factors that influence the choice of college or getting a job.

Teens also need to develop morals, values, and attitudes for living in society. They need to develop a sense about good and bad, right and wrong, and the important and unimportant. Parents, peers, culture, religion, TV, school, and movies are some influencing factors. Drug abuse, unwanted pregnancy, alcoholism, and criminal acts are common among troubled teens.

# YOUNG ADULTHOOD (18 TO 40 YEARS)

Mental and social development continue during young adulthood. There is little physical growth. Adult height has been reached. Body systems are fully developed. Developmental tasks of young adulthood include:

- Choosing education and a career
- Selecting a partner
- Learning to live with a partner
- Becoming a parent and raising children
- Developing a satisfactory sex life

Education and career are closely related. Most jobs require certain knowledge and skills. The education needed depends on the career choice. Education usually increases job choices. Employment is needed for economic independence and to support a family.

Most adults marry at least once. Others choose to remain single. They may live alone or with friends of the same or opposite sex. Gay and lesbian persons may commit to a partner.

People marry for many reasons. They include love, emotional security, wanting a family, and sex. Some want to leave an unhappy home life. Some marry for social status, money, and companionship. Some marry to feel wanted, needed, and desirable.

Many factors also affect the selection of a partner. They include age, religion, interests, education, race, personality, and love. Some marriages or partnerships are happy and successful. Others are not. There are no guarantees that a relationship will work. Therefore partners must work together to build a relationship based on trust, respect, caring, and friendship.

Partners must learn to live together. Habits, routines, meals, and pastimes are changed or adjusted to "fit" the other person's needs. They must learn to solve problems and make decisions together. They need to work toward the same goals. Open and honest communication is needed for a successful partnership (Fig. 8-17, p. 130).

Adults also need to develop a satisfactory sex life. Sexual frequency, desires, practices, and preferences vary. For a satisfying and intimate relationship, a partner must understand and accept the other's needs.

With modern birth control methods, couples can plan when to have children and how many to have. Some pregnancies are unplanned. Some couples decide not to have children. Some have problems or cannot have children. The man or woman may have physical problems that prevent or interfere with pregnancy.

Most couples have a child early in their marriage. Some wait several years to start a family. Parents must agree on child-rearing practices and discipline methods. They need to adjust to the child and to the child's needs for parental time, energy, and attention.

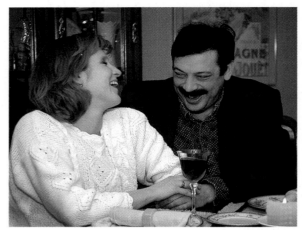

FIG. **8-17** Communication is needed for a successful partnership and satisfactory sex life.

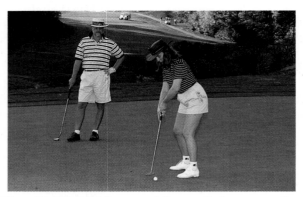

FIG. **8-18** Middle-age adults usually have more time for leisure activities.

## MIDDLE ADULTHOOD (40 TO 65 YEARS)

This stage is more stable and comfortable. Children usually are grown and have moved away. Partners have time to spend together. Worries about children and money are fewer. Developmental tasks relate to:
- Adjusting to physical changes
- Having grown children
- Developing leisure-time activities
- Adjusting to aging parents

Several physical changes occur. Many are gradual and go unnoticed. Others are seen early. Energy and endurance begin to slow down. So do metabolism and physical activities. Therefore weight control becomes a problem. Facial wrinkles and gray hair appear. It is common to need eyeglasses. Hearing loss may begin. Menstruation stops, and menstrual cycles end. This is called **menopause.** It occurs between the ages of 40 and 55 years. Ovaries stop secreting hormones. The woman cannot have children.

Many diseases and illnesses can develop. The disorders can become chronic or threaten life.

Children leave home for college, marry, move to their own homes, and start families. Adults have to cope with letting children go and being in-laws and grandparents. Parents must let children lead their own lives. However, they provide emotional support when needed.

These adults often have spare time as the demands of parenthood decrease. Hobbies and pastimes bring pleasure. They include gardening, fishing, painting, golfing, volunteer work, and being part of clubs and organizations (Fig. 8-18). These activities are even more important after retirement and during late adulthood.

Some middle-age adults have parents who are aging and in poor health. Responsibility for aging parents may begin during this stage. Many middle-age adults deal with the death of parents.

## LATE ADULTHOOD (65 YEARS AND OLDER)

Chapter 9 describes the many changes that occur in older persons. Developmental tasks of this stage are:
- Adjusting to decreased strength and loss of health
- Adjusting to retirement and reduced income
- Coping with a partner's death
- Developing new friends and relationships
- Preparing for one's own death

# ■ REVIEW QUESTIONS ■

Circle the **BEST** answer.

1 Changes in mental, emotional, and social function are called
   a Growth
   b Development
   c A reflex
   d A stage

2 Which is *false?*
   a Growth and development occur from the simple to the complex.
   b Growth and development occur in an orderly pattern.
   c Growth and development occur at a set pace.
   d Each stage has its own characteristics.

3 Which reflexes are needed for feeding in the infant?
   a The Moro and startle reflexes
   b The rooting and sucking reflexes
   c The grasping and Moro reflexes
   d The rooting and grasping reflexes

4 Which occurs first in infants?
   a Holding the head up
   b Rolling from front to back
   c Rolling from back to front
   d The pincer grasp

5 An infant can stand alone at about
   a 9 months
   b 10 months
   c 11 months
   d 12 months

6 Infants point and use gestures to communicate at around
   a 5 months
   b 7 months
   c 9 months
   d 11 months

7 Toilet training begins
   a During infancy
   b During the toddler years
   c When the primary caregiver is ready
   d At the age of 3 years

8 The toddler can
   a Use a spoon and cup
   b Ride a bike
   c Help set the table
   d Name parts of the body

9 Playing with other children begins during
   a Infancy
   b The toddler years
   c The preschool years
   d Middle childhood

10 Loss of baby teeth usually begins at the age of
   a 4 years
   b 5 years
   c 6 years
   d 7 years

11 Peer groups become important to
   a Toddlers
   b Preschool children
   c School-age children
   d Adolescents

12 Reproductive organs begin to function, and secondary sex characteristics appear. This is called
   a Late childhood
   b Adolescence
   c Puberty
   d Adulthood

13 Which is *false?*
   a Boys reach puberty earlier than girls.
   b Girls reach puberty between the ages of 9 and 15 years.
   c Menarche marks the onset of puberty in girls.
   d A growth spurt occurs during adolescence.

14 Dating usually begins
   a During late childhood
   b With group dating
   c With "pairing off"
   d During late adolescence

15 Adolescence is a time when parents and children
   a Talk openly about sex
   b Express love and affection
   c Disagree
   d Do things as a family

**16** Which is *not* a developmental task of young adulthood?
  a Adjusting to changes in the body and appearance
  b Selecting a partner
  c Choosing a career
  d Becoming a parent

**17** Middle adulthood is from about
  a 25 to 35 years
  b 30 to 40 years
  c 40 to 50 years
  d 40 to 65 years

**18** Middle adulthood is a time when
  a Families are started
  b Physical energy and free time increase
  c Children are grown and leave home
  d People need to prepare for death

*Answers to these questions are on p. 816.*

# 9

# Care of the
# Older Person

## OBJECTIVES

- Define the key terms listed in this chapter
- Describe the effects of retirement
- Identify the social changes common in older adulthood
- Describe the physical changes from aging and the care required
- Describe housing options for older persons
- Describe resident rights

## KEY TERMS

**geriatrics** The care of aging people

**gerontology** The study of the aging process

**involuntary seclusion** Separating a person from others against his or her will; keeping the person confined to a certain area or away from his or her room without consent

**old** Persons between 75 and 84 years of age

**old-old** Persons 85 years of age and older

**ombudsman** Someone who supports or promotes the needs and interests of another person

**young-old** Persons between 65 and 74 years of age

People live longer than ever before. They are healthier and more active. Today, one of every eight Americans is 65 years old or older. The U.S. Government reported that there were 34,500,000 older people in 1999. That is 3,300,000 more people than in 1990.

In 1998, a 65-year-old woman could expect to live 19 more years. A 65-year-old man could expect to live 16 more years. As you can see, women live longer than men. In 1999, there were 20,200,000 older women. There were 14,300,000 older men.

Most older people live in a family setting. They live with a partner, children, or other family. Some live alone or with friends. Others live in nursing centers. The need for nursing center care increases with aging. In 1997, only 1,470,000 (4.3%) of the people age 65 years or older lived in nursing centers.

Late adulthood involves these age ranges:
- **Young-old**—people between 65 and 74 years of age
- **Old**—people between 75 and 84 years of age
- **Old-old**—people 85 years of age and older

**Gerontology** is the study of the aging process. **Geriatrics** is the care of aging people. Aging is normal. Normal changes occur in body structure and function. They increase the risk for illness, injury, and disability. Psychological and social changes also occur. Most changes are slow. Most people adjust well to these changes. They lead happy, meaningful lives.

As stated in Chapter 8, the developmental tasks of late adulthood are:
- Adjusting to decreased strength and loss of health
- Adjusting to retirement and reduced income
- Coping with a partner's death
- Developing new friends and relationships
- Preparing for one's own death

## PSYCHOLOGICAL AND SOCIAL CHANGES

Graying hair, wrinkles, and slow movements are physical reminders of growing old. Retirement and deaths of loved ones are social reminders. Physical and social changes have psychological effects. They affect love and belonging and self-esteem needs.

People cope with aging in their own way. How they cope depends on:
- Health status
- Life experiences
- Finances
- Education
- Social support systems

## RETIREMENT

Age 65 is the usual retirement age. Some retire earlier. Others work into their 70s. Retirement is a reward for a lifetime of work. The person can relax and enjoy life (Fig. 9-1). Travel, leisure, and doing what one wants to are retirement "benefits." Many people enjoy retirement. Others are not so lucky. They may be ill or disabled. Poor health and medical bills can make retirement very hard.

Work helps meet love, belonging, and self-esteem needs. The person feels fulfilled and useful. Friendships form. Co-workers share daily events. Leisure time, recreation, and companionship often involve co-workers. Some retired people want to work. They have part-time jobs or do volunteer work (Fig. 9-2).

**REDUCED INCOME.** Retirement usually means reduced income. Social Security may provide the only income.

The retired person still has expenses. Rent or house payments continue. Food, clothing, utility bills, and taxes are other expenses. Car expenses, home repairs, drugs, and health care are other costs. So are entertainment and gifts.

Reduced income may force life-style changes. Examples include:
- Limiting social and leisure events
- Buying cheaper food, clothes, and household items
- Moving to cheaper housing
- Living with children or other family
- Avoiding health care or needed drugs
- Relying on children or other family for money or needed items

Severe money problems can result. Some people plan for retirement. They have savings, investments, retirement plans, and insurance. They are financially comfortable during retirement.

## SOCIAL RELATIONSHIPS

Social relationships change throughout life. *See Caring About Culture: Foreign-Born Persons.* Children grow up and leave home. They have their own families. Many live far away from parents. Older family and friends die, move away, or are disabled. Yet most older people have regular contact with children, grandchildren, family, and friends. Others are lonely. Separation from children is a common cause. So is lack of companionship with people their own age (Fig. 9-3).

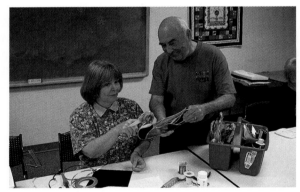

**FIG. 9-1** A retired couple enjoying arts and crafts together.

### CARING ABOUT CULTURE
#### FOREIGN-BORN PERSONS
Some older persons speak and understand a foreign language. Communication occurs with family and friends who speak the same language. They also share cultural values and practices. These relatives and friends may move away or die. The person may not have anyone to talk to. He or she may not be understood by others. The person feels greater loneliness and isolation.

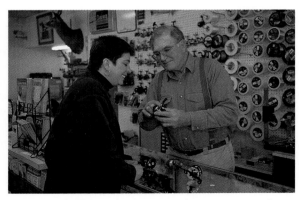

**FIG. 9-2** This retired man works at a sports shop.

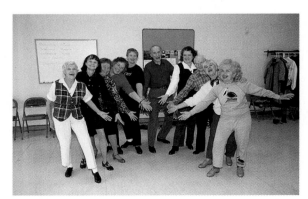

**FIG. 9-3** Older people enjoy being with people their own age.

Many older people adjust to these changes. Hobbies, church and community events, and new friends help prevent loneliness. Some communities and groups sponsor bus trips to ball games, shopping, plays, and concerts.

Grandchildren can bring great love and joy (Fig. 9-4). Family times help prevent loneliness. They help the older person feel useful and wanted (Fig. 9-5).

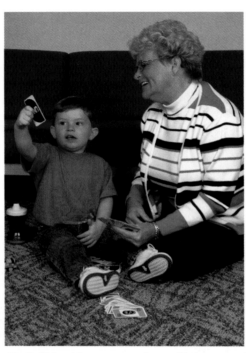

**FIG. 9-4** This older woman plays with her grandchild.

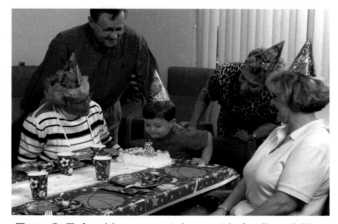

**FIG. 9-5** An older woman takes part in family activities.

## CHILDREN AS CAREGIVERS

Some children care for older parents. Parents and children change roles. The child cares for the parent. This helps some older persons feel more secure. Others feel unwanted, in the way, and useless. Some lose dignity and self-respect. Tensions may occur among the child, parent, and other household members. Lack of privacy is a cause. So are disagreements and criticisms about housekeeping, child rearing, cooking, and friends.

## DEATH OF A PARTNER

As couples age, the chances increase that a partner will die. Women usually live longer than men. Therefore many women become widows.

A person may try to prepare for a partner's death. When death occurs, the loss is crushing. No amount of preparation is ever enough for the emptiness and changes that result. The person loses a friend, lover, companion, and confidant. Grief may be very great. Serious physical and mental health problems can result. Some lose the will to live. Some attempt suicide.

## PHYSICAL CHANGES

Physical changes occur with aging. They happen to everyone (Box 9-1). Body processes slow down. Energy level and body efficiency decline. The rate and degree of change vary with each person. Influencing factors include diet, health, exercise, stress, environment, and heredity. The changes are slow and occur over many years. Often they are not seen for a long time. Some changes are caused by disease, illness, or injury.

## THE INTEGUMENTARY SYSTEM

The skin loses its elasticity, strength, and fatty tissue layer. The skin thins and sags. Folds, lines, and wrinkles appear. Oil and sweat secretions decrease. Dry skin occurs. The skin is fragile and easily injured. Skin breakdown, skin tears, and pressure ulcers are risks (Chapter 28). So are bruising and delayed healing. This is because blood vessels decrease in number.

Brown spots appear on the skin. They are called "age spots" or "liver spots." They are common on the wrists and hands.

The skin has fewer nerve endings. This affects the ability to sense heat, cold, and pain. Loss of the skin's fatty tissue layer also makes the person more sensitive to cold. Protect the person from drafts and cold. Sweaters, lap blankets, socks, and extra blankets are helpful. So are higher thermostat settings.

Dry skin causes itching. It is easily damaged. A shower or bath twice a week is enough for hygiene. Partial baths are taken at other times. Mild soaps or soap substitutes are used to clean the underarms,

## BOX 9-1 PHYSICAL CHANGES DURING THE AGING PROCESS

### INTEGUMENTARY SYSTEM

- Skin becomes less elastic
- Skin loses its strength
- Brown spots ("age spots" or "liver spots") on the wrists and hands
- Fewer nerve endings
- Fewer blood vessels
- Fatty tissue layer is lost
- Skin thins and sags
- Skin is fragile and easily injured
- Folds, lines, and wrinkles appear
- Decreased secretion of oil and sweat glands
- Dry skin
- Itching
- Increased sensitivity to heat and cold
- Decreased sensitivity to pain
- Nails become thick and tough
- Whitening or graying hair
- Facial hair in some women
- Loss or thinning of hair
- Drier hair

### MUSCULOSKELETAL SYSTEM

- Muscle atrophy
- Strength decreases
- Bone mass decreases
- Bone strength decreases
- Bones become brittle; can break easily
- Vertebrae shorten
- Joints become stiff and painful
- Hip and knee joints become flexed
- Gradual loss of height
- Decreased mobility

### NERVOUS SYSTEM

- Fewer nerve cells
- Slower nerve conduction
- Reflexes slow
- Reduced blood flow to the brain
- Progressive loss of brain cells
- Shorter memory
- Forgetfulness
- Slower ability to respond
- Confusion
- Dizziness
- Sleep patterns change
- Reduced sensitivity to touch
- Reduced sensitivity to pain

- Smell and taste decrease
- Eyelids thin and wrinkle
- Less tear secretion
- Pupils less responsive to light
- Decreased vision at night or in dark rooms
- Problems seeing green and blue colors
- Poor vision
- Changes in auditory nerve
- Eardrums atrophy
- High-pitched sounds not heard
- Decreased ear wax secretion
- Hearing loss

### CARDIOVASCULAR SYSTEM

- Heart pumps with less force
- Arteries narrow and are less elastic
- Less blood flows through narrowed arteries
- Weakened heart works harder to pump blood through narrowed vessels

### RESPIRATORY SYSTEM

- Respiratory muscles weaken
- Lung tissue becomes less elastic
- Difficulty breathing
- Decreased strength for coughing

### DIGESTIVE SYSTEM

- Decreased saliva production
- Difficulty in swallowing
- Decreased appetite
- Decreased secretion of digestive juices
- Difficulty digesting fried and fatty foods
- Indigestion
- Loss of teeth
- Decreased peristalsis causing flatulence and constipation

### URINARY SYSTEM

- Kidney function decreases
- Reduced blood supply to kidneys
- Kidneys atrophy
- Urine becomes concentrated
- Bladder muscles weaken
- Urinary frequency
- Urinary urgency may occur
- Urinary incontinence may occur
- Nighttime urination may occur

### REPRODUCTIVE SYSTEM

- See Chapter 37

genitals, and under breasts. Often soap is not used on the arms, legs, back, chest, and abdomen. Lotions, oils, and creams prevent drying and itching. Deodorants usually are not needed. Sweat gland secretion is decreased. See Chapter 16 for hygiene.

Nails become thick and tough. Feet usually have poor circulation. A nick or cut can lead to a serious infection. See Chapter 17 for nail and foot care.

Older persons often complain of cold feet. Socks provide warmth. Hot water bottles and heating pads are not used. Burns are great risks. Fragile skin, poor circulation, and decreased sensitivity to heat and cold increase the risk of burns.

White or gray hair is common. Hair loss occurs in men. Hair thins on men and women. Thinning occurs on the head, in the pubic area, and under the arms. Facial hair (lip and chin) may occur in women.

Hair is drier from decreases in scalp oils. Brushing promotes circulation and oil production. Shampoo frequency depends on personal choice. Usually it decreases with age. It is done as needed for hygiene and comfort.

Skin changes can be seen. Gray hair, hair loss, brown spots, and sagging skin are some examples. These changes can affect self-esteem and body image.

## THE MUSCULOSKELETAL SYSTEM

Muscle cells decrease in number. Muscles atrophy (shrink). They decrease in strength. Bones lose strength, become brittle, and break easily. Joints become stiff and painful. Sometimes just turning in bed can cause fractures (broken bones).

Vertebrae shorten. Hip and knee joints flex (bend) slightly. These changes cause gradual loss of height and strength. Mobility also decreases.

Older persons need to stay active. Activity, exercise, and diet help prevent bone loss and loss of muscle strength. Walking is good exercise. Exercise groups and range-of-motion exercises are helpful (Chapter 22). A diet high in protein, calcium, and vitamins is needed.

Bones can break easily. Protect the person from injury and prevent falls (Chapter 10). Turn and move the person gently and carefully. Some persons need help and support getting out of bed. Some need help walking.

## THE NERVOUS SYSTEM

Nerve cells are lost. Nerve conduction and reflexes slow. Responses are slower. For example, an older person slips. The message telling the brain of the slip travels slowly. The message from the brain to prevent the fall also travels slowly. The person falls.

Blood flow to the brain is reduced. Dizziness may occur. It increases the risk for falls. Practice measures to prevent falls (Chapter 10). Remind the person to get up slowly from the bed or chair. This helps prevent dizziness (Chapter 22).

Brain cells are lost over time. This affects personality and mental function. So does reduced blood flow to the brain. Memory is shorter. Forgetfulness increases. Responses slow. Confusion, dizziness, and fatigue may occur. Older people often remember events from long ago better than recent events. Many older people are mentally active and involved in current events. They show fewer personality and mental changes. (See Chapter 35 for a discussion of confusion and dementia.)

Sleep patterns change. Older persons have a harder time falling asleep. Sleep periods are shorter. They wake often during the night, and have less deep sleep. Less sleep is needed. Loss of energy and decreased blood flow cause fatigue. They may rest or nap during the day. They may go to bed early and get up early.

**THE SENSES.** Aging affects touch, smell, taste, sight, and hearing. Touch and sensitivity to pain and pressure are reduced. So is sensing heat and cold. These changes increase the risk for injury. The person may not notice painful injuries or diseases. Or the person feels minor pain. You need to:
- Protect older persons from injury (Chapter 10)
- Follow safety measures for heat and cold (Chapter 29)
- Check for signs of skin breakdown (Chapters 16 and 28)
- Give good skin care (Chapter 16)
- Prevent pressure ulcers (Chapter 28)

Taste and smell dull. Appetite decreases. Taste buds decrease in number. The tongue senses sweet, salty, bitter, and sour tastes. Sweet and salty tastes are lost first. Older people often complain that food has no taste. They like more salt and sugar on food.

**The eye.** Eyelids thin and wrinkle. Tear secretion is less. Therefore dust and pollutants can irritate the eyes.

The pupil becomes smaller and responds less to light. Vision is poor at night or in dark rooms. The eye takes longer to adjust to lighting changes. Vision problems occur when going from a dark to a bright room. They also occur when going from a bright to a dark room.

Clear vision is reduced. Eyeglasses are needed. The lens of the eye yellows. Therefore greens and blues are harder to see.

Older persons become more farsighted. The lens becomes more rigid with age. It is harder for the eye to shift from far to near vision and from near to far vision. These changes increase the risk of falls and accidents. The risk is greater on stairs and where lighting is poor. Eyeglasses are worn as needed. Keep rooms well lit. Night-lights help at night.

**The ear.** Changes occur in the auditory nerve. Eardrums atrophy (shrink). High-pitched sounds are hard to hear. Severe hearing loss occurs if these changes progress. A hearing aid may be needed. It must be clean and correctly placed in the ear.

Wax secretion decreases. Wax becomes harder and thicker. It is easily impacted (wedged in the ear). This can cause hearing loss. A doctor or nurse removes the wax.

## THE CARDIOVASCULAR SYSTEM

The heart muscle weakens. It pumps blood with less force. Problems may not occur at rest. Activity, exercise, excitement, and illness increase the body's need for oxygen and nutrients. A damaged or weak heart cannot meet these needs.

Arteries narrow and are less elastic. Less blood flows through them. Poor circulation occurs in many body parts. A weak heart must work harder to pump blood through narrowed vessels.

Exercise helps maintain health and well-being. Many older persons exercise daily. They walk, jog, golf, and bicycle. They also hike, ski, play tennis, swim, and play other sports. Older persons need to be as active as possible.

Sometimes circulatory changes are severe. Rest is needed during the day. Overexertion is avoided. The person should not walk far, climb many stairs, or carry heavy things. Personal care items, TV, phone, and other needed items are kept nearby. Some exercise helps circulation. It also prevents blood clots in leg veins. Some persons need to stay in bed. They need range-of-motion exercises (Chapter 22). Doctors may order certain exercises and activity limits.

## THE RESPIRATORY SYSTEM

Respiratory muscles weaken. Lung tissue becomes less elastic. Often lung changes are not noted at rest. Difficulty breathing may occur with activity. The person may lack strength to cough and clear the airway of secretions. Respiratory infections and diseases may develop. These can threaten the older person's life.

Normal breathing is promoted. Avoid heavy bed linens over the chest. They prevent normal chest expansion. Turning, repositioning, and deep breathing are important. They help prevent respiratory complications from bedrest. Breathing usually is easier in semi-Fowler's position (Chapter 13). The person should be as active as possible.

## THE DIGESTIVE SYSTEM

Salivary glands produce less saliva. This can cause difficulty swallowing. Taste and smell dull. This decreases appetite.

Secretion of digestive juices decreases. As a result, fried and fatty foods are hard to digest. They may cause indigestion.

Loss of teeth and ill-fitting dentures cause chewing problems. This causes digestion problems. Hard-to-chew foods are avoided. Ground or chopped meat is easier to chew.

Peristalsis decreases. The stomach and colon empty slower. Flatulence and constipation can occur (Chapter 19).

Dry, fried, and fatty foods are avoided. This helps swallowing and digestion problems. Oral hygiene and denture care improve taste. Some people do not have teeth or dentures. Their food is pureed or ground.

High-fiber foods help prevent constipation. However, they are hard to chew and can irritate the intestines. They include apricots, celery, and fruits and vegetables with skins and seeds. Persons with chewing problems or constipation often need foods that provide soft bulk. They include whole-grain cereals and cooked fruits and vegetables.

Fewer calories are needed. Energy and activity levels decline. More fluids are needed for chewing, swallowing, digestion, and kidney function. Foods are needed to prevent constipation and bone changes. High-protein foods are needed for tissue growth and repair. However, some older persons lack protein in their diets. High-protein foods (meat and fish) are costly.

## THE URINARY SYSTEM

Kidney function decreases. The kidneys shrink (atrophy). Blood flow to the kidneys is reduced. Waste removal is less efficient. Urine is more concentrated.

Bladder muscles weaken. Bladder size decreases. It holds less urine. Urinary frequency or urgency may occur. Many older persons have to urinate during the night. Urinary incontinence (inability to control the passage of urine from the bladder) may occur (Chapter 18).

In men, the prostate gland enlarges. This puts pressure on the urethra. Difficulty urinating or frequent urination occurs.

Urinary tract infections are risks. Adequate fluids are needed. The person needs water, juices, milk, and gelatin. Personal choice in fluids is important. Most fluids should be taken before 1700 (5:00 PM). This reduces the need to urinate during the night.

Persons with incontinence may need bladder training programs. Sometimes catheters are needed. See Chapter 18.

## THE REPRODUCTIVE SYSTEM

Changes occur in the reproductive system. See Chapter 37.

## FOCUS ON HOME CARE
### HOME CHANGES

Simple changes can make a home safe and easy to use. The nurse will discuss needed changes with the patient and family.

#### FOR LIMITED REACH

- Shelves lowered 3 inches or pull-down shelves
- Appliances within reach—side-by-side refrigerator/freezer, cook-top range, wall-mounted oven, dishwasher 8 inches off the floor
- Hand-held shower nozzle
- Peepholes or view panels at the correct height for the person
- Closet rods that adjust for height
- Pull-out drawers, bins, and baskets in closets and kitchens
- Electrical outlets 27 inches above the floor

#### FOR SMALL HANDS; FOR LIMITED FLEXIBILITY AND LIFTING

- Easy-to-grasp cabinet and drawer handles
- Grab bars by showers, tubs, and toilets
- Elevated toilet seats—17 to 18 inches high
- Shower seat; tub seat with transfer bench
- Lever faucet and door handles that operate with a push
- Keyless locking system
- Shelves near outside doors—the person can set items down to open the door
- Automatic garage door opener
- Rocker light switches that turn on and off with a push
- Spray attachment to kitchen sink—the person can fill pots after placing them on the stove

#### FOR POOR EYESIGHT

- Increase light bulb wattage
- Stove controls clearly marked and easy to see
- Lights in closets and stairways
- Outside lights by sidewalks, stairs, and doors
- Task lighting under cabinets and over counters
- Night-lights in bedrooms, bathrooms, and hallways
- Phone with a large keypad

#### FOR HEARING LOSS

- Increase phone volume
- Smoke detectors with strobe lights
- Text teletypewriters (TTYs) or Telecommunications Devices for the Deaf (TDDs). They are obtained from the phone company. The hearing-impaired person receives written messages (Fig. 9-6)
- Amplified phone handset—increases sound and makes the caller's voice louder
- Extension bells make the phone ring louder
- Doorbells are heard throughout the house

#### OTHER

- Handrails on stairways and outside steps
- No scatter or throw rugs
- Nonskid surfaces in showers and tubs
- Bathroom phone
- Rounded counter-tops
- Anti-scald devices on faucets and showerheads

From The American Association of Retired Persons.

## HOUSING OPTIONS

Most older persons live in their own homes. Many function without help. Others need help from family or community agencies. *See Focus on Home Care: Home Changes.*

There are many in-home and community-based services for older persons. Many are free. Others have a small fee. *See Focus on Home Care: In-Home and Community-Based Services.*

Some older persons choose to give up their homes. Others have to. Reduced income, taxes, home repairs, and yard work are factors. Some older people move to warmer climates. Others do not want a large home when children are gone. Some cannot care for themselves.

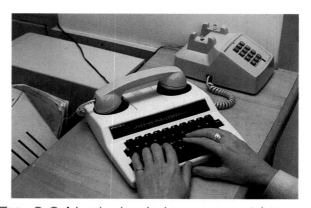

**FIG. 9-6** A hearing-impaired person uses a teletypewriter to communicate with a caller. The Americans With Disabilities Act of 1990 requires that every state must provide access to Telecommunications Relay Services (TRS). A communications assistant relays messages between the caller and the hearing-impaired person. Messages are typed to the hearing-impaired person. They are relayed orally to the caller. The communications assistant must relay everything that is said and maintain the confidentiality of all conversations.

## FOCUS ON HOME CARE
### IN-HOME AND COMMUNITY-BASED SERVICES

In-home and community-based services assist older persons with activities of daily living. Bathing, dressing, meals, housekeeping, shopping, and transportation are examples. Many services also provide social contact. These services are available in most areas:

- *Adult day care.* A program for those who cannot be alone during the day.
- *Case management.* A case manager assesses the needs of the older person and family. Arrangements are made for needed services.
- *Meal programs.* Meals are provided in-home or in a senior center. Home delivery programs are often called *Meals-on-Wheels.*
- *Financial counseling.* Help is given with checking accounts, paying bills, income taxes, and insurance forms and claims.
- *Companionship services.* A volunteer visits the older person at home. Supervision and support services are provided as needed.
- *Home health care.* Nursing and physical, occupational, and speech therapies are provided. So are housekeeping and medical equipment services.
- *Homemaker services.* Help is given with household tasks. Cleaning, laundry, shopping, and preparing meals are examples. Some people need help with personal care.
- *Hospice care.* See Chapter 1. Nursing, comfort, and homemaker services are provided.
- *Personal care.* Help is given with eating, bathing, oral care, grooming, and dressing.
- *Rehabilitation.* Therapies are given to assist the person to regain or maintain his or her highest level of functioning.
- *Senior centers.* These centers offer many social and recreational activities. Classes, day trips, travel groups, performing arts, and nature activities are examples. Services also include meals, counseling, legal help, health screening, and transportation.
- *Telephone reassurance.* Regular phone contact is provided. The person is called at various times during the day. If the person does not answer, someone is sent to the person's home. Also, the older person can call the service when help is needed.
- *Transportation.* Older persons are given rides to and from doctor visits, appointments, shopping, church, and other places.
- *Wellness programs.* Blood pressure, blood sugar, and other tests are done to promote health. Sessions are held about fitness, nutrition, and other health topics.

---

Leaving a home is often very hard. Family, memories, gardens, neighbors, friends, churches, parks, and shopping provide close ties to one's home and neighborhood. Moving, whether a short or long distance, brings many losses. When a person must move, losses are even greater.

There are many housing options for older persons. A new home setting should maintain or improve the person's quality of life.

## LIVING WITH FAMILY

Sometimes older brothers, sisters, and cousins live together. They:
- Provide companionship
- Share living expenses
- Provide care during illness or disability

Living with adult children is an option. The older parent (or parents) moves in with the child. Or the child moves to the parent's home. The parent may be healthy, may need some help, or may be ill or disabled. Some adult children give care to avoid nursing center care. A nursing center is an option if they cannot give needed care.

Living with an adult child is a social change. Everyone in the home must adjust. Sleeping plans may change if there is no spare bedroom. The parent may need a hospital bed. It can go in a living room, dining room, or bedroom.

The adult child's family needs time alone. Other family members may help give care. *Respite care* is an option. Respite means a break, rest, or lull. The person receives nursing center care or home care for weekends and vacations. Many community and church groups have volunteers who help give care.

**ADULT DAY CARE CENTERS.** Many adult children need to work even though the parent cannot stay alone. Adult day care centers provide meals, supervision, and activities. Some provide rides to and from the center. Some serve persons with Alzheimer's disease (Chapter 35).

Requirements vary. Some require that the person be able to walk. A cane or walker is used if needed. Others allow wheelchairs. Most require that the person perform some self-care.

Many activities are offered. Cards, board games,

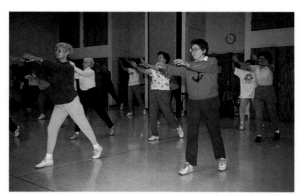

FIG. 9-7 This adult day care center has an exercise class.

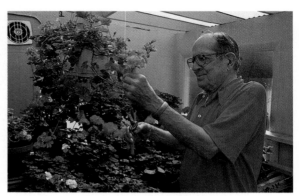

FIG. 9-8 This man enjoys gardening. Apartment living usually does not allow for gardening or yard work.

movies, crafts, dancing, walks, and lectures are common (Fig. 9-7). Some provide bowling and swimming. All activities are supervised. Needed help is given.

## ELDER COTTAGE HOUSING OPPORTUNITY (ECHO)

Elder Cottage Housing Opportunity (ECHO) homes are small homes designed for older and disabled persons. The portable home is placed in the yard of a single-family home. The older person lives independently but near family or friends.

## APARTMENTS

Some older persons like apartments. The owner provides maintenance, yard work, snow removal, and appliance repair. Older persons remain independent. They can keep personal items. However, rent and utility bills are costly. Many people enjoy gardening and yard work (Fig. 9-8). Apartment living usually does not provide those activities.

An *accessory apartment* is in a home. A home is built or remodeled to include a separate living area. It has a kitchen, bedroom, and bathroom. Some have a small living room. The older person lives independently but near other people. Some children have these apartments for older parents. Or the older person's home may have an apartment. Renting other living space gives the older person more income.

## CONGREGATE HOUSING

Congregate means a group, a gathering, or a cluster. Older people live in apartments near people of the same age. Buildings have wheelchair access, handrails, elevators, and other safety measures. Some apartments are furnished. Appliances are arranged to meet the needs of older persons.

There are many services. A doctor or nurse is on call. Someone checks on each person daily. A dining room is common. Rides are provided to church, the doctor, or shopping areas. Tenants pay monthly rent. If government funds are involved, rents are lower than for standard apartments.

## HOMESHARING

Two or more people share a house or apartment. Each person has a bedroom. They share other living space—kitchen, bathroom, living room. They share household chores and expenses. Or cooking, cleaning, and yard work are exchanged for rent.

Shared housing is a way to avoid living alone. It provides companionship. Some people feel safer when living with another person.

## ASSISTED LIVING

Assisted living facilities are for persons who need help with daily living (Chapter 39). They have their own apartments or rooms. They share dining and living room areas. They usually can walk. Some need help with meals, personal care, drugs, laundry, and housekeeping. The person has social contact with others in a homelike setting. Health care and 24-hour oversight are provided. Nursing care is not provided.

## BOARD AND CARE HOMES

Board and care homes provide a room, meals, laundry, and supervision. Each person has a room. They share common areas and eat meals together.

Some homes are for older persons. Others are for people with certain problems. Dementia, mental health problems, and developmental disabilities are examples.

## FOSTER CARE

Some families take older persons into their homes. The family provides help with daily living. A room, meals, and laundry are provided. Help is given with shopping and transportation. The person receives needed health care.

## CONTINUING CARE RETIREMENT COMMUNITIES

Continuing care retirement communities (CCRCs) offer many services. They range from independent living units to 24-hour nursing care. A CCRC has housing, activity, and health care services. It meets the changing needs of older persons living alone or with a partner. CCRCs usually provide:

- Nursing care and other health care services
- Meals (including special diets)
- Housekeeping
- Transportation
- Personal assistance
- Recreational and educational activities

Independent living units are small apartments. Residents perform self-care and take their own drugs. Food service is offered. Help is nearby if needed. Many people have their own cars. They travel or drive about as desired. Rides are provided for those who need them.

Services are added as the person's needs change. Over time, some persons need nursing care. They move into the nursing center within the CCRC. Many older couples find comfort in this plan. One partner needs nursing care. The other is close by and can visit often.

The person signs a contract with the CCRC. The contract is for a certain time or for the person's lifetime. The contract lists the services provided and the required fees.

## NURSING CENTERS

Some older persons cannot care for themselves. Nursing centers are options for them. Nursing centers provide nursing, rehabilitation, dietary, recreational, social, and religious services.

Some people stay in nursing centers until death. Others stay until they can return home. The nursing center is the person's temporary or permanent home. The setting is as homelike as possible (Fig. 9-9).

Nursing centers meet the needs of older and disabled persons. Physical changes of aging are considered in the center's design. So are safety needs (Chapter 10). Programs and services meet the person's basic needs. Box 9-2 lists the features of a quality nursing center.

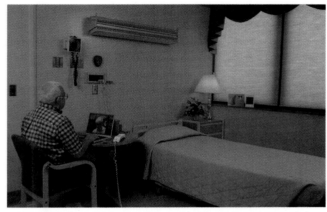

**FIG. 9-9** A nursing center is as homelike as possible.

---

**BOX 9-2 FEATURES OF A GOOD NURSING CENTER**

- The center has a current operating state license.
- The administrator has a current state license.
- The center is Medicare- and Medicaid-certified.
- The location suits the resident. Family and friends can visit easily.
- The center has safety features (Chapter 10). For example, hallways have handrails. Bathrooms and showers have grab bars.
- Exits are clearly marked. They are not obstructed.
- State and/or Federal fire codes are met.
- Resident rooms open to the hallway.
- Resident rooms have windows.
- A doctor is available for emergencies.
- No heavy odors are present. Scented sprays are not used to mask odors.
- Hallways are wide enough for 2 wheelchairs to pass with ease.
- Wheelchair ramps provide easy access into and out of the home.

- The kitchen has separate areas for food preparation, garbage, and dishwashing.
- There is enough refrigerator space for food.
- Toilet facilities allow wheelchair use.
- Dining rooms are attractive.
- Dining rooms allow wheelchair use.
- Food looks, smells, and tastes good.
- Residents receive needed help with eating if required.
- Residents look clean.
- Residents are dressed properly for a full day of activity and social interaction.
- There are attractive gardens and landscaping.
- There is an activity area for resident use.
- Staff is friendly and available to residents and visitors.
- There is a volunteer program.
- There is an active resident council.
- There is a residents' stated policy that identifies residents' individual rights.

Used with permission from the American Association of Homes and Services for the Aging.

---

**BOX 9-3** **OBRA ENVIRONMENT REQUIREMENTS**

**SUFFICIENT SPACE AND EQUIPMENT**

- Dining space with easy access. Tables and chairs are appropriate.
- Program areas with easy access. Equipment is appropriate.
- Recreational areas have easy access. There is enough space for movement and to store equipment and supplies.
- Toilet facilities have easy access. They are nearby.
- Furniture is comfortable and functional for residents, families, and visitors.
- Tables are of proper height.
- Chairs provide comfort. They allow ease of sitting and standing.
- Halls have handrails.
- Halls allow easy access for wheelchairs, walkers, and other space and safety needs.

**QUALITY OF LIFE AND COMFORT**

- The center is clean and orderly. This includes halls, dining rooms, health services, program and recreational areas, and bathrooms.

- The setting is odor-free.
- Temperature is between 71° and 81° F.
- Noise level is acceptable.
- Ventilation and humidity are adequate.
- There are no glares.
- There is music and TV as requested by the person or family.
- Paint color or wallpaper appeals to residents.
- The setting is pest-free and hazard-free.
- The person's needs are met.
- Linens are clean and soft. There is an adequate supply.
- Posted signs identify nonsmoking areas.

**RESIDENT ROOMS**

- See Chapter 14.

**SAFETY**

- See Chapter 10.

From Jaffe MS: *The OBRA guidelines for quality improvement,* ed 2, Aurora, Colo, 1996, Skidmore-Roth.

---

Federal and state agencies monitor the care given (Chapter 1). The center must follow standards required by law.

Most nursing centers receive Medicare or Medicaid funds. Such centers must meet the requirements of the Omnibus Budget Reconciliation Act of 1987 (OBRA). Funding is lost if they are not met. OBRA requirements are described throughout this book. Box 9-3 lists the OBRA requirements for a center's physical environment.

**HOSPITAL LONG-TERM CARE UNITS.** Many hospitals have long-term care units. They are for persons who need skilled care but not at the level once required. In time, some go home. Others transfer to nursing centers.

---

## RESIDENT'S RIGHTS

OBRA is a federal law. It applies to all 50 states. Nursing centers must provide care in a manner and in a setting that maintains or improves each person's quality of life, health, and safety. Resident rights are a major part of OBRA.

Nursing center residents have rights as United States citizens. They also have rights relating to their everyday lives and care in a nursing center. Nursing centers must protect and promote their rights. The center cannot interfere with their rights. Some residents are not competent (not able). They cannot exercise their rights. A responsible party (spouse or adult child) or legal representatives does so for them.

Nursing centers must inform residents of their rights. This is done orally and in writing. Such information is given before or during admission to the center. It is given in the language the person uses and understands. The following resident rights relate to your work.

### INFORMATION

The right to information means access to all records about the person. They include the medical record, contracts, incident reports, and financial records. The request for any record can be oral or written. The record is provided within 24 hours of the request. The center has 2 working days to provide requested photocopies.

The person has the right to be fully informed of his or her total health condition. Information is given in language the person can understand. Interpreters are used as needed. Sign language or other aids are used for those with hearing losses.

The person must also have information about his or her doctor. This includes the doctor's name, specialty, and how to contact the doctor.

Report any request for information to the nurse. You *do not* give the information described above to the person or family (Chapter 2).

## REFUSING TREATMENT

The person has the right to refuse treatment or to take part in research. Treatment means the care provided to relieve symptoms, improve function, or maintain or restore health. If a person does not give consent or refuses treatment, it cannot be given. The center must find out what the person is refusing and why. The center should try to teach the person about the treatment, problems from not having it, and other treatment choices. If a person refuses a certain treatment, the center must provide all other services.

Advance directives are part of the right to refuse treatment. They include living wills or instructions about life support. See Chapter 41.

Report any treatment refusal to the nurse. Care plan changes may be needed.

## PRIVACY AND CONFIDENTIALITY

Privacy and confidentiality are discussed in Chapters 2 and 3. They also are part of the AHA's *Patient Care Partnership: Understanding Expectations, Rights, and Responsibilities* (Chapter 6). They are rights under OBRA.

Residents have the right to personal privacy. The person's body is not exposed unnecessarily. Only staff directly involved in care and treatments are present. The person must give consent for others to be present. For example, a student wants to observe a treatment. The person's consent is needed for the student to observe.

A person has the right to use the bathroom in private. Privacy also is maintained for personal care measures.

Residents have the right to visit with others in private—in areas where others cannot see or hear them. If requested, the center must provide private space. Offices, chapels, dining rooms, and meeting rooms are used as needed.

The right to visit in private also involves mail and phone calls (Fig. 9-10). The person has the right to send and receive mail without others interfering. No one can open mail the person sends or receives without his or her consent. Mail is given to the person within 24 hours of its delivery to the center.

Information about the person's care, treatment, and condition is kept confidential. So are medical and financial records. Consent is needed to release them to other agencies or persons.

You must provide privacy and confidentiality. Doing so shows respect for the person. It also protects the person's dignity.

## PERSONAL CHOICE

Residents can choose their own doctors. They also have the right to take part in planning and deciding about their care and treatment. They have the right to choose activities, schedules, and care based on their preferences. They can decide when to get up and go to bed, what to wear, how to spend time, and what to eat (Fig. 9-11). They can choose friends and visitors inside and outside the center.

Personal choice promotes quality of life, dignity, and self-respect. You must allow personal choice whenever safely possible.

## DISPUTES AND GRIEVANCES

Residents have the right to voice concerns, questions, and complaints about treatment or care. The problem may involve another person. It may be about treatment or care that was not given. The center must promptly try to correct the matter. No one can punish the person in any way for voicing the dispute or grievance.

## WORK

The person does not work for care, care items, or other things or privileges. The person is not required to perform services for the center.

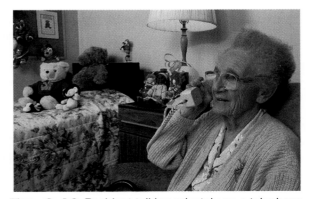

**FIG. 9-10** Resident talking privately on a telephone.

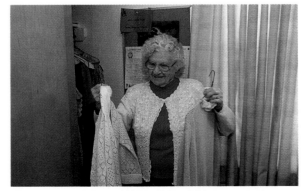

**FIG. 9-11** Resident choosing what clothing to wear.

However, the person *can* work or perform services if he or she wants to. A person may want to garden, repair or build things, sew, mend, or cook. Other persons need work for rehabilitation or activity reasons. The desire or need for work is part of the person's care plan. The care plan states:

- The reason for the work—desire or need
- What work will be done
- If services are paid or voluntary

## PARTICIPATION IN RESIDENT AND FAMILY GROUPS

Residents have the right to form and take part in resident and family groups. A person's family has the right to meet with other families. These groups can discuss concerns and suggest center improvements. They also can plan activities. They can provide support and comfort to group members.

Residents have the right to take part in social, cultural, religious, and community events. They have the right to help in getting to and from events of their choice.

## CARE AND SECURITY OF PERSONAL POSSESSIONS

Residents have the right to keep and use personal items. This includes clothing and some furnishings. The type and amount of personal items allowed depend on available space and the health and safety of others.

Treat the person's property with care and respect. The items may not have value to you. However, they are important to the person. They also relate to personal choice, dignity, and quality of life.

The center must protect the person's property. Items are labeled with the person's name. The center must investigate reports of lost, stolen, or damaged items. Police help is sometimes needed. The person and family are advised not to keep jewelry and other costly items in the center.

Protect yourself and the center from being accused of stealing a person's property. Do not go through a person's closet, drawers, purse, or other space without the person's knowledge and consent. A nurse may ask you to inspect closets and drawers. If so, have another worker with you and the person or legal representative. The worker is a witness to your activities.

## FREEDOM FROM ABUSE, MISTREATMENT, AND NEGLECT

Residents have the right to be free from verbal, sexual, physical, or mental abuse (Chapter 2). They also have the right to be free from involuntary seclusion. **Involuntary seclusion** is:

- Separating a person from others against his or her will
- Keeping the person confined to a certain area
- Keeping the person away from his or her room without consent.

No one can abuse, neglect, or mistreat a resident. This includes center staff, volunteers, staff from other agencies or groups, other residents, family members, visitors, and legal representatives. Nursing centers must investigate suspected or reported cases of abuse. Also, nursing centers cannot employ persons who were convicted of abusing, neglecting, or mistreating others.

## FREEDOM FROM RESTRAINT

Residents have the right not to have body movements restricted. Restraints and certain drugs can restrict body movements. Some drugs can restrain the person because they affect mood, behavior, and mental function. Sometimes residents are restrained to protect them from harming themselves or others. A doctor's order is needed for restraint use. Restraints are not used for staff convenience or to discipline a person. Restraints are discussed in Chapter 11.

## QUALITY OF LIFE

Nursing centers must care for residents in a manner that promotes dignity and self-esteem. It must also promote physical, psychological, and mental well-being. Protecting resident rights promotes quality of life. It shows respect for the person.

The person is spoken to in a polite and courteous manner (Chapter 6). Good, honest, and thoughtful care enhances the person's quality of life. Box 9-4 lists OBRA-required actions that promote dignity and privacy. Surveyors check for these actions in the person's care.

**ACTIVITIES.** Nursing centers provide activity programs that allow personal choice. They must promote physical, intellectual, social, spiritual, and emotional well-being. Many centers provide religious services for spiritual health. You assist residents to and from activity programs. You may need to help them with activities.

**ENVIRONMENT.** The center's environment must promote quality of life. It must be clean, safe, and as homelike as possible (Chapters 10 and 14). Letting the person have personal items enhances quality of life. It allows personal choice. It also promotes a homelike setting.

## OMBUDSMAN PROGRAM

The Older Americans Act is a federal law. It requires a long-term care ombudsman program in every state. An **ombudsman** is someone who supports or promotes the needs and interests of another person. Long-term care ombudsmen are employed by a state agency. Some are volunteers. They do not work at a nursing center. They act on behalf of nursing center and assisted-living residents.

Ombudsmen protect the health, safety, welfare, and rights of residents. They:
- Investigate and resolve complaints
- Provide services to assist residents
- Provide information about long-term care services
- Monitor nursing center care
- Monitor nursing center conditions
- Provide support to resident and family groups
- Educate residents, families, and the public about long-term care issues and concerns
- Represent residents' interests before local, state, and federal governments

Residents have the right to voice grievances and disputes. They also have the right to communicate privately with anyone of their choice. They can share concerns with anyone outside the center. Nursing centers must post the names, addresses, and phone numbers of local and state ombudsmen. This information must be posted where residents can easily see it.

A resident or family may share a concern with you. You must know state and center policies and procedures for contacting an ombudsman. Ombudsman services are useful when:
- There is concern about a person's care or treatment
- Someone interferes with a person's rights, health, safety, or welfare

---

**BOX 9-4  OBRA-REQUIRED ACTIONS TO PROMOTE THE RESIDENT'S DIGNITY AND PRIVACY**

### COURTEOUS AND DIGNIFIED INTERACTIONS
- Use the right tone of voice.
- Use good eye contact.
- Stand or sit close enough as needed.
- Use the person's proper name and title.
- Gain the person's attention before interacting with him or her.
- Use touch if the person approves.
- Respect the person's social status.
- Listen with interest to what the person is saying.
- Do not yell, scold, or embarrass the person.

### COURTEOUS AND DIGNIFIED CARE
- Groom hair, beards, and nails as the person wishes.
- Assist with dressing in the right clothing for time of day and personal choice.
- Promote independence and dignity in dining.
- Respect private space and property.
- Assist with walking and transfers without interfering with independence.
- Assist with bathing and hygiene preferences without interfering with independence:
  —Neat and clean appearance
  —Clean shaven or groomed beard
  —Nails trimmed and clean
  —Dentures, hearing aid, glasses, and other prostheses used correctly
  —Clothing is clean
  —Clothing is properly fitted and fastened
  —Shoes, hose, and socks are properly applied and fastened
  —Extra clothing for warmth as needed, such as sweater or lap blanket

### PRIVACY AND SELF-DETERMINATION
- Drape properly during care and procedures to avoid exposure and embarrassment.
- Drape properly in chair.
- Use curtains or screens during care and procedures.
- Close the door to room during care and procedures or as person desires.
- Knock on the door before entering. Wait to be asked in.
- Close the bathroom door when person uses the bathroom.

### MAINTAIN PERSONAL CHOICE AND INDEPENDENCE
- Person smokes in designated areas.
- Person takes part in activities according to interests.
- Person is involved in scheduling activities and care.
- Person gives input into care plan about preferences and independence.
- Person is involved in room or roommate change.

# ■ REVIEW QUESTIONS ■

Circle the **BEST** answer.

1  Retirement usually means
   a  Lowered income
   b  Changes from aging
   c  Companionship and usefulness
   d  Financial security

2  Which does *not* cause loneliness in older persons?
   a  Children moving away
   b  The death of family and friends
   c  Problems communicating with others
   d  Contact with other older persons

3  Older people living with their children often feel
   a  Independent
   b  Wanted and a part of things
   c  Useless
   d  Dignified

4  These statements are about a partner's death. Which is *false?*
   a  The person loses a lover, friend, companion, and confidant.
   b  Preparing for the event lessens grief.
   c  The survivor may develop health problems.
   d  The survivor's life will likely change.

5  Changes occur in the skin with aging. Care should include the following *except*
   a  Providing for warmth
   b  Applying lotion
   c  Using soap daily
   d  Providing good skin care

6  An older person has cold feet. You should
   a  Provide socks
   b  Apply a hot water bottle
   c  Soak the feet in hot water
   d  Apply a heating pad

7  Aging causes changes in the musculoskeletal system. Which is *false?*
   a  Bones become brittle and can break easily.
   b  Bedrest is needed for loss of strength.
   c  Joints become stiff and painful.
   d  Exercise slows musculoskeletal changes.

8  Reduced blood supply to the brain can result in the following *except*
   a  Confusion
   b  Dizziness
   c  Improved memory
   d  Fatigue

9  Changes occur in the nervous system. Which is *true?*
   a  Less sleep is needed than when younger.
   b  The person forgets recent events.
   c  Sensitivity to pain increases.
   d  Confusion occurs in all older persons.

10  Arteries lose their elasticity and become narrow. These changes result in
   a  A slower heart rate
   b  Lower blood pressure
   c  Poor circulation to many body parts
   d  Less blood in the body

11  An older person has cardiovascular changes. Care includes the following *except*
   a  Placing needed items nearby
   b  A moderate amount of daily exercise
   c  Avoiding exertion
   d  Walking long distances

12  Respiratory changes occur with aging. Which is *false?*
   a  Heavy bed linens are avoided.
   b  The person is turned often if on bedrest.
   c  The side-lying position is best for breathing.
   d  The person should be as active as possible.

13  Older persons should avoid dry foods because of
   a  Decreases in saliva
   b  Loss of teeth or ill-fitting dentures
   c  Decreased amounts of digestive juices
   d  Decreased peristalsis

14  Changes occur in the digestive system. Older persons should eat
   a  Fruits and vegetables with skins and seeds
   b  Dry and fatty foods
   c  Raw apricots and celery
   d  Protein foods

**15** The doctor ordered increased fluid intake for an older person. You should
  **a** Give most of the fluid before 1700 (5:00 PM)
  **b** Provide mostly water
  **c** Start a bladder training program
  **d** Insert a catheter

**16** You are working in a nursing center. You must
  **a** Open a person's mail
  **b** Choose what the person wears
  **c** Provide for the person's privacy
  **d** Search the person's closet and drawers

**17** Who decides how to style a person's hair?
  **a** The person
  **b** The nurse
  **c** You
  **d** The ombudsman

**18** Residents can do the following *except*
  **a** Choose their nursing team
  **b** Contact an ombudsman
  **c** Voice concerns
  **d** Make personal choices

*Answers to these questions are on p. 816.*

# Safety

## OBJECTIVES

- Define the key terms listed in this chapter
- Describe accident risk factors
- Identify safety measures for infants and children
- Explain why you identify a person before giving care
- Explain how to accurately identify a person
- Describe the safety measures to prevent falls, burns, poisoning, and suffocation
- Explain how to prevent equipment accidents
- Explain how to handle hazardous substances
- Describe safety measures for fire prevention and oxygen use
- Explain what to do during a fire
- Give examples of natural and human-made disasters
- Explain how to protect yourself from workplace violence
- Describe your role in risk management
- Perform the procedure described in this chapter

## KEY TERMS

**coma** A state of being unaware of one's surroundings and being unable to react or respond to people, places, or things

**disaster** A sudden catastrophic event in which many people are injured and killed and property is destroyed

**electric shock** When electrical current passes through the body

**ground** That which carries leaking electricity to the earth and away from an electrical item

**hazardous substance** Any chemical in the workplace that can cause harm

**hemiplegia** Paralysis on one side of the body

**paraplegia** Paralysis from the waist down

**quadriplegia** Paralysis from the neck down

**suffocation** When breathing stops from the lack of oxygen

**workplace violence** Violent acts (including assault or threat of assault) directed toward persons at work or while on duty

Safety is a basic need. Patients and residents are at great risk for falls and other accidents. Falls can cause serious injury. Some accidents and injuries cause death.

Common sense and simple safety measures can prevent most accidents. You must protect patients and residents, yourself, and co-workers. The safety measures in this chapter apply to everyday life. They apply to hospital, long-term care, and home settings. The nursing care plan lists other safety measures needed by the person.

## THE SAFE ENVIRONMENT

In a safe setting, a person has little risk of illness or injury. The person feels safe and secure physically and mentally. The risk of infection, falls, burns, poisoning, or other injuries is low. Temperature and noise levels are comfortable. Smells are pleasant. There is enough room and light to move about safely. The person and the person's property are safe from fire and intruders. The person is not afraid. He or she has few worries and concerns.

# ACCIDENT RISK FACTORS

Some people cannot protect themselves. They rely on others for safety. You need to know the factors that increase a person's risk of accidents and injuries. Follow the person's care plan.

- *Awareness of surroundings.* People need to know their surroundings to protect themselves from injury. A coma can occur from illness or injury. **Coma** is a state of being unaware of one's surroundings or being unable to react or respond to people, places, or things. The person relies on others for protection. Confused and disoriented persons may not understand what is happening to and around them (Chapter 35). They can harm themselves and others.
- *Impaired vision.* Poor vision can lead to falls. A person may not see toys, rugs, furniture, or cords. Some have problems reading labels on cleaners and other containers. Poisoning can result. It can also result from taking the wrong drug or the wrong dose.
- *Impaired hearing.* Persons with impaired hearing have problems hearing explanations and instructions. They may not hear warning signals or fire alarms. Some cannot hear approaching meal carts, drug carts, stretchers, or people in wheelchairs. They do not know to move to safety.
- *Impaired smell and touch.* Illness and aging affect smell and touch. The person may not detect smoke or gas odors. When touch is reduced, burns are a risk. The person has problems sensing heat and cold. Some people have a decreased pain sense. They may be unaware of injury. For example, Mrs. Jones does not feel a blister from new shoes. She has poor circulation to her legs and feet. The blister can become a serious wound.

---

### FOCUS ON CHILDREN
#### ACCIDENT RISK FACTORS

Infants are helpless. Young children have not learned the difference between safety and danger. They explore their surroundings, put objects in their mouths, and touch and feel new things. They are at risk for falls, poisoning, choking, burns, and other accidents. Practice the safety measures in Box 10-1.

---

### FOCUS ON OLDER PERSONS
#### ACCIDENT RISK FACTORS

Changes from aging increase the risk for falls and other injuries. Movements are slower and less steady. Balance may be affected. Older persons are less sensitive to heat and cold. Poor vision, hearing problems, and dulled sense of smell are common. Confusion, poor judgment, memory problems, and disorientation may occur (Chapter 35).

---

- *Impaired mobility.* Some diseases and injuries affect mobility. A person may be aware of danger but cannot move to safety. Some persons cannot walk or propel wheelchairs. Some persons are paralyzed. **Paraplegia** is paralysis from the waist down. **Quadriplegia** is paralysis from the neck down. **Hemiplegia** is paralysis on one side of the body.
- *Drugs.* Drugs have side effects. They include loss of balance, drowsiness, and lack of coordination. Reduced awareness, confusion, and disorientation also can occur. The person may be fearful and uncooperative. Report behavior changes to the nurse. Also report the person's complaints.
- *Age.* Children and older persons are at risk for injuries. *See Focus on Children: Accident Risk Factors. See Focus on Older Persons: Accident Risk Factors.*

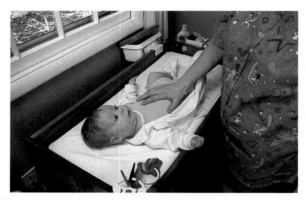

**FIG. 10-1** Keep one hand on a child lying in a crib or on a scale, bed, table, or other furniture.

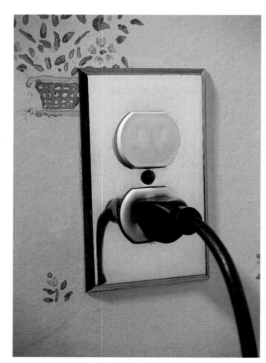

**FIG. 10-2** Safety plug in an outlet.

## BOX 10-1  SAFETY MEASURES FOR INFANTS AND CHILDREN

### GENERAL SAFETY

- Do not leave infants and children unattended. Supervise them at all times.
- Avoid baby walkers on wheels.
- Use the safety strap to fasten a child in a highchair or infant carrier seat.
- Lock the highchair tray after putting the child in the chair.
- Keep highchairs away from stoves, tables, and counters.
- Do not hang items with strings, cords, or elastic cords around cribs or playpens.
- Keep childproof caps on drugs and other harmful substances.
- Store knives (including kitchen knives), razor blades, matches, guns, tools, and other dangerous items where children cannot reach them. Keep them in locked storage areas.
- Do not prop baby bottles on a rolled towel or blanket. Hold the baby and bottle during feedings.
- Use safety gates at the top and bottom of stairs. They prevent small children from climbing up and down stairs. Make sure the child cannot get caught in the gate slats.
- Keep one hand on a child lying in a crib or on a scale, bed, table, or other furniture (Fig. 10-1).
- Keep one hand on the baby when changing a diaper.
- Read all package and label instructions. Follow the manufacturer's instructions.

### BEDROOM SAFETY

- Check infants often when in cribs.
- Make sure crib rails are up and locked in place when the baby is in the crib.
- Do not use a crib with loose, broken, or missing parts. This includes screws, nuts, and bolts.
- Make sure bunk beds and ladders are fastened and supported properly.
- Do not let children younger than 6 years sleep on the top bunk.
- Check bunk bed guardrails. Spaces between the slats should be less than 3.5 inches. Guardrails should raise at least 5 inches above the mattress.
- Keep bedroom doors closed. Bedrooms of older children and parents may contain toys, perfumes, and other items that present hazards to young children. Choking, poisoning, burns, and suffocation are risks.

### ELECTRICAL SAFETY

- Keep electrical items away from sinks, tubs, toilets, and other water sources.
- Unplug electrical items when not in use.
- Place safety plugs in outlets (Fig. 10-2). This includes electrical strips and surge protectors. Children cannot stick fingers or small objects into the openings.
- Keep electrical cords and electrical items out of the reach of children.

### WINDOW SAFETY

- Install safety guards on windows.
- Keep cords for window drapes, blinds, and shades out of the reach of children. Be careful where you place cribs and playpens.
- Keep children away from open windows. Do not let them sit on windowsills. Window screens are not strong enough to prevent children from falling out of windows.
- Do not place a crib or furniture near windows. This prevents children from climbing from furniture onto a window seat or sill.

### WATER SAFETY

- Supervise any child who is in or near water. This includes tubs, toilets, sinks, buckets and containers, wading pools, swimming pools, hot tubs, spas, and whirlpools.
- Keep bathroom doors closed to prevent drowning in toilets or bathtubs.
- Keep sinks, tubs, and basins empty when not in use.
- Keep buckets, containers, and wading pools empty and upside down when not in use.
- Keep toilet lids down. Use toilet safety locks.
- Keep diaper pails locked.
- Keep a locked safety cover on spas, hot tubs, and whirlpools when not in use.
- Remove pool, spa, hot tub, and whirlpool covers before use. The cover must be completely off. If not, the child can get trapped under the cover.
- Remove steps to above-ground pools when not in use.
- Have a phone by the pool, spa, hot tub, and whirlpool.
- Keep rescue equipment near pools.
- Do not let children dive into above-ground pools. They are too shallow. For safe diving, water must be 9 feet deep or greater.
- Have children enter an in-ground pool feet first. The water is shallow.
- Teach safe diving. Children should dive only from the diving board. They should dive with their hands in front of them.
- Do not let children slide down a pool slide head first. Head injuries can occur.
- Prevent hair entanglement or body part entrapment in pools, spas, hot tubs, and whirlpools. They can occur in suction and drain covers. If hair is caught, the head is kept underwater. Trapped body parts can keep the person underwater or cause serious injury. Have suction and drain covers installed that meet current safety standards. Replace missing or broken covers. Do not let children play near drain or suction covers.
- Know where to find the power cut-off switch for pools, spas, hot tubs, and whirlpools. You must quickly turn off the electricity in an emergency.
- Keep hot tub, spa, and whirlpool temperatures no higher than 104° F. Higher temperatures can cause drowsiness, which can lead to drowning. Heat stroke and death are other risks.

*Continued.*

## BOX 10-1 SAFETY MEASURES FOR INFANTS AND CHILDREN—CONT'D

### VEHICLE SAFETY

- Lock your vehicle doors and trunk. Keep keys where children cannot see or reach them. They can open a door or trunk with a remote control key.
- Do not let children play in vehicles. They like to play hide-and-seek in cars and car trunks. They can easily suffocate and die from high temperatures in the car or trunk.
- Keep any access to the trunk closed. Some vehicles have fold-down seats that give more trunk space. Children can get into the trunk from inside the car.
- Do not leave children unattended in a car, truck, van, or other motor vehicle. They can develop heat-related illness, suffocate, and die very quickly from high temperatures in the vehicle. It takes only a few minutes.
- Use federally approved car restraints that fit the child's size and weight (Fig. 10-3). Follow the manufacturer's instructions.
- Do not use a car safety seat that does not have manufacturer's instructions.
- Use a car safety seat that has a label with the manufacturer's name, model number, or the date it was made.
- Install infant car safety seats rear-facing only (Fig. 10-4). Infants ride this way until they are at least 20 pounds and at least 1 year old.
- Do not use a rear-facing car or convertible seat in the front seat of a vehicle with an air bag.
- Do not use a car safety seat that is more than 10 years old. Check the label for the date it was made.
- Do not use a car safety seat that was involved in a crash.
- Do not use a car safety seat that has cracks, missing parts, or torn or loose harnesses and buckles.
- Use booster seats for children between the ages of 4 and 8 years. Secure them with lap and shoulder belts.
- Have children younger than 12 years ride in the back seat.
- Follow seat-belt laws.

### CLOTHING SAFETY

- Do not use pins on children's clothing.
- Remove drawstrings from jackets, coats, sweaters, and other clothing. This includes drawstrings on the hood, at the neckline, and at the waist. Drawstrings can get tangled or caught in play equipment, furniture, handrails, car or bus doors, elevators, escalators, and other moving devices.
- Do not dress children in loose clothing or clothing with drawstrings, fringe, strings, or ties if they will use playground equipment. The clothing can get caught on the equipment.
- Do not let children wear necklaces, strings, cords, or other items around the neck. These can get caught on furniture, doorknobs, and playground equipment.

### TOY AND PLAY SAFETY

- Do not let children play on curbs or behind parked cars.
- Do not let children play in piles of leaves or snow near heavy traffic.
- Keep children away from exercise bikes and equipment.
- Read all warning labels on toys.
- Check age recommendations on toys. Give children only age-appropriate toys.
- Check toys and other play equipment regularly. Look for cracks, chips, breaks, sharp edges, loose parts, and other damage. This includes playground equipment.
- Do not let children play with toys that shoot objects into the air.
- Do not let children play with toys that make loud, sharp, or shrill noises. They could damage hearing.
- Do not let children play with toys that have long strings, straps, or cords. Strings, straps, and cords should be less than 7 inches long.
- Keep older children's toys away from infants and younger children.
- Make sure toys are too large to fit into the child's mouth.
- Do not let children use riding toys near stairs, pools, or traffic.
- Make sure children wear safety gear as needed. This includes helmets, elbow and knee pads, wrist guards, and reflective shoes and clothing.

### FURNITURE SAFETY

- Prevent furniture from tipping over. Injuries and deaths can occur from children falling on, leaning on, climbing on, pulling on, sitting on, or trying to move poorly secured furniture. TV carts, bookcases, stands, chests-of-drawers, and tables present dangers.
- Make sure TVs are placed on low stands and are as far back on the stand as possible.
- Make sure that angle-braces or anchors are used to secure furniture to walls.
- Do not use tablecloths and placemats. This prevents infants and young children from pulling things off the table and onto themselves. Center pieces, items on the table, and hot food and liquids can injure the child.
- Do not use toy chests with free-falling lids. Such a lid can fall on the child's head or neck. The lid should have a spring-loaded lid-support or sliding panels.

### OTHER

- Protect the child from falls (Box 10-3).
- Protect the child from burns (p. 161).
- Protect the child from poisoning (p. 161).
- Protect the child from choking and suffocating (p. 163).
- See Chapter 38 for other infant safety measures.

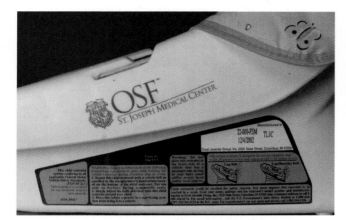

**FIG. 10-3** Federally approved car safety seats carry this label.

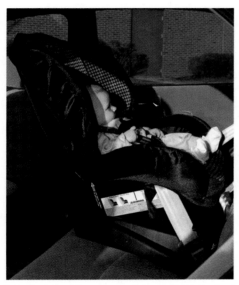

**FIG. 10-4** Infant in a car safety seat. Note that the seat is rear-facing.

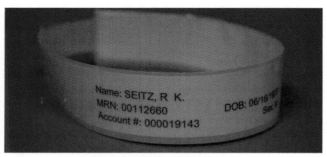

**FIG. 10-5** ID bracelet.

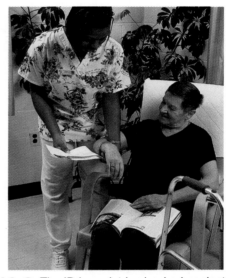

**FIG. 10-6** The ID bracelet is checked against the assignment sheet to accurately identify the person.

> **FOCUS ON LONG-TERM CARE**
> IDENTIFYING THE PERSON
>
> Alert and oriented nursing center residents may choose not to wear ID bracelets. This is noted on the person's care plan. Follow center policy and the care plan to identify the person.
>
> Some nursing centers have a photograph ID system. The person's photo is taken on admission. Then it is placed in the person's medical record. If your center uses such a system, learn to use it safely.

# IDENTIFYING THE PERSON

You will care for many people. Each has different treatments, therapies, and activity limits. You must give the right care to the right person. Life and health are threatened if the wrong care is given.

The person receives an identification (ID) bracelet when admitted to the agency (Fig. 10-5). The bracelet has the person's name, room and bed number, birth date, age, and doctor. Known allergies and the agency's name are included. Some agencies include the person's religion.

You use the ID bracelet to identify the person before giving care. The assignment sheet or treatment card states what care to give. To identify the person:

- Compare identifying information on the assignment sheet or treatment card with that on the ID bracelet

(Fig. 10-6). Carefully check the person's full name. Some people have the same first and last names. For example, John Smith is a very common name.

- Call the person by name when checking the ID bracelet. This is a courtesy given as you touch the person and before giving care. However, just calling the person by name is not enough to identify him or her. Confused, disoriented, drowsy, hearing-impaired, or distracted persons may answer to any name.

*See Focus on Long-Term Care: Identifying the Person.*

# PREVENTING FALLS

Most falls occur in bedrooms and bathrooms. Throw rugs, poor lighting, cluttered floors, out-of-place furniture, and pets underfoot are causes. So are slippery floors, bathtubs, and showers. Needing to urinate also is a major cause of falls. For example, Mrs. Ford has an urgent need to urinate. She falls trying to get to the bathroom.

The risk of falling increases with age. Persons older than 65 years are at high risk. A history of falls increases the risk of falling again.

Most falls occur in the evening, between 1800 (6:00 PM) and 2100 (9:00 PM). Falls also are more likely during shift changes. During shift changes, staff are busy going off and coming on duty. Confusion can occur about who gives care and answers signal lights. Shift change times vary among agencies. They often occur between these hours:

- 0600 (6:00 AM) and 0800 (8:00 AM)
- 1400 (2:00 PM) and 1600 (4:00 PM)
- 2200 (10:00 PM) and 2400 (midnight)

Besides the accident risk factors (p. 152), other problems can increase a person's risk of falling (Box 10-2). Therefore agencies have fall prevention programs. Box 10-3 lists measures that are part of fall prevention programs and care plans. The care plan also lists measures for the person's risk factors.

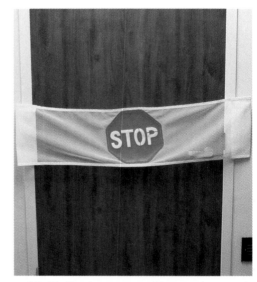

**FIG. 10-7** Barriers are used to prevent wandering.

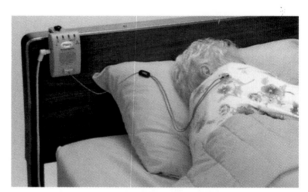

**FIG. 10-8** Bed alarm.

| BOX 10-2 FACTORS INCREASING THE RISK OF FALLS | |
|---|---|
| • A history of falls<br>• Weakness<br>• Slow reaction time<br>• Poor vision<br>• Confusion<br>• Disorientation<br>• Decreased mobility<br>• Foot problems<br>• Shoes that fit poorly<br>• Elimination needs<br>• Urinary incontinence<br>• Dizziness and lightheadedness<br>• Dizziness on standing<br>• Joint pain and stiffness<br>• Muscle weakness<br>• Low blood pressure<br>• Balance problems | • Drug side effects:<br>—Low blood pressure when standing or sitting<br>—Drowsiness<br>—Fainting<br>—Dizziness<br>—Poor coordination<br>—Unsteadiness<br>—Frequent urination<br>—Confusion and disorientation<br>• Vision problems<br>• Overuse of alcohol<br>• Depression<br>• Strange setting<br>• Poor judgment<br>• Memory problems<br>• Care equipment (IV poles, drainage tubes and bags, and others)<br>• Improper use of wheelchairs, walkers, canes, and crutches |

**BOX 10-3** **SAFETY MEASURES TO PREVENT FALLS**

## BASIC NEEDS

- Fluid needs are met.
- Glasses and hearing aids are worn as needed. Reading glasses are not worn when up and about.
- Help is given with elimination needs. It is given at regular times and whenever requested. Assist the person to the bathroom. Or provide the bedpan, urinal, or commode.
- The bedpan, urinal, or commode is kept within easy reach if the person can use the device without help.
- A warm drink, soft lights, or a back massage is used to calm the person who is agitated.
- Barriers are used to prevent wandering (Fig. 10-7).
- The person is properly positioned when in bed, a chair, or a wheelchair. Use pillows, wedge pads, or seats as the nurse and care plan direct (Chapter 13).
- Correct procedures are used for transfers (Chapter 13).

## BATHROOMS

- Tubs and showers have nonslip surfaces or nonslip bath mats.
- Safety rails and grab bars are in showers. They are by tubs and toilets.
- Bathrooms have hand rails.
- Shower chairs are used (Chaper 16).
- Safety measures for tub baths and showers are followed (Chapter 16).

## FLOORS

- Floors have wall-to-wall carpeting or carpeting that is tacked down.
- Scatter, area, and throw rugs are not used.
- Floor coverings are one color. Bold designs can cause dizziness in older persons.
- Floors have nonglare, nonslip surfaces.
- Nonskid wax is used on hardwood, tiled, or linoleum floors.
- Report loose floor boards and tiles. Report frayed rugs and carpets.
- Floors and stairs are free of clutter. They are free of items that can cause tripping—toys, cords, and other items.
- Floors are free of spills. Wipe up spills at once.
- Floors are free of excess furniture and equipment.
- Electric and extension cords are out of the way.
- Equipment and supplies are kept on one side of the hallway.

## FURNITURE

- Furniture is placed for easy movement.
- Furniture is not rearranged.
- Chairs have armrests. Armrests give support when sitting and standing.
- A telephone and lamp are at the bedside.

## HOSPITAL BEDS AND OTHER EQUIPMENT

- The bed is in the lowest horizontal position, except when giving bedside care. The distance from the bed to the floor is reduced if the person falls or gets out of bed.
- Bed rails are used according to the care plan.
- Wheelchairs, walkers, and canes fit properly. Another person's equipment is not used.
- Crutches, canes, and walkers have nonskid tips.
- Correct equipment is used for transfers (Chapter 13). Follow the care plan.
- Wheel locks on beds, wheelchairs, and stretchers are in working order.
- Bed wheels are locked for transfers.
- Wheelchair and stretcher safety measures are followed (p. 166).

## LIGHTING

- Rooms, hallways, stairways, and bathrooms have good lighting.
- Light switches (including in bathrooms) are within reach and easy to find.
- Night-lights are in bedrooms, hallways, and bathrooms.

## SHOES AND CLOTHING

- Nonskid footwear is worn. Socks, bedroom slippers, and long shoelaces are avoided.
- Clothing fits properly. Clothing is not loose. It does not drag on the floor. Belts are tied or secured in place.

## SIGNAL LIGHTS AND ALARMS

- The person is taught how to use the signal light (Chapter 14).
- The signal light is always within the person's reach.
- The person is asked to call for assistance when help is needed in getting out of bed or a chair or when walking.
- Signal lights are answered promptly. The person may need help right away. He or she may not wait for help.
- Bed and chair alarms are used. They sense when the person tries to get up (Fig. 10-8).
- Respond to bed and chair alarms at once.

## OTHER

- The person is checked often. Careful and frequent observation is important.
- Frequent checks are made on persons with poor judgment or memory.
- Persons at risk for falling are in rooms close to the nurses' station.
- Hand rails are on both sides of stairs and hallways. They also are in bathrooms.
- Family and friends are asked to visit during busy times. They are asked to visit during the evening and night shifts.
- Companions are provided. Sitters, companions, or volunteers are with the person.
- Tasks and procedures are explained before and while performing them.
- Nonslip strips are on the floor next to the bed and in the bathroom. They are intact.
- Caution is used when turning corners, entering corridor intersections, and going through doors. You could injure a person coming from the other direction.
- Pull (do not push) wheelchairs, stretchers, carts, and other wheeled equipment through doorways. This allows you to lead the way and to see where you are going.
- A safety check is made of the room after visitors leave. They may have lowered a bed rail, removed the signal light, or moved a walker out of reach. Or they may have brought an item that could harm the person.

## BED RAILS

Bed rails (side rails) on hospital beds are raised and lowered. They lock in place with levers, latches, or buttons. Bed rails are half, three quarters, or the full length of the bed. When half-length rails are used, each side may have two rails. One is for the upper part of the bed and the other for the lower part.

The nurse and care plan tell you when to raise bed rails. They are needed by persons who are unconscious or sedated with drugs. Some confused or disoriented people need them. If a person needs bed rails, keep them up at all times except when giving bedside care.

Bed rails present hazards. The person can fall when trying to climb over them. Or the person cannot get out of bed to use the bathroom. Entrapment is a risk (Fig. 10-9). That is, a person can get caught, trapped, or entangled in bed rail bars or bed rail gaps. Gaps occur:

- Between half-length rails
- Between the rail and the headboard or footboard
- Between the bed rail and mattress

Injury or death can occur if the person's head, neck, chest, arm, or leg is trapped. Persons at greatest risk are those who:

- Are confused or disoriented
- Are restrained (Chapter 11)
- Are small in size
- Have poor muscle control

For an adult's safety, it is recommended that gaps should be 4 inches or less between:

- The bed rail bars
- An upper and lower bed rail
- The bed rail and the mattress
- The upper bed rail and the headboard
- The lower bed rail and the footboard

Always check for the "4-inch rule" when giving care (Fig. 10-10). Report any concerns to the nurse at once.

Bed rails prevent the person from getting out of bed. They are considered restraints by OBRA and the Centers for Medicare & Medicaid Services (CMS). Bed rails cannot be used unless they are needed to treat a person's medical symptoms. Some people feel safer with bed rails up. Others use them to change positions in bed. The person or legal representative must give consent for raised bed rails. The need for bed rails must be carefully noted in the person's medical record and care plan.

Accrediting agencies and many states have standards for bed rail use. They are allowed when the person's condition requires them. Bed rail use must be in the person's best interests.

The procedures in this book include using bed rails. This helps you learn how to use them correctly. The nurse, the care plan, and your assignment sheet tell you which people use bed rails. If a person does not use bed rails, omit the "raise bed rails" or "lower bed rails" steps.

If a person uses bed rails, check the person often. Report to the nurse that you checked the person. If you are allowed to chart, record when you checked the person and your observations.

---

**SAFETY ALERT:** *Bed Rails*

You will raise the bed to give care. Follow these safety measures to prevent the person from falling:

- If the person uses bed rails, always raise the far bed rail if you are working alone. Raise both bed rails if you need to leave the bedside for any reason.
- If the person does not use bed rails, ask a co-worker to help you. The co-worker stands on the far side of the bed. This protects the person from falling off the bed.
- Never leave the person alone when the bed is raised.

---

*See Focus on Children: Bed Rails.*

---

▶ **FOCUS ON CHILDREN**
**BED RAILS**

The space between crib rail slats must be no more than 2⅜ inches. If the space is larger, the baby's head can get caught between the slats. The baby can suffocate and die.

The mattress and crib must be the same size. If the mattress is smaller than the crib, gaps occur between:

- The crib rail and the mattress
- The crib rail and the headboard
- The crib rail and the footboard

Two adult fingers should fit between these spaces. Larger spaces can trap the baby. The baby can suffocate and die.

Never leave the crib rails down when the baby is in the crib.

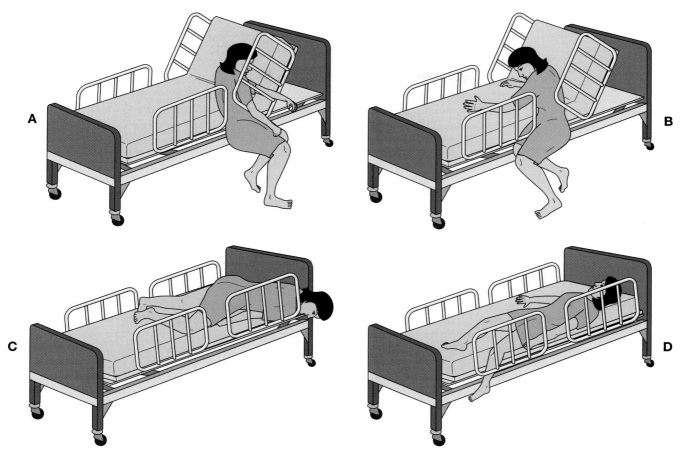

**FIG. 10-9** Entrapment is a safety risk with bed rails. **A,** The person is trapped between the bed rail bars. **B,** The person is trapped between the bed rail gaps. **C,** The person is trapped between the bed rail and the headboard. **D,** The person is caught between the mattress and the bed rail.

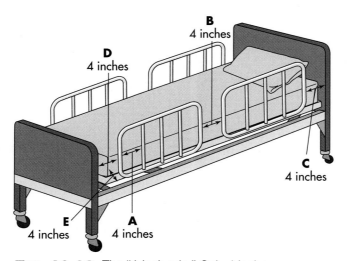

**FIG. 10-10** The "4-inch rule." Only 4 inches are recommended **A,** between bed rails bars, **B,** between the upper and lower bed rails, **C,** between the upper bed rail and the headboard, **D,** between the lower bed rail and the footboard, and **E,** between the bed rail and the mattress.

## HAND RAILS AND GRAB BARS

Hand rails are in hallways, stairways, and bathrooms (Fig. 10-11). They give support to persons who are weak or unsteady when walking. They also provide support for sitting down on or getting up from a toilet. Grab bars are along bathtubs for use in getting in and out of the tub.

## WHEEL LOCKS

Bed legs have wheels. They let the bed move easily. Each wheel has a lock to prevent the bed from moving (Fig. 10-12). Wheels are locked at all times except when moving the bed. Make sure bed wheels are locked:
- When giving bedside care
- When you transfer a person to and from the bed

Wheelchair and stretcher wheels also are locked during transfers (p. 166). You or the person can be injured if the bed, wheelchair, or stretcher moves.

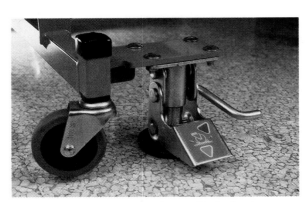

**FIG. 10-12** Lock on a bed wheel.

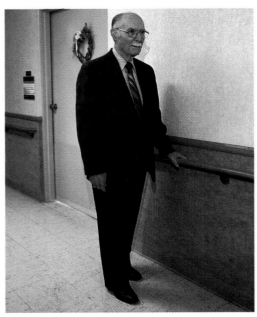

**FIG. 10-11** Hand rails provide support when walking.

# PREVENTING BURNS

Burns are a leading cause of death. Children and older persons are at great risk. Smoking in bed, spilling hot liquids, children playing with matches, barbecue grills, fireplaces, and stoves are common causes. So is very hot bath water. The safety measures in Box 10-4 can prevent burns.

# PREVENTING POISONING

Poisoning also is a major cause of death. Children and older adults are at risk. Drugs and household products are common poisons. Poisoning in adults may be from carelessness, confusion, or poor vision when reading labels. As a result, the person may take too much of a drug. Sometimes poisoning is a suicide attempt.

## BOX 10-4 SAFETY MEASURES TO PREVENT BURNS

**CHILDREN**

- Do not leave children home alone.
- Supervise young children at all times.
- Store matches and lighters where children cannot reach them.
- Do not let children near stoves, space heaters, fireplaces, barbecue grills, radiators, registers, and other heat sources.
- Keep space heaters and materials that can catch fire away from children.
- Teach children fire safety and fire prevention measures. Also teach the dangers of fire.
- Use the stove's back burners when infants and children are in the kitchen.
- Do not let children help you cook at the stove.
- Check metal playground equipment before children play on it. Metal surfaces exposed to sunlight can heat to high temperatures. They can burn hands, arm, legs, and buttocks.
- Check car seats, seat belts, and seat belt buckles. If hot, they can burn children.
- Cover car seats with towels if you park in the sun.

**COOKING**

- Turn pot and pan handles so they point inward. They point away from where people stand and walk.
- Do not leave cooking utensils in pots and pans.
- Do not wear clothing with long, loose sleeves when cooking.
- Do not put wet food into frying pans or deep-fryers. The water causes the oil to splatter.
- Use dry oven mitts and potholders. Water conducts heat.
- Stay near the stove, microwave, and barbecue grill when cooking. Do not leave them unattended.
- Keep hot food and liquids away from counter and table edges.
- Turn the oven and stove burners off when not in use.

**EATING AND DRINKING**

- Assist with eating and drinking as needed. Spilled hot foods and fluids can cause burns.

- Do not carry or eat hot foods and fluids near infants and young children.

**WATER**

- Turn on cold water first, then hot water. Turn off hot water first, then cold water.
- Measure bath water temperature (Chapter 16). Check it before a person gets into a tub.
- Have anti-scald devices installed on faucets and showerheads.
- Check for "hot spots" in bath water. Move your hand back and forth.
- Do not leave children unattended in bathtubs.
- Position the child facing away from faucets when bathing a child in a tub or at a sink.
- Do not let children touch faucet handles.
- Place knob covers over faucets to prevent children from turning on the water.

**APPLIANCES**

- Follow safety guidelines when applying heat and cold (Chapter 29).
- Do not let the person sleep with a heating pad.
- Do not use electric blankets.
- Do not leave irons unattended. Keep them off when not in use.
- Keep curling irons and electric rollers out of the reach of children. Turn them off when not in use.

**SMOKING**

- Be sure people smoke only in smoking areas.
- Do not leave smoking materials at the bedside. They are left at the bedside if the person is trusted to smoke alone in smoking areas. Follow the care plan.
- Supervise the smoking of persons who cannot protect themselves.
- Do not allow smoking in bed.
- Do not allow smoking where oxygen is used or stored (Chapter 30).

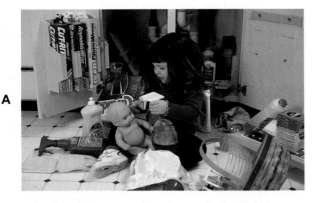

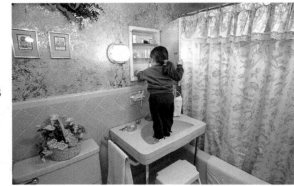

FIG. 10-13 Harmful substances must be kept in locked areas out of the reach of children. **A,** Household cleaners are within a child's reach when in low cabinets. **B,** The bathroom medicine chest holds many hazardous substances.

Common poisons include:
- Drugs (including aspirin) and vitamins
- Household products—detergents, sprays, furniture polish, window cleaners, bleach, paint, paint thinner, toilet bowl cleaners, drain cleaners, gasoline, kerosene, glue, and so on
- Personal care products—shampoos, hair conditioners, bath oils, powders, lotions, nail polish remover, sprays, make-up, perfumes, after-shave lotions, deodorants, mouthwash, and so on
- Fertilizers, insecticides, bug sprays, and so on
- Lead
- House plants
- Alcohol
- Carbon monoxide

To prevent poisoning, follow the safety measures in Box 10-5.

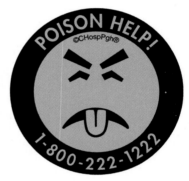

FIG. 10-14 The "Mr. Yuk" warning sticker is placed on hazardous products. (Courtesy Children's Hospital, Pittsburgh Poison Center, Pittsburgh, Pa.)

---

**BOX 10-5 SAFETY MEASURES TO PREVENT POISONING**

- Keep all harmful substances in high, locked areas (Fig. 10-13). Children and confused persons cannot see or reach them.
- Keep childproof caps on all harmful substances.
- Store harmful substances according to the manufacturer's instructions (p. 168).
- Make sure all harmful substances are labeled (p. 168).
- Do not mix cleaning products.
- Read labels carefully. Have good lighting.
- Use products according to the manufacturer's instructions.
- Keep harmful products in their original containers. Do not store them in food containers.
- Do not store harmful substances near food.
- Discard harmful substances that are outdated (p. 169).
- Use safety latches on kitchen, bathroom, garage, basement, and workshop cabinets.
- Keep drugs out of purses, backpacks, briefcases, luggage, and other items where children may find them.

- Family and friends may keep drugs in such places. Keep children away from such items.
- Never call drugs or vitamins "candy."
- Keep plants where persons at risk cannot reach them.
- Teach children not to eat plants and unknown foods. Teach them not to eat leaves, stems, seeds, berries, nuts, or bark.
- Place poison warning stickers ("Mr. Yuk") on harmful substances (Fig. 10-14).
- Keep all baby products and diaper-changing supplies out of the child's reach.
- Do not let children play near walls with chipped paint. The paint may contain lead.
- Keep emergency numbers by the telephone: poison control center, police, ambulance, hospital, and doctor.
- Supervise children when visiting family and friends. Look for harmful substances on kitchen counters, kitchen tables, or bathroom counters.

# PREVENTING SUFFOCATION

**Suffocation** is when breathing stops from the lack of oxygen. Death occurs if the person does not start breathing. Common causes include choking, drowning, inhaling gas or smoke, strangulation, and electrical shock.

Follow safety measures in Box 10-6 to prevent suffocation.

## CARBON MONOXIDE POISONING

Carbon monoxide is a colorless, odorless, and tasteless gas. It is produced by the burning of fuel. Motor vehicles, furnaces, gas water heaters, fireplaces, space heaters, gas stoves, wood-burning stoves, and gas dryers use fuel. So do barbecue grills, lawn mowers, snow blowers, chain saws, and other equipment.

All fuel-burning devices must be in working order and be used correctly. Otherwise, dangerous levels of carbon monoxide can result. Instead of breathing in oxygen, the person breathes in air filled with carbon monoxide. Headache, nausea, and dizziness are common. So are confusion, breathing problems, sleepiness, and cherry-pink skin. Death can occur.

Faulty exhaust systems on cars are common causes of carbon monoxide poisoning. So are damaged furnaces and chimneys.

Follow these safety measures:
- Have car exhaust systems checked regularly.
- Follow the manufacturer's instructions when using fuel-burning devices.
- Use the correct fuel when using fuel-burning devices.
- Do not idle a vehicle, lawn mower, snow blower, weed trimmer, or other device in an open or closed garage. Fumes can leak into the home.
- Have fuel-burning devices and chimneys checked when people in the same building show signs and symptoms.
- Open doors and windows if you or others have signs and symptoms.
- Open doors and windows if you notice gas odors.
- Have gas odors checked by trained professionals.
- Do not use a gas oven to heat a home.
- Do not use barbecue grills indoors or in a garage.

---

**BOX 10-6  SAFETY MEASURES TO PREVENT SUFFOCATION**

**ALL AGE-GROUPS**
- Unplug appliances when not in use.
- Check equipment for frayed cords and proper working order (p. 164). Make sure they are in good repair.
- Do not use the person's electrical items until they are safety-checked. The maintenance department does this.
- Use electrical appliances correctly.
- Cut food into small, bite-size pieces for persons who cannot do so themselves.
- Make sure dentures fit properly and are in place.
- Make sure the person can chew and swallow the food served.
- Report loose teeth or dentures.
- Check the care plan for swallowing problems before serving snacks or fluids. The person may ask for something that he or she cannot swallow.
- Tell the nurse at once if the person has problems swallowing.
- Do not give oral food or fluids to persons with feeding tubes (Chapter 20).
- Follow aspiration precautions (Chapter 20).
- Do not leave a person unattended in a bathtub or shower.
- Move all persons from the area if you smell smoke.
- Position the person in bed properly (Chapter 13).
- Use bed rails correctly (p. 158).
- Use restraints correctly (Chapter 11).

**CHILDREN**
- Keep plastic bags, covers, and dry-cleaning bags away from children.
- Place safety plugs in outlets. This includes electrical strips and surge protectors.
- Keep electrical cords and electrical items out of the reach of children.
- Position infants on their backs for sleep.
- Do not use pillows to position infants.
- Do not use pillows to prevent infants from falling off of beds and furniture.
- Remove pillows, comforters, quilts, sheepskin, stuffed toys, and other soft items from the crib when the baby is sleeping.
- Do not give infants and young children hot dogs, peanuts, popcorn, grapes, raisins, hard candy, or gum.
- Report loose teeth.
- Use Mylar balloons instead of latex ones.
- Store latex balloons where children cannot see or reach them.
- Do not let children inflate or deflate latex balloons.
- Deflate and discard latex balloons after use.
- Pick up and discard broken balloon pieces at once. Do not let children near them.
- Check floors for small objects—buttons, coins, beads, marbles, pins, tacks, nails, screws, and so on. Children can choke on them.

## PREVENTING EQUIPMENT ACCIDENTS

All equipment is unsafe if broken, not used correctly, or not working properly. Inspect all equipment before use. Check glass and plastic items for cracks, chips, and sharp or rough edges. They can cause cuts, stabs, or scratches. Follow the Bloodborne Pathogen Standard (Chapter 12). Do not use or give damaged items to patients or residents. Take the item to the nurse. The nurse will have you do one of the following:

- Discard the item following agency policy.
- Tag the item and send it for repair following agency policy.

Electric items must work properly and be in good repair. Frayed cords (Fig. 10-15) and overloaded electrical outlets (Fig. 10-16) can cause fires and electrical shocks. **Electrical shock** is when electrical current passes through the body. It can burn the skin, muscles, nerves, and other tissues. It can affect the heart and cause death.

Three-pronged plugs (Fig. 10-17) are used on all electrical items. Two prongs carry electrical current. The third prong is the ground. A **ground** carries leaking electricity to the earth and away from an electrical item. If a ground is not used, leaking electricity can be conducted to a person. It can cause electrical shocks and possible death. If you receive a shock, report it at once. Tag the item, and send it for repair.

Warning signs of a faulty electrical item include:

- Shocks
- Loss of power or a power outage
- Dimming or flickering lights
- Sparks
- Sizzling or buzzing sounds
- Burning odor
- Loose plugs

Practice the safety measures in Box 10-7 when using equipment. An incident report (p. 178) is completed if a patient, resident, visitor, or staff member has an equipment-related accident. The Safe Medical Devices Act requires that agencies report equipment-related illnesses, injuries, and deaths.

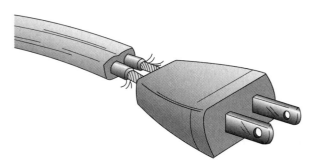

**FIG. 10-15** A frayed electrical cord.

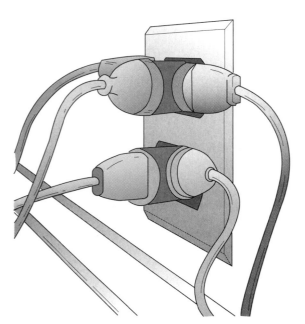

**FIG. 10-16** An overloaded electrical outlet.

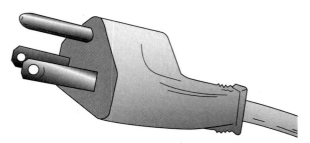

**FIG. 10-17** A three-pronged plug.

## BOX 10-7 SAFETY MEASURES TO PREVENT EQUIPMENT ACCIDENTS

- Follow agency policies and procedures.
- Follow the manufacturer's instruction.
- Read all caution and warning labels.
- Do not use an unfamiliar item. Ask for needed training. Also ask a nurse to supervise you the first time you use the item.
- Use equipment only for its intended purpose.
- Make sure the item works before you begin.
- Make sure you have all needed equipment. For example, you need to plug in an item. There must be an outlet.
- Place a "Do Not Use" sticker on broken items. Complete a repair request form and explain the problem.
- Tell the nurse about broken items.
- Do not try to repair broken items.
- Do not run electrical cords under rugs.
- Keep electrical items away from water.
- Keep work areas clean and dry. Wipe up spills right away.
- Do not touch electrical items if you are wet, if your hands are wet, or if you are standing in water.

- Do not put a finger or any item into an outlet.
- Turn off equipment before unplugging it. Sparks occur when electrical items are unplugged while turned on.
- Hold onto the plug (not the cord) when removing it from an outlet (Fig. 10-18).
- Do not give showers or tub baths during electrical storms. Lightening can travel through pipes.
- Do not use electrical items or phones during storms.
- Do not use water to put out an electrical fire. If possible, turn off or unplug the item.
- Do not touch a person who is experiencing an electrical shock. If possible, turn off or unplug the item. Call for help at once.
- Keep electrical cords away from heating vents and other heat sources.
- Turn off equipment when done using the item.

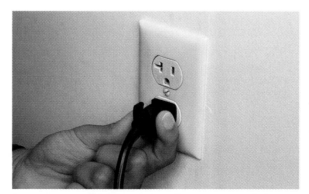

**FIG. 10-18** Hold onto the plug to remove it from an electrical outlet.

## WHEELCHAIR AND STRETCHER SAFETY

Some people cannot walk or they have severe problems walking. A wheelchair may be useful (Fig. 10-19). If able, the person propels the chair using the handrims. Some use their feet to move the chair. Other wheelchairs are propelled by motors. The person moves the chair with hand, chin, mouth, or other controls. If the person cannot propel the wheelchair, another person pushes it using the handgrips/push handles.

Stretchers are used to transport persons who cannot use wheelchairs. They cannot sit up or must lie down. A stretcher is used to move the person from one area of the agency to another.

Follow the safety measures in Box 10-8 when using wheelchairs and stretchers. The person can fall from the chair or stretcher. Or the person can fall during transfers to and from the chair or stretcher.

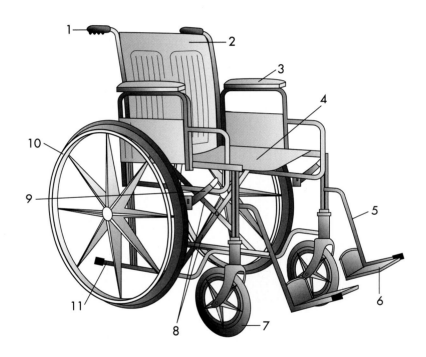

1. Handgrip/push handle
2. Back upholstery
3. Armrest
4. Seat upholstery
5. Front rigging
6. Footplate
7. Caster
8. Crossbrace
9. Wheel lock
10. Wheel and handrim
11. Tipping lever

**FIG. 10-19** Parts of a wheelchair.

## BOX 10-8 WHEELCHAIR AND STRETCHER SAFETY

### WHEELCHAIR SAFETY

- Check the brakes. Make sure you can lock and unlock them.
- Check for flat or loose tires. A brake will not lock onto a flat or loose tire.
- Make sure that wheel spokes are intact. Damaged, broken, or loose spokes can interfere with moving the wheelchair or locking the brakes.
- Make sure casters point forward. This keeps the wheelchair balanced and stable.
- Position the person's feet on the footplates.
- Make sure the person's feet are on the footplates before pushing or repositioning the chair. The person's feet must not touch or drag on the floor when the chair is moving.
- Push the chair forward when transporting the person. Do not pull the chair backward.
- Lock both brakes before you transfer a person to or from the wheelchair.
- Remind the person to keep the brakes locked when not moving the wheelchair. The brakes prevent the chair from moving if the person wants to move to or from the chair.
- Do not let the person stand on the footplates.
- Do not let the footplates fall back onto the person's legs.
- Make sure the person has needed wheelchair accessories—safety belt, pouches, trays, lapboards, cushions.
- Remove the armrests (if removable) when the person transfers to the bed, commode, tub, or car (Chapter 13).
- Remove the armrests (if removable) when lifting the person from the chair (Chapter 13).
- Swing front rigging out of the way for transfers to and from the wheelchair. Some front riggings detach for transfers.
- Clean the wheelchair according to agency policy.
- Ask a nurse or physical therapist to show you how to propel wheelchairs up steps and ramps and over curbs.
- Follow measures to prevent equipment accidents (p. 164).

### STRETCHER SAFETY

- Ask two co-workers to help with the transfer (Chapter 13).
- Lock the stretcher wheels before the transfer.
- Fasten the safety straps when the person is properly positioned on the stretcher.
- Ask a co-worker to help with the transport.
- Raise the side rails. Keep them up during the transport.
- Make sure the person's arms and hands do not dangle through the side rail bars.
- Stand at the head of the stretcher. Your co-worker stands at the foot of the stretcher.
- Move the stretcher feet first (Fig. 10-20).
- Do not leave the person alone.
- Follow measures to prevent equipment accidents (p. 164).

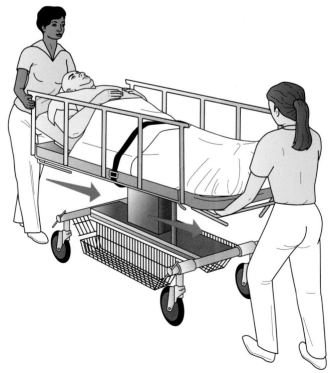

**FIG. 10-20** A person is transported by stretcher. The stretcher is moved feet first.

# HANDLING HAZARDOUS SUBSTANCES

A **hazardous substance** is any chemical in the workplace that can cause harm. The Occupational Safety and Health Administration (OSHA) requires that health care employees:

- Understand the risks of hazardous substances
- Know how to safely handle them

Physical hazards can cause fires or explosions. Health hazards are chemicals that can cause acute or chronic health problems. Acute problems occur rapidly and last a short while. They usually occur from a short-term exposure. Chronic problems usually result from long-term exposure. They occur over a long period.

Health hazards can:

- Cause cancer
- Affect blood cell formation and function
- Damage the kidneys, nervous system, lungs, skin, eyes, or mucous membranes
- Cause birth defects, miscarriages, and fertility problems from reproductive system damage

Exposure to hazardous substances can occur under normal working conditions. It also can happen during certain emergencies. Such emergencies include equipment failures, container ruptures, or the uncontrolled release of a hazard into the workplace. Hazardous substances include:

- Drugs used in cancer therapy (chemotherapy, anti-cancer drugs)
- Anesthesia gases
- Gases used to sterilize equipment
- Oxygen
- Disinfectants and cleaning solutions
- Radiation used for x-rays and cancer treatments
- Mercury (found in thermometers and blood pressure devices)

To protect employees, OSHA requires a hazard communication program. The program includes container labeling, material safety data sheets (MSDSs), and employee training.

## LABELING

Hazardous substance containers include bags, barrels, bottles, boxes, cans, cylinders, drums, and storage tanks. All need warning labels (Fig. 10-21). The manufacturer applies the labels. Warning labels identify:

- Physical and health hazards (Health hazards include the organs affected and potential health problems.)
- Precaution measures (for example, "Do not use near open flame" or "Avoid skin contact")
- What personal protective equipment to wear (Chapter 12)
- How to use the substance safely
- Storage and disposal information

Words, pictures, and symbols communicate the warnings. A container must have a label. It must not be removed or damaged in any way. If a warning label is removed or damaged, do not use the substance. Take the container to the nurse, and explain the problem. Do not leave the container unattended.

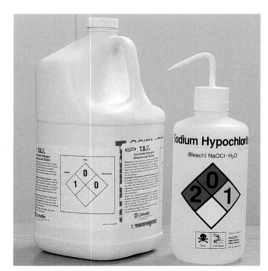

**FIG. 10-21** Warning labels on hazardous substances.

## MATERIAL SAFETY DATA SHEETS

Every hazardous substance has an MSDS. It provides detailed information about the hazardous substance:

- The chemical name and any common names
- The ingredients in the substance
- Physical and chemical characteristics (appearance, color, odor, boiling point, and others)
- Potential physical effects (fire, explosion)
- Conditions that could cause a chemical reaction
- How the chemical enters the body (inhalation, ingestion, skin contact, or absorption)
- Health hazards including signs and symptoms
- Protective measures (how to use, handle, and store the substance)
- Emergency and first-aid procedures
- Explosion information and fire-fighting measures (including what type of fire extinguisher to use [p. 170]).
- How to clean up a spill or leak
- Personal protective equipment needed during clean up
- How to dispose of the hazardous material
- Manufacturer information (name, address, and a telephone number for information)

Employees must have ready access to MSDSs. They are in a binder at a certain place on each unit (Fig. 10-22). Many agencies also have them on computer. Check the MSDS before using a hazardous substance, cleaning up a leak or spill, or disposing of the substance. Tell the nurse about a leak or spill right away. Do not leave a leak or spill unattended.

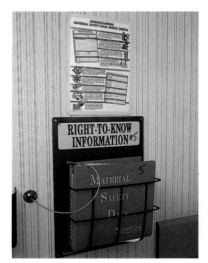

**FIG. 10-22** Material safety data sheets (MSDSs) are in a binder. The binder is placed for staff use.

## EMPLOYEE TRAINING

Your employer provides hazardous substance training. You are told about hazards, exposure risks, and protection measures. You learn to read and use warning labels and MSDSs.

Each hazardous substance requires certain protection measures. Box 10-9 lists general rules to safely handle hazardous substances.

---

**BOX 10-9 SAFETY MEASURES FOR HAZARDOUS SUBSTANCES**

- Read all warning labels.
- Follow the safety measures on the warning label and MSDS.
- Make sure each container has a warning label that is not damaged.
- Use a leak-proof container to carry or transport a hazardous substance.
- Wear personal protective equipment to clean spills and leaks. The warning label or MSDS tells you what to wear (mask, gown, gloves, eye protection, safety boots).
- Clean up spills at once. Work from clean to dirty using circular motions.
- Dispose of hazardous waste in sealed bags or containers.
- Stand behind a lead shield during x-ray or radiation therapy procedures.
- Do not enter a room while a person is having x-rays or radiation therapy.
- Wash your hands after handling hazardous substances.
- Work in well-ventilated areas to avoid inhaling gases.
- Store hazardous substances according to the MSDS.

## FIRE SAFETY

Fire is a constant danger. Faulty electrical equipment and wiring, overloaded electrical circuits, and smoking are major causes. The entire health team must prevent fires. They must act quickly and responsibly during a fire.

### FIRE AND THE USE OF OXYGEN

Three things are needed for a fire:
- A spark or flame
- A material that will burn
- Oxygen

Air has some oxygen. However, some people need extra oxygen. Doctors order oxygen therapy for them (Chapter 30). Safety measures are needed where oxygen is used and stored:

- "No Smoking" signs are placed on the door and near the bed.
- The person and visitors are reminded not to smoke in the room.
- Smoking materials (cigarettes, cigars, and pipes), matches, and lighters are removed from the room.
- Electrical items are turned off *before* being unplugged.

---

**BOX 10-10   FIRE PREVENTION MEASURES**

- Follow the safety measures for oxygen use.
- Smoke only where allowed to do so. Do not smoke in patients' homes.
- Be sure all ashes, cigars, cigarettes, and other smoking materials are out before emptying ashtrays.
- Provide ashtrays to persons who are allowed to smoke.
- Empty ashtrays into a metal container partially filled with sand or water. Do not empty ashtrays into plastic containers or wastebaskets lined with paper or plastic bags.
- Supervise persons who smoke. This is very important for persons who are confused, disoriented, or sedated.
- Follow safety practices when using electrical items.
- Supervise the play of children. Keep matches out of their reach.
- Do not leave cooking unattended on stoves, in ovens or microwave ovens, or on barbecue grills.
- Store flammable liquids in their original containers. Keep the containers where children cannot reach them.
- Do not light matches or lighters or smoke around flammable liquids or materials.
- Do not leave candles unattended.
- Keep candles away from flammable liquids or materials.
- Keep materials that will burn away from space heaters, fireplaces, radiators, registers, and other heat sources.

---

- Wool blankets and synthetic fabrics that cause static electricity are removed from the person's room. The person wears a cotton gown or pajamas.
- Electrical items are in good working order. This includes shavers, TVs, and radios.
- Lit candles and incense are not allowed.
- Materials that ignite easily are removed from the room. They include oil, grease, alcohol, nail polish remover, and so on.

Agencies have no-smoking policies and are smoke-free settings. No smoking is allowed inside buildings. Signs are posted on all entry doors. Some people ignore such rules. Remind them about the no-smoking rules.

### PREVENTING FIRES

Fire prevention measures were described in relation to children, burns, equipment-related accidents, and oxygen use. Other measures are listed in Box 10-10.

### WHAT TO DO DURING A FIRE

Know your agency's policies and procedures for fire emergencies. Know where to find fire alarms, fire extinguishers, and emergency exits. Fire drills are held to practice emergency fire procedures. Remember the word *RACE* when a fire occurs:

- R—for *rescue*. Rescue persons in immediate danger. Move them to a safe place.
- A—for *alarm*. Sound the nearest fire alarm. Notify the switchboard operator.
- C—for *confine*. Close doors and windows to confine the fire. Turn off oxygen or electrical items used in the general area of the fire.
- E—for *extinguish*. Use a fire extinguisher on a small fire that has not spread to a larger area.

Clear equipment from all normal and emergency exists. *Do not use elevators if there is a fire.*

**USING A FIRE EXTINGUISHER.** Agencies require that all employees demonstrate use of a fire extinguisher. Different extinguishers are used for different kinds of fires:
- Oil and grease fires
- Electrical fires
- Paper and wood fires

A general procedure for using a fire extinguisher follows.

**EVACUATING.** Agencies have evacuation procedures. If evacuation is necessary, people closest to danger are taken out first. Those who can walk are given blankets to wrap around themselves. A staff member escorts them to a safe place. Figures 10-24 and 10-25, pp. 172-173 show how to rescue persons who cannot walk. Once firefighters arrive, they direct rescue efforts.

*See Focus on Home Care: Fire Safety*, p. 172.

## USING A FIRE EXTINGUISHER

### PROCEDURE

1 Pull the fire alarm.
2 Get the nearest fire extinguisher.
3 Carry it upright.
4 Take it to the fire.
5 Remove the safety pin (Fig. 10-23, *A*).

6 Direct the hose at the base of the fire (Fig. 10-23, *B*).
7 Push the top handle down (Fig. 10-23, *C*).
8 Sweep the hose slowly back and forth at the base of the fire.

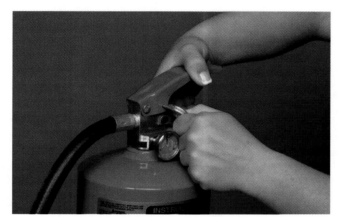

A

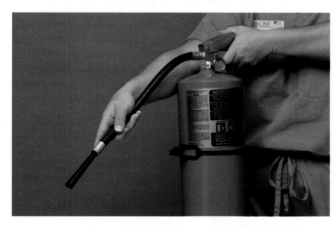

B

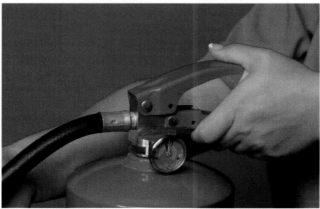

C

**FIG. 10-23** Using a fire extinguisher. **A,** Remove the safety pin. **B,** Direct the hose at the base of the fire. **C,** Push the top handle down.

## FOCUS ON HOME CARE

### FIRE SAFETY

#### FIRE AND THE USE OF OXYGEN

Home care patients may need oxygen therapy. Remind the patient, family, and visitors about needed safety measures. See Chapter 30.

#### PREVENTING FIRES

Smoke detectors save lives. Always locate them in patients' homes. Make sure they are working. Tell the nurse and family if a smoke detector does not work.

Space heaters present fire hazards. Electric and fuel-burning heaters are common. Practice these safety measures:

- Follow the manufacturer's instructions. Use the recommended fuel.
- Keep heaters at least 3 feet away from curtains, drapes, furniture, and anything that will burn.
- Do not place heaters on stairs, in doorways, or where people walk.
- Protect yourself and others from burns. Heaters are hot. Do not touch them. Keep them away from children and persons who cannot protect themselves.
- Prevent electrocution. Keep electric heaters away from water. (Water conducts electricity.) Make sure the cord is in good repair.
- Do not leave heaters unattended.
- Store fuel in its original container. Keep the container outside.
- Refill the heater outside.
- Do not fill the heater while it is running or hot. Do not overfill the heater.

#### WHAT TO DO DURING A FIRE

Know two exit routes from the home or building. Get the patient, family, and yourself out as fast as possible. Do not use elevators. In an apartment building, alert others to the fire. Use the fire alarm system and yell "FIRE" in the hallways. Call 911 or the fire department from a nearby phone. Do not go back into the building.

Touch doors before opening them. Do not open a hot door. Use another way out.

If your clothing is on fire, do not run. Drop to the floor or ground. Cover your face. Roll to smother the flames. If another person's clothing is on fire, get the person to the floor or ground. Roll the person, or cover the person with a blanket or coat. This smothers the flames.

If smoke is present, cover your nose and mouth with a damp cloth. Do the same for the patient and family. Have everyone crawl to the nearest exit.

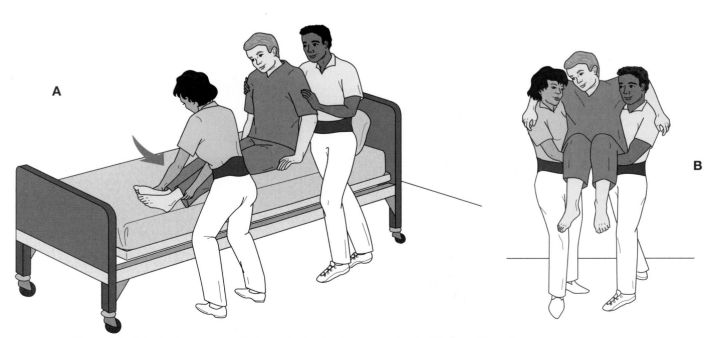

**FIG. 10-24** Swing-carry technique. **A,** Assist the person to a sitting position. A co-worker grasps the person's ankles as you both turn the person so that he sits on the side of the bed. **B,** Pull the person's arm over your shoulder. With one arm, reach across the person's back to your co-worker's shoulder. Reach under the person's knees and grasp your co-worker's arm. Your co-worker does the same.

## FOCUS ON HOME CARE
### FIRE SAFETY—CONT'D

If you cannot get out of the building because of flames or smoke:

- Call 911 or the fire department. Tell the operator where you are. Give exact information: address, phone number, and where you are in the home.
- Cover your nose and mouth with a damp cloth. Do the same for the patient and family.
- Move away from the fire. Go to a room with a window. Close the door to the room. Stuff wet towels, blankets, or sheets at the bottom of the door.

- Open the window.
- Hang something from the window (towel, sheet, blanket, clothing). This helps the firefighters find you.

### USING A FIRE EXTINGUISHER

Locate fire extinguishers in the patient's home. Read the manufacturer's instructions. Make sure the device works. Tell the nurse and the family if a fire extinguisher does not work.

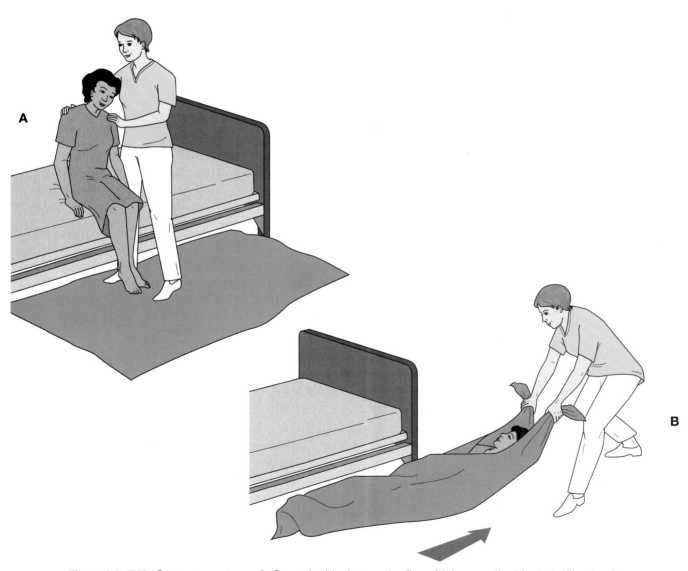

**FIG. 10-25** One-rescuer carry. **A,** Spread a blanket on the floor. Make sure the blanket will extend beyond the person's head. Assist the person to sit on the side of the bed. Grasp the person under the arms, and cross your hands over her chest. Lower the person to the floor by sliding her down one of your legs. **B,** Wrap the blanket around the person. Grasp the blanket over the head area. Pull the person to a safe area.

# DISASTERS

A **disaster** is a sudden catastrophic event. Many people are injured and killed. Property is destroyed. Natural disasters include tornadoes, hurricanes, blizzards, earthquakes, volcanic eruptions, floods, and some fires. Human-made disasters include auto, bus, train, and airplane accidents. They also include fires, bombings, nuclear power plant accidents, riots, explosions, gas or chemical leaks, and wars.

The agency has procedures for disasters that could occur in your area. Follow them to keep patients, residents, visitors, and staff safe.

Communities, fire and police departments, and agencies have disaster plans. They include policies and procedures to deal with great numbers of people needing treatment. The plan generally provides for:

- Discharging persons who can go home.
- Assigning staff and equipment to emergency areas
- Assigning staff to transport persons from the treatment areas
- Calling off-duty staff to work

A disaster may damage the agency. The disaster plan includes policies and procedures to evacuate the agency.

## BOMB THREATS

Agencies have polices and procedures for bomb threats. You must follow them if a caller makes a bomb threat or if you find an item that looks or sounds strange. Often bomb threats are sent by phone. However, they can be sent by mail, e-mail, messenger, or other means. Or the person can leave a bomb in the agency.

# WORKPLACE VIOLENCE

**Workplace violence** is violent acts (including assault or threat of assault) directed toward persons at work or while on duty. It includes:

- Murders
- Beatings, stabbings, and shootings
- Rapes
- Use of weapons—firearms, bombs, or knives
- Kidnapping
- Robbery
- Threats—obscene phone calls; threatening oral, written, or body language; and harassment of any nature (being followed, sworn at, or shouted at)

Workplace violence can occur in any place where an employee performs a work-related duty. It can be a permanent or temporary place. This includes buildings, parking lots, field sites, homes, and travel to and from work assignments. Workplace violence can occur anywhere in the agency. However, it is most frequent in mental health units, emergency rooms, waiting rooms, and geriatric units.

According to OSHA, more assaults occur in health care settings than in other industries. Nurses and nursing assistants are at risk. They have the most contact with patients, residents, and visitors. Risk factors include:

- People with weapons
- Patients as police holds (persons arrested or convicted of crimes)
- Acutely disturbed and violent persons seeking health care
- Alcohol and drug abuse
- Mentally ill persons who do not take needed drugs, do not have follow-up care, and are not in hospitals unless they are an immediate threat to themselves or others
- Pharmacies have drugs and are a target for robberies
- Gang members and substance abusers are in agencies as patients or visitors
- Upset, agitated, and disturbed family and visitors
- Long waits for emergency or other services
- Being alone with patients and residents during care or transport to other areas
- Low staff levels during meals, emergencies, and at night
- Poor lighting in hallways, rooms, parking lots, and other areas
- Lack of training in recognizing and managing potentially violent situations

OSHA has guidelines for violence prevention programs. The goal is to prevent or reduce employee exposure to situations that can cause death or injury. Work-site hazards are identified. Prevention measures are developed and followed. Also, employees receive safety and health training. You need to:

- Understand and follow your agency's workplace violence prevention program
- Understand and follow safety and security measures
- Voice safety and security concerns
- Report violent incidents promptly and accurately
- Serve on health and safety committees that review workplace violence
- Attend training programs that help you recognize and manage agitation, assaultive behavior, and criminal intent

Box 10-11 lists some measures that can prevent or control workplace violence. Box 10-12, p. 176 lists personal safety practices. Follow them all the time. Also practice these measures when dealing with agitated or aggressive persons:

- Stand away from the person. Judge the length of the person's arms and legs. Stand far enough away so the person cannot hit or kick you.
- Stand close to the door. Do not become trapped in the room.

## BOX 10-11 MEASURES TO PREVENT OR CONTROL WORKPLACE VIOLENCE

- Alarm systems, closed-circuit video monitoring, panic buttons, hand-held alarms, cellular phones, two-way radios, and telephone systems are installed (Fig. 10-26). These systems have a direct line to security staff or the police.
- Metal detectors are at entrances to identify guns, knives, or other weapons.
- Curved mirrors are at hallway intersections and hard-to-see areas.
- Bullet-resistant, shatter-proof glass is at nurses' stations, reception areas, and admitting areas.
- Waiting rooms are comfortable and reduce stress.
- Family and visitors are informed in a timely manner.
- Furniture is placed to prevent entrapment.
- Pictures, vases, and other items that can serve as weapons are few in number.
- Staff restrooms lock and prevent access to visitors.
- Unused doors are locked.
- Bright lights are inside and outside buildings.
- Burned-out lights are replaced or repaired.
- Broken lights, windows, and door locks are replaced or repaired.
- Security escort services are used for walking to cars, bus stops, or train stations.
- Vehicles are locked and in good repair.
- Security officers deal with agitated, aggressive, or disruptive persons.
- Restraints are used if persons are a threat to themselves or others.
- Visitors sign in and receive a pass to access patient or resident areas.
- Visiting hours and policies are enforced.
- A list of "restricted visitors" is made for patients or residents with a history of violence or who are victims of violence.
- Mental health patients are supervised as they move throughout the agency.
- Access to the pharmacy and drug storage areas is controlled.
- The RN assesses the behavioral history of new and transferred patients and residents.
- Aggressive and agitated persons are treated in open areas. Privacy and confidentiality are maintained.
- Staff is not alone when caring for persons with agitated or aggressive behaviors.
- Jewelry that can serve as weapons is not worn (grabbing earrings and bracelets, strangulating with necklaces).
- Long hair is worn up and off the collar (Chapter 3). A person can pull long hair and cause head injuries.
- Keys, scissors, pens, or other items that can serve as weapons are not visible.
- Tools or items left by maintenance staff or visitors are removed if they can serve as weapons.
- Staff wear ID badges that prove employment.
- A "buddy system" is used when using elevators, restrooms, and low traffic areas.
- Uniforms fit well. Tight uniforms limit running. An attacker can grab loose uniforms.
- Shoes have good soles. Shoes that cause slipping limit running.

---

- Know where to find panic buttons, signal lights, alarms, closed-circuit monitors, and other security devices.
- Keep your hands free.
- Stay calm. Talk to the person in a calm manner. Do not raise your voice or argue, scold, or interrupt the person.
- Do not touch the person.
- Tell the person that you will get a nurse to speak to him or her.
- Leave the room as soon as you can. Make sure the person is safe.
- Tell the nurse or security officer about the matter.
- Complete an incident report according to agency policy (p. 178).
  *See Focus on Home Care: Workplace Violence, p. 177.*

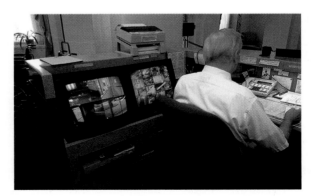

**FIG. 10-26** People entering and leaving the agency are monitored on closed-circuit TV.

## BOX 10-12  PERSONAL SAFETY PRACTICES

### GENERAL MEASURES

- Be careful when getting on elevators.
- Let someone know where you are at all times. Let someone know when you leave and when you arrive at your destination. If you do not call in when expected, the person knows something is wrong.
- Make it known that you do not carry drugs, needles, or syringes.
- Do not carry valuables. Leave them at home or in the car trunk. If someone wants what you have, give it. The only thing of value is *you.*
- Carry wallets, purses, and backpacks safely. Men should carry wallets in inside coat or pants pockets. Never carry a wallet in the rear pocket. Keep a firm grip on a purse. Keep it close to your body.
- Carry a whistle or shriek alarm.
- Avoid ATM machines at night.
- Do not hitchhike or pick up hitchhikers.

### HOME SETTINGS

- Keep doors and windows to the home locked at all times.
- Do not open doors to strangers. Ask for identification.
- Do not let a stranger into the home to use a phone. Offer to make the call.
- Do not give personal information to callers or people at the door.
- Know the area you will visit. Ask questions about the area.
- Make a "dry run" of the area. Know your route. The shortest route may not be the safest.

### CAR SAFETY

- Have plenty of gas in your car.
- Keep your car in good working order.
- Keep these in your car—local map, flashlight with working batteries, flares, a fire extinguisher, and a first-aid kit.
- Raise the hood and use the flares if the car breaks down. Stay in the car. Call the police if you have a wireless phone. If someone stops by to help, ask that person to call the police.
- Lock your car. Sometimes you may want to leave it unlocked. If you need to get in the car fast, you do not want to fumble with keys. Use your judgment. Do not leave anything in the car if you leave it unlocked.
- Have your car key ready so you can get into the car quickly. Do not fumble for keys on the way to or at the car.
- Check the back seat before getting into the car. Make sure no one is in the car. Leave at once if someone is in the car.
- Check under the car. A person hiding under the car can grab your ankle or leg. Leave at once if someone is under the car.
- Lock car doors when you get in the car. Keep windows rolled up.

- Keep purses, backpacks, and other valuables under the seat or near your side. Do not leave them on the seat. They are easy targets for smash-and-grab robberies.

### PARKING YOUR CAR

- Check for places to park. Choose a well-lit area. If using a parking garage, park near entrances, exits, and on the lower level. Try to get close to the attendant if possible. The closest space to your destination is not always the safest for parking.
- Park your car so that you can leave quickly and easily. Park at street corners so no one can park in front of you. In parking lots, back in. You can see more from the front windshield than from the back window.

### WALKING

- Do not wear headphones when walking. They keep you from hearing cars and people around you.
- Use well-lit and busy streets if you have to walk. Avoid vacant lots, alleys, wooded areas, and construction sites. Again, the shortest way is not always the safest.
- Walk near the curb. Stay away from doorways, shrubs, and bushes.
- Note the location of phone booths. Or carry a wireless phone. Know your location, and keep phone calls simple.
- Go to a police or fire station or a store if you think someone is following you.

### PUBLIC TRANSPORTATION

- Carry money for phone calls and for bus, train, or taxi fares. Have money in your pocket to avoid fumbling with a purse or wallet.
- Stand with others and near the ticket booth if using public transportation. Sit near the driver or conductor.

### IF YOU ARE THREATENED OR ATTACKED

- Scream as loud and as long as you can. Keep screaming. Men and women should scream.
- Yell "FIRE," not "HELP." Most people will respond to "FIRE."
- Use your car keys as a weapon. Carry them in your strong hand. Have one key extended (Fig. 10-27). Hold the key firmly. If you are attacked, go for the person's face. Slash the person's face with the key. Do not use poking motions. Do not try for a certain target because you might miss. Do not be shy—your attacker will not be.
- Remember, you have two arms, two hands, two feet, and two knees. You can attack from four directions at once. Do not be shy—your attacker will not be. Push, pull, yank, and so on. You can attack a man's or woman's genital area.
- Use your thumbs as weapons. Go for the eyes and push hard.
- Carry a travel size of aerosol hair spray. Go for the face.

## FOCUS ON HOME CARE
### WORKPLACE VIOLENCE

More measures are needed for home safety. Always keep doors locked. Do not let strangers into the home or building. Do not give information over the phone (Chapter 4). Do not let any stranger know that you are with an older, ill, or disabled person.

Physical, emotional, verbal, and sexual abuse can occur in home settings. If you feel uncomfortable or threatened in any way, report the matter to the nurse. Give as much information as you can. Failing to report the matter does not help you or the patient. Leave the home and call your supervisor if you feel an immediate threat to your health or well-being.

The following can threaten your safety. Report these and other threats to the nurse:

- Sexual abuse or harassment by the patient or by any person in the home (husband, wife, sister, brother, boyfriend, girlfriend, son, daughter, family, and friends). See Chapter 2.
- Hitting, kicking, slapping, spitting, biting, scratching, pinching, pushing, or other attacks by the patient or anyone in the home.
- Attacks or threatened attacks with any weapon (knife, gun, bat, rope, tool [hammer, screwdriver, and so on], razor, scissors, spray, pot, pan, cane, chair, and so on).
- Denial of meal breaks, water, bathroom use, toilet paper, or hand washing facilities.
- Denial of adequate sleeping conditions for a live-in situation.
- Inadequate heating or ventilation.
- Name calling, obscene language, or racial or cultural slurs.
- Exposure to unsafe conditions (blocked fire escapes, broken stairways, vermin infestations, and so on).

## RISK MANAGEMENT

Risk management involves identifying and controlling risks and safety hazards affecting the agency. The intent is to:
- Protect everyone in the agency (patients, residents, visitors, and staff)
- Protect agency property from harm or danger
- Protect the person's valuables
- Prevent accidents and injuries

Risk management deals with these and other issues:
- Accident and fire prevention
- Negligence and malpractice
- Patient and resident abuse
- Workplace violence
- Federal and state requirements

Risk managers work with all agency departments. They look for patterns and trends in incident reports, patient and resident complaints, staff complaints, and accident and injury investigations. Risk managers look for and correct unsafe situations. They also make procedure changes and training recommendations as needed.

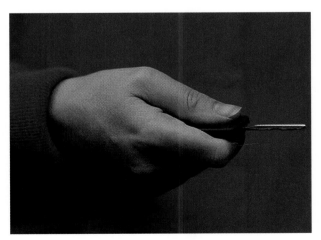

**FIG. 10-27** A car key is used as a weapon.

## PERSONAL BELONGINGS

The person's belongings must be kept safe. Often they are sent home with the family. A personal belongings list is completed. Each item is listed and described. The staff member and person sign the completed list.

A valuables envelope is used for money and jewelry. Each jewelry item is listed and described on the envelope. Describe what you see. For example, describe a ring as having a white stone with six prongs in a yellow setting. Do not assume the stone is a diamond in a gold setting. For valuables:

- Count money with the person.
- Put money and each jewelry item in the envelope with the person watching. Sign the envelope like the personal belongings list.
- Give the envelope to the nurse. The nurse puts it in a safe or gives it to the family.

Dentures, eyeglasses, hearing aids, watches, and radios are kept at the bedside. Items kept at the bedside are listed in the person's record. Some people keep money for newspapers and gift cart items. The amount kept is noted in the person's record. *See Focus on Long-Term Care: Personal Belongings.*

> ### FOCUS ON LONG-TERM CARE
> #### PERSONAL BELONGINGS
> Clothing and shoes are labeled with the person's name. So are radios, blankets, and other items brought from home.

## REPORTING ACCIDENTS AND ERRORS

Report accidents and errors at once. This includes:

- Accidents involving patients, residents, visitors, or staff
- Errors in care; includes giving the wrong care, giving care to the wrong person, or not giving care
- Broken or lost items owned by the person; for example, dentures, hearing aids, and eyeglasses
- Lost money or clothing
- Hazardous substance accidents
- Workplace violence incidents

An *incident report* is completed as soon as possible after the incident. The following information is required:

- Names of those involved
- Date and time of the accident or error
- Location of the accident or error
- A complete description of what happened
- Names of witnesses
- Any other requested information

Incident reports are reviewed by risk management and a committee of health care workers. They look for patterns and trends of accidents or errors. For example, are falls occurring on the same shift and on the same unit? Are lost or missing items being reported on the same shift or same unit? There may be new policies or procedures to prevent future incidents.

# ■ REVIEW QUESTIONS ■

Circle **T** if the statement is true and **F** if it is false.

1   T F   Childproof caps are kept on drugs and harmful products.
2   T F   Harmful products are kept in locked areas where children cannot reach them.
3   T F   Safety plugs in outlets protect children from electrical shocks.
4   T F   The "Mr. Yuk" sticker signals a poison.
5   T F   Keeping electrical cords and appliances in good repair prevents suffocation.
6   T F   To correctly identify a person, call him or her by name.
7   T F   Children have the greatest risk for falling.
8   T F   Falls are more likely to occur during the evening.
9   T F   Older persons are at risk for accidents because of changes in the body.
10  T F   Needing to urinate is a major cause of falls.
11  T F   Socks and bedroom slippers help prevent falls.
12  T F   Good lighting helps prevent falls.
13  T F   Bed rails are always raised when the bed is raised.
14  T F   The signal light must always be within the person's reach.
15  T F   Hazardous substances must have warning labels.
16  T F   Many people are injured and killed and property is destroyed in a disaster.
17  T F   Smoking is allowed where oxygen is used.

Circle the **BEST** answer.

18  Who provides a safe setting for patients and residents?
    a   The nursing team
    b   The health team
    c   The administrator
    d   The risk manager

19  Which is *not* a risk for accidents?
    a   Needing eyeglasses
    b   Hearing impairment
    c   Memory problems
    d   Being of middle age

20  A person in a coma
    a   Has suffered an electrical shock
    b   Has dementia
    c   Is unaware of his or her surroundings
    d   Has stopped breathing

21  You are caring for infants. Which is *unsafe?*
    a   Checking them in cribs often
    b   Laying them on their backs for sleep
    c   Propping a baby bottle on a rolled towel
    d   Keeping plastic bags away from them

22  A paraplegic is paralyzed
    a   From the waist down
    b   From the neck down
    c   On the right side of the body
    d   On the left side of the body

23  Mrs. Ford is 86 years old. Which is *unsafe* for her?
    a   Nonglare, waxed floors
    b   One-color floor coverings
    c   Safety rails and grab bars in the bathroom
    d   Nonskid shoes

24  To prevent falls, you should do the following *except*
    a   Wipe up spills right away
    b   Turn on night-lights
    c   Encourage the use of hand rails and grab bars
    d   Keep bed rails up

25  Which does *not* prevent falls?
    a   Meeting elimination needs
    b   Answering signal lights promptly
    c   Keeping persons at risk for falls in their rooms
    d   Using bed rails according to the care plan

26  These statements are about bed rails. Which is *true?*
    a   The person can get caught in bed rails.
    b   Bed rails are kept up when the person is in bed.
    c   OBRA requires the use of bed rails.
    d   Gaps between bed rails should be 4 inches or more.

27  Burns are caused by the following *except*
    a   Smoking
    b   Leaving children unattended or home alone
    c   Very hot bath water
    d   Oxygen

28  Mrs. Ford often tries to get up without help. You should do the following *except*
    a   Remind her to use the signal light
    b   Check on her often
    c   Help her to the bathroom at regular intervals
    d   Keep her bed rails up

**29** To prevent equipment accidents, you should
a Fix broken items
b Use two-pronged plugs
c Check glass and plastic items for damage
d Complete an incident report

**30** Mr. Wallace is a new resident. You need to shave him. Before using his electric shaver
a You need to inspect it
b The maintenance staff needs to do a safety check
c You need to check for a frayed cord
d You need an outlet

**31** You are using equipment. Which is *unsafe?*
a Following the manufacturer's instructions
b Keeping electrical items away from water and spills
c Pulling on the cord to remove a plug from an outlet
d Turning off electrical items after using them

**32** Mr. Wallace uses a wheelchair. Which measure is *unsafe?*
a The brakes are locked for transfers.
b He can stand on the footplates.
c The brakes are locked when he is watching TV.
d The casters point forward.

**33** Stretcher safety involves the following *except*
a Locking the wheels for transfers
b Fastening the safety straps
c Raising the side rails
d Moving the stretcher head first

**34** You spilled a hazardous substance. You should do the following *except*
a Read the material safety data sheet
b Cover the spill and go tell the nurse
c Wear any needed personal protective equipment to clean up the spill
d Complete an incident report

**35** The following are needed to start a fire *except*
a A spark or flame
b A material that will burn
c Oxygen
d Carbon monoxide

**36** The fire alarm sounds. The following are done *except*
a Turning off oxygen
b Using elevators
c Closing doors and windows
d Moving patients and residents to a safe place

**37** Your clothing is on fire. You should do the following *except*
a Run to get help
b Drop to the floor or ground
c Cover your face
d Roll to smother the flames

**38** To help prevent workplace violence, you need to do the following *except*
a Follow safety and security measures
b Take part in training programs
c Wear personal protective equipment
d Report safety and security concerns

**39** A person is agitated and aggressive. You should do the following *except*
a Stand away from the person
b Stand close to the door
c Use touch to show you care
d Talk to the person without raising your voice

**40** You work the night shift. Which is *unsafe?*
a Parking in a well-lit area
b Locking your car
c Finding your keys after getting into the car
d Checking the backseat and under your car

**41** Mr. Wallace is a new resident. Which helps prevent property loss?
a Sending personal belongings home with his family
b Labeling items with his name
c Putting personal items in a safe
d Giving him a wheelchair pouch for his things

**42** You gave Mrs. Ford the wrong treatment. Which is *true?*
a Report the error at the end of the shift.
b Take action only if Mrs. Ford was injured.
c You are guilty of negligence.
d You must complete an incident report.

*Answers to these questions are on p. 816.*

# 11

# Restraint Alternatives and Safe Restraint Use

## OBJECTIVES

- Define the key terms listed in this chapter
- Describe the purpose and complications of restraints
- Identify restraint alternatives
- Explain how to use restraints safely
- Perform the procedure described in this chapter

## KEY TERMS

**active physical restraint** A restraint attached to the person's body and to a fixed (immovable) object; it restricts movement or body access

**passive physical restraint** A restraint near but not directly attached to the person's body; it does not totally restrict freedom of movement and allows access to certain body parts

**restraint** Any item, object, device, garment, material, or drug that limits or restricts a person's freedom of movement or access to one's body

Many safety measures are presented in Chapter 10. However, some persons need extra protection. They may present dangers to themselves or others. For example:

- Ms. Perez needs help with getting up and with walking. She forgets to call for help. Falling is a risk.
- Ms. Wilson tries to pull out her feeding tube. The tube is part of her treatment.
- Ms. Walsh scratches and picks at a wound. This can damage the skin or the wound.
- Mr. Ross wanders. He may wander into traffic or get lost in neighborhoods, parks, forests, or other areas. Exposure to hot or cold weather presents other dangers.
- Mr. Winters tries to hit, pinch, and bite the staff. They are at risk for harm.

The RN uses the nursing process to decide how to best meet the person's safety needs. In nursing centers, a resident care conference is held. The health team reviews and updates the person's care plan. Every attempt is made to protect the person without using restraints. Sometimes they are needed.

A **restraint** is any item, object, device, garment, material, or drug that limits or restricts a person's freedom of movement or access to one's body. Restraints are used only as a *last resort* to protect persons from harming themselves or others.

## HISTORY OF RESTRAINT USE

Until the late 1980s, restraints were thought to *prevent* falls. Research shows that restraints *cause* falls. Falls occur when persons try to get free of the restraints.

Injuries are more serious from falls in restrained persons than in those not restrained.

Restraints also were used to prevent wandering or interfering with treatment. They were often used for persons who showed confusion, poor judgment, or behavior problems. Older persons were restrained more often than younger persons were. Restraints were viewed as necessary protective devices. Their purpose was to protect a person. However, they can cause serious harm (Box 11-1). They can even cause death.

OBRA, the Centers for Medicare & Medicaid Services (CMS), and the federal Food and Drug Administration (FDA) have guidelines about restraint use in hospitals and nursing centers. So do states and accrediting agencies. They do not forbid restraint use. *However, all other appropriate alternatives must be tried first.*

Every agency has policies and procedures for restraint use. They include identifying persons at risk for harm, harmful behaviors, restraint alternatives, and proper restraint use. Staff training is required.

## RESTRAINT ALTERNATIVES

Often there are causes and reasons for harmful behaviors. Knowing and treating the cause can prevent restraint use. The RN tries to find out what the behavior means. This is very important for persons who have speech or cognitive problems. The focus is on these questions:

- Is the person in pain?
- Is the person ill or injured?

(See Chapter 30.)

## BOX 11-1  RISKS OF RESTRAINT USE

- Agitation
- Anger
- Bruises
- Constipation
- Cuts
- Dehydration
- Depression
- Embarrassment
- Fecal incontinence (Chapter 19)
- Fractures
- Humiliation
- Mistrust
- Nerve injuries
- Nosocomial infection (Chapter 12)
- Pneumonia
- Pressure ulcers (Chapter 28)
- Strangulation
- Urinary incontinence (Chapter 18)
- Urinary tract infection

- Is the person short of breath? Are cells getting enough oxygen? (See Chapter 30.)
- Is the person afraid in a new setting?
- Does the person need to urinate or have a bowel movement?
- Is a dressing, bandage, or binder tight or causing other discomfort? (See Chapter 28.)
- Is clothing tight or causing other discomfort?
- Is the person's position uncomfortable?
- Is the person too hot or too cold?
- Is the person hungry?
- Is the person thirsty?
- Are body fluids, secretions, or excretions causing skin irritation?
- Is the person seeing, hearing, or feeling things that are not real? (See Chapter 34.)
- Is the person confused or disoriented? (See Chapter 35.)
- Are drugs causing the behaviors?

Restraint alternatives for the person are identified (Box 11-2). They become part of the care plan. The health team follows the care plan. Care plan changes are made as needed. Restraint alternatives may not protect the person. Then the doctor may need to order restraints.

## BOX 11-2  ALTERNATIVES TO RESTRAINTS

- Diversion is provided. This includes TV, videos, music, games, books, relaxation tapes, and so on.
- Lifelong habits and routines are in the care plan. For example, showers before breakfast; reads in the bathroom; walks outside before lunch; watches TV after lunch; and so on.
- Family and friends make videos of themselves for the person to watch.
- Videos are made of visits with family and friends for the person to watch.
- Time is spent in supervised areas (dining room, lounge, near nurses' station).
- Pillows, wedge cushions, posture, and positioning aids are used.
- The signal light is within reach.
- Signal lights are answered promptly.
- Food, fluid, and elimination needs are met.
- The bedpan, urinal, or commode is within the person's reach.
- Back massages are given.
- Family, friends, and volunteers visit.
- The person has companions and sitters.
- Time is spent with the person.
- Extra time is spent with a person who is restless.
- Reminiscing is done with the person.
- A calm, quiet setting is provided.
- The person wanders in safe areas.
- The entire staff is aware of persons who tend to wander. This includes staff in housekeeping, maintenance, business office, dietary, and so on.

- Exercise programs are provided.
- Outdoor time is planned during nice weather.
- The person does jobs or tasks he or she consents to.
- Warning devices are used on beds, chairs, and doors.
- Knob guards are used on doors.
- Padded hip protectors are worn under clothing (Fig. 11-1, p. 184).
- Floor cushions are placed next to beds (Fig. 11-2, p. 184).
- Roll guards are attached to the bed frame (Fig. 11-3, p. 184).
- Falls are prevented (Chapter 10).
- The person's furniture meets his or her needs (lower bed, reclining chair, rocking chair).
- Walls and furniture corners are padded.
- Observations and visits are made at least every 15 minutes.
- The person is moved closer to the nurses' station.
- Procedures and care measures are explained.
- Frequent explanations are given about required equipment or devices.
- Persons who are confused are oriented to person, time, and place. Calendars and clocks are provided.
- Light is adjusted to meet the person's needs and preferences.
- Staff assignments are consistent.
- Uninterrupted sleep is promoted.
- Noise levels are reduced.

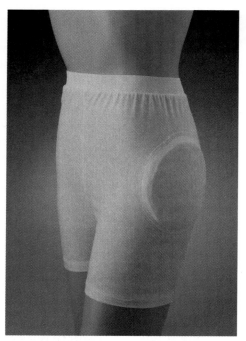

**FIG. 11-1** Hip protector. (Courtesy J. T. Posey Co., Arcadia, Calif.)

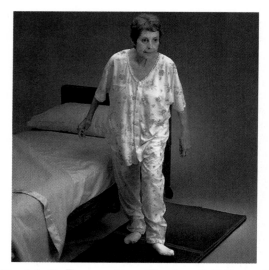

**FIG. 11-2** Floor cushion. (Courtesy J. T. Posey Co., Arcadia, Calif.)

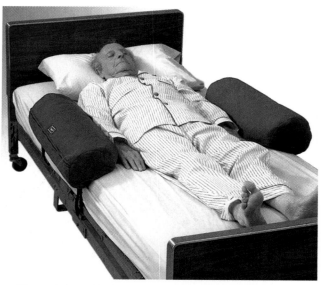

**FIG. 11-3** Roll guard. (Courtesy J. T. Posey Co., Arcadia, Calif.)

## SAFE RESTRAINT USE

Restraints can cause serious injury and even death. To protect the person, federal and state guidelines are followed. So are accrediting agency guidelines. They are part of your agency's policies and procedures for restraint use.

Restraints are not used to discipline a person. They are not used for staff convenience. *Discipline* is any action that punishes or penalizes a person. *Convenience* is any action that:
- Controls the person's behavior
- Requires less effort by the agency
- Is not in the person's best interests

Restraints are used only when necessary to treat a person's medical symptoms. Symptoms may relate to physical, emotional, or behavioral problems. Sometimes restraints are needed to protect the person or others. That is, patients and residents may behave in ways that are harmful to themselves or others (p. 182).

Imagine what it is like to be restrained:
- Your nose itches. But your hands and arms are restrained. You cannot scratch your nose.
- You need to use the bathroom. Your hands and arms are restrained. You cannot get up. You cannot reach your signal light. You soil yourself with urine or a bowel movement.
- Your phone is ringing. You cannot answer it because your hands and arms are restrained.
- You are not wearing your eyeglasses. You cannot identify people coming into and going out of your room. And you cannot speak because of a stroke. You have a vest restraint. You cannot move or turn in bed.
- You are thirsty. The water glass is within your reach but your hands and arms are restrained.
- You hear the fire alarm. You have on a restraint. You cannot get up to move to a safe place. You must wait until someone rescues you.

What would you try to do? Would you calmly lie or sit there? Would you try to get free from the restraint? Would you cry out for help? What would the nursing staff think? Would they think that you are uncomfortable? Or would they think that you are agitated and uncooperative? Would they think your behavior is improving or getting worse? Would you feel anger, embarrassment, or humiliation?

Try to put yourself in the person's situation. Then you can better understand how the person feels. Treat the person like you would want to be treated—with kindness, caring, respect, and dignity.

## PHYSICAL AND DRUG RESTRAINTS

According to OBRA and CMS, *physical restraints* includes these points:
- May be any manual method, physical or mechanical device, material or equipment
- Is attached to or next to the person's body
- Cannot be easily removed by the person
- Restricts freedom of movement or access to one's body

Physical restraints are applied to the chest, waist, elbows, wrists, hands, or legs. They confine the person to a bed or chair. Or they prevent movement of a body part. Some furniture or barriers also prevent free movement:
- Geriatric chairs (Geri-chairs) or chairs with attached trays are examples (Fig. 11-4). Such chairs are often used for persons needing support to sit up.
- Placing any chair so close to a wall that the person cannot move.
- Bed rails (Chapter 10).
- Sheets tucked in so tightly that they restrict movement.
  Drugs are restraints if they:
- Control behavior or restrict movement
- Are not standard treatment for the person's condition

Drugs cannot be used for discipline or staff convenience. They cannot be used if not required for the person's treatment. They cannot be used if they affect physical or mental function.

Sometimes drugs can help persons who are confused or disoriented. They may become anxious, agitated, or aggressive. The doctor may order drugs to control these behaviors. The goal is to control the behavior without making the person sleepy and unable to function at his or her highest level.

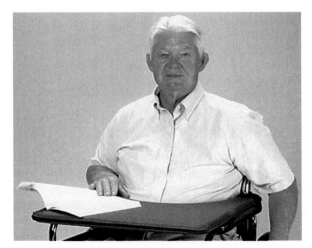

**FIG. 11-4** This lap-top tray is a restraint alternative. It is considered a restraint when used to prevent freedom of movement. (Courtesy J. T. Posey Co., Arcadia, Calif.)

## COMPLICATIONS OF RESTRAINT USE

Box 11-1 lists complications from restraints. Injuries occur as the person tries to get free of the restraint. Cuts, bruises, and fractures are common. Injuries also occur from using the wrong restraint, applying it wrong, or keeping it on too long. *The most serious risk is death from strangulation.*

There are also mental effects. Restraints affect dignity and self-esteem. Depression, anger, and agitation are common. So are embarrassment, humiliation, and mistrust.

Restraints are medical devices. The Safe Medical Device Act applies if a restraint causes illness, injury, or death. Also, CMS requires that the agency report any death that occurs while a person is in restraints.

## SAFETY GUIDELINES

*If a restraint is used, the least restrictive method is used.* While providing protection, it allows the greatest amount of movement or body access possible. Follow the safety measures listed in Box 11-3. Also remember the following:

- *Restraints are used to protect the person. They are not used for staff convenience or to discipline a person.* Restraining someone is not easier than properly supervising and observing the person. A restrained person requires more staff time for care, supervision, and observation. A restraint is used only when it is the best safety measure for the person. It is not used to punish or penalize uncooperative persons.
- *Restraints require a doctor's order.* If restraints are needed for medical reasons, a written doctor's order is required. The doctor gives the reason for the restraint, what body part to restrain, what to use, and how long to use it. This information is on the care plan and your assignment sheet.

*Text continued on p. 191.*

---

**BOX 11-3** **SAFETY MEASURES FOR USING RESTRAINTS**

- Use the restraint noted in the care plan. The least-restrictive device is used.
- Apply a restraint only after being instructed about its proper use.
- Demonstrate proper application of the restraint to the nurse before applying it.
- Use the correct size. The nurse and care plan tell you what size to use. Small restraints are tight. They cause discomfort and agitation. They also restrict breathing and circulation. Strangulation is a risk from big or loose restraints.
- Use only restraints that have the manufacturer's instructions and warning labels.
- Read the manufacturer's warning labels. Note the front and back of the restraint.
- Follow the manufacturer's instructions. Some restraints are safe for bed, chair, and wheelchair use. Others are used only with certain equipment.
- Do not use sheets, towels, tape, rope, straps, bandages, or other items to restrain a person.
- Use intact restraints. Look for tears, cuts, or frayed fabric or straps. Look for missing or loose hooks, loops, or straps or other damage.
- Do not use restraints to position a person on a toilet.
- Do not use restraints to position a person on furniture that does not allow for correct application. Follow the manufacturer's instructions.

- Follow agency policies and procedures.
- Position the person in good body alignment before applying the restraint (Chapter 13).
- Pad bony areas and skin. This prevents pressure and injury from the restraint.
- Secure the restraint. It should be snug but allow some movement of the restrained part.
  —*If applied to the chest or waist:* Make sure that the person can breathe easily. A flat hand should slide between the restraint and the person's body (Fig. 11-5).
  —*For wrist and mitt restraints:* You should be able to slide one or two fingers under the restraint.
- Follow the manufacturer's instructions to check for snugness.
- Criss-cross vest restraints in front (Fig. 11-6). Do not criss-cross restraints in the back unless part of the manufacturer's instructions (Fig. 11-7). Criss-crossing vests in the back can cause death from strangulation.
- Tie restraints according to agency policy. The policy should follow the manufacturer's instructions. Quick-release buckles or airline-type buckles are used (Fig. 11-8). So are quick-release ties (Fig. 11-9, p. 188).
- Secure straps out of the person's reach.
- Leave 1 to 2 inches of slack in the straps. This allows some movement of the part.

*Continued.*

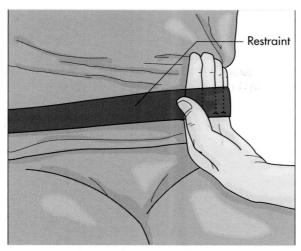

**FIG. 11-5** A flat hand slides between the restraint and the person.

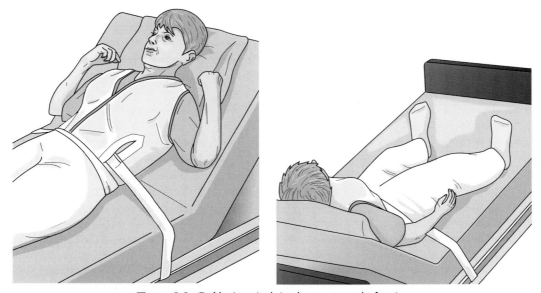

**FIG. 11-6** Vest restraint criss-crosses in front.

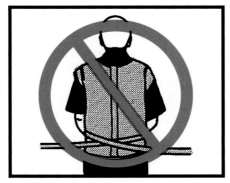

**FIG. 11-7** Never criss-cross vest or jacket straps in back. (Courtesy J. T. Posey Co., Arcadia, Calif.)

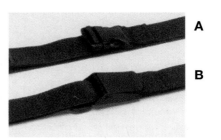

**FIG. 11-8 A,** Quick release buckle. **B,** Airline-type buckle. (Courtesy J. T. Posey Co., Arcadia, Calif.)

---

**BOX 11-3** **SAFETY MEASURES FOR USING RESTRAINTS—CONT'D**

- Secure the restraint to the movable part of the bed frame at waist level (see Fig. 11-9). For chairs, secure straps to the wheelchair or the chair frame (Fig. 11-10).
- Make sure that straps will not slide in any direction. If straps slide, they change the restraint's position. The person can get suspended off the mattress or chair (Figs. 11-11 and 11-12). Strangulation can result.
- Never secure restraints to the bed rails. The person can reach bed rails to release knots or buckles. Also, injury to the person is likely when raising or lowering bed rails.
- Use bed rail covers or gap protectors according to the nurse's instructions (Fig. 11-13, p. 190). They prevent entrapment between the rails or the bed rail bars (see Fig. 11-11). Entrapment can occur between:
  —The bars of a bed rail
  —The space between half-length (split) bed rails
  —The bed rail and mattress
  —The headboard or footboard and mattress
- Keep full bed rails up when using a vest, jacket, or belt restraint. Also use bed rail covers or gap protectors. Otherwise the person could fall off the bed and strangle on the restraint. If half-length bed rails are used, the person can get caught between them.

- Position the person in semi-Fowler's position when using a vest, jacket, or belt restraint.
- Position the person in a chair so the hips are well to the back of the chair.
- Apply a belt restraint at a 45-degree angle over the hips (Fig. 11-14, p. 191).
- Do not use back cushions when a person is restrained in a chair. If the cushion moves out of place, slack occurs in the straps. Strangulation could result if the person slides forward or down from the extra slack (see Fig. 11-12).
- Do not cover the restraint with a sheet, blanket, bedspread, or other covering. The restraint must be within plain view at all times.
- Check the person's circulation at least every 15 minutes if mitt, wrist, or ankle restraints are applied. You should feel a pulse at a pulse site below the restraint. Fingers or toes should be warm and pink. Tell the nurse at once if:
  —You cannot feel a pulse
  —Fingers or toes are cold, pale, or blue in color
  —The person complains of pain, numbness, or tingling in the restrained part
  —The skin is red or damaged

*Continued.*

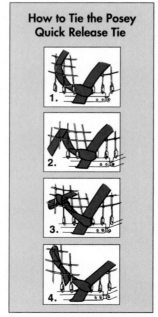

**FIG. 11-9** The Posey quick release tie. (Courtesy J. T. Posey Co., Arcadia, Calif.)

**How to Tie the Posey Quick Release Tie**

1.
2.
3.
4.

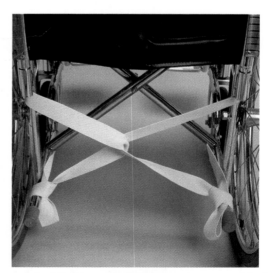

**FIG. 11-10** The restraint straps are secured to the wheelchair frame with quick release ties. (Courtesy J. T. Posey Co., Arcadia, Calif.)

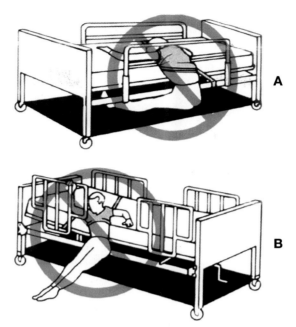

**FIG. 11-11 A,** A person can get suspended and caught between bed rail bars. **B,** The person can get suspended and caught between half-length bed rails. (Courtesy J. T. Posey Co., Arcadia, Calif.)

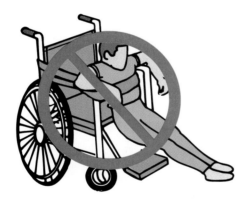

**Straps to prevent sliding should always be over the thighs—NOT around the waist or chest.** Straps should be at a 45° angle and secured to the chair under the seat, not behind the back. They should be snug but comfortable and not restrict breathing. If a belt or vest is too loose or applied around the waist, the person may slide partially off the seat—resulting in the possible suffocation and death.

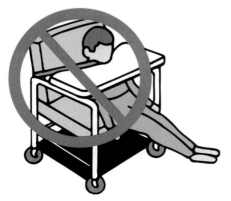

**Tray tables (with or without a belt or vest) pose potential danger if the person should slide partly under the table and become caught.** This could result in suffocation and death. Make sure the person's hips are positioned at the back of the chair—this may necessitate the use of an anti-slide material (Posey Grip), a pommel cushion, or a restrictive device if the person shows any tendency to slide forward.

**FIG. 11-12** Strangulation could result if the person slides forward or down because of extra slack in the restraint. (Courtesy J. T. Posey Co., Arcadia, Calif.)

**BOX 11-3 SAFETY MEASURES FOR USING RESTRAINTS—CONT'D**

- Check the person at least every 15 minutes if a belt, jacket, or vest restraint is used. The person should be able to breathe easily. Also check the position of the restraint, especially in the front and back.
- Check the person at least every 15 minutes for safety and comfort.
- Monitor persons in the supine position constantly. They are at great risk for aspiration if vomiting occurs (Chapter 20). Call for the nurse at once.
- Do not use a restraint near a fire, flame, or smoking materials. Restraint fabrics may ignite easily.
- Keep scissors in your pocket. In an emergency, cutting the tie may be faster than untying the knot. Never leave scissors at the bedside or where the person can reach them.

- Remove the restraint and reposition the person every 2 hours. Meet the person's basic needs:
  —Meet elimination needs.
  —Offer food and fluids.
  —Meet hygiene needs.
  —Give skin care.
  —Perform range-of-motion exercises or ambulate the person (Chapter 22). Follow the care plan.
  —Chart what was done, the care given, your observations, and when and what you reported to the nurse.
- Keep the signal light within the person's reach.
- Report to the nurse every time you checked the person and released the restraint. Report your observations and the care given. Follow center policy for recording.

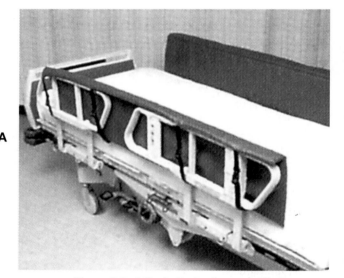
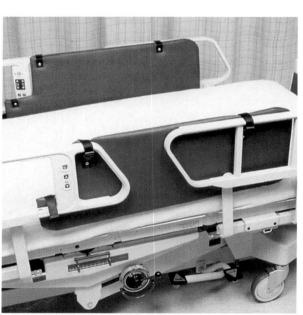

**FIG. 11-13 A,** Bed rail covers. **B,** Gap protectors. (Courtesy J. T. Posey Co., Arcadia, Calif.)

- *The least restrictive method is used.* An **active physical restraint** attaches to the person's body and to a fixed (immovable) object. It restricts movement or body access. Vest, jacket, leg, arm, wrist, hand, and some belt restraints are active physical restraints. A **passive physical restraint** is near but not directly attached to the person's body (bed rails or wedge cushions). It does not totally restrict freedom of movement. It allows access to certain body parts. Passive physical restraints are the least restrictive.

- *Restraints are used only after trying other ways to protect the person.* Some people can harm themselves or others. The care plan must include measures to protect the person and prevent harm to others. Restraints lessen the person's dignity. They are allowed only after other measures fail to protect the person (see Box 11-2). Many fall prevention measures are restraint alternatives (Chapter 10).

- *Unnecessary restraint is false imprisonment* (Chapter 2). If told to apply a restraint, you must clearly understand the need. If not, politely ask about its use. If you apply a restraint that is not needed, you could face false imprisonment charges.

- *Informed consent is required.* The person must understand the reason for the restraint. The person is told how the restraint will help the planned medical treatment. The person is told about risks of restraint use. If the person cannot give informed consent, his or her legal representative is given the information. Either the person or legal representative must give consent. Restraints cannot be used without consent. The doctor or nurse provides the necessary information and obtains informed consent.

- *The manufacturer's instructions are followed.* The manufacturer gives instructions about applying and securing the restraint. Failure to follow them could affect the person's safety. You could be negligent for improperly applying or securing a restraint.

- *The person's basic needs must be met.* The restraint must be snug and firm, but not tight. Tight restraints affect circulation and breathing. The person must be comfortable and able to move the restrained part to a limited and safe extent. The person is checked at least every 15 minutes or as often as required by the person's needs. Food, fluid, comfort, safety, exercise, hygiene, and elimination needs must be met.

- *Restraints are applied with enough help to protect the person and staff from injury.* Persons in immediate danger of harming themselves or others are restrained quickly. Combative and agitated people can hurt themselves and the staff when restraints are applied. Enough staff members are needed to complete the task safely and quickly.

- *Restraints can increase confusion and agitation.* Whether confused or alert, people are aware of restricted movements. They may try to get out of the restraint or struggle or pull at it. Many restrained persons beg anyone who passes by to free or to help release them. These behaviors often are viewed as signs of confusion. Confusion increases in some persons because they do not understand what is happening to them. Restrained persons need repeated explanations and reassurance. Spending time with them has a calming effect.

- *Quality of life must be protected.* Restraints are used for as short a time as possible. The care plan must show how restraint use is reduced. The goal is to meet the person's needs with as little restraint as possible. You must meet the person's physical and psychosocial needs. Visit with the person and explain the reason for restraints.

- *The person is observed at least every 15 minutes or more often as required by the care plan.* Restraints are dangerous. Injuries and deaths can occur from improper restraint use and poor observation. Complications from restraints are prevented. Interferences with breathing and circulation are examples. Practice the safety measures in Box 11-3, p. 186.

- *The restraint is removed, the person repositioned, and basic needs met at least every 2 hours.* This includes food, fluid, hygiene, and elimination needs and giving skin care. Range-of-motion exercises are done. Or the person is ambulated according to the care plan.

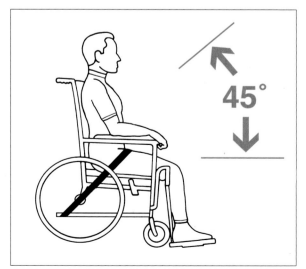

**FIG. 11-14** The safety belt is at a 45-degree angle over the hips. (Courtesy J. T. Posey Co., Arcadia, Calif.)

## Reporting and Recording

Information about restraints is recorded in the person's medical record (Fig. 11-15). You might apply restraints or care for a restrained person. Report the following to the nurse. If you are allowed to chart, include this information:

- The type of restraint applied
- The body part or parts restrained
- The reason for the application
- Safety measures taken (for example, bed rails padded and up)
- The time you applied the restraint
- The time you removed the restraint
- The care given when the restraint was removed
- Skin color and condition
- The pulse felt in the restrained part
- Changes in the person's behavior
- Complaints of a tight restraint, difficulty breathing, and pain, numbness, or tingling in the restrained part (report these complaints to the nurse at once)

## Applying Restraints

Restraints are made of cloth or leather. Cloth restraints (soft restraints) are mitts, belts, straps, jackets, and vests. They are applied to the wrists, ankles, hands, waist, and chest. Leather restraints are applied to the wrists and ankles. They are used for extreme agitation and combativeness.

*See Focus on Older Persons: Applying Restraints.*

**Wrist restraints.** Wrist restraints (limb holders) limit arm movement (Fig. 11-16). They may be used when a person continually tries to pull out tubes used for treatment (IV, feeding tube, catheter, wound drainage tubes, or monitoring lines). Or the person tries to scratch, pick at, pull at, or peel the skin, a wound, or a dressing. This can damage the skin or the wound.

**Mitt restraints.** Hands are placed in mitt restraints. They prevent finger use. They do not prevent hand, wrist, or arm movements. They are used for the same reasons as wrist restraints are. Most mitts are padded (Fig. 11-17).

**RESTRAINT RELEASE RECORD**

*(Reference tag: F221)*

**PLEASE NOTE: Restrained individuals must be checked at least every 15 minutes. In addition, restraints must be released for the purpose of exercise, toileting, etc. at least every two hours.**

| REASON FOR RESTRAINT | RESTRAINT ORDERED (Circle) | REMOVAL REASON CODES | |
|---|---|---|---|
| *Is nonweight bearing and attempts to rise when in W/C.* | Waist, Pelvic, Siderails 2 Full, 1 Full, 2 Half, 1 Half; Wrist, Belt (circled); Geri Chair, Vest; Ankle, Bar; Other___ | A- Supervised meals<br>B- Supervised group activities<br>C- Care provided by CNA<br>D- One-to-one with volunteer<br>E- One-to-one with social worker | F- 2-3 hrs. with periodic evaluation<br>G- Total elimination of restraint<br>H- *off when in bed*<br>I- ___<br>J- ___ |

| DATE *7/18* Month/Year | 15 MINUTE CHECK WHEN RESTRAINED — Shift Initials 11-7 | 7-3 | 3-11 | RELEASE EVERY TWO HOURS FOR PERSONAL CARE — Shift Initials 11-7 | 7-3 | 3-11 | TOTAL HOURS RELEASED PER SHIFT AND REASONS (USE REASON CODES ABOVE) 11-7 | 7-3 | 3-11 | COMMENTS/ RESIDENT'S RESPONSE (Negative or Positive) |
|---|---|---|---|---|---|---|---|---|---|---|
| 1 | Lg | BG | MM | Lg | BG | MM | 8(H) | 4(A,B, C,H) | 5(A,C, D,H) | *No agitation – no falls no attempts to rise* |
| 2 | Lg | BG | MM | Lg | BG | MM | 8(H) | 5(A,B, C,F,H) | 6(A,C, F,H) | *Doing well – no falls –* |
| 3 | DL | RD | DL | ML | RD | ML | 8(H) | 6(A,B, C,F,H) | 8(A,C, F,H) | No falls - Resident wants belt removed |
| 4 | | | | | | | | | | |
| 5 | | | | | | | | | | |
| 6 | | | | | | | | | | |

**Fig. 11-15** Charting sample. (Courtesy Briggs Corp., Des Moines, Iowa.)

**BELT RESTRAINTS.** The belt restraint (Fig. 11-18) is used when injuries from falls are risks. The person cannot get out of bed or out of a chair. However, the person can turn from side to side or sit up in bed.

The belt is applied around the waist and secured to the bed or chair. It is applied over a garment. The person can release the quick-release type. It is less restrictive than those that only staff members can release.

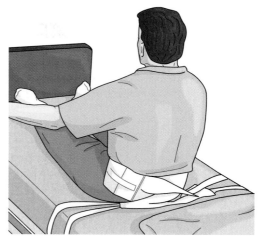

> ### FOCUS ON OLDER PERSONS
> #### APPLYING RESTRAINTS
> Some older persons have dementia. Restraints may increase their confusion and agitation. They do not understand what you are doing. They may resist staff efforts to apply a restraint and actively try to get free from it. This can cause serious injury and even death. It decreases quality of life.
>
> Never use force to apply a restraint. Always ask a co-worker to help apply a restraint to a person who is confused and agitated. Report any problems to the nurse at once.

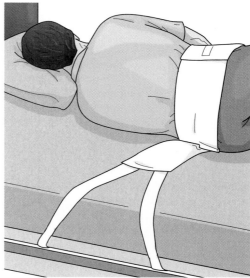

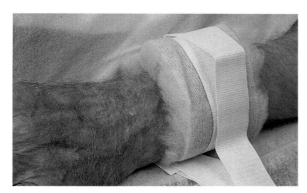

**FIG. 11-16** Limb restraint. Note the soft part is toward the skin.

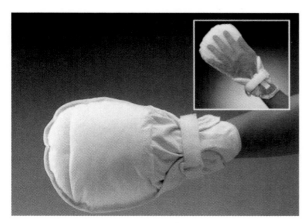

**FIG. 11-17** Mitt restraint. (Courtesy J. T. Posey Co., Arcadia, Calif.)

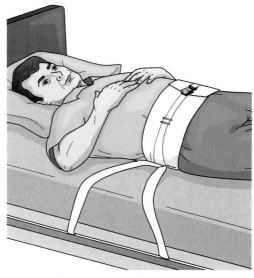

**FIG. 11-18** Belt restraint.

**VEST RESTRAINTS AND JACKET RESTRAINTS.**
Vest and jacket restraints are applied to the chest. They may be used to prevent injuries from falls. And they may be used for persons who need positioning for a medical treatment. The person cannot turn in bed or get out of bed or a chair.

A jacket restraint is applied with the opening in the back. For a vest restraint, the vest crosses in front (see Fig. 11-6). *The straps of vest and jacket restraints always cross in the front.* They must *never* cross in the back. Vest and jacket restraints are never worn backward. Strangulation or other injury could occur if the person slides down in the bed or chair. The restraint is always applied over a garment. *(Note: A vest or jacket restraint may have a positioning slot in the back. Criss-cross the straps following the manufacturer's instructions.)*

Vest and jacket restraints have life-threatening risks. Death can occur from strangulation. If the person gets caught in the restraint, it can become so tight that the person's chest cannot expand to inhale air. The person quickly suffocates and dies. Restraints must be applied correctly. For vest and jacket restraints, this is critical. You are advised to only assist the nurse in applying them. The nurse should assume full responsibility for applying a vest or jacket restraint.

*See Focus on Children: Applying Restraints.*

---

**DELEGATION GUIDELINES:** *Applying Restraints*
Before applying any restraint, you need this information from the nurse and the care plan:
- Why the doctor ordered the restraint
- What type and size to use
- Where to apply the restraint
- How to safely apply the restraint (Have the nurse show you how to apply it. Then demonstrate correct application back to the nurse.)
- How to correctly position the person
- What bony areas to pad and how to pad them
- If bed rail covers or gap protectors are needed
- If bed rails are up or down
- What special equipment is needed
- If the person needs to be checked more often than every 15 minutes
- When to apply and release the restraint

---

**SAFETY ALERT:** *Applying Restraints*
Restraints can cause serious harm, even death. Always follow the manufacturer's instructions. Check the person at least every 15 minutes or more often as instructed by the nurse and the care plan.

---

**FOCUS ON CHILDREN**
**APPLYING RESTRAINTS**
Elbow restraints limit arm movements. They prevent infants and children from bending their elbows (Fig. 11-19). They are used to prevent scratching and touching incisions or pulling out tubes. Both arms are restrained to achieve the desired effect.

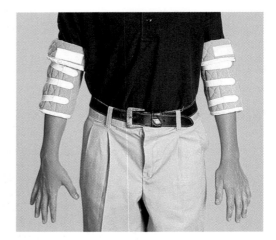
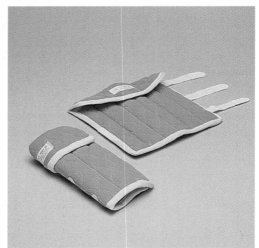

**FIG. 11-19** Elbow restraints. (Courtesy J. T. Posey Co., Arcadia, Calif.)

## APPLYING RESTRAINTS

### QUALITY OF LIFE

Remember to:
- Knock before entering the person's room
- Address the person by name
- Introduce yourself by name and title

### PRE-PROCEDURE

1 Follow *Delegation Guidelines: Applying Restraints.* See *Safety Alert: Applying Restraints.*
2 Collect the following as instructed by the nurse:
   - Correct type and size of restraints
   - Padding for bony areas
   - Bed rail pads or gap protectors
3 Practice hand hygiene.
4 Identify the person. Check the ID bracelet against the assignment sheet. Call the person by name.
5 Explain the procedure to the person.
6 Provide for privacy.

### PROCEDURE

7 Make sure the person is comfortable and in good body alignment (Chapter 13).
8 Put the bed rail pads or gap protectors on the bed if the person is in bed, if needed. Follow the manufacturer's instructions.
9 Pad bony areas according to the nurse's instructions.
10 Read the manufacturer's instructions. Note the front and back of the restraint.
11 *For wrist restraints:*
   a Apply the restraint following the manufacturer's instructions. Place the soft part toward the skin.
   b Secure the restraint so it is snug but not tight. Make sure you can slide one or two fingers under the restraint (Fig. 11-20). Follow the manufacturer's instructions.
   c Tie the straps to the movable part of the bed frame out of the person's reach. Use an agency-approved tie. Leave 1 to 2 inches of slack in the straps.
   d Repeat step 11 (a, b, and c) for the other wrist.
12 *For mitt restraints:*
   a Make sure the person's hands are clean and dry.
   b Apply the mitt restraint. Follow the manufacturer's instructions.
   c Tie the straps to the movable part of the bed frame. Use an agency-approved tie. Leave 1 to 2 inches of slack in the straps.
   d Make sure the restraint is snug. Slide one or two fingers between the restraint and the wrist. Adjust the straps if it is too loose or too tight. Check for snugness again.
   e Repeat step 12 (b, c, and d) for the other hand.

*Continued.*

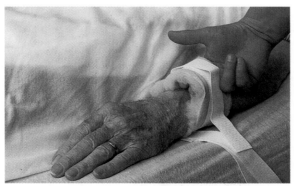

**FIG. 11-20** Two fingers fit between the restraint and the wrist.

## APPLYING RESTRAINTS

### PROCEDURE—CONT'D

**13** *For a belt restraint:*
  **a** Assist the person to a sitting position.
  **b** Apply the restraint with your free hand. Follow the manufacturer's instructions.
  **c** Remove wrinkles or creases from the front and back of the restraint.
  **d** Bring the ties through the slots in the belt.
  **e** Help the person lie down if he or she is in bed.
  **f** Make sure the person is comfortable and in good body alignment (Chapter 13).
  **g** Secure the straps to the movable part of the bed frame out of the person's reach or to the chair or wheelchair. Use an agency-approved tie. Leave 1 to 2 inches of slack in the straps.

**14** *For a vest restraint:*
  **a** Assist the person to a sitting position.
  **b** Apply the restraint with your free hand. Follow the manufacturer's instructions. The "V" part of the vest crosses in front.
  **c** Make sure the vest is free of wrinkles in the front and back.
  **d** Help the person lie down if he or she is in bed.
  **e** Bring the straps through the slots.
  **f** Make sure the person is comfortable and in good body alignment (Chapter 13).
  **g** Secure the straps to the chair or to the movable part of the bed frame. If secured to the bed frame, the straps are secured at waist level out of the person's reach. Use an agency-approved tie. Leave 1 to 2 inches of slack in the straps.
  **h** Make sure the vest is snug. Slide an open hand between the restraint and the person. Adjust the restraint if it is too loose or too tight. Check for snugness again.

**15** *For a jacket restraint:*
  **a** Assist the person to a sitting position.
  **b** Apply the restraint with your free hand. Follow the manufacturer's instructions. Remember, the jacket opening goes in the back.
  **c** Close the back with the zipper, ties, or hook and loop closures.
  **d** Make sure the side seams are under the arms. Remove any wrinkles in the front and back.
  **e** Help the person lie down if he or she is in bed.
  **f** Make sure the person is comfortable and in good body alignment (Chapter 13).
  **g** Secure the straps to the chair or to the movable part of the bed frame. If secured to the bed frame, the straps are secured at waist level out of the person's reach. Use an agency-approved knot. Leave 1 to 2 inches of slack in the straps.
  **h** Make sure the jacket is snug. Slide an open hand between the restraint and the person. Adjust the restraint if it is too loose or too tight. Check for snugness again.

**16** *For elbow restraints:*
  **a** Wrap the restraint around the child's elbow. Follow the manufacturer's instructions.
  **b** Secure the restraint. Follow the manufacturer's instructions. Leave 1 to 2 inches of slack in the straps.
  **c** Repeat step 16 (a and b) for the other arm.

### POST-PROCEDURE

**17** Position the person as the nurse directs.
**18** Place the signal light within the person's reach.
**19** Raise or lower bed rails. Follow the care plan and the manufacturer's instructions for the restraint.
**20** Unscreen the person.
**21** Decontaminate your hands.
**22** Check the person and the restraints at least every 15 minutes. Report and record your observations.
  **a** For wrist and mitt restraints: check the pulse, color, and temperature of the restrained parts.
  **b** For vest, jacket, and belt restraints: check the person's breathing. *Call for the nurse at once if the person is not breathing or is having difficulty breathing.* Make sure the restraint is properly positioned in the front and back.
**23** Do the following at least every 2 hours:
  ■ Remove the restraint.
  ■ Reposition the person.
  ■ Meet food, fluid, hygiene, and elimination needs.
  ■ Give skin care.
  ■ Perform range-of-motion exercises, or ambulate the person. Follow the care plan.
  ■ Reapply the restraints.
**24** Report and record your observations and the care given (see Fig. 11-15).

# ■ REVIEW QUESTIONS ■

Circle **T** if the statement is true and **F** if it is false.

1   T F   Restraint alternatives fail to protect a person. The nurse can order a restraint.
2   T F   Restraints can be used for staff convenience.
3   T F   A device is a restraint only if it is attached to the person's body.
4   T F   Bed rails are restraints.
5   T F   Restraints are used only for specific medical symptoms.
6   T F   Restraints can be used to protect the person from harming others.
7   T F   Unnecessary restraint is false imprisonment.
8   T F   Informed consent is needed for restraint use.
9   T F   You can apply restraints when you think they are needed.
10  T F   Restraint straps are secured within the person's reach.
11  T F   You can use a vest restraint to position a person on the toilet.
12  T F   Restraints are removed every 2 hours to reposition the person and give skin care.
13  T F   Restraint straps are tied to bed rails.
14  T F   Some drugs are restraints.
15  T F   A vest restraint crosses in front.
16  T F   Bed rails are left down when vest restraints are used.

Circle the **BEST** answer.

17  These statements are about restraints. Which is *false*?
a   A restraint can be an object, device, garment, or material.
b   A restraint limits or restricts a person's movement.
c   Some drugs are restraints.
d   A restraint is used when the nurse thinks it is needed.

18  Which is *not* a restraint alternative?
a   Positioning the person's chair close to a wall
b   Answering signal lights promptly
c   Taking the person outside in nice weather
d   Padding walls and corners of furniture

19  Physical restraints
a   Control mental function
b   Control a behavior
c   Confine a person to a bed or chair
d   Decrease care needs

20  The following can occur because of restraints. Which is the *most* serious?
a   Fractures
b   Strangulation
c   Pressure ulcers
d   Urinary tract infection

21  A belt restraint is applied to a person in bed. Where should you tie the straps?
a   To the bed rails
b   To the head board
c   To the movable part of the bed frame
d   To the foot board

22  Mrs. Hall has a restraint. You should check her and the position of the restraint at least
a   Every 15 minutes
b   Every 30 minutes
c   Every hour
d   Every 2 hours

23  Mrs. Hall has mitt restraints. Which of these is especially important to report to the nurse?
a   Her heart rate
b   Her respiratory rate
c   Why the restraints were applied
d   If you felt a pulse in the restrained extremities

24  Which are *not* used to prevent falls?
a   Wrist restraints
b   Jacket restraints
c   Belt restraints
d   Vest restraints

25  The doctor ordered mitt restraints for Mrs. Hall. You need the following information from the nurse *except*
a   What size to use
b   What other equipment is needed
c   What drugs Mrs. Hall is taking
d   When to apply and release the restraints

**26** Mr. Boyd has a vest restraint. It is not too tight or too loose if you can slide
    **a** A fist between the vest and the person
    **b** One finger between the vest and the person
    **c** An open hand between the vest and the person
    **d** Two fingers between the vest and the person

**27** The correct way to apply any restraint is to follow the
    **a** Nurse's directions
    **b** Doctor's orders
    **c** Care plan
    **d** Manufacturer's instructions

*Answers to these questions are on p. 817.*

# Preventing Infection

## OBJECTIVES

- Define the key terms listed in this chapter
- Identify what microbes need to live and grow
- List the signs and symptoms of infection
- Explain the chain of infection
- Describe nosocomial infection and the persons at risk
- Describe the practices of medical asepsis
- Describe disinfection and sterilization methods
- Explain how to care for equipment and supplies
- Explain Standard and Transmission-Based Precautions and the Bloodborne Pathogen Standard
- Explain the principles and practices of surgical asepsis
- Perform the procedures described in this chapter

## KEY TERMS

**asepsis** Being free of disease-producing microbes

**biohazardous waste** Items contaminated with blood, body fluids, secretions, or excretions; *bio* means life, and *hazardous* means dangerous or harmful

**carrier** A human or animal that is a reservoir for microbes but does not have signs and symptoms of infection

**clean technique** Medical asepsis

**communicable disease** A disease caused by pathogens that spread easily; a contagious disease

**contagious disease** Communicable disease

**contamination** The process of becoming unclean

**disinfection** The process of destroying pathogens

**germicide** A disinfectant applied to the skin, tissues, or non-living objects

**immunity** Protection against a certain disease

**infection** A disease resulting from the invasion and growth of microbes in the body

**medical asepsis** Practices used to remove or destroy pathogens and to prevent their spread from one person or place to another person or place; clean technique

**microbe** A microorganism

**microorganism** A small *(micro)* living plant or animal *(organism)* seen only with a microscope; a microbe

**non-pathogen** A microbe that does not usually cause an infection

**normal flora** Microbes that live and grow in a certain area

**nosocomial infection** An infection acquired during a stay in a health agency

**pathogen** A microbe that is harmful and can cause an infection

**reservoir** The environment in which a microbe lives and grows

**spore** A bacterium protected by a hard shell

**sterile** The absence of *all* microbes

**sterile field** A work area free of *all* pathogens and non-pathogens (including spores)

**sterile technique** Surgical asepsis

**sterilization** The process of destroying *all* microbes

**surgical asepsis** The practices that keep items free of *all* microbes; sterile technique

**vaccination** The administration of a vaccine to produce immunity against an infectious disease

**vaccine** A preparation containing dead or weakened microbes

Infection is a major safety and health hazard. Minor infections cause short illnesses. Some infections are serious and can cause death. Infants and older persons are at risk. So are disabled persons. The health team protects patients, residents, visitors, and themselves from infection. They prevent the cause of the infection from spreading.

# MICROORGANISMS

A **microorganism (microbe)** is a small *(micro)* living plant or animal *(organism)*. It is seen only with a microscope. Microbes are everywhere. They are in the mouth, nose, respiratory tract, stomach, intestines, and on the skin. They are in the air, soil, water, and food. They are on animals, clothing, and furniture.

Some microbes are harmful and can cause infections. They are called **pathogens. Non-pathogens** are microbes that do not usually cause an infection.

## TYPES OF MICROBES

There are five types of microbes:
- *Bacteria*—plant life that multiplies rapidly. Often called *germs,* they are one cell. They can cause infection in any body system.
- *Fungi*—plants that live on other plants or animals. Mushrooms, yeasts, and molds are common fungi. Fungi can infect the mouth, vagina, skin, feet, and other body areas.
- *Protozoa*—one-celled animals. They can infect the blood, brain, intestines, and other body areas.
- *Rickettsiae*—found in fleas, lice, ticks, and other insects. They are spread to humans by insect bites. Rocky Mountain spotted fever is an example. The person has fever, chills, headache, rash, and other signs and symptoms.
- *Viruses*—grow in living cells. They cause many diseases. The common cold, herpes, and hepatitis are examples.

## REQUIREMENTS OF MICROBES

Microbes need a reservoir to live and grow. The **reservoir** *(host)* is the environment in which a microbe lives and grows. People, plants, animals, the soil, food, and water are common reservoirs. Microbes need *water* and *nourishment* from the reservoir. Most need *oxygen* to live. A *warm* and *dark* environment is needed. Most grow best at body temperature. They are destroyed by heat and light.

## NORMAL FLORA

**Normal flora** are microbes that live and grow in a certain area. Certain microbes are in the respiratory tract, in the intestines, and on the skin. They are non-pathogens when in or on a natural reservoir. When a non-pathogen is transmitted from its natural site to another site or host, it becomes a pathogen. *Escherichia coli* is in the colon. If it enters the urinary system, it can cause an infection.

# DRUG-RESISTANT ORGANISMS

*Drug-resistant organisms* are microbes that are able to resist the effects of antibiotics. Antibiotics are drugs that kill microbes that cause infections. Some microbes can change their structures. This makes them more difficult to kill. They can survive in the presence of antibiotics. Therefore the infections they cause are difficult to treat. There are two main causes of drug-resistant organisms—doctors prescribing antibiotics when they are not needed (over-prescribing) and people not taking antibiotics for the amount of time prescribed. Two common types of drug-resistant organisms are:
- *Methicillin-resistant Staphylococcus aureas (MRSA): Staphylococcus aureas* (commonly called "staph") is normally found in the nose and on the skin. It can cause serious wound infections and pneumonia. This microbe has become resistant to methicillin, a type of penicillin.
- *Vancomycin-resistant Enterococcus (VRE): Enterococcus* is normally found in the intestines and is present in feces. It can be transmitted to others by contaminated hands, toilet seats, care equipment, and other items that the hands touch. When not in its natural site (the intestines), it can cause an infection. It can cause urinary tract, wound, pelvic, and other infections. This microbe is resistant to many antibiotics.

# INFECTION

An **infection** is a disease resulting from the invasion and growth of microbes in the body. A *local infection* is in a body part. A *systemic infection* involves the whole body. (Systemic means entire.) The person has some or all of the signs and symptoms listed in Box 12-1, p. 202. *See Focus on Older Persons: Infection, p. 202.*

## THE CHAIN OF INFECTION

The chain of infection (Fig. 12-1, p. 202) is a process involving a:
- Source
- Reservoir
- Portal of exit
- Method of transmission
- Portal of entry
- Susceptible host

## BOX 12-1 SIGNS AND SYMPTOMS OF INFECTION

- Fever
- Increased pulse and respiratory rates
- Pain or tenderness
- Fatigue and loss of energy
- Loss of appetite *(anorexia)*
- Nausea
- Vomiting
- Diarrhea
- Rash
- Sores on mucous membranes
- Redness and swelling of a body part
- Discharge or drainage from the infected area

### FOCUS ON OLDER PERSONS
#### INFECTION

The immune system protects the body from disease and infection (Chapter 7). Like other body systems, changes occur in the immune system with aging. When an older person has an infection, he or she may not show the signs and symptoms listed in Box 12-1. The person may have only a slight fever or no fever at all. Redness and swelling may be very slight. The person may not complain of pain. Confusion and delirium may occur (Chapter 35).

An infection can become life-threatening before the older person has obvious signs and symptoms. You must be alert to the most minor changes in a person's behavior or condition. Report any concerns to the nurse at once.

The *source* is a pathogen. It must have a *reservoir* where it can grow and multiply. Humans and animals are reservoirs. If they do not have signs and symptoms of infection, they are **carriers.** Carriers can pass the pathogen to others. The pathogen must leave the reservoir. That is, it needs a *portal of exit.* Exits are the respiratory, gastrointestinal, urinary, and reproductive tracts, breaks in the skin, and the blood.

After leaving the reservoir, the pathogen must be *transmitted* to another host (Fig. 12-2). The pathogen enters the body through a *portal of entry.* Portals of entry and exit are the same. A *susceptible host* (a person at risk for infection) is needed for the microbe to grow and multiply.

The human body can protect itself from infection. The ability to resist infection relates to age, nutrition, stress, fatigue, and health. Drugs, disease, and injury also are factors.

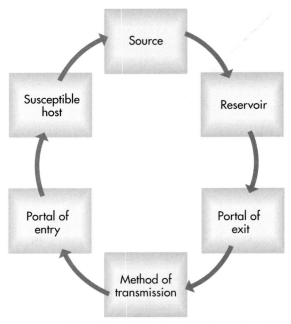

**FIG. 12-1** The chain of infection. (Redrawn from Potter PA, Perry AG: *Fundamentals of nursing: concepts, process, and practice,* ed 4, St Louis, 1997, Mosby.)

## NOSOCOMIAL INFECTION

A **nosocomial infection** is an infection acquired during a stay in a health agency. (*Nosocomial* comes from the Greek word for hospital.) Nosocomial infections are caused by normal flora. Or they are caused by microbes transmitted to the person from another source.

For example, *E. coli* is normally in the colon. Feces (bowel movements) contain *E. coli.* Poor wiping after bowel movements can cause *E. coli* to enter the urinary system. The hands can transmit *E. coli* to other body areas. If hand washing is poor, *E. coli* spreads to any body part or anything the hands touch. It also can be transmitted to other people.

Microbes can enter the body through equipment used in treatments, therapies, and tests. Such items must be free of microbes. Staff can transfer microbes from one person to another and from themselves to others. Common sites for nosocomial infections are:
- The urinary system
- The respiratory system
- Wounds
- The bloodstream

Patients and residents are weak from disease or injury. Some have wounds or open skin areas. Infants and older persons have a hard time fighting infections. The health team must prevent the spread of infection. Nosocomial infections are prevented by:
- Medical asepsis
- Surgical asepsis
- Isolation Precautions
- The Bloodborne Pathogen Standard

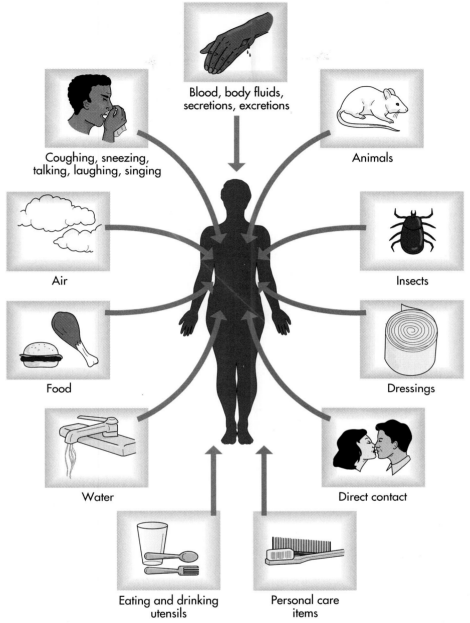

**FIG. 12-2** Methods of transmitting microbes.

## MEDICAL ASEPSIS

**Asepsis** is being free of disease-producing microbes. Microbes are everywhere. Measures are needed to achieve asepsis. **Medical asepsis (clean technique)** is the practices used to:

- Remove or destroy pathogens. The number of pathogens is reduced.
- Prevent pathogens from spreading from one person or place to another person or place.

Microbes cannot be present during surgery or when instruments are inserted into the body. Open wounds (cuts, burns, incisions) require the absence of microbes. They are portals of entry for microbes. **Surgical asepsis (sterile technique)** is the practices that keep items free of *all* microbes. **Sterile** means the absence of *all* microbes—pathogens and non-pathogens. **Sterilization** is the process of destroying *all* microbes (pathogens and non-pathogens).

**Contamination** is the process of becoming unclean. In medical asepsis, an item or area is *clean* when it is free of pathogens. The item or area is contaminated if pathogens are present. A sterile item or area is contaminated when pathogens or non-pathogens are present.

# FOCUS ON HOME CARE

## ASEPTIC PRACTICES

You must prevent the spread of microbes in the home. Also, protect the person from microbes brought into the home. The measures listed above and others are needed.

To prevent foodborne illnesses:

- Buy packaged and canned foods first when shopping.
- Do not buy cans that are bulging or dented.
- Do not buy jars that are cracked or have loose or bulging lids.
- Do not buy produce that is bruised or damaged.
- Check the expiration, "use by," and "sell by" dates on food. Do not buy outdated food.
- Buy food that will stay fresh the longest.
- Open egg cartons before buying them. Do not buy eggs that are dirty or cracked.
- Buy frozen and fresh meat, fish, seafood, and poultry last.
- Keep raw meat, poultry, fish, seafood, and eggs away from other foods in your shopping cart.
- Take groceries home right away. Place them in the car, not the trunk, during hot weather.
- Do not buy any package that is open, torn, or crushed on the edges.
- Store fresh and frozen foods promptly.
- Store eggs in their original carton. Use them within 3 weeks.
- Wash your hands before preparing food. Wash your hands after handling raw meat, fish, seafood, poultry, and eggs.
- Wear gloves if you have a cut or sore on your hands.
- Handle food safely. Follow instructions on safe-handling labels (Fig. 12-3).
- Use smooth cutting boards made of hard maple or plastic. Do not use cutting boards with cracks or crevices.
- Wash cutting boards with soap, hot water, and a scrub brush. Then sanitize them in the dishwasher. Or use a bleach solution—1 tablespoon of bleach to 1 gallon of water.
- Wash and sanitize cutting boards after using them for raw food. This includes produce.
- Wash and sanitize cutting boards before using them for ready-to-eat foods.
- Use one cutting board for produce. Use another cutting board for meat, poultry, fish, and seafood.
- Wash and sanitize surfaces after contact with produce or raw meat, poultry, fish, or seafood.
- Use clean utensils. Wash them between cutting different foods.
- Wash the lids of canned food before opening them. This keeps dirt from the food.
- Clean the can opener blade after each use.
- Take apart and clean food processors and meat grinders after using them. Do this as soon as possible.
- Cook meats, poultry, fish, and seafood adequately. Use a meat thermometer.

- Cook eggs until the white and yolk are firm.
- Do not put cooked meat, poultry, fish, or seafood on an unwashed plate or platter that held raw meat, poultry, fish, or seafood.
- Wash fresh fruits and vegetables thoroughly. Rinse them in warm water. Use a scrub brush if necessary.
- Place leftover food in small containers. Cover containers with lids, foil, or plastic wrap. Date the containers. Use the food within 3 to 5 days.
- Refrigerate leftover food as soon as possible. It should be within 2 hours after cooking.
- Thaw food in the refrigerator or microwave. Or put the package in a water-tight plastic bag. Submerge the bag in cold water. Change the water every 30 minutes.
- Do not use or taste food that looks or smells bad. Discard it at once.
- Wash dishes and other eating and cooking utensils. Use liquid detergent and hot water. Wash glasses and cups first. Follow with silverware, plates, bowls, and then pots and pans. Rinse items well with hot water. Place them in a drainer to dry. Air-drying is more aseptic than towel drying.
- Rinse dishes before loading them into the dishwasher. Use dishwasher soap. Do not wash pots and pans and cast iron, wood, and most plastic items in a dishwasher.
- Clean appliances, counters, tables, and other surfaces after each meal. Use a sponge or dishcloth moistened with warm water and detergent. Thoroughly remove grease, spills, and splashes. Use a liquid surface cleaner. Clean sinks with scouring powder.
- Wash dishcloths and sponges in the washing machine. Use hot water.
- Dispose of garbage, leftover food, and other soiled supplies after each meal. Place paper, boxes, and cans in a paper or plastic bag or in recycle bins. A garbage disposal is best for food and liquid garbage. Or put food or wet items in a container lined with a plastic bag. Do not put bones in the garbage disposal. Some homes have trash compactors. Some cities recycle paper, glass, plastic, and other items. Follow recycling procedures.
- Empty garbage at least once a day.

Microbes easily grow and spread in bathrooms. The entire family must help keep the bathroom clean. Aseptic measures are needed whenever the bathroom is used:

- Flush the toilet after each use.
- Rinse the sink after washing, shaving, or oral hygiene.
- Wipe out the tub or shower after each use.
- Remove and dispose of hair from the sink, tub, or shower.
- Hang towels out to dry, or place them in a hamper.
- Wipe up water spills.
- Your job may include cleaning bathrooms every day. Wear utility gloves for this task. Use a disinfectant or water and detergent to clean all surfaces:
  —The toilet bowl, seat, and outside areas
  —The floor

## FOCUS ON HOME CARE
### ASEPTIC PRACTICES—CONT'D

—The sides, walls, and curtain or door of the shower or tub
—Towel racks
—Toilet tissue, toothbrush, and soap holders
—The mirror
—The sink
—Windowsills
- For bathroom cleaning you also need to:
  —Mop uncarpeted floors. Vacuum carpeted floors.
  —Empty wastebaskets.
  —Put out clean towels and washcloths.
  —Open bathroom windows for a short time and use air fresheners. These help reduce odors and give a fresh smell to the bathroom.

—Wash bath mats, the wastebasket, and the laundry hamper every week.
—Replace toilet and facial tissue as needed.
  For general housekeeping:
- Wipe up spills right away.
- Dust furniture.
- Vacuum or mop floors. Damp-mop uncarpeted floors at least weekly.
- Use a dust mop or broom to sweep. Use a dustpan to collect dust and crumbs. Sweep daily or more often if needed.
- Wash clothes and linens.

## COMMON ASEPTIC PRACTICES

Aseptic practices break the chain of infection. To prevent the spread of microbes, wash your hands:
- After urinating or having a bowel movement.
- After changing tampons or sanitary pads.
- After contact with your own or another person's blood, body fluids, secretions, or excretions. This includes saliva, vomitus, urine, feces, vaginal discharge, mucus, semen, wound drainage, pus, and respiratory secretions.
- After coughing, sneezing, or blowing your nose.
- Before and after handling, preparing, or eating food.
  Also do the following:
- Provide all persons with their own toothbrush, drinking glass, towels, washcloths, and other personal care items.

- Cover your nose and mouth when coughing, sneezing, or blowing your nose.
- Bathe, wash hair, and brush your teeth regularly.
- Wash fruits and raw vegetables before eating or serving them.
- Wash cooking and eating utensils with soap and water after use.

  *See Focus on Home Care: Aseptic Practices. See Focus on Older Persons: Aseptic Practices.*

## FOCUS ON OLDER PERSONS
### ASEPTIC PRACTICES

Persons with dementia do not understand aseptic practices. Others must protect them from infection. Assist them with hand washing:
- After elimination
- After coughing, sneezing, or blowing the nose
- Before or after they eat or handle food
- Any time their hands are soiled
  Check and clean their hands and fingernails often. They may not or cannot tell you when soiling occurs.

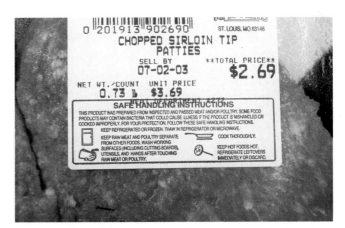

**FIG. 12-3** Safe-handling instructions required by the U.S. Department of Agriculture.

# HAND HYGIENE

*Hand hygiene is the easiest and most important way to prevent the spread of infection.* Your hands are used for almost everything. They are easily contaminated. They can spread microbes to other persons or items. *Practice hand hygiene before and after giving care.* See Box 12-2 for the rules of hand hygiene.

> **SAFETY ALERT:** *Hand Hygiene*
> You use your hands in almost every task. They can pick up microbes from one person, place, or thing. They transfer them to other people, places, and things. That is why hand hygiene is so very important. You must practice hand hygiene before and after giving care.

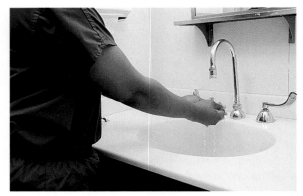

**FIG. 12-4** The uniform does not touch the sink. Soap and water are within reach. Hands are lower than the elbows.

---

## BOX 12-2    RULES OF HAND HYGIENE

- Wash your hands (with soap and water) when they are visibly dirty or soiled with blood, body fluids, secretions, or excretions.
- Wash your hands (with soap and water) before eating and after using a restroom.
- Wash your hands (with soap and water) if exposure to the anthrax spore is suspected or proven.
- Use an alcohol-based hand rub to decontaminate your hands if they are not visibly soiled. (If an alcohol-based hand rub is not available, wash your hands with soap and water.) Follow this rule in the following clinical situations:
  —Before having direct contact with a person.
  —After contact with the person's intact skin (for example, after taking a pulse or blood pressure or after lifting and moving a person).
  —After contact with body fluids or excretions, mucous membranes, non-intact skin, and wound dressings if hands are not visibly soiled.
  —When moving from a contaminated body site to a clean body site during care activities.
  —After contact with objects (including equipment) in the person's care setting.
  —After removing gloves.
- Follow these rules for washing your hands with soap and water. See *Hand washing* procedure.
  —Wash your hands under warm running water. Do not use hot water.
  —Stand away from the sink. Do not let your hands, body, or uniform touch the sink. The sink is contaminated. (See Fig. 12-4.)
  —Keep your hands and forearms lower than your elbows. Your hands are dirtier than your elbows and forearms. If you hold your hands and forearms up, dirty water runs from hands to elbows. Those areas become contaminated.

  —Rub your palms together to work up a good lather (Fig. 12-5). The rubbing action helps remove microbes and dirt.
  —Pay attention to areas often missed during hand washing—thumbs, knuckles, sides of the hands, little fingers, and under the nails.
  —Clean fingernails by rubbing the tips against your palms (Fig. 12-6).
  —Use a nail file or orange stick to clean under fingernails (Fig. 12-7). Microbes easily grow under the fingernails.
  —Wash your hands for at least 15 seconds. Wash your hands longer if they are dirty or soiled with blood, body fluids, secretions, or excretions. Use your judgment.
  —Dry your hands starting at the fingers. Work up to your forearms. You will dry the cleanest area first.
  —Use a clean paper towel for each faucet to turn water off (Fig. 12-8). Faucets are contaminated. The paper towels prevent clean hands from becoming contaminated again.
- Follow these rules when decontaminating your hands with an alcohol-based hand rub:
  —Apply the product to the palm of one hand. Follow the manufacturer's instructions for the amount to use.
  —Rub your hands together.
  —Make sure you cover all surfaces of your hands and fingers.
  —Continue rubbing your hands together until your hands are dry.
- Apply hand lotion or cream after hand hygiene. This prevents skin chapping and drying. Skin breaks can occur in chapped and dry skin. Skin breaks are portals of entry for microbes.

---

Modified from Centers for Disease Control and Prevention: Guideline for hand hygiene in health-care settings, *Morbidity and Mortality Report*, October 25, 2002, Vol 51, No. RR-16.

## HAND WASHING

**NNAAP™**

### PROCEDURE

1 See *Safety Alert: Hand Hygiene.*
2 Make sure you have soap, paper towels, orange stick or nail file, and a wastebasket. Collect missing items.
3 Push your watch up 4 to 5 inches. Also push up uniform sleeves.
4 Stand away from the sink so your clothes do not touch the sink. Stand so the soap and faucet are easy to reach (see Fig. 12-4).
5 Turn on and adjust the water until it feels warm.
6 Wet your wrists and hands. Keep your hands lower than your elbows.
7 Apply about 1 teaspoon of soap to your hands.
8 Rub your palms together and interlace your fingers to work up a good lather (see Fig. 12-5). This step should last at least 15 seconds.
9 Wash each hand and wrist thoroughly. Clean well between the fingers.
10 Clean under the fingernails. Rub your fingertips against your palms (see Fig. 12-6).
11 Clean under fingernails with a nail file or orange stick (see Fig. 12-7). This step is done for the first hand washing of the day and when your hands are highly soiled.
12 Rinse your wrists and hands well. Water flows from the arms to the hands.
13 Repeat steps 7 through 12, if needed.
14 Dry your wrists and hands with paper towels. Pat dry starting at your fingertips.
15 Discard the paper towels.
16 Turn off faucets with clean paper towels. This prevents you from contaminating your hands (see Fig. 12-8). Use a clean paper towel for each faucet.
17 Discard paper towels.

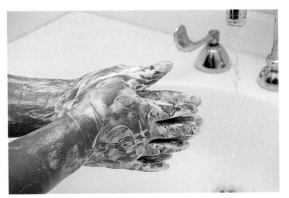

**FIG. 12-5** The palms are rubbed together to work up a good lather.

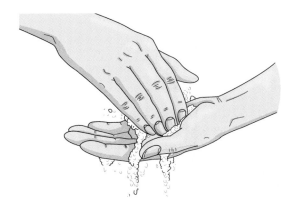

**FIG. 12-6** The fingertips are rubbed against the palms to clean under the fingernails.

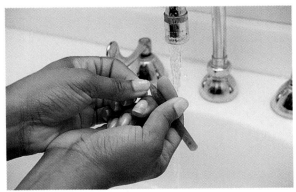

**FIG. 12-7** A nail file is used to clean under the fingernails.

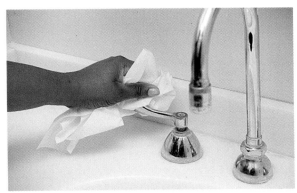

**FIG. 12-8** A paper towel is used to turn off the faucet.

## SUPPLIES AND EQUIPMENT

Supply departments disinfect, sterilize, and distribute equipment. Many single-use and multi-use items are disposable. Single-use items are discarded after use. A person uses multi-use items many times. They include bedpans, urinals, wash basins, water pitchers, and drinking cups. Do not "borrow" them for another person. Disposable items help prevent the spread of infection.

Non-disposable items are cleaned and then disinfected. Then they are sterilized.

**CLEANING.** Cleaning reduces the number of microbes present. It also removes organic matter such as blood, body fluids, secretions, and excretions. When cleaning equipment:

- Wear personal protective equipment—gloves, mask, gown, and eyewear—when cleaning items contaminated with blood, body fluids, secretions, or excretions.
- Rinse the item in cold water first. Rinsing removes organic matter. Heat causes organic matter to become thick, sticky, and hard to remove.
- Wash the item with soap and hot water.
- Scrub thoroughly. Use a brush if necessary.
- Rinse the item in warm water.
- Dry the item.
- Disinfect or sterilize the item.
- Disinfect equipment and the sink used in the cleaning procedure.
- Discard personal protective equipment.
- Practice hand hygiene.

**DISINFECTION.** **Disinfection** is the process of destroying pathogens. Spores are not destroyed. **Spores** are bacteria protected by a hard shell. Spores are killed by extremely high temperatures.

**Germicides** are disinfectants applied to skin, tissues, and nonliving objects. Alcohol is a common germicide.

Reusable items are cleaned with *chemical disinfectants.* Such items include:

- Blood pressure cuffs
- Commodes and metal bedpans
- Counter tops
- Wheelchairs and stretchers
- Furniture

Chemical disinfectants can burn and irritate the skin. Wear utility gloves or rubber household gloves to prevent skin irritation. These gloves are *waterproof.* Do not wear disposable gloves. Some chemical disinfectants have special measures for use or storage (Chapter 10). *See Focus on Home Care: Disinfection.*

**STERILIZATION.** Sterilizing destroys all nonpathogens and pathogens, including spores. Very high temperatures are used. Microbes are destroyed by heat.

### FOCUS ON HOME CARE
#### DISINFECTION

Detergent and hot water are used for eating and drinking utensils, linens, and clothes. Many commercial products disinfect household surfaces—sinks, counters, floors, toilets, tubs, and showers. Use the products preferred by the family or as instructed by the nurse.

Vinegar is a good, cheap disinfectant. You can use it to clean bedpans, urinals, commodes, and toilets. To make a vinegar solution, mix 1 cup of white vinegar and 3 cups of water. Label the container as "vinegar solution." Include the date and your name on the label.

Boiling water, radiation, liquid or gas chemicals, dry heat, and *steam under pressure* are sterilization methods. An *autoclave* (Fig. 12-9) is a pressure steam sterilizer. Glass, surgical items, and metal objects are autoclaved. High temperatures destroy plastic and rubber items. They are not autoclaved. Steam under pressure usually sterilizes objects in 30 to 45 minutes.

*See Focus on Home Care: Sterilization.*

## OTHER ASEPTIC MEASURES

Hand hygiene, cleaning, disinfection, and sterilization are important aseptic measures. So are the measures listed in Box 12-3. They are useful in home, work, and everyday life.

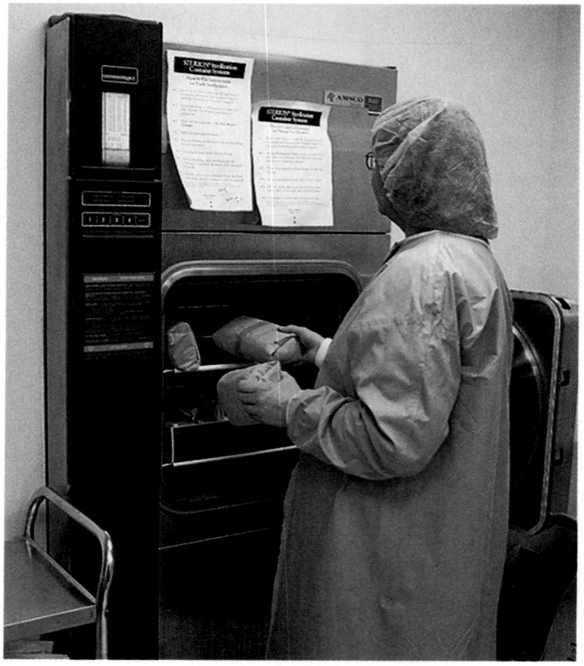


**FIG. 12-9** An autoclave.

## FOCUS ON HOME CARE
### STERILIZATION

You can use boiling water to sterilize items in the home (Fig. 12-10).

- Use a pot with a lid. The pot must be large enough to hold the items.
- Place the items in the pot.
- Fill the pot with cold water. Completely cover all items with water.
- Put the lid on the pot.
- Bring the water to a full boil. Steam will escape from under the lid.
- Boil the items for at least 15 minutes.
- Turn off the heat.
- Let the water and items cool.
- Remove the items onto a clean towel. Use tongs.
- Let the items air-dry.
- Put the items away as the family prefers or the nurse instructs.

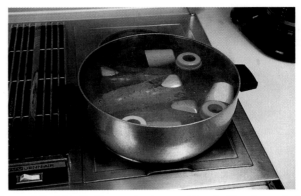

**FIG. 12-10** Boiling water is used to sterilize these baby bottles.

## BOX 12-3 ASEPTIC MEASURES

**CONTROLLING RESERVOIRS (HOSTS—YOU OR THE PERSON)**

- Provide for the person's hygiene needs (Chapter 16).
- Wash contaminated areas with soap and water. Feces, urine, and blood can contain microbes. So can body fluids, secretions, and excretions.
- Use leak-proof plastic bags for soiled tissues, linen, and other materials.
- Keep tables, counters, wheelchair trays, and other surfaces clean and dry.
- Label bottles with the person's name and the date the bottle was opened.
- Keep bottles and fluid containers tightly capped or covered.
- Keep drainage containers below the drainage site (Chapter 28).
- Empty drainage containers and dispose of drainage following agency policy. Usually drainage containers are emptied every shift. Follow the nurse's instructions.

**CONTROLLING PORTALS OF EXIT**

- Cover your nose and mouth when coughing or sneezing.
- Provide the person with tissues to use when coughing or sneezing.
- Wear personal protective equipment as needed (p. 213).

**CONTROLLING TRANSMISSION**

- Make sure all persons have their own personal care equipment. This includes wash basins, bedpans, urinals, commodes, and eating and drinking utensils.

- Do not take equipment from one person's room to use for another person. Even if the item is unused, do not take it from one room to another.
- Hold equipment and linens away from your uniform (Fig. 12-11, p. 210).
- Practice hand hygiene:
  —Before and after contact with every person
  —Whenever your hands are soiled
  —After contact with blood, body fluids, secretions, or excretions
  —After removing gloves
  —Before assisting with any sterile procedure
- Assist the person with hand washing:
  —Before and after eating
  —After elimination
  —After changing tampons, sanitary napkins, or other personal hygiene products
  —After contact with blood, body fluids, secretions, or excretions
- Prevent dust movement. Do not shake linens or equipment. Use a damp cloth for dusting.
- Clean from the cleanest area to the dirtiest. This prevents soiling a clean area.
- Clean away from your body. Do not dust, brush, or wipe toward yourself. Otherwise you transmit microbes to your skin, hair, and clothing.
- Flush urine and feces down the toilet. Avoid splatters and splashes.
- Pour contaminated liquids directly into sinks or toilets. Avoid splashing onto other areas.

*Continued.*

---

**ASEPTIC MEASURES—CONT'D**

### CONTROLLING TRANSMISSION—CONT'D

- Do not sit on a person's bed. You will pick up microbes. You will transfer them to the next surface that you sit on.
- Do not use items that are on the floor. The floor is contaminated.
- Clean tubs, showers, and shower chairs after each use. Follow the agency's disinfection procedures.
- Clean bedpans, urinals, and commodes after each use. Follow the agency's disinfection procedures.
- Report pests—ants, spiders, mice, and so on.

### CONTROLLING PORTALS OF ENTRY

- Provide for good skin care (Chapter 16). This promotes intact skin.
- Provide for good oral hygiene (Chapter 16). This promotes intact mucous membranes.
- Do not let the person lie on tubes or other items. This protects the skin from injury.

- Make sure linens are dry and wrinkle-free (Chapter 15). This protects the skin from injury.
- Turn and reposition the person as directed by the nurse. This protects the skin from injury.
- Assist with or clean the genital area after elimination (Chapter 16). Wipe and clean from the urethra (the cleanest area) to the rectum (the dirtiest area). This helps prevent urinary tract infections.
- Make sure drainage tubes are properly connected. Otherwise microbes can enter the drainage system.

### PROTECTING THE SUSCEPTIBLE HOST

- Follow the care plan to meet hygiene needs. This protects the skin and mucous membranes.
- Follow the care plan to meet nutrition and fluid needs. This helps prevent infection.
- Assist with coughing and deep-breathing exercises as directed. This helps prevent respiratory infections.

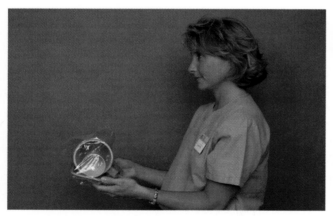

**FIG. 12-11** Hold equipment away from your uniform.

## ISOLATION PRECAUTIONS

Blood, body fluids, secretions, and excretions can transmit pathogens. Sometimes barriers are needed to prevent their escape. The pathogens are kept within a certain area. Usually the area is the person's room. This requires isolation procedures. The Centers for Disease Control and Prevention (CDC) has guidelines for two types of Isolation Precautions:

- Standard Precautions
- Transmission-Based Precautions

Isolation Precautions prevent the spread of **contagious** or **communicable diseases.** They are diseases caused by pathogens that are spread easily. Examples include measles, mumps, chickenpox, and sexually transmitted diseases. Some respiratory, gastrointestinal, wound, skin, and blood infections also are highly contagious.

Isolation Precautions are based on *clean* and *dirty. Clean* areas or objects are free of pathogens. They are not contaminated. *Dirty* areas or objects are contaminated with pathogens. If a *clean* area or object has contact with something *dirty*, the clean item is now dirty. *Clean* and *dirty* also depend on how the pathogen is spread.

## STANDARD PRECAUTIONS

Standard Precautions (Box 12-4) reduce the risk of spreading pathogens and known and unknown infections. *Standard Precautions are used for all persons.* They prevent the spread of infection from:

- Blood
- All body fluids, secretions, and excretions (except sweat) even if blood is not visible
- Non-intact skin (skin with open breaks)
- Mucous membranes

## BOX 12-4 STANDARD PRECAUTIONS

### HAND HYGIENE

- Wash your hands after touching blood, body fluids, secretions, excretions, and contaminated items.
- Decontaminate your hands right away after removing gloves.
- Decontaminate your hands between patient or resident contacts.
- Practice hand hygiene whenever needed to avoid spreading microbes to other persons or areas.
- Decontaminate your hands between tasks and procedures on the same person. This prevents cross-contamination of different body sites.
- Use soap for routine hand washing. (The nurse tells you when other agents are needed. The nurse also tells you what to use.)

### GLOVES

- Wear gloves when touching blood, body fluids, secretions, and excretions.
- Wear gloves when touching contaminated items.
- Put on clean gloves just before touching mucous membranes and non-intact skin.
- Change gloves between tasks and procedures on the same person.
- Change gloves after contacting matter that may be highly contaminated.
- Remove gloves promptly after use.
- Remove gloves before touching uncontaminated items and surfaces.
- Remove gloves before going to another person.
- Decontaminate your hands at once after removing gloves. This prevents the transfer of microbes to other persons or areas.

### MASKS, EYE PROTECTION, AND FACE SHIELDS

- Wear masks, eye protection, and face shields during procedures and tasks that are likely to cause splashes or sprays of blood, body fluids, secretions, and excretions. They protect the mucous membranes of the mouth, eyes, and nose from splashes or sprays (Fig. 12-12, p. 212).

### GOWNS

- Wear a gown during tasks that are likely to cause splashes or sprays of blood, body fluids, secretions, or excretions. The gown protects the skin and prevents soiling of clothing.
- Remove a soiled gown as soon as possible.
- Decontaminate your hands after gown removal. This prevents spreading microbes to other persons or areas.

### CARE EQUIPMENT

- Handle used care equipment carefully. Equipment may be soiled with blood, body fluids, secretions, and excretions. Prevent skin and mucous membrane exposure and clothing contamination. Also prevent the transfer of microbes to other persons and areas.
- Do not use reusable items for another person. The item must be cleaned and disinfected or sterilized.
- Discard disposable (single-use) items properly.

### ENVIRONMENTAL CONTROL

- Follow agency procedures for the routine care, cleaning, and disinfection of surfaces. This includes environmental surfaces, bed rails, bedside equipment, and other surfaces.

### LINENS

- Follow agency policy for linen that is soiled with blood, body fluids, secretions, or excretions. The policy describes how to handle, transport, and process soiled linen.
- Prevent skin and mucous membrane exposures and clothing contamination when handling linens.
- Prevent the transfer of microbes to other persons and areas when handling linens.

### OCCUPATIONAL HEALTH AND BLOODBORNE PATHOGENS

- Prevent injuries when handling needles, scalpels, and other sharp instruments or devices.
- Prevent injuries when handling sharp instruments after procedures.
- Prevent injuries when cleaning instruments.
- Prevent injuries when disposing of needles.
- Never recap used needles. Do not handle them with both hands. Do not use any method that involves directing the needle point toward any body part. Follow agency policy for handling and disposing of needles.
- Do not remove used needles from disposable syringes by hand.
- Do not bend, break, or otherwise handle used needles by hand.
- Place used syringes and needles, scalpel blades, and other sharp items in puncture-resistant containers.
- Use barrier devices for rescue breathing (Chapter 40).

### PATIENT OR RESIDENT PLACEMENT

- A private room is used if the person:
  —Contaminates the area
  —Does not or cannot assist in maintaining hygiene or environmental control
- Follow the nurse's instructions if a private room is not available.

Modified to comply with *Guideline for Hand Hygiene in Health-Care Settings,* Centers for Disease Control and Prevention, October 25, 2002.

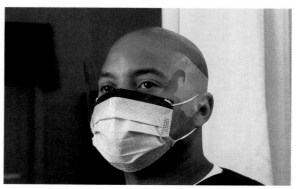

**FIG. 12-12** This mask has an eye shield. The eyes and mucous membranes of the mouth and nose are protected.

---

### BOX 12-5   TRANSMISSION-BASED PRECAUTIONS

#### AIRBORNE PRECAUTIONS

For known or suspected infections involving microbes transmitted by airborne droplets—measles, chickenpox, tuberculosis (TB)

**PRACTICES**

- Standard Precautions are followed.
- A private room is preferred.
- Keep the room door closed and the person in the room.
- Wear respiratory protection (tuberculosis respirator) when entering the room of a person with known or suspected TB.
- Do not enter the room of a person with known or suspected measles or chickenpox if you are susceptible to these diseases.
- Wear respiratory protection (mask) if you must enter the room of a person with known or suspected measles or chickenpox if you are susceptible to these diseases. (Respiratory protection is not needed for persons immune to measles or chickenpox.)
- Limit moving and transporting the person from the room. The person wears a mask if moving or transporting from the room is necessary.

#### DROPLET PRECAUTIONS

For known or suspected infections involving microbes transmitted by droplets produced by coughing, sneezing, talking, or procedures—meningitis, pneumonia, epiglottitis, diphtheria, pertussis (whooping cough), influenza, mumps, rubella, streptococcal pharyngitis, scarlet fever

**PRACTICES**

- Standard Precautions are followed.
- A private room is preferred.
- Wear a mask when working within 3 feet of the person. (Wear a mask on entering the room if required by agency policy.)

- Limit moving and transporting the person from the room. The person wears a mask if moving or transporting from the room is necessary.

#### CONTACT PRECAUTIONS

For known or suspected infections involving microbes transmitted by:
- Direct contact with the person (hand or skin-to-skin contact that occurs during care)
- Indirect contact (touching surfaces or care items in the person's room)—gastrointestinal, respiratory, skin, or wound infections

**PRACTICES**

- Standard Precautions are followed.
- A private room is preferred.
- Wear gloves when entering the room.
- Change gloves after having contact with infective matter that may contain high concentrations of microbes.
- Remove gloves before leaving the person's room.
- Practice hand hygiene immediately after removing gloves. The nurse tells you what agent to use.
- Do not touch potentially contaminated surfaces or items after removing gloves and hand hygiene.
- Wear a gown on entering the room if you will have substantial contact with the person, surfaces, or items in the room.
- Wear a gown on entering the room if the person is incontinent or has diarrhea, an ileostomy, a colostomy, or wound drainage not contained by a dressing.
- Remove the gown before leaving the person's room. Make sure your clothing does not contact potentially contaminated surfaces in the person's room.
- Limit moving or transferring the person from the room. Maintain precautions if the person is moved or transferred from the room.

# TRANSMISSION-BASED PRECAUTIONS

Some infections require Transmission-Based Precautions (Box 12-5). You must understand how certain infections are spread (see Fig. 12-2). This helps you understand the three types of Transmission-Based Precautions.

---

**DELEGATION GUIDELINES:** *Transmission-Based Precautions*

You may assist in the care of persons who require Transmission-Based Precautions. If so, review the type used with the nurse (Airborne, Droplet, or Contact Precautions). You also need this information from the nurse and the care plan:

- What agent to use for hand hygiene (Contact Precautions)
- What personal protective equipment to use
- What special safety measures are needed

---

**SAFETY ALERT:** *Transmission-Based Precautions*

Preventing the spread of infection is important. Standard Precautions and Transmission-Based Precautions protect everyone—patients, residents, visitors, staff, and you. If you are careless, everyone's safety is at risk.

---

# PROTECTIVE MEASURES

Agency policies may differ from those in this text. The rules in Box 12-6 are a guide for giving safe care when using Isolation Precautions.

Isolation Precautions involve wearing gloves, a gown, a mask, or protective eyewear. Removing linens, trash, and equipment from the room may require double-bagging. Special measures are needed to collect specimens and to transport persons on Isolation Precautions.

---

**BOX 12-6  RULES FOR ISOLATION PRECAUTIONS**

- Collect all needed items before entering the room.
- Prevent contamination of equipment and supplies. Floors are contaminated. So is any object on the floor or that falls to the floor.
- Use mops wetted with a disinfectant solution to clean floors. Floor dust is contaminated.
- Prevent drafts. Pathogens are carried in the air by drafts.
- Use paper towels to handle contaminated items.
- Remove items from the room in leak-proof plastic bags.
- Double bag items if the outer part of the bag is or can be contaminated (p. 220).
- Follow agency policy for removing and transporting disposable and reusable items.
- Return reusable dishes, eating utensils, and trays to the food service department. Discard disposable dishes, eating utensils, and trays in the waste container in the person's room.
- Do not touch your hair, nose, mouth, eyes, or other body parts.
- Do not touch any clean area or object if your hands are contaminated.
- Wash your hands if they are visibly dirty or contaminated with blood, body fluids, secretions, or excretions.
- Place clean items on paper towels.
- Do not shake linen.
- Use paper towels to turn faucets on and off.
- Use a paper towel to open the door to the person's room. Discard it as you leave.
- Tell the nurse if you have any cuts, open skin areas, a sore throat, vomiting, or diarrhea.

**GLOVES.** The skin is a natural barrier. It prevents microbes from entering the body. Small skin breaks on the hands and fingers are common. Some are very small and hard to see. Disposable gloves protect you from pathogens in the person's blood, body fluids, secretions, and excretions. They also protect the person from microbes on your hands.

Wear gloves whenever contact with blood, body fluids, secretions, excretions, mucous membranes, and non-intact skin is likely. Contact may be direct. Or contact may be with items or surfaces contaminated with blood, body fluids, secretions, or excretions.

Do not tear gloves when putting them on. Carelessness, long fingernails, and rings can tear gloves. Blood, body fluids, secretions, and excretions can enter the glove through the tear. This contaminates the hand. Remember the following:

- Gloves are easier to put on when your hands are dry.
- You need a new pair for every person.
- Remove and discard torn, cut, or punctured gloves at once. Practice hand hygiene. Then put on a new pair.
- Wear gloves once. Discard them after use.
- Put on clean gloves just before touching mucous membranes or non-intact skin.

- Put on new gloves whenever gloves become contaminated with blood, body fluids, secretions, or excretions. A task may require more than one pair of gloves.
- Change gloves when moving from a contaminated body site to a clean body site.
- Make sure gloves cover your wrists. If you wear a gown, gloves cover the cuffs (Fig. 12-13).
- Remove gloves so the inside part is on the outside. The inside is *clean.*
- Decontaminate your hands after removing gloves.

---

**SAFETY ALERT:** *Gloves*
Some gloves are made of latex (a rubber product). Latex allergies are common. They can cause skin rashes. Asthma and shock are more serious problems. Report skin rashes and breathing problems to the nurse at once.

If you have a latex allergy, wear latex-free gloves. Some patients and residents are allergic to latex. This information is on the care plan and your assignment sheet.

---

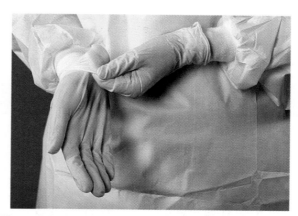

**FIG. 12-13** The gloves cover the cuffs of the gown.

## REMOVING GLOVES

### PROCEDURE

1 Make sure that glove touches only glove.
2 Grasp a glove just below the cuff (Fig. 12-14, *A*). Grasp it on the outside.
3 Pull the glove down over your hand so it is inside out (Fig. 12-14, *B*).
4 Hold the removed glove with your other gloved hand.
5 Reach inside the other glove. Use the first two fingers of the ungloved hand (Fig. 12-14, *C*).
6 Pull the glove down (inside out) over your hand and the other glove (Fig. 12-14, *D*).
7 Discard the gloves. Follow agency policy.
8 Decontaminate your hands.

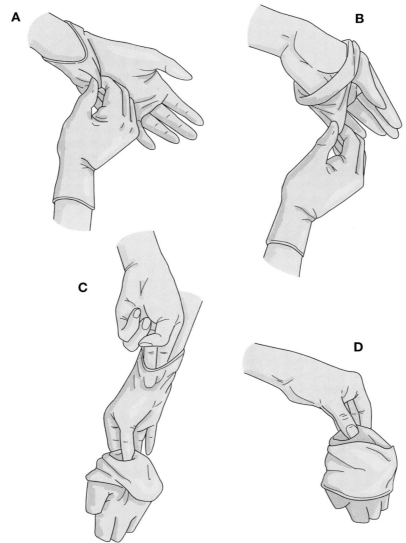

**FIG. 12-14** Removing gloves. **A,** Grasp the glove below the cuff. **B,** Pull the glove down over the hand. The glove is inside out. **C,** Insert the fingers of the ungloved hand inside the other glove. **D,** Pull the glove down and over the hand and glove. The glove is inside out.

■ **MASKS AND RESPIRATORY PROTECTION.**
Masks prevent the spread of microbes from the respiratory tract. They are used for Airborne and Droplet Precautions. Patients, residents, visitors, and staff wear them.

Masks are disposable. A wet or moist mask is contaminated. Breathing can cause masks to become wet or moist. Apply a new mask when contamination occurs.

A mask fits snugly over your nose and mouth. Practice hand hygiene before putting on a mask. When removing a mask, touch only the ties. The front of the mask is contaminated.

Tuberculosis respirators (Fig. 12-15) are worn when caring for persons with tuberculosis (TB) (Chapter 33). They are worn for Airborne Precautions.

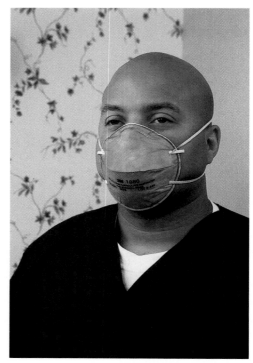

**FIG. 12-15** Tuberculosis respirator.

## WEARING A MASK

### PROCEDURE

1 Practice hand hygiene.
2 Pick up the mask by its upper ties. Do not touch the part that will cover your face.
3 Place the mask over your nose and mouth (Fig. 12-16, *A*).
4 Place the upper strings above your ears. Tie them at the back of your head (Fig. 12-16, *B*).
5 Tie the lower strings at the back of your neck (Fig. 12-16, *C*). The lower part of the mask is under your chin.
6 Pinch the metal band around your nose. The top of the mask must be snug over your nose. If you wear glasses, the mask must be snug under the bottom of the glasses.
7 Decontaminate your hands. Put on gloves.

8 Provide care. Avoid coughing, sneezing, and unnecessary talking.
9 Change the mask if it becomes moist or contaminated.
10 Remove the mask as follows:
  a Remove the gloves.
  b Decontaminate your hands.
  c Untie the lower strings.
  d Untie the top strings.
  e Hold the top strings. Remove the mask.
  f Bring the strings together. The inside of the mask folds together (Fig. 12-16,*D*). Do not touch the inside of the mask.
11 Discard the mask. Follow agency policy.
12 Decontaminate your hands.

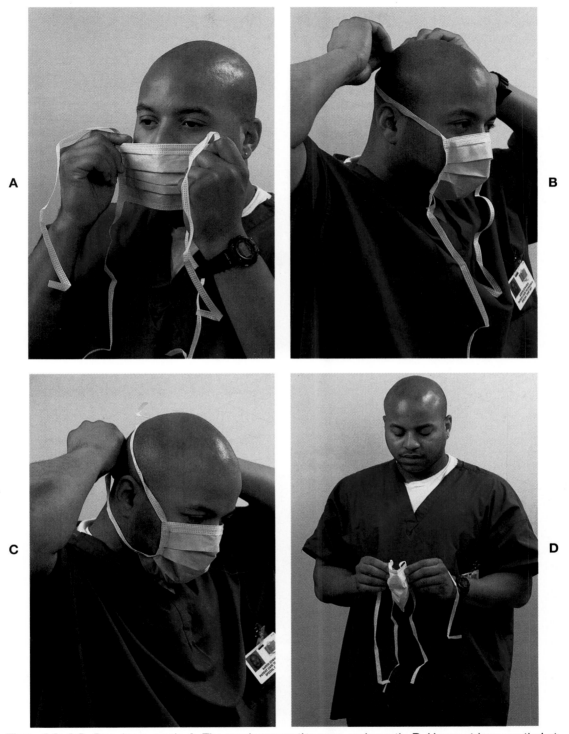

**FIG. 12-16** Donning a mask. **A,** The mask covers the nose and mouth. **B,** Upper strings are tied at the back of the head. **C,** Lower strings are tied at the back of the neck. **D,** The inside of the mask is folded together after removal.

**PROTECTIVE APPAREL.** Gowns, aprons, shoe covers, boots, and leg coverings prevent the spread of microbes. They protect your clothes and body from contact with blood, body fluids, secretions, and excretions. They also protect against splashes and sprays.

Gowns must completely cover clothing. The long sleeves have tight cuffs. The gown opens at the back. It is tied at the neck and waist. The inside and neck are *clean.* The outside and waist strings are *contaminated.*

Gowns are used once. A wet gown is contaminated. It is removed and a dry one put on. Disposable gowns are made of paper. They are discarded after use.

**EYEWEAR AND FACE SHIELDS.** Goggles and face shields protect your eyes, mouth, and nose from splashing or spraying of blood, body fluids, secretions, and excretions (see Fig. 12-12). Splashes and sprays can occur when giving care, cleaning items, or disposing of fluids.

Discard disposable eyewear after use. Reusable eyewear is cleaned before reuse. It is washed with soap and water. Then a disinfectant is used.

## DONNING AND REMOVING A GOWN

### PROCEDURE

1 Remove your watch and all jewelry.
2 Roll up uniform sleeves.
3 Practice hand hygiene.
4 Put on a mask if required. (See *Wearing a Mask*, p. 216.)
5 Hold a clean gown out in front of you. Let it unfold. Do not shake the gown.
6 Put your hands and arms through the sleeves (Fig. 12-17, *A*).
7 Make sure the gown covers the front of your uniform. It should be snug at the neck.
8 Tie the strings at the back of the neck (Fig. 12-17, *B*).
9 Overlap the back of the gown. Make sure it covers your uniform. The gown should be snug, not loose (Fig. 12-17, *C*).
10 Tie the waist strings at the back.
11 Put on the gloves.
12 Provide care.
13 Remove and discard the gloves. Decontaminate your hands.
14 Remove the face mask. Discard it following agency policy.
15 Decontaminate your hands.
16 Remove the gown:
   a Untie the waist strings.
   b Decontaminate your hands.
   c Untie the neck strings. Do not touch the outside of the gown.
   d Pull the gown down from the shoulder.
   e Turn the gown inside out as it is removed. Hold it at the inside shoulder seams, and bring your hands together (Fig. 12-17, *D*).
17 Roll up the gown away from you. Keep it inside out.
18 Discard the gown. Follow agency policy.
19 Decontaminate your hands.
20 Open the door using a paper towel. Discard it as you leave.

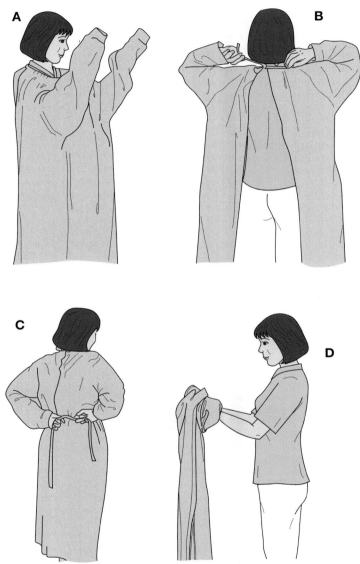

**FIG. 12-17** Gowning. **A,** The arms and hands are put through the sleeves. **B,** The strings are tied at the back of the neck. **C,** The gown is overlapped in the back to cover the entire uniform. **D,** The gown is turned inside out as it is removed.

■ **BAGGING ITEMS.** Contaminated items are bagged to remove them from the person's room. Leak-proof plastic bags are used. They have the *BIOHAZARD* symbol (Fig. 12-18). **Biohazardous waste** is items contaminated with blood, body fluids, secretions, or excretions. (*Bio* means life. *Hazardous* means dangerous or harmful.)

Bag and transport linens following agency policy. All linen bags need a *BIOHAZARD* symbol. Melt-away bags are common. They dissolve in hot water. Once soiled linen is bagged, no one needs to handle it. Do not overfill the bag. Tie the bag securely. Then place it in a laundry hamper lined with a biohazard plastic bag.

Trash is placed in a container labeled with the *BIOHAZARD* symbol. Follow agency policy for bagging and transporting trash, equipment, and supplies. Usually one bag is needed. Double bagging involves two bags. Double bagging is not needed unless the outside of the bag is soiled.

**COLLECTING SPECIMENS.** Blood, body fluids, secretions, and excretions often require laboratory testing (Chapter 26). Specimens are transported to the laboratory in biohazard specimen bags. To collect a specimen:

- Label the specimen container and biohazard specimen bag. Apply warning labels according to agency policy.
- Don personal protective equipment as required. Gloves are worn.
- Put the specimen container and lid in the person's bathroom. Put them on a paper towel.
- Collect the specimen. Do not contaminate the outside of the container. Also avoid contamination when transferring the specimen from the collecting vessel to the specimen container.
- Put the lid on securely.
- Remove the gloves. Decontaminate your hands.
- Use a paper towel to pick up and take the container outside the room.
- Put the container in a biohazard bag.
- Discard the paper towels.
- Follow agency policy for transporting the specimen to the laboratory.
- Decontaminate your hands.

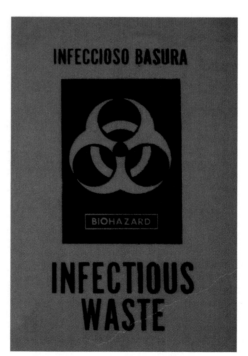

**FIG. 12-18** *BIOHAZARD* symbol.

## DOUBLE BAGGING

### PROCEDURE

1 Ask a co-worker to help you. The co-worker stands outside the room.
2 Placed soiled linen, reusable items, disposable supplies, and trash in the right containers. Containers are lined with leak-proof biohazard bags.
3 Seal the bags securely with ties.
4 Ask your co-worker to make a wide cuff on the clean bag. It is held wide open. The cuff protects the hands from contamination (Fig. 12-19).

5 Place the contaminated bag into the clean bag (Fig. 12-20). Do not touch the outside of the clean bag.
6 Ask your co-worker to seal the bag. Have the bag labeled according to agency policy.
7 Repeat steps 4, 5, and 6 as needed for other contaminated bags.
8 Ask your co-worker to take or send the bags to the appropriate department for disposal, disinfection, or sterilization.

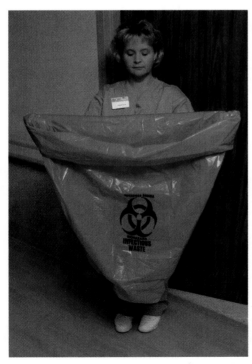

**FIG. 12-19** A cuff is made on a clean bag.

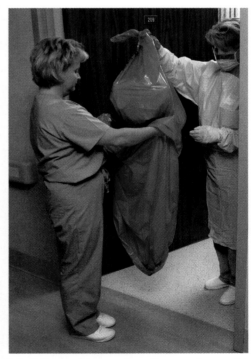

**FIG. 12-20** Double bagging. One nursing assistant is in the room by the doorway. The other is outside the doorway. The "dirty" bag is placed inside the "clean" bag.

**TRANSPORTING PERSONS.** Persons on Isolation Precautions usually do not leave their rooms. Sometimes they go to other areas for treatments or tests.

Transporting procedures vary among agencies. Some require transport by bed. This prevents contaminating wheelchairs and stretchers. Others use wheelchairs and stretchers.

A safe transport means that other persons are protected from the infection. Follow agency procedures and these guidelines:
- The person wears a clean gown or pajamas and an isolation gown.
- The person wears a mask for Airborne or Droplet Precautions.
- Cover any draining wounds.
- Give the person tissues and a leak-proof bag. Used tissues are placed in the bag.
- Wear a gown, mask, and gloves as required.
- Place an extra layer of sheets and absorbent pads on the stretcher or wheelchair. This protects against draining body fluids.
- Do not let anyone else on the elevator. This reduces exposure to the infection.
- Alert staff in the receiving area about the Isolation Precautions. They wear gloves and personal protective equipment as needed.
- Disinfect the stretcher or wheelchair after use.

## MEETING BASIC NEEDS

The person has love, belonging, and self-esteem needs. Often they are unmet when Transmission-Based Precautions are used. Visitors and staff often avoid the person. They may need gowns, masks, eyewear, and gloves. These take extra effort before entering the room. Some are not sure what they can touch. They may fear getting the disease.

The person may feel lonely, unwanted, and rejected. Self-esteem suffers. The person knows the disease can be spread to others. He or she may feel dirty and undesirable. Without intending to, visitors and staff can make the person feel ashamed and guilty for having a contagious disease.

The nurse helps the person, visitors, and staff understand the need for isolation precautions and how they affect the person. You can help meet love, belonging, and self-esteem needs. The following actions are helpful. Remember to disinfect or discard items that become contaminated.
- Remember, the *pathogen* is undesirable, not the *person.*
- Treat the person with respect, kindness, and dignity.
- Provide newspapers, magazines, and other reading matter.
- Provide hobby materials if possible.
- Place a clock in the room.
- Encourage the person to phone family and friends.
- Provide a current TV guide.
- Organize your work so you can stay to visit with the person.
- Say "hello" from the doorway often.

See Focus on Children: Isolation Precautions. See Focus on Older Persons: Isolation Precautions. See Focus on Home Care: Isolation Precautions.

### FOCUS ON CHILDREN
#### ISOLATION PRECAUTIONS

Infants and children do not understand isolation. Eyewear, masks, and gowns may scare them. Parents and staff look different. Gloves and gowns prevent skin-to-skin contact with parents. Because of likely contamination, toys and comfort items (blankets and stuffed animals) may be kept from the child. This adds to the child's distress.

The nurse prepares the child and family for isolation. Simple explanations are given to the child. If appropriate for his or her age, the child is given a mask, eyewear, and a gown to touch and play with.

Children need to see the faces of people entering the room. Let the child see your face before putting on a mask and eyewear. Say "hello" to the child, and state your name.

### FOCUS ON OLDER PERSONS
#### ISOLATION PRECAUTIONS

Persons with poor vision, confusion, or dementia need to know who you are. Let them see your face. State your name and what you are going to do. Then put on personal protective equipment.

### FOCUS ON HOME CARE
#### ISOLATION PRECAUTIONS

Always practice Standard Precautions in home settings. Sometimes Transmission-Based Precautions are needed. The nurse tells you what measures are needed.

# BLOODBORNE PATHOGEN STANDARD

HIV and the hepatitis B virus (HBV) are major health concerns (Chapter 33). The health team is at risk for exposure to the viruses. The Bloodborne Pathogen Standard is intended to protect them from exposure. It is a regulation of the Occupational Safety and Health Administration (OSHA). See Box 12-7 for terms used in the standard.

HIV and HBV are found in blood. They are bloodborne pathogens. They exit the body through blood. They are spread to others by blood. Other potentially infectious materials (OPIM) also spread the viruses (see Box 12-7).

## EXPOSURE CONTROL PLAN

The agency must have an exposure control plan. It identifies staff at risk for exposure to blood or OPIM. All caregivers are at risk. So are the surgical, central supply, laundry, housekeeping, and laboratory staffs. The plan includes actions to take for an exposure incident.

---

### BOX 12-7 BLOODBORNE PATHOGEN STANDARD DEFINITIONS

- *Blood.* Human blood, human blood components, and products made from human blood
- *Bloodborne pathogens.* Pathogens present in human blood and that can cause disease in humans; they include but are not limited to hepatitis B virus (HBV) and human immunodeficiency virus (HIV)
- *Contaminated.* The presence or reasonably anticipated presence of blood or other potentially infectious materials on an item or surface
- *Contaminated laundry.* Laundry soiled with blood or other potentially infectious materials or that may contain sharps
- *Contaminated sharps.* Any contaminated object that can penetrate the skin—needles, scalpels, broken glass, broken capillary tubes, exposed ends of dental wires, and so on
- *Decontamination.* The use of physical or chemical means to remove, inactivate, or destroy bloodborne pathogens on a surface or item to the point where infectious particles can no longer be transmitted and the surface or item is safe for handling, use, or disposal
- *Engineering controls.* Controls that isolate or remove the bloodborne pathogen hazard from the workplace (sharps disposal containers, self-sheathing needles)
- *Exposure incident.* Eye, mouth, other mucous membrane, non-intact skin, or parenteral contact with blood or other potentially infectious materials that results from an employee's duties
- *Hand washing facilities.* The adequate supply of running water, soap, single-use towels, or hot-air drying machines
- *HBV.* Hepatitis B virus
- *HIV.* Human immunodeficiency virus
- *Occupational exposure.* Reasonably anticipated skin, eye, mucous membrane, or parenteral contact with blood or other potentially infectious materials that may result from an employee's duties
- *Other potentially infectious materials (OPIM):*
  —Human body fluids: semen, vaginal secretions, cerebrospinal fluid, synovial fluid, pleural fluid, pericardial fluid, peritoneal fluid, amniotic fluid, saliva in dental procedures, any body fluid that is visibly contaminated with blood, and all body fluids when it is difficult or impossible to differentiate between them
  —Any tissue or organ (other than intact skin) from a human (living or dead)
  —HIV-containing cell or tissue cultures, organ cultures, and HIV- or HBV-containing culture medium or other solutions; blood, organs, or other tissues from experimental animals infected with HIV or HBV
- *Parenteral.* Piercing mucous membranes or the skin barrier through needle-sticks, human bites, cuts, abrasions, and so on
- *Personal protective equipment (PPE).* The clothing or equipment worn by an employee for protection against a hazard
- *Regulated waste:*
  —Liquid or semi-liquid blood or OPIM
  —Contaminated items that would release blood or OPIM in a liquid or semi-liquid state if compressed
  —Items caked with dried blood or OPIM that can release these materials during handling
  —Contaminated sharps; pathological and microbiological wastes containing blood or OPIM
- *Source individual.* Any person (living or dead) whose blood or OPIM may be a source of occupational exposure to employees; examples include but are not limited to:
  —Hospital and clinic patients
  —Clients in agencies for the developmentally disabled
  —Trauma victims
  —Clients of drug and alcohol treatment agencies
  —Hospice and nursing center residents
  —Human remains
  —Persons who donate or sell blood or blood components
- *Sterilize.* The use of a physical or chemical procedure to destroy all microbes, including spores
- *Work practice controls.* Controls that reduce the likelihood of exposure by changing the way the task is performed

Staff at risk receive free training. Training occurs upon employment and yearly. Training is also required for new or changed tasks involving exposure to bloodborne pathogens. Training must include:

- An explanation of the standard and where to get a copy
- The causes, signs, and symptoms of bloodborne diseases
- How bloodborne pathogens are spread
- An explanation of the exposure control plan and where to get a copy
- How to know which tasks might cause exposure
- The use and limits of safe work practices, engineering controls, and personal protective equipment
- Information on the hepatitis B vaccination
- Who to contact and what to do in an emergency
- Information on reporting an exposure incident, postexposure evaluation, and follow-up
- Information on warning labels and color-coding

## PREVENTIVE MEASURES

Preventive measures reduce the risk of exposure. Such measures follow.

**HEPATITIS B VACCINATION.** Hepatitis B is a liver disease. It is caused by the hepatitis B virus (HBV). HBV is spread by blood and sexual contact.

The hepatitis B vaccine produces immunity against hepatitis B. **Immunity** means that a person has protection against a certain disease. He or she will not get the disease.

A **vaccination** involves giving a vaccine to produce immunity against an infectious disease. A **vaccine** is a preparation containing dead or weakened microbes. The hepatitis B vaccination involves three injections (shots). The second injection is given 1 month after the first. The third injection is given 6 months after the second one. The vaccination can be given before or after exposure to HBV.

You can receive the hepatitis B vaccination within 10 working days of being hired. The agency pays for it. You can refuse the vaccination. If so, you must sign a statement refusing the vaccine. You can have the vaccination at a later time.

**ENGINEERING AND WORK PRACTICE CONTROLS.**
*Engineering controls* reduce employee exposure in the workplace. Special containers for contaminated sharps (needles, broken glass) and specimens remove and isolate the hazard from staff. Containers are puncture-resistant, leak-proof, and color-coded in red. They have the *BIOHAZARD* symbol.

*Work practice controls* also reduce exposure risks. All tasks involving blood or OPIM are done in ways to limit splatters, splashes, and sprays. Producing droplets also is avoided. OSHA requires these work practice controls:

- Do not eat, drink, smoke, apply cosmetics or lip balm, or handle contact lenses in areas of occupational exposure.
- Do not store food or drinks where blood or OPIM are kept.
- Practice hand hygiene after removing gloves.
- Wash hands as soon as possible after skin contact with blood or OPIM.
- Never recap, bend, or remove needles by hand. When recapping, bending, or removing contaminated needles is required, use mechanical means (forceps) or a one-handed method.
- Never shear or break contaminated needles.
- Discard contaminated needles and sharp instruments in containers that are closable, puncture-resistant, and leak-proof. Containers are color-coded red and have the *BIOHAZARD* symbol. Containers must be upright and not allowed to overfill.

**PERSONAL PROTECTIVE EQUIPMENT (PPE).**
This includes gloves, goggles, face shields, masks, laboratory coats, gowns, shoe covers, and surgical caps. Blood or OPIM must not pass through them. They protect your clothes, undergarments, skin, eyes, and mouth.

PPE is free to employees. Correct sizes are available. The agency makes sure that PPE is cleaned, laundered, repaired, replaced, or discarded. You must safely handle and use PPE. Follow these OSHA required measures:

- Remove PPE before leaving the work area.
- Remove PPE when a garment becomes contaminated.
- Place used PPE in marked areas or containers when being stored, washed, decontaminated, or discarded.
- Wear gloves when you expect contact with blood or OPIM.
- Wear gloves when handling or touching contaminated items or surfaces.
- Replace worn, punctured, or contaminated gloves.
- Never wash or decontaminate disposable gloves for reuse.
- Discard utility gloves that show signs of cracking, peeling, tearing, or puncturing. Utility gloves are decontaminated for reuse if the process will not ruin them.

**EQUIPMENT.** Contaminated equipment is cleaned and decontaminated. Decontaminate work surfaces with a proper disinfectant:
- Upon completing tasks
- At once when there is obvious contamination
- After any spill of blood or OPIM
- At the end of the work shift when surfaces became contaminated since the last cleaning

Use a brush and dustpan or tongs to clean up broken glass. Never pick up broken glass with your hands, not even with gloves. Discard broken glass into a puncture-resistant container.

**WASTE.** Special measures are required when discarding regulated waste:
- Liquid or semi-liquid blood or OPIM
- Items contaminated with blood or OPIM
- Items caked with blood or OPIM
- Contaminated sharps

Closable, puncture-resistant, and leak-proof containers are used. Containers are color-coded in red. They have the *BIOHAZARD* symbol. *See Focus on Home Care: Waste.*

**HOUSEKEEPING.** The agency must be kept clean and sanitary. A cleaning schedule is required. It includes decontamination methods and the tasks and procedures to be done.

**LAUNDRY.** OSHA requires these measures for contaminated laundry:
- Handle it as little as possible.
- Wear gloves or other needed PPE.
- Bag contaminated laundry where it was used.
- Mark laundry bags or containers with the *BIOHAZARD* symbol for laundry sent offsite.
- Place wet, contaminated laundry in leak-proof containers before transport. The containers are color-coded in red or labeled with the *BIOHAZARD* symbol.

## EXPOSURE INCIDENTS

An *exposure incident* is any eye, mouth, other mucous membrane, non-intact skin, or parenteral contact with blood or OPIM. *Parenteral* means piercing the mucous membranes or the skin barrier. Piercing occurs through needle-sticks, human bites, cuts, and abrasions.

Report exposure incidents at once. Medical evaluation and follow-up are free. This includes required tests. Your blood is tested for HBV and HIV. If you refuse testing, the blood sample is kept for at least 90 days. Testing is done later if you change your mind.

Confidentiality is important. You are told of evaluation results. You also are told of any medical conditions that may need treatment. You receive a written opinion of the medical evaluation within 15 days after its completion.

The *source individual* is the person whose blood or body fluids are the source of an exposure incident. His or her blood is tested for HIV or HBV. State laws vary about releasing the results. The agency informs you about laws affecting the source's identity and test results.

### FOCUS ON HOME CARE
#### WASTE

Dressings, gloves, syringes, needles, and other sharps are used for home care. You will not use syringes, needles, and other sharps. However, you assist the family in disposing of these items. Proper disposal is needed to protect trash handlers from infection. The Environmental Protection Agency (EPA) suggests that you:
- Place needles, syringes, and other sharp items into hard plastic or metal containers. They should have a screw-on lid or other secure lid. A plastic detergent bottle and lid are examples. Do not use glass or clear plastic containers.
- Tape the lid in place with a heavy tape. This gives added protection.
- Keep the sharps container out of the reach of children and pets.
- Place dressings, gloves, soiled bed protectors, disposable sheets, and other care items in plastic bags. Close the bags securely.
- Label containers and plastic bags with a "Not for Recycling" label.
- Place plastic bags and sharps containers in a garbage can with a lid.
- Make sure animals cannot get into the garbage can. Trash scents can attract animals.

## SURGICAL ASEPSIS

**Surgical asepsis (sterile technique)** is the practices that keep equipment and supplies free of *all* microbes. **Sterile** means the absence of *all* microbes, including spores. Surgical asepsis is required any time the skin or sterile tissues are entered.

Surgery and labor and delivery areas require surgical asepsis. So do many tests and nursing procedures. If a break occurs in sterile technique, microbes can enter the body. Infection is a risk.

You can assist nurses with sterile procedures. Some states let nursing assistants perform certain sterile procedures. Examples include sterile dressing changes and suctioning.

---

**SAFETY ALERT:** *Sterile Procedures*
Do not perform a sterile procedure unless:
- Your state allows you to perform the procedure
- The procedure is in your job description
- You received the necessary education and training
- You review the procedure with the nurse
- A nurse is available for questions and guidance

---

## PRINCIPLES OF SURGICAL ASEPSIS

All items in contact with the person are kept sterile. If an item is contaminated, infection is a risk. A sterile field is needed. A **sterile field** is a work area free of all pathogens and non-pathogens (including spores). Box 12-8 lists the principles and practices of surgical asepsis. Follow them to maintain a sterile field. *See Focus on Home Care: Surgical Asepsis.*

---

**DELEGATION GUIDELINES:** *Assisting With Sterile Procedures*
Before performing or assisting with a sterile procedure, you need this information from the nurse:
- The name of the procedure and the reason for it
- What gloves to wear—sterile or disposable (if assisting)
- If assisting, what you are expected to do
- What observations to report at once
- What you can and cannot touch

---

### FOCUS ON HOME CARE
SURGICAL ASEPSIS
You may need to clean a work surface before you practice surgical asepsis. Use soap and water. Practice Standard Precautions. Clean from the cleanest area to the dirtiest. Also clean away from your body and uniform. Dry the surface after cleaning.

## BOX 12-8 PRINCIPLES AND PRACTICES FOR SURGICAL ASEPSIS

- A sterile item can touch only another sterile item:
  - —If a sterile item touches a clean item, the sterile item is contaminated.
  - —If a clean item touches a sterile item, the sterile item is contaminated.
  - —A sterile package that is open, torn, punctured, wet, or moist is contaminated.
  - —A sterile package is contaminated when the expiration date has passed.
  - —Place only sterile items on a sterile field.
  - —Use sterile gloves or sterile forceps to handle other sterile items (Fig. 12-21).
  - —Consider any item as contaminated if unsure of its sterility.
  - —Do not use contaminated items. They are discarded or re-sterilized.
- A sterile field or sterile items are always kept within your vision and above your waist:
  - —If you cannot see an item, the item is contaminated.
  - —If the item is below your waist, the item is contaminated.
  - —Keep sterile-gloved hands above your waist and within your sight.
  - —Do not leave a sterile field unattended.
  - —Do not turn your back on a sterile field.
- Airborne microbes can contaminate sterile items or a sterile field:
  - —Prevent drafts. Close the door, and avoid extra movements. Ask other staff in the room to avoid extra movements.
  - —Avoid coughing, sneezing, talking, or laughing over a sterile field. Turn your head away from the sterile field if you must talk.

- —Wear a mask if you need to talk during the procedure.
- —Do not perform or assist with sterile procedures if you have a respiratory infection.
- —Do not reach over a sterile field.
- Fluid flows downward, in the direction of gravity:
  - —Hold wet items down (see Fig. 12-21). If held up, fluid flows down into a contaminated area. The contaminated fluid flows back into the sterile field when the item is held down.
- The sterile field is kept dry, unless the area below it is sterile:
  - —The sterile field is contaminated if it gets wet and the area below it is not sterile.
  - —Avoid spilling and splashing when pouring sterile fluids into sterile containers.
- The edges of a sterile field are contaminated:
  - —A 1-inch (2.5 cm) margin around the sterile field is considered contaminated (Fig. 12-22).
  - —Place all sterile items inside the 1-inch (2.5 cm) margin of the sterile field.
  - —Items outside the 1-inch (2.5 cm) margin are contaminated.
- Honesty is essential to sterile technique:
  - —You know when you contaminate an item or sterile field. Be honest with yourself even if other staff members are not present.
  - —Remove the contaminated item, and correct the matter. If necessary, start over with sterile supplies.
  - —Report the contamination to the nurse.

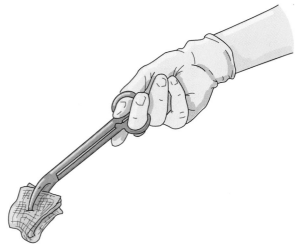

**FIG. 12-21** Sterile forceps are used to handle sterile items.

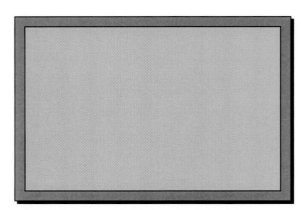

**FIG. 12-22** A 1-inch (2.5 cm) margin around the sterile filed is considered contaminated.

## STERILE GLOVING

The sterile field is set up first. Then sterile gloves are put on. After sterile gloves are on, you can handle sterile items within the sterile field. Do not touch anything outside the sterile field.

Sterile gloves are disposable. They come in many sizes so they fit snugly. The insides are powdered for ease in donning the gloves. The right and left gloves are marked on the package.

**SAFETY ALERT:** *Sterile Gloving*

Always keep sterile gloved hands above your waist and within your vision. Touch only items within the sterile field. If you contaminate the gloves, remove them. Decontaminate your hands, and put on a new pair. Replace gloves that are torn, cut, or punctured.

## STERILE GLOVING

### PROCEDURE

1 Follow *Delegation Guidelines: Assisting With Sterile Procedures*, p. 226. See *Safety Alerts: Sterile Procedures*, p. 226 *and Sterile Gloving*.
2 Practice hand hygiene.
3 Set up a sterile field.
4 Inspect the package for sterility:
   a Check the expiration date.
   b See if the package is dry.
   c Check for tears, holes, punctures, and water-marks.
5 Arrange a work surface.
   a Make sure you have enough room.
   b Arrange the work surface at waist level and within your vision.
   c Clean and dry the work surface.
   d Do not reach over or turn your back on the work surface.
6 Open the package. Grasp the flaps. Gently peel them back.
7 Remove the inner package. Place it on your work surface.
8 Read the manufacturer's instructions on the inner package. It may be labeled with *left, right, up,* and *down.*
9 Arrange the inner package for left, right, up, and down. The left glove is on your left. The right glove is on your right. The cuffs are near you with the fingers pointing away.
10 Grasp the folded edges of the inner package. Use the thumb and index finger of each hand.
11 Fold back the inner package to expose the gloves (Fig. 12-23, *A*). Do not touch or otherwise contaminate the inside of the package or the gloves. The inside of the inner package is a sterile field.

12 Note that each glove has a cuff about 2 to 3 inches wide. The cuffs and insides of the gloves are *not considered sterile.*
13 Put on the right glove if you are right-handed. Put on the left glove if you are left-handed.
   a Pick up the glove with your other hand. Use your thumb and index and middle fingers (Fig. 12-23, *B*).
   b Touch only the cuff and the inside of the glove.
   c Turn the hand to be gloved palm side up.
   d Lift the cuff up. Slide your fingers and hand into the glove (Fig. 12-23, *C*).
   e Pull the glove up over your hand. If some fingers get stuck, leave them that way until the other glove is on. *Do not use your ungloved hand to straighten the glove. Do not let the outside of the glove touch any non-sterile surface.*
   f Leave the cuff turned down.
14 Put on the other glove. Use your gloved hand.
   a Reach under the cuff of the second glove. Use the four fingers of your gloved hand (Fig. 12-23, *D*). Keep your gloved thumb close to your gloved palm.
   b Pull on the second glove (Fig. 12-23, *E*). Your gloved hand cannot touch the cuff or any surface. Hold the thumb of your first gloved hand away from your gloved palm.
15 Adjust each glove with the other hand. The gloves should be smooth and comfortable (Fig. 12-23, *F*).
16 Slide your fingers under the cuffs to pull them up (Fig. 12-23, *G*).
17 Touch only sterile items.
18 Remove the gloves. See Figure 12-14.
19 Decontaminate your hands.

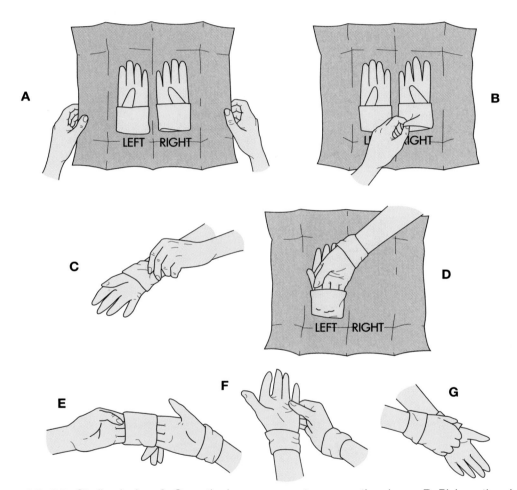

**FIG. 12-23** Sterile gloving. **A,** Open the inner wrapper to expose the gloves. **B,** Pick up the glove at the cuff with your thumb and index and middle fingers. **C,** Slide your fingers and hand into the glove. **D,** Reach under the cuff of the other glove with your fingers. **E,** Pull on the second glove. **F,** Adjust each glove for comfort. **G,** Slide your fingers under the cuffs to pull them up.

## CROSS-TRAINING OPPORTUNITIES

Central supply and housekeeping staffs help prevent infection. You may be asked to cross-train for one or both areas:

- *Central supply.* The staff disinfect and sterilize supplies and equipment. They stock nursing units with care items. They bring special equipment to nursing units as requested.
- *Housekeeping.* The staff clean patient or resident rooms, nursing units, hallways, bathrooms, and other areas. They have methods and procedures for cleaning and disinfecting floors, furniture, bathrooms, and equipment.

Circle **T** if the statement is true and **F** if it is false.

1   **T F** Microbes are pathogens in their natural sites.

2   **T F** A pathogen can cause an infection.

3   **T F** An item is sterile if non-pathogens are present.

4   **T F** You hold your hands and forearms up during hand washing.

5   **T F** Unused items in a person's room are used for another person.

6   **T F** A person received the hepatitis B vaccine. The person will develop the disease.

7   **T F** The 1-inch edge around a sterile field is considered contaminated.

8   **T F** A sterile package has a watermark. The package is contaminated.

9   **T F** The inside and cuffs of sterile gloves are considered contaminated.

Circle the **BEST** answer.

10 Most pathogens need the following to grow *except*
  a Water
  b Light
  c Oxygen
  d Nourishment

11 Signs and symptoms of infection include the following *except*
  a Fever, nausea, vomiting, rash, and/or sores
  b Pain or tenderness, redness, and/or swelling
  c Fatigue, loss of appetite, and/or a discharge
  d A wound and/or bleeding

12 Which is *not* a portal of exit?
  a Respiratory tract
  b Blood
  c Reproductive system
  d Intact skin

13 Which does *not* prevent nosocomial infections?
  a Hand hygiene before and after giving care
  b Sterilizing all care items
  c Surgical asepsis
  d Standard Precautions

14 When cleaning equipment, do the following *except*
  a Rinse the item in cold water before cleaning
  b Wash the item with soap and hot water
  c Use a brush if necessary
  d Work from dirty to clean areas

15 Isolation Precautions
  a Prevent infection
  b Destroy pathogens
  c Keep pathogens within a certain area
  d Destroy all microbes

16 Standard Precautions
  a Are used for all persons
  b Prevent the spread of pathogens through the air
  c Require gowns, masks, gloves, and eyewear
  d Involve medical and surgical asepsis

17 You wear utility gloves for contact with
  a Blood
  b Body fluids
  c Secretions and excretions
  d Cleaning solutions

18 A mask
  a Can be reused
  b Is clean on the inside
  c Is contaminated when moist
  d Should fit loosely for breathing

19 These statements are about personal protective equipment (PPE). Which is *false*?
  a Wash disposable gloves for reuse.
  b Remove PPE before leaving the work area.
  c Discard cracked or torn utility gloves.
  d Wear gloves when touching contaminated items or surfaces.

20 Contaminated work surfaces are cleaned at the following times *except*
  a After completing a task
  b When there is obvious contamination
  c After blood is spilled
  d After removing gloves

21 The Bloodborne Pathogen Standard involves the following *except*
  a Wearing gloves
  b Discarding sharp items into a biohazard container
  c Storing food and blood in different places
  d Eating and drinking in areas of occupational exposure

22 You were exposed to a bloodborne pathogen. Which is *true?*
  a You do not have to report the incident.
  b You pay for required tests.
  c You can refuse HBV and HIV testing.
  d The source individual can refuse testing.

23 These statements are about surgical asepsis. Which is *false?*
  a A sterile item can touch only another sterile item.
  b Wet items are held up.
  c If you cannot see an item, it is considered contaminated.
  d Sterile items are kept above your waist.

24 You have on sterile gloves. You can touch
  a Anything on the sterile field
  b Anything on your work surface
  c Anything below your waist
  d Any part of your uniform

*Answers to these questions are on p. 817.*

# 13

# Body Mechanics

## OBJECTIVES

- Define the key terms in this chapter
- Explain the purpose and rules of body mechanics
- Explain how ergonomics can prevent workplace accidents
- Identify the causes, signs, and symptoms of back injuries
- Identify comfort and safety measures for lifting, turning, and moving persons in bed
- Explain how to safely perform transfers
- Explain why body alignment and position changes are important
- Identify the comfort and safety measures for positioning a person
- Position persons in the basic bed positions and in a chair
- Perform the procedures described in this chapter

## KEY TERMS

**base of support**   The area on which an object rests

**body alignment**   The way the head, trunk, arms, and legs are aligned with one another; posture

**body mechanics**   Using the body in an efficient and careful way

**dorsal recumbent position**   The back-lying or supine position

**ergonomics**   The science of designing a job to fit the worker

**Fowler's position**   A semi-sitting position; the head of the bed is raised between 45 and 90 degrees

**friction**   The rubbing of one surface against another

**gait belt**   A transfer belt

**lateral position**   The side-lying position

**logrolling**   Turning the person as a unit, in alignment, with one motion

**posture**   Body alignment

**prone position**   Lying on the abdomen with the head turned to one side

**shearing**   When skin sticks to a surface while muscles slide in the direction the body is moving

**side-lying position**   The lateral position

**Sims' position**   A left side-lying position in which the upper leg is sharply flexed so it is not on the lower leg and the lower arm is behind the person

**supine position**   The back-lying or dorsal recumbent position

**transfer belt**   A belt used to support persons who are unsteady or disabled; a gait belt

You will turn and reposition persons often. You move them in bed. You transfer them to and from chairs, wheelchairs, stretchers, and toilets. During these and other tasks, you must use your body correctly. This protects you and the person from injury.

See Box 13-1 for a review of the musculoskeletal system. Or review Chapter 7.

## BODY MECHANICS

**Body mechanics** means using the body in an efficient and careful way. It involves good posture, balance, and using your strongest and largest muscles for work. Fatigue, muscle strain, and injury can result from improper use and positioning of the body during activity or rest. Focus on the person's and your own body mechanics. Good body mechanics reduce the risk of injury.

## BOX 13-1 | MUSKULOSKELETAL SYSTEM: REVIEW OF BODY STRUCTURE AND FUNCTION

The musculoskeletal system:
- Provides the framework for the body
- Allows the body to move
- Protects the body
- Gives the body shape

### BONES

Bones are hard, rigid structures made up of living cells. *Long bones* (leg bones) bear the weight of the body. *Short bones* allow skill and ease in movement. Bones in the wrists, fingers, ankles, and toes are short bones. *Flat bones* protect the organs. Such bones include the ribs, skull, pelvic bones, and shoulder blades. *Irregular bones* are the vertebrae in the spinal column. They allow various degrees of movement and flexibility.

### JOINTS

A *joint* is the point at which two or more bones meet (Fig. 13-1). Joints allow movement. A *ball-and-socket* joint allows movement in all directions. The joints of the hips and shoulders are ball-and-socket joints. A *hinge joint* allows movement in one direction. The elbow and knee are hinge joints. A *pivot joint* allows turning from side to side. The skull is connected to the spine by a pivot joint.

### MUSCLES

There are more than 500 muscles in the human body (Fig. 13-2, p. 236). *Voluntary* muscles can be consciously controlled. Muscles that are attached to bones *(skeletal muscles)* are voluntary. Arm muscles do not work unless you move your arm. Likewise for leg muscles.

*Involuntary muscles* work automatically and cannot be consciously controlled. Involuntary muscles control the action of the stomach, intestines, blood vessels, and other body organs. *Cardiac muscle* is in the heart. It is an involuntary muscle.

Muscles perform three important body functions:
- Movement of body parts
- Maintenance of posture
- Production of body heat

Some muscles constantly contract to maintain the body's posture. When muscles contract, they burn food for energy. This results in the production of heat. The greater the muscular activity, the more heat produced in the body. When exposed to cold, the body shivers to produce heat. The shivering sensation is from rapid, general muscle contractions.

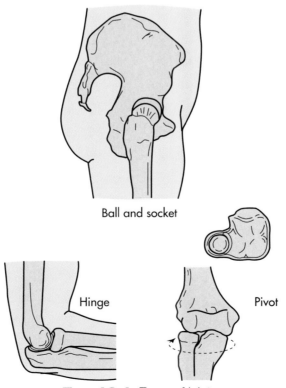

Ball and socket

Hinge

Pivot

**FIG. 13-1** Types of joints.

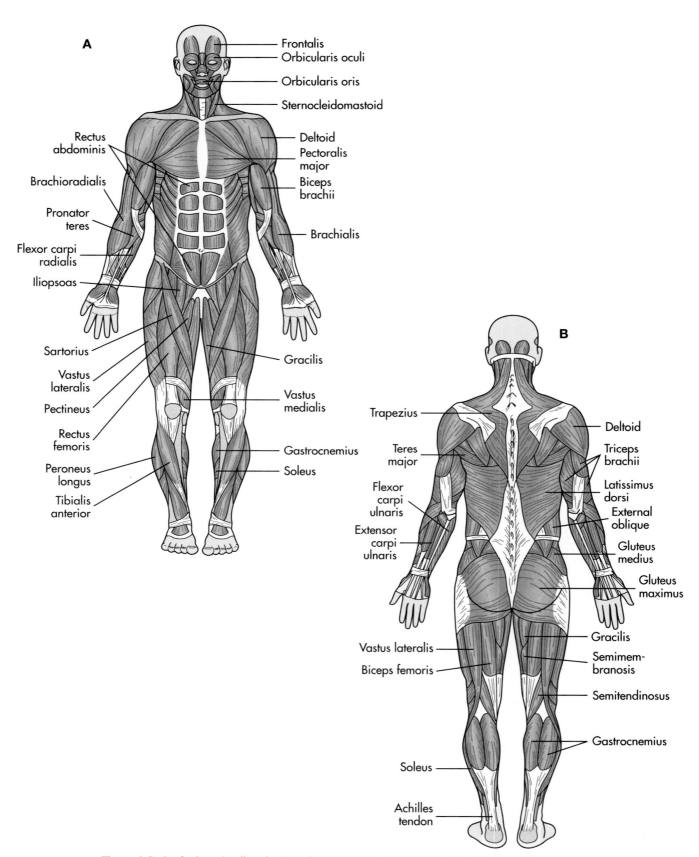

**FIG. 13-2  A,** Anterior (front) view of the muscles. **B,** Posterior (back) view of the muscles.

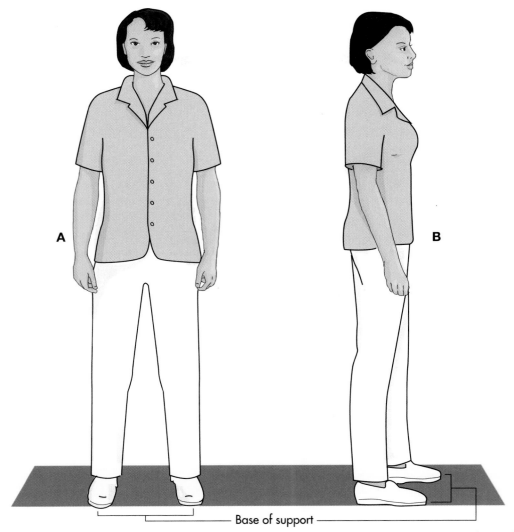

**FIG. 13-3 A,** Anterior (front) view of an adult in good body alignment. The feet are apart for a wide base of support. **B,** Lateral (side) view of an adult with good posture and alignment.

**Body alignment (posture)** is the way the head, trunk, arms, and legs are aligned with one another. Good alignment lets the body move and function with strength and efficiency. Standing, sitting, and lying down require good alignment.

**Base of support** is the area on which an object rests. A good base of support is needed for balance (Fig. 13-3). When standing, your feet are your base of support. Stand with your feet apart for a wider base of support and more balance.

Your strongest and largest muscles are in the shoulders, upper arms, hips, and thighs. Use these muscles to lift and move heavy objects. Otherwise, you place strain and exertion on smaller and weaker muscles. This causes fatigue and injury. *Back injuries are a major risk.* For good body mechanics:

- Bend your knees and squat to lift a heavy object (Fig. 13-4, p. 238). Do not bend from your waist. Bending from the waist places strain on small back muscles.
- Hold items close to your body and base of support (see Fig. 13-4). This involves upper arm and shoulder muscles. Holding objects away from your body places strain on small muscles in your lower arms.

All activities require good body mechanics. You must safely and efficiently lift and move persons and heavy objects. Follow the rules in Box 13-2, p. 238.

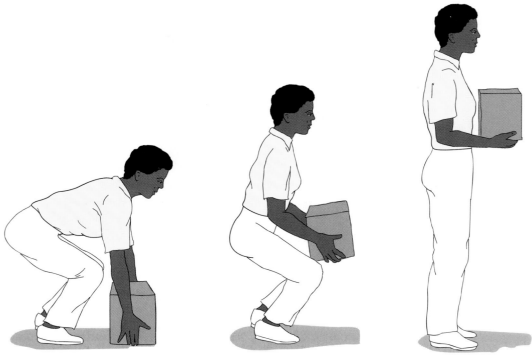

**FIG. 13-4** Picking up a box using good body mechanics.

---

**BOX
13-2** **RULES FOR BODY MECHANICS**

- Keep your body in good alignment with a wide base of support.
- Use the stronger and larger muscles in your shoulders, upper arms, thighs, and hips.
- Keep objects close to your body when you lift, move, or carry them (see Fig. 13-4).
- Avoid unnecessary bending and reaching. Raise the bed so it is close to your waist. Adjust the overbed table so it is at your waist level.
- Face your work area. This prevents unnecessary twisting.
- Push, slide, or pull heavy objects whenever you can, rather than lifting them. Pushing is better than pulling.
- Widen your base of support when pushing or pulling. Move your front leg forward when pushing. Move your rear leg back when pulling (Fig. 13-5).
- Use both hands and arms to lift, move, or carry heavy objects.

- Turn your whole body when changing the direction of your movement. Move and turn your feet in the direction of the turn, instead of twisting your body.
- Work with smooth and even movements. Avoid sudden or jerky motions.
- *Get help from a co-worker if the person cannot assist with turning or moving.*
- *Get help from a co-worker to move heavy objects or persons. Do not lift or move them by yourself.*
- Bend your hips and knees to lift heavy objects from the floor (see Fig. 13-4). Straighten your back as the object reaches thigh level. Your leg and thigh muscles work to raise the item off the floor and to waist level.
- Do not lift objects higher than chest level. Do not lift above your shoulders. Use a step stool to reach an object higher than chest level.

# ERGONOMICS

**Ergonomics** is the science of designing the job to fit the worker. (*Ergo* means work. *Nomos* means law.) The task, work station, equipment, and tools are changed to reduce stress on the worker's body. The goal is to prevent a serious and disabling work-related musculoskeletal disorder (MSD).

MSDs are injuries and disorders of the muscles, tendons, ligaments, joints, and cartilage. They also involve the nervous system. The arms and back are often affected. MSDs are painful. They can develop slowly over weeks, months, and years. Or they can occur from one event. Pain, numbness, tingling, stiff joints, difficulty moving, and muscle loss can occur.

MSDs are workplace health hazards. Time off work is often needed. According to the U.S. Department of Labor, nursing assistants are at great risk. Back injuries are a major threat.

## BACK INJURIES

Back injuries can occur from repeated activities over time or from one event. Signs and symptoms include:
- Pain when trying to assume a normal posture
- Decreased mobility
- Pain when standing or rising from a seated position

According to the Occupational Safety and Health Administration (OSHA), these factors lead to back disorders:
- Reaching while lifting
- Poor posture when sitting or standing
- Staying in one position too long
- Poor body mechanics when lifting, pushing, pulling, or carrying objects
- Poor physical condition—not having the strength or endurance to perform tasks without strain
- Repeated lifting of awkward items, equipment, or persons
- Twisting while lifting
- Bending while lifting
- Maintaining a bent posture
- Heavy lifting
- Fatigue
- Poor footing such as on slippery floors
- Lifting with forceful movement

Follow the rules in Box 13-2. They help prevent back injuries.

> **SAFETY ALERT:** *Back Injuries*
> According to OSHA, these activities are associated with back injury in nursing centers:
> - Moving a person who totally depends on others for care
> - Moving a person who is combative
> - Transferring a person who is on the floor to the bed or a chair
> - Repositioning a person in bed or chair
> - Transferring a person from bed to chair or from chair to bed
> - Transferring a person from one chair to another chair (includes transfers to and from the wheelchair and toilet)
> - Bending to bathe a person or to change linens
> - Weighing a person
> - Changing an incontinence product
> - Trying to stop a person from falling
>
> Use good body mechanics to protect yourself and others from injury. Do not work alone. Have a co-worker help you lift, move, turn, or transfer a person.

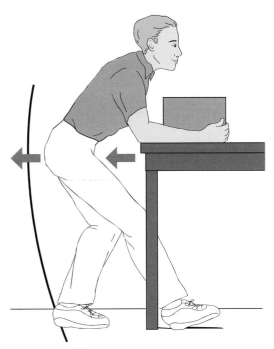

**FIG. 13-5** Move your rear leg back when pulling an item.

# LIFTING AND MOVING PERSONS IN BED

Some persons can move and turn in bed. Others need help from at least one person. Those who are weak, unconscious, paralyzed, on complete bed rest, or in casts need help. Sometimes two or three people or a mechanical lift is needed.

## COMFORT AND SAFETY

Protect the person's skin during lifting and moving. Friction and shearing injure the skin. Both cause infection and pressure ulcers (Chapter 28).

- **Friction** is the rubbing of one surface against another. When moved in bed, the person's skin rubs against the sheet.
- **Shearing** is when the skin sticks to a surface while muscles slide in the direction the body is moving (Fig. 13-6). It occurs when the person slides down in bed or is moved in bed.

Reduce friction and shearing by rolling or lifting the person. A cotton drawsheet (Chapter 15) serves as a *lift sheet (turning sheet)* to move the person in bed and reduce friction. Some agencies use turning pads for this purpose (p. 247).

These are other comfort and safety measures for moving persons:

- Ask co-workers to help *before* starting the procedure.
- Cover and screen the person to protect the right to privacy.
- Protect tubes or drainage containers connected to the person.

See *Focus on Older Persons: Lifting and Moving Persons in Bed.*

---

### FOCUS ON OLDER PERSONS
#### LIFTING AND MOVING PERSONS IN BED

Older persons are at great risk for shearing. Their skin is fragile and easily torn. Many have arthritis and osteoporosis (Chapter 33). They have fragile bones and joints. Protect them from pain and injury.

Ask a co-worker to help you lift and move older persons. Use a lift sheet. Move them carefully and gently. Persons with dementia may try to resist your efforts. Do not force the person. Proceed slowly. Use a calm voice. Divert the person's attention if necessary.

---

**DELEGATION GUIDELINES:** *Lifting and Moving Persons in Bed*

Many delegated tasks involve lifting and moving the person in bed. Before lifting or moving a person, you need this information from the nurse and the care plan:

- Position limits and restrictions
- How far you can lower the head of the bed
- Any limits in the person's ability to move or be repositioned
- What procedure to use
- How many workers are needed to safely lift and move the person
- What equipment is needed—trapeze, lift sheet, mechanical lift
- How to position the person (p. 272)
- If the person uses bed rails
- What observations to report and record

---

**SAFETY ALERT:** *Lifting and Moving Persons in Bed*

For safety and efficiency, decide how you will move the person before starting the procedure. If you need help from a co-worker, ask someone to help before you begin. Also plan how to protect drainage tubes or containers connected to the person.

Beds are raised horizontally to lift and move persons in bed (Chapter 14). This reduces bending and reaching. You must:

- Use the bed correctly
- Protect the person from falling when the bed is raised
- Follow the rules of body mechanics
- Keep the person in good alignment
- Position the person in good alignment after lifting or moving (p. 272)

---

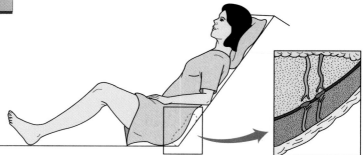

**FIG. 13-6** When the head of the bed is raised to a sitting position, skin on the buttocks stays in place. However, internal structures move forward as the person slides down in bed. This causes skin to be pinched between the mattress and the hip bones.

## ◼ RAISING THE PERSON'S HEAD AND SHOULDERS

You may have to raise a person's head and shoulders to give care. Simply turning or removing a pillow requires this procedure. You can raise the person's head and shoulders easily and safely by locking arms with the person. It is best to have help with older persons and those who are heavy or hard to move. This protects the person and you from injury.

*Text continued on p. 244.*

## RAISING THE PERSON'S HEAD AND SHOULDERS

### QUALITY OF LIFE

Remember to:
- Knock before entering the person's room
- Address the person by name
- Introduce yourself by name and title

### PRE-PROCEDURE

1 Follow *Delegation Guidelines: Lifting and Moving Persons in Bed.* See *Safety Alert: Lifting and Moving Persons in Bed.*
2 Ask a co-worker to assist if you need help.
3 Practice hand hygiene.
4 Identify the person. Check the ID bracelet against the assignment sheet. Call the person by name.
5 Explain what you are going to do.
6 Provide for privacy.
7 Lock the bed wheels.
8 Raise the bed for body mechanics. Bed rails are up if used.

### PROCEDURE

9 Ask your co-worker to stand on the other side of the bed. Lower the bed rails if up.
10 Ask the person to put the near arm under your near arm and behind your shoulder. His or her hand rests on top of your shoulder. If you are standing on the right side, the person's right hand rests on your right shoulder (Fig. 13-7, *A*, p. 242). The person does the same with your co-worker. The person's left hand rests on your co-workers left shoulder (Fig. 13-8, *A*, p. 243).
11 Put your arm nearest to the person under his or her arm. Your hand is on the person's shoulder. Your co-worker does the same.
12 Put your free arm under the person's neck and shoulders (Fig. 13-7, *B*, p. 242). Your co-worker does the same (Fig. 13-8, *B*, p. 243).
13 Help the person pull up to a sitting or semi-sitting position on the count of "3" (Figs. 13-7, *C*, p. 242 and 13-8, *C*, p. 243).
14 Use the arm and hand that supported the person's neck and shoulders to give care (Fig. 13-7, *D*, p. 242). Your co-worker supports the person (Fig. 13-8, *D*, p. 243).
15 Help the person lie down. Provide support with your locked arms. Support the person's neck and shoulders with your other arm.

### POST-PROCEDURE

16 Provide for comfort. Position the person in good alignment (p. 272).
17 Place the signal light within reach.
18 Raise or lower bed rails. Follow the care plan.
19 Lower the bed to its lowest position.
20 Unscreen the person.
21 Decontaminate your hands.
22 Report and record your observations.

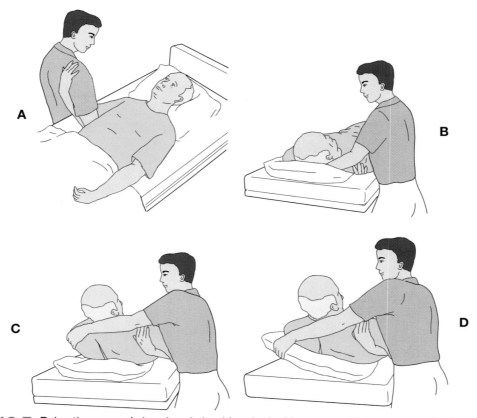

**FIG. 13-7** Raise the person's head and shoulders by locking arms with the person. **A,** The person's near arm is under the nursing assistant's near arm and behind the shoulder. **B,** The nursing assistant's far arm is under the person's neck and shoulders, with the near arm under the person's nearest arm. **C,** The person is raised to a semi-sitting position by locking arms. **D,** The nursing assistant lifts the pillow while the person is in a semi-sitting position.

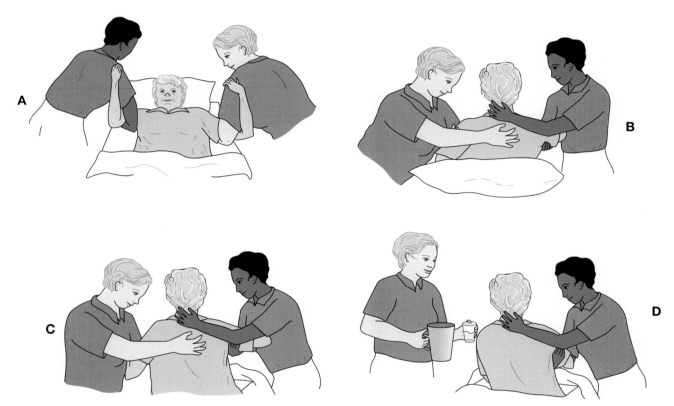

**FIG. 13-8** Raising the person's head and shoulders with assistance. **A,** Two nursing assistants lock arms with the person. **B,** The nursing assistants have their arms under the person's head and neck. **C,** The nursing assistants raise the person to a semi-sitting position. **D,** One nursing assistant supports the person in the semi-sitting position while the other gives care.

## ◼ MOVING THE PERSON UP IN BED

When the bed is raised, it is easy to slide down toward the middle and foot of the bed (Fig. 13-9). The person is moved up in bed for good alignment and comfort.

You can usually move children up in bed alone. You can sometimes move lightweight adults up in bed alone if they use a trapeze. However, it is best to have help and to use a lift sheet. At least two workers are needed to move heavy, weak, and very old persons up in bed. Always protect the person and yourself from injury.

## MOVING THE PERSON UP IN BED

### QUALITY OF LIFE

Remember to:
- Knock before entering the person's room
- Address the person by name
- Introduce yourself by name and title

### PRE-PROCEDURE

1 Follow *Delegation Guidelines: Lifting and Moving Persons in Bed*, p. 240. See *Safety Alert: Lifting and Moving Persons in Bed*, p. 240.
2 Ask a co-worker to assist you if you need help.
3 Practice hand hygiene.
4 Identify the person. Check the ID bracelet against the assignment sheet. Call the person by name.

5 Explain what you are going to do.
6 Provide for privacy.
7 Lock the bed wheels.
8 Raise the bed for body mechanics. Bed rails are up if used.

### PROCEDURE

9 Lower the head of the bed to a level appropriate for the person. It is as flat as possible.
10 Stand on one side of the bed. Your co-worker stands on the other side.
11 Lower the bed rail near you. Your co-worker does the same.
12 Place the pillow against the headboard if the person can be without it. This prevents the person's head from hitting the headboard when being moved up.
13 Stand with a wide base of support. Point the foot near the head of the bed toward the head of the bed. Face the head of the bed.
14 Bend your hips and knees. Keep your back straight.

15 Place one arm under the person's shoulder and one arm under the thighs. Your co-worker does the same. Grasp each other's forearms (Fig. 13-10).
16 Ask the person to grasp the trapeze if he or she has one (Fig. 13-11).
17 Have the person flex both knees.
18 Explain that you will move on the count of "3." The person pushes against the bed with the feet if able.
19 Move the person to the head of the bed on the count of "3." Shift your weight from your rear leg to your front leg (see Figs. 13-10 and 13-11).
20 Repeat steps 13 through 19 if necessary.

### POST-PROCEDURE

21 Put the pillow under the person's head and shoulders. Straighten linens.
22 Provide for comfort. Position the person in good alignment (p. 272).
23 Place the signal light within reach.
24 Raise or lower bed rails. Follow the care plan.

25 Raise the head of the bed to a level appropriate for the person.
26 Lower the bed to its lowest position.
27 Unscreen the person.
28 Decontaminate your hands.
29 Report and record your observations.

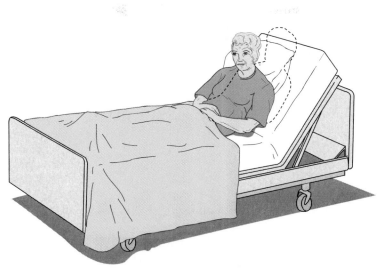

FIG. 13-9 A person in poor alignment after sliding down in bed.

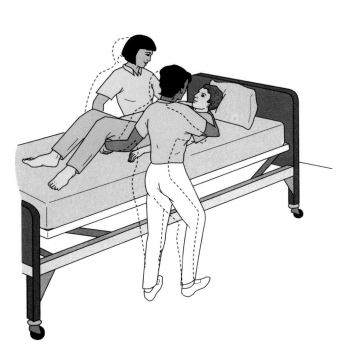

FIG. 13-10 A person is moved up in bed by two nursing assistants. Each has one arm under the person's shoulders and the other under the thighs. They have locked arms under the person. The person's knees are flexed. The nursing assistants shift their weight from the rear leg to the front leg as the person is moved up in bed.

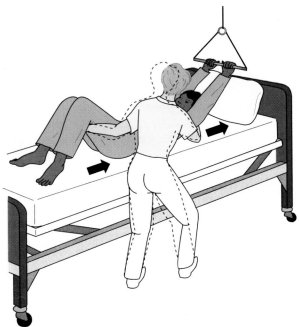

FIG. 13-11 The person grasps a trapeze and flexes the knees. The nursing assistant shifts her body weight from the rear leg to the front leg as she moves the person up in bed. *NOTE* Although you can move children and lightweight adults alone with this method, it is best to have help.

## MOVING THE PERSON UP IN BED WITH A LIFT SHEET

With a co-worker's help, you can easily and safely move a person up in bed with a *lift sheet*. (It is called a *turning sheet* when used to turn the person. See p. 240.) Friction and shearing are reduced. The person is lifted more evenly. Use a flat sheet folded in half, a drawsheet, or a turning pad (Fig. 13-12). Place it under the person from the head to above the knees.

Use this procedure for:
- Most nursing center residents, particularly those who cannot move themselves
- Persons who are unconscious or paralyzed
- Persons recovering from spinal cord surgery or spinal cord injuries
- Older persons

---

### MOVING THE PERSON UP IN BED WITH A LIFT SHEET

#### QUALITY OF LIFE

Remember to:
- Knock before entering the person's room
- Address the person by name
- Introduce yourself by name and title

#### PRE-PROCEDURE

1 Follow *Delegation Guidelines: Lifting and Moving Persons in Bed*, p. 240. See *Safety Alert: Lifting and Moving Persons in Bed*, p. 240.
2 Ask a co-worker to help you.
3 Practice hand hygiene.
4 Identify the person. Check the ID bracelet against the assignment sheet. Call the person by name.
5 Explain what you are going to do.
6 Provide for privacy.
7 Lock the bed wheels.
8 Raise the bed for body mechanics. Bed rails are up if used.

#### PROCEDURE

9 Lower the head of the bed to a level appropriate for the person. It is as flat as possible.
10 Stand on one side of the bed. Your co-worker stands on the other side.
11 Lower the bed rails if up.
12 Place the pillow against the headboard if the person can be without it.
13 Stand with a broad base of support. Point the foot near the head of the bed toward the head of the bed. Face that direction.
14 Roll the sides of the lift sheet up close to the person.
15 Grasp the rolled-up lift sheet firmly near the person's shoulders and buttocks (Fig. 13-13). Support the head.
16 Bend your hips and knees.
17 Move the person up in bed on the count of "3." Shift your weight from your rear leg to your front leg.
18 Repeat steps 13 through 17 if necessary.
19 Unroll the lift sheet.

#### POST-PROCEDURE

20 Put the pillow under the person's head and shoulders. Straighten linens.
21 Provide for comfort. Position the person in good alignment (p. 272).
22 Place the signal light within reach.
23 Raise or lower bed rails. Follow the care plan.
24 Raise the head of the bed to a level appropriate for the person.
25 Lower the bed to its lowest position.
26 Unscreen the person.
27 Decontaminate your hands.
28 Report and record your observations.

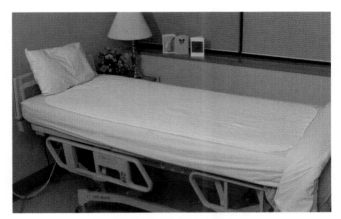

**FIG. 13-12** Turning pad.

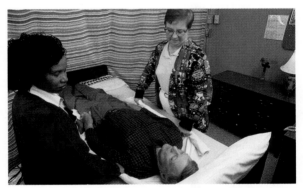

**FIG. 13-13** A lift sheet is used to move the person up in bed. The lift sheet extends from the person's head to above the knees. The lift sheet is rolled close to the person and held near the shoulders and buttocks.

# MOVING THE PERSON TO THE SIDE OF THE BED

Repositioning and care procedures require moving the person to the side of the bed. The person is moved to the side of the bed before turning. Otherwise, after turning, the person lies on the side of the bed—not in the middle.

Sometimes you have to reach over the person. Giving a bed bath is an example. You reach less if the person is close to you.

One method involves moving the person in segments. One person can sometimes do this. The lift sheet method is used for persons recovering from spinal cord injuries or spinal cord surgery.

Using a lift shift helps prevent pain, skin damage, and injury to the bones, joints, and spinal cord. When using a lift sheet, you need a co-worker to help you. *See Focus on Older Persons: Moving the Person to the Side of the Bed.*

---

**SAFETY ALERT:** *Moving the Person to the Side of the Bed*

You need to know which method to use. Get this information from the nurse whenever delegated tasks involve moving the person to the side of the bed. Such tasks include repositioning, bed-making, bathing, and range-of-motion exercises.

The wrong method could seriously injure a person. This is very important for persons who are very old, have arthritis, or have spinal cord involvement.

---

## FOCUS ON OLDER PERSONS
### MOVING THE PERSON TO THE SIDE OF THE BED

A lift sheet is used to move older persons in bed. It is also used to move persons with arthritis. The lift sheet helps prevent pain and bone and joint injuries.

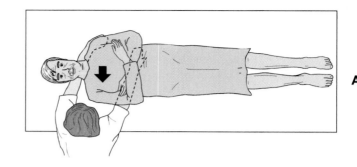
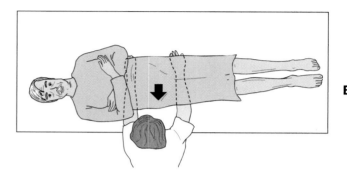
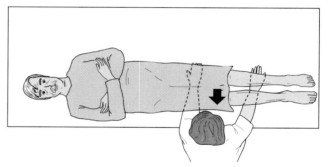

**FIG. 13-14** The person is moved to the side of the bed in segments. **A,** The upper part of the body is moved. **B,** The lower part of the body is moved. **C,** The legs and feet are moved.

## MOVING THE PERSON TO THE SIDE OF THE BED

### QUALITY OF LIFE

Remember to:
- Knock before entering the person's room
- Address the person by name
- Introduce yourself by name and title

### PRE-PROCEDURE

1 Follow *Delegation Guidelines: Lifting and Moving Persons in Bed*, p. 240. See *Safety Alerts: Lifting and Moving Persons in Bed*, p. 240, and *Moving the Person to the Side of the Bed*.
2 Ask a co-worker to help if using a lift sheet.
3 Practice hand hygiene.
4 Identify the person. Check the ID bracelet against the assignment sheet. Call the person by name.
5 Explain the procedure to the person.
6 Provide for privacy.
7 Lock the bed wheels.
8 Raise the bed for body mechanics. Bed rails are up if used.

### PROCEDURE

9 Lower the head of the bed to a level appropriate for the person. It is as flat as possible.
10 Stand on the side of the bed to which you will move the person.
11 Lower the bed rail near you if bed rails are used. (Both bed rails are lowered for step 15).
12 Stand with your feet about 12 inches apart. One foot is in front of the other. Flex your knees.
13 Cross the person's arms over the person's chest.
14 *Method 1: Moving the person in segments:*
  a Place your arm under the person's neck and shoulders. Grasp the far shoulder.
  b Place your other arm under the mid-back.
  c Move the upper part of the person's body toward you. Rock backward and shift your weight to your rear leg (Fig. 13-14, *A*).
  d Place one arm under the person's waist and one under the thighs.

  e Rock backward to move the lower part of the person toward you (Fig. 13-14, *B*).
  f Repeat the procedure for the legs and feet (Fig. 13-14, *C*). Your arms should be under the person's thighs and calves.
15 *Method 2: Moving the person with a lift sheet:*
  a Roll the lift sheet up close to the person (see Fig. 13-13).
  b Grasp the rolled-up lift sheet near the person's shoulders and buttocks. Your co-worker does the same. Support the head.
  c Rock backward on the count of "3," moving the person toward you. Your co-worker rocks backward slightly and then forward toward you while keeping the arms straight.
  d Unroll the lift sheet. Remove any wrinkles.

### POST-PROCEDURE

16 Provide for comfort.
17 Position the person in good alignment. Follow the nurse's directions and the care plan.
18 Place the signal light within reach.
19 Raise or lower bed rails. Follow the care plan.
20 Lower the bed to its lowest position.
21 Unscreen the person.
22 Decontaminate your hands.
23 Report and record your observations.

# TURNING PERSONS

Certain procedures require the side-lying position. The person is turned toward or away from you. The direction depends on the person's condition and the situation.

Turning persons onto their sides helps prevent complications from bedrest (Chapter 22). After the person is turned, position him or her in good alignment. Pillows are used to support the person in the side-lying position.

Some persons turn and reposition themselves in bed. Others need help. Some totally depend on the nursing staff for care.

*See Focus on Older Persons: Turning Persons.*

> ### ► FOCUS ON OLDER PERSONS
> #### TURNING PERSONS
> Many older persons suffer from arthritis in their spines and knees. When turning these persons it is best to use the logrolling procedure using a turning sheet (lift sheet). Logrolling is less painful for these persons (p. 252).

**DELEGATION GUIDELINES:** *Turning Persons*
Before turning and repositioning a person, you need this information from the nurse and the care plan:
- How much help the person needs
- The person's comfort level and what body parts are painful
- Which procedure to use
- What supportive devices are needed for positioning (Chapter 22)
- Where to place pillows
- What observations to report and record

**SAFETY ALERT:** *Turning Persons*
Use good body mechanics when turning a person in bed. The person must be in good alignment. Otherwise, musculoskeletal injuries, skin breakdown, or pressure ulcers could occur.

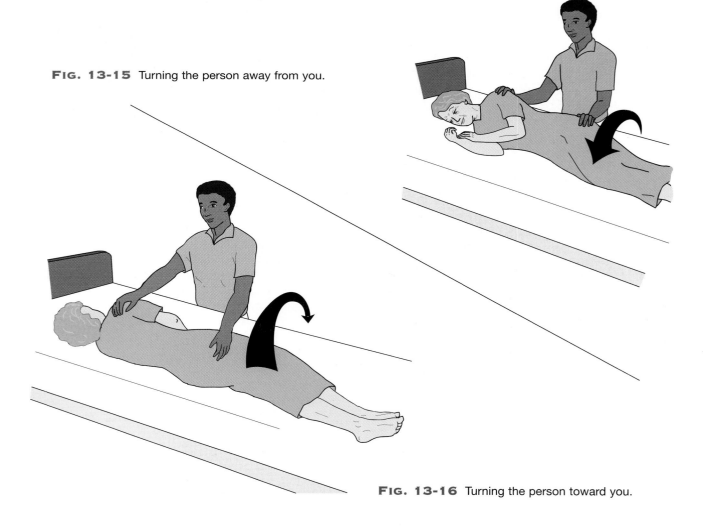

**FIG. 13-15** Turning the person away from you.

**FIG. 13-16** Turning the person toward you.

# TURNING AND POSITIONING THE PERSON

NNAAP™

## QUALITY OF LIFE

Remember to:
- Knock before entering the person's room
- Address the person by name
- Introduce yourself by name and title

## PRE-PROCEDURE

1 Follow *Delegation Guidelines: Turning Persons.* See *Safety Alert: Turning Persons.*
2 Practice hand hygiene.
3 Identify the person. Check the ID bracelet against the assignment sheet. Call the person by name.
4 Explain the procedure to the person.
5 Provide for privacy.
6 Lock the bed wheels.
7 Raise the bed for body mechanics. Bed rails are up if used.

## PROCEDURE

8 Lower the head of the bed to a level appropriate for the person. It is as flat as possible.
9 Stand on the side of the bed opposite to where you will turn the person. The far bed rail is up if used.
10 Lower the bed rail near you if used.
11 Move the person to the side near you. (See procedure: *Moving the Person to the Side of the Bed,* p. 249.)
12 Cross the person's arms over the person's chest. Cross the leg near you over the far leg.
13 *Moving the person away from you:*
   a Stand with a wide base of support. Flex your knees.
   b Place one hand on the person's shoulder. Place the other on the buttock near you.
   c Push the person gently toward the other side of the bed (Fig. 13-15). Shift your weight from your rear leg to your front leg.

14 *Moving the person toward you:*
   a Raise the bed rail if used.
   b Go to the other side. Lower the bed rail if used.
   c Stand with a wide base of support. Flex your knees.
   d Place one hand on the person's far shoulder. Place the other on the far hip.
   e Roll the person toward you gently (Fig. 13-16).
15 Position the person. Follow the nurse's directions and the care plan. The following is common:
   a Place a pillow under the head and neck.
   b Adjust the shoulder. The person should not lie on an arm.
   c Place a small pillow under the upper hand and arm.
   d Position a pillow against the back.
   e Flex the upper knee. Position the upper leg in front of the lower leg.
   f Support the upper leg and thigh on pillows.

## POST-PROCEDURE

16 Provide for comfort.
17 Place the signal light within reach.
18 Raise or lower bed rails. Follow the care plan.
19 Lower the bed to its lowest position.
20 Unscreen the person.
21 Decontaminate your hands.
22 Report and record your observations.

# LOGROLLING

**Logrolling** is turning the person as a unit, in alignment, with one motion. The spine is kept straight. The procedure is used to turn:

- Older persons with arthritic spines or knees
- Persons recovering from hip fractures
- Persons with spinal cord injuries (the spine is kept straight at all times after spinal cord injury)
- Persons recovering from spinal surgery (the spine is kept straight at all times after spinal surgery)

Two or three staff members are needed to logroll a person. Three are needed if the person is tall or heavy. Sometimes a turning sheet is used.

> **SAFETY ALERT:** *Logrolling*
> After spinal cord injury or surgery, a pillow under the head and neck is usually not allowed. Follow the nurse's directions and the care plan.

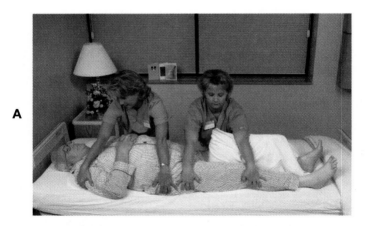

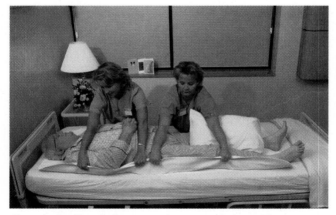

**FIG. 13-17** Logrolling. **A,** A pillow is between the person's legs. The arms are crossed on the chest. The person is on the far side of the bed. **B,** A turning sheet is used to logroll a person.

## LOGROLLING THE PERSON

### QUALITY OF LIFE

Remember to:
- Knock before entering the person's room
- Address the person by name
- Introduce yourself by name and title

### PRE-PROCEDURE

1 Follow *Delegation Guidelines: Turning Persons.* See *Safety Alerts: Turning Persons* and *Logrolling Persons.*
2 Ask a co-worker to help you.
3 Practice hand hygiene.
4 Identify the person. Check the ID bracelet against the assignment sheet. Call the person by name.
5 Explain the procedure to the person.
6 Provide for privacy.
7 Lock the bed wheels.
8 Raise the bed for body mechanics. Bed rails are up if used.

### PROCEDURE

9 Make sure the bed is flat.
10 Stand on the side opposite to which you will turn the person. Your co-worker stands on the other side.
11 Lower the bed rails if used.
12 Move the person as a unit to the side of the bed near you. Use the turn sheet.
13 Place the person's arms across the chest. Place a pillow between the knees.
14 Raise the bed rail if used.
15 Go to the other side.
16 Stand near the shoulders and chest. Your co-worker stands near the buttocks and thighs.
17 Stand with a broad base of support. One foot is in front of the other.
18 Ask the person to hold his or her body rigid.
19 Roll the person toward you (Fig. 13-17, *A*). Or use a turn sheet (Fig. 13-17, *B*). Turn the person as a unit.

### POST-PROCEDURE

20 Provide for comfort. Position the person in good alignment. Use pillows as directed by the nurse and care plan. The following is common (unless the person has spinal cord involvement):
   a One pillow against the back for support
   b One pillow under the head and neck if allowed
   c One pillow or folded bath blanket between the legs
   d A small pillow under the arm and hand
21 Place the signal light within reach.
22 Raise or lower bed rails. Follow the care plan.
23 Lower the bed to its lowest position.
24 Unscreen the person.
25 Decontaminate your hands.
26 Report and record your observations.

# SITTING ON THE SIDE OF THE BED (DANGLING)

Persons sit on the side of the bed *(dangle)* for many reasons. Some increase activity in stages—bed rest, to sitting on the side of the bed, and then to sitting in a chair. Walking is the next step. Surgical patients sit on the side of the bed some time after surgery.

While dangling the legs, the person coughs and deep breathes. He or she moves the legs back and forth and in circles. This stimulates circulation.

Two staff members may be needed. Persons with balance and coordination problems need support. If dizziness or fainting occurs, lay the person down.

See *Focus on Older Persons: Sitting on the Side of the Bed (Dangling).*

---

**FOCUS ON OLDER PERSONS**

**SITTING ON THE SIDE OF THE BED (DANGLING)**

Many older persons have circulatory changes. They may become dizzy or faint when getting up too fast. They may need to sit on the side of the bed for a few minutes before a transfer or walking.

---

**DELEGATION GUIDELINES:** *Dangling*

The nurse may ask you to help a person sit on the side of the bed. The procedure is part of other tasks—assisting the person to stand, transferring from bed to chair, partial bath, and others. When delegated the dangling procedure or tasks that involve dangling, you need this information from the nurse and the care plan:

- Areas of weakness. For example, if the person's arms are weak, he or she cannot hold onto the side of the mattress for support. If the left side is weak, you need to turn the person onto the stronger right side. The person can use the right arm to help move from the lying to sitting position.
- The amount of help the person needs.
- If you need a co-worker to help you.
- How long the person needs to sit on the side of the bed.
- What exercises the person needs to perform while dangling:
  —Leg and foot exercises (Chapter 22)
  —Coughing and deep breathing (Chapter 30)
- If the person will walk or transfer to a chair after dangling.
- What observations to report and record (Fig. 13-18).

---

**SAFETY ALERT:** *Dangling*

Problems with sitting and balance often occur after illness, injury, surgery, and bedrest. Some persons who are disabled also have problems sitting and with balance. Provide support when the person is sitting on the side of the bed. This protects the person from falling and other injuries.

---

| Date | Time | |
|------|------|---|
| 9/9 | 0900 | Assisted to sit on the side of the bed with assistance of one. |
| | | Active leg exercises performed. Tolerated procedure without |
| | | complaints of pain or discomfort. No c/o dizziness. BP 130/78 (L) |
| | | arm sitting, P=74 regular rate and rhythm, R=20 unlabored. Color |
| | | good. Assisted to lie down after 5 minutes. Positioned on (L) side. |
| | | Bed in low position, signal light within reach. Adam Aims, CNA ———— |

FIG. 13-18 Charting sample.

# HELPING THE PERSON SIT ON THE SIDE OF THE BED (DANGLE)

## QUALITY OF LIFE

Remember to:
- Knock before entering the person's room
- Address the person by name
- Introduce yourself by name and title

## PRE-PROCEDURE

1 Follow *Delegation Guidelines: Dangling.* See *Safety Alert: Dangling.*
2 Explain the procedure to the person.
3 Practice hand hygiene.
4 Identify the person. Check the ID bracelet against the assignment sheet. Call the person by name.
5 Decide what side of the bed to use.
6 Move furniture to provide moving space.
7 Provide for privacy.
8 Position the person in a side-lying position facing you. The person lies on the strong side.
9 Lock the bed wheels.
10 Raise the bed for body mechanics. Bed rails are up if used.

## PROCEDURE

11 Raise the head of the bed to a sitting position.
12 Lower the bed rail if up.
13 Stand by the person's hips. Face the foot of the bed.
14 Stand with your feet apart. The foot near the head of the bed is in front of the other foot.
15 Slide one arm under the person's neck and shoulders. Grasp the far shoulder. Place your other hand over the thighs near the knees (Fig. 13-19, *A*).
16 Pivot toward the foot of the bed while moving the person's legs and feet over the side of the bed. As the legs go over the edge of the mattress, the trunk is upright (Fig. 13-19, *B*).
17 Ask the person to hold onto the edge of the mattress. This supports the person in the sitting position.
18 Do not leave the person alone. Provide support if necessary.
19 Check the person's condition:
   a Ask how the person feels. Ask if the person feels dizzy or lightheaded.
   b Check pulse and respirations.
   c Check for difficulty breathing.
   d Note if the skin is pale or bluish in color (*cyanosis*).
20 Help the person lie down if necessary.
21 Reverse the procedure to return the person to bed.
22 Lower the head of the bed after the person returns to bed. Help him or her move to the center of the bed.

## POST-PROCEDURE

23 Provide for comfort. Position the person in good alignment.
24 Place the signal light within reach.
25 Lower the bed to its lowest position.
26 Raise or lower bed rails. Follow the care plan.
27 Return furniture to its proper places.
28 Unscreen the person.
29 Decontaminate your hands.
30 Report and record your observations.

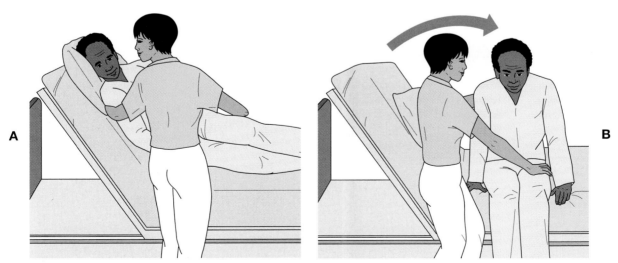

**FIG. 13-19** Helping the person sit on the side of the bed. **A,** The person's shoulders and thighs are supported. **B,** The person sits upright as the legs and feet are pulled over the edge of the bed.

# TRANSFERRING PERSONS

To *transfer* a person means moving the person from one place to another. Persons are often moved from beds to chairs, wheelchairs, shower chairs, commodes, toilets, or stretchers. Some transfer themselves or need little help. Some persons are transferred by one, two, or three people.

The rules of body mechanics apply to transfers. Arrange the room so there is enough space for a safe transfer. Correct chair, wheelchair, commode, shower chair, or stretcher placement is needed for a safe transfer.

---

**DELEGATION GUIDELINES:** *Transferring Persons*
When you are delegated transferring procedures, you need this information from the nurse and the care plan:
- What procedure to use:
  —Transferring the Person To a Chair or Wheelchair
  —Transferring the Person To a Wheelchair With Assistance
  —Transferring the Person From Wheelchair to Bed
  —Transferring the Person Using a Mechanical Lift
  —Transferring the Person To a Stretcher
  —Transferring the Person To and From the Toilet
- Areas of weakness. For example, if the person's arms are weak, the person cannot hold the side of the mattress for support. If the person has a weak left side, he or she gets out of bed on the stronger right side. The person can use the right arm to help move from the lying to sitting position.
- What equipment is needed—transfer belt, wheelchair, mechanical lift, stretcher, positioning devices, wheelchair cushion, and so on.
- The amount of help the person needs.
- How many co-workers need to help you.
- What observations to report and record:
  —Pulse rate before and after the transfer
  —Complaints of lightheadedness, pain, discomfort, difficulty breathing, weakness, or fatigue
  —The amount of help needed to transfer the person
  —How the person helped with the transfer

---

**SAFETY ALERT:** *Transferring Persons*
The person wears nonskid footwear for transfers. Such footwear protects the person from falls. Slipping and sliding are prevented. Remember to securely tie shoelaces. Otherwise the person can trip and fall.

The bed and stretcher wheels must be locked. And wheelchair and shower chair brakes must be on. Both measures prevent the bed, stretcher, wheelchair, or shower chair from moving during the transfer. Otherwise, the person can fall. You also are at risk for injury.

---

## APPLYING TRANSFER BELTS

A **transfer belt** is used to support persons who are unsteady or disabled. It helps prevent falls and other injuries. The belt goes around the person's waist. You grasp underneath the belt to support the person during the transfer. The belt is called a **gait belt** when used for walking with a person. Many agencies require staff to use these belts when transferring or walking a person.

---

**SAFETY ALERT:** *Transfer Belts*
Transfer belts are used routinely in nursing centers. If the person needs help, a transfer belt is required. To use one safely, always follow the manufacturer's instructions.

A transfer belt is always applied over clothing. It is never applied over bare skin. Also, it is applied under the breasts. Breasts must not be caught under the belt.

## APPLYING A TRANSFER BELT

### QUALITY OF LIFE

Remember to:
- Knock before entering the person's room
- Address the person by name
- Introduce yourself by name and title

### PROCEDURE

1 See *Safety Alert: Transfer Belts*.
2 Practice hand hygiene.
3 Identify the person. Check the ID bracelet against the assignment sheet. Call the person by name.
4 Explain the procedure to the person.
5 Provide for privacy.
6 Assist the person to a sitting position.
7 Apply the belt around the person's waist over clothing. Do not apply it over bare skin.

8 Tighten the belt so it is snug. It should not cause discomfort or impair breathing. You should be able to slide four fingers (your open, flat hand) under the belt.
9 Make sure that a woman's breasts are not caught under the belt.
10 Place the buckle off center in the front or in the back for the person's comfort (Fig. 13-20). The buckle is not over the spine.

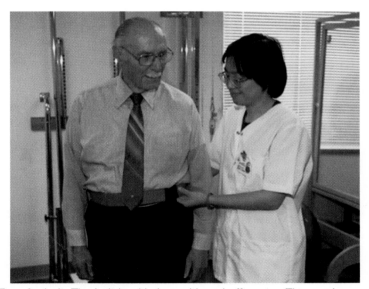

**FIG. 13-20** Transfer belt. The belt buckle is positioned off center. The nursing assistant grasps the belt from underneath.

# BED TO CHAIR OR WHEELCHAIR TRANSFERS

Safety is important for chair, wheelchair, commode, or shower chair transfers. The procedure used depends on the person's abilities, condition, and size. If the person cannot assist, a mechanical lift is used (p. 266).

Help the person out of bed on his or her strong side. If the left side is weak and the right side strong, get the person out of bed on the right side. In transferring, the strong side moves first. It pulls the weaker side along. Transfers from the weak side are awkward and unsafe.

Most wheelchairs and bedside chairs have vinyl seats and backs. Vinyl holds body heat. The person becomes warm and perspires more. You can cover the back and seat with a folded bath blanket. This increases the person's comfort in the chair. Some people have wheelchair cushions or positioning devices. They prevent pressure ulcers, maintain posture, or prevent sliding forward. Ask the nurse how to use and place the devices.

See *Focus on Long-Term Care: Bed to Chair or Wheelchair Transfers.*

---

**FOCUS ON LONG-TERM CARE**
**BED TO CHAIR OR WHEELCHAIR TRANSFERS**

Some residents cannot assist in transfers to or from chairs or wheelchairs. For those residents, a mechanical lift is used (p. 266).

---

**SAFETY ALERT:** *Chair or Wheelchair Transfers*
The chair or wheelchair must support the person's weight. The number of staff members needed for a transfer depends on the person's abilities, condition, and size.

During the procedure, the person must not put his or her arms around your neck. Otherwise the person can pull you forward or cause you to lose your balance. Neck, back, and other injuries from falls are possible.

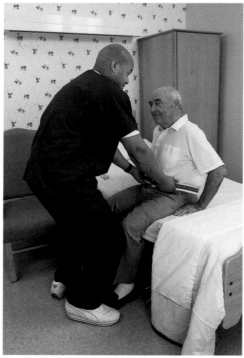

**FIG. 13-21** Transferring the person to a chair using a transfer belt. The person's feet and knees are blocked by the nursing assistant's feet and knees. This prevents the person from sliding or falling.

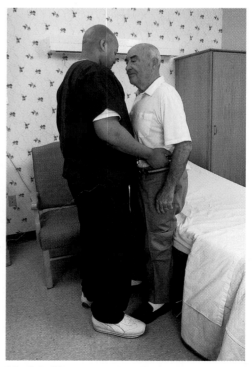

**FIG. 13-22** The person is pulled up to a standing position and supported by holding the transfer belt and blocking the person's knees and feet.

# TRANSFERRING THE PERSON TO A CHAIR OR WHEELCHAIR

NNAAP™

## QUALITY OF LIFE

Remember to:
- Knock before entering the person's room
- Address the person by name
- Introduce yourself by name and title

## PRE-PROCEDURE

1 Follow *Delegation Guidelines: Transferring Persons*, p. 256. See *Safety Alerts:*
  - *Transferring Persons*, p. 256
  - *Transfer Belts*, p. 256
  - *Chair or Wheelchair Transfers*
2 Explain the procedure to the person.
3 Collect:
  - Wheelchair or arm chair
  - Bath blanket
  - Lap blanket
  - Robe and nonskid footwear
  - Paper or sheet
  - Transfer belt if needed
  - Seat cushion if needed
4 Practice hand hygiene.
5 Identify the person. Check the ID bracelet against the assignment sheet. Call the person by name.
6 Provide for privacy.
7 Decide which side of the bed to use. Move furniture for moving space.

## PROCEDURE

8 Place the chair at the head of the bed. The chair is even with the headboard.
9 Place a folded bath blanket or cushion on the seat (if needed).
10 Lock wheelchair wheels. Raise the footplates. Remove or swing the front rigging out of the way.
11 Lower the bed to its lowest position. Lock the bed wheels.
12 Fanfold top linens to the foot of the bed.
13 Place the paper or sheet under the person's feet. Put footwear on the person.
14 Help the person sit on the side of the bed. His or her feet touch the floor.
15 Help the person put on a robe.

16 Apply the transfer belt if needed.
17 *Method 1: Using a transfer belt:*
  a Stand in front of the person.
  b Have the person hold onto the mattress.
  c Make sure the person's feet are flat on the floor.
  d Have the person lean forward.
  e Grasp the transfer belt at each side. Grasp the belt from underneath.
  f Brace your knees against the person's knees. Block his or her feet with your feet (Fig. 13-21). Or use the knee and foot of one leg to block the person's weak foot. Place your other foot slightly behind you for balance.
  g Ask the person to push down on the mattress and to stand on the count of "3." Pull the person into a standing position as you straighten your knees (Fig. 13-22).

*Continued.*

## TRANSFERRING THE PERSON TO A CHAIR OR WHEELCHAIR—CONT'D

NNAAP™

### PROCEDURE—CONT'D

**18** *Method 2: No transfer belt:*
  **a** Follow step 17, a-c.
  **b** Place your hands under the person's arms. Your hands are around the person's shoulder blades (Fig. 13-23).
  **c** Have the person lean forward.
  **d** Brace your knees against the person's knees. Block his or her feet with your feet. Or use the knee and foot of one leg to block the person's weak foot. Place your other foot slightly behind you for balance.
  **e** Ask the person to push down on the mattress and to stand on the count of "3." Pull the person up into a standing position as you straighten your knees.

**19** Support the person in the standing position. Hold the transfer belt, or keep your hands around the person's shoulder blades. Continue to block the person's feet and knees with your feet and knees. This helps prevent falling.

**20** Turn the person so he or she can grasp the far arm of the chair. The legs will touch the edge of the chair (Fig. 13-24).

**21** Continue to turn the person until the other arm-rest is grasped.

**22** Lower him or her into the chair as you bend your hips and knees. The person assists by leaning forward and bending the elbows and knees (Fig. 13-25).

**23** Make sure the buttocks are to the back of the seat. Position the person in good alignment.

**24** Attach the wheelchair front rigging. Position the person's feet on the wheelchair footplates.

**25** Cover the person's lap and legs with a lap blanket. Keep the blanket off the floor and the wheels.

**26** Remove the transfer belt if used.

**27** Position the chair as the person prefers. Lock the wheelchair wheels.

### POST-PROCEDURE

**28** Place the signal light and other needed items within reach.

**29** Unscreen the person.

**30** Decontaminate your hands.

**31** Report and record your observations.

**32** See procedure: *Transferring the Person from the Chair or Wheelchair to Bed*, p. 263, to return the person to bed.

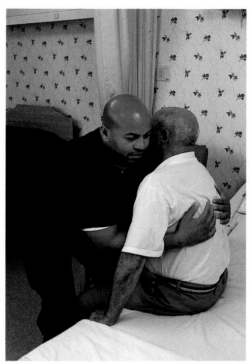

**FIG. 13-23** The person is being prepared to stand. The hands are placed under the person's arms and around the shoulder blades.

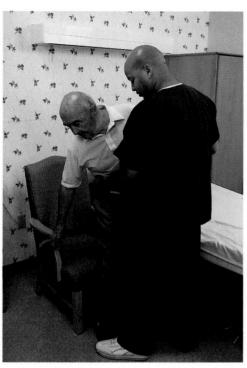

**FIG. 13-24** The person is supported as he grasps the far arm of the chair. The legs are against the chair.

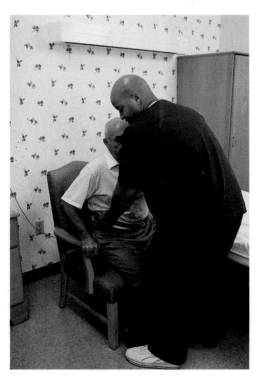

**FIG. 13-25** The person holds the arm rests, leans forward, and bends the elbows and knees while being lowered into the chair.

## CHAIR OR WHEELCHAIR TO BED TRANSFERS

Chair or wheelchair to bed transfers have the same rules as bed to chair transfers. If the person is weak on one side, transfer the person so that the strong side moves first. Therefore the person is transferred to bed on the opposite side from which the person transferred out of bed.

For example, Mrs. Lee's right side is weak. Her left side is strong. To transfer her from bed to chair, the chair was on the left side of the bed. This allowed her left side (strong side) to move first. Now you will transfer Mrs. Lee back to bed. If you leave the chair on the left side of the bed, her right side—the weak side—is near the bed. The weak side will move first. This is unsafe. Therefore you need to move the chair to the other side of the bed. Mrs. Lee's stronger left side will be near the bed. The stronger left side moves first for a safe transfer.

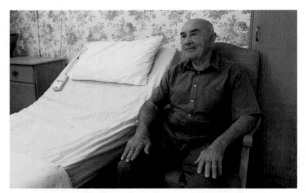

**FIG. 13-26** To transfer the person from chair to bed, the chair is positioned so the person's strong side is near the bed.

# TRANSFERRING THE PERSON FROM THE CHAIR OR WHEELCHAIR TO BED

## QUALITY OF LIFE

Remember to:
- Knock before entering the person's room
- Address the person by name
- Introduce yourself by name and title

## PRE-PROCEDURE

1 Follow *Delegation Guidelines: Transferring Persons*, p. 256. See *Safety Alerts:*
  - *Transferring Persons*, p. 256
  - *Transfer Belts*, p. 256
  - *Chair or Wheelchair Transfers*, p. 258
2 Explain the procedure to the person.
3 Collect paper or sheet and a transfer belt (if needed).
4 Practice hand hygiene.
5 Identify the person. Check the ID bracelet against the assignment sheet. Call the person by name.
6 Provide for privacy.

## PROCEDURE

7 Move furniture for moving space.
8 Raise the head of the bed to a sitting position. The bed is in the lowest position.
9 Move the signal light so it is on the strong side when the person is in bed.
10 Position the chair or wheelchair so the person's strong side is next to the bed (Fig. 13-26). Have a co-worker help you if necessary.
11 Lock the wheelchair and bed wheels.
12 Remove and fold the lap blanket.
13 Remove the person's feet from the footplates. Raise the footplates. Remove or swing the front rigging out of the way.
14 Apply the transfer belt (if needed).
15 Make sure the person's feet are flat on the floor.
16 Stand in front of the person.
17 Ask the person to hold onto the armrests. Or place your arms under the person's arms. Your hands are around the shoulder blades.
18 Have the person lean forward.
19 Grasp the transfer belt on each side if using it. Grasp underneath the belt.
20 Brace your knees against the person's knees. Block his or her feet with your feet. Or use the knee and foot of one leg to block the person's weak foot. Place your other foot slightly behind you for balance.
21 Ask the person to push down on the armrests on the count of "3." Pull the person into a standing position as you straighten your knees.
22 Support the person in the standing position. Hold the transfer belt, or keep your hands around the person's shoulder blades. Continue to block the person's knees and feet with your knees and feet.
23 Turn the person so he or she can reach the edge of the mattress. The legs will touch the mattress.
24 Continue to turn the person until he or she can reach the mattress with both hands.
25 Lower him or her onto the bed as you bend your hips and knees. The person assists by leaning forward and bending the elbows and knees.
26 Remove the transfer belt.
27 Remove the robe and footwear.
28 Help the person lie down.

## POST-PROCEDURE

29 Provide for comfort. Cover the person as needed.
30 Place the signal light and other needed items within reach.
31 Arrange furniture to meet the person's needs.
32 Unscreen the person.
33 Decontaminate your hands.
34 Report and record your observations.

# WHEELCHAIR TRANSFERS WITH ASSISTANCE

Some wheelchair transfers involve lifting the person from the bed to the chair. To return the person to bed, he or she is lifted from the chair to the bed. Such transfers are done when the person cannot stand or assist in the transfer.

The procedure has risks. Because the person is lifted, back injuries are major threats. Using a mechanical lift is preferred. However, sometimes the health team must do the lifting. Two people are needed for the procedure. Do not perform this procedure unless the nurse instructs you to do so. When deciding to use this procedure, the nurse considers:
- The person's height and weight
- The person's physical condition
- The amount of room for the transfer
- The skills and strength of staff members

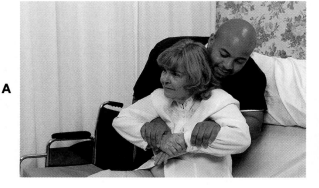

A

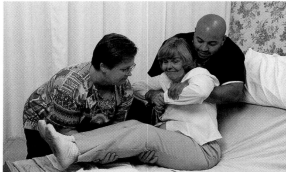

B

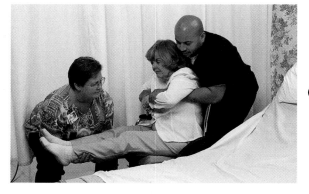

C

**FIG. 13-27** Transferring the person to a wheelchair. **A,** Grasp the person's forearms by putting your arms under the person's arms. **B,** Hold the thighs and calves to support the lower extremities during a transfer. **C,** Lower the person into the chair.

## TRANSFERRING THE PERSON TO A WHEELCHAIR WITH ASSISTANCE

### QUALITY OF LIFE

Remember to:
- Knock before entering the person's room
- Address the person by name
- Introduce yourself by name and title

### PRE-PROCEDURE

1 Follow *Delegation Guidelines: Transferring Persons,* p. 256. See *Safety Alerts:*
  - *Transferring Persons,* p. 256
  - *Chair or Wheelchair Transfers,* p. 258
  - *Wheelchair Transfers with Assistance*
2 Ask a co-worker to help you.
3 Explain the procedure to the person.
4 Collect:
  - Wheelchair with removable armrests
  - Bath blanket
  - Lap blanket
  - Nonskid footwear
  - Cushion if used
5 Practice hand hygiene.
6 Identify the person. Check the ID bracelet against the assignment sheet. Call the person by name.
7 Provide for privacy.
8 Decide which side of the bed to use. Move furniture for moving space.

### PROCEDURE

9 Fanfold top linens to the foot of the bed.
10 Assist the person to the side of the bed near you. Raise the head of the bed to help him or her to a sitting position.
11 Place the wheelchair at the side of the bed, even with the person's hips.
12 Remove the front rigging.
13 Remove the armrest near the bed.
14 Put the cushion or a folded bath blanket on the seat.
15 Lock wheelchair and bed wheels.
16 Stand behind the wheelchair. Put your arms under the person's arms and grasp the person's forearms (Fig. 13-27, *A*).
17 Have your co-worker grasp the person's thighs and calves (Fig. 13-27, *B*).
18 Bring the person toward the chair on the count of "3." Lower him or her into the chair (Fig. 13-27, *C*).
19 Make sure the person's buttocks are to the back of the seat. Position the person in good alignment.
20 Put the armrest and front rigging on the wheelchair.
21 Put footwear on the person. Position the person's feet on the footplates.
22 Cover the person's lap and legs with a lap blanket. Keep the blanket off the floor and wheels.
23 Position the chair as the person prefers. Lock the wheelchair wheels.

### POST-PROCEDURE

24 Place the signal light and other needed items within reach.
25 Unscreen the person.
26 Decontaminate your hands.
27 Report and record your observations.
28 Reverse the procedure to return the person to bed.

# USING MECHANICAL LIFTS

Persons who cannot help themselves are transferred with mechanical lifts. So are persons too heavy for the staff to transfer. Lifts are used for transfers to chairs, stretchers, tubs, shower chairs, toilets, commodes, whirlpools, or vehicles.

There are manual and electric lifts. Before using a lift:
- Make sure you are trained in its use.
- Make sure the lift works.
- Make sure the sling, straps, hooks, and chains are in good repair.
- Compare the person's weight and the lift's weight limit. Do not use the lift if a person's weight exceeds the lift's capacity.

At least two staff members are needed. The following procedure is used as a guide.

> **SAFETY ALERT:** *Mechanical Lifts*
> Mechanical lifts vary among manufacturers. Also, manufacturers have different models. Knowing how to use one lift does not mean that you know how to use others. Always follow the manufacturer's instructions.
>
> If you have questions, ask the nurse. If you have not used a certain lift before, ask the nurse to show you how to use it safely. Also ask the nurse to help you use it the first time and until you are comfortable using it.

**A**
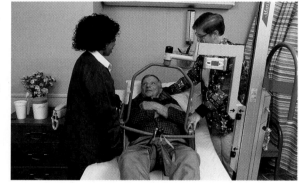

**B**
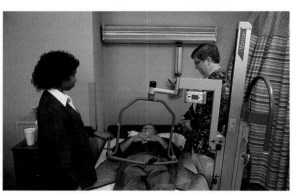

**C**
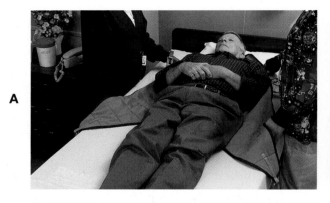

**D**
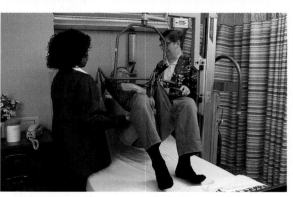

**E**
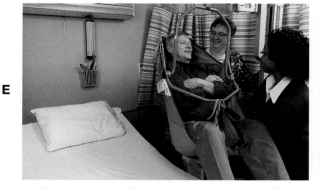

**F**
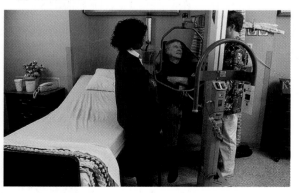

**FIG. 13-28** Using a mechanical lift. **A,** The sling is positioned under the person. The lower edge is behind the person's knees. **B,** The lift is over the person. **C,** The sling is attached to a swivel bar. **D,** The lift is raised until the sling and person are off of the bed. **E,** The person's legs are supported as the person and lift are moved away from the bed. **F,** The person is guided into a chair.

## TRANSFERRING THE PERSON USING A MECHANICAL LIFT

### QUALITY OF LIFE

Remember to:
- Knock before entering the person's room
- Address the person by name
- Introduce yourself by name and title

### PRE-PROCEDURE

1 Follow *Delegation Guidelines: Transferring Persons*, p. 256. See *Safety Alerts: Transferring Persons*, p. 256 and *Mechanical Lifts*.
2 Ask a co-worker to help you.
3 Explain the procedure to the person.
4 Collect:
- Mechanical lift
- Arm chair or wheelchair
- Footwear
- Bath blanket or cushion
- Lap blanket
5 Practice hand hygiene.
6 Identify the person. Check the ID bracelet against the assignment sheet. Call the person by name.
7 Provide for privacy.

### PROCEDURE

8 Center the sling under the person (Fig. 13-28, *A*). To position the sling, turn the person from side to side as if making an occupied bed (Chapter 15). Position the sling according to the manufacturer's instructions.
9 Place the chair at the head of the bed. It should be even with the headboard and about 1 foot away from the bed. Place a folded bath blanket or cushion in the chair.
10 Lock the bed wheels. Lower the bed to its lowest position.
11 Raise the lift so you can position it over the person.
12 Position the lift over the person (Fig. 13-28, *B*).
13 Lock the lift wheels in position.
14 Attach the sling to the swivel bar (Fig. 13-28, *C*).
15 Raise the head of the bed to a sitting position.
16 Cross the person's arms over the chest. He or she can hold onto the straps or chains but not the swivel bar.
17 Raise the lift high enough until the person and sling are free of the bed (Fig. 13-28, *D*).

18 Have your co-worker support the person's legs as you move the lift and person away from the bed (Fig. 13-28, *E*).
19 Position the lift so that the person's back is toward the chair.
20 Position the chair so you can lower the person into it.
21 Lower the person into the chair. Guide the person into the chair (Fig. 13-28, *F*).
22 Lower the swivel bar to unhook the sling. Leave the sling under the person unless otherwise indicated.
23 Put footwear on the person. Position the person's feet on wheelchair footplates.
24 Cover the person's lap and legs with a lap blanket. Keep it off the floor and wheels.
25 Position the chair as the person prefers. Lock the wheelchair wheels.

### POST-PROCEDURE

26 Place the signal light and other needed items within reach.
27 Unscreen the person.
28 Decontaminate your hands.
29 Report and record your observations.
30 Reverse the procedure to return the person to bed.

# ◼ TRANSFERRING THE PERSON TO AND FROM A TOILET

Using the bathroom for elimination promotes dignity, self-esteem, and independence. It also is more private than using a bedpan, urinal, or bedside commode. However, getting to the toilet is hard for persons who use wheelchairs. Bathrooms are often small. There is little room for you and a wheelchair. Therefore transfers involving wheelchairs and toilets are often hard. The risk of falls is great.

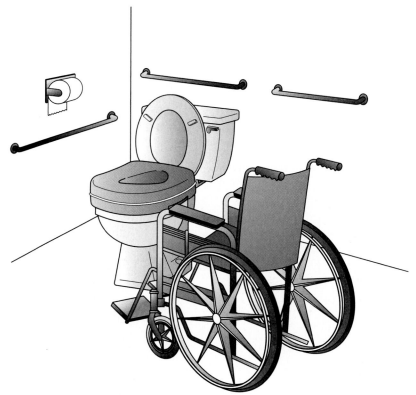

**FIG. 13-29** The wheelchair is placed at a right (90-degree) angle to the toilet.

## TRANSFERRING THE PERSON TO AND FROM THE TOILET

### QUALITY OF LIFE

Remember to:
- Knock before entering the person's room
- Address the person by name
- Introduce yourself by name and title

### PRE-PROCEDURE

1 Follow *Delegation Guidelines: Transferring Persons*, p. 256. See *Safety Alerts: Transfer Belts*, p. 256 and *Chair or Wheelchair Transfers*, p. 258.
2 Practice hand hygiene.
3 Make sure the person has an elevated toilet seat. The toilet seat and wheelchair are at the same level.

4 Check the grab bars by the toilet. If they are loose, tell the nurse. Do not transfer the person to the toilet if the grab bars are not secure.

### PROCEDURE

5 Have the person wear nonskid footwear.
6 Position the wheelchair next to the toilet if there is enough room. If not, position the wheelchair at a right (90-degree) angle to the toilet (Fig. 13-29). It is best if the person's strong side is near the toilet.
7 Lock the wheelchair wheels.
8 Raise the footplates. Remove or swing the front rigging out of the way.
9 Apply the transfer belt.
10 Help the person unfasten clothing.
11 Use the transfer belt to help the person stand and to turn to the toilet. (See procedure: *Transferring the Person to a Chair or Wheelchair*, p. 259.) The person uses the grab bars to turn to the toilet.
12 Support the person with the transfer belt while he or she lowers clothing. Or have the person hold onto the grab bars for support. Lower the person's pants and undergarments.
13 Use the transfer belt to lower the person onto the toilet seat.
14 Remove the transfer belt.
15 Tell the person you will stay nearby. Remind the person to use the signal light or call for you when help is needed.

16 Close the bathroom door to provide for privacy.
17 Stay near the bathroom. Complete other tasks in the person's room.
18 Knock on the bathroom door when the person calls for you.
19 Help with wiping, perineal care (Chapter 16), flushing, and hand washing as needed.
20 Apply the transfer belt.
21 Use the transfer belt to help the person stand.
22 Help the person raise and secure clothing.
23 Use the transfer belt to transfer the person to the wheelchair. (See procedure: *Transferring the Person to a Chair or Wheelchair*, p. 259.)
24 Make sure the person's buttocks are to the back of the seat. Position the person in good alignment.
25 Position the person's feet on the footplates.
26 Cover the person's lap and legs with a lap blanket. Keep the blanket off the floor and wheels.
27 Position the chair as the person prefers. Lock the wheelchair wheels.

### POST-PROCEDURE

28 Place the signal light and other needed items within reach.
29 Unscreen the person.

30 Practice hand hygiene.
31 Report and record your observations.

# ■ MOVING THE PERSON TO A STRETCHER

Stretchers are used to transport persons to other areas. They are used for persons who:

- Cannot sit up
- Must stay in a lying position
- Are seriously ill

The stretcher is covered with a folded flat sheet or bath blanket. A pillow and extra blankets are on hand. With the nurse's permission, raise the head of the stretcher to Fowler's or semi-Fowler's position (Chapter 14). This increases the person's comfort.

A drawsheet or lift sheet is used. At least three workers are needed for a safe transfer.

Safety straps are used when the person is on the stretcher. The stretcher's side rails are kept up during the transport. The stretcher is moved feet first. This is so the co-worker at the head of the stretcher can watch the person's breathing and color during the transport. Never leave a person on a stretcher alone.

> **SAFETY ALERT:** *Moving the Person to a Stretcher*
> Follow the rules for stretcher safety (Chapter 10). Make sure the bed and stretcher wheels are locked. Also practice good body mechanics to protect yourself from injury. Protect the person by making sure he or she is in good alignment. Also make sure you have enough help and that you hold the person securely. You must not drop the person onto the floor.

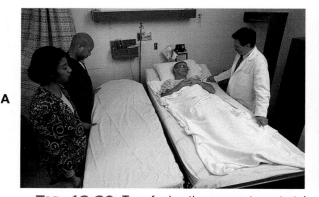
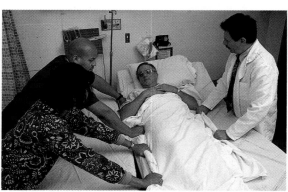

**A**    **B**

**FIG. 13-30** Transferring the person to a stretcher. **A,** The stretcher is against the bed and is held in place. **B,** A drawsheet is used to transfer the person from the bed to a stretcher.

## TRANSFERRING THE PERSON TO A STRETCHER

### QUALITY OF LIFE

Remember to:
- Knock before entering the person's room
- Address the person by name
- Introduce yourself by name and title

### PRE-PROCEDURE

1 Follow *Delegation Guidelines: Transferring Persons*, p. 256. See *Safety Alert: Stretcher Transfers*.
2 Ask two co-workers to help you.
3 Explain the procedure to the person.
4 Collect:
- Stretcher covered with a sheet or bath blanket
- Bath blanket
- Pillow(s) if needed

5 Practice hand hygiene.
6 Identify the person. Check the ID bracelet against the assignment sheet. Call the person by name.
7 Provide for privacy.
8 Raise the bed to its highest level.

### PROCEDURE

9 Position yourself and co-workers. Two workers stand on the side of the bed where the stretcher will be. The third worker stands on the other side of the bed.
10 Cover the person with a bath blanket. Fanfold top linens to the foot of the bed.
11 Loosen the cotton drawsheet on each side.
12 Lower the head of the bed. It is as flat as possible.
13 Lower the bed rails if used.
14 Move the person to the side of the bed. The drawsheet serves as your lift sheet.
15 Protect the person from falling. Hold the far arm and leg.
16 Have your co-workers position the stretcher next to the bed. They stand behind the stretcher (Fig. 13-30, *A*).

17 Lock the bed and stretcher wheels.
18 Roll up and grasp the drawsheet as shown in Figure 13-30, *B*. This supports the entire length of the person's body.
19 Transfer the person to the stretcher on the count of "3" by lifting and pulling him or her. The person is centered on the stretcher.
20 Place a pillow or pillows under the person's head and shoulders if allowed. Raise the head of the stretcher if allowed.
21 Cover the person. Provide for comfort.
22 Fasten safety straps. Raise the side rails.
23 Unlock the stretcher's wheels. Transport the person.

### POST-PROCEDURE

24 Decontaminate your hands.
25 Report and record:
- The time of the transport
- Where the person was transported to

- Who went with him or her
- How the transfer was tolerated

26 Reverse the procedure to return the person to bed.

# POSITIONING

The person must be properly positioned at all times. Regular position changes and good alignment promote comfort and well-being. Breathing is easier. Circulation is promoted. Proper positioning also helps prevent pressure ulcers and contractures.

You move and turn when in bed or a chair for your comfort. Many patients and residents do too. Some need reminding to adjust their positions. Others need help. Still others depend entirely on the nursing team for position changes.

Whether in bed or chair, the person is repositioned at least every 2 hours. Some people are repositioned more often. You must follow the nurse's instructions and the care plan.

The doctor may order certain positions or position limits. This is common after some surgeries and tests. Follow these guidelines to safely position a person:

- Use good body mechanics.
- Ask a co-worker to help you if needed.
- Explain the procedure to the person.
- Be gentle when moving the person.
- Provide for privacy.
- Place the signal light within reach after positioning.
- Use pillows as directed for support and alignment.

---

**DELEGATION GUIDELINES:** *Positioning*

You are often delegated tasks that involve positioning and repositioning. You need this information from the nurse and the care plan:

- Position or positioning limits ordered by the doctor
- How often to turn and reposition the person
- How many co-workers need to help you
- What skin care measures to perform (Chapter 16)
- What range-of-motion exercises to perform (Chapter 22)
- Where to place pillows
- What positioning devices are needed and how to use them
- What observations to report and record

---

**SAFETY ALERT:** *Positioning*

Pressure ulcers (Chapter 28) are serious threats from lying or sitting too long in one place. Wet, soiled, and wrinkled linens are other causes. Whenever you reposition a person, make sure linens are clean, dry, and wrinkle-free. Change or straighten linens as needed.

Contractures can develop from staying in one position too long (Chapter 22). A contracture is the lack of joint mobility caused by abnormal shortening of a muscle. Repositioning, exercise, and activity help prevent contractures.

---

## FOWLER'S POSITION

**Fowler's position** is a semi-sitting position. The head of the bed is raised between 45 and 90 degrees (Fig. 13-31). For good alignment:

- Keep the spine straight.
- Support the head with a small pillow.
- Support the arms with pillows.

The nurse may ask you to place a small pillow under the lower back, thighs, and ankles. Persons with heart and respiratory disorders usually breathe easier in Fowler's position.

## SUPINE POSITION

The **supine (dorsal recumbent) position** is the back-lying position (Fig. 13-32). For good alignment:

- The bed is flat.
- The head and shoulders are supported on a pillow.
- Arms and hands are at the sides. You can support the arms with regular pillows. Or you can support the hands on small pillows with the palms down.

The nurse may ask you to place a folded or rolled towel under the lower back and a small pillow under the thighs. A pillow under the lower legs lifts the heels off of the bed. This prevents them from rubbing on the sheets.

## PRONE POSITION

A person in the **prone position** lies on the abdomen with the head turned to one side. Small pillows are placed under the head, abdomen, and lower legs (Fig. 13-33). Arms are flexed at the elbows with the hands near the head.

You also can position a person with the feet hanging over the end of the mattress (Fig. 13-34). If that is done, a pillow is not needed under the feet.

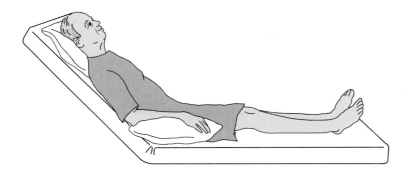

**FIG. 13-31** Fowler's position.

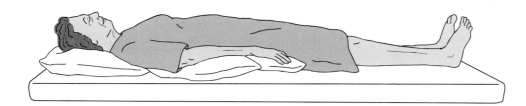

**FIG. 13-32** Supine position.

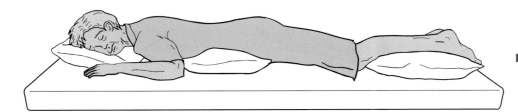

**FIG. 13-33** Prone position.

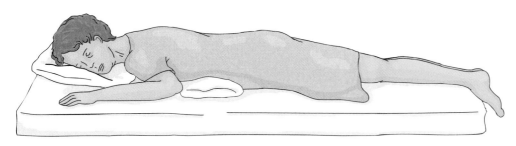

**FIG. 13-34** Prone position with the feet hanging over the edge of the mattress.

## LATERAL POSITION

A person in the **lateral (side-lying) position** lies on one side or the other (Fig. 13-35):

- A pillow is under the head and neck.
- The upper leg is in front of the lower leg. (The nurse may ask you to position the upper leg behind the lower leg, not on top of it.)
- The upper leg and thigh are supported with pillows.
- A small pillow is positioned against the person's back. The person rolls back against the pillow so that his or her back is at a 45-degree angle with the mattress.
- A small pillow is under the upper hand and arm.

## SIMS' POSITION

The **Sims' position** is a left side-lying position. The upper leg is sharply flexed so it is not on the lower leg. The lower arm is behind the person (Fig. 13-36). For good alignment:

- Place a pillow under the person's head and shoulder.
- Support the upper leg with a pillow.
- Place a pillow under the upper arm and hand.
   *See Focus on Older Persons: Positioning.*

### FOCUS ON OLDER PERSONS
#### POSITIONING

Most older persons cannot tolerate the prone position. They have limited range of motion in their necks. The Sims' position usually is not comfortable for them. Check with the nurse before positioning any older person in the prone or Sims' position.

## CHAIR POSITION

Persons who sit in chairs must hold their upper bodies and heads erect. If not, poor alignment results. For good alignment:

- The person's back and buttocks are against the back of the chair.
- Feet are flat on the floor or wheelchair footplates. Never leave the feet unsupported.
- Backs of the knees and calves are slightly away from the edge of the seat (Fig. 13-37).

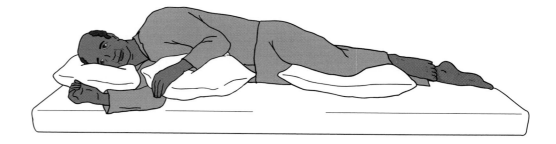

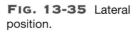

**FIG. 13-35** Lateral position.

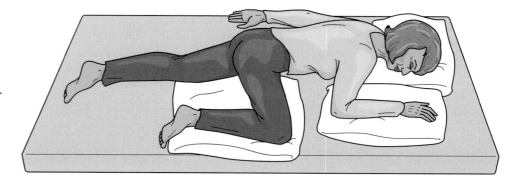

**FIG. 13-36** Sims' position.

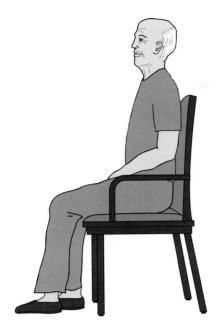

FIG. 13-37 The person is positioned in a chair. The person's feet are flat on the floor, the calves do not touch the chair, and the back is straight and against the back of the chair.

The nurse may ask you to put a small pillow between the person's lower back and the chair. This supports the lower back. *Remember, a pillow is not used behind the back if restraints are used (Chapter 11).*

Paralyzed arms are supported on pillows. Some residents have positioners (Fig. 13-38). Ask the nurse about their proper use. Wrists are positioned at a slight upward angle.

Some people require postural supports if they cannot keep their upper bodies erect (Fig. 13-39). Postural supports help keep them in good alignment. The health team selects the best product for the person's needs. The person's safety, dignity, and function are considered.

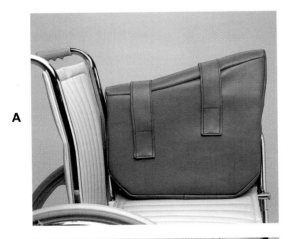

A

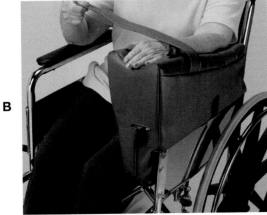

B

FIG. 13-38 Elevated armrest. (Courtesy J. T. Posey Co., Arcadia, Calif.)

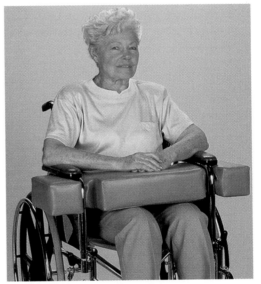

A

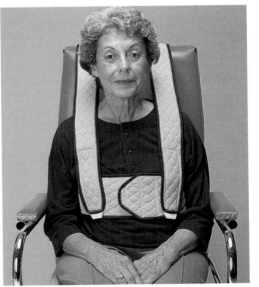

B

FIG. 13-39 Postural supports. **A,** Pelvic holder. **B,** Torso support. (Courtesy J. T. Posey Co., Arcadia, Calif.)

**REPOSITIONING IN A CHAIR OR WHEELCHAIR.**
The person can slide down into the chair. For good alignment and safety, the person's back and buttocks must be against the back of the chair.

Some persons can help with repositioning. Others need help. Use this method if the person is alert, cooperative, can follow instructions, and has the strength to help:

- Lock the wheelchair wheels.
- Stand in front of the person. Block his or her knees and feet with your knees and feet.
- Apply a transfer belt.
- Position the person's feet flat on the floor.
- Position the person's arms on the armrests.
- Grasp the transfer belt on each side while the person leans forward.
- Ask the person to push with his or her feet and arms on the count of "3."
- Lift the person back into the chair on the count of "3" as the person pushes with his or her feet and arms (Fig. 13-40).

This method is used if the person cannot assist with repositioning. Two staff members are needed (Fig. 13-41):

- Ask a co-worker to help you. Decide who is the tallest. The tallest worker stands behind the wheelchair. The other stands in front of the person.
- Lock the wheelchair wheels.
- Apply a transfer belt.
- Ask the person to place folded hands in his or her lap.
- The worker behind the wheelchair grasps the transfer belt on each side.
- The other worker stands in front of the person. The hands and arms are placed under the person's knees.
- On the count of "3," lift the person to the back of the chair. Support the legs (worker in front) and use the transfer belt (worker in back).

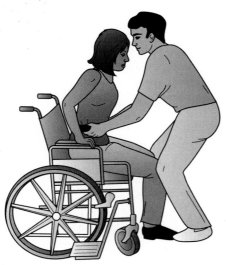

**FIG. 13-40** Repositioning the person in a wheelchair. A transfer belt is used to lift the person to the back of the chair.

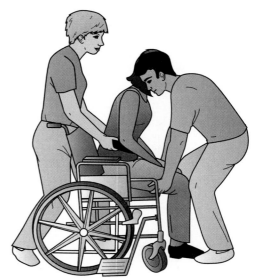

**FIG. 13-41** Two workers reposition a person in a wheelchair. The tallest worker stands behind the chair and lifts with the transfer belt. The other worker stands in front of the person. Hands and arms are under the knees to support the legs during repositioning.

# ■ REVIEW QUESTIONS ■

Circle the **BEST** answer.

1 Good body mechanics involves the following *except*
   a Good posture
   b Balance
   c Using the strongest and largest muscles
   d Having the job fit the worker

2 Good body alignment means
   a The area on which an object rests
   b Having the head, trunk, arms, and legs aligned with one another
   c Using muscles, tendons, ligaments, joints, and cartilage correctly
   d The back-lying or supine position

3 These actions are about body mechanics. Which is *incorrect*?
   a Hold objects away from your body when lifting, moving, or carrying them.
   b Face the direction you are working to prevent twisting.
   c Push, pull, or slide heavy objects.
   d Use both hands and arms to lift, move, or carry heavy objects.

4 Nursing assistants are at great risk for
   a Friction and shearing
   b Arm and hand injuries
   c Back injuries
   d Falls

5 Which helps prevent work-related injuries?
   a Using a mechanical lift at all times
   b Avoiding work that involves lifting, moving, or carrying people or items
   c Having a co-worker help you with lifting, moving, turning, or transfer activities
   d Using a transfer belt at all times

6 A person's skin rubs against the sheet. This is called
   a Shearing
   b Friction
   c Ergonomics
   d Posture

7 Which occurs when a person slides down in bed?
   a Shearing
   b Friction
   c Ergonomics
   d Posture

8 Which protects the skin when moving the person in bed?
   a Rolling or lifting the person
   b Sliding the person up in bed
   c Moving the mattress
   d Using ergonomics

9 Whenever you lift, move, turn, transfer, or reposition a person, you must
   a Allow personal choice
   b Protect the person's privacy
   c Use pillows for support
   d Get help from a co-worker

10 You are delegated tasks that involve lifting and moving persons in bed. Which is *true*?
   a The nurse tells you how to position the person.
   b You decide which procedure to use.
   c Bed rails are used at all times.
   d Three workers are needed to complete the task safely.

11 A lift sheet is placed so that it
   a Covers the person's body
   b Is under the person from the head to above the knees
   c Extends from the mid-back to mid-thigh level
   d Covers the entire mattress

12 Before turning a person onto his or her side, you
   a Move the person to the side of the bed
   b Move the person to the middle of the bed
   c Lock arms with the person
   d Position pillows for comfort

13 The logrolling procedure
   a Is used after spinal cord injuries or surgery
   b Requires a transfer belt
   c Requires a mechanical lift
   d Involves a stretcher and a lift sheet

**14** When getting ready to dangle a person, you need to know
   a Which side is stronger
   b If bed rails are used
   c If a mechanical lift is needed
   d If a transfer belt is needed

**15** For chair and wheelchair transfers, the person must
   a Wear nonskid footwear
   b Have the bed rails up
   c Use a mechanical lift
   d Have a lift sheet

**16** Before transferring a person to or from a bed, you must
   a Have the person wear nonskid footwear
   b Lock the bed wheels
   c Apply a transfer belt
   d Position pillows for support

**17** A transfer belt is applied
   a To the skin
   b Over clothing
   c Over breasts
   d Under the robe

**18** When transferring a person to bed, a chair, or the toilet
   a The person's strong side moves first
   b The weak side moves first
   c Pillows are used for support
   d The transfer belt is removed

**19** You are going to use a mechanical lift. You must do the following *except*
   a Follow the manufacturer's instructions
   b Make sure the lift works
   c Compare the person's weight to the lift's weight limit
   d Use a transfer belt

**20** To safely transfer a person with a mechanical lift, at least
   a One worker is needed
   b Two workers are needed
   c Three workers are needed
   d Four workers are needed

**21** These statements are about transfers to and from a toilet. Which is *false?*
   a The person wears nonskid footwear.
   b Wheelchair wheels must be locked.
   c The person uses the towel bars for support.
   d A transfer belt is used.

**22** These statements are about transfers to and from a stretcher. Which is *false?*
   a The bed and stretcher wheels must be locked.
   b The stretcher's side rails are raised when the person is on the stretcher.
   c Once on the stretcher, the person can be left alone.
   d At least three workers are needed for a safe transfer.

**23** Patients and residents are repositioned at least every
   a 30 minutes
   b 1 hour
   c 2 hours
   d 3 hours

**24** The back-lying position is called
   a Fowler's position
   b The supine position
   c The prone position
   d Sims' position

**25** A person is positioned in a chair. The feet
   a Must be flat on the floor
   b Are positioned on footplates
   c Dangle
   d Are positioned on pillows

*Answers to these questions are on p. 817.*

# The Person's Unit

## OBJECTIVES

- Define the key terms listed in this chapter
- Identify comfortable temperature ranges and those required by OBRA
- Describe how to protect the person from drafts
- List ways to prevent or reduce odors and noise
- Explain how lighting affects comfort
- Describe the basic bed positions
- Describe how to use furniture and equipment in the person's unit
- Describe how a bathroom is equipped
- Explain how to maintain the person's unit
- Describe the OBRA requirements for resident rooms

## KEY TERMS

**Fowler's position** A semi-sitting position; the head of the bed is raised between 45 and 90 degrees

**full visual privacy** Having the means to be completely free from public view while in bed

**reverse Trendelenburg's position** The head of the bed is raised, and the foot of the bed is lowered

**semi-Fowler's position** The head of the bed is raised 30 degrees; or the head of the bed is raised 30 degrees, and the knee portion is raised 15 degrees

**Trendelenburg's position** The head of the bed is lowered, and the foot of the bed is raised

Patients and residents spend a lot of time in their rooms (Fig. 14-1). Private rooms are for one person. Semi-private rooms are for two people. Some rooms are for four people. Rooms are designed to provide comfort, safety, and privacy.

temperatures for comfort. Therefore hospitals usually have higher room temperatures. *See Focus on Long-Term Care: Temperature and Ventilation,* p. 281.

Stale room air and lingering odors affect comfort and rest. Ventilation systems provide fresh air and

## COMFORT

Age, illness, and activity affect comfort. So do temperature, ventilation, noise, odors, and lighting. These factors are controlled to meet the person's needs.

### TEMPERATURE AND VENTILATION

Heating and air conditioning systems maintain a comfortable temperature. Most healthy people are comfortable when the temperature is 68° F to 74° F. This range may be too hot or too cold for others. Infants, older persons, and those who are ill may need higher

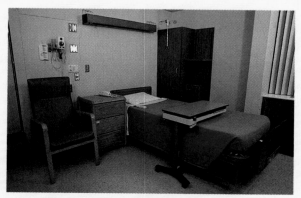

**FIG. 14-1** Furniture and equipment in a typical unit.

move room air. Drafts occur as air moves. Infants, older persons, and those who are ill are sensitive to drafts. To protect them from drafts:

- Make sure they wear the correct clothing.
- Cover them with blankets. Some people like extra blankets.
- Offer lap blankets to those in chairs or wheelchairs. Lap blankets cover the legs.
- Move them from drafty areas.

*See Focus on Older Persons: Temperature and Ventilation.*

## ODORS

Many odors occur in health care agencies. Food aromas and flower scents are pleasant. Bowel movements and urine have embarrassing odors. So do draining wounds and vomitus. Body, breath, and smoking odors may offend others.

Some people are very sensitive to odors. They may become nauseated. Good nursing care, ventilation, and housekeeping practices help prevent odors. To reduce odors:

- Empty and clean bedpans, urinals, commodes, and kidney (emesis) basins promptly.
- Change soiled linens and clothing promptly.
- Follow agency policy for soiled linens and clothing.
- Check incontinent persons often (Chapters 18 and 19).
- Clean persons who are wet or soiled from urine, feces, vomitus, or wound drainage.
- Dispose of incontinence and ostomy products promptly (Chapters 18 and 19).
- Keep laundry containers closed.
- Provide good hygiene to prevent body and breath odors (Chapter 16).

- Use room deodorizers as needed. Sometimes odors remain after removing the cause. Do not use sprays around persons with breathing problems. Ask the nurse if you are unsure.

Be aware of smoke odors. If you smoke, follow the agency's policy. Practice hand hygiene after handling smoking materials and before giving care. Give careful attention to your uniforms, hair, and breath because of clinging smoke odors.

## NOISE

Ill people are sensitive to noises and sounds. Common health care sounds may disturb them. The clanging of bedpans, urinals, and wash basins is annoying. So is the clatter of dishes and trays. Loud TVs, radios, phones, and intercoms are irritating. So is noise from equipment needing repair or oil. Wheels on stretchers, wheelchairs, carts, and other items must be oiled properly.

Loud talking and laughter in hallways and at the nurses' station are common. Patients and residents may think that the staff are talking and laughing about them.

People want to know the cause and meaning of new sounds. This relates to safety and security needs. Patients and residents may find sounds dangerous, frightening, or irritating. They may become upset, anxious, and uncomfortable. What is noise to one person may not be noise to another. For example, a teenager plays loud music. It may bother adults.

Health care agencies are designed to reduce noise. Drapes, carpeting, and acoustical tiles absorb noise. Plastic items make less noise than metal equipment (bedpans, urinals, and wash basins). To decrease noise:

- Control your voice.
- Handle equipment carefully.
- Keep equipment working properly.
- Answer phones, signal lights, and intercoms promptly.

## LIGHTING

Good lighting is needed for safety and comfort. Glares, shadows, and dull lighting can cause falls, headaches, and eyestrain. A bright room is cheerful. Dim light is better for relaxing and rest.

Adjust lighting to meet the person's changing needs. Shades and drapes are adjusted as needed. The overbed light can provide soft, medium, and bright lighting. Some agencies have ceiling lights. They provide soft to very bright light.

Persons with poor vision need bright light. This is very important at mealtimes and when moving about. Bright lighting also helps the staff perform procedures.

Keep light controls within the person's reach. This protects the right to personal choice.

# ROOM FURNITURE AND EQUIPMENT

Rooms are furnished and equipped to meet basic needs. There are furniture and equipment for comfort, sleep, elimination, nutrition, hygiene, and activity. There is equipment to communicate with staff, family, and friends. The right to privacy is also considered.

*See Focus on Long-Term Care: Room Furniture and Equipment.*

## THE BED

Beds have electrical or manual controls. Beds are raised horizontally to give care. This reduces bending and reaching. The lowest horizontal position lets the person get out of bed with ease (Fig. 14-2). The head of the bed is flat or raised varying degrees.

Electric beds are common. Controls are on a side panel, bed rail, or the footboard (Fig. 14-3). Patients and residents are taught how to use the controls safely. They are warned not to raise the bed to the high position and not to adjust the bed to harmful positions. They are told of any position limits or restrictions.

Most electric beds "lock" into any position by the staff. The person cannot adjust the bed to unsafe positions. Persons restricted to certain positions may need their beds locked. The locking feature is useful for persons with confusion or dementia.

Manual beds have cranks at the foot of the bed (Fig. 14-4):
- Left crank—raises or lowers the head of the bed
- Right crank—adjusts the knee portion
- Center crank—raises or lowers the entire bed horizontally

The cranks are pulled up for use. They are kept down at all other times. Cranks in the "up" position are safety hazards. Anyone walking past may bump into them.

*See Focus on Home Care: The Bed.*

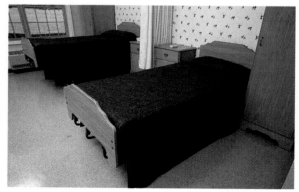

**FIG. 14-2** One bed is in the highest horizontal position. The other bed is in the lowest horizontal position.

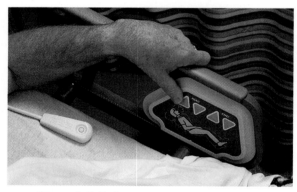

**FIG. 14-3** Controls for an electric bed.

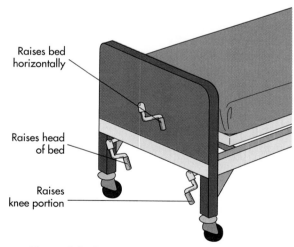

Raises bed horizontally

Raises head of bed

Raises knee portion

**FIG. 14-4** Manually operated hospital bed.

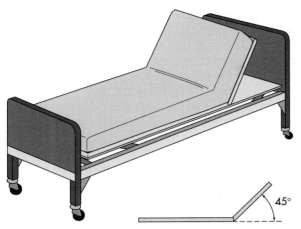

**FIG. 14-5** Fowler's position.

**BED POSITIONS.** There are five basic bed positions:

- *Flat*—This is the usual sleeping position. The position is used after spinal cord injury or surgery and for cervical traction.
- *Fowler's position*—**Fowler's position** is a semi-sitting position. The head of the bed is raised 45 to 90 degrees (Fig. 14-5). See Chapter 13.
- *Semi-Fowler's position*—In **semi-Fowler's position,** the head of the bed is raised 30 degrees (Fig. 14-6). Some agencies define semi-Fowler's position as when the head of the bed is raised 30 degrees and the knee portion is raised 15 degrees. To give safe care, know the definition your agency uses.
- *Trendelenburg's position*—In **Trendelenburg's position,** the head of the bed is lowered and the foot of the bed is raised (Fig. 14-7). A doctor orders the position. Blocks are placed under the legs at the foot of the bed. Or the bed frame is tilted.
- *Reverse Trendelenburg's position*—In **reverse Trendelenburg's position,** the head of the bed is raised and the foot of the bed is lowered (Fig. 14-8). Blocks are placed under the legs at the head of the bed. Or the bed frame is tilted. This position requires a doctor's order.

*See Focus on Home Care: Bed Positions, p. 284.*

> **SAFETY ALERT:** *The Bed*
> Beds have bed rails and wheels. See Chapter 10. Bed wheels are locked at all times except when moving the bed. They must be locked when you:
> - Give bedside care
> - Transfer a person to and from the bed. The person can be injured if the bed moves.
>
> Use bed rails as the nurse and care plan direct. Otherwise the person could suffer injury or other harm.

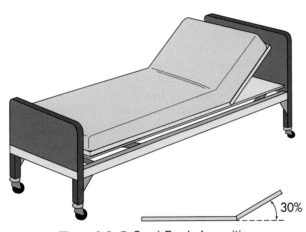

**FIG. 14-6** Semi-Fowler's position.

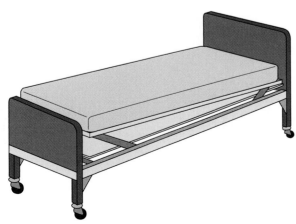

**FIG. 14-7** Trendelenburg's position.

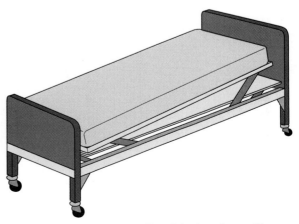

**FIG. 14-8** Reverse Trendelenburg's position.

## THE OVERBED TABLE

The overbed table (see Fig. 14-1) is placed over the bed by sliding the base under the bed. It is raised or lowered for the person in bed or in a chair. Turn the handle or lever to adjust the table. It is used for meals, writing, reading, and other activities.

Many overbed tables have a storage area under the top. The storage area often is used for beauty, hair care, shaving, or other personal items. Many also have a flip-up mirror.

The nursing team uses the overbed table as a work area. Only clean and sterile items are placed on the table. Never place bedpans, urinals, or soiled linen on the overbed table. Clean the table after using it for a work surface.

## THE BEDSIDE STAND

The bedside stand is next to the bed. It is used to store personal items and personal care equipment. It has a top and a lower cabinet with a shelf (Fig. 14-10). The top drawer is used for money, eyeglasses, books, and other items.

The top shelf is used for the wash basin, which can hold personal care items. These include soap and soap dish, powder, lotion, deodorant, towels, washcloth, bath blanket, and a clean gown or pajamas. An emesis or kidney basin (shaped like a kidney) can hold oral hygiene items. The kidney basin is stored on the top shelf or in the top drawer. The bedpan and its cover, the urinal, and toilet paper are on the lower shelf.

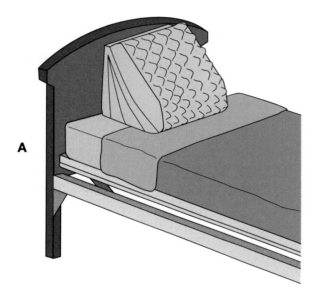

**A**

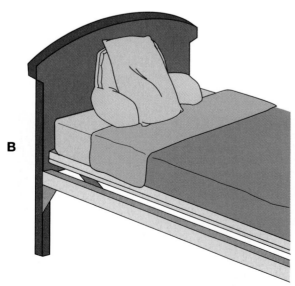

**B**

**FIG. 14-9** Backrests for regular beds. **A,** Wedge pillow. **B,** Study pillow with armrests.

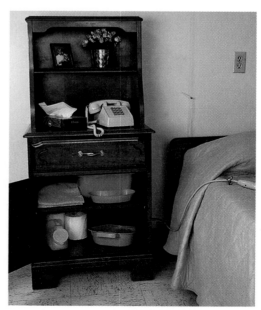

**FIG. 14-10** The bedside stand.

The top of the stand is often used for tissues and the phone. The person may put a radio, flowers, gifts, cards, and other items there. Some stands have a side or back rod for towels and washcloths.

## CHAIRS

The person's unit has at least one chair. It is usually upholstered with armrests. It must be comfortable and sturdy. It must not move or tip during transfers. The person should be able to get in and out of it with ease. It should not be too low or too soft. Nursing center residents may bring chairs from home (Fig. 14-11).

## PRIVACY CURTAINS

Rooms have privacy curtains. The curtain is pulled around the bed to provide privacy for the person (Chapter 2). *Always* pull it completely around the bed when giving care. Privacy curtains prevent others from seeing the person. They do not block sound or conversations. *See Focus on Long-Term Care: Privacy Curtains. See Focus on Home Care: Privacy Curtains.*

## PERSONAL CARE ITEMS

Personal care items are used for hygiene and elimination. A bedpan and urinal are provided. Also, the agency provides a *patient pack.* It has a wash basin, kidney basin, water pitcher and glass, and soap and soap dish (Fig. 14-13). Some provide powder, lotion, toothbrush, toothpaste, mouthwash, tissues, and a comb.

Some persons bring items from home. Oral hygiene equipment, hair care supplies, and deodorant are examples. Some prefer their own soap, lotion, and powder. You must respect the person's choice of personal care products.

### FOCUS ON LONG-TERM CARE
**PRIVACY CURTAINS**

According to OBRA, residents have the right to full visual privacy. **Full visual privacy** is having the means to be completely free from public view while in bed. The privacy curtain is a means to full visual privacy.

### FOCUS ON HOME CARE
**PRIVACY CURTAINS**

Portable screens help provide privacy in the home setting (Fig. 14-12).

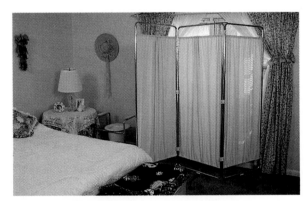

FIG. 14-12 Portable screen provides privacy in the home.

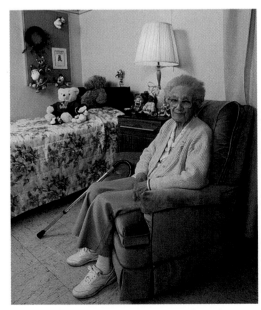

FIG. 14-11 Resident's chair from home.

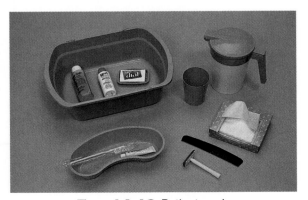

FIG. 14-13 Patient pack.

## THE CALL SYSTEM

The call system lets the person signal for help. The signal light is at the end of a long cord (Fig. 14-14). It attaches to the bed or chair. Always keep the signal light within the person's reach—in the room, bathroom, and shower or tub room.

To get help, the person presses a button at the end of the signal light. The signal light connects to a light above the room door. The signal light also connects to a light panel or intercom system at the nurses' station (Fig. 14-15). These tell the nursing team that the person needs help. The staff member turns off the signal light at the bedside when responding to the call for help.

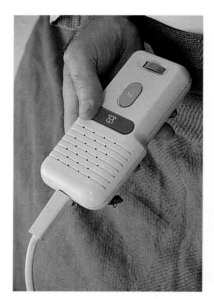

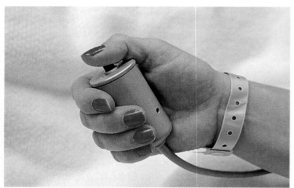

**FIG. 14-14** The signal light button is pressed when help is needed. *NOTE:* There are different types of signal lights.

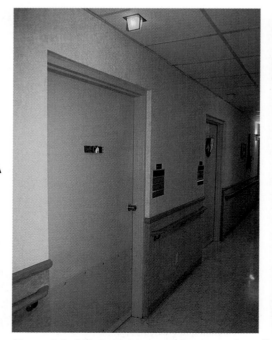

A

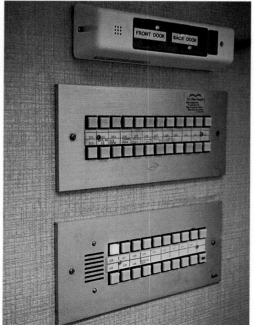

B

**FIG. 14-15 A,** Light above the room door. **B,** Light panel or intercom at the nurses' station.

An intercom system lets a nursing team member talk with the person from the nurses' station. The person tells what is needed. Then the light is turned off at the station. Hearing-impaired persons may have problems using an intercom. Be careful when using an intercom. Remember confidentiality. Persons nearby can hear what you and the person say.

Some people have limited hand mobility. They may need a special signal light that is turned on by tapping it with a hand or fist (Fig. 14-16).

The person learns how to use the call system when admitted to the agency. Some people cannot use signal lights. Examples are persons who are confused or in a coma. Check the care plan for special communication measures. Check these persons often. Make sure their needs are met.

The phrase "signal light" is used in this book when referring to the call system. You must:
- Keep the signal light within the person's reach. Even if the person cannot use the signal light, keep it within reach for use by visitors and staff. They may need to signal for help.
- Place the signal light on the person's strong side.
- Remind the person to signal when help is needed.
- Answer signal lights promptly. The person signals when help is needed. The person may have an urgent need to use the bathroom. You can prevent embarrassing problems by promptly helping the person to the bathroom. You also help prevent infection, skin breakdown, pressure ulcers, and falls.
- Answer bathroom and shower or tub room signal lights at once.

*See Focus on Home Care: The Call System.*

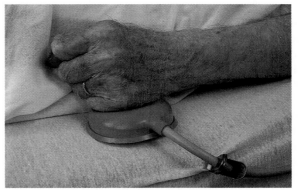

**FIG. 14-16** Signal light for a person with limited hand mobility.

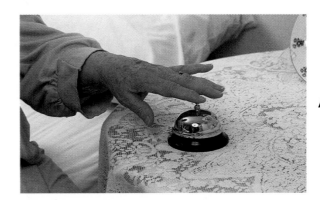

**A**

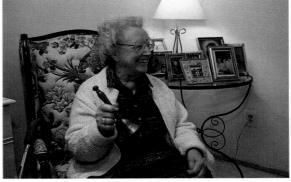

**B**

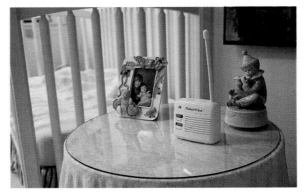

**C**

**FIG. 14-17 A,** Tap bell. **B,** Dinner bell. **C,** Baby monitor.

## FOCUS ON HOME CARE
### THE CALL SYSTEM

Some home care patients stay in bed or in a certain part of the home. They need a way to call for help. Tap bells, dinner bells, baby monitors, and other devices are useful (Fig. 14-17). Or you can give the person a small can with a few coins inside. Children's toys with bells, horns, and whistles may be useful.

## THE BATHROOM

Many agencies have a bathroom in each room. Some have a bathroom between two rooms. A toilet, sink, call system, and mirror are standard equipment (Fig. 14-18). Some bathrooms have showers.

Grab bars are by the toilet for the person's safety. The person uses them for support when lowering to or raising from the toilet. Some agencies have raised toilet seats. The higher toilets make wheelchair transfers easier. They also are helpful for persons with joint problems.

Towel racks, toilet paper, soap, a paper towel dispenser, and wastebasket are in the bathroom. They are placed within easy reach of the person.

Usually the signal light is next to the toilet. Pressing a button or pulling a cord turns on the signal light. When the bathroom signal light is used, the light flashes above the room door and at the nurses' station. The sound at the nurses' station is different from signal lights in rooms. These differences alert the nursing team that the person is in the bathroom. Someone must respond at once when a person needs help in a bathroom.

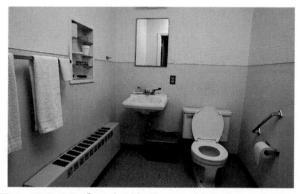

**FIG. 14-18** Standard bathroom. Note the grab bar by the toilet.

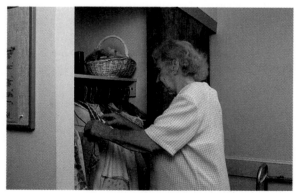

**FIG. 14-19** The resident can reach items in her closet.

## CLOSET AND DRAWER SPACE

Closet and drawer space are provided for clothing. OBRA (Chapter 9) requires closet space for each nursing center resident. Such closet space must have shelves and a clothes rack (Fig. 14-19). The person must have free access to the closet and its contents.

Items in the closet or drawers are the person's private property. You must not search the closet or drawers without the person's permission.

Sometimes people hoard items—napkins, straws, sugar, salt and pepper, and food. Hoarding can cause safety or health risks. Agency representatives can inspect a person's closet or drawers if hoarding is suspected. The person is informed of the inspection. He or she is present when it takes place.

> **SAFETY ALERT:** *Closet and Drawer Space*
> The nurse may ask you to inspect a person's closet, drawers, or personal property. If so, the person must be present. Also have a co-worker with you. Your co-worker is a witness to what you are doing. This protects you if the person claims that something was stolen or damaged.

## OTHER EQUIPMENT

Many agencies furnish rooms with other equipment. A TV, radio, and clock provide comfort and relaxation. Many rooms have phones. Residents may bring favorite furniture and items from home.

> ### ▶ FOCUS ON LONG-TERM CARE
> **OTHER EQUIPMENT**
>
> Nursing center residents have left their homes. Each had furniture, appliances, a private bathroom, and many personal belongings and treasures. Now the person lives in a strange place. He or she probably shares a room with another person. Leaving one's home is a hard part of growing old with poor health. It is important to make the person's unit as homelike as possible.
>
> Residents may bring some furniture and personal items. A chair, footstool, lamp, and small table are often allowed. They can bring family photos, religious items, and books. Some may have plants to care for.
>
> The resident is allowed personal choice in arranging items. The choices must be safe and not cause falls or other accidents. Also, the person's choices must not interfere with the rights of others. You may have to help the person choose the best place for personal items.
>
> The center is now the person's home. You must help the person feel safe, secure, and comfortable. A homelike setting is important for quality of life. OBRA serves to promote quality of life. Box 14-1 lists OBRA's requirements for resident rooms.

---

**BOX 14-1  OBRA REQUIREMENTS FOR RESIDENTS' ROOMS**

- Designed for one to four residents
- Direct access to exit corridor
- Full visual privacy— privacy curtain that extends around the bed, movable screens, doors
- At least one window to the outside
- Closet space with racks and shelves for each person
- Toilet facilities in the room or nearby (includes bathing facilities)
- Call system in the room and in toilet/bathing areas
- Bed of proper height and size
- Clean, comfortable mattress
- Bedding appropriate to the weather and climate
- Furniture for clothing and personal items; a chair for visitors
- Clean and orderly room
- Odor-free room
- Room temperature between 71° and 81° F
- Acceptable noise level

- Adequate ventilation and room humidity
- Appropriate lighting
- No glares from floors, windows, and lighting
- Clean, orderly drawers, shelves, and personal items
- Pest-free room
- Hand rails in needed areas
- Bed rails only if needed
- Clean, dry floor
- Pathways free of clutter and furniture
- Bed in low position and locked
- Personal supplies and items labeled and stored appropriately
- Drawers free of unwrapped food
- Items within reach for use in bed or bathroom
- Space for wheelchair or walker use
- Raised toilet seat
- Stool and skid-proof tub or shower

---

**BOX 14-2  MAINTAINING THE PERSON'S UNIT**

- Make sure the person can reach the overbed table and the bedside stand.
- Arrange personal items as the person prefers. Make sure they are easily reached.
- Keep the signal light within the person's reach at all times.
- Make sure the person can reach the phone, TV, and light controls.
- Provide the person with enough tissues and toilet paper.
- Adjust lighting, temperature, and ventilation for the person's comfort.
- Handle equipment carefully to prevent noise.

- Explain the causes of strange noises.
- Empty the person's wastebasket as often as needed. It is emptied at least once a day.
- Respect the person's belongings. An item may not be important or valuable to you. Yet it has great meaning for the person. Even a scrap of paper can have great meaning to the person.
- Do not throw away any items belonging to the person.
- Do not move furniture or the person's belongings. Persons with poor vision rely on memory or feel for the location of items.
- Straighten bed linens as often as needed.

---

Blood pressure equipment is often mounted on walls. There are also wall outlets for oxygen and suction (Fig. 14-20). Oxygen tanks and portable suction equipment are common in long-term care and home care settings. An IV pole (IV standard) is used to hang IV bags or feeding bags.

*See Focus on Long-Term Care: Other Equipment.*

## GENERAL RULES

The person's unit is kept clean, neat, and safe. This is a responsibility of everyone involved in the person's care. The rules in Box 14-2 are followed to maintain the person's unit.

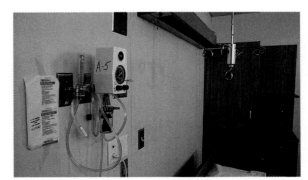

**FIG. 14-20** This room has an IV pole and oxygen and suction outlets.

# ■ REVIEW QUESTIONS ■

Circle the **BEST** answer.

1  Which is a comfortable temperature range for most people?
   a  60° F to 66° F
   b  68° F to 74° F
   c  74° F to 80° F
   d  80° F to 86° F

2  Which does *not* protect a person from drafts?
   a  Wearing enough clothing
   b  Being covered with enough blankets
   c  Being moved out of a drafty area
   d  Sitting by the air conditioner

3  Which does *not* prevent or reduce odors?
   a  Placing fresh flowers in the room
   b  Emptying bedpans promptly
   c  Using room deodorizers
   d  Practicing good hygiene

4  To prevent odors, you need to do the following *except*
   a  Check incontinent persons often
   b  Dispose of incontinence and ostomy products at the end of your shift
   c  Keep laundry containers closed
   d  Clean persons who are wet or soiled

5  Which does *not* control noise?
   a  Using plastic items
   b  Handling dishes with care
   c  Speaking softly
   d  Talking with others in the hallway

6  Beds are raised horizontally to
   a  Prevent bending and reaching when giving care
   b  Let the person get in and out of bed with ease
   c  Raise the head of the bed
   d  Lock the bed in position

7  The head of the bed is raised 30 degrees. This is called
   a  Fowler's position
   b  Semi-Fowlers position
   c  Trendelenburg's position
   d  Reverse Trendelenburg's position

8  The overbed table is *not* used
   a  For eating
   b  As a working surface
   c  For the urinal
   d  To store shaving articles

9  The bedpan is stored
   a  In the closet
   b  In the bedside stand
   c  In the overbed table
   d  Under the bed

10  Signal lights are answered
    a  When you have time
    b  At the end of your shift
    c  Promptly
    d  When you are by the person's room

11  To maintain a person's unit, you can do the following *except*
    a  Save items that do not look important
    b  Provide enough tissues and toilet paper
    c  Place personal items as you choose
    d  Straighten bed linens as needed

Circle **T** if the statement is true and **F** if it is false.

12  T F  Soft, dim lighting is relaxing.
13  T F  The privacy curtain prevents others from hearing conversations.
14  T F  The signal light must always be within the person's reach except in the bathroom.
15  T F  The overbed table and bedside stand should be within the person's reach.
16  T F  You should explain the cause of strange noises.
17  T F  Nursing center residents must be able to reach items in their closets.
18  T F  You can adjust the person's room temperature for your comfort.

*Answers to these questions are on p. 817.*

# Bedmaking

## OBJECTIVES

- Define the key terms listed in this chapter
- Describe open, closed, occupied, and surgical beds
- Explain how to use drawsheets
- Handle linens following the rules of medical asepsis
- Perform the procedures described in this chapter

## KEY TERMS

**drawsheet**   A small sheet placed over the middle of the bottom sheet; it helps keep the mattress and bottom linens clean and dry; the cotton drawsheet

**plastic drawsheet**   A drawsheet placed between the bottom sheet and the cotton drawsheet to protect the mattress and bottom linens from dampness and soiling; waterproof drawsheet

Beds are made every day. A clean, dry, and wrinkle-free bed increases comfort. It also helps prevent skin breakdown and pressure ulcers (Chapter 28).

Beds are usually made in the morning after baths. Or they are made while the person is in the shower or out of the room. Beds are made and rooms straightened before visitors arrive.

Do the following to keep beds neat and clean:
- Straighten linens whenever loose or wrinkled.
- Straighten loose or wrinkled linens at bedtime.
- Check for and remove food and crumbs after meals.
- Check linens for dentures, eyeglasses, hearing aids, sharp objects, and other items.
- Change linens whenever they become wet, soiled, or damp.
- Follow Standard Precautions and the Bloodborne Pathogen Standard. Contact with blood, body fluids, secretions, or excretions is likely.

## TYPES OF BEDS

Beds are made in these ways:
- A *closed bed* is not in use. Top linens are not folded back. The bed is ready for a new patient or resident (Fig. 15-1).
- An *open bed* is in use. Top linens are folded back so the person can get into bed. A closed bed becomes an open bed by folding back the top linens (Fig. 15-2).
- An *occupied bed* is made with the person in it (Fig. 15-3).
- A *surgical bed* is made to transfer a person from a stretcher to the bed. It also is called a *postoperative bed* or *recovery bed* (Fig. 15-4).

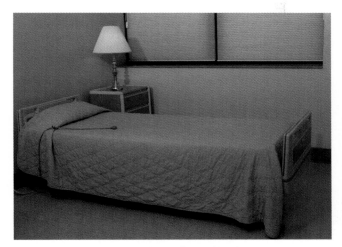

FIG. 15-1 Closed bed.

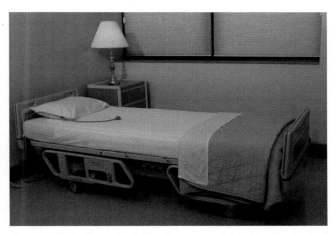

FIG. 15-2 Open bed. Top linens are folded to the foot of the bed.

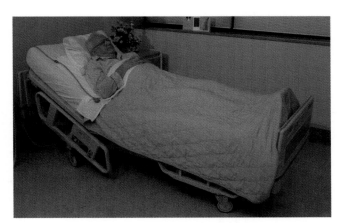

FIG. 15-3 Occupied bed.

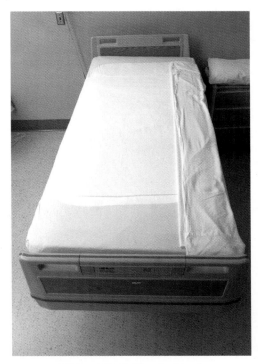

FIG. 15-4 Surgical bed.

# LINENS

When handling linens and making beds, practice medical asepsis. Your uniform is considered dirty. Always hold linens away from your body and uniform (Fig. 15-5). Never shake linens in the air. Shaking them spreads microbes. Clean linens are placed on a clean surface. Never put clean or dirty linens on the floor.

Collect enough linens. If the person has two pillows, get two pillowcases. The person may need extra blankets for warmth. Do not bring unneeded linens to a person's room. Once in the person's room, extra linen is considered contaminated. It is not used for another person.

Collect linens in the order you will use them:
- Mattress pad (if needed)
- Bottom sheet (flat or fitted)
- Plastic drawsheet, waterproof drawsheet, or waterproof pad (optional)
- Cotton drawsheet (if needed)
- Top sheet (if needed)
- Blanket
- Bedspread
- Pillowcase(s)
- Bath towel(s)
- Hand towel
- Washcloth
- Gown
- Bath blanket

Use one arm to hold the linens. Use your other hand to pick them up. The item you will use first is at the bottom of your stack. (You picked up the mattress pad first. It is at the bottom. The bath blanket is on top.) You need the mattress pad first. To get it on top, place your arm over the bath blanket. Then turn the stack over onto the arm on the bath blanket (Fig. 15-6). The arm that held the linens is now free. Place the clean linens on a clean surface.

Remove dirty linen one piece at a time. Roll each piece away from you. The side that touched the person is inside the roll and away from you (Fig. 15-7).

In hospitals, top and bottom sheets and pillowcases are changed daily. The mattress pad, drawsheets, blanket, and bedspread are reused for the same person. They are not reused if soiled, wet, or wrinkled. *Wet, damp, or soiled linens are changed right away. Wear gloves and follow Standard Precautions and the Bloodborne Pathogen Standard.*

*See Focus on Long-Term Care: Linens. See Focus on Home Care: Linens.*

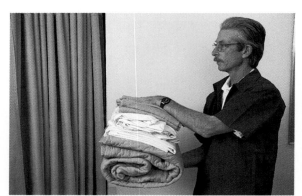

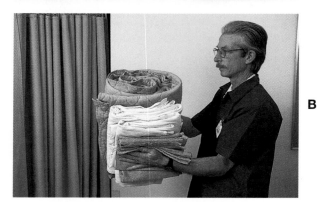

**FIG. 15-6** Collecting linens. **A,** The arm is placed over the top of the stack of linens. **B,** The stack of linens is turned over onto the arm. Note that linens are held away from the body.

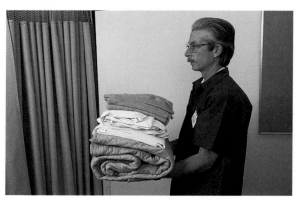

**FIG. 15-5** Hold linens away from your body and uniform.

## DRAWSHEETS

A **drawsheet** is a small sheet placed over the middle of the bottom sheet. It helps keep the mattress and bottom linens clean and dry. It is also called the *cotton drawsheet* because it is made of cotton. A **plastic drawsheet** is waterproof. It is placed between the bottom sheet and cotton drawsheet. It protects the mattress and bottom linens from dampness and soiling. In some agencies, it is called a *waterproof drawsheet.*

The cotton drawsheet protects the person from contact with the plastic and absorbs moisture. However, discomfort and skin breakdown may occur. Plastic retains heat. Plastic drawsheets are hard to keep tight and wrinkle-free. Many agencies use incontinence products (Chapter 18) to keep the person and linens dry. Others use waterproof pads.

Cotton drawsheets are often used without plastic drawsheets. Plastic-covered mattresses cause some persons to perspire heavily. This increases discomfort. A cotton drawsheet reduces heat retention and absorbs moisture. Cotton drawsheets are often used as lift or turning sheets (Chapter 13). When used for this purpose, do not tuck them in at the sides.

The bedmaking procedures that follow include plastic and cotton drawsheets. This is so you learn how to use them. Ask the nurse about their use in your agency.

*See Focus on Home Care: Drawsheets.*

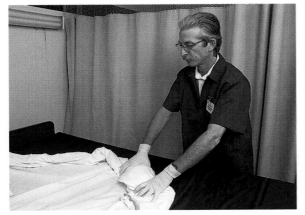

**FIG. 15-7** Roll linens away from you when removing them from the bed.

## MAKING BEDS

When making beds, safety and medical asepsis are important. Follow the rules in Box 15-1. *See Focus on Home Care: Making Beds. See Focus on Children: Making Beds.*

---

**DELEGATION GUIDELINES:** *Making Beds*

Before making a bed, you need this information from the nurse and the care plan:

- What type of bed to make—closed, open, occupied, or surgical.
- If you need to use a plastic drawsheet, waterproof pad, or incontinence product.
- Position restrictions or limits in the person's movement.
- If the person uses bed rails.
- The person's treatment, therapy, and activity schedule. For example, Mr. Smith needs a treatment in bed. Change linens after the treatment. Mrs. Jones goes to physical therapy. Make the bed while she is out of the room.
- If the bed needs to be locked into a certain position (Chapter 14).
- How to position the person and the positioning devices needed.

---

**SAFETY ALERT:** *Making Beds*

You need to raise the bed for body mechanics. The bed also must be flat. If the bed is locked, unlock it. Then reposition the bed. Return the bed to the desired position when you are done. Then lock the bed.

Wear gloves when removing linen from the person's bed. Also follow the other aspects of Standard Precautions and the Bloodborne Pathogen Standard. Linens may contain blood, body fluids, secretions, or excretions.

After making a bed, lower the bed to its lowest position. Lock the bed wheels. For an occupied bed, raise or lower bed rails according to the care plan.

---

**FOCUS ON HOME CARE**
**MAKING BEDS**

Many home care patients do not have hospital beds. You will see twin-, regular-, queen-, and king-size beds. Water beds, sofa sleepers, cots, and recliners are common. Make the bed as the person wishes. Follow the rules in Box 15-1. If the person's wishes are unsafe, contact the nurse.

Your assignment may include doing laundry. Wash linen when soiling is fresh to help prevent staining. Urine, feces, vomit, and blood can stain linens. Follow these guidelines:

- Wear gloves. Linen may contain blood, body fluids, secretions, or excretions.
- Rinse the item with cold water to remove the substance.
- Treat the stain. The person may use a stain-removing agent. Read and follow the manufacturer's instructions. Or the nurse may direct you to soak the item for 30 minutes in an ammonia solution:
  —1 quart warm water
  —½ teaspoon liquid dishwashing detergent
  —1 tablespoon ammonia
- Rinse the item with cool water after soaking.
- Machine-wash it with a detergent.

Ammonia is a poison. Do not inhale the fumes or let the ammonia have contact with your skin or eyes. Follow the manufacturer's instructions. *Do not mix ammonia with bleach or other chemicals. Deadly fumes will result.*

## FOCUS ON CHILDREN
### MAKING BEDS

Cribs and crib linens present safety hazards. Mattresses, linens, and bumper pads pose many dangers. They can cause strangulation and suffocation. Report any safety hazard to the nurse. Follow these safety rules and the safety measures in Chapter 10:

- The crib mattress must be firm. A soft mattress can cover the baby's nose and mouth. This prevents breathing.
- The mattress and crib must be the same size. The mattress must fit snugly in the crib frame. If not, the baby's head can get caught between the mattress and the frame.
- No more than 2 adult fingers should fit between the mattress and crib sides. If more than 2 fingers fit, the mattress is too small. It must be replaced.
- The mattress must be at least 26 inches lower than the top of the crib rails. This prevents falling out of the crib. The mattress is lowered when the baby starts to stand in the crib.
- Do not use plastic trash bags and dry-cleaning bags to protect the mattress.
- Bumper pads are used until the baby starts to stand. Then they are removed.
- Bumper pads must cover the entire inside of the crib.
- Bumper pads must fit snugly against the slats. If not, the baby's head can get caught between the bumper pads and the slats.
- Bumper pads snap or tie in place. At least six straps or ties are needed.
- Bumper pad straps or ties must be away from the baby. Avoid long straps or ties. The baby can get entangled in them.
- The mattress is covered with a crib sheet that fits well.
- Check the crib sheet for loose threads or stitching.
- Pillows, blankets, and comforters are not used for babies.

## BOX 15-1  RULES FOR BEDMAKING

- Use good body mechanics at all times.
- Follow the rules of medical asepsis.
- Follow Standard Precautions and the Bloodborne Pathogen Standard.
- Practice hand hygiene before handling clean linen.
- Practice hand hygiene after handling dirty linen.
- Bring enough linen to the person's room.
- Bring only the linens that you will need. Extra linens cannot be used for another person.
- Do not use torn linen.
- Never shake linens. Shaking linens spreads microbes.
- Extra linen in a person's room is considered contaminated. Do not use it for other people. Put it with the dirty laundry.
- Hold linens away from your uniform. Dirty and clean linen must not touch your uniform.
- Never put dirty linens on the floor or on clean linens. Follow agency policy for dirty linen.
- Keep bottom linens tucked in and wrinkle-free.
- Cover a plastic drawsheet with a cotton drawsheet. A plastic drawsheet must not touch the person's body.
- Straighten and tighten loose sheets, blankets, and bedspreads as needed.
- Make as much of one side of the bed as possible before going to the other side. This saves time and energy.
- Change wet, damp, and soiled linens right away.

# THE CLOSED BED

A closed bed is made after a person is discharged. It is made for a new patient or resident. The bed is made after the bed frame and mattress are cleaned and disinfected. *See Focus on Long-Term Care: The Closed Bed. See Focus on Home Care: The Closed Bed.*

*Text continued on p. 304.*

## FOCUS ON LONG-TERM CARE
### THE CLOSED BED

In long-term care, closed beds are made for residents who are up for most or all of the day. Top linens are folded back at bedtime. Clean linens are used as needed.

## FOCUS ON HOME CARE
### THE CLOSED BED

In home care, a closed bed also means that linens are not folded back. Closed beds are made for patients who are up for most or all of the day. Clean linens are used as needed.

## MAKING A CLOSED BED

### QUALITY OF LIFE

Remember to:
- Knock before entering the person's room
- Address the person by name
- Introduce yourself by name and title

### PRE-PROCEDURE

1 Follow *Delegation Guidelines: Making Beds*, p. 296. See *Safety Alert: Making Beds*, p. 296.
2 Practice hand hygiene.
3 Collect clean linen:
- Mattress pad (if needed)
- Bottom sheet (flat sheet or fitted sheet)
- Plastic drawsheet or waterproof pad (if needed)
- Cotton drawsheet (if needed)
- Top sheet
- Blanket
- Bedspread
- Two pillowcases
- Bath towel(s)
- Hand towel
- Washcloth
- Gown
- Bath blanket
- Gloves
- Laundry bag

4 Place linen on a clean surface.
5 Raise the bed for body mechanics.

### PROCEDURE

6 Put on the gloves.
7 Remove linen. Roll each piece away from you. Place each piece in a laundry bag. (*NOTE:* Discard disposable bed protectors in the trash. Do not put them in the laundry bag.)
8 Clean the bed frame and mattress if this is part of your job.
9 Remove and discard the gloves. Decontaminate your hands.
10 Move the mattress to the head of the bed.
11 Put the mattress pad on the mattress. It is even with the top of the mattress.
12 Place the bottom sheet on the mattress pad (Fig. 15-8):
  a Unfold it lengthwise.
  b Place the center crease in the middle of the bed.
  c Position the lower edge even with the bottom of the mattress.
  d Place the large hem at the top and the small hem at the bottom.
  e Face hem-stitching downward, away from the person.
13 Open the sheet. Fanfold it to the other side of the bed (Fig. 15-9).
14 Tuck the top of the sheet under the mattress. The sheet is tight and smooth.
15 Make a mitered corner if using a flat sheet (Fig. 15-10).

*Continued.*

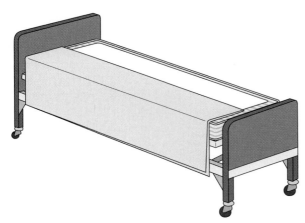

**FIG. 15-8** The bottom sheet is on the bed with the center crease in the middle. The lower edge of the sheet is even with the bottom of the mattress.

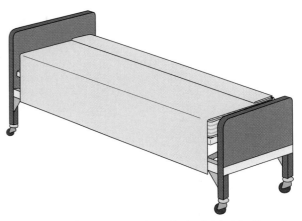

**FIG. 15-9** The bottom sheet is fanfolded to the other side of the bed.

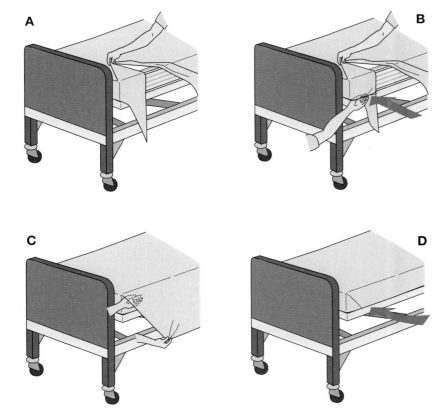

**FIG. 15-10** Making a mitered corner. **A,** The bottom sheet is tucked under the mattress. The side of the sheet is raised onto the mattress. **B,** The remaining portion of the sheet is tucked under the mattress. **C,** The raised portion of the sheet is brought off the mattress. **D,** The entire side of the sheet is tucked under the mattress.

## MAKING A CLOSED BED—CONT'D

### PROCEDURE—CONT'D

16 Place the plastic drawsheet on the bed. It is about 14 inches from the top of the mattress. Or put the waterproof pad on the bed.

17 Open the plastic drawsheet. Fanfold it to the other side of the bed.

18 Place a cotton drawsheet over the plastic drawsheet. It covers the entire plastic drawsheet (Fig. 15-11).

19 Open the cotton drawsheet. Fanfold it to the other side of the bed.

20 Tuck both drawsheets under the mattress. Or tuck each in separately.

21 Go to the other side of the bed.

22 Miter the top corner of the flat bottom sheet.

23 Pull the bottom sheet tight so there are no wrinkles. Tuck in the sheet.

24 Pull the drawsheets tight so there are no wrinkles. Tuck both in together or separately (Fig. 15-12).

25 Go to the other side of the bed.

26 Put the top sheet on the bed:
   a Unfold it lengthwise.
   b Place the center crease in the middle.
   c Place the large hem even with the top of the mattress.
   d Open the sheet. Fanfold it to the other side.
   e Face hem-stitching outward, away from the person.
   f Do not tuck the bottom in yet.
   g Never tuck top linens in on the sides.

27 Place the blanket on the bed:
   a Unfold it so the center crease is in the middle.
   b Put the upper hem about 6 to 8 inches from the top of the mattress.
   c Open the blanket. Fanfold it to the other side.
   d If steps 33 and 34 are not done, turn the top sheet down over the blanket. Hem-stitching is down, away from the person.

28 Place the bedspread on the bed:
   a Unfold it so the center crease is in the middle.
   b Place the upper hem even with the top of the mattress.
   c Open and fanfold the spread to the other side.
   d Make sure the spread facing the door is even. It covers all top linens.

29 Tuck in top linens together at the foot of the bed. They should be smooth and tight. Make a mitered corner.

30 Go to the other side.

31 Straighten all top linen. Work from the head of the bed to the foot.

32 Tuck in the top linens together at the foot of the bed. Make a mitered corner.

33 Turn the top hem of the spread under the blanket to make a cuff (Fig. 15-13).

34 Turn the top sheet down over the spread. Hem-stitching is down. (Steps 33 and 34 are not done in some agencies. The spread covers the pillow. If so, tuck the spread under the pillow.)

35 Put the pillowcase on the pillow as in Figure 15-14, p. 302 or Figure 15-15, p. 303. Fold extra material under the pillow at the seam end of the pillowcase.

36 Place the pillow on the bed. The open end of the pillowcase is away from the door. The seam is toward the head of the bed.

### POST-PROCEDURE

37 Attach the signal light to the bed.

38 Lower the bed to its lowest position. Lock the bed wheels.

39 Put towels, washcloth, gown, and bath blanket in the bedside stand.

40 Follow agency policy for dirty linen.

41 Decontaminate your hands.

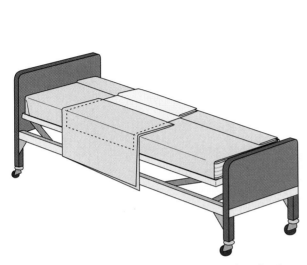

FIG. 15-11 A cotton drawsheet is over the plastic drawsheet. The cotton drawsheet completely covers the plastic drawsheet.

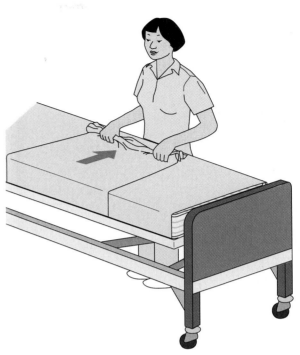

FIG. 15-12 The drawsheet is pulled tight to remove wrinkles.

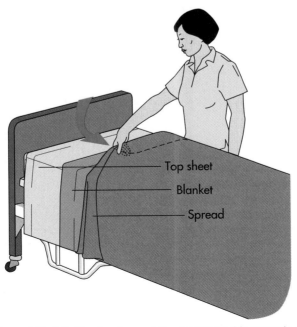

FIG. 15-13 The top hem of the bedspread is turned under the top hem of the blanket to make a cuff.

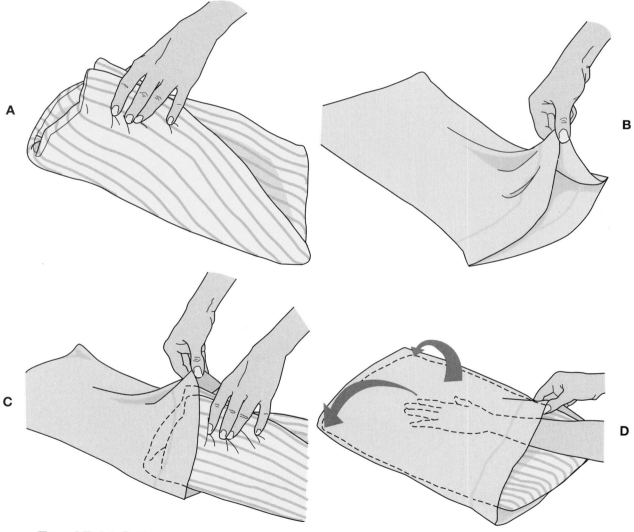

**FIG. 15-14** Putting a pillowcase on a pillow. **A,** Open the pillowcase so it is flat on the bed. Grasp the corners of the pillow at the seam end and form a "∨" with the pillow. **B,** The pillowcase is opened with the free hand. **C,** The "∨" end of the pillow is guided into the pillowcase. **D,** The "∨" end of the pillow falls into the corners of the pillowcase.

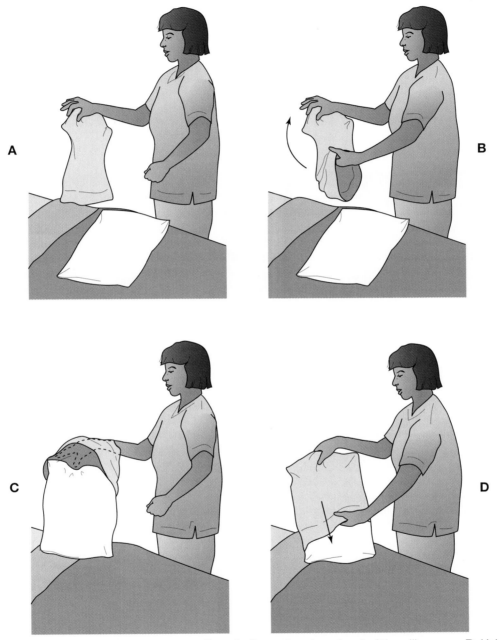

**FIG. 15-15** Putting a pillowcase on a pillow. **A,** Grasp the closed end of the pillowcase. **B,** Using your other hand, gather up the pillowcase. The pillowcase should cover your hand holding the closed end. **C,** Grasp the pillow with the hand covered by the pillowcase. **D,** Pull the pillowcase down over the pillow with your other hand.

# THE OPEN BED

A closed bed becomes an open bed by folding the top linens back. Open beds are made for newly admitted persons arriving by wheelchair. They are also made for persons who are out of bed. The open bed lets the person get into bed with ease.

## MAKING AN OPEN BED

### QUALITY OF LIFE

Remember to:
- Knock before entering the person's room
- Address the person by name
- Introduce yourself by name and title

### PROCEDURE

1 Follow *Delegation Guidelines: Making Beds,* p. 296. See *Safety Alert: Making Beds,* p. 296.
2 Practice hand hygiene.
3 Collect linen for a closed bed.
4 Make a closed bed.
5 Fanfold top linens to the foot of the bed (see Fig. 15-2).
6 Attach the signal light to the bed.
7 Lower the bed to its lowest position.
8 Put towels, washcloth, gown, and bath blanket in the bedside stand.
9 Follow agency policy for dirty linen.
10 Decontaminate your hands.

# THE OCCUPIED BED

An occupied bed is made when a person stays in bed. When making an occupied bed, keep the person in good alignment. You must know about restrictions or limits in the person's movement or position.

Explain each procedure step to the person before it is done. This is important even if the person cannot respond to you or is in a coma.

*Text continued on p. 309.*

**SAFETY ALERT:** *The Occupied Bed*

You need to raise the bed for body mechanics. This limits reaching and bending. Back injuries are prevented.

The person's safety is important. The person lies on one side of the bed and then the other. Protect the person from falling out of bed. If the person uses bed rails, the far bed rail is up. If the person does not use bed rails, have another person help you. You work on one side of the bed. Your co-worker works on the other.

After making the bed, lower it to its lowest position and lock the bed wheels. Raise or lower bed rails according to the care plan.

---

## MAKING AN OCCUPIED BED

NNAAP™

### QUALITY OF LIFE

Remember to:
- Knock before entering the person's room
- Address the person by name
- Introduce yourself by name and title

### PRE-PROCEDURE

1 Follow *Delegation Guidelines: Making Beds*, p. 296. See *Safety Alerts: Making Beds*, p. 296 and *The Occupied Bed*.
2 Explain the procedure to the person.
3 Practice hand hygiene.
4 Collect the following:
   - Gloves
   - Laundry bag
   - Clean linen (see procedure: *Making a Closed Bed*, p. 298)

5 Place linen on a clean surface.
6 Identify the person. Check the ID bracelet against the assignment sheet. Call the person by name.
7 Provide for privacy.
8 Remove the signal light.
9 Raise the bed for body mechanics. Bed rails are up if used.
10 Lower the head of the bed. It is as flat as possible.

### PROCEDURE

11 Lower the bed rail near you.
12 Put on gloves.
13 Loosen top linens at the foot of the bed.
14 Remove the bedspread. Then remove the blanket (Fig. 15-16, p. 307). Place each over the chair.
15 Cover the person with a bath blanket. It provides warmth and privacy.
   a Unfold a bath blanket over the top sheet.
   b Ask the person to hold onto the bath blanket. If he or she cannot, tuck the top part under the person's shoulders.
   c Grasp the top sheet under the bath blanket at the shoulders. Bring the sheet down to the foot of the bed. Remove the sheet from under the blanket (Fig. 15-17, p. 307).
16 Move the mattress to the head of the bed.

17 Position the person on the side of the bed away from you. Adjust the pillow for comfort.
18 Loosen bottom linens from the head to the foot of the bed.
19 Fanfold bottom linens one at a time toward the person. Start with the cotton drawsheet (Fig. 15-18, p. 308). If reusing the mattress pad, do not fanfold it.
20 Place a clean mattress pad on the bed. Unfold it lengthwise. The center crease is in the middle. Fanfold the top part toward the person. If reusing the mattress pad, straighten and smooth any wrinkles.
21 Place the bottom sheet on the mattress pad. Hemstitching is away from the person. Unfold the sheet so the crease is in the middle. The small hem is even with the bottom of the mattress. Fanfold the top part toward the person.

*Continued.*

## MAKING AN OCCUPIED BED—CONT'D

NNAAP™

### PROCEDURE—CONT'D

22 Make a mitered corner at the head of the bed. Tuck the sheet under the mattress from the head to the foot.

23 Pull the plastic drawsheet toward you over the bottom sheet. Tuck excess material under the mattress. Do the following for a clean plastic drawsheet (Fig. 15-19, p. 308).
   a Place the plastic drawsheet on the bed. It is about 14 inches from the mattress top.
   b Fanfold the top part toward the person.
   c Tuck in the excess fabric.

24 Place the cotton drawsheet over the plastic drawsheet. It covers the entire plastic drawsheet. Fanfold the top part toward the person. Tuck in excess fabric.

25 Raise the bed rail if used. Go to the other side, and lower the bed rail.

26 Explain to the person that he or she will roll over a bump. Assure the person that he or she will not fall.

27 Help the person turn to the other side. Adjust the pillow for comfort.

28 Loosen bottom linens. Remove one piece at a time. Place each piece in the laundry bag. (*NOTE:* Discard disposable bed protectors in the trash. Do not put them in the laundry bag.)

29 Remove and discard the gloves. Decontaminate your hands.

30 Straighten and smooth the mattress pad.

31 Pull the clean bottom sheet toward you. Make a mitered corner at the top. Tuck the sheet under the mattress from the head to the foot of the bed.

32 Pull the drawsheets tightly toward you. Tuck both under together or separately.

33 Position the person supine in the center of the bed. Adjust the pillow for comfort.

34 Put the top sheet on the bed. Unfold it lengthwise. The crease is in the middle. The large hem is even with the top of the mattress. Hem-stitching is on the outside.

35 Ask the person to hold onto the top sheet so you can remove the bath blanket. Or tuck the top sheet under the person's shoulders. Remove the bath blanket.

36 Place the blanket on the bed. Unfold it so the crease is in the middle and it covers the person. The upper hem is 6 to 8 inches from the top of the mattress.

37 Place the bedspread on the bed. Unfold it so the center crease is in the middle and it covers the person. The top hem is even with the mattress top.

38 Turn the top hem of the spread under the blanket to make a cuff.

39 Bring the top sheet down over the spread to form a cuff.

40 Go to the foot of the bed.

41 Make a toe pleat. Make a 2-inch pleat across the foot of the bed. The pleat is about 6 to 8 inches from the foot of the bed.

42 Lift the mattress corner with one arm. Tuck all top linens under the mattress together. Make a mitered corner.

43 Raise the bed rail if used. Go to the other side, and lower the bed rail if used.

44 Straighten and smooth top linens.

45 Tuck the top linens under the bottom of the mattress. Make a mitered corner.

46 Change the pillowcase(s).

### POST-PROCEDURE

47 Place the signal light within reach.

48 Raise or lower bed rails. Follow the care plan.

49 Raise the head of the bed to a level appropriate for the person. Provide for comfort.

50 Lower the bed to its lowest position. Lock the bed wheels.

51 Put towels, washcloth, gown, and bath blanket in the bedside stand.

52 Unscreen the person. Thank him or her for cooperating.

53 Follow agency policy for dirty linen.

54 Decontaminate your hands.

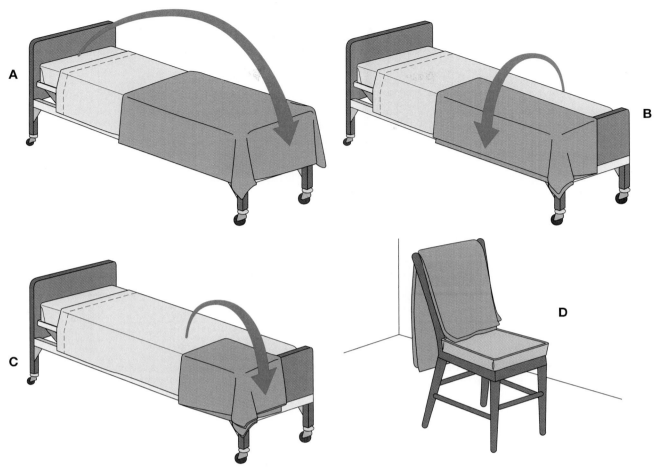

**FIG. 15-16** Folding linen for reuse. **A,** The top edge of the blanket is folded down to the bottom edge. **B,** The blanket is folded from the far side of the bed to the near side. **C,** The top edge of the blanket is folded down to the bottom edge again. **D,** The folded blanket is placed over the back of a chair.

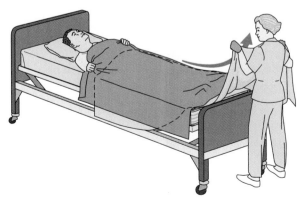

**FIG. 15-17** The person holds onto the bath blanket. The top sheet is removed from under the bath blanket.

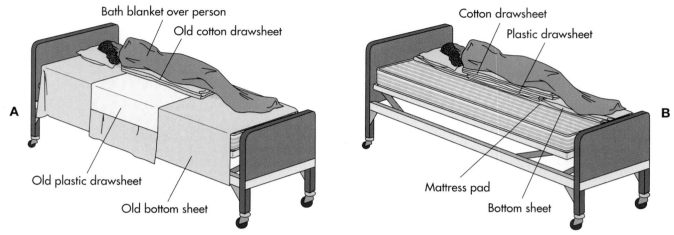

**FIG. 15-18** Occupied bed. **A,** The cotton drawsheet is fanfolded and tucked under the person. **B,** All bottom linens are tucked under the person.

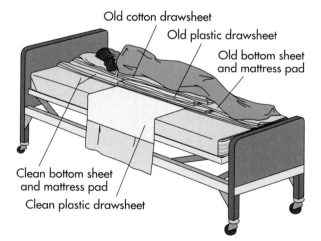

**FIG. 15-19** A clean bottom sheet and plastic drawsheet are on the bed with both fanfolded and tucked under the person.

# THE SURGICAL BED

The surgical bed also is called a *recovery bed* or *postoperative bed*. It is a form of the open bed. Top linens are folded to transfer the person from a stretcher to the bed.

Surgical beds are made for persons who arrive at the agency by ambulance. They also are used for persons who are taken by stretcher to treatment or therapy areas. Surgical beds are made when portable tubs are used.

If the bed is made for a postoperative (surgical) patient, a complete linen change is done.

SAFETY ALERT: *Surgical Beds*
To safely transfer a person from a stretcher to a surgical bed, see *Moving the Person to a Stretcher* in Chapter 13. After the transfer, lower the bed to its lowest position and lock the bed wheels. Raise or lower bed rails according to the care plan.

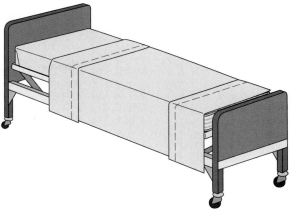

FIG. 15-20 Surgical bed. The bottom of the top linens is folded back onto the bed. The fold is even with the edge of the mattress.

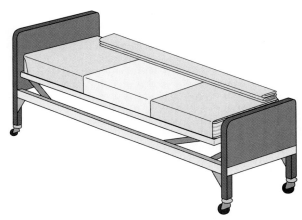

FIG. 15-21 A surgical bed with the top linens fanfolded lengthwise to the opposite side of the bed.

## MAKING A SURGICAL BED

### PROCEDURE

1 Follow *Delegation Guidelines: Making Beds*, p. 296. See *Safety Alerts: Making Beds*, p. 296 and *Surgical Beds*.
2 Practice hand hygiene.
3 Collect the following:
 - Clean linen (see procedure: *Making a Closed Bed*, p. 298)
 - Gloves
 - Laundry bag
 - Equipment requested by the nurse
4 Place linen on a clean surface.
5 Remove the signal light.
6 Raise the bed for body mechanics.
7 Remove all linen from the bed. Wear gloves.
8 Make a closed bed (See procedure: *Making a Closed Bed*, p. 298). Do not tuck the top linens under the mattress.

9 Fold all top linens at the foot of the bed back onto the bed. The fold is even with the edge of the mattress (Fig. 15-20).
10 Fanfold linen lengthwise to the side of the bed farthest from the door (Fig. 15-21).
11 Put the pillowcase(s) on the pillow(s).
12 Place the pillow(s) on a clean surface.
13 Leave the bed in its highest position.
14 Leave both bed rails down.
15 Put the towels, washcloth, gown, and bath blanket in the bedside stand.
16 Move furniture away from the bed. Allow room for the stretcher and for the staff.
17 Do not attach the signal light to the bed.
18 Follow agency policy for soiled linen.
19 Decontaminate your hands.

# ■ REVIEW QUESTIONS ■

Circle the **BEST** answer.

1 Which requires a linen change?
   a The person will have visitors
   b Wet linen
   c Wrinkled linen
   d Crumbs in the bed

2 You will transfer a person from a stretcher to the bed. Which bed should you make?
   a A closed bed
   b An open bed
   c An occupied bed
   d A surgical bed

3 When handling linens
   a Put dirty linens on the floor
   b Hold linens away from your body and uniform
   c Shake linens to remove crumbs
   d Take extra linen to another person's room

4 A resident is out of the room most of the day. What type of bed should you make?
   a A closed bed
   b An open bed
   c An occupied bed
   d A surgical bed

5 A complete linen change is done when
   a The bottom linens are wet or soiled
   b The bed is made for a new person
   c The person will transfer from a stretcher to the bed
   d Linens are loose or wrinkled

6 You are using a plastic drawsheet. Which is *true*?
   a A cotton drawsheet must completely cover the plastic drawsheet.
   b Disposable bed protectors are needed.
   c The person's consent is needed.
   d The plastic is in contact with the person's skin.

7 When making an occupied bed, you do the following *except*
   a Cover the person with a bath blanket
   b Screen the person
   c Raise the far bed rail if bed rails are used
   d Fanfold top linens to the foot of the bed

8 A surgical bed is kept
   a In Fowler's position
   b In the lowest position
   c In the highest position
   d In the supine position

*Answers to these questions are on p. 817.*

# Personal Hygiene

## OBJECTIVES

- Define the key terms listed in this chapter
- Explain why personal hygiene is important
- Describe the care given before and after breakfast, after lunch, and in the evening
- Describe the rules for bathing
- Identify safety measures for tub baths and showers
- Explain the purposes of a back massage
- Explain the purposes of perineal care
- Identify the observations to make while assisting with hygiene
- Perform the procedures described in this chapter

## KEY TERMS

**AM care** Routine care before breakfast; early morning care

**aspiration** Breathing fluid or an object into the lungs

**early morning care** AM care

**evening care** HS care or PM care

**HS care** Care given at bedtime (hour of sleep [HS]); evening care or PM care

**morning care** Care given after breakfast; hygiene measures are more thorough at this time

**oral hygiene** Mouth care

**pericare** Perineal care

**perineal care** Cleaning the genital and anal areas; pericare

**plaque** A thin film that sticks to the teeth; it contains saliva, microbes, and other substances

**PM care** HS care or evening care

**tartar** Hardened plaque

Hygiene promotes comfort, safety, and health. The skin is the body's first line of defense against disease. Intact skin prevents microbes from entering the body and causing an infection. Likewise, mucous membranes of the mouth, genital area, and anus must be clean and intact. Besides cleansing, good hygiene prevents body and breath odors. It is relaxing and increases circulation. (Review the structures and functions of the teeth and skin in Box 16-1.)

Culture and personal choice affect hygiene. *See Caring About Culture: Personal Hygiene.* Some people take showers. Others take tub baths. Some bathe at bedtime. Others bathe in the morning. Bathing fre-quency also varies. Some bathe one or two times a day—before work and after work or exercise. Some people do not have water for bathing. Others cannot afford soap, deodorant, shampoo, toothpaste, or other hygiene products.

Many factors affect hygiene needs—perspiration, vomiting, elimination, drainage from wounds or body openings, bedrest, and activity. Illness and aging changes can affect self-care abilities. Some people need help with hygiene. The RN uses the nursing process to meet the person's hygiene needs. Follow the nurse's directions and the care plan. *See Focus on Older Persons: Personal Hygiene.*

## BOX 16-1 REVIEW OF BODY STRUCTURE AND FUNCTION

### THE TEETH AND GUMS

The teeth cut, chop, and grind food into small bits for digestion and swallowing. A tooth has three main parts: the crown, neck, and root (Fig. 16-1). The crown is the outer part. It is covered by enamel. The neck is surrounded by the gums (gingivae). The root fits into the bone of the lower or upper jaw.

### THE SKIN

The skin is the largest system. It is the body's natural covering. There are two layers: the epidermis and the dermis (Fig. 16-2, p. 314). The *epidermis* is the outer layer. It contains living and dead cells. Dead cells constantly flake off and are replaced by living cells. Living cells also die and flake off. The epidermis has no blood vessels and few nerve endings. The *dermis* is the inner layer. It is made up of connective tissue. Blood vessels, nerves, sweat and oil glands, and hair roots are found in the dermis.

Sweat glands help regulate body temperature. Sweat is secreted through the skin's pores. The body is cooled as sweat evaporates. Oil glands secrete an oily substance into the space near the hair shaft. Oil travels to the skin surface. The oil helps keep the hair and skin soft and shiny.

The skin has these functions:

- Provides the body's protective covering. Intact skin prevents bacteria and other substances from entering the body.
- Prevents large amounts of water from leaving the body.
- Protects organs from injury.
- Nerve endings in the skin sense both pleasant and unpleasant stimulation. Cold, pain, touch, and pressure are sensed.
- Helps regulate body temperature. Blood vessels dilate (widen) when temperature outside the body is high. More blood is brought to the body surface for cooling during evaporation. When blood vessels constrict (narrow), the body retains heat because less blood reaches the skin.

## CARING ABOUT CULTURE

### PERSONAL HYGIENE

Personal hygiene is very important to *East Indian Hindus.* Their religion requires at least one bath a day. Some believe it is harmful to bathe after a meal. Another Hindu belief is that a cold bath prevents blood disease. Some believe that eye injuries can occur if a bath is too hot. Hot water can be added to cold water. However, cold water is not added to hot water. After bathing, the body is carefully dried with a towel.

From Giger JN, Davidhizar RE: *Transcultural nursing: assessment and intervention,* ed 3, St Louis, 1999, Mosby.

## FOCUS ON OLDER PERSONS

### PERSONAL HYGIENE

Some older persons resist your efforts to assist with hygiene. Illness, disability, dementia, and personal choice are common reasons. Follow the care plan to meet the person's needs.

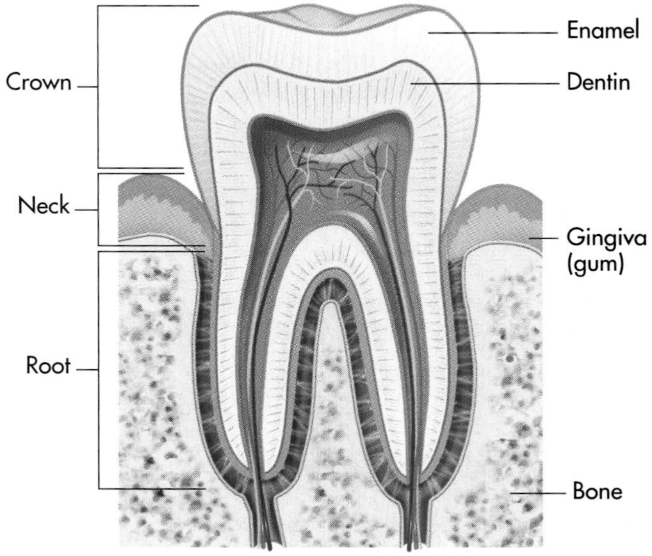

**FIG. 16-1** Parts of the tooth. (From Thibodeau GA, Patton KT: *The human body in health & disease,* ed 3, St Louis, 2002, Mosby.)

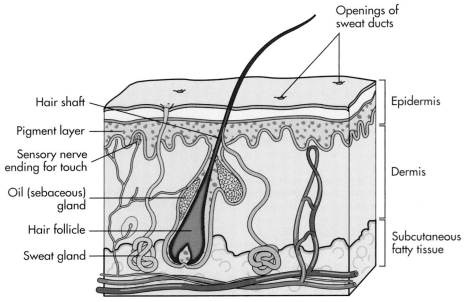

**FIG. 16-2** Structures of the skin.

## DAILY CARE

Most people have hygiene routines and habits. For example, teeth are brushed and face and hands washed on awakening. These and other hygiene measures are often done before and after meals and at bedtime.

Infants and young children need help with hygiene. So do some weak and disabled adults. Routine care is given at certain times. You assist with hygiene whenever it is needed.

### BEFORE BREAKFAST

Routine care before breakfast is **early morning care** or **AM care.** Night shift or day shift staff members give AM care. They prepare patients and residents for breakfast or morning tests. AM care includes:
- Assisting with elimination
- Cleaning incontinent persons
- Changing wet or soiled linens
- Assisting with hygiene—face and hand washing and oral hygiene
- Assisting with dressing and hair care
- Positioning persons for breakfast—dining room, bedside chair, or in bed
- Making beds and straightening units

### AFTER BREAKFAST

**Morning care** is given after breakfast. Hygiene measures are more thorough at this time. They usually involve:
- Assisting with elimination
- Cleaning incontinent persons
- Changing wet or soiled linens
- Assisting with hygiene—face and hand washing, oral hygiene, bathing, back massage, and perineal care
- Assisting with grooming—hair care, shaving, dressing, or changing gowns or pajamas
- Assisting with activity—range-of-motion exercises and ambulation
- Making beds and straightening units

### AFTERNOON CARE

Routine hygiene is done after lunch and the evening meal. If done before visitors arrive, the person is refreshed and can visit without interruption. Afternoon care involves:
- Assisting with elimination
- Cleaning incontinent persons
- Changing wet or soiled linens and garments
- Assisting with hygiene and grooming—face and hand washing, oral hygiene, hair care, changing garments
- Assisting with activity—range-of-motion exercises and ambulation
- Brushing or combing hair if needed
- Straightening beds and units
  *See Focus on Long-Term Care: Afternoon Care.*

> ### FOCUS ON LONG-TERM CARE
> #### AFTERNOON CARE
> Residents often nap in the afternoon. You help them lie down for the nap and with getting up afterwards. Before and after naps you assist with elimination, clean incontinent persons, and change wet or soiled garments and linens.

## EVENING CARE

Care given at bedtime is **HS care, evening care,** or **PM care.** (*HS* means hour of sleep.) HS care is relaxing and promotes comfort. Measures performed before sleep include:
- Assisting with elimination
- Cleaning incontinent persons
- Changing wet or soiled linens and garments
- Assisting with hygiene—face and hand washing, oral hygiene, and back massages
- Helping persons change into sleepwear
- Straightening beds and units

## ORAL HYGIENE

**Oral hygiene** (mouth care) does the following:
- Keeps the mouth and teeth clean
- Prevents mouth odors and infections
- Increases comfort
- Makes food taste better
- Reduces the risk for *cavities (dental caries)* and *periodontal disease*

Periodontal disease *(gum disease, pyorrhea)* is an inflammation of tissues around the teeth. Plaque and tartar build up from poor oral hygiene. **Plaque** is a thin film that sticks to teeth. It contains saliva, microbes, and other substances. Plaque causes tooth decay *(cavities)*. When plaque hardens, it is called **tartar.** Tartar builds up at the gum line near the neck of the tooth. Tartar buildup causes periodontal disease. The gums are red and swollen and bleed easily. As the disease progresses, bone is destroyed and teeth loosen. Tooth loss is common.

Illness, disease, and some drugs often cause a bad taste in the mouth. They may cause a whitish coating in the mouth and on the tongue. Others cause redness and swelling in the mouth and on the tongue. Dry mouth is common from oxygen, smoking, decreased fluid intake, and anxiety. Some drugs cause dry mouth.

The nurse assesses the person's need for mouth care. The speech/language pathologist and the dietitian may also do so. Oral hygiene is given on awakening, after meals, and at bedtime. Many people practice oral hygiene before meals. Some persons need mouth care every 2 hours or more often. Always follow the care plan. *See Focus on Children: Oral Hygiene.*

### EQUIPMENT

A toothbrush, toothpaste, dental floss, and mouthwash are needed. The toothbrush should have soft bristles. Persons with dentures need a denture cleaner, denture cup, and denture brush or toothbrush. Use only denture cleaning products. Otherwise, you could damage dentures.

Sponge swabs are used for persons with sore, tender mouths. They also are used for unconscious persons. Use sponge swabs with care. Check the foam pad to make sure it is tight on the stick. The person could choke on the foam pad if it comes off the stick.

---

**DELEGATION GUIDELINES:** *Oral Hygiene*
To assist with oral hygiene, you need this information from the nurse and the care plan:
- The type of oral hygiene to give (pp. 316-323)
- If flossing is needed (p. 318)
- What cleaning agent and equipment to use
- If lubricant is applied to the lips; if so, what lubricant to use
- How often to give oral hygiene
- How much help the person needs
- What observations to report and record:
  —Dry, cracked, swollen, or blistered lips
  —Mouth or breath odor
  —Redness, swelling, irritation, sores, or white patches in the mouth or on the tongue
  —Bleeding, swelling, or redness of the gums
  —Loose teeth
  —Rough, sharp, or chipped areas on dentures

---

### FOCUS ON CHILDREN
#### ORAL HYGIENE

Infants need mouth care to remove food and bacteria. This helps prevent "baby bottle tooth decay." Wipe their gums with a clean gauze pad after each feeding. After the first baby tooth erupts, begin brushing with a child's soft toothbrush.

---

**SAFETY ALERT:** *Oral Hygiene*
Follow Standard Precautions and the Bloodborne Pathogen Standard when giving oral hygiene. You have contact with the person's mucous membranes. Gums may bleed during mouth care. Also, the mouth has many microbes. Pathogens spread through sexual contact may be in the mouths of some persons.

## BRUSHING TEETH

Many people perform oral hygiene themselves. Others need help gathering and setting up equipment. You may have to brush the teeth of persons who:

- Are very weak
- Cannot use or move their arms
- Are too confused to brush their teeth

*See Focus on Children: Brushing Teeth.*

> ### FOCUS ON CHILDREN
> BRUSHING TEETH
>
> Children learn to brush their teeth around 3 years of age. They may not be thorough. They need help brushing. Older children can do a thorough job. Remind them when to brush.

## ASSISTING THE PERSON TO BRUSH THE TEETH

### QUALITY OF LIFE

Remember to:
- Knock before entering the person's room
- Address the person by name
- Introduce yourself by name and title

### PRE-PROCEDURE

1 Follow *Delegation Guidelines: Oral Hygiene*, p. 315. See *Safety Alert: Oral Hygiene*, p. 315.
2 Explain the procedure to the person.
3 Practice hand hygiene.
4 Collect the following:
   - Toothbrush
   - Toothpaste
   - Mouthwash (or solution noted on the care plan)
   - Dental floss (if used)
   - Water glass with cool water
   - Straw
   - Kidney basin
   - Hand towel
   - Paper towels
5 Place the paper towels on the overbed table. Arrange items on top of them.
6 Identify the person. Check the ID bracelet against the assignment sheet. Call the person by name.
7 Provide for privacy.
8 Position the person so he or she can brush with ease.

### PROCEDURE

9 Lower the bed rail (if used).
10 Place the towel over the person's chest. This protects garments and linens from spills.
11 Adjust the overbed table in front of the person.
12 Let the person perform oral hygiene. This includes brushing the teeth, rinsing the mouth, flossing, and using mouthwash or other solution.
13 Remove the towel when the person is done.
14 Adjust the overbed table next to the bed.

### POST-PROCEDURE

15 Provide for comfort.
16 Place the signal light within reach.
17 Raise or lower bed rails. Follow the care plan.
18 Clean and return items to their proper place. Wear gloves.
19 Wipe off the overbed table with the paper towels. Discard the paper towels.
20 Remove the gloves. Decontaminate your hands.
21 Unscreen the person.
22 Follow agency policy for dirty linen.
23 Decontaminate your hands.
24 Report and record your observations.

## BRUSHING THE PERSON'S TEETH

*NNAAP™*

### QUALITY OF LIFE

Remember to:
- Knock before entering the person's room
- Address the person by name
- Introduce yourself by name and title

### PRE-PROCEDURE

1 Follow *Delegation Guidelines: Oral Hygiene*, p. 315. See *Safety Alert: Oral Hygiene*, p. 315.
2 Explain the procedure to the person.
3 Practice hand hygiene.
4 Collect gloves and items listed in procedure: *Assisting the Person to Brush the Teeth.*
5 Place the paper towels on the overbed table. Arrange items on top of them.
6 Identify the person. Check the ID bracelet against the assignment sheet. Call the person by name.
7 Provide for privacy.
8 Raise the bed for body mechanics. Bed rails are up if used.

### PROCEDURE

9 Lower the bed rail near you if up.
10 Assist the person to a sitting position or to a side-lying position near you.
11 Place the towel over the person's chest.
12 Adjust the overbed table so you can reach it with ease.
13 Put on the gloves.
14 Apply toothpaste to the toothbrush.
15 Hold the toothbrush over the kidney basin. Pour some water over the brush.
16 Brush the teeth gently (Fig. 16-3, p. 318).
17 Brush the tongue gently.
18 Let the person rinse the mouth with water. Hold the kidney basin under the person's chin (Fig. 16-4, p. 318). Repeat this step as needed.
19 Floss the person's teeth (p. 318).
20 Let the person use mouthwash or other solution. Hold the kidney basin under the chin.
21 Remove the towel when done.
22 Remove and discard the gloves. Decontaminate your hands.

### POST-PROCEDURE

23 Provide for comfort.
24 Place the signal light within reach.
25 Lower the bed to its lowest position.
26 Raise or lower bed rails. Follow the care plan.
27 Clean and return equipment to its proper place. Wear gloves.
28 Wipe off the overbed table with the paper towels. Discard the paper towels.
29 Remove the gloves. Decontaminate your hands.
30 Adjust the overbed table for the person.
31 Unscreen the person.
32 Follow agency policy for dirty linen.
33 Decontaminate your hands.
34 Report and record your observations.

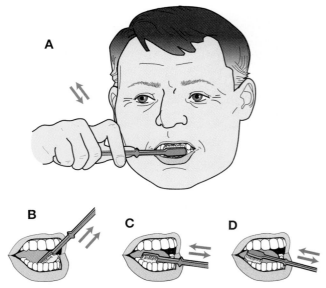

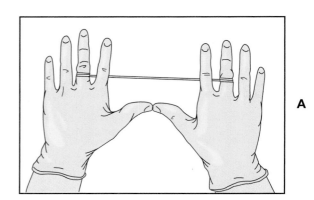

FIG. 16-3 Brushing teeth. **A,** The brush is at a 45-degree angle to the gums. Teeth are brushed with short strokes. **B,** The brush is at a 45-degree angle against the inside of the front teeth. Teeth are brushed from the gum to the crown of the tooth with short strokes. **C,** The brush is held horizontally against the inner surfaces of the teeth. The teeth are brushed back and forth. **D,** The brush is positioned on the biting surfaces of the teeth. The teeth are brushed back and forth.

## FLOSSING

Flossing removes plaque and tartar from the teeth. These substances cause periodontal disease (p. 315). Flossing also removes food from between the teeth. Usually done after brushing, it can be done at other times. Some people floss after meals. If done once a day, bedtime is the best time to floss.

You need to floss for persons who cannot do so. *See Focus on Children: Flossing. See Focus on Older Persons: Flossing.*

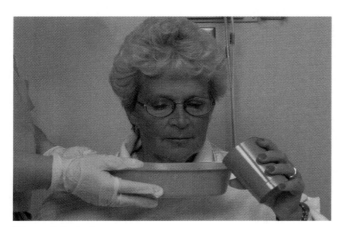

FIG. 16-4 The kidney basin is held under the person's chin.

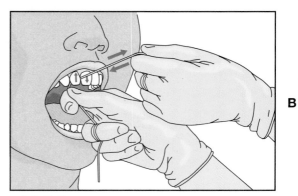

FIG. 16-5 Flossing. **A,** Floss is held between the middle fingers to floss the upper teeth. **B,** Floss is moved in up-and-down motions between the teeth. Floss is moved up and down from the crown to the gum line.

By age 2½ years, all baby teeth have erupted. Flossing begins at this time. You need to floss for preschoolers. Older children can floss themselves. They may need reminding and some supervision.

Flossing was not a common oral hygiene measure many years ago. Therefore some older persons do not floss their teeth. Others do. Follow the person's care plan.

## FLOSSING THE PERSON'S TEETH

### QUALITY OF LIFE

Remember to:
- Knock before entering the person's room
- Address the person by name
- Introduce yourself by name and title

### PRE-PROCEDURE

1 Follow *Delegation Guidelines: Oral Hygiene*, p. 315. See *Safety Alert: Oral Hygiene*, p. 315.
2 Explain the procedure to the person.
3 Practice hand hygiene.
4 Collect the following:
   - Kidney basin
   - Water glass with cool water
   - Floss
   - Hand towel
   - Paper towels
   - Gloves
5 Place the paper towels on the overbed table. Arrange items on top of them.
6 Identify the person. Check the ID bracelet against the assignment sheet. Call the person by name.
7 Provide for privacy.
8 Raise the bed for body mechanics. Bed rails are up if used.

### PROCEDURE

9 Lower the bed rail near you if up.
10 Assist the person to a sitting position or a side-lying position near you.
11 Place the towel over the person's chest.
12 Adjust the overbed table so you can reach it with ease.
13 Put on the gloves.
14 Break off an 18-inch piece of floss from the dispenser.
15 Hold the floss between the middle fingers of each hand (Fig. 16-5, *A*).
16 Stretch the floss with your thumbs.
17 Start at the upper back tooth on the right side. Work around to the left side.
18 Move the floss gently up and down between the teeth (Fig. 16-5, *B*). Move floss up and down against the side of the tooth. Work from the top of the crown to the gum line.
19 Move to a new section of floss after every second tooth.
20 Floss the lower teeth. Use up-and-down motions as for the upper teeth. Start on the right side. Work around to the left side.
21 Let the person rinse his or her mouth. Hold the kidney basin under the chin. Repeat rinsing as necessary.
22 Remove the towel when done.
23 Remove and discard the gloves. Decontaminate your hands.

### POST-PROCEDURE

24 Follow steps 23 through 34 for procedure: *Brushing the Person's Teeth*, p. 317.

# MOUTH CARE FOR THE UNCONSCIOUS PERSON

Unconscious persons cannot eat or drink. They may breathe with their mouths open. Many receive oxygen. These factors cause mouth dryness. They also cause crusting on the tongue and mucous membranes. Oral hygiene keeps the mouth clean and moist. It also helps prevents infection.

The care plan tells you what cleaning agent to use. Use sponge swabs to apply the cleaning agent. Apply a lubricant (check the care plan) to the lips after cleaning. It prevents cracking of the lips.

Unconscious persons usually cannot swallow. Protect them from choking and aspiration. **Aspiration** is breathing fluid or an object into the lungs. It can cause pneumonia and death. To prevent aspiration:

- Position the person on one side with the head turned well to the side (Fig. 16-6). In this position, excess fluid runs out of the mouth.
- Use only a small amount of fluid. Sometimes oral suctioning (Chapter 30) is needed.

Keep the person's mouth open with a padded tongue blade (Fig. 16-7). Do not use your fingers. The person can bite down on them. The bite breaks the skin and creates a portal of entry for microbes. Infection is a risk.

Unconscious persons cannot speak or respond to you. However, some can hear. Always assume that unconscious persons can hear. Explain what you are doing step by step. Also tell the person when you are done and when you are leaving the room.

Mouth care is given at least every 2 hours. Follow the nurse's directions and the care plan. Unconscious persons are also repositioned at least every 2 hours. Combine mouth care, skin care, and comfort measures to promote comfort and safety.

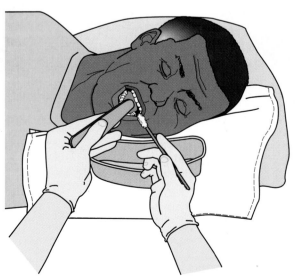

**FIG. 16-6** The head of the unconscious person is turned well to the side to prevent aspiration. A padded tongue blade is used to keep the mouth open while cleaning the mouth with swabs.

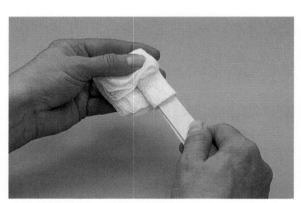

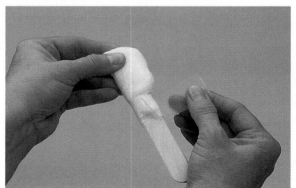

**FIG. 16-7** Making a padded tongue blade. **A,** Place two wooden tongue blades together. Wrap gauze around the top half. **B,** Tape the gauze in place.

## PROVIDING MOUTH CARE FOR AN UNCONSCIOUS PERSON

### QUALITY OF LIFE

Remember to:
- Knock before entering the person's room
- Address the person by name
- Introduce yourself by name and title

### PRE-PROCEDURE

1 Follow *Delegation Guidelines: Oral Hygiene*, p. 315. See *Safety Alert: Oral Hygiene*, p. 315.
2 Practice hand hygiene.
3 Collect the following:
- Cleaning agent (check the care plan)
- Sponge swabs
- Padded tongue blade
- Water glass with cool water
- Hand towel
- Kidney basin
- Lip lubricant
- Paper towels
- Gloves

4 Place the paper towels on the overbed table. Arrange items on top of them.
5 Identify the person. Check the ID bracelet against the assignment sheet. Call the person by name.
6 Explain the procedure to the person.
7 Provide for privacy.
8 Raise the bed for body mechanics. Bed rails are up if used.

### PROCEDURE

9 Lower the bed rail near you if up.
10 Put on the gloves.
11 Position the person in a side-lying position near you. Turn his or her head well to the side.
12 Place the towel under the person's face.
13 Place the kidney basin under the chin.
14 Adjust the overbed table so you can reach it with ease.
15 Separate the upper and lower teeth. Use the padded tongue blade. Be gentle. Never use force. If you have problems, ask the nurse for help.
16 Clean the mouth using sponge swabs moistened with the cleaning agent (see Fig. 16-6):
  a Clean the chewing and inner surfaces of the teeth.
  b Clean the outer surfaces of the teeth.
  c Swab the roof of the mouth, inside of the cheeks, and the lips.
  d Swab the tongue.
  e Moisten a clean swab with water. Swab the mouth to rinse.
  f Place used swabs in the kidney basin.
17 Apply lubricant to the lips.
18 Remove the towel.
19 Remove and discard the gloves. Decontaminate your hands.
20 Explain that the procedure is done. Explain that you will reposition him or her.
21 Reposition the person. Provide for comfort.
22 Raise or lower bed rails. Follow the care plan.

### POST-PROCEDURE

23 Place the signal light within reach.
24 Lower the bed to its lowest position.
25 Clean and return equipment to its proper place. Discard disposable items. (Wear gloves.)
26 Wipe off the overbed table with paper towels. Discard the paper towels.
27 Remove the gloves. Decontaminate your hands.
28 Unscreen the person.
29 Tell the person that you are leaving the room.
30 Follow agency policy for dirty linen.
31 Decontaminate your hands.
32 Report and record observations.

# DENTURE CARE

Mouth care is given and dentures cleaned as often as natural teeth are. Dentures are slippery when wet. They easily break or chip if dropped onto a hard surface (floors, sinks). Hold them firmly. During cleaning, firmly hold them over a basin of water lined with a towel. This prevents them from falling onto a hard surface.

The cleaning agent has the manufacturer's instructions. They explain how to use the cleaner and what water temperature to use. Hot water causes dentures to loose their shape (warp). If not worn after cleaning, store dentures in a container with cool water or a denture soaking solution. Otherwise they can dry out and warp.

Dentures are usually removed at bedtime. Some people do not wear their dentures. Others wear dentures for eating and remove them after meals. Remind them not to wrap dentures in tissues or napkins. Otherwise, they are easily discarded.

Many people clean their own dentures. Some need help collecting and cleaning items. They may need help getting to the bathroom. You clean dentures for those who cannot do so.

Many people do not like being seen without their dentures. Privacy is important. Allow privacy when the person cleans dentures. If you clean dentures, return them to the person as quickly as possible.

---

**SAFETY ALERT:** *Denture Care*

Dentures are the person's property. They are costly. Handle them very carefully. Label the denture cup with the person's name and room number. Report lost or damaged dentures to the nurse at once. Losing or damaging dentures is negligent conduct.

---

## PROVIDING DENTURE CARE

NNAAP™

### QUALITY OF LIFE

Remember to:
- Knock before entering the person's room
- Address the person by name
- Introduce yourself by name and title

### PRE-PROCEDURE

1 Follow *Delegation Guidelines: Oral Hygiene*, p. 315. See *Safety Alerts: Oral Hygiene*, p. 315, and *Denture Care*.
2 Explain the procedure to the person.
3 Practice hand hygiene.
4 Collect the following:
   - Denture brush or soft-bristle toothbrush
   - Denture cup labeled with the person's name and room number
   - Cleaning agent
   - Water glass with cool water
   - Straw
   - Mouthwash (or other noted solution)
   - Kidney basin
   - Two hand towels
   - Gauze squares
   - Gloves
5 Identify the person. Check the ID bracelet against the assignment sheet. Call the person by name.
6 Provide for privacy.

## PROVIDING DENTURE CARE—CONT'D

NNAAP™

### PROCEDURE

7 Lower the bed rail near you if used.

8 Place a towel over the person's chest.

9 Put on the gloves.

10 Ask the person to remove the dentures. Carefully place them in the kidney basin.

11 Remove the dentures if the person cannot do so. Use gauze squares to get a good grip on the slippery dentures:

  **a** Grasp the upper denture with your thumb and index finger (Fig. 16-8, p. 324). Move it up and down slightly to break the seal. Gently remove the denture. Place it in the kidney basin.

  **b** Grasp and remove the lower denture with your thumb and index finger. Turn it slightly, and lift it out of the mouth. Place it in the kidney basin.

12 Follow the care plan for raising bed rails.

13 Take the kidney basin, denture cup, brush, and cleaning agent to the sink.

14 Line the sink with a towel. Fill the sink with water.

15 Rinse each denture under warm running water. (Some states require cool water.) Rinse out the denture cup.

16 Return dentures to the denture cup.

17 Apply the cleaning agent to the brush.

18 Brush the dentures as in Figure 16-9, p. 324.

19 Rinse dentures under running water. Use warm or cool water as directed by the cleaning agent manufacturer. (Some states require cool water.)

20 Place dentures in the denture cup. Cover the dentures with cool water.

21 Clean the kidney basin.

22 Take the denture cup and kidney basin to the bedside table.

23 Lower the bed rail if up.

24 Position the person for oral hygiene.

25 Have the person use mouthwash (or noted solution). Hold the kidney basin under the chin.

26 Ask the person to insert the dentures. Insert them if the person cannot:

  **a** Hold the upper denture firmly with your thumb and index finger. Raise the upper lip with the other hand. Insert the denture. Gently press on the denture with your index fingers to make sure it is in place.

  **b** Hold the lower denture with your thumb and index finger. Pull the lower lip down slightly. Insert the denture. Gently press down on it to make sure it is in place.

27 Place the denture cup in the top drawer of the bedside stand if the dentures are not worn. The dentures must be in water or in a denture soaking solution.

28 Remove the towel.

29 Remove the gloves. Decontaminate your hands.

### POST-PROCEDURE

30 Assist with hand washing.

31 Provide for comfort.

32 Place the signal light within reach.

33 Raise or lower bed rails. Follow the care plan.

34 Unscreen the person.

35 Clean and return equipment to its proper place. Discard disposable items. Wear gloves for this step.

36 Follow agency policy for dirty linen.

37 Decontaminate your hands.

38 Report and record your observations.

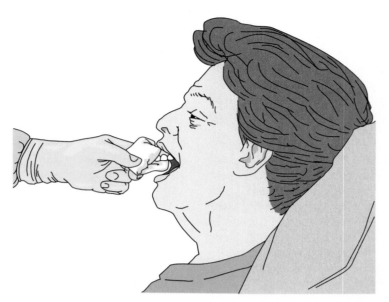

**FIG. 16-8** Remove the upper denture by grasping it with the thumb and index finger of one hand. Use a piece of gauze to grasp the slippery denture.

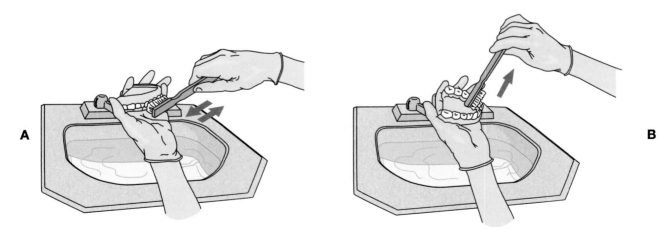

**FIG. 16-9** Cleaning dentures. **A,** Outer surfaces of the upper denture are brushed with back-and-forth motions. Note that the denture is held over the sink. The sink is filled halfway with water and is lined with a towel. **B,** Position the brush vertically to clean the inner surfaces of the denture. Use upward strokes.

# BATHING

Bathing cleans the skin. It also cleans the mucous membranes of the genital and anal areas. Microbes, dead skin, perspiration, and excess oils are removed. A bath is refreshing and relaxing. Circulation is stimulated and body parts exercised. Observations are made, and you have time to talk to the person.

Complete or partial bed baths, tub baths, or showers are given. The method depends on the person's condition, self-care abilities, and personal choice. Bathing is common after breakfast. However, the person's choice of bath time is respected whenever possible.

Bathing frequency is a personal matter. Some people bathe daily. Others bathe twice a week. Personal choice, weather, activity, and illness affect bathing frequency. Ill persons may have fevers and perspire heavily. They need frequent bathing. Other illnesses and dry skin may limit bathing to every 2 or 3 days.

The rules for bed baths, showers, and tub baths are in Box 16-2. Table 16-1, p. 326, describes common skin care products.

*See Focus on Children: Bathing. See Focus on Older Persons: Bathing,* p. 326.

---

### ▶ FOCUS ON CHILDREN
#### BATHING

The nurse collects information about the child's bathing practices on admission. The care plan reflects the child's normal practices and needs during illness.

## DELEGATION GUIDELINES: *Bathing*

To assist with bathing, you need this information from the nurse and the care plan:

- What bath to give—complete bed bath, partial bath, tub bath, shower, towel bath, or bag bath.
- How much help the person needs.
- The person's activity or position limits.
- What water temperature to use. Bath water cools rapidly. Therefore water temperature for a complete bed bath is usually between 110° and 115° F (43.3° and 46.1° C) for adults. Infants and older persons have fragile skin. They need lower water temperatures.
- What skin care products to use and what the person prefers.
- What observations to report and record:
  - The color of the skin, lips, nail beds, and sclera (whites of the eyes)
  - The location and description of rashes
  - Dry skin
  - Bruises or open skin areas
  - Pale or reddened areas, particularly over bony parts
  - Drainage or bleeding from wounds or body openings
  - Swelling of the feet and legs
  - Corns or calluses on the feet
  - Skin temperature
  - Complaints of pain or discomfort

---

### BOX 16-2    RULES FOR BATHING

- Follow the care plan for bathing method and skin care products.
- Allow personal choice whenever possible.
- Follow Standard Precautions and the Bloodborne Pathogen Standard.
- Collect needed items before starting the procedure.
- Provide for privacy. Screen the person. Close doors, shades, and drapes.
- Assist the person with elimination. Bathing stimulates the need to urinate. Comfort and relaxation increase if urination needs are met.
- Cover the person for warmth and privacy.
- Reduce drafts. Close doors and windows.
- Protect the person from falling.
- Use good body mechanics at all times.

- Know what water temperature to use. See *Delegation Guidelines: Bathing.*
- Keep bar soap in the soap dish between latherings. This prevents soapy water.
- Wash from the cleanest to the dirtiest areas.
- Encourage the person to help as much as is safely possible.
- Rinse the skin thoroughly. You must remove all soap.
- Pat the skin dry to avoid irritating or breaking the skin. Do not rub the skin.
- Dry under the breasts, between skin folds, in the perineal area, and between the toes.
- Bathe the skin whenever feces or urine is present. This prevents skin breakdown and odors.

*Safety Alert: Bathing*

Hot water can burn delicate and fragile skin. Measure water temperature according to agency policy. If unsure if the water is too hot, ask the nurse to check it.

Protect the person from falls. Practice the measures presented in Chapter 10.

Use caution when applying powder. Do not use powders near persons with respiratory disorders. Inhaling powder can irritate the airway and lungs. Before applying powder, check with the nurse and the care plan. To safely apply powder:

- Do not shake or sprinkle powder onto the person
- Turn away from the person
- Sprinkle a small amount of powder onto your hands or a cloth
- Apply the powder in a thin layer

Beds are made after baths. After making the bed, lower the bed to its lowest position. Then lock the bed wheels. For an occupied bed, raise or lower bed rails according to the care plan.

Protect the person and yourself from infection. When giving baths and making beds, contact with blood, body fluids, secretions, and excretions is likely. Follow Standard Precautions and the Bloodborne Pathogen Standard.

## FOCUS ON OLDER PERSONS
### BATHING

Dry skin occurs with aging. Soap also dries the skin. Dry skin is easily damaged. Therefore older persons usually need a complete bath or shower two times a week. Partial baths are taken the other days. Some bathe daily but not with soap. Thorough rinsing is needed when using soap. Lotions and oils help keep the skin soft.

Some older persons have dementia. Bathing may scare or frighten them. They do not understand what is happening or why. They may fear harm or danger. Therefore they may resist care and become agitated and combative. They may shout at the caregiver and cry out for help.

The rules in Box 16-2 apply when bathing persons with dementia. The care plan includes measures to help the person through the bathing procedure. Such measures include:

- Complete pre-procedure activities—ready supplies and linens, increase room temperature, and so on.
- Do not rush the person.
- Use a calm, pleasant voice.
- Divert the person's attention (Chapter 35).
- Be gentle.
- Calm the person.
- Try the bath later if the person continues to resist care.

| TABLE 16-1 | SKIN CARE PRODUCTS | |
| --- | --- | --- |
| **Type** | **Purpose** | **Care Considerations** |
| Soaps | Clean the skin<br>Remove dirt, dead skin, skin oil, some microbes, and perspiration | Tend to dry and irritate the skin<br>Dry skin is easily injured and causes itching and discomfort<br>Skin must be rinsed well to remove all soap<br>Not needed for every bath; plain water can clean the skin<br>Plain water is often used for older persons because of dry skin<br>People with dry skin may prefer soaps containing bath oils<br>Not used if a person has very dry skin |
| Bath oils | Keep the skin soft and prevent drying | Some soaps contain bath oil<br>Liquid bath oil can be added to bath water<br>Showers and tubs become slippery from bath oils; safety precautions are needed to prevent falls |
| Creams and lotions | Protect the skin from the drying effect of air and evaporation | Do not feel greasy but leave an oily film on the skin<br>Most are scented |
| Powders | Absorb moisture and prevent friction when two skin surfaces rub together | Usually applied under the breasts, under the arms, and in the groin area, and sometimes between the toes<br>Applied to dry skin in a thin, even layer<br>Excessive amounts cause caking and crusts that can irritate skin |
| Deodorants | Mask and control body odors | Applied to the underarms<br>Not applied to irritated skin<br>Do not take the place of bathing |
| Antiperspirants | Reduce the amount of perspiration | Applied to the underarms<br>Not applied to irritated skin<br>Do not take the place of bathing |

## THE COMPLETE BED BATH

The *complete bed bath* involves washing the person's entire body in bed. Persons who are unconscious, paralyzed, in a cast or traction, or weak from illness or surgery may need bed baths.

A bed bath is new to some people. Some are embarrassed to have others see their bodies. Some fear exposure. Explain how the bed bath is given. Also explain how you cover the body for privacy.

*See Focus on Children: The Complete Bed Bath. See Focus on Older Persons: The Complete Bed Bath.*

### FOCUS ON CHILDREN
#### THE COMPLETE BED BATH

See Chapter 38 for bathing infants. Follow the adult procedure for bathing toddlers and older children. Infants and young children have fragile skin. Lower water temperatures are used. Ask the nurse about what water temperature to use.

### FOCUS ON OLDER PERSONS
#### THE COMPLETE BED BATH

Older persons have fragile skin. Lower water temperatures are used. Ask the nurse about what water temperature to use.

## TOWEL BATHS

For the towel bath, an over-sized towel is used. It covers the body from the neck to the feet. The towel is saturated with a cleansing solution. The solution contains water, a cleaning agent, and a skin-softening agent. It also has a drying agent so the person's body dries quickly. To give a towel bath, follow agency procedures. *See Focus on Older Persons: Towel Baths.*

## BAG BATHS

Bag baths are commercially prepared or prepared at the agency. There are 8 to 10 washcloths in a plastic bag. They are moistened with a cleaning agent that does not need rinsing. The washcloths are warmed in a microwave. (The nurse and manufacturer's instructions tell you what microwave setting to use.) A new washcloth is used for each body part. The skin air-dries. Towels are not needed.

*Text continued on p. 332.*

### FOCUS ON OLDER PERSONS
#### TOWEL BATHS

The towel bath is quick, soothing, and relaxing. Persons with dementia often respond well to this type of bath. The nurse and care plan tell you when to use the towel bath.

## GIVING A COMPLETE BED BATH

NNAAP™

### QUALITY OF LIFE

Remember to:
- Knock before entering the person's room
- Address the person by name
- Introduce yourself by name and title

### PRE-PROCEDURE

1 Follow *Delegation Guidelines: Bathing*, p. 325. See *Safety Alert: Bathing.*
2 Identify the person. Check the ID bracelet against the assignment sheet. Call the person by name.
3 Explain the procedure to the person.
4 Offer the bedpan or urinal (Chapter 18). Provide for privacy.
5 Practice hand hygiene.
6 Collect clean linen for a closed bed (see procedure: *Making a Closed Bed*, p. 298). Place linen on a clean surface.
7 Collect the following:
   - Wash basin
   - Soap
   - Bath thermometer
   - Orange stick or nail file
   - Washcloth
   - Two bath towels and two hand towels
   - Bath blanket
   - Clothing, gown, or pajamas
   - Items for oral hygiene
   - Lotion
   - Powder
   - Deodorant or antiperspirant
   - Brush and comb
   - Other grooming items if requested
   - Paper towels
   - Gloves
8 Arrange items on the overbed table. Adjust the height as needed.
9 Close doors and windows to prevent drafts.
10 Provide for privacy.
11 Raise the bed for body mechanics. Bed rails are up if used.

*Continued.*

## GIVING A COMPLETE BED BATH—CONT'D

### PROCEDURE

12 Remove the signal light. Lower the bed rail near you if up.
13 Put on gloves.
14 Provide oral hygiene.
15 Cover the person with a bath blanket. Remove top linens (see procedure: *Making an Occupied Bed,* p. 305).
16 Lower the head of the bed. It is as flat as possible. The person has at least one pillow.
17 Cover the overbed table with paper towels.
18 Raise the bed rail near you if bed rails are used. Both bed rails must be up.
19 Fill the wash basin two-thirds full with water. Water temperature is usually 110° to 115° F (43.3° to 46.1° C) for adults. Measure water temperature. Use a bath thermometer. Or test the water by dipping your elbow or inner wrist into the basin.
20 Place the basin on the overbed table.
21 Lower the bed rail if up.
22 Place a hand towel over the person's chest.
23 Make a mitt with the washcloth (Fig. 16-10). Use a mitt for the entire bath.
24 Wash around the person's eyes with water. Do not use soap. Gently wipe from the inner to the outer aspect of the eye with a corner of the mitt (Fig. 16-11, p. 330). Clean around the far eye first. Repeat this step for the near eye. Use a clean part of the washcloth for each stroke.
25 Ask the person if you should use soap to wash the face.
26 Wash the face, ears, and neck. Rinse and pat dry with the towel on the chest.
27 Help the person move to the side of the bed near you.
28 Remove the gown. Do not expose the person. (Waiting to remove the gown at this time helps the person feel less exposed and more comfortable with the bath.)
29 Place a bath towel lengthwise under the far arm.
30 Support the arm with your palm under the person's elbow. His or her forearm rests on your forearm.
31 Wash the arm, shoulder, and underarm. Use long, firm strokes (Fig. 16-12, p. 330). Rinse and pat dry.
32 Place the basin on the towel. Put the person's hand into the water (Fig. 16-13, p. 330). Wash it well. Clean under fingernails with an orange stick or nail file.
33 Have the person exercise the hand and fingers.

34 Remove the basin. Dry the hand well. Cover the arm with the bath blanket.
35 Repeat steps 29 to 34 for the near arm.
36 Place a bath towel over the chest crosswise. Hold the towel in place. Pull the bath blanket from under the towel to the waist.
37 Lift the towel slightly, and wash the chest (Fig. 16-14, p. 330). Do not expose the person. Rinse and pat dry, especially under breasts.
38 Move the towel lengthwise over the chest and abdomen. Do not expose the person. Pull the bath blanket down to the pubic area.
39 Lift the towel slightly, and wash the abdomen (Fig. 16-15, p. 331). Rinse and pat dry.
40 Pull the bath blanket up to the shoulders, covering both arms. Remove the towel.
41 Change soapy or cool water. Measure bath water as in step 19. If bed rails are used, raise the bed rail near you before leaving the bedside. Lower it when you return.
42 Uncover the far leg. Do not expose the genital area. Place a towel lengthwise under the foot and leg.
43 Bend the knee, and support the leg with your arm. Wash it with long, firm strokes. Rinse and pat dry.
44 Place the basin on the towel near the foot.
45 Lift the leg slightly. Slide the basin under the foot.
46 Place the foot in the basin (Fig. 16-16, p. 331). Use an orange stick or nail file to clean under toenails if necessary. If the person cannot bend the knees:
   a Wash the foot. Carefully separate the toes. Rinse and pat dry.
   b Clean under the toenails with an orange stick or nail file if necessary.
47 Remove the basin. Dry the leg and foot. Cover the leg with the bath blanket. Remove the towel.
48 Repeat steps 42 to 47 for the near leg.
49 Change the water. Measure water temperature as in step 19. If bed rails are used, raise the bed rail near you before leaving the bedside. Lower it when you return.
50 Turn the person onto the side away from you. The person is covered with the bath blanket.
51 Uncover the back and buttocks. Do not expose the person. Place a towel lengthwise on the bed along the back.
52 Wash the back. Work from the back of the neck to the lower end of the buttocks. Use long, firm, continuous strokes (Fig. 16-17, p. 331). Rinse and dry well.

## GIVING A COMPLETE BED BATH—CONT'D

### PROCEDURE—CONT'D

53 Give a back massage (p. 339). The person may want the back massage after the bath.
54 Turn the person onto his or her back.
55 Change the water for perineal care. Measure water temperature as in step 19. (Some states also require changing gloves and hand hygiene at this time.) If bed rails are used, raise the bed rail near you before leaving the bedside. Lower it when you return.
56 Let the person wash the genital area. Adjust the overbed table so he or she can reach the wash basin, soap, and towels with ease. Place the signal light within reach. Ask the person to signal when finished. Make sure the person understands what to do.

57 Remove the gloves. Decontaminate your hands.
58 Answer the signal light promptly. Provide perineal care if the person cannot do so (p. 342). (Decontaminate your hands and wear gloves for perineal care.)
59 Give a back massage if you have not already done so.
60 Apply deodorant or antiperspirant. Apply lotion and powder as requested. See *Safety Alert: Bathing*, p. 326.
61 Put clean garments on the person.
62 Comb and brush the hair (Chapter 17).
63 Make the bed. Attach the signal light.

### POST-PROCEDURE

64 Provide for comfort.
65 Lower the bed to its lowest position.
66 Raise or lower bed rails. Follow the care plan.
67 Empty and clean the wash basin. Return it and other supplies to their proper place.
68 Wipe off the overbed table with the paper towels. Discard the paper towels.

69 Unscreen the person.
70 Follow agency policy for dirty linen.
71 Decontaminate your hands.
72 Report and record your observations.

**A**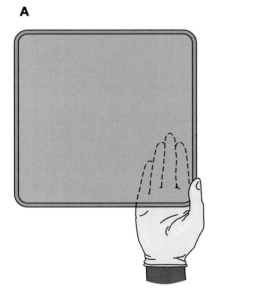

**B**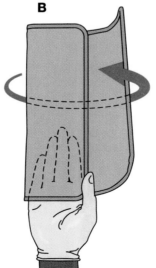

**C**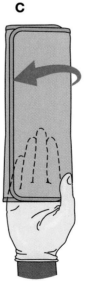

**D**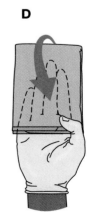

FIG. 16-10 Making a mitted washcloth. **A,** Grasp the near side of the washcloth with your thumb. **B,** Bring the washcloth around and behind your hand. **C,** Fold the side of the washcloth over your palm as you grasp it with your thumb. **D,** Fold the top of the washcloth down and tuck it under next to your palm.

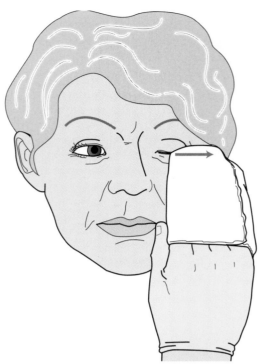

FIG. 16-11 Wash around the person's eyes with a mitted washcloth. Wipe from the inner to the outer aspect of the eye.

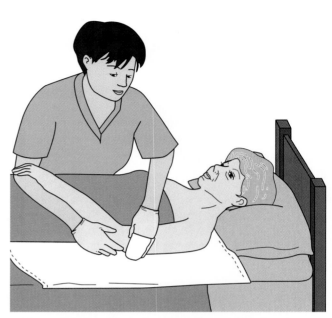

FIG. 16-12 Wash the person's arm with firm, long strokes using a mitted washcloth.

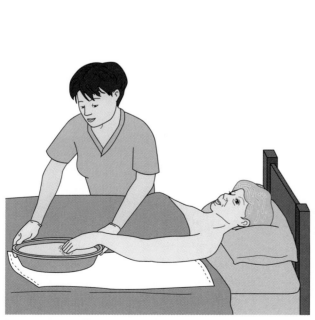

FIG. 16-13 The person's hands are washed by placing the wash basin on the bed.

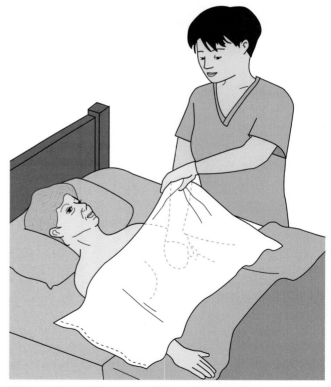

FIG. 16-14 The person's breasts are not exposed during the bath. A bath towel is placed horizontally over the chest area. The towel is lifted slightly to reach under to wash the breasts and chest.

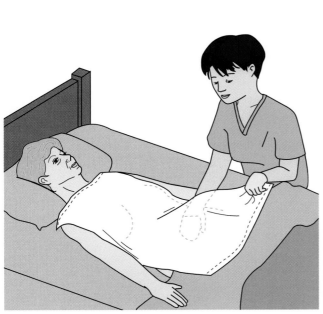

FIG. 16-15 The bath towel is turned so that it is vertical to cover the breasts and abdomen. The towel is lifted slightly to bathe the abdomen. The bath blanket covers the pubic area.

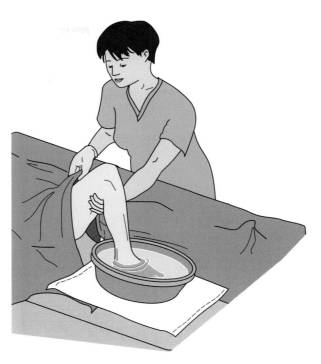

FIG. 16-16 The foot is washed by placing it in the wash basin on the bed.

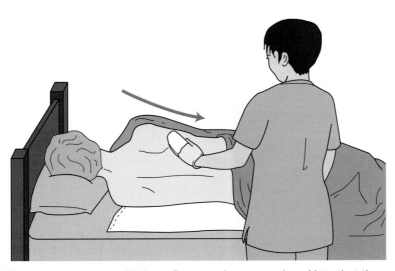

FIG. 16-17 The back is washed with long, firm, continuous strokes. Note that the person is in a side-lying position. A towel is placed lengthwise on the bed to protect the linens from water.

## ◼ THE PARTIAL BATH

The *partial bath* involves bathing the face, hands, axillae (underarms), back, buttocks, and perineal area. Odors or discomfort occurs if these areas are not clean. Some persons bathe themselves in bed or at the sink. You assist as needed. Most need help washing the back. You give partial baths to persons who cannot bathe themselves.

The rules for bathing apply (see Box 16-2). So do the complete bed bath considerations.

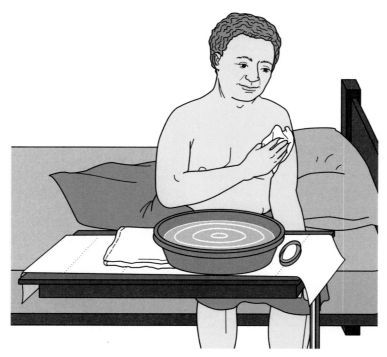

**FIG. 16-18** The person is bathing himself in bed. Necessary equipment is within his reach.

## GIVING A PARTIAL BATH

### QUALITY OF LIFE

Remember to:
- Knock before entering the person's room
- Address the person by name
- Introduce yourself by name and title

### PRE-PROCEDURE

1 Follow *Delegation Guidelines: Bathing*, p. 325. See *Safety Alert: Bathing*, p. 326.

2 Follow steps 2 through 10 in procedure: *Giving a Complete Bed Bath*, p. 327.

### PROCEDURE

3 Make sure the bed is in the lowest position.
4 Assist with oral hygiene. (Wear gloves.) Adjust the overbed table as needed.
5 Remove top linen. Cover the person with a bath blanket.
6 Cover the overbed table with paper towels.
7 Fill the wash basin with water. Water temperature is 110° to 115° F (43.3° to 46.1° C) for adults or as directed by the nurse. Measure water temperature with the bath thermometer. Or test bath water by dipping your elbow or inner wrist into the basin.
8 Place the basin on the overbed table.
9 Position the person in Fowler's position. Or assist him or her to sit at the bedside.
10 Adjust the overbed table so the person can reach the basin and supplies.
11 Help the person undress.
12 Ask the person to wash easy-to-reach body parts (Fig. 16-18). Explain that you will wash the back and areas the person cannot reach.
13 Place the signal light within reach. Ask him or her to signal when help is needed or bathing is complete.
14 Leave the room after decontaminating your hands.
15 Return when the signal light is on. Knock before entering. Decontaminate your hands.
16 Change the bath water. Measure bath water temperature as in step 7.
17 Raise the bed for body mechanics. The far bed rail is up if used.
18 Ask what was washed. Put on gloves. Wash and dry areas the person could not reach. The face, hands, underarms, back, buttocks, and perineal area are washed for the partial bath.
19 Remove the gloves. Decontaminate your hands.
20 Give a back massage.
21 Apply lotion, powder, and deodorant or antiperspirant as requested.
22 Help the person put on clean garments.
23 Assist with hair care and other grooming needs.
24 Assist the person to a chair. (Lower the bed if the person transfers to a chair.) Otherwise, turn the person onto the side away from you.
25 Make the bed.
26 Lower the bed to its lowest position.

### POST-PROCEDURE

27 Provide for comfort.
28 Place the signal light within reach.
29 Raise or lower bed rails. Follow the care plan.
30 Empty and clean the basin. Return the basin and supplies to their proper place.
31 Wipe off the overbed table with the paper towels. Discard the paper towels.
32 Unscreen the person.
33 Follow agency policy for dirty linen.
34 Decontaminate your hands.
35 Report and record your observations.

# TUB BATHS AND SHOWERS

Many people like tub baths or showers. Falls, chilling, and burns from hot water are risks. Safety is important (Box 16-3). The measures in Box 16-2 also apply.

Some bathrooms have showers. If not, reserve the tub or shower room for the person.

**TUB BATHS.** Many people find tub baths relaxing. A tub bath can cause a person to feel faint, weak, or tired. These are greater risks for persons who were on bedrest. A bath lasts no longer than 20 minutes.

Some agencies have portable tubs. The sides are lowered to transfer the person from bed to the tub (Fig. 16-19). The sides are raised after the transfer. Then the person is transported to the tub room. The tub is filled, and the bath proceeds in the usual manner.

Whirlpool tubs have special lifts (Fig. 16-20). The person is transported to the tub room in a special wheelchair or stretcher. The chair or stretcher and person are lifted into the tub (Fig. 16-21). The tub has a whirlpool action that cleanses. You wash the upper body. Carefully wash under breasts, between skin folds, and in the perineal area. Dry the person after the bath.

---

**BOX 16-3**    **SAFETY MEASURES FOR TUB BATHS AND SHOWERS**

- Know what water temperature to use. See *Delegation Guidelines: Tub Baths and Showers*, p. 336.
- Clean the tub or shower before and after use.
- Dry the tub or shower room floor.
- Check handrails, grab bars, hydraulic lifts, and other safety aids. They must be in working order.
- Place a bath mat in the tub or on the shower floor. This is not needed if there are nonskid strips or a nonskid surface.
- Cover the person for warmth and privacy. This includes during transport to and from the shower room or tub room.
- Place needed items within the person's reach.
- Place the signal light within the person's reach.
- Show the person how to use the signal light in the shower or tub room.
- Have the person use grab bars when getting in and out of the tub. The person must not use towel bars for support.
- Turn cold water on first; then hot water. Turn hot water off first; then cold water.
- Adjust water temperature and pressure to prevent chilling or burns. Do this before the person gets into the shower. If a shower chair is used, position it first.

- Direct water away from the person while adjusting water temperature and pressure.
- Fill the tub before the person gets into it.
- Measure water temperature. For showers and tub baths, use the digital display. Or you can use a bath thermometer for a tub bath.
- Keep the water spray directed toward the person during the shower. This helps keep him or her warm.
- Keep bar soap in the soap dish between latherings. This prevents soapy water. It reduces the risk of slipping and falls in showers and tubs.
- Avoid using bath oils. They make tub and shower surfaces slippery.
- Do not leave weak or unsteady persons unattended.
- Stay within hearing distance if the person can be left alone. Wait outside the shower curtain or door. You will be nearby if the person calls for you or has an accident.
- Drain the tub before the person gets out of the tub. Cover him or her to protect from exposure and chilling.

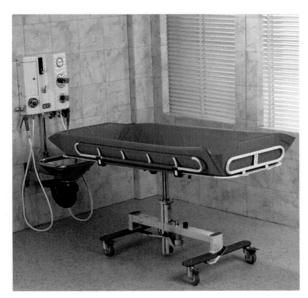

FIG. 16-19 Portable tub. (Courtesy Arjo, Inc, Morton Grove, Ill.)

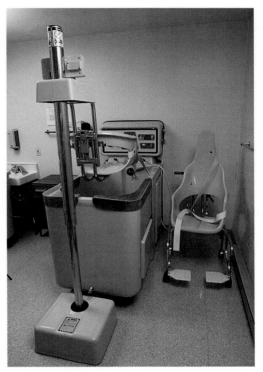

FIG. 16-20 Whirlpool tub with a hydraulic lift.

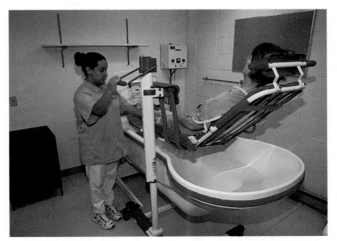

FIG. 16-21 The stretcher and person are lowered into the tub.

**SHOWERS.** Some patients and residents use shower chairs (Fig. 16-22). Water drains through an opening in the seat. The chair is used to transport the person to and from the shower stall or cabinet (Fig. 16-23). The wheels are locked during the shower to prevent the chair from moving.

Some people can stand in the shower. Have them use the grab bars for support during the shower. Like tubs, showers have nonskid surfaces. If not, a bath mat is used. Never let weak or unsteady persons stand in the shower. They need to use a shower chair.

Some shower rooms have two or more stalls or cabinets. Protect the person's privacy. The person has the right not to have his or body seen by others. Properly screen and cover the person. Also, close doors and the shower curtain.

Shower stalls and cabinets are easier to get into than a shower that is a bathtub-shower unit. The person does not have to step over the tub to get into the shower. *See Focus on Home Care: Showers*, p. 338. *See Focus on Children: Showers*, p. 338.

---

**DELEGATION GUIDELINES:** *Tub Baths and Showers*
Before helping a person with a tub bath or shower, you need this information from the nurse and the care plan:
- If the person takes a tub bath or shower
- What water temperature to use (usually 105° F; 40.5° C)
- If any special equipment is needed
- How much help the person needs
- Can the person bathe unattended
- What observations to report and record (p. 325)

---

**SAFETY ALERT:** *Tub Baths and Showers*
Some persons are very weak or large. Two staff members are needed to safely assist them with tub baths and showers.

You may use portable tubs, whirlpool equipment, and shower chairs. Always follow the manufacturer's instructions. Also, protect the person from falls, chilling, and burns. Follow the safety measures in Chapter 10. Remember to measure water temperature.

Clean the tub or shower before and after use. This prevents the spread of microbes and infection.

---

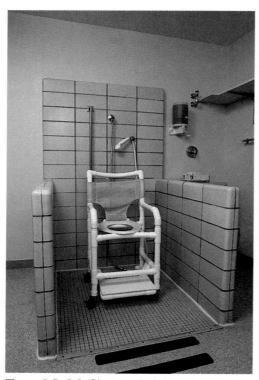

**FIG. 16-22** Shower chair in a shower stall.

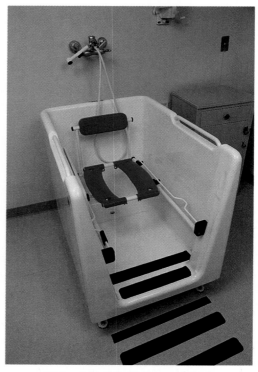

**FIG. 16-23** Shower cabinet.

## ASSISTING WITH A TUB BATH OR SHOWER

### QUALITY OF LIFE

Remember to:
- Knock before entering the person's room
- Address the person by name
- Introduce yourself by name and title

### PRE-PROCEDURE

1 Follow *Delegation Guidelines: Tub Baths and Showers*. See *Safety Alert: Tub Baths and Showers*.
2 Reserve the bathtub or shower.
3 Identify the person. Check the ID bracelet against the assignment sheet. Call the person by name.
4 Explain the procedure to the person.
5 Practice hand hygiene.
6 Collect the following:
   - Washcloth and two bath towels
   - Soap
   - Bath thermometer (for a tub bath)
   - Clothing, gown, or pajamas
   - Grooming items as requested
   - Robe and nonskid footwear
   - Rubber bath mat if needed
   - Disposable bath mat
   - Gloves
   - Wheelchair or shower chair

### PROCEDURE

7 Place items in the tub or shower room. Use the space provided or a chair.
8 Clean the tub or shower.
9 Place a rubber bath mat in the tub or on the shower floor. Do not block the drain.
10 Place the disposable bath mat on the floor in front of the tub or shower.
11 Put the *Occupied* sign on the door.
12 Return to the person's room. Provide for privacy.
13 Help the person sit on the side of the bed.
14 Help the person put on a robe and nonskid footwear.
15 Assist or transport the person to the tub or shower room.
16 *For a tub bath:*
   a Have the person sit on a chair.
   b Fill the tub halfway with warm water (105° F; 40.5° C). See Figure 16-24, p. 338. Measure water temperature with the bath thermometer. Or check the digital display (Fig. 16-25, p. 338).
17 *For a shower:*
   a Turn on the shower.
   b Adjust water temperature and pressure.
18 Help the person undress and remove footwear.
19 Help the person into the tub or shower. Position the shower chair, and lock the wheels.
20 Assist with washing if necessary. Wear gloves.

21 Ask the person to use the signal light when done or when help is needed. Remind the person that a tub bath lasts no longer than 20 minutes.
22 Place a towel across the chair.
23 Leave the room if the person can bathe unattended. If not, stay in the room or remain nearby. Remove the gloves and decontaminate your hands if you will leave the room.
24 Check the person every 5 minutes.
25 Return when he or she signals for you. Knock before entering. Decontaminate your hands.
26 Turn off the shower, or drain the tub. Cover the person while the tub drains.
27 Help the person out of the tub or shower and onto the chair.
28 Help the person dry off. Pat gently. Dry under breasts, between skin folds, in the perineal area, and between the toes.
29 Assist with lotion and other grooming items as needed.
30 Help the person dress and put on footwear.
31 Help the person return to the room. Provide for privacy.
32 Assist the person to a chair or into bed.
33 Provide a back massage if the person returns to bed.
34 Assist with hair care and other grooming needs.

### POST-PROCEDURE

35 Make the bed. Provide for comfort.
36 Raise or lower bed rails. Follow the care plan.
37 Place the signal light within reach.
38 Unscreen the person.
39 Clean the tub or shower. Remove soiled linen. Wear gloves for this step.
40 Discard disposable items. Put the *Unoccupied* sign on the door. Return supplies to their proper place.
41 Follow agency policy for dirty linen.
42 Decontaminate your hands.
43 Report and record your observations.

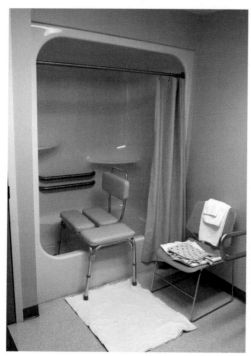

**FIG. 16-24** A bath mat is in the tub, the tub is filled halfway with water, and a floor mat is in front of the tub.

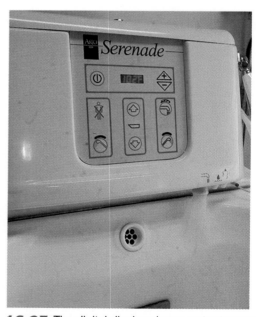

**FIG. 16-25** The digital display shows water temperature.

# THE BACK MASSAGE

The back massage (back rub) relaxes muscles and stimulates circulation. Massages are given after the bath and with HS care. You can also give back massages at other times. Examples include after repositioning or helping the person relax.

Back massages last 3 to 5 minutes. Observe the skin before the massage. Look for breaks in the skin, bruises, reddened areas, and other signs of skin breakdown.

Lotion reduces friction during the massage. It is warmed before being applied. To warm lotion, do one of the following:

- Place the bottle in the bath water.
- Hold the bottle under warm water.
- Rub some lotion between your hands.

The prone position is best for a massage. The side-lying position is often used. Use firm strokes. Always keep your hands in contact with the person's skin. After the massage, apply some lotion to the elbows, knees, and heels. This keeps the skin soft. These bony areas are at risk for skin breakdown.

**DELEGATION GUIDELINES:** *Back Massage*

Before giving a back massage, you need this information from the nurse and the care plan:

- Can the person have a back massage (see *Safety Alert: Back Massage*)
- How to position the person
- Does the person have position limits
- When the person should receive a back massage
- Does the person need frequent back massages for comfort and to relax
- What observations to report and record:
  —Bruising
  —Reddened areas
  —Signs of skin breakdown

**SAFETY ALERT:** *Back Massage*

Back massages are dangerous for persons with certain heart diseases, back injuries, back surgeries, skin diseases, and some lung disorders. Check with the nurse and care plan before giving back massages to persons with these conditions.

Do not massage bony areas that are reddened. Reddened areas signal skin breakdown and pressure ulcers. Massage can lead to further tissue damage.

Wear gloves if the person's skin is not intact. Always follow Standard Precautions and the Bloodborne Pathogen Standard.

# GIVING A BACK MASSAGE

## QUALITY OF LIFE

Remember to:
- Knock before entering the person's room
- Address the person by name
- Introduce yourself by name and title

## PRE-PROCEDURE

1 Follow *Delegation Guidelines: Back Massage*, p. 339. See *Safety Alert: Back Massage*, p. 339.
2 Identify the person. Check the ID bracelet against the assignment sheet. Call the person by name.
3 Explain the procedure to the person.
4 Practice hand hygiene.

5 Collect the following:
- Bath blanket
- Bath towel
- Lotion
6 Provide for privacy.
7 Raise the bed for body mechanics. Bed rails are up if used.

## PROCEDURE

8 Lower the bed rail near you if up.
9 Position the person in the prone or side-lying position. The back is toward you.
10 Expose the back, shoulders, upper arms, and buttocks. Cover the rest of the body with the bath blanket.
11 Lay the towel on the bed along the back.
12 Warm the lotion.
13 Explain that the lotion may feel cool and wet.
14 Apply lotion to the lower back area.
15 Stroke up from the buttocks to the shoulders. Then stroke down over the upper arms. Stroke up the upper arms, across the shoulders, and down the back to the buttocks (Fig. 16-26). Use firm strokes. Keep your hands in contact with the person's skin.

16 Repeat step 15 for at least 3 minutes.
17 Knead by grasping skin between your thumb and fingers (Fig. 16-27). Knead half of the back. Start at the buttocks and move up to the shoulder. Then knead down from the shoulder to the buttocks. Repeat on the other half of the back.
18 Apply lotion to bony areas. Use circular motions with the tips of your index and middle fingers. (Do not massage reddened bony areas.)
19 Use fast movements to stimulate. Use slow movements to relax the person.
20 Stroke with long, firm movements to end the massage. Tell the person you are finishing.
21 Cover the person. Remove the towel and bath blanket.

## POST-PROCEDURE

22 Provide for comfort.
23 Lower the bed to its lowest position.
24 Raise or lower bed rails. Follow the care plan.
25 Place the signal light within reach.
26 Return lotion to its proper place.

27 Unscreen the person.
28 Follow agency policy for dirty linen.
29 Decontaminate your hands.
30 Report and record your observations.

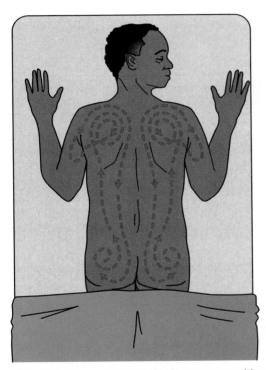

**FIG. 16-26** The person lies in the prone position for a back massage. Stroke upward from the buttocks to the shoulders, down over the upper arms, back up the upper arms, across the shoulders, and down the back to the buttocks.

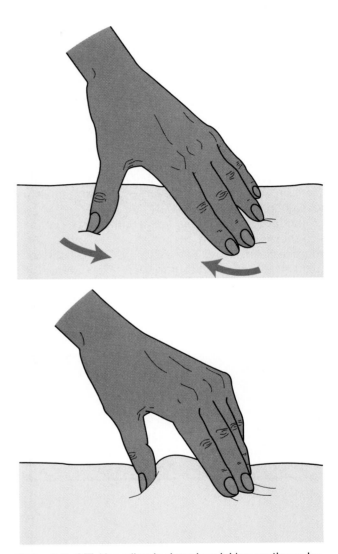

**FIG. 16-27** Kneading is done by picking up tissue between the thumb and fingers.

# PERINEAL CARE

**Perineal care (pericare)** involves cleaning the genital and anal areas. These areas provide a warm, moist, and dark place for microbes to grow. Cleaning prevents infection and odors, and it promotes comfort.

Perineal care is done daily during the bath. It also is done whenever the area is soiled with urine or feces. Persons with certain disorders need perineal care more often. It is given before and after some surgeries and after childbirth.

The person does perineal care if able. Otherwise, it is given by nursing staff. The procedure embarrasses many people and nursing staff, especially when it involves the other sex. *Perineum* and *perineal* are not common terms. Most people understand *privates, private parts, crotch, genitals,* or the *area between the legs.* Use terms the person understands. The term must also be in good taste professionally.

Standard Precautions, medical asepsis, and the Bloodborne Pathogen Standard are followed. Work from the cleanest area to the dirtiest. This is commonly called cleaning from "front to back." The urethral area (the front) is the cleanest. The anal area (the back) is the dirtiest. Therefore clean from the urethra to the anal area.

---

## FOCUS ON CHILDREN
### PERINEAL CARE

All children need perineal care. When diapers are worn, the perineal area is exposed to urine and feces. Poor wiping after urinating and bowel movements is a common problem in younger children. Older children may hesitate to clean the genital and anal areas.

---

The perineal area is delicate and easily injured. Use warm water, not hot. Use washcloths, towelettes, cotton balls, or swabs according to agency policy. Rinse thoroughly. Pat dry after rinsing. This reduces moisture and promotes comfort. *See Focus on Children: Perineal Care.*

---

**DELEGATION GUIDELINES:** *Perineal Care*

Before giving perineal care, you need this information from the nurse and the care plan:

- When perineal care needs to be done
- What terms the person understands—perineum, privates, private parts, crotch, genitals, area between the legs, and so on
- How much help the person needs
- What water temperature to use—usually 105° to 109° F (40.5° to 42.7° C)
- Any position restrictions or limits
- What observations to report and record:
  —Odors
  —Redness, swelling, discharge, or irritation
  —Complaints of pain, burning, or other discomfort
  —Signs of urinary or fecal incontinence (Chapters 18 and 19)

---

**SAFETY ALERT:** *Perineal Care*

Hot water can burn delicate perineal tissues. To prevent burns, measure water temperature according to agency policy. If the water seems too hot, ask the nurse to check it.

Protect yourself and the person from infection. Contact with blood, body fluids, secretions, and excretions is likely during perineal care. Follow Standard Precautions and the Bloodborne Pathogen Standard.

*Text continued on p. 346.*

---

## GIVING FEMALE PERINEAL CARE

NNAAP™

### QUALITY OF LIFE

Remember to:
- Knock before entering the person's room
- Address the person by name
- Introduce yourself by name and title

### PRE-PROCEDURE

1 Follow *Delegation Guidelines: Perineal Care.* See *Safety Alert: Perineal Care.*
2 Explain the procedure to the person.
3 Practice hand hygiene.

4 Collect the following:
- Soap
- At least 4 washcloths
- Bath towel

## GIVING FEMALE PERINEAL CARE—CONT'D

### PRE-PROCEDURE—CONT'D

- Bath blanket
- Bath thermometer
- Wash basin
- Waterproof pad
- Gloves
- Paper towels

5 Cover the overbed table with paper towels. Arrange items on top of them.
6 Identify the person. Check the ID bracelet against the assignment sheet. Call her by name.
7 Provide for privacy.
8 Raise the bed for body mechanics. Bed rails are up if used.

### PROCEDURE

9 Lower the bed rail near you if up.
10 Cover the person with a bath blanket. Move top linens to the foot of the bed.
11 Position the person on her back.
12 Drape her as in Figure 16-28, p. 344.
13 Raise the bed rail if used.
14 Fill the wash basin. Water temperature is about 105° to 109° F (40.5° to 42.7° C). Measure water temperature according to agency policy.
15 Place the basin on the overbed table.
16 Lower the bed rail if up.
17 Put on the gloves.
18 Help the person flex her knees and spread her legs. Or help her spread her legs as much as possible with her knees straight.
19 Place a waterproof pad under her buttocks.
20 Fold the corner of the bath blanket between her legs onto her abdomen.
21 Wet the washcloths. Squeeze out excess water before using them.
22 Apply soap to a washcloth.
23 Separate the labia. Clean downward from front to back with one stroke (Fig. 16-29, p. 344).
24 Repeat steps 22 and 23 until the area is clean. Use a clean part of the washcloth for each stroke. Use more than one washcloth if needed.

25 Rinse the perineum with a clean washcloth. Separate the labia. Stroke downward from front to back. Repeat as necessary. Use a clean part of the washcloth for each stroke. Use more than one washcloth if needed.
26 Pat the area dry with the towel.
27 Fold the blanket back between her legs.
28 Help the person lower her legs and turn onto her side away from you.
29 Apply soap to a washcloth.
30 Clean the rectal area. Clean from the vagina to the anus with one stroke (Fig. 16-30, p. 344).
31 Repeat steps 29 and 30 until the area is clean. Use a clean part of the washcloth for each stroke. Use more than one washcloth if needed.
32 Rinse the rectal area with a washcloth. Stroke from the vagina to the anus. Repeat as necessary. Use a clean part of the washcloth for each stroke. Use more than one washcloth if needed.
33 Pat the area dry with the towel.
34 Remove the waterproof pad.
35 Remove and discard the gloves. Decontaminate your hands.

### POST-PROCEDURE

36 Provide for comfort.
37 Cover the person. Remove the bath blanket.
38 Lower the bed to its lowest position.
39 Raise or lower bed rails. Follow the care plan.
40 Place the signal light within reach.
41 Empty and clean the wash basin. Wear gloves.
42 Return the basin and supplies to their proper place.

43 Wipe off the overbed table with the paper towels. Discard the paper towels.
44 Remove the gloves. Decontaminate your hands.
45 Unscreen the person.
46 Follow agency policy for dirty linen.
47 Decontaminate your hands.
48 Report and record your observations.

A

B

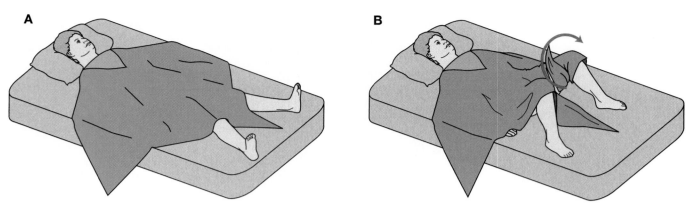

**FIG. 16-28** Draping for perineal care. **A,** Position the bath blanket like a diamond: one corner is at the neck, there is a corner at each side, and one corner is between the person's legs. **B,** Wrap the blanket around the leg by bringing the corner around under the leg and over the top. Tuck the corner under the hip.

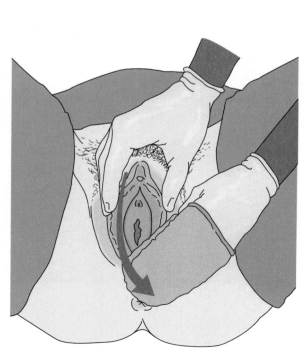

**FIG. 16-29** Separate the labia with one hand. Use a mitted washcloth to cleanse between the labia with downward strokes.

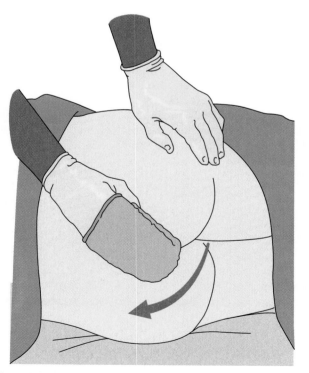

**FIG. 16-30** The rectal area is cleaned by wiping from the vagina to the anus. The side-lying position allows the anal area to be cleaned more thoroughly.

## GIVING MALE PERINEAL CARE

### QUALITY OF LIFE

Remember to:
- Knock before entering the person's room
- Address the person by name
- Introduce yourself by name and title

### PROCEDURE

1 Follow steps 1 through 22 in procedure: *Giving Female Perineal Care*, p. 343.
2 Retract the foreskin if the person is uncircumcised (Fig. 16-31).
3 Grasp the penis.
4 Clean the tip. Use a circular motion. Start at the meatus, and work outward (Fig. 16-32). Repeat as needed. Use a clean part of the washcloth each time.
5 Rinse the area with another washcloth.
6 Return the foreskin to its natural position.
7 Clean the shaft of the penis. Use firm, downward strokes. Rinse the area.
8 Help the person flex his knees and spread his legs. Or help him spread his legs as much as possible with his knees straight.
9 Clean the scrotum. Rinse well. Observe for redness and irritation in the skin folds.
10 Pat dry the penis and scrotum.
11 Fold the bath blanket back between his legs.
12 Help him lower his legs and turn onto his side away from you.
13 Clean the rectal area (see procedure: *Giving Female Perineal Care*, p. 343). Rinse and dry well.
14 Remove the waterproof pad.
15 Remove and discard the gloves. Decontaminate your hands.

### POST-PROCEDURE

16 Follow steps 36 through 48 in procedure: *Giving Female Perineal Care*, p. 343

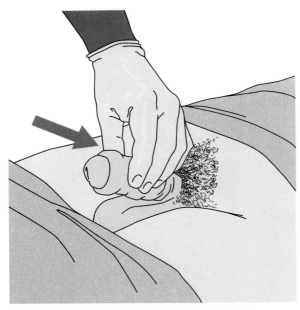

**FIG. 16-31** The foreskin of the uncircumcised male is pulled back for perineal care. It is returned to the normal position immediately after cleaning.

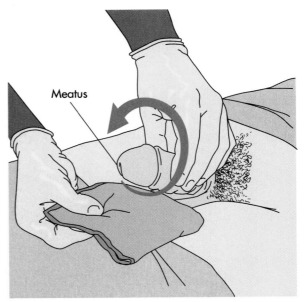

**FIG. 16-32** The penis is cleaned with circular motions starting at the meatus.

Meatus

# REPORTING AND RECORDING

You make many observations while assisting with hygiene. The nurse tells you what to report at once. Report bleeding and changes from prior observations right away.

Also report and record the care given (Fig. 16-33). If care is not recorded, it is assumed that care was not given. This can cause serious legal problems.

Activities of Daily Living Flow Sheet

JAN  FEB  MAR  APR  MAY  JUN  JUL  AUG  SEP  (OCT)  NOV  DEC

| ORDER/INSTRUCTION | TIME | 1 | 2 | 3 | 4 | 5 | 6 | 7 | 8 | 9 | 10 | 11 | 12 | 13 | 14 | 15 | 16 | 17 | 18 | 19 | 20 | 21 | 22 | 23 | 24 | 25 | 26 | 27 | 28 | 29 | 30 | 31 |
|---|---|---|---|---|---|---|---|---|---|---|---|---|---|---|---|---|---|---|---|---|---|---|---|---|---|---|---|---|---|---|---|---|---|
| Oral Care<br>Own (Dentures) None<br>I=Independent S=Set up<br>A=Assist | 11-7 | | | | | | | | | | | | | | | | | | | | | | | | | | | | | | | |
| | 7-3 | S | S | S | | | | | | | | | | | | | | | | | | | | | | | | | | | | |
| | 3-11 | S | S | S | | | | | | | | | | | | | | | | | | | | | | | | | | | | |
| Hygiene, Washing Face and Hands<br>I=Independent S=Set up<br>A=Assist T=Total Care | 11-7 | / | / | / | | | | | | | | | | | | | | | | | | | | | | | | | | | | |
| | 7-3 | / | / | / | | | | | | | | | | | | | | | | | | | | | | | | | | | | |
| | 3-11 | / | / | / | | | | | | | | | | | | | | | | | | | | | | | | | | | | |
| Bath and Shampoo every _Monday_ and _Thurs_<br>on _7-3_ shift<br>T=Tub S=Shower<br>B=Bed bath | 11-7 | | | | | | | | | | | | | | | | | | | | | | | | | | | | | | | |
| | 7-3 | T | | | | | | | | | | | | | | | | | | | | | | | | | | | | | | |
| | 3-11 | | | | | | | | | | | | | | | | | | | | | | | | | | | | | | | |
| Back massage daily | 11-7 | | | | | | | | | | | | | | | | | | | | | | | | | | | | | | | |
| | 7-3 | | | | | | | | | | | | | | | | | | | | | | | | | | | | | | | |
| | 3-11 | √ | √ | √ | | | | | | | | | | | | | | | | | | | | | | | | | | | | |
| Pericare<br>I=Independent S=Set up<br>A=Assist T=Total Care | 11-7 | A | A | A | | | | | | | | | | | | | | | | | | | | | | | | | | | | |
| | 7-3 | | | | | | | | | | | | | | | | | | | | | | | | | | | | | | | |
| | 3-11 | A | A | A | | | | | | | | | | | | | | | | | | | | | | | | | | | | |

**FIG. 16-33** Charting sample.

# ■ REVIEW QUESTIONS ■

**Circle T if the statement is true and F if it is false.**

1  **T F**  Hygiene is needed for comfort, safety, and health.
2  **T F**  After lunch Mrs. Bell asks for a back massage. You can give her a back massage then.
3  **T F**  Mrs. Bell's toothbrush has hard bristles. They are good for oral hygiene.
4  **T F**  Unconscious persons are supine for mouth care.
5  **T F**  You use your fingers to keep an unconscious person's mouth open for oral hygiene.
6  **T F**  Mrs. Bell has a lower denture. It is washed over a counter.
7  **T F**  Bath oils cleanse and soften the skin.
8  **T F**  Powders absorb moisture and prevent friction.
9  **T F**  Deodorants reduce the amount of perspiration.
10  **T F**  A tub bath lasts 30 minutes.
11  **T F**  You can give permission for showers but not for tub baths.
12  **T F**  Weak persons are left alone in the shower if they are sitting.
13  **T F**  A back massage relaxes muscles and stimulates circulation.
14  **T F**  Perineal care helps prevent infection.
15  **T F**  Foreskin is returned to its normal position immediately after cleaning.

**Circle the BEST answer.**

16  You brush Mrs. Bell's teeth and note the following. Which is *not* reported to the nurse?
  a  Bleeding, swelling, or redness of the gums
  b  Irritations, sores, or white patches in the mouth or on the tongue
  c  Lips that are dry, cracked, swollen, or blistered
  d  Food between the teeth

17  Which is *not* a purpose of bathing?
  a  Increasing circulation
  b  Promoting drying of the skin
  c  Exercising body parts
  d  Refreshing and relaxing the person

18  Soaps do the following *except*
  a  Remove dirt and dead skin
  b  Soften the skin
  c  Remove skin oil and perspiration
  d  Dry the skin

19  Which action is *wrong* when bathing Mrs. Bell?
  a  Covering her for warmth and privacy
  b  Rinsing her skin thoroughly to remove all soap
  c  Washing from the dirtiest to cleanest area
  d  Patting her skin dry

20  What is a safe water temperature for a complete bed bath?
  a  95° F
  b  100° F
  c  110° F
  d  120° F

21  You are going to give a back massage. Which is *false?*
  a  It should last 3 to 5 minutes.
  b  Lotion is warmed before being applied.
  c  Your hands are always in contact with the skin.
  d  The side-lying position is best.

*Answers to these questions are on p. 817.*

# 17

# Grooming

# OBJECTIVES

- Define the key terms listed in this chapter
- Explain why grooming is important
- Identify the factors that affect hair care
- Explain how to care for matted and tangled hair
- Describe how to shampoo hair
- Describe the measures practiced when shaving a person
- Explain why nail and foot care are important
- Describe the rules for changing gowns and clothing
- Perform the procedures described in this chapter

# KEY TERMS

**alopecia** Hair loss

**dandruff** Excessive amount of dry, white flakes from the scalp

**hirsutism** Excessive body hair in women and children

**pediculosis (lice)** Infestation with lice

**pediculosis capitis** Infestation of the scalp *(capitis)* with lice

**pediculosis corporis** Infestation of the body *(corporis)* with lice

**pediculosis pubis** Infestation of the pubic *(pubis)* hair with lice

Hair care, shaving, and nail and foot care are important to many people. Like hygiene, these grooming measures prevent infection and promote comfort. They also affect love, belonging, and self-esteem needs.

People differ in their grooming measures. Some want only clean hair. Others want a certain hair style. Some want only clean hands. Others want clean, manicured, and polished nails. Many men shave and groom their beards. Likewise, many women shave their legs and underarms. Some women have facial hair. They may shave or use other hair removal methods.

## HAIR CARE

How the hair looks and feels affects mental well-being. Some people cannot perform hair care. You assist with hair care whenever necessary. *See Focus on Long-Term Care: Hair Care*, p. 350.

The nursing process reflects the person's culture, personal choice, skin and scalp condition, health history, and self-care ability. These terms are common in care plans:

- **Alopecia** means hair loss. Hair loss may be complete or partial. Male pattern baldness occurs with aging and is the result of heredity. Hair also thins in some women with aging. Cancer treatments (radiation therapy to the head and chemotherapy) often cause alopecia in males and females. Skin disease is another cause. Stress, poor nutrition, pregnancy, some drugs, and hormone changes are other causes. Except for hair loss from aging, hair usually grows back.
- **Hirsutism** is excessive body hair in women and children. It results from heredity and abnormal amounts of male hormones.
- **Dandruff** is the excessive amount of dry, white flakes from the scalp. Itching often occurs. Sometimes eyebrows and ear canals are involved. Medicated shampoos correct the problem.
- **Pediculosis (lice)** is the infestation with lice. (*Infestation* means being in or on a host.) Lice are parasites. Lice bites cause severe itching in the affected area. **Pediculosis capitis** is the infestation of the scalp *(capitis)* with lice. **Pediculosis pubis** is the infestation of the pubic *(pubis)* hair with lice. Head and pubic lice attach their eggs to hair shafts. **Pediculosis corporis** is the infestation of the body *(corporis)* with lice. Lice eggs attach to clothing and furniture. Lice easily spread to others through clothing, furniture, bed linen, and sexual contact. They also are spread by sharing combs and brushes. Medicated shampoos, lotions, and creams are used to treat lice. Thorough bathing is needed. So is washing clothing and linen in hot water. Report signs of lice to the nurse at once.

# BRUSHING AND COMBING HAIR

Brushing and combing hair are part of early morning care, morning care, and afternoon care. They also are done whenever needed. Many people want hair care done before visitors arrive. Encourage patients and residents to do their own hair care. Assist as needed. Perform hair care for those who cannot do so. The person chooses how to brush, comb, and style hair.

Brushing increases blood flow to the scalp. It also brings scalp oils along the hair shaft. Scalp oils help keep hair soft and shiny. Brushing and combing prevent tangled and matted hair. When brushing and combing hair, start at the scalp. Then brush or comb to the hair ends.

Long hair easily mats and tangles. Daily brushing and combing prevent the problem. So does braiding. Do not braid hair without the person's consent. *Never cut matted or tangled hair.* Tell the nurse if the person has matted or tangled hair. The nurse may have you comb or brush through the matting and tangling. To do this:

- Take a small section of hair near the ends.
- Comb or brush through to the hair ends.
- Working up to the scalp, add small sections of hair.
- Comb or brush through each longer section to the hair ends.
- Brush or comb from the scalp to the hair ends.

Special measures are needed for curly, coarse, and dry hair. Use a wide-tooth comb for curly hair. Start at the neckline. Working upward, lift and fluff hair outward. Continue to the forehead. Wet hair or apply a conditioner or petroleum jelly as directed. This makes combing easier. The person may have certain practices or hair care products. They are part of the care plan. Also, the person can guide you when giving hair care. *See Caring About Culture: Braiding Hair.*

When giving hair care, place a towel across the shoulders to protect the person's garments. If the person is in bed, give hair care before changing the pillowcase. If done after a linen change, place a towel across the pillow to collect falling hair. *See Focus on Children: Brushing and Combing Hair.*

**DELEGATION GUIDELINES:** *Brushing and Combing Hair*
You need this information from the nurse and care plan before brushing and combing hair:

- How much help the person needs
- What to do if hair is matted and tangled
- What measures are needed for curly, coarse, or dry hair
- What hair care products to use
- The person's preferences and routine hair care measures
- What observations to report and record:
  —Scalp sores
  —Flaking
  —Presence of lice
  —Patches of hair loss
  —Very dry or very oily hair

**SAFETY ALERT:** *Brushing and Combing Hair*
Sharp brush bristles can injure the scalp. So can a comb with sharp or broken teeth. Tell the nurse if you have concerns about the person's brush or comb.

## CARING ABOUT CULTURE
### BRAIDING HAIR
Styling hair in small braids is a common practice of some cultural groups. The braids are left intact for shampooing. To undo these braids, the nurse obtains the person's consent.

## FOCUS ON LONG-TERM CARE
### HAIR CARE
Many nursing centers have beauty and barber shops for residents. Residents can have their hair shampooed, cut, and styled. Men also can have their mustaches and beards groomed.

## FOCUS ON CHILDREN
### BRUSHING AND COMBING HAIR
Hairstyles are important to older children and teenagers. Do not make judgments about the child's hairstyle. Style hair in a way that pleases the child and parents. Do not style hair according to your standards or customs.

# BRUSHING AND COMBING THE PERSON'S HAIR

## QUALITY OF LIFE

Remember to:
- Knock before entering the person's room
- Address the person by name
- Introduce yourself by name and title

## PRE-PROCEDURE

1 Follow *Delegation Guidelines: Brushing and Combing Hair.* See *Safety Alert: Brushing and Combing Hair.*
2 Identify the person. Check the ID bracelet against the assignment sheet. Call the person by name.
3 Explain the procedure to the person. Ask the person how to style hair.
4 Collect the following:
- Comb and brush
- Bath towel
- Hair care items as requested
5 Arrange items on the bedside stand.
6 Practice hand hygiene.
7 Provide for privacy.

## PROCEDURE

8 Lower the bed rail if used.
9 Help the person to the chair. The person puts on a robe and nonskid footwear when up. (If the person is in bed, raise the bed for body mechanics. Bed rails are up if used. Lower the near bed rail. Assist the person to semi-Fowler's position if allowed.)
10 Place a towel across the shoulders or across the pillow.
11 Ask the person to remove eyeglasses. Put them in the eyeglass case. Put the case inside the bedside stand.
12 Part hair into two sections (Fig. 17-1, *A*, p. 352). Divide one side into two sections (Fig. 17-1, *B*, p. 352).
13 Brush the hair. Start at the scalp, and brush toward the hair ends (Fig. 17-2, p. 352).
14 Style the hair as the person prefers.
15 Remove the towel.
16 Let the person put on the eyeglasses.

## POST-PROCEDURE

17 Provide for comfort.
18 Lower the bed to its lowest position.
19 Raise or lower bed rails. Follow the care plan.
20 Place the signal light within reach.
21 Unscreen the person.
22 Clean and return items to their proper place.
23 Follow agency policy for dirty linen.
24 Decontaminate your hands.

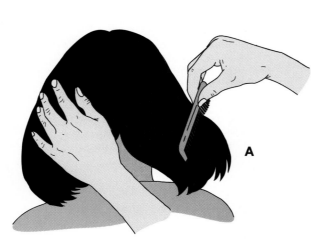

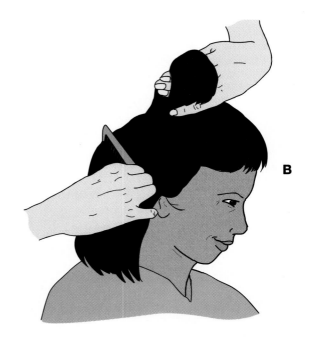

FIG. 17-1 Parting hair. **A,** Part hair down the middle. Divide it into two main sections. **B,** Then part the main section into two smaller sections.

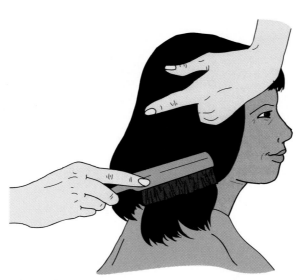

FIG. 17-2 Brush hair by starting at the scalp. Brush down to the hair ends.

# SHAMPOOING

Most people shampoo at least once a week. Some shampoo two or three times a week. Others shampoo every day. Many factors affect frequency. They include the condition of the hair and scalp, hairstyle, and personal choice.

Some persons use certain shampoos and conditioners. Others use medicated shampoo ordered by the doctor.

The person may need help shampooing. After shampooing, dry and style hair as quickly as possible. Women may want hair curled or rolled up before drying. Check with the nurse before doing so.

Tell the nurse if a shampoo is requested. Do not wash a person's hair unless a nurse asks you to do so. The shampooing method used depends on the person's condition, safety factors, and personal choice. The nurse tells you what method to use:

- *Shampoo during the shower or tub bath.* The person shampoos in the shower. A hand-held nozzle is used for those using shower chairs or taking tub baths. A spray of water is directed to the hair. Place an extra towel, shampoo, and hair conditioner within the person's reach. Assist as needed.
- *Shampoo at the sink.* The person sits facing away from the sink. A folded towel is placed over the sink edge to protect the neck. The person's head is tilted back over the edge of the sink. A water pitcher or hand-held nozzle is used to wet and rinse the hair.

- *Shampoo on a stretcher.* The stretcher is front of the sink. A towel is placed under the neck. The head is tilted over the edge of the sink (Fig. 17-3). A water pitcher or hand-held nozzle is used to wet and rinse the hair. Remember to lock the stretcher wheels and use the safety straps and side rails.
- *Shampoo in bed.* The person's head and shoulders are moved to the edge of the bed if possible. A shampoo tray is placed under the head to protect the linens and mattress from water. The tray also drains water into a basin placed on a chair by the bed (Fig. 17-4, p. 354). Use a water pitcher to wet and rinse the hair.

See Focus on Children: Shampooing, p. 354. See Focus on Older Persons: Shampooing, p. 354. See Focus on Home Care: Shampooing, p. 354. See Focus on Long-Term Care: Shampooing, p. 354.

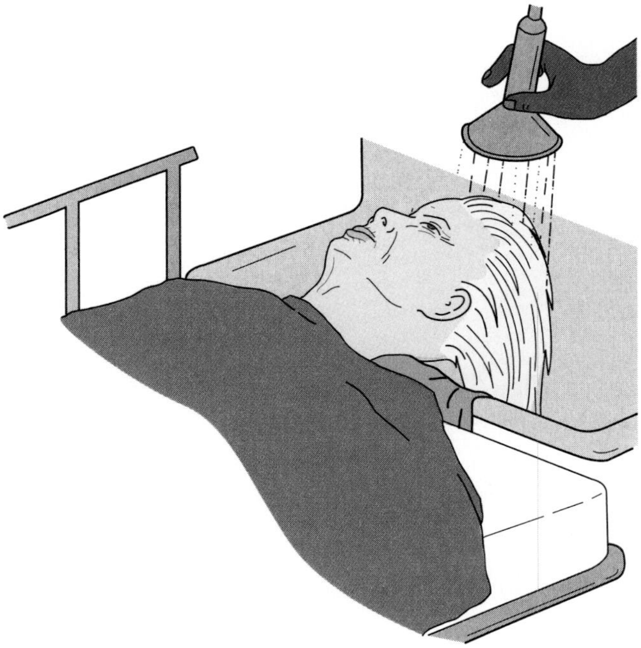

**FIG. 17-3** Shampooing while the person is on a stretcher. The stretcher is in front of the sink.

---

**DELEGATION GUIDELINES:** *Shampooing*

Before shampooing hair, you need this information from the nurse and the care plan:
- When to shampoo the person's hair
- What method to use
- What shampoo and conditioner to use
- The person's position restrictions or limits
- What water temperature to use—usually 105° F (40.5° C)
- If hair is curled or rolled up before drying
- What observations to report and record:
  —Scalp sores
  —Hair falling out in patches
  —The presence of lice
  —How the person tolerated the procedure

---

**SAFETY ALERT:** *Shampooing*

You must keep shampoo out of the eyes. The person holds a hand towel or washcloth over the eyes. Do not let shampoo get near the eyes. When rinsing, cup your hand at the person's forehead. This keeps soapy water from running down the person's forehead and into the eyes.

If a medicated shampoo or conditioner is used, return it to the nurse. Never leave it at the bedside unless instructed to do so.

Follow Standard Precautions if the person has scalp lesions. Also follow the Bloodborne Pathogen Standard.

## FOCUS ON OLDER PERSONS
### SHAMPOOING

Oil gland secretion decreases with aging. Therefore older persons have dry hair. They may shampoo less often than younger adults.

When shampooing during the tub bath or shower, the person tips his or her head back to keep shampoo and water out of the eyes. Support the back of the head with one hand as you shampoo with the other. Some older people cannot tip their heads back. They lean forward and hold a washcloth over the eyes. Support the forehead with one hand as you shampoo with the other. Make sure the person can breathe easily.

Many older people have limited range of motion in their necks. They cannot tolerate shampooing at the sink or on a stretcher.

## FOCUS ON CHILDREN
### SHAMPOOING

Oil gland secretion increases during puberty. Therefore adolescents tend to have oily hair. Frequent shampooing is often necessary.

## FOCUS ON HOME CARE
### SHAMPOOING

You can make a trough from a plastic shower curtain or tablecloth. Or use a plastic drop cloth for painting. (Avoid plastic trash bags. They slip and slide easily and are not sturdy.) Place the plastic under the person's head. Make a raised edge around the plastic to prevent water from spilling over the sides. Direct the ends of the plastic into the basin. Water flows into the basin.

## FOCUS ON LONG-TERM CARE
### SHAMPOOING

Shampooing is usually done weekly on the person's bath or shower day. If a woman's hair is done in the beauty shop, do not shampoo her hair. She wears a shower cap during the tub bath or shower.

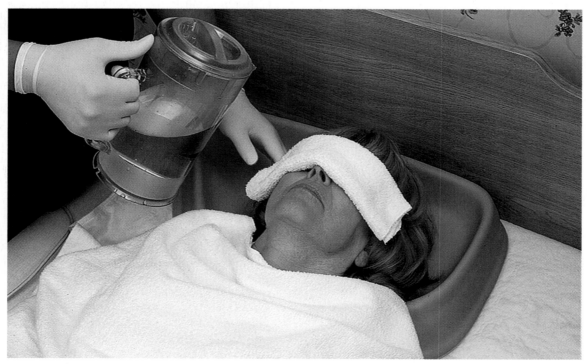

**FIG. 17-4** A shampoo tray is used to shampoo a person in bed. The tray is directed to the side of the bed so water drains into a collecting basin.

## SHAMPOOING THE PERSON'S HAIR

NNAAP™

### QUALITY OF LIFE

Remember to:
- Knock before entering the person's room
- Address the person by name
- Introduce yourself by name and title

### PRE-PROCEDURE

1. Follow *Delegation Guidelines: Shampooing*, p. 353. See *Safety Alert: Shampooing*, p. 353.
2. Explain the procedure to the person.
3. Practice hand hygiene.
4. Collect the following:
   - Two bath towels
   - Hand towel or washcloth
   - Shampoo
   - Hair conditioner (if requested)
   - Bath thermometer
   - Pitcher or nozzle (if needed)
   - Shampoo tray (if needed)
   - Basin or pan (if needed)
   - Waterproof pad (if needed)
   - Gloves (if needed)
   - Comb and brush
   - Hair dryer
5. Arrange items nearby.
6. Identify the person. Check the ID bracelet against the assignment sheet. Call the person by name.
7. Provide for privacy.
8. Raise the bed for body mechanics for a shampoo in bed. The far bed rail is up if bed rails are used.

### PROCEDURE

9. Position the person for the method you will use. Place the waterproof pad and shampoo tray under the head and shoulders if needed.
10. Place a bath towel across the shoulders or across the pillow.
11. Brush and comb the hair to remove snarls and tangles.
12. Raise the bed rail if used.
13. Obtain water. Water temperature should be about 105° F (40.5° C). Test temperature according to agency policy.
14. Lower the bed rail (if used).
15. Put on gloves (if needed).
16. Ask the person to hold a dampened hand towel or washcloth over the eyes. It should not cover the nose and mouth. (A damp towel or washcloth is easier to hold. It will not slip.)
17. Use the pitcher or nozzle to wet the hair.
18. Apply a small amount of shampoo.
19. Work up a lather with both hands. Start at the hairline. Work toward the back of the head.
20. Massage the scalp with your fingertips. Do not scratch the scalp.
21. Rinse the hair.
22. Repeat steps 18 through 21.
23. Apply conditioner. Follow directions on the container.
24. Squeeze water from the person's hair.
25. Cover hair with a bath towel.
26. Dry the person's face with a towel.
27. Help the person raise the head if appropriate.
28. Rub the hair and scalp with the towel. Use the second towel if the first is wet.
29. Comb the hair to remove snarls and tangles.
30. Dry and style hair as quickly as possible.

### POST-PROCEDURE

31. Remove and discard the gloves (if used). Decontaminate your hands.
32. Provide for comfort.
33. Lower the bed to its lowest position.
34. Raise or lower bed rails. Follow the care plan.
35. Place the signal light within reach.
36. Unscreen the person.
37. Clean and return equipment to its proper place. Discard disposable items.
38. Follow agency policy for dirty linen.
39. Decontaminate your hands.

# SHAVING

Many men shave for comfort and mental well-being. Many women shave their legs and underarms. Women with coarse facial hair may shave. Or they may use other hair removal methods. See Box 17-1 for shaving rules.

Blade and electric shavers are used. If the agency's electric shaver is used, clean it between each use. Follow agency policy.

Safety razors (blade razors) involve razor blades. They can cause nicks or cuts. They are not used for persons who take anticoagulant drugs. An *anticoagulant* prevents or slows down (*anti*) blood clotting (*coagulate*). Bleeding occurs easily. A nick or cut can cause serious bleeding. Electric shavers are used for persons taking such drugs.

Soften the beard and skin before using a safety razor. Apply a warm washcloth or towel to the face for a few minutes. Then lather the face with soap and water or a shaving cream.

*See Focus on Older Persons: Shaving.*

---

**DELEGATION GUIDELINES:** *Shaving*

You need this information from the nurse and care plan when delegated shaving tasks:

- What shaver to use—electric or safety razor
- If the person takes anticoagulant drugs
- When to shave the person

---

**SAFETY ALERT:** *Shaving*

Safety razors are very sharp. Protect the person and yourself from nick or cuts. Prevent contact with blood.

You will rinse the razor often during the shaving procedure. Then you will wipe the razor with tissues or paper towels. To protect yourself from cuts, place the tissues or paper towels on the overbed table. Do not hold them in your hand.

Follow Standard Precautions and the Bloodborne Pathogen Standard. Discard used razor blades and disposable shavers in the sharps container.

---

**FOCUS ON OLDER PERSONS**

SHAVING

Some older persons have dementia. Do not use safety razors to shave them. They may not understand what you are doing. They may resist care and move quickly. Serious nicks and cuts can occur. Use electric shavers.

---

**BOX 17-1   RULES FOR SHAVING**

- Use electric shavers for persons taking anticoagulant drugs. Never use safety razors.
- Protect bed linens. Place a towel under the part being shaved. Or place a towel across the shoulders to protect clothing.
- Soften the skin before shaving.
- Encourage the person to do as much as safely possible.
- Hold the skin taut as needed.
- Shave in the direction of hair growth when shaving the face and underarms.
- Shave up from the ankles when shaving legs. This is against hair growth.
- Do not cut, nick, or irritate the skin.
- Rinse the body part thoroughly.
- Apply direct pressure to nicks or cuts.
- Report nicks, cuts, or irritation to the nurse at once.

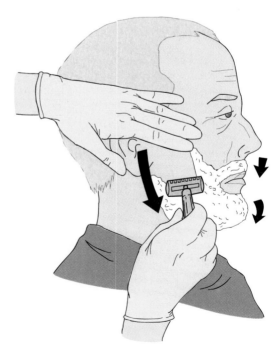

**FIG. 17-5** Shave in the direction of hair growth. Use longer strokes on the larger areas of the face. Use short strokes around the chin and lips.

## SHAVING THE PERSON

### QUALITY OF LIFE

Remember to:
- Knock before entering the person's room
- Address the person by name
- Introduce yourself by name and title

### PRE-PROCEDURE

1 Follow *Delegation Guidelines: Shaving.* See *Safety Alert: Shaving.*
2 Explain the procedure to the person.
3 Practice hand hygiene.
4 Collect the following:
  - Wash basin
  - Bath towel
  - Hand towel
  - Washcloth
  - Safety razor
  - Mirror
  - Shaving cream, soap, or lotion
  - Shaving brush
  - After-shave lotion (men only)
  - Tissues or paper towels
  - Paper towels
  - Gloves
5 Arrange paper towels and supplies on the overbed table.
6 Identify the person. Check the ID bracelet against the assignment sheet. Call the person by name.
7 Provide for privacy.
8 Raise the bed for body mechanics. Bed rails are up if used.

### PROCEDURE

9 Fill the basin with warm water.
10 Place the basin on the overbed table.
11 Lower the bed rail near you if up.
12 Assist the person to semi-Fowler's position if allowed or to the supine position.
13 Adjust lighting to clearly see the person's face.
14 Place the bath towel over the chest.
15 Adjust the overbed table for easy reach.
16 Tighten the razor blade to the shaver.
17 Wash the person's face. Do not dry.
18 Wet the washcloth or towel. Wring it out.
19 Apply the washcloth or towel to the face for a few minutes.
20 Put on gloves.
21 Apply shaving cream with your hands. Or use a shaving brush to apply lather.
22 Hold the skin taut with one hand.
23 Shave in the direction of hair growth. Use shorter strokes around the chin and lips (Fig. 17-5).
24 Rinse the razor often. Wipe it with tissues or paper towels.
25 Apply direct pressure to any bleeding areas.
26 Wash off any remaining shaving cream or soap. Dry with a towel.
27 Apply after-shave lotion if requested.
28 Remove the towel and gloves. Decontaminate your hands.
29 Move the overbed table to the side of the bed.

### POST-PROCEDURE

30 Provide for comfort.
31 Place the signal light within reach.
32 Lower the bed to its lowest position.
33 Raise or lower bed rails. Follow the care plan.
34 Clean and return equipment and supplies to their proper place. Discard disposable items. Wear gloves.
35 Wipe off the overbed table with the paper towels. Discard the paper towels.
36 Remove the gloves. Decontaminate your hands.
37 Position the table for the person.
38 Unscreen the person.
39 Follow agency policy for dirty linen.
40 Decontaminate your hands.
41 Report nicks or bleeding to the nurse.

## CARING FOR BEARDS AND MUSTACHES

Beards and mustaches need daily care. Food can collect in hair. So can mouth and nose drainage. Daily washing and combing are needed. Ask the person how to groom his beard or mustache. *Never trim or shave a beard or mustache without the person's consent.*

## SHAVING FEMALE LEGS AND UNDERARMS

Many women shave their legs and underarms. This practice varies among cultures. Some women shave only the lower legs. Others shave to mid-thigh or the entire leg.

Legs and underarms are shaved after bathing. The skin is soft at this time. Soap and water, shaving cream, or lotion is used for lather. Collect shaving items with bath items. Use the kidney basin to rinse the razor. Do not use the bath water. Follow the rules in Box 17-1.

---

**SAFETY ALERT:** *Nail and Foot Care*

You do not cut or trim toenails if a person:
- Has diabetes
- Has poor circulation to the legs and feet
- Takes drugs that affect blood clotting
- Has very thick nails or ingrown toenails

The RN or podiatrist (foot [*pod*] doctor) cuts toenails and provides foot care for these persons.

Check between the toes for cracks and sores. These areas often are overlooked. If left untreated, a serious infection could occur.

The feet are easily burned. Persons with decreased sensation or circulatory problems may not feel hot temperatures.

Breaks in the skin and bleeding can occur. Follow Standard Precautions and the Bloodborne Pathogen Standard.

---

## ■ NAIL AND FOOT CARE

Nail and foot care prevents infection, injury, and odors. Hangnails, ingrown nails (nails that grow in at the side), and nails torn away from the skin cause skin breaks. These breaks are portals of entry for microbes. Long or broken nails can scratch skin or snag clothing.

The feet are easily infected and injured. Dirty feet, socks, or stockings harbor microbes and cause odors. Shoes and socks provide a warm, moist environment for the growth of microbes. Injuries occur from stubbing toes, stepping on sharp objects, or being stepped on. Shoes that fit poorly cause blisters.

Poor circulation prolongs healing. Diabetes and vascular disease are common causes of poor circulation. Infections or foot injuries are very serious for older persons and persons with circulatory disorders. Gangrene and amputation are serious complications (Chapter 33). Trimming and clipping toenails can easily result in injuries.

Nails are easier to trim and clean after soaking or bathing. Use nail clippers to cut fingernails. *Never use scissors.* Use extreme caution to prevent damage to nearby tissues.

Some agencies do not let nursing assistants cut or trim toenails. Follow agency policy.

*See Focus on Home Care: Nail and Foot Care.*

---

**DELEGATION GUIDELINES:** *Nail and Foot Care*

Before giving nail and foot care, you need this information from the nurse and the care plan:
- What water temperature to use
- How long to soak fingernails (usually 5 to 10 minutes)
- How long to soak feet (usually 15 to 20 minutes)
- What observations to report and record:
  —Reddened, irritated, or callused areas
  —Breaks in the skin
  —Corns on top of and between toes
  —Very thick nails
  —Loose nails

---

### FOCUS ON HOME CARE
#### NAIL AND FOOT CARE

The feet soak during a tub bath. Or the person can sit on the side of the tub and soak the feet. Make sure the person can step into and out of the tub. Otherwise, soak the feet in a basin or a whirlpool foot bath.

If comfortable for the person, he or she can soak fingers in the sink. Or use a bowl if a small basin is not available.

## GIVING NAIL AND FOOT CARE

NNAAP™

### QUALITY OF LIFE

Remember to:
- Knock before entering the person's room
- Address the person by name
- Introduce yourself by name and title

### PRE-PROCEDURE

1 Follow *Delegation Guidelines: Nail and Foot Care.* See *Safety Alert: Nail and Foot Care.*
2 Explain the procedure to the person.
3 Practice hand hygiene.
4 Collect the following:
- Wash basin or whirlpool foot bath
- Soap
- Bath thermometer
- Bath towel
- Hand towel
- Washcloth
- Kidney basin
- Nail clippers
- Orange stick
- Emery board or nail file
- Lotion for hands
- Lotion or petroleum jelly for feet
- Paper towels
- Disposable bath mat
- Gloves
5 Arrange paper towels and other items on the overbed table.
6 Identify the person. Check the ID bracelet against the assignment sheet. Call the person by name.
7 Provide for privacy.
8 Assist the person to the bedside chair. Place the signal light within reach.

### PROCEDURE

9 Place the bath mat under the feet.
10 Fill the wash basin or whirlpool foot bath. The nurse tells you what water temperature to use. (Measure water temperature with a bath thermometer. Or test it by dipping your elbow or inner wrist into the basin.)
11 Place the basin or foot bath on the bath mat.
12 Help the person put the feet into the basin or foot bath.
13 Adjust the overbed table in front of the person.
14 Fill the kidney basin. See step 10 for water temperature.
15 Place the kidney basin on the overbed table.
16 Place the person's fingers into the basin. Position the arms for comfort (Fig. 17-6, p. 360).
17 Let the fingers soak for 5 to 10 minutes. Let the feet soak for 15 to 20 minutes. Rewarm water as needed.
18 Put on gloves.
19 Clean under the fingernails with the orange stick. Use a towel to wipe the orange stick after each nail.
20 Remove the kidney basin. Dry the hands and between the fingers thoroughly.
21 Clip fingernails straight across with the nail clippers (Fig. 17-7, p. 360).
22 Shape nails with an emery board or nail file.
23 Push cuticles back with the orange stick or a washcloth (Fig. 17-8, p. 360).
24 Apply lotion to the hands.
25 Move the overbed table to the side.
26 Wash the feet with soap and a washcloth. Wash between the toes.
27 Remove the feet from the basin or foot bath. Dry thoroughly, especially between the toes.
28 Apply lotion or petroleum jelly to the tops and soles of the feet. Do not apply between the toes. Warm lotion before applying it.
29 Remove and discard the gloves. Decontaminate your hands.
30 Help the person put on socks and nonskid footwear.

### POST-PROCEDURE

31 Provide for comfort.
32 Place the signal light within reach.
33 Raise or lower bed rails. Follow the care plan.
34 Clean and return equipment and supplies to their proper place. Discard disposable items. Wear gloves for this step.
35 Remove the gloves. Decontaminate your hands.
36 Unscreen the person.
37 Follow agency policy for dirty linen.
38 Decontaminate your hands.
39 Report and record your observations.

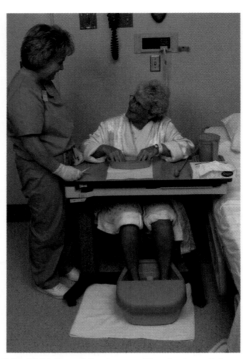

**FIG. 17-6** Nail and foot care. The feet soak in a whirlpool footbath, and the fingers soak in a kidney basin.

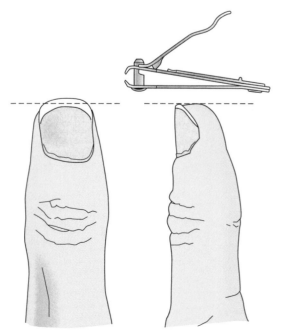

**FIG. 17-7** Clip fingernails straight across. Use a nail clipper.

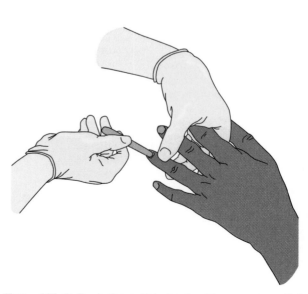

**FIG. 17-8** Push the cuticle back with an orange stick.

# CHANGING GOWNS AND CLOTHING

Gowns or pajamas are changed after the bath and when wet or soiled. Some persons wear regular clothes. They dress in the morning and change into sleepwear for bed. Incontinent persons may change more often.

Some persons need help with these activities. Follow these rules:

- Provide for privacy. Do not expose the person.
- Encourage the person to do as much as possible.
- Let the person choose what to wear. Make sure the right undergarments are chosen.
- Remove clothing from the strong or "good" side first.
- Put clothing on the weak side first.
- Support the arm or leg when removing or putting on a garment.

## CHANGING GOWNS

Many hospital patients wear gowns. If there is injury or paralysis, the gown is removed from the strong arm first. Support the weak arm while removing the gown. Put the clean gown on the weak arm first and then on the strong arm.

Some agencies have special gowns for IV therapy. They open along the entire sleeve and close with ties, snaps, or Velcro. Sometimes standard hospital gowns are used.

---

**DELEGATION GUIDELINES:** *Changing Gowns*

Before changing a gown, you need this information from the nurse and the care plan:
- Which arm has the IV
- If the person has an IV pump (see *Safety Alert: Changing Gowns*)
- If you or the nurse will check the flow rate (If you check the flow rate, find out what it should be [Chapter 20].)

---

**SAFETY ALERT:** *Changing Gowns*

IV pumps control the rate of infusion. If the person has an IV pump and a standard gown, do not use the following procedure. The arm with the IV is not put through the sleeve.

---

*Text continued on p. 364.*

## CHANGING THE GOWN OF THE PERSON WITH AN IV

### QUALITY OF LIFE

Remember to:
- Knock before entering the person's room
- Address the person by name
- Introduce yourself by name and title

### PRE-PROCEDURE

1 Follow *Delegation Guidelines: Changing Gowns*, p. 361. See *Safety Alert: Changing Gowns*, p. 361.
2 Explain the procedure to the person.
3 Practice hand hygiene.
4 Get a clean gown and a bath blanket.

5 Identify the person. Check the ID bracelet against the assignment sheet. Call the person by name.
6 Provide for privacy.
7 Raise the bed for body mechanics. Bed rails are up if used.

### PROCEDURE

8 Lower the bed rail near you (if up).
9 Cover the person with a bath blanket. Fanfold linens to the foot of the bed.
10 Untie the gown. Free parts that the person is lying on.
11 Remove the gown from the arm with no IV.
12 Gather up the sleeve of the arm with the IV. Slide it over the IV site and tubing. Remove the arm and hand from the sleeve (Fig. 17-9, *A*).
13 Keep the sleeve gathered. Slide your arm along the tubing to the bag (Fig. 17-9, *B*).
14 Remove the bag from the pole. Slide the bag and tubing through the sleeve (Fig. 17-9, *C*).

Do not pull on the tubing. Keep the bag above the person.
15 Hang the IV bag on the pole.
16 Gather the sleeve of the clean gown that will go on the arm with the IV infusion.
17 Remove the bag from the pole. Slip the sleeve over the bag at the shoulder part of the gown (Fig. 17-9, *D*). Hang the bag.
18 Slide the gathered sleeve over the tubing, hand, arm, and IV site. Then slide it onto the shoulder.
19 Put the other side of the gown on the person. Fasten the gown.
20 Cover the person. Remove the bath blanket.

### POST-PROCEDURE

21 Provide for comfort.
22 Place the signal light within reach.
23 Lower the bed to its lowest position.
24 Raise or lower bed rails. Follow the care plan.

25 Unscreen the person.
26 Follow agency policy for dirty linen.
27 Decontaminate your hands.
28 Check the flow rate. Or ask the nurse to check it.

**FIG. 17-9**
Changing a gown.

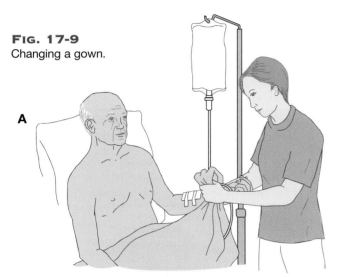

**A,** The gown is removed from the arm with no IV. The sleeve on the arm with the IV is gathered up, slipped over the IV site and tubing, and removed from the arm and hand.

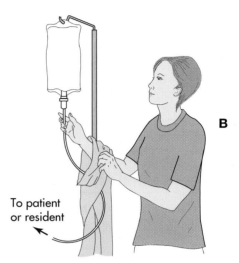

To patient
or resident

**B,** The gathered sleeve is slipped along the IV tubing to the bag.

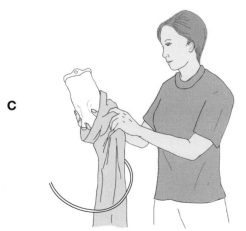

**C,** The IV bag is removed from the pole and passed through the sleeve.

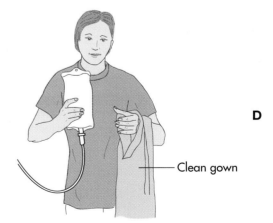

Clean gown

**D,** The gathered sleeve of the clean gown is slipped over the IV bag at the shoulder part of the gown.

# DRESSING AND UNDRESSING

Clothing changes are usually necessary on admission and discharge. Some people enter and leave the agency in a gown or pajamas. Most wear street clothes. The rules listed on p. 361 are followed for dressing and undressing. *See Focus on Long-Term Care: Dressing and Undressing. See Focus on Home Care: Dressing and Undressing.*

**DELEGATION GUIDELINES: *Dressing and Undressing***
Before changing clothing, you need this information from the nurse and the care plan:
- How much help the person needs
- If the person needs to wear certain garments
- What observations to report and record:
  —How much help was given
  —How the person tolerated the procedure
  —Any complaints by the person

## UNDRESSING THE PERSON

### QUALITY OF LIFE

Remember to:
- Knock before entering the person's room
- Address the person by name
- Introduce yourself by name and title

### PRE-PROCEDURE

1 Follow *Delegation Guidelines: Dressing and Undressing.*
2 Explain the procedure to the person.
3 Practice hand hygiene.
4 Get a bath blanket.
5 Identify the person. Check the ID bracelet against the assignment sheet. Call the person by name.
6 Provide for privacy.
7 Raise the bed for body mechanics. Bed rails are up if used.
8 Lower the bed rail on the person's weak side.
9 Position him or her supine.
10 Cover the person with the bath blanket. Fanfold linens to the foot of the bed.

### PROCEDURE

11 Remove garments that open in the back:
  a Raise the head and shoulders. Or turn him or her onto the side away from you.
  b Undo buttons, zippers, ties, or snaps.
  c Bring the sides of the garment to the sides of the person (Fig. 17-10). If he or she is in a side-lying position, tuck the far side under the person. Fold the near side onto the chest (Fig. 17-11).
  d Position the person supine.
  e Slide the garment off the shoulder on the strong side. Remove it from the arm (Fig. 17-12, p. 366).
  f Repeat step 11e for the weak side.

12 Remove garments that open in the front:
  a Undo buttons, zippers, snaps, or ties.
  b Slide the garment off the shoulder and arm on the strong side.
  c Raise the head and shoulders. Bring the garment over to the weak side (Fig. 17-13, p. 366). Lower the head and shoulders.
  d Remove the garment from the weak side.
  e If you cannot raise the head and shoulders:
    (1) Turn the person toward you. Tuck the removed part under the person.

## UNDRESSING THE PERSON—CONT'D

### PROCEDURE

(2) Turn him or her onto the side away from you.
(3) Pull the side of the garment out from under the person. Make sure he or she will not lie on it when supine.
(4) Return the person to the supine position.
(5) Remove the garment from the weak side.
13 Remove pullover garments:
  a Undo any buttons, zippers, ties, or snaps.
  b Remove the garment from the strong side.
  c Raise the head and shoulders. Or turn the person onto the side away from you. Bring the garment up to the person's neck (Fig. 17-14, p. 366).
  d Remove the garment from the weak side.
  e Bring the garment over the person's head.
  f Position him or her in the supine position.
14 Remove pants or slacks:
  a Remove footwear.
  b Position the person supine.
  c Undo buttons, zippers, ties, snaps, or buckles.

  d Remove the belt.
  e Ask the person to lift the buttocks off the bed. Slide the pants down over the hips and buttocks (Fig. 17-15, p. 367). Have the person lower the hips and buttocks.
  f If the person cannot raise the hips off the bed:
    (1) Turn the person toward you.
    (2) Slide the pants off the hip and buttock on the strong side (Fig. 17-16, p. 367).
    (3) Turn the person away from you.
    (4) Slide the pants off the hip and buttock on the weak side (Fig. 17-17, p. 367).
  g Slide the pants down the legs and over the feet.
15 Dress the person. See procedure: *Dressing the Person*, p. 368.
16 Help the person get out of bed if he or she is to be up. If the person will stay in bed:
  a Cover the person, and remove the bath blanket.
  b Provide for comfort.
  c Lower the bed to its lowest position.
  d Raise or lower bed rails. Follow the care plan.

### POST-PROCEDURE

17 Place the signal light within reach.
18 Unscreen the person.
19 Follow agency policy for soiled clothing.

20 Decontaminate your hands.
21 Report and record your observations.

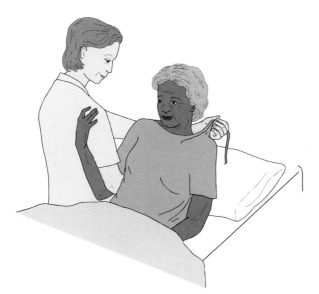

**FIG. 17-10** The sides of the garment are brought from the back to the sides of the person.

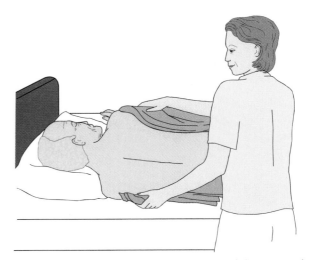

**FIG. 17-11** A garment that opens in back is removed from the person in the side-lying position. The far side of the garment is tucked under the person. The near side is folded onto the person's chest.

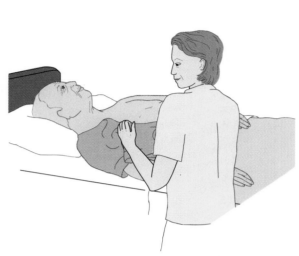

**FIG. 17-12** The garment is removed from the strong side first.

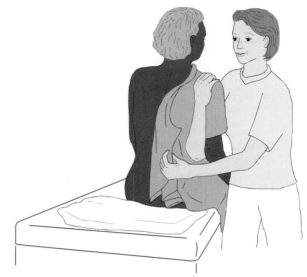

**FIG. 17-13** A front-opening garment is removed with the person's head and shoulders raised. The garment is removed from the strong side first. Then it is brought around the back to the weak side.

**FIG. 17-14** A pullover garment is removed from the strong side first. Then the garment is brought up to the person's neck so that it can be removed from the weak side.

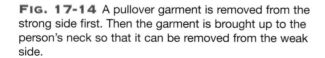
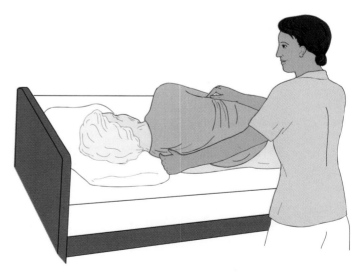

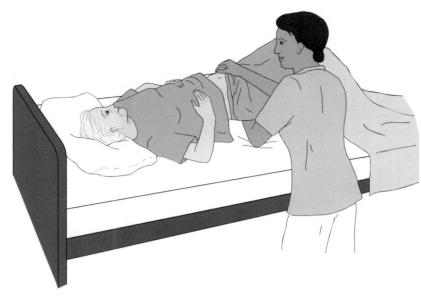

**FIG. 17-15** The person lifts the hips and buttocks for removing the pants. The pants are slid down over the hips and buttocks.

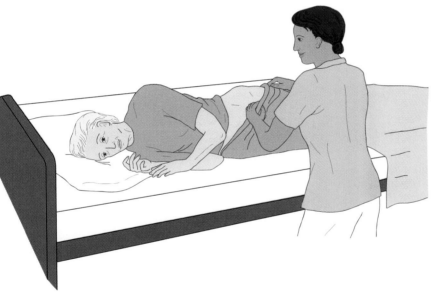

**FIG. 17-16** Pants are removed in the side-lying position. They are removed from the strong side first. They are slid over the hips and buttocks.

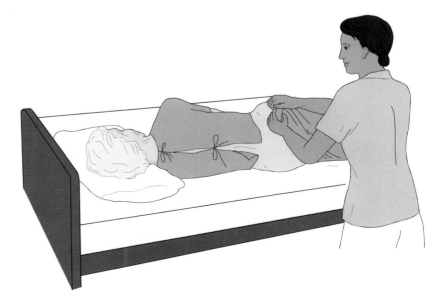

**FIG. 17-17** The person is turned onto the other side. The pants are removed from the weak side.

# DRESSING THE PERSON

## QUALITY OF LIFE

Remember to:
- Knock before entering the person's room
- Address the person by name
- Introduce yourself by name and title

## PRE-PROCEDURE

1 Follow *Delegation Guidelines: Dressing and Undressing*, p. 364.
2 Explain the procedure to the person.
3 Practice hand hygiene.
4 Get a bath blanket and clothing requested by the person.
5 Identify the person. Check the ID bracelet against the assignment sheet. Call the person by name.

6 Provide for privacy.
7 Raise the bed for body mechanics. Bed rails are up if used.
8 Lower the bed rail (if up) on the person's strong side.
9 Undress the person. See procedure: *Undressing the Person*, p. 364.
10 Position the person supine.

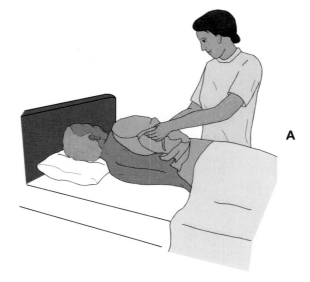

**FIG. 17-18** Dressing a person.
**A,** The side-lying position can be used to put on garments that open in the back. Turn the person toward you after the garment is put on the arms. The side of the garment is brought to the person's back.

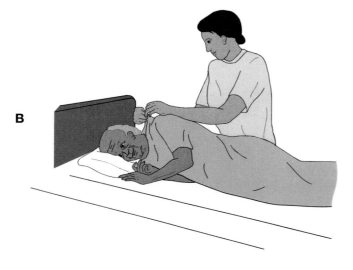

**B,** Then turn the person away from you. The other side of the garment is brought to the back and fastened.

## DRESSING THE PERSON—CONT'D

NNAAP™

## PROCEDURE

11 Cover the person with the bath blanket. Fanfold linens to the foot of the bed.
12 Put on garments that open in the back:
   a Slide the garment onto the arm and shoulder of the weak side.
   b Slide the garment onto the arm and shoulder of the strong side.
   c Raise the person's head and shoulders.
   d Bring the sides to the back.
   e If the person is in a side-lying position:
      (1) Turn the person toward you.
      (2) Bring one side of the garment to the person's back (Fig. 17-18, A).
      (3) Turn the person away from you.
      (4) Bring the other side to the person's back (Fig. 17-18, B).
   f Fasten buttons, snaps, ties, or zippers.
   g Position the person supine.
13 Put on garments that open in the front:
   a Slide the garment onto the arm and shoulder on the weak side.
   b Raise the head and shoulders. Bring the side of the garment around to the back. Lower the person down. Slide the garment onto the arm and shoulder of the strong arm.
   c If the person cannot raise the head and shoulders:
      (1) Turn the person toward you.
      (2) Tuck the garment under him or her.
      (3) Turn the person away from you.
      (4) Pull the garment out from under him or her.
      (5) Turn the person back to the supine position.
      (6) Slide the garment over the arm and shoulder of the strong arm.
   d Fasten buttons, snaps, ties, or zippers.
14 Put on pullover garments:
   a Position the person supine.
   b Bring the neck of the garment over the head.

   c Slide the arm and shoulder of the garment onto the weak side.
   d Raise the person's head and shoulders.
   e Bring the garment down.
   f Slide the arm and shoulder of the garment onto the strong side.
   g If the person cannot assume a semi-sitting position:
      (1) Turn the person toward you.
      (2) Tuck the garment under the person.
      (3) Turn the person away from you.
      (4) Pull the garment out from under him or her.
      (5) Position the person supine.
      (6) Slide the arm and shoulder of the garment onto the strong side.
   h Fasten buttons, snaps, ties, or zippers.
15 Put on pants or slacks:
   a Slide the pants over the feet and up the legs.
   b Ask the person to raise the hips and buttocks off the bed.
   c Bring the pants up over the buttocks and hips.
   d Ask the person to lower the hips and buttocks.
   e If the person cannot raise the hips and buttocks:
      (1) Turn the person onto the strong side.
      (2) Pull the pants over the buttock and hip on the weak side.
      (3) Turn the person onto the weak side.
      (4) Pull the pants over the buttock and hip on the strong side.
      (5) Position the person supine.
   f Fasten buttons, ties, snaps, zipper, and the belt buckle.
16 Put socks and footwear on the person.
17 Help the person get out of bed. If the person will stay in bed:
   a Cover the person, and remove the bath blanket.
   b Provide for comfort.
   c Lower the bed to its lowest position.
   d Raise or lower bed rails. Follow the care plan.

## POST-PROCEDURE

18 Place the signal light within reach.
19 Unscreen the person.
20 Follow agency policy for soiled clothing.

21 Decontaminate your hands.
22 Report and record your observations.

# ■ REVIEW QUESTIONS ■

Circle the **BEST** answer.

**1** Mr. Lee has *alopecia*. This is
  **a** Excessive body hair
  **b** Dry, white flakes from the scalp
  **c** An infestation of lice
  **d** Hair loss

**2** Which prevents hair from matting and tangling?
  **a** Bedrest
  **b** Daily brushing and combing
  **c** Daily shampooing
  **d** Cutting hair

**3** Mrs. Clark's hair is not matted or tangled. When brushing the hair, start at
  **a** The forehead
  **b** The hair ends
  **c** The scalp
  **d** The back of the neck

**4** Brushing keeps the hair
  **a** Soft and shiny
  **b** Clean
  **c** Free of lice
  **d** Long

**5** Mr. Lee wants his hair washed. You should
  **a** Wash his hair during his shower
  **b** Wash his hair at the sink
  **c** Shampoo him in bed
  **d** Follow the care plan

**6** When shaving Mr. Lee, do the following *except*
  **a** Practice Standard Precautions
  **b** Follow the Bloodborne Pathogen Standard
  **c** Shave in the direction of hair growth
  **d** Shave when the skin is dry

**7** Mr. Lee is nicked during shaving. Your first action is to
  **a** Wash your hands
  **b** Apply direct pressure
  **c** Tell the nurse
  **d** Use an electric razor

**8** Fingernails are cut with
  **a** Toenail clippers
  **b** Scissors
  **c** A nail file
  **d** Nail clippers

**9** Fingernails are trimmed
  **a** Before soaking
  **b** After soaking
  **c** Before trimming toenails
  **d** After trimming toenails

Circle **T** if the statement is true and **F** if it is false.

**10** **T F** Mr. Lee has a mustache and beard. You think he would be more comfortable without facial hair. You can shave his beard and mustache.
**11** **T F** Mr. Lee has poor circulation in his legs and feet. You can cut and trim his toenails.
**12** **T F** Clothing is removed from the strong side first.
**13** **T F** The person chooses what to wear.
**14** **T F** You can cut matted hair.

*Answers to these questions are on p. 817.*

# Urinary Elimination

## OBJECTIVES

- Define the key terms listed in this chapter
- Describe normal urine
- Describe the rules for normal urination
- Describe urinary incontinence and the care required
- Explain why catheters are used
- Explain how to care for persons with catheters
- Describe straight, indwelling, and condom catheters
- Describe two methods of bladder training
- Perform the procedures described in this chapter

## KEY TERMS

**catheter** A tube used to drain or inject fluid through a body opening

**catheterization** The process of inserting a catheter

**dysuria** Painful or difficult *(dys)* urination *(uria)*

**Foley catheter** An indwelling or retention catheter

**functional incontinence** The person has bladder control but cannot use the toilet in time

**hematuria** Blood *(hemat)* in the urine *(uria)*

**indwelling catheter** A catheter left in the bladder so urine drains constantly into a drainage bag; retention or Foley catheter

**micturition** Urination or voiding

**nocturia** Frequent urination *(uria)* at night *(noct)*

**oliguria** Scant amount *(olig)* of urine *(uria);* less than 500 ml in 24 hours

**overflow incontinence** Urine leaks when the bladder is too full

**polyuria** Abnormally large amounts *(poly)* of urine *(uria)*

**reflex incontinence** The loss of urine at predictable intervals when the bladder is full

**retention catheter** A Foley or indwelling catheter

**straight catheter** A catheter that drains the bladder and then is removed

**stress incontinence** When urine leaks during exercise and certain movements

**urge incontinence** The loss of urine in response to a sudden, urgent need to void; the person cannot get to a toilet in time

**urinary frequency** Voiding at frequent intervals

**urinary incontinence** The loss of bladder control

**urinary urgency** The need to void at once

**urination** The process of emptying urine from the bladder; micturition or voiding

**voiding** Urination or micturition

Eliminating waste is a physical need. The respiratory, digestive, integumentary, and urinary systems remove body wastes. The digestive system rids the body of solid wastes. The lungs remove carbon dioxide. Sweat contains water and other substances. Blood contains waste products from body cells burning food for energy. The urinary system removes waste products from the blood. It also maintains the body's water balance. See Box 18-1 for a review of the urinary system.

## NORMAL URINATION

The healthy adult produces about 1500 ml (milliliters) (3 pints) of urine a day. Many factors affect urine production. They include age, disease, the amount and kinds of fluid ingested, dietary salt, body temperature, perspiration, and drugs. Some substances increase urine production—coffee, tea, alcohol, and some drugs. A diet high in salt causes the body to retain water. When water is retained, less urine is produced.

**Urination, micturition,** and **voiding** mean the process of emptying urine from the bladder. The amount of fluid intake, habits, and available toilet facilities affect frequency. So do activity, work, and illness. People usually void at bedtime, after getting up, and before meals. Some people void every 2 to 3 hours. The need to void at night disturbs sleep.

Some persons need help getting to the bathroom. Others use bedpans, urinals, or commodes. Follow the rules in Box 18-2 and the person's care plan.

*See Focus on Children: Normal Urination, p. 374.*

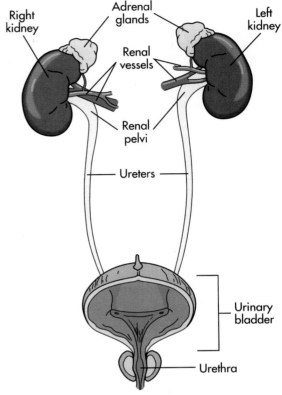

**FIG. 18-1** The urinary system.

| BOX 18-1 | THE URINARY SYSTEM: BODY STRUCTURE AND FUNCTION |
|---|---|

The two kidneys (Fig. 18-1) lie in the upper abdomen against the muscles of the back on each side of the spine. Blood passes through the two kidneys. Urine is formed in the kidneys.

Urine consists of wastes and excess fluids filtered out of the blood. Urine flows through the two ureters to the urinary bladder. Urine is stored in the bladder. The urethra connects the bladder to the outside of the body. Urine passes from the body through the urethra. *Urination, micturition,* and *voiding* mean the process of emptying the bladder.

See Chapter 7 for more information.

| BOX 18-2 | RULES FOR NORMAL ELIMINATION |
|---|---|

- Practice medical asepsis.
- Follow Standard Precautions and the Bloodborne Pathogen Standard.
- Provide fluids as the nurse and care plan direct.
- Follow the person's voiding routines and habits. Check with the nurse and the care plan.
- Help the person to the bathroom when the request is made. Or provide the commode, bedpan, or urinal. The need to void may be urgent.
- Help the person assume a normal position for voiding if possible. Women sit or squat. Men stand.
- Warm the bedpan or urinal.
- Cover the person for warmth and privacy.
- Provide for privacy. Pull the curtain around the bed, close room and bathroom doors, and pull drapes or window shades. Leave the room if the person can be alone.

- Tell the person that running water, flushing the toilet, or playing music can mask voiding sounds. Voiding with others close by embarrasses some people.
- Stay nearby if the person is weak or unsteady.
- Place the signal light and toilet tissue within reach.
- Allow enough time to void. Do not rush the person.
- Promote relaxation. Some people like to read.
- Run water in a sink if the person cannot start the stream. Or place the person's fingers in warm water.
- Provide perineal care as needed (Chapter 16).
- Assist with hand washing after voiding. Provide a wash basin, soap, washcloth, and towel.
- Assist the person to the bathroom or offer the bedpan, urinal, or commode at regular times. Some people are embarrassed or are too weak to ask for help.

## OBSERVATIONS

Normal urine is pale yellow, straw-colored, or amber. It is clear with no particles. A faint odor is normal. Observe urine for color, clarity, odor, amount, and particles.

Some foods affect urine color. Red food dyes, beets, blackberries, and rhubarb cause red-colored urine. Carrots and sweet potatoes cause bright yellow urine. Certain drugs change urine color. Asparagus causes a urine odor.

Ask the nurse to observe urine that looks or smells abnormal. Report complaints of urgency, burning on urination, or painful or difficult urination. Also report the problems in Table 18-1. The nurse uses the information for the nursing process.

**TABLE 18-1 COMMON URINARY ELIMINATION PROBLEMS**

| Problem | Definition | Causes |
|---|---|---|
| Dysuria | Painful or difficult (dys) urination (uria) | Urinary tract infection, trauma, urinary tract obstruction |
| Hematuria | Blood (hemat) in the urine (uria) | Kidney disease, urinary tract infection, trauma |
| Nocturia | Frequent urination (uria) at night (noct) | Excess fluid intake, kidney disease, prostate disease |
| Oliguria | Scant amount (olig) of urine (uria), less than 500 ml in 24 hours | Poor fluid intake, shock, burns, kidney disease, heart failure |
| Polyuria | Abnormally large amounts (poly) of urine (uria) | Drugs, excess fluid intake, diabetes, hormone imbalance |
| Urinary frequency | Voiding at frequent intervals | Excess fluid intake, bladder infections, pressure on the bladder, drugs |
| Urinary incontinence | The loss of bladder control | Trauma, disease, urinary tract infections, reproductive or urinary tract surgeries, aging, fecal impaction, constipation, not getting to the bathroom |
| Urinary urgency | The need to void at once | Urinary tract infection, fear of incontinence, full bladder, stress |

# BEDPANS

Bedpans are used by persons who cannot be out of bed. Women use bedpans for voiding and bowel movements. Men use them only for bowel movements. Bedpans are made of plastic or metal. Metal bedpans are often cold. They are warmed with water and dried before use.

A *fracture pan* has a thin rim. It is only about ½-inch deep at one end (Fig. 18-2). The smaller end is placed under the buttocks (Fig. 18-3). Fracture pans are used:
- By persons with casts
- By persons in traction
- By persons with limited back motion
- After spinal cord injury or surgery
- After a hip fracture
- After hip replacement surgery
  See Focus on Older Persons: Bedpans.

*Text continued on p. 378.*

**DELEGATION GUIDELINES:** *Bedpans*

Before assisting with a bedpan, you need this information from the nurse and care plan:
- What bedpan to use—standard bedpan or fracture pan
- Position or activity limits
- If the nurse needs to observe the results before disposing of the contents
- What observations to report and record:
  —Urine color, clarity, and odor
  —Amount
  —Presence of particles
  —Complaints of urgency, burning, dysuria, or other problems
  —For bowel movements, see Chapter 19

**SAFETY ALERT:** *Bedpans*

Urine and bowel movements may contain blood and microbes. Microbes can live and grow in dirty bedpans. Follow Standard Precautions and the Bloodborne Pathogen Standard when handling bedpans and their contents. Thoroughly clean bedpans after use.

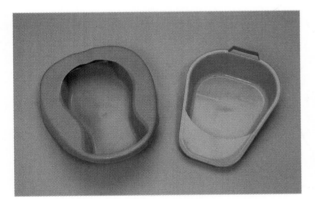

**FIG. 18-2** Standard bedpan *(left)* and the fracture pan *(right)*.

**FOCUS ON OLDER PERSONS**

BEDPANS

Some older persons have fragile bones from osteoporosis or painful joints from arthritis (Chapter 33). Fracture pans provide more comfort for them than do standard bedpans.

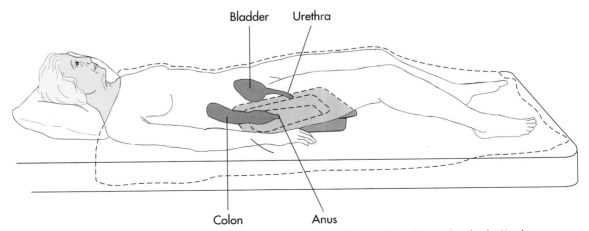

Bladder    Urethra

Colon    Anus

**FIG. 18-3** A person positioned on a fracture pan. The small end is under the buttocks.

# GIVING THE BEDPAN

NNAAP™

## QUALITY OF LIFE

Remember to:
- Knock before entering the person's room
- Address the person by name
- Introduce yourself by name and title

## PRE-PROCEDURE

1 Follow *Delegation Guidelines: Bedpans*, p. 375. See *Safety Alert: Bedpans*, p. 375.
2 Provide for privacy.
3 Practice hand hygiene.
4 Put on gloves.
5 Collect the following:
   - Bedpan

- Bedpan cover
- Toilet tissue
6 Arrange equipment on the chair or bed.
7 Explain the procedure to the person.

## PROCEDURE

8 Warm and dry the bedpan if necessary.
9 Lower the bed rail near you if up.
10 Position the person supine. Raise the head of the bed slightly.
11 Fold the top linens and gown out of the way. Keep the lower body covered.
12 Ask the person to flex the knees and raise the buttocks by pushing against the mattress with his or her feet.
13 Slide your hand under the lower back. Help raise the buttocks.
14 Slide the bedpan under the person (Fig. 18-4).
15 If the person cannot assist in getting on the bedpan:
   a Turn the person onto the side away from you.
   b Place the bedpan firmly against the buttocks (Fig. 18-5, *A*).
   c Push the bedpan down and toward the person (Fig. 18-5, *B*).
   d Hold the bedpan securely. Turn the person onto the back.
   e Make sure the bedpan is centered under the person.
16 Cover the person.
17 Raise the head of the bed so the person is in a sitting position.
18 Make sure the person is correctly positioned on the bedpan (Fig. 18-6).
19 Raise the bed rail if used.
20 Place the toilet tissue and signal light within reach.

21 Ask the person to signal when done or when help is needed.
22 Remove the gloves. Decontaminate your hands.
23 Leave the room, and close the door.
24 Return when the person signals. Knock before entering.
25 Decontaminate your hands. Put on gloves.
26 Raise the bed for body mechanics. Lower the bed rail (if used) and the head of the bed.
27 Ask the person to raise the buttocks. Remove the bedpan. Or hold the bedpan and turn him or her onto the side away from you.
28 Clean the genital area if the person cannot do so. Clean from front (urethra) to back (anus) with toilet tissue. Use fresh tissue for each wipe. Provide perineal care if needed.
29 Cover the bedpan. Take it to the bathroom. Lower the bed and raise the bed rail (if used) before leaving the bedside.
30 Note the color, amount, and character of urine or feces.
31 Empty and rinse the bedpan. Clean it with a disinfectant.
32 Remove soiled gloves. Practice hand hygiene, and put on clean gloves.
33 Return the bedpan and clean cover to the bedside stand.
34 Help the person with hand washing.
35 Remove the gloves. Decontaminate your hands.

## POST-PROCEDURE

36 Provide for comfort.
37 Place the signal light within reach.
38 Raise or lower bed rails. Follow the care plan.
39 Unscreen the person.

40 Follow agency policy for soiled linen.
41 Decontaminate your hands.
42 Report and record your observations.

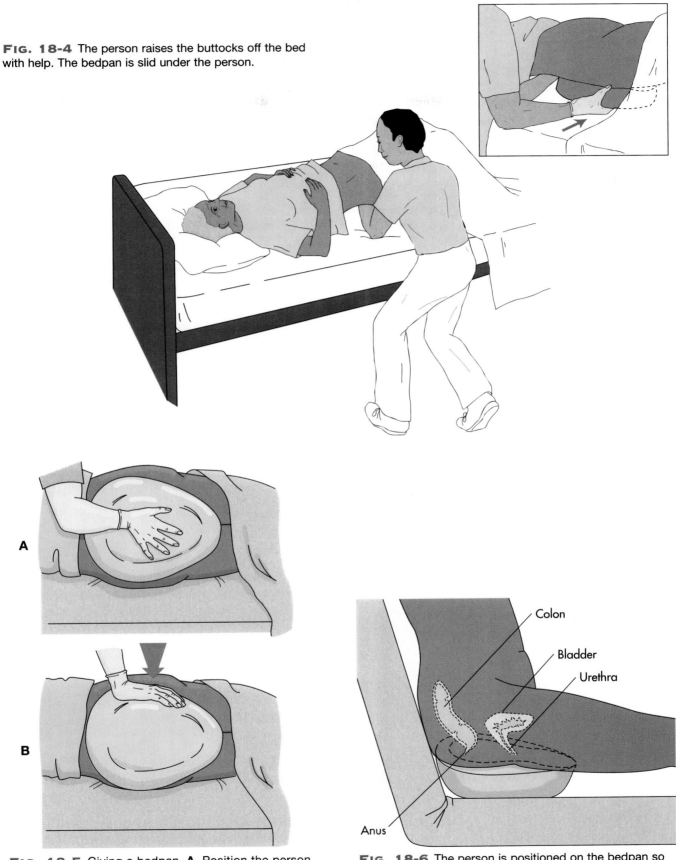

FIG. 18-4 The person raises the buttocks off the bed with help. The bedpan is slid under the person.

A

B

FIG. 18-5 Giving a bedpan. **A,** Position the person on one side. Place the bedpan firmly against the buttocks. **B,** Push downward on the bedpan and toward the person.

Colon

Bladder

Urethra

Anus

FIG. 18-6 The person is positioned on the bedpan so the urethra and anus are directly over the opening.

# URINALS

Men use urinals to void (Fig. 18-7). Plastic urinals have caps and hook-type handles. The urinal hooks to the bed rail within the man's reach. He stands to use the urinal if possible. Or he sits on the side of the bed or lies in bed to use it. Some men need support when standing. You may have to place and hold the urinal for some men.

After voiding, the cap is closed. This prevents urine spills. Remind men to hang urinals on bed rails and to signal after using them. Remind them not to place urinals on overbed tables and bedside stands. The overbed table is used for eating and as a work surface. Bedside stands are used for supplies. Table surfaces must not be contaminated with urine.

Some agencies do not use bed rails. Follow agency policy for where to place urinals.

**DELEGATION GUIDELINES:** *Urinals*

Before assisting with urinals, you need this information from the nurse and care plan:

- How the urinal is used—standing, sitting, or lying in bed
- If help is needed with placing or holding the urinal
- If the man needs support to stand (If yes, how many staff members are needed.)
- If the nurse needs to observe the urine before its disposal
- What observations to report and record (See *Delegation Guidelines: Bedpans*, p. 375.)

**SAFETY ALERT:** *Urinals*

Follow Standard Precautions and the Bloodborne Pathogen Standard when handling urinals and their contents. Empty them promptly to prevent odors and the spread of microbes. A filled urinal spills easily, causing safety hazards. Also, it is an unpleasant sight and a source of odor. Urinals are cleaned like bedpans.

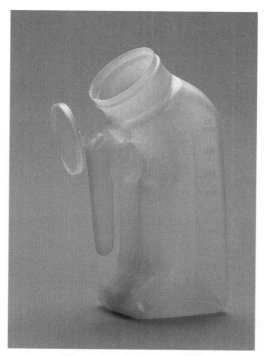

**FIG. 18-7** Male urinal.

## GIVING THE URINAL

### QUALITY OF LIFE

Remember to:
- Knock before entering the person's room
- Address the person by name
- Introduce yourself by name and title

### PRE-PROCEDURE

1 Follow *Delegation Guidelines: Urinals.* See *Safety Alert: Urinals.*
2 Provide for privacy.
3 Determine if the man will stand, sit, or lie in bed.
4 Practice hand hygiene.
5 Put on gloves.

### PROCEDURE

6 Give him the urinal if he is in bed. Remind him to tilt the bottom down to prevent spills.
7 If he is going to stand:
   a Help him sit on the side of the bed.
   b Put nonskid footwear on him.
   c Help him stand. Provide support if he is unsteady.
   d Give him the urinal.
8 Position the urinal if necessary. Position his penis in the urinal if he cannot do so.
9 Provide for privacy.
10 Place the signal light within reach. Ask him to signal when done or when he needs help.
11 Remove the gloves. Decontaminate your hands.
12 Leave the room, and close the door.
13 Return when he signals for you. Knock before entering.
14 Decontaminate your hands. Put on gloves.
15 Close the cap on the urinal. Take it to the bathroom.
16 Note the color, amount, and character of the urine.
17 Empty the urinal. Rinse it with cold water. Clean it with a disinfectant.
18 Return the urinal to its proper place.
19 Remove soiled gloves. Practice hand hygiene, and put on clean gloves.
20 Assist with hand washing.
21 Remove the gloves. Decontaminate your hands.

### POST-PROCEDURE

22 Provide for comfort.
23 Place the signal light within reach.
24 Raise or lower bed rails. Follow the care plan.
25 Unscreen him.
26 Follow agency policy for soiled linen.
27 Decontaminate your hands.
28 Report and record your observations.

# COMMODES

A commode is a chair or wheelchair with an opening for a bedpan or container (Fig. 18-8). Persons unable to walk to the bathroom often use commodes. The commode allows a normal position for elimination. The commode arms and back provide support and help prevent falls.

Some commodes are wheeled into bathrooms and placed over toilets. They are useful for persons who need support when sitting. The container is removed if the commode is used with the toilet. Wheels are locked after the commode is positioned over the toilet.

---

**DELEGATION GUIDELINES:** *Commodes*

You need this information from the nurse and care plan when assisting with commodes:
- If the commode is used at the bedside or over the toilet
- How much help the person needs
- If the person can be left alone
- If the nurse needs to observe urine or bowel movements
- What observations to report and record (See *Delegation Guidelines: Bedpans*, p. 375.)

---

**SAFETY ALERT:** *Commodes*

To use a commode, the person is transferred to or from bed or a chair or wheelchair. Practice safe transfer procedures (Chapter 13). Use the transfer belt.

Urine and feces may contain blood and microbes. Follow Standard Precautions and the Bloodborne Pathogen Standard. Thoroughly clean the commode container after use.

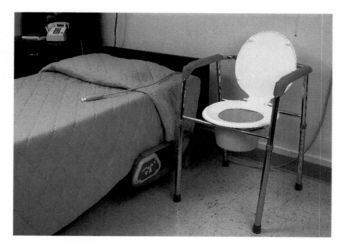

**FIG. 18-8** The commode has a toilet seat with a container. The container slides out from under the seat for emptying.

## HELPING THE PERSON TO THE COMMODE

### QUALITY OF LIFE

Remember to:
- Knock before entering the person's room
- Address the person by name
- Introduce yourself by name and title

### PRE-PROCEDURE

1 Follow *Delegation Guidelines: Commodes*. See *Safety Alert: Commodes*.
2 Explain the procedure to the person.
3 Provide for privacy.
4 Practice hand hygiene.
5 Put on gloves.
6 Collect the following:
- Commode
- Toilet tissue
- Bath blanket
- Transfer belt

### PROCEDURE

7 Bring the commode next to the bed. Remove the chair seat and container lid.
8 Help the person sit on the side of the bed.
9 Help him or her put on a robe and nonskid footwear.
10 Assist the person to the commode. Use the transfer belt.
11 Cover the person with a bath blanket for warmth.
12 Place the toilet tissue and signal light within reach.
13 Ask him or her to signal when done or when help is needed. (Stay with the person if necessary. Be respectful. Provide as much privacy as possible.)
14 Remove the gloves. Decontaminate your hands.
15 Leave the room. Close the door.
16 Return when the person signals. Knock before entering.
17 Decontaminate your hands. Put on the gloves.
18 Help the person clean the genital area as needed. Remove the gloves, and practice hand hygiene.
19 Help the person back to bed using the transfer belt. Remove the robe, transfer belt, and footwear. Raise the bed rail if used.
20 Put on clean gloves. Remove and cover the commode container. Clean the commode.
21 Take the container to the bathroom.
22 Check urine and feces for color, amount, and character.
23 Clean and disinfect the container.
24 Return the container to the commode. Return other supplies to their proper place.
25 Return the commode to its proper place.
26 Remove soiled gloves. Practice hand hygiene, and put on clean gloves.
27 Assist with hand washing.
28 Remove the gloves. Decontaminate your hands.

### POST-PROCEDURE

29 Provide for comfort.
30 Place the signal light within reach.
31 Raise or lower bed rails. Follow the care plan.
32 Unscreen the person.
33 Follow agency policy for soiled linen.
34 Decontaminate your hands.
35 Report and record your observations.

# URINARY INCONTINENCE

Urinary incontinence is the loss of bladder control. It may be temporary or permanent. There are basic types of incontinence:

- **Stress incontinence.** Urine leaks during exercise and certain movements. Urine loss is small (less than 50 ml). Often called *dribbling,* it occurs with laughing, sneezing, coughing, lifting, or other activities. Late pregnancy and obesity are other causes. The problem is common in women. Pelvic muscles weaken from pregnancies and with aging.
- **Urge incontinence.** Urine is lost in response to a sudden, urgent need to void. The person cannot get to a toilet in time. Urinary frequency, urinary urgency, and nighttime voidings are common. Causes include urinary tract infections, nervous system disorders, bladder cancer, and an enlarged prostate.
- **Overflow incontinence.** Urine leaks when the bladder is too full. The person feels like the bladder is not empty. The person only dribbles or has a weak urine stream. Diabetes, enlarged prostate, and some drugs are causes.
- **Functional incontinence.** The person has bladder control but cannot use the toilet in time. Immobility, restraints, unanswered signal lights, no signal light within reach, and not knowing where to find the bathroom are causes. So is difficulty removing clothing. Confusion and disorientation are other causes.
- **Reflex incontinence.** Urine is lost at predictable intervals. Urine is lost when the bladder is full. The person does not feel the need to void. Nervous system disorders and injuries are common causes.

Sometimes incontinence results from intestinal, rectal, and reproductive system surgeries. More than one type of incontinence can be present. This is called *mixed incontinence.*

Incontinence is embarrassing. Garments get wet, and odors develop. The person is uncomfortable. Skin irritation, infection, and pressure ulcers are risks. Falling is a risk when trying to get to the bathroom quickly. The person's pride, dignity, and self-esteem are affected. Loss of independence, social isolation, and depression are common.

The nurse uses the nursing process to meet the person's needs. Follow the nurse's instructions and the care plan. Nursing measures depend on the type of incontinence. The care plan may include some of the measures in Box 18-3. *Good skin care and dry clothing and linens are essential.* Following the rules for normal urinary elimination prevents incontinence in some people. Others need bladder training (p. 394). Sometimes catheters are ordered (p. 384).

Incontinence products help keep the person dry (Fig. 18-9). They have two layers and a waterproof back. Fluid passes through the first layer. It is absorbed by the lower layer. The nurse selects products that best meet the person's needs. Follow agency procedures when using them.

Incontinence is linked to abuse, mistreatment, and neglect. Caring for persons with incontinence is stressful. They need frequent care. They may wet again right after skin care and changing wet garments and linens. Remember, incontinence is beyond the person's control. It is not something the person chooses to do. Be patient. The person's needs are great. If you find yourself becoming short-tempered and impatient, talk to the nurse at once. The person has the right to be free from abuse, mistreatment, or neglect. Kindness, empathy, understanding, and patience are needed.

*See Focus on Older Persons: Urinary Incontinence. See Focus on Home Care: Urinary Incontinence.*

### FOCUS ON OLDER PERSONS
#### URINARY INCONTINENCE

Urinary incontinence is common in older persons. They are at risk for nervous, endocrine, and reproductive system disorders. Dementia, tumors, and poor mobility are other risks. Complications from incontinence pose serious problems for older persons. These include falls, pressure ulcers, and urinary tract infections. Long hospital or long-term care stays are often necessary. The resulting health care costs are high.

Persons with dementia may void in the wrong places. Trash cans, planters, heating vents, and closets are examples. Some persons remove incontinence products and throw them on the floor or in the toilet. Other persons resist staff efforts to keep them clean and dry. Check with the nurse and the care plan for measures to help the person.

### FOCUS ON HOME CARE
#### URINARY INCONTINENCE

Incontinence is stressful for the family. They often have problems coping with the person's incontinence. It is a common reason for long-term care.

## BOX 18-3 NURSING MEASURES FOR PERSONS WITH URINARY INCONTINENCE

- Record the person's voidings. This includes incontinent times and successful use of the toilet, commode, bedpan, or urinal.
- Answer signal lights promptly. The need to void may be urgent.
- Promote normal urinary elimination (Box 18-2).
- Promote normal bowel elimination (Chapter 19).
- Encourage voiding at scheduled intervals.
- Follow the person's bladder training program (p. 394).
- Have the person wear easy-to-remove clothing. Incontinence can occur while trying to deal with buttons, zippers, and undergarments.
- Encourage the person to do pelvic muscle exercises as instructed by the nurse.
- Help prevent urinary tract infections:
  —Promote fluid intake as the nurse directs.
  —Have the person wear cotton underwear.
  —Keep the perineal area clean and dry.
- Decrease fluid intake before bedtime.
- Provide good skin care.
- Provide dry garments and linens.
- Observe for signs of skin breakdown.
- Use incontinence products as the nurse directs. Follow the manufacturer's instructions.
- Provide perineal care as needed (Chapter 16). Remember to:
  —Use a safe and comfortable water temperature.
  —Follow Standard Precautions and the Bloodborne Pathogen Standard.
  —Protect the person and dry garments and linen from the wet incontinence product.
  —Expose only the perineal area.
  —Wash, rinse, and dry the perineal area and buttocks.
  —Remove wet incontinence products, garments, and linen. Apply clean, dry ones.

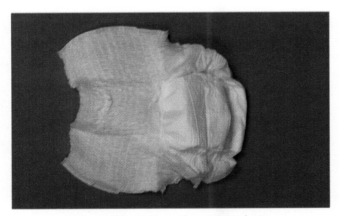

**FIG. 18-9** Incontinence product.

# CATHETERS

A **catheter** is a tube used to drain or inject fluid through a body opening. Inserted through the urethra into the bladder, a urinary catheter drains urine.

- A **straight catheter** drains the bladder and then is removed.
- An **indwelling catheter (retention or Foley catheter)** is left in the bladder. Urine drains constantly into a drainage bag. A balloon near the tip is inflated after the catheter is inserted. The balloon prevents the catheter from slipping out of the bladder (Fig. 18-10). Tubing connects the catheter to the drainage bag.

**Catheterization** is the process of inserting a catheter. It is done by a doctor or nurse. With the proper education and supervision, some states and agencies let nursing assistants insert catheters.

Catheters often are used before, during, and after surgery. They keep the bladder empty. This reduces the risk of bladder injury during surgery. After surgery, a full bladder causes pressure on nearby organs.

Some people are too weak or disabled to use the bedpan, urinal, commode, or toilet. Dying persons are an example. For them, catheters can promote comfort and prevent incontinence. Catheters can protect wounds and pressure ulcers from contact with urine. They also allow hourly urinary output measurements. However, they are a last resort for incontinence. Catheters do not treat the cause of incontinence.

Catheters also have diagnostic uses:
- To collect sterile urine specimens.
- To measure the amount of urine left in the bladder after the person voids. This is called *residual urine.*

You will care for persons with indwelling catheters. The risk of infection is high. Follow the rules in Box 18-4 to promote comfort and safety.

---

**DELEGATION GUIDELINES:** *Catheters*
The nurse may delegate catheter care to you. If so, you need this information from the nurse and the care plan:
- When to give catheter care—daily, twice a day, after bowel movements, or when vaginal discharge is present
- Where to secure the catheter—thigh or abdomen
- How to secure drainage tubing—clip, tape, safety pin and rubber band, or other device
- What observations to report and record:
  —Complaints of pain, burning, irritation, or the need to void
  —Crusting, abnormal drainage, or secretions
  —The color, clarity, and odor of urine
  —Particles in the urine
  —Drainage system leaks

---

**SAFETY ALERT:** *Catheters*
Urine may contain microbes and blood. Follow Standard Precautions and the Bloodborne Pathogen Standard.

*Text continued on p. 388.*

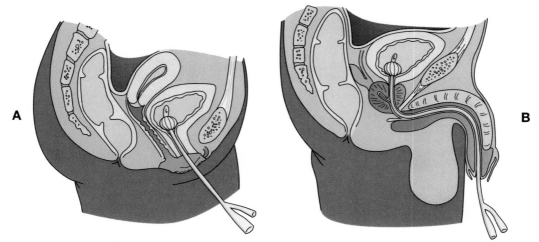

**FIG. 18-10** Indwelling catheter. **A,** Indwelling catheter in the female bladder. The inflated balloon at the tip prevents the catheter from slipping out through the urethra. **B,** Indwelling catheter with the balloon inflated in the male bladder.

## BOX 18-4    CARING FOR PERSONS WITH INDWELLING CATHETERS

- Follow the rules of medical asepsis.
- Follow Standard Precautions and the Bloodborne Pathogen Standard.
- Allow urine to flow freely through the catheter or tubing. Tubing should not have kinks. The person should not lie on the tubing.
- Keep the catheter connected to the drainage tubing. Follow the measures on p. 388 if the catheter and drainage tube are disconnected.
- Keep the drainage bag below the bladder. This prevents urine from flowing backward into the bladder.
- Attach the drainage bag to the bed frame, back of the chair, or lower part of an IV pole. *Never attach the drainage bag to the bed rail.* Otherwise it is higher than the bladder when the bed rail is raised.
- Do not let the drainage bag rest on the floor. This can contaminate the system.
- Coil the drainage tubing on the bed. Secure it to the bottom linen (Fig. 18-11). Follow agency policy. Use a clip, tape, safety pin with rubber band, or other device as directed by the nurse. Tubing must not loop below the drainage bag.
- Secure the catheter to the inner thigh (see Fig. 18-11). Or secure it to the man's abdomen. This prevents excess catheter movement and friction at the insertion site.
- Secure the catheter with tape or other devices as the nurse directs.
- Check for leaks. Check the site where the catheter connects to the drainage bag. Report any leaks to the nurse at once.
- Provide catheter care daily or twice a day (see procedure: *Giving Catheter Care,* p. 386). Some agencies consider perineal care to be sufficient. Follow the care plan.
- Provide perineal care daily, after bowel movements, and when there is vaginal drainage. Follow the care plan.
- Empty the drainage bag at the end of the shift or as the nurse directs. Measure and record the amount of urine (see procedure: *Emptying a Urinary Drainage Bag,* p. 391). Report increases or decreases in the amount of urine.
- Use a separate measuring container for each person. This prevents the spread of microbes from one person to another.
- Do not let the drain on the drainage bag touch any surface.
- Report complaints to the nurse at once—pain, burning, the need to void, or irritation. Also report the color, clarity, and odor of urine and the presence of particles.
- Encourage fluid intake as instructed by the nurse.

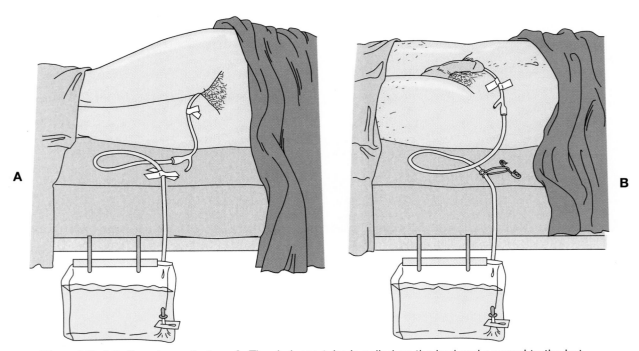

**FIG. 18-11** Securing catheters. **A,** The drainage tube is coiled on the bed and secured to the bottom linens. The catheter is taped to the inner thigh. Enough slack is left on the catheter to prevent friction at the urethra. **B,** The catheter is secured to the man's abdomen.

## GIVING CATHETER CARE

NNAAP™

### QUALITY OF LIFE

Remember to:
- Knock before entering the person's room
- Address the person by name
- Introduce yourself by name and title

### PRE-PROCEDURE

1 Follow *Delegation Guidelines: Catheters*, p. 384. See *Safety Alert: Catheters*, p. 384.
2 Explain the procedure to the person.
3 Practice hand hygiene.
4 Collect the following:
   - Items for perineal care (Chapter 16)
   - Gloves
   - Bed protector
   - Bath blanket
5 Identify the person. Check the ID bracelet against the assignment sheet. Call the person by name.
6 Provide for privacy.
7 Raise the bed for body mechanics. Bed rails are up if used.

### PROCEDURE

8 Lower the bed rail near you if up.
9 Put on the gloves.
10 Cover the person with a bath blanket. Fanfold top linens to the foot of the bed.
11 Drape the person for perineal care. (See Fig. 16-28, p. 344.)
12 Fold back the bath blanket to expose the genital area.
13 Place the bed protector under the buttocks. Ask the person to flex the knees and raise the buttocks off the bed.
14 Give perineal care. (See procedures: *Giving Female Perineal Care* or *Giving Male Perineal Care* in Chapter 16.)
15 Apply soap to a clean, wet washcloth.
16 Separate the labia (female). In an uncircumcised male, retract the foreskin (Fig. 18-12). Check for crusts, abnormal drainage, or secretions.
17 Hold the catheter near the meatus.
18 Clean the catheter from the meatus down the catheter about 4 inches (Fig. 18-13). Clean downward, away from the meatus with 1 stroke. Do not tug or pull on the catheter. Repeat as needed with a clean area of the washcloth. Use a clean washcloth if needed.
19 Rinse the catheter with a clean washcloth. Rinse from the meatus down the catheter about 4 inches. Rinse downward, away from the meatus with 1 stroke. Do not tug or pull on the catheter. Repeat as needed with a clean area of the washcloth. Use a clean washcloth if needed.
20 Secure the catheter. Coil and secure tubing (see Fig. 18-11).
21 Remove the bed protector.
22 Cover the person. Remove the bath blanket.
23 Remove the gloves. Decontaminate your hands.

### POST-PROCEDURE

24 Provide for comfort.
25 Place the signal light within reach.
26 Raise or lower bed rails. Follow the care plan.
27 Lower the bed to its lowest position.
28 Clean and return equipment to its proper place. Discard disposable items. (Wear gloves for this step.)
29 Remove the gloves. Decontaminate your hands.
30 Unscreen the person.
31 Follow agency policy for soiled linen.
32 Decontaminate your hands.
33 Report and record your observations (Fig. 18-14).

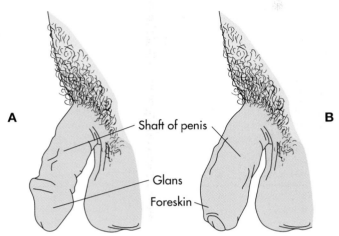

FIG. 18-12 **A,** Circumcised male. **B,** Uncircumcised male.

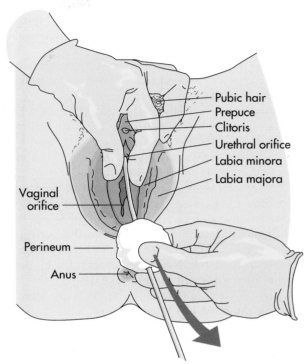

FIG. 18-13 The catheter is cleaned starting at the meatus. About 4 inches of the catheter is cleaned.

| Date | Time | |
|------|------|---|
| 12/21 | 0900 | Catheter care given. No drainage from around the catheter. Resident denies discomfort. Clear amber urine flowing freely. Catheter secured to abdomen with tape. Drainage tubing attached to bed with clip. Resident positioned on (L) side. Bed in low position. Signal light within reach. Adam Aims, CNA |

FIG. 18-14 Charting sample.

# DRAINAGE SYSTEMS

A closed drainage system is used for indwelling catheters. Nothing can enter the system from the catheter to the drainage bag. The urinary system is sterile. Infection can occur if microbes enter the drainage system. The microbes travel up the tubing or catheter into the bladder and kidneys. A urinary infection can threaten health and life.

The drainage system has tubing and a drainage bag. Tubing attaches at one end to the catheter. At the other end, it attaches to the drainage bag.

The bag hangs from the bed frame, chair, or wheelchair. It must not touch the floor. The bag is always kept lower than the person's bladder (see Fig. 18-11). Some people wear leg bags when up. The leg bag attaches to the thigh or calf (p. 392).

Microbes can grow in urine. If the drainage bag is higher than the bladder, urine can flow back into the bladder. An infection can occur. Therefore do not hang the drainage bag on a bed rail. When the bed rail is raised, the bag is higher than bladder level. When the person walks, the bag is held lower than the bladder.

Sometimes drainage systems are disconnected accidentally. If that happens, tell the nurse at once. Do not touch the ends of the catheter or tubing. Do the following:

- Practice hand hygiene. Put on gloves.
- Wipe the end of the tube with an antiseptic wipe.
- Wipe the end of the catheter with another antiseptic wipe.
- Do not put the ends down. Do not touch the ends after you clean them.
- Connect the tubing to the catheter.
- Discard the wipes into a biohazard bag.
- Remove the gloves. Practice hand hygiene.

Leg bags are changed to drainage bags when the person is in bed. This drainage bag stays lower than bladder level. You will have to open the closed drainage system. You must prevent microbes from entering the system.

Drainage bags are emptied and urine measured:

- At the end of every shift
- When changing from a leg bag to a drainage bag
- When changing from a drainage bag to a leg bag
- When the bag is becoming full

*Text continued on p. 392.*

---

**DELEGATION GUIDELINES:** *Drainage Systems*

Your delegated tasks may involve urinary drainage systems. If so, you need this information from the nurse and the care plan:

- When to empty the drainage bag
- If the person uses a leg bag
- When to switch drainage bags and leg bags
- If you should clean or discard the drainage bag
- What observations to report and record:
  —The amount of urine measured
  —The color, clarity, and odor of urine
  —Particles in the urine
  —Complaints of pain, burning, irritation, or the need to urinate
  —Drainage system leaks

---

**SAFETY ALERT:** *Drainage Systems*

Urine may contain microbes and blood. Follow Standard Precautions and the Bloodborne Pathogen Standard.

The procedure: *Changing a Leg Bag to a Drainage Bag*, involves opening sterile packages and keeping sterile items free from contamination. Review "Surgical Asepsis" in Chapter 12.

Leg bags hold less than 1000 ml of urine. Most drainage bags hold at least 2000 ml of urine. Therefore leg bags fill faster than drainage bags. Check leg bags often. Empty the leg bag if it is becoming half full. Measure the contents.

## CHANGING A LEG BAG TO A DRAINAGE BAG

### QUALITY OF LIFE

Remember to:
- Knock before entering the person's room
- Address the person by name
- Introduce yourself by name and title

### PRE-PROCEDURE

1 Follow *Delegation Guidelines: Drainage Systems*. See *Safety Alert: Drainage Systems*.
2 Explain the procedure to the person.
3 Practice hand hygiene.
4 Collect the following:
- Gloves
- Drainage bag and tubing
- Antiseptic wipes
- Bed protector
- Sterile cap and plug
- Catheter clamp
- Paper towels
- Bedpan
- Bath blanket

5 Arrange paper towels and equipment on the overbed table.
6 Identify the person. Check the ID bracelet against the assignment sheet. Call the person by name.
7 Provide for privacy.

### PROCEDURE

8 Have the person sit on the side of the bed.
9 Put on the gloves
10 Expose the catheter and leg bag.
11 Clamp the catheter (Fig. 18-15, p. 390). This prevents urine from draining from the catheter into the drainage tubing.
12 Let urine drain from below the clamp site into the drainage tubing. This empties the lower end of the catheter.
13 Help the person lie down.
14 Raise the bed rails if used. Raise the bed for body mechanics.
15 Lower the bed rail near you if up.
16 Cover the person with a bath blanket. Expose the catheter and leg bag.
17 Place the bed protector under the person's leg.
18 Open the antiseptic wipes. Set them on the paper towels.
19 Open the package with the sterile cap and plug. Set the package on the paper towels. Do not let anything touch the sterile cap or plug (Fig. 18-16, p. 390).
20 Open the package with the drainage bag and tubing.
21 Attach the drainage bag to the bed frame.
22 Disconnect the catheter from the drainage tubing. Do not let anything touch the ends.
23 Insert the sterile plug into the catheter end (Fig. 18-17, p. 390). Touch only the end of the plug. Do not touch the part that goes inside the catheter. (If you contaminate the end of the catheter, wipe the end with an antiseptic wipe. Do so before you insert the sterile plug.)
24 Place the sterile cap on the end of the leg bag drainage tube (see Fig. 18-17, p. 390). (If you contaminate the tubing end, wipe the end with an antiseptic wipe. Do so before you put on the sterile cap.)
25 Remove the cap from the new drainage tubing.
26 Remove the sterile plug from the catheter.
27 Insert the end of the drainage tubing into the catheter.
28 Remove the clamp from the catheter.
29 Loop the drainage tubing on the bed. Secure the tubing to the mattress.
30 Remove the leg bag. Place it in the bedpan.
31 Remove and discard the bed protector.
32 Cover the person. Remove the bath blanket.
33 Take the bedpan to the bathroom.
34 Remove the gloves. Practice hand hygiene.

*Continued.*

## CHANGING A LEG BAG TO A DRAINAGE BAG—CONT'D

### POST-PROCEDURE

**35** Provide for comfort.

**36** Place the signal light within reach.

**37** Raise or lower bed rails. Follow the care plan.

**38** Lower the bed to its lowest position.

**39** Unscreen the person.

**40** Put on clean gloves. Discard disposable supplies.

**41** Empty the drainage bag. (See procedure: *Emptying a Urinary Drainage Bag*).

**42** Discard the drainage tubing and bag following agency policy. Or clean the bag following agency policy.

**43** Clean the bedpan. Place it in a clean cover.

**44** Return the bedpan and other supplies to their proper place.

**45** Remove the gloves. Decontaminate your hands.

**46** Report and record your observations.

**47** Reverse the procedure to attach a leg bag to the catheter.

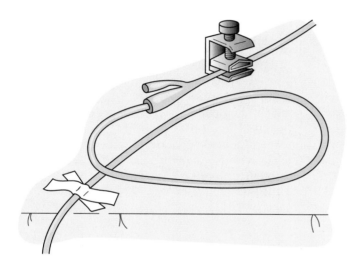

**FIG. 18-15** The clamped catheter prevents urine from draining out of the bladder. The clamp is applied directly to the catheter—not to the drainage tubing.

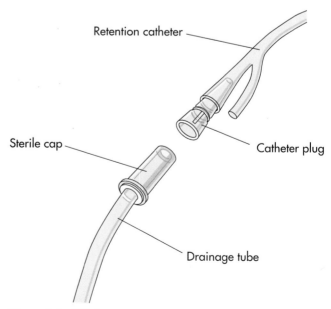

**FIG. 18-17** Sterile plug inserted into the end of the catheter. The sterile cap is on the end of the drainage tube.

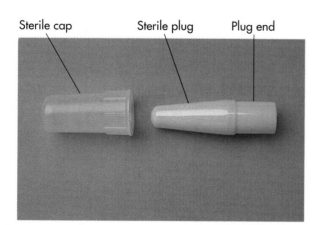

**FIG. 18-16** Sterile cap and catheter plug. The inside of the cap is sterile. Touch only the end of the plug.

# EMPTYING A URINARY DRAINAGE BAG

## QUALITY OF LIFE

Remember to:
- Knock before entering the person's room
- Address the person by name
- Introduce yourself by name and title

### PRE-PROCEDURE

1 Follow *Delegation Guidelines: Drainage Systems,* p. 388. See *Safety Alert: Drainage Systems,* p. 388.
2 Collect equipment:
- Graduate (measuring container)
- Gloves
- Paper towels
3 Practice hand hygiene.
4 Explain the procedure to the person.
5 Identify the person. Check the ID bracelet against the assignment sheet. Call the person by name.
6 Provide for privacy.

### PROCEDURE

7 Put on the gloves.
8 Place a paper towel on the floor. Place the graduate on top of it.
9 Position the graduate under the collection bag.
10 Open the clamp on the drain.
11 Let all urine drain into the graduate. Do not let the drain touch the graduate (Fig. 18-18).
12 Close and position the clamp (see Fig. 18-11).
13 Measure urine.
14 Remove and discard the paper towel.
15 Rinse the graduate. Return it to its proper place.
16 Remove the gloves. Practice hand hygiene.
17 Record the time and amount on the intake and output (I&O) record (Chapter 20).

### POST-PROCEDURE

18 Unscreen the person.
19 Report and record the amount and other observations.

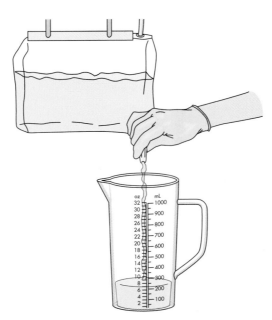

**FIG. 18-18** The clamp on the drainage bag is opened. The drain is directed into the graduate. The drain must not touch the inside of the graduate.

# CONDOM CATHETERS

Condom catheters are often used for incontinent men. They also are called *external catheters, Texas catheters,* and *urinary sheaths.* A condom catheter is a soft sheath that slides over the penis. Tubing connects the condom catheter and drainage bag. Many men prefer leg bags (Fig. 18-19).

To apply a condom catheter, follow the manufacturer's instructions. Thoroughly wash the penis with soap and water. Then dry it before applying the catheter.

Elastic tape secures the catheter in place. Use the elastic tape packaged with the catheter. Elastic tape expands when the penis changes size. This allows blood flow to the penis. *Never use adhesive tape to secure catheters. It does not expand. Blood flow to the penis is cut off, injuring the penis.*

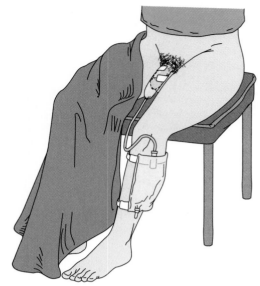

**FIG. 18-19** Condom catheter attached to a leg bag.

---

**DELEGATION GUIDELINES:** *Condom Catheters*

Before removing or applying a condom catheter, you need this information from the nurse and the care plan:

- What size to use—small, medium, or large
- When to remove the catheter and apply a new one
- If a leg bag or standard drainage system is used
- What observations to report and record:
  —Reddened or open areas on the penis
  —Swelling of the penis
  —Color, clarity, and odor of urine
  —Particles in the urine

---

**SAFETY ALERT:** *Condom Catheters*

Do not apply a condom catheter if the penis is red, irritated, or shows signs of skin breakdown. Report your observations to the nurse at once.

If you are not familiar with the condom catheters used at the agency, ask the nurse to show correct application to you. Then ask the nurse to observe you applying the catheter.

Blood must flow to the penis. Use elastic tape. Apply it in a spiral fashion.

Urine may contain microbes and blood. Follow Standard Precautions and the Bloodborne Pathogen Standard.

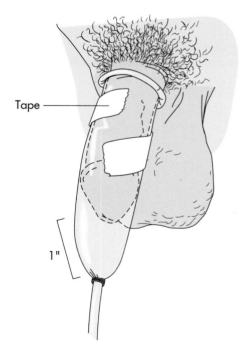

Tape

1"

**FIG. 18-20** A condom catheter applied to the penis. There is a 1-inch space between the penis and the end of the catheter. Tape is applied in a spiral fashion to secure the condom catheter to the penis.

## APPLYING A CONDOM CATHETER

### QUALITY OF LIFE

Remember to:
- Knock before entering the person's room
- Address the person by name
- Introduce yourself by name and title

### PRE-PROCEDURE

1 Follow *Delegation Guidelines: Condom Catheters.* See *Safety Alert: Condom Catheters.*
2 Explain the procedure to the man.
3 Practice hand hygiene.
4 Collect the following:
   - Condom catheter
   - Elastic tape
   - Drainage bag or leg bag
   - Cap for the drainage bag
   - Basin of warm water
   - Soap
   - Towel and washcloths
   - Bath blanket
   - Gloves
   - Bed protector
   - Paper towels
5 Arrange paper towels and equipment on the overbed table.
6 Provide for privacy.
7 Identify the person. Check the ID bracelet against the assignment sheet. Call the person by name.
8 Raise the bed for body mechanics. Bed rails are up if used.

### PROCEDURE

9 Lower the bed rail near you if up.
10 Cover the person with a bath blanket. Lower top linens to the knees.
11 Ask the person to raise his buttocks off the bed. Or turn him onto his side away from you.
12 Slide the bed protector under his buttocks.
13 Have the person lower his buttocks. Or turn him onto his back.
14 Secure the drainage bag to the bed frame. Or have a leg bag ready. Close the drain.
15 Expose the genital area.
16 Put on the gloves.
17 Remove the condom catheter.
   a Remove the tape. Roll the sheath off the penis.
   b Disconnect the drainage tubing from the condom. Cap the drainage tube.
   c Discard the tape and condom.
18 Provide perineal care (see procedure: *Giving Male Perineal Care*, p. 345). Observe the penis for reddened areas and skin breakdown or irritation.
19 Remove the protective backing from the condom. This exposes the adhesive strip.
20 Hold the penis firmly. Roll the condom onto the penis. Leave a 1-inch space between the penis and the end of the catheter (Fig. 18-20).
21 Secure the condom with elastic tape. Apply tape in a spiral (see Fig. 18-20). Do not apply tape completely around the penis.
22 Connect the condom to the drainage tubing. Coil excess tubing on the bed. Or attach a leg bag.
23 Remove the bed protector and gloves. Discard them. Practice hand hygiene.
24 Cover the person. Remove the bath blanket.

### POST-PROCEDURE

25 Provide for comfort.
26 Place the signal light within reach.
27 Raise or lower bed rails. Follow the care plan.
28 Lower the bed to its lowest position.
29 Unscreen the person.
30 Decontaminate your hands. Put on clean gloves.
31 Measure and record the amount of urine in the bag. Clean or discard the collection bag.
32 Clean and return the wash basin and other equipment. Return items to their proper place.
33 Remove the gloves. Decontaminate your hands.
34 Report and record your observations.

## BLADDER TRAINING

Bladder training programs help some persons with urinary incontinence. Some persons need bladder training after indwelling catheter removal. Control of urination is the goal. Bladder control promotes comfort and quality of life. It also increases self-esteem. You assist with bladder training as directed by the nurse and the care plan.

There are two basic methods for bladder training:

- The person uses the toilet, commode, bedpan, or urinal at certain times. The person is given 15 or 20 minutes to start voiding. The rules for normal urination are followed. The normal position for urination is assumed if possible. Privacy is important.
- The person has a catheter. The catheter is clamped to prevent urine flow from the bladder (see Fig. 18-15). It is usually clamped for 1 hour at first. Over time, it is clamped for 3 to 4 hours. Urine drains when the catheter is unclamped. When the catheter is removed, voiding is encouraged every 3 to 4 hours or as directed by the nurse and the care plan.

# ■ REVIEW QUESTIONS ■

Circle the **BEST** answer.

1 Which is *false?*
   a Urine is normally clear and yellow or amber in color.
   b Urine normally has an ammonia odor.
   c Micturition usually occurs before going to bed and upon rising.
   d A person normally voids about 1500 ml a day.

2 Which is *not* a rule for normal urinary elimination?
   a Help the person assume a normal position for voiding.
   b Provide for privacy.
   c Help the person to the bathroom or commode. Or provide the bedpan or urinal as soon as requested.
   d Always stay with the person who is on a bedpan.

3 The best position for using a bedpan is
   a Fowler's position
   b The supine position
   c The prone position
   d The side-lying position

4 After using the urinal, the man should
   a Put it on the bedside stand
   b Use the signal light
   c Put it on the overbed table
   d Empty it

5 Urinary incontinence
   a Is always permanent
   b Requires good skin care
   c Is treated with a catheter
   d Requires bladder training

6 A person has an indwelling catheter. Which action is *incorrect?*
   a Keep the drainage bag above the level of the bladder.
   b Keep drainage tubing free of kinks.
   c Coil the drainage tubing on the bed.
   d Secure the catheter according to agency policy.

7 A person has an indwelling catheter. Which action is *incorrect?*
   a Tape any leaks at the connection site.
   b Follow Standard Precautions and the Bloodborne Pathogen Standard.
   c Empty the drainage bag at the end of each shift.
   d Report complaints of pain, burning, the need to urinate, or irritation at once.

8 Mr. Powers has a condom catheter. You apply elastic tape
   a Completely around the penis
   b To the inner thigh
   c To the abdomen
   d In a spiral fashion

9 The goal of bladder training is to
   a Remove the catheter
   b Allow the person to walk to the bathroom
   c Gain control of urination
   d Void every 3 or 4 hours

10 Which is *not* a cause of functional incontinence?
   a Unanswered signal light
   b No signal light within reach
   c Problems removing clothing
   d Urinary tract infection

*Answers to these questions are on p. 818.*

# Bowel Elimination

# OBJECTIVES

- Define the key terms listed in this chapter
- Describe normal defecation
- List the observations to make about defecation
- Identify the factors that affect bowel elimination
- Describe common bowel elimination problems
- Explain how to promote comfort and safety during defecation
- Describe bowel training
- Explain why enemas are given
- Describe the common enema solutions
- Describe the rules for giving enemas
- Explain the purpose of rectal tubes
- Describe how to care for a person with an ostomy
- Perform the procedures described in this chapter

# KEY TERMS

**colostomy**  A surgically created opening *(stomy)* between the colon *(colo)* and abdominal wall

**constipation**  The passage of a hard, dry stool

**defecation**  The process of excreting feces from the rectum through the anus; a bowel movement

**dehydration**  The excessive loss of water from tissues

**diarrhea**  The frequent passage of liquid stools

**enema**  The introduction of fluid into the rectum and lower colon

**fecal impaction**  The prolonged retention and buildup of feces in the rectum

**fecal incontinence**  The inability to control the passage of feces and gas through the anus

**feces**  The semi-solid mass of waste products in the colon that are expelled through the anus

**flatulence**  The excessive formation of gas in the stomach and intestines

**flatus**  Gas or air passed through the anus

**ileostomy**  A surgically created opening *(stomy)* between the ileum (small intestine *[ileo]*) and the abdominal wall

**ostomy**  A surgically created artificial opening

**peristalsis**  The alternating contraction and relaxation of intestinal muscles

**stoma**  An opening; see *colostomy* and *ileostomy*

**stool**  Excreted feces

**suppository**  A cone-shaped, solid drug that is inserted into a body opening; it melts at body temperature

Bowel elimination is a basic physical need. It is affected by many factors. They include privacy, habits, age, diet, exercise and activity, fluids, and drugs. Problems easily occur. Promoting normal bowel elimination is important. You will assist patients and residents in meeting their elimination needs. See Box 19-1 for a review of the gastrointestinal system.

---

**BOX 19-1 THE GASTROINTESTINAL TRACT: BODY STRUCTURE AND FUNCTION**

The gastointestinal (GI) tract is part of the digestive system (Chapter 7). Bowel elimination is the excretion of wastes from the GI tract. Foods and fluids are normally taken in through the mouth. They are partially digested in the stomach. The partially digested foods and fluids are called *chyme.*

Chyme passes from the stomach into the small intestine. Further digestion and absorption of nutrients occur as the chyme passes through the small bowel. Then chyme enters the large intestine (large bowel or colon) where fluid is absorbed. Chyme becomes less fluid and more solid in consistency. **Feces** refer to the semi-solid mass of waste products in the colon that are expelled through the anus.

Feces move through the intestines by peristalsis. **Peristalsis** is the alternating contraction and relaxation of intestinal muscles. The feces move through the large intestine to the rectum. Feces are stored in the rectum until excreted from the body (Fig. 19-1). **Defecation** (bowel movement) is the process of excreting feces from the rectum through the anus. **Stool** refers to excreted feces.

See Chapter 7 for more information.

---

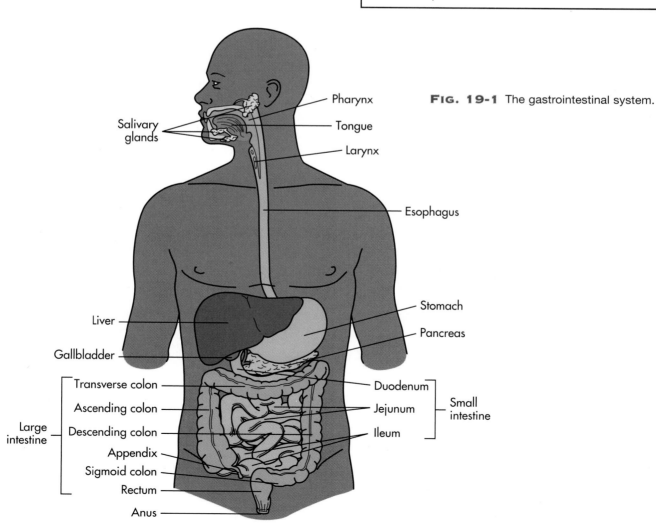

**FIG. 19-1** The gastrointestinal system.

Pharynx
Tongue
Larynx
Esophagus
Salivary glands
Stomach
Pancreas
Liver
Gallbladder
Transverse colon
Ascending colon
Descending colon
Appendix
Sigmoid colon
Rectum
Anus
Duodenum
Jejunum
Ileum
Small intestine
Large intestine

# NORMAL BOWEL MOVEMENTS

Some people have a bowel movement every day. Others have one every 2 to 3 days. Some people have two or three bowel movements a day. Many people defecate after breakfast. Others do so in the evening.

Stools are normally brown. Bleeding in the stomach and small intestine causes black or tarry stools. Bleeding in the lower colon and rectum causes red-colored stools. So do beets. A diet high in green vegetables can cause green stools. Diseases and infection can cause clay-colored or white, pale, orange-colored, or green-colored stools.

Stools are normally soft, formed, moist, and shaped like the rectum. They have a normal odor caused by bacterial action in the intestines. Certain foods and drugs also cause odors.

See *Focus on Children: Normal Bowel Movements.*

## OBSERVATIONS

Your observations are used for the nursing process. Carefully observe stools before disposing of them. Observe and report the following to the nurse. Ask the nurse to observe abnormal stools.

- Color
- Amount
- Consistency
- Odor
- Shape
- Frequency of defecation
- Complaints of pain or discomfort

> ### FOCUS ON CHILDREN
> #### NORMAL BOWEL MOVEMENTS
> Breast-fed infants have yellow stools. Stool consistency ranges from thick liquid to very soft. Bottle-fed infants can have liquid-like stools that are yellowish brown or greenish brown, pasty stools. Stool color and consistency change with solid foods.
>
> Newborns usually have a bowel movement with every feeding. Frequency changes as they grow older. Some infants have two or three bowel movements a day. Others have just one.

# FACTORS AFFECTING BOWEL ELIMINATION

These factors affect stool frequency, consistency, color, and odor. The nurse considers them when using the nursing process to meet the person's elimination needs. Normal, regular elimination is the goal.

- *Privacy.* Bowel elimination is a private act. Odors and sounds are embarrassing. Lack of privacy can prevent defecation despite having the urge. Some people ignore the urge when others are present.
- *Habits.* Many people have a bowel movement after breakfast. Some drink a hot beverage, read, or take a walk. These activities are relaxing. Defecation is easier when a person is relaxed, not tense.
- *Diet.* A well-balanced diet and bulk are needed. High-fiber foods leave a residue for needed bulk. Fruits, vegetables, and whole grain cereals and breads are high in fiber. Milk and milk products cause constipation in some people and diarrhea in others. Chocolate and other foods cause similar reactions. Spicy foods can irritate the intestines. Frequent stools or diarrhea can result. Gas-forming foods stimulate peristalsis, which aids defecation. They include onions, beans, cabbage, cauliflower, radishes, and cucumbers.
- *Fluids.* Feces contain water. Stool consistency depends on the amount of water absorbed in the colon. The amounts of fluid intake, urine output, and vomiting are factors. Feces harden and dry when large amounts of water are absorbed or when fluid intake is poor. Hard, dry feces move slowly through the colon. Constipation can occur. Drinking 6 to 8 glasses of water daily promotes normal bowel elimination. Warm fluids—coffee, tea, hot cider, and warm water—increase peristalsis.
- *Activity.* Exercise and activity maintain muscle tone and stimulate peristalsis. Irregular elimination and constipation often occur from inactivity and bedrest. Inactivity may result from disease, surgery, injury, and aging.
- *Drugs.* Drugs can prevent constipation or control diarrhea. Other drugs have diarrhea or constipation as side effects. Drugs for pain relief often cause constipation. Antibiotics (used to fight or prevent infection) often cause diarrhea. Diarrhea occurs when the antibiotics kill normal flora in the colon. Normal flora is needed to form stools.
- *Disability.* Some people cannot control bowel movements. They defecate whenever feces enter the rectum. A bowel training program is needed (p. 405).
- *Age.* Age affects bowel elimination. See *Focus on Children: Factors Affecting Bowel Elimination*, p. 400. See *Focus on Older Persons: Factors Affecting Bowel Elimination*, p. 400.

## FOCUS ON CHILDREN
### FACTORS AFFECTING BOWEL ELIMINATION

Infants and toddlers do not have control of bowel movements. They defecate whenever feces enter the rectum. Bowel training is learned between 2 and 3 years of age.

## FOCUS ON OLDER PERSONS
### FACTORS AFFECTING BOWEL ELIMINATION

Aging causes changes in the gastrointestinal system. Feces pass through the intestine at a slower rate. Constipation is a risk. Some older persons lose bowel control. Older persons are at risk for intestinal tumors and disorders.

Older persons may not completely empty the rectum. They often need to defecate again 30 to 45 minutes after the first bowel movement.

Many older persons expect to have a bowel movement every day. The slightest irregularity concerns them. The nurse teaches them about normal elimination.

## COMFORT AND SAFETY

The care plan includes measures to meet the person's elimination needs. It may involve diet, fluids, and exercise. Follow the measures in Box 19-2 to promote comfort and safety.

## COMMON PROBLEMS

Common problems include constipation, fecal impaction, diarrhea, fecal incontinence, and flatulence.

### CONSTIPATION

**Constipation** is the passage of a hard, dry stool. The person usually strains to have a bowel movement. Stools are large or marble-size. Large stools cause pain as they pass through the anus. Constipation occurs when feces move slowly through the bowel. This allows more time for water absorption. Common causes include a low-fiber diet, ignoring the urge to defecate, decreased fluid intake, inactivity, drugs, aging, and certain diseases. Dietary changes, fluids, and activity prevent or relieve constipation. So do drugs and enemas.

---

## BOX 19-2   COMFORT AND SAFETY DURING BOWEL ELIMINATION

- Help the person to the toilet or commode. Or provide the bedpan as soon as requested.
- Wheel the person into the bathroom on the commode if possible. Place the commode over the toilet. This provides privacy.
- Provide for privacy. Ask visitors to leave the room. Close doors, and pull privacy curtains. Also close window curtains, blinds, or shades.
- Make sure the bedpan is warm.
- Position the person in a normal sitting or squatting position.
- Cover the person for warmth and privacy.

- Allow enough time for defecation.
- Place the signal light and toilet tissue within reach.
- Leave the room if the person can be alone.
- Stay nearby if the person is weak or unsteady.
- Provide perineal care.
- Dispose of feces promptly. This reduces odors and prevents the spread of microbes.
- Assist the person with hand washing after elimination.
- Follow the care plan if the person has fecal incontinence. The care plan tells you when to assist with elimination.
- Follow Standard Precautions and the Bloodborne Pathogen Standard.

# FECAL IMPACTIONS

A **fecal impaction** is the prolonged retention and buildup of feces in the rectum. Feces are hard or putty-like. Fecal impaction results if constipation is not relieved. The person cannot defecate. More water is absorbed from already hard feces. Liquid feces pass around the hardened fecal mass in the rectum. The liquid feces seep from the anus.

The person tries many times to have a bowel movement. Abdominal discomfort, nausea, cramping, and rectal pain are common. Report these signs and symptoms to the nurse.

A digital (finger) exam is done to check for an impaction. A lubricated, gloved finger is inserted into the rectum to feel for a hard mass (Fig. 19-2). The mass is felt in the lower rectum. Sometimes it is higher in the colon and out of reach. The digital exam often produces the urge to defecate. The doctor may order drugs and enemas to remove the impaction.

Sometimes the fecal mass is removed with a gloved finger. This is called *digital removal of an impaction.* A finger is hooked around a piece of feces. Then the finger and stool are removed. The stool is dropped into the bedpan. The process is repeated as needed. Most people find the procedure uncomfortable and embarrassing.

Checking for and removing impactions are very dangerous. The vagus nerve in the rectum can be stimulated. This nerve also affects the heart. Stimulation of the vagus nerve slows the heart rate. The heart rate can slow to dangerous levels in some persons.

**DELEGATION GUIDELINES:** *Fecal Impactions*
Before you check for and remove impactions, make sure that:
- Your state allows you to perform such procedures
- The procedures are in your job description
- You have the necessary education and training
- You review the procedures with a nurse
- A nurse is available to answer questions and to supervise you

Also make sure you have the following information from the nurse:
- What the doctor's order says
- When to take the person's pulse
- What pulse rates to report at once
- What observations to report and record

**SAFETY ALERT:** *Fecal Impactions*
You must be very careful and gentle. Rectal bleeding can occur. Contact with feces is likely. They may contain microbes or blood. Follow Standard Precautions and the Bloodborne Pathogen Standard.

*Text continued on p. 404*

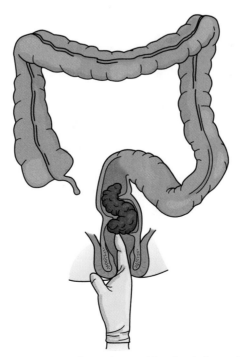

**FIG. 19-2** An index finger is used to check for an impaction.

# CHECKING FOR A FECAL IMPACTION

## QUALITY OF LIFE

Remember to:
- Knock before entering the person's room
- Address the person by name
- Introduce yourself by name and title

## PRE-PROCEDURE

1 Follow *Delegation Guidelines: Fecal Impactions,* p. 401. See *Safety Alert: Fecal Impactions,* p. 401.
2 Explain the procedure to the person.
3 Practice hand hygiene.
4 Collect the following:
   - Bedpan and cover
   - Bath blanket
   - Toilet tissue
   - Gloves
   - Lubricant
   - Waterproof pad
   - Basin of warm water
   - Soap
   - Washcloth
   - Bath towel
5 Identify the person. Check the ID bracelet against the assignment sheet. Call the person by name.
6 Provide for privacy.
7 Raise the bed for body mechanics. Bed rails are up if used.

## PROCEDURE

8 Lower the bed rail near you if up.
9 Cover the person with a bath blanket. Fanfold top linens to the foot of the bed.
10 Position the person in Sims' position or in a left side-lying position.
11 Put on the gloves.
12 Place the waterproof pad under the buttocks.
13 Expose the anal area.
14 Lubricate your gloved index finger.
15 Ask the person to take a deep breath through his or her mouth.
16 Insert the gloved finger while the person is taking a deep breath.
17 Check for a fecal mass.
18 Remove your finger.
19 Help the person onto the bedpan or to the bathroom or commode if needed. Provide for privacy.
20 Remove and discard the gloves. Practice hand hygiene.
21 Put on clean gloves.
22 Wash the person's anal area with soap and water. Pat dry.
23 Remove the waterproof pad and your gloves. Decontaminate your hands.
24 Provide for comfort.

## POST-PROCEDURE

25 Cover the person. Remove the bath blanket.
26 Place the signal light within reach.
27 Lower the bed to its lowest position.
28 Raise or lower bed rails. Follow the care plan.
29 Unscreen the person.
30 Clean and return equipment to its proper place. Discard disposable items. (Wear gloves.)
31 Follow agency policy for soiled linen.
32 Remove the gloves. Practice hand hygiene.
33 Report and record your observations.

# REMOVING A FECAL IMPACTION

## QUALITY OF LIFE

Remember to:
- Knock before entering the person's room
- Address the person by name
- Introduce yourself by name and title

## PROCEDURE

1 Follow steps 1 through 12 in procedure: *Checking for a Fecal Impaction.*
2 Check the person's pulse. Note the rate and rhythm.
3 Expose the anal area.
4 Lubricate your gloved index finger.
5 Ask the person to take a deep breath through the mouth.
6 Insert your lubricated, gloved index finger.
7 Hook your index finger around a small piece of feces.
8 Remove your finger and the feces.
9 Drop the stool into the bedpan.
10 Clean your finger with toilet tissue. Place the toilet tissue in the bedpan.
11 Reapply lubricant as needed.
12 Repeat steps 5 through 10 until you no longer feel feces.
13 Check the person's pulse at intervals. Use your clean gloved hand. Note the rate and rhythm.

Stop the procedure if the pulse rate has slowed or if the rhythm is irregular.
14 Wipe the anal area with toilet tissue.
15 Cover the person with the bath blanket.
16 Cover the bedpan.
17 Remove and discard the gloves. Practice hand hygiene, and put on clean gloves.
18 Raise the bed rail if used. Take the bedpan to the bathroom.
19 Empty, clean, and disinfect the bedpan.
20 Return the bedpan to the bedside stand.
21 Remove and discard the gloves. Practice hand hygiene.
22 Fill the wash basin with warm water.
23 Lower the bed rail near you if up.
24 Put on clean gloves.
25 Wash the buttocks, and give perineal care.
26 Remove the waterproof pad and your gloves. Practice hand hygiene.

## POST-PROCEDURE

27 Provide for comfort.
28 Cover the person, and remove the bath blanket.
29 Place the signal light within reach.
30 Lower the bed to its lowest position.
31 Raise or lower bed rails. Follow the care plan.
32 Unscreen the person.

33 Clean and return equipment to its proper place. Discard disposable items. (Wear gloves.)
34 Follow agency policy for soiled linen.
35 Remove the gloves. Decontaminate your hands.
36 Report and record your observations.

## RHEA

ea is the frequent passage of liquid stools. Feces
ve through the intestines rapidly. This reduces the
me for fluid absorption. The need to defecate is urgent.
Some people cannot get to a bathroom in time.
Abdominal cramping, nausea, and vomiting may occur.

Causes of diarrhea include infections, some drugs,
irritating foods, and microbes in food and water. Diet
and drugs reduce peristalsis. You need to:

- Assist with elimination needs promptly.
- Dispose of stools promptly. This prevents odors and
  the spread of microbes.
- Give good skin care. Liquid feces irritate the skin. So
  does frequent wiping with toilet tissue. Skin breakdown and pressure ulcers are risks.

Fluid lost through diarrhea is replaced. Otherwise
dehydration occurs. **Dehydration** is the excessive loss
of water from tissues. The person has pale or flushed
skin, dry skin, coated tongue, and oliguria (scant
amount of urine). Thirst, weakness, dizziness, and
confusion also occur. Falling blood pressure and increased pulse and respirations are serious signs. Death
can occur. The nursing process is used to meet the person's fluid needs. The doctor may order IV fluids.

Microbes often cause diarrhea. Preventing the
spread of infection is important. Always follow
Standard Precautions and the Bloodborne Pathogen
Standard when in contact with stools.

*See Focus on Children: Diarrhea. See Focus on Older
Persons: Diarrhea.*

## FECAL INCONTINENCE

**Fecal incontinence** is the inability to control the passage of feces and gas through the anus. Causes include:

- Intestinal diseases
- Nervous system diseases and injuries
- Fecal impaction
- Diarrhea
- Some drugs
- Mental health problems or dementia (Chapters 34
  and 35)—the person may not recognize the need or
  act of defecating
- Unanswered signal lights when help is needed with
  elimination
- Not finding the bathroom when in a new setting

Fecal incontinence affects the person emotionally.
Frustration, embarrassment, anger, and humiliation
are common. The person may need:

- Bowel training
- Help with elimination after meals and every 2 to 3
  hours
- Incontinence products to keep garments and linens
  clean
- Good skin care

*See Focus on Children: Fecal Incontinence. See Focus on
Older Persons: Fecal Incontinence.*

### FOCUS ON CHILDREN
#### DIARRHEA

Infants and young children have large amounts of body
water. They are at risk for dehydration. Death can be
rapid. Report any liquid or watery stool at once. Ask
the nurse to observe the stool. Note the number of wet
diapers. Infants wet less when dehydrated.

### FOCUS ON CHILDREN
#### FECAL INCONTINENCE

Infants and toddlers normally have fecal incontinence
until toilet trained.

### FOCUS ON OLDER PERSONS
#### DIARRHEA

Older persons are at risk for dehydration. The amount
of body water decreases with aging. Many diseases
common in older persons affect body fluids. So do
many drugs. Report signs of diarrhea at once. Ask the
nurse to observe the stool. Death is a risk if dehydration is not recognized and treated.

### FOCUS ON OLDER PERSONS
#### FECAL INCONTINENCE

Some older persons have dementia. They may smear
feces on themselves, furniture, and walls. Some are not
aware of having bowel movements. Some resist care.
Follow the person's care plan. Talk to the nurse if you
have problems keeping the person clean.

## FLATULENCE

Gas and air are normally in the stomach and intestines. They are expelled through the mouth (belching, eructing) and anus. Gas and air passed through the anus is called **flatus. Flatulence** is the excessive formation of gas or air in the stomach and intestines. Causes include:

- Swallowing air while eating and drinking (This includes chewing gum, eating fast, drinking through a straw, and drinking carbonated beverages. Tense or anxious people may swallow large amounts of air when drinking.)
- Bacterial action in the intestines
- Gas-forming foods (onions, beans, cabbage, cauliflower, radishes, and cucumbers)
- Constipation
- Bowel and abdominal surgeries
- Drugs that decrease peristalsis

If flatus is not expelled, the intestines distend. That is, they swell or enlarge from the pressure of the gases. Abdominal cramping or pain, shortness of breath, and a swollen abdomen occur. "Bloating" is a common complaint. Walking, moving in bed, and the left side-lying position often produce flatus. Doctors may order enemas, drugs, or rectal tubes to relieve flatulence.

## BOWEL TRAINING

Bowel training has two goals:

- To gain control of bowel movements.
- To develop a regular pattern of elimination. Fecal impaction, constipation, and fecal incontinence are prevented.

Meals, especially breakfast, stimulate the urge to defecate. The person's usual time of day for defecation is noted on the care plan. Toilet, commode, or bedpan use is offered at this time. Factors that promote elimination are part of the care plan and bowel training program. These include a high-fiber diet, increased fluids, warm fluids, activity, and privacy. The nurse tells you about a person's bowel training program.

The doctor may order a suppository to stimulate defecation. A **suppository** is a cone-shaped, solid drug that is inserted into a body opening. It melts at body temperature. A nurse inserts a rectal suppository into the rectum (Fig. 19-3). A bowel movement occurs about 30 minutes later.

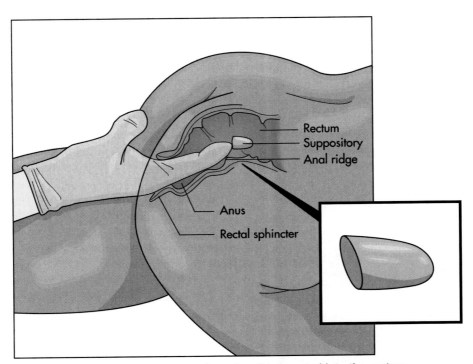

Rectum
Suppository
Anal ridge
Anus
Rectal sphincter

**FIG. 19-3** The suppository *(inset)* is inserted into the rectum.

# ENEMAS

An **enema** is the introduction of fluid into the rectum and lower colon. Doctors order enemas:

- To remove feces
- To relieve constipation, fecal impaction, or flatulence
- To clean the bowel of feces before certain surgeries and diagnostic procedures

Comfort and safety measures for bowel elimination are practiced when giving an enema (see Box 19-2). So are the rules in Box 19-3.

The doctor orders the enema solution. The solution depends on the enema's purpose:

- *Tap-water* enema—obtained from a faucet.
- *Soapsuds enema (SSE)*—add 3 to 5 ml of castile soap to 500 to 1000 ml of tap water.
- *Saline enema*—a solution of salt and water. Add 1 to 2 teaspoons of table salt to 500 to 1000 ml of tap water.
- *Oil-retention enema*—mineral, olive, or cottonseed oil. Usually commercially prepared.
- *Small-volume enema*—contains about 120 ml (4 ounces) of solution. Usually commercially prepared.

Other enema solutions may be ordered. Consult with the nurse and use the agency procedure manual to safely prepare and give enemas. Do not give enemas that contain drugs. Nurses give these enemas.

---

| BOX 19-3 | COMFORT AND SAFETY MEASURES FOR GIVING ENEMAS |
|---|---|

- Have the person void first. This increases the person's comfort during the enema procedure.
- Measure solution temperature with a bath thermometer. See *Delegation Guidelines: Enemas.*
- Give the amount of solution ordered.
- Position the person as the nurse directs. The Sims' position or the left side-lying position is preferred.
- Ask the nurse and check the procedure manual to see how far to insert the enema tubing. It is usually inserted 3 to 4 inches in adults.
- Lubricate the enema tip before inserting it.
- Stop tube insertion if you feel resistance, the person complains of pain, or bleeding occurs.
- Ask the nurse how high to raise the enema bag. For adults, it is usually held 12 inches above the anus.
- Give the solution slowly. Usually it takes 10 to 15 minutes to give 750 to 1000 ml.
- Hold the enema tube in place while giving the solution.
- Ask the nurse how long the person should retain the solution. The length of time depends on the amount and type of solution.
- Make sure the bathroom will be vacant when the person needs to defecate. Make sure that another person will not use the bathroom.
- Ask the nurse to observe the enema results.

---

**DELEGATION GUIDELINES:** *Enemas*

Some states and agencies let nursing assistants give enemas. Others do not. Before giving an enema, make sure that:

- Your state allows you to perform the procedure
- The procedure is in your job description
- You have the necessary education and training
- You review the procedure with a nurse
- A nurse is available to answer questions and to supervise you

If the above conditions are met, you need this information from the nurse:

- What type of enema to give—cleansing, small-volume, or oil-retention
- What size enema tube to use
- How many times to repeat the enema
- The amount of solution ordered by the doctor—usually 500 to 1000 ml for a cleansing enema
- How much castile soap to use for an SSE
- How much salt to use for a saline enema
- What the solution temperature should be—usually 105° F (40.5° C) for adults; 100° F (37.7° C) for children
- How to position the person—Sims' or the left side-lying position
- How far to insert the enema tubing—usually 3 to 4 inches for adults
- How high to hold the solution container
- How fast to give the solution—750 to 1000 ml is usually given over 10 to 15 minutes
- How long the person should try to retain the solution
- What to report and record (Fig. 19-4)

---

**SAFETY ALERT:** *Enemas*

Enemas are usually safe procedures. Many people give themselves enemas at home. However, enemas are dangerous for older persons and those with certain heart and kidney diseases.

Contact with stools is likely when giving enemas. They may contain microbes and blood. Follow Standard Precautions and the Bloodborne Pathogen Standard.

| Date | Time | |
|------|------|---|
| 7/8 | 1700 | 750 ml tap water enema given with the resident in the (L) side-lying position. |
| | | The resident was asked to retain the enema for at least 15 minutes. Bed in low |
| | | position. Signal light within reach. No resident complaints at this time. Resident |
| | | informed that I would return in 15 minutes or when the signal light was used. |
| | | Angie Martinez, CNA ———— |
| | 1715 | Assisted resident to the bedside commode. Privacy curtain pulled. Signal light and |
| | | toilet tissue within reach. Resident reminded to signal when finished expelling the |
| | | enema or if she needs assistance. Angie Martinez, CNA ———— |
| | 1722 | Resident assisted from the commode to bed. Assisted with perineal care and hand- |
| | | washing. States she feels tired. Denies pain or discomfort. Positioned in semi- |
| | | Fowler's position. Bed in low position. Signal light within reach. Large amt. soft, |
| | | brown stool emptied from the commode. No unusual odor noted. Mary Smith, RN |
| | | asked to observe results. Angie Martinez, CNA ———— |

**FIG. 19-4** Charting sample.

# THE CLEANSING ENEMA

Cleansing enemas clean the bowel of feces and flatus. They relieve constipation and fecal impaction. They are needed before certain surgeries and diagnostic procedures.

The doctor orders a soapsuds, tap-water, or saline enema. The doctor may order *enemas until clear.* This means that enemas are given until the return solution is clear and free of feces. Ask the nurse how many enemas to give. Agency policy may allow repeating them 2 or 3 times.

Tap-water enemas can be dangerous. The colon may absorb some of the water into the bloodstream. This creates a fluid imbalance. Only one tap-water enema is given. Do not repeat the enema. Repeated enemas increase the risk of excessive fluid absorption. The tap-water enema takes effect in about 15 to 20 minutes.

Soapsuds enemas irritate the bowel's mucous lining. Repeated enemas can damage the bowel. So can using more than 3 to 5 ml of castile soap or stronger soaps. The SSE takes effect in about 10 to 15 minutes.

The saline enema solution is similar to body fluid. However, some of the salt solution may be absorbed. This too can cause a fluid imbalance. When excess salt is in the body, the body retains water. The saline enema takes effect in about 15 to 20 minutes.

*See Focus on Children: The Cleansing Enema.*

---

### FOCUS ON CHILDREN
#### THE CLEANSING ENEMA

Only saline enemas are used for cleansing enemas in children. Check with the nurse for the amount of solution to give. These are guidelines:
- Infants—50 to 200 ml
- Toddlers—200 to 300 ml
- School-age children—300 to 500 ml
- 12 years and older—500 to 1000 ml

In infants, the enema tube is inserted 1 inch. In toddlers, the tube is inserted 2 inches. For school-age children, it is inserted 3 inches. It is inserted 3 to 4 inches in older children.

---

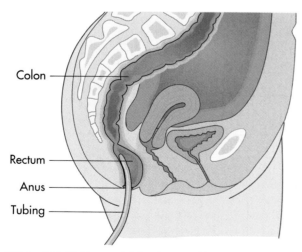

**FIG. 19-5** Enema tubing inserted into the adult rectum.

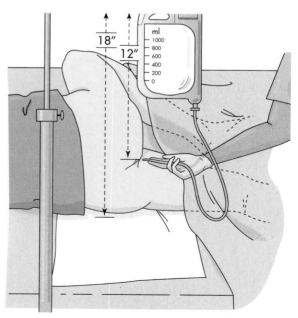

**FIG. 19-6** Giving an enema. The person is in Sims' position. The enema bag hangs from an IV pole. The bag is 12 inches above the anus and 18 inches above the mattress.

## GIVING A CLEANSING ENEMA

### QUALITY OF LIFE

Remember to:
- Knock before entering the person's room
- Address the person by name
- Introduce yourself by name and title

### PRE-PROCEDURE

1 Follow *Delegation Guidelines: Enemas*, p. 406. See *Safety Alert: Enemas*, p. 406.
2 Explain the procedure to the person.
3 Practice hand hygiene.
4 Collect the following:
   - Bedpan or commode
   - Disposable enema kit as directed by the nurse (enema bag, tube, clamp, and waterproof pad)
   - Bath thermometer
   - Waterproof pad
   - Water-soluble lubricant
   - Gloves
   - 3 to 5 ml (1 teaspoon) castile soap or 1 to 2 teaspoons of salt
   - Toilet tissue
   - Bath blanket
   - IV pole
   - Robe and nonskid footwear
   - Paper towels
5 Identify the person. Check the ID bracelet with the assignment sheet. Call the person by name.
6 Provide for privacy.
7 Raise the bed for body mechanics. Bed rails are up if used.

### PROCEDURE

8 Lower the bed rail near you if up.
9 Cover the person with a bath blanket. Fanfold top linens to the foot of the bed.
10 Position the IV pole so the enema bag is 12 inches above the anus. Or it is at a height directed by the nurse.
11 Raise the bed rail if used.
12 Prepare the enema:
   a Close the clamp on the tube.
   b Adjust water flow until it is lukewarm.
   c Fill the enema bag for the amount ordered.
   d Measure water temperature with the bath thermometer. It is usually 105° F (40.5° C) for adults; 100° F (37.7° C) for children.
   e Prepare the enema solution as directed by the nurse, (p. 406):
      (1) Saline enema: add salt as directed.
      (2) Soapsuds enema: add castile soap as directed.
      (3) Tap-water enema: add nothing to the water.
   f Stir the solution with the bath thermometer. Scoop off any suds (SSE).
   g Seal the bag.
   h Hang the bag on the IV pole.
13 Lower the bed rail near you.
14 Position the person in Sims' position or in a left side-lying position.
15 Put on the gloves.
16 Place a waterproof pad under the buttocks.
17 Expose the anal area.
18 Place the bedpan behind the person.
19 Position the enema tube in the bedpan. Remove the cap from the tubing.
20 Open the clamp. Let solution flow through the tube to remove air. Clamp the tube.
21 Lubricate the tube 3 to 4 inches from the tip.
22 Separate the buttocks to see the anus.
23 Ask the person to take a deep breath through the mouth.
24 Insert the tube gently 3 to 4 inches into the adult's rectum (Fig. 19-5). Do this when the person is exhaling. Stop if the person complains of pain, you feel resistance, or bleeding occurs.
25 Check the amount of solution in the bag.
26 Unclamp the tube. Give the solution slowly (Fig. 19-6).
27 Ask the person to take slow, deep breaths. This helps the person relax.
28 Clamp the tube if the person needs to defecate, has cramping, or starts to expel solution. Unclamp when symptoms subside.
29 Give the amount of solution ordered. Stop if the person cannot tolerate the procedure.
30 Clamp the tube before it is empty. This prevents air from entering the bowel.
31 Hold toilet tissue around the tube and against the anus. Remove the tube.
32 Discard the toilet tissue into the bedpan.
33 Wrap the tubing tip with paper towels. Place it inside the enema bag.

*Continued.*

## GIVING A CLEANSING ENEMA—CONT'D

### PROCEDURE—CONT'D

34 Help the person onto the bedpan. Raise the head of the bed, and raise the bed rail if used. Or assist the person to the bathroom or commode. The person wears a robe and nonskid footwear when up. The bed is in the lowest position.
35 Place the signal light and toilet tissue within reach. Remind the person not to flush the toilet.
36 Discard disposable items.
37 Remove the gloves. Decontaminate your hands.
38 Leave the room if the person can be left alone.
39 Return when the person signals. Knock before entering.
40 Decontaminate your hands, and put on gloves. Lower the bed rail if up.

41 Observe enema results for amount, color, consistency, and odor. Call for the nurse to observe the results.
42 Provide perineal care as needed.
43 Remove the bed protector.
44 Empty, clean, and disinfect the bedpan or commode. Flush the toilet after the nurse observes the results. Return items to their proper place.
45 Remove the gloves. Practice hand hygiene.
46 Assist with hand washing. Wear gloves if needed.
47 Cover the person. Remove the bath blanket.

### POST-PROCEDURE

48 Provide for comfort.
49 Place the signal light within reach.
50 Lower the bed to its lowest position.
51 Raise or lower bed rails. Follow the care plan.
52 Unscreen the person.

53 Follow agency policy for soiled linen and used supplies.
54 Decontaminate your hands.
55 Report and record your observations.

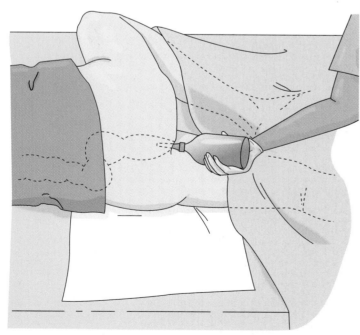

**FIG. 19-7** The small-volume enema tip is inserted 2 inches into the rectum.

## THE SMALL-VOLUME ENEMA

Small-volume enemas irritate and distend the rectum. This causes defecation. They are often ordered for constipation or when the bowel does not need complete cleansing.

These enemas are ready to give. The solution is usually given at room temperature. To give the enema, squeeze and roll up the plastic bottle from the bottom. Do not release pressure on the bottle. Otherwise, solution is drawn from the rectum back into the bottle.

Urge the person to retain the solution until there is a need to defecate. This usually takes about 5 to 10 minutes. Staying in the Sims' or left side-lying position helps to retain the enema.

## GIVING A SMALL-VOLUME ENEMA

### QUALITY OF LIFE

Remember to:
- Knock before entering the person's room
- Address the person by name
- Introduce yourself by name and title

### PRE-PROCEDURE

1 Follow *Delegation Guidelines: Enemas*, p. 406. See *Safety Alert: Enemas*, p. 406.
2 Explain the procedure to the person.
3 Practice hand hygiene.
4 Collect the following:
   - Small-volume enema
   - Bedpan or commode
   - Waterproof pad
   - Toilet tissue
   - Gloves
   - Robe and nonskid footwear
   - Bath blanket
5 Identify the person. Check the ID bracelet against the assignment sheet. Call the person by name.
6 Provide for privacy.
7 Raise the bed for body mechanics. Bed rails are up if used.

### PROCEDURE

8 Lower the bed rail near you if up.
9 Cover the person with a bath blanket. Fanfold top linens to the foot of the bed.
10 Position the person in Sims' or a left side-lying position.
11 Put on the gloves.
12 Place the waterproof pad under the buttocks.
13 Expose the anal area.
14 Position the bedpan near the person.
15 Remove the cap from the enema tip.
16 Separate the buttocks to see the anus.
17 Ask the person to take a deep breath through the mouth.
18 Insert the enema tip 2 inches into the rectum (Fig. 19-7). Do this when the person is exhaling. Insert the tip gently. Stop if the person complains of pain, you feel resistance, or bleeding occurs.
19 Squeeze and roll the bottle gently. Release pressure on the bottle after you remove the tip from the rectum.
20 Put the bottle into the box, tip first.
21 Help the person onto the bedpan; raise the head of the bed. Raise or lower bed rails according to the care plan. Or assist the person to the bathroom or commode. The person wears a robe and nonskid footwear when up. The bed is in the lowest position.
22 Place the signal light and toilet tissue within reach. Remind the person not to flush the toilet.
23 Discard disposable items.
24 Remove the gloves. Decontaminate your hands.
25 Leave the room if the person can be left alone.
26 Return when the person signals. Knock before entering.
27 Decontaminate your hands. Lower the bed rail if up.
28 Put on gloves.
29 Observe enema results for amount, color, consistency, and odor.
30 Help the person with perineal care.
31 Remove the bed protector.
32 Empty, clean, and disinfect the bedpan or commode. Flush the toilet after the nurse observes the results.
33 Return equipment to its proper place.
34 Remove the gloves. Practice hand hygiene.
35 Assist with hand washing. Wear gloves if necessary.
36 Return top linens. Remove the bath blanket.

### POST-PROCEDURE

37 Follow steps 48 through 55 in procedure: *Giving a Cleansing Enema.*

## ◼ THE OIL-RETENTION ENEMA

Oil-retention enemas relieve constipation and fecal impactions. The oil is retained for 30 to 60 minutes or longer (1 to 3 hours). Retaining oil softens feces and lubricates the rectum. This lets feces pass with ease. Most oil-retention enemas are commercially prepared.

---

### GIVING AN OIL-RETENTION ENEMA

#### QUALITY OF LIFE

Remember to:
- Knock before entering the person's room
- Address the person by name
- Introduce yourself by name and title

#### PRE-PROCEDURE

1 Follow *Delegation Guidelines: Enemas,* p. 406. See *Safety Alert: Enemas,* p. 406.
2 Explain the procedure to the person.
3 Practice hand hygiene.
4 Collect the following:
 - Oil-retention enema
 - Waterproof pads
 - Gloves
 - Bath blanket
5 Identify the person. Check the ID bracelet against the assignment sheet. Call the person by name.
6 Provide for privacy.
7 Raise the bed for body mechanics. Bed rails are up if used.

#### PROCEDURE

8 Follow steps 8 through 20 in procedure: *Giving a Small-Volume Enema,* p. 411.
9 Cover the person. Leave him or her in the Sims' or left side-lying position.
10 Encourage him or her to retain the enema for the time ordered.
11 Place more waterproof pads on the bed if needed.
12 Remove the gloves. Decontaminate your hands.
13 Lower the bed to its lowest position.
14 Raise or lower bed rails. Follow the care plan.
15 Provide for comfort.
16 Place the signal light within reach.
17 Unscreen the person.
18 Decontaminate your hands.
19 Check the person often.

#### POST-PROCEDURE

20 Follow steps 48 through 55 in procedure: *Giving a Cleansing Enema,* p. 410.

# RECTAL TUBES

A rectal tube is inserted into the rectum. Its purpose is to relieve flatulence and intestinal distention. Flatus passes without effort or straining.

The rectal tube is inserted 4 inches into the adult rectum. It is left in place for 20 to 30 minutes. This helps prevent rectal irritation. It can be reinserted every 2 to 3 hours. *Rectal tubes are not used after rectal surgery.*

Often the tube is connected to a flatus bag or to a water container (Fig. 19-8). The bag inflates as gas passes into it. If connected to a water container, the water bubbles as gas passes through the tube into the water. For this system, the rectal tube is attached to connecting tubing. The connecting tubing attaches to the water container.

Feces may be expelled along with flatus. If a flatus bag is not used, place the open end of the tube in a folded, waterproof pad.

*See Focus on Children: Rectal Tubes.*

## FOCUS ON CHILDREN
### RECTAL TUBES
The tube is inserted 2 to 4 inches into the child's rectum. The nurse tells you what size tube to use and how far to insert the tube.

**DELEGATION GUIDELINES:** *Rectal Tubes*
Before inserting a rectal tube, you need this information from the nurse and the care plan:
- What size tube to use
- When to insert the tube
- How long to leave it in place
- If you should connect the tube to a flatus bag or a water container
- What observations to report and record:
  —The person's report of passing flatus and how much
  —Complaints of pain or discomfort

**SAFETY ALERT:** *Rectal Tubes*
Do not force the tube into the rectum. Stop and call for the nurse if you feel resistance, the person complains of pain, or bleeding occurs.

Contact with feces is likely. They may contain microbes and blood. Follow Standard Precautions and the Bloodborne Pathogen Standard.

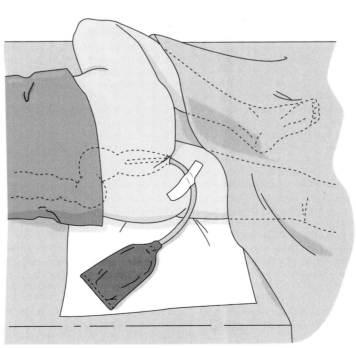

**FIG. 19-8** Inserting a rectal tube. The tube is inserted 4 inches into the adult rectum. The rectal tube is taped to the thigh. The flatus bag rests on the bed.

## INSERTNG A RECTAL TUBE

### QUALITY OF LIFE

Remember to:
- Knock before entering the person's room
- Address the person by name
- Introduce yourself by name and title

### PRE-PROCEDURE

1 Follow *Delegation Guidelines: Rectal Tubes*, p. 413. See *Safety Alert: Rectal Tubes*, p. 413.
2 Explain the procedure to the person.
3 Practice hand hygiene.
4 Collect the following:
  - Disposable rectal tube with flatus bag
  - Water-soluble lubricant
  - Tape
  - Gloves
  - Waterproof pad
5 Identify the person. Check the ID bracelet against the assignment sheet. Call the person by name.
6 Provide for privacy.
7 Raise the bed for body mechanics. Bed rails are up if used.

### PROCEDURE

8 Lower the bed rail near you if up.
9 Position the person in Sims' or a left side-lying position.
10 Put on the gloves.
11 Place the waterproof pad under the buttocks.
12 Expose the anal area.
13 Lubricate 4 inches from the tube tip.
14 Separate the buttocks to see the anus.
15 Ask the person to take a deep breath through the mouth.
16 Insert the tube 4 inches into the adult rectum. Do this when the person is exhaling. Insert the tube gently. Stop if the person complains of pain, you feel resistance, or bleeding occurs.
17 Tape the rectal tube to the thigh (see Fig 19-8).
18 Position the flatus bag so it rests on the bed protector (see Fig. 19-8).
19 Cover the person.
20 Leave the tube in place for the time directed by the nurse. It is left in place no longer than 30 minutes.
21 Lower the bed to its lowest position.
22 Place the signal light within reach.
23 Raise or lower bed rails. Follow the care plan.
24 Remove the gloves. Decontaminate your hands.
25 Leave the room. Check the person often. Knock before entering the room.
26 Return to the room when it is time to remove the tube. Knock before entering the room.
27 Decontaminate your hands. Put on gloves.
28 Remove the tube. Wipe the rectal area.
29 Wrap the rectal tube and flatus bag in the bed protector. Remove the bed protector and your gloves. Decontaminate your hands.
30 Ask the person about the amount of gas expelled.

### POST-PROCEDURE

31 Provide for comfort.
32 Place the signal light within reach.
33 Unscreen the person.
34 Discard disposable items. Follow agency policy for soiled linen. Wear gloves.
35 Remove the gloves. Decontaminate your hands.
36 Report and record your observations.

# THE PERSON WITH AN OSTOMY

Sometimes part of the intestines is removed surgically. Cancer, bowel disease, and trauma (stab or bullet wounds) are common reasons. An ostomy is sometimes necessary. An **ostomy** is a surgically created artificial opening. The opening is called a **stoma.** The person wears a pouch over the stoma to collect feces and flatus. Stomas do not have nerve endings. Therefore they are not painful. You will not hurt the person when touching the stoma.

## COLOSTOMY

A **colostomy** is a surgically created opening *(stomy)* between the colon *(colo)* and abdominal wall. Part of the colon is brought out onto the abdominal wall and a stoma made. Feces and flatus pass through the stoma instead of through the anus. With a permanent colostomy, the diseased part of the colon is removed. A temporary colostomy gives the diseased or injured bowel time to heal. After healing, surgery is done to re-connect the bowel.

The colostomy site depends on the site of disease or injury (Fig. 19-9). Stool consistency depends on the colostomy site. Consistency ranges from liquid to formed. The more colon remaining to absorb water, the more solid and formed the stool. If the colostomy is near the start of the colon, stools are liquid. A colostomy near the end of the colon results in formed stools.

Feces irritate the skin. Skin care prevents skin breakdown around the stoma. The skin is washed and dried. Then a skin barrier is applied around the stoma. It prevents feces from having contact with the skin. The skin barrier is part of the pouch or a separate device.

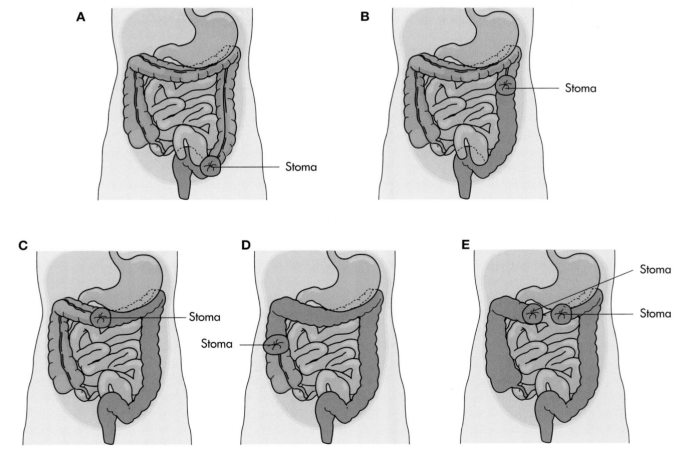

**FIG. 19-9** Colostomy sites. *Shading* shows the part of the bowel surgically removed. **A,** Sigmoid colostomy. **B,** Descending colostomy. **C,** Transverse colostomy. **D,** Ascending colostomy. **E,** Double-barrel colostomy has two stomas. One allows for the excretion of feces. The other is for the introduction of drugs to help the bowel heal. This type of colostomy is usually temporary.

## ILEOSTOMY

An **ileostomy** is a surgically created opening (*stomy*) between the ileum (small intestine [*ileo*]) and the abdominal wall. Part of the ileum is brought out onto the abdominal wall, and a stoma is made. The entire colon is removed (Fig. 19-10). Liquid feces drain constantly from an ileostomy. Water is not absorbed because the colon was removed. Feces in the small intestine contain digestive juices that are very irritating to the skin. The ileostomy pouch must fit well. Feces must not touch the skin. Good skin care is required.

**OSTOMY POUCHES.** The pouch has an adhesive backing that is applied to the skin. Sometimes pouches are secured to ostomy belts (Fig. 19-11). Many pouches have a drain at the bottom that closes with clips, clamps, or wire closures. The drain is opened to empty the pouch. The pouch is emptied when feces are present. It is opened when it balloons or bulges with flatus. The drain is wiped with toilet tissue before it is closed.

The pouch is changed every 3 to 7 days and when it leaks. Some people change the pouch daily and whenever soiling occurs. However, frequent pouch changes can damage the skin.

Odors are prevented by:
- Good hygiene
- Emptying the pouch
- Avoiding gas-forming foods
- Putting deodorants into the pouch (The nurse tells you what to use.)

The person can wear normal clothes. However, tight garments can prevent feces from entering the pouch. Also, bulging from feces and flatus can be seen with tight clothes.

Peristalsis increases after eating. Therefore stomas are usually quiet before breakfast. That is, expelling feces is less likely at this time. If the person showers or bathes with the pouch off, it is best done before breakfast. Showers and baths are delayed 1 to 2 hours after applying a new pouch. This gives adhesive time to stick to the skin.

Do not flush pouches down the toilet. Follow agency policy for disposing of them.

*See Focus on Children: Ostomy Pouches.*

> ### FOCUS ON CHILDREN
> #### OSTOMY POUCHES
> Children of all ages can have ostomies, even premature infants. If changing a child's ostomy pouch is delegated to you, the nurse gives you the necessary instructions.

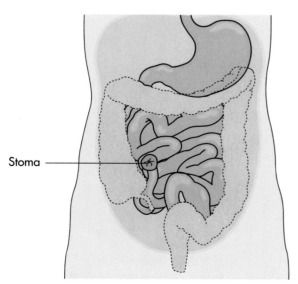

**FIG. 19-10** An ileostomy. The entire large intestine is surgically removed.

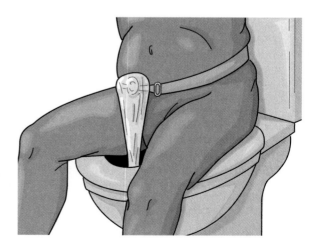

**FIG. 19-11** The ostomy pouch is secured to an ostomy belt. The pouch is emptied by directing it into the toilet and unclamping the end.

**DELEGATION GUIDELINES:** *Ostomy Pouches*

Many people manage their ostomies without help. Others need assistance. When the nurse delegates changing an ostomy pouch to you, make sure that:

- Your state allows you to perform the procedure
- The procedure is in your job description
- You have the necessary education and training
- You review the procedure with the nurse
- The nurse is available to answer questions and to supervise you

If the above conditions are met, you need this information from the nurse and the care plan:

- What kind of ostomy the person has—colostomy or ileostomy
- What equipment and supplies to use
- What observations to report and record:
  —Signs of skin breakdown (normally the stoma is red like mucous membranes)
  —Color, amount, consistency, and odor of feces
  —Complaints of pain or discomfort

**SAFETY ALERT:** *Ostomy Pouches*

When changing an ostomy pouch, contact with feces is likely. They may contain microbes or blood. Follow Standard Precautions and the Bloodborne Pathogen Standard.

Tell the nurse if you observe signs of skin breakdown. Do this before you apply a new pouch.

## CHANGING AN OSTOMY POUCH

### QUALITY OF LIFE

Remember to:
- Knock before entering the person's room
- Address the person by name
- Introduce yourself by name and title

### PRE-PROCEDURE

1 Follow *Delegation Guidelines: Ostomy Pouches.* See *Safety Alert: Ostomy Pouches.*
2 Explain the procedure to the person.
3 Practice hand hygiene.
4 Collect the following:
  - Clean pouch with skin barrier
  - Skin barrier (if not part of the pouch)
  - Pouch clamp, clip, or wire closure
  - Clean ostomy belt (if used)
  - Skin barrier as ordered
  - Gauze squares or washcloths
  - Adhesive remover
  - Cotton balls
  - Bedpan with cover
  - Waterproof pad
  - Bath blanket
  - Toilet tissue
  - Wash basin
  - Bath thermometer
  - Prescribed soap or cleansing agent
  - Pouch deodorant
  - Paper towels
  - Gloves
  - Disposable bag
5 Arrange your work area.
6 Identify the person. Check the ID bracelet against the assignment sheet. Call the person by name.
7 Provide for privacy.
8 Raise the bed for body mechanics. Bed rails are up if used.

*Continued.*

## CHANGING AN OSTOMY POUCH—CONT'D

### PROCEDURE

9 Lower the bed rail near you if up.

10 Cover the person with a bath blanket. Fanfold linens to the foot of the bed.

11 Put on the gloves.

12 Place the waterproof pad under the buttocks.

13 Disconnect the pouch from the belt if one is worn. Remove the belt.

14 Remove the pouch gently. Gently push the skin down and away from the skin barrier. Place the pouch in the bedpan.

15 Wipe around the stoma with toilet tissue or a gauze square. This removes mucus and feces. Place soiled tissue in the bedpan. Discard gauze squares in the bag.

16 Moisten a cotton ball with adhesive remover. Clean around the stoma to remove any remaining skin barrier. Clean from the stoma outward.

17 Cover the bedpan. Take it to the bathroom. (If the person uses bed rails, they are up before you leave the bedside.)

18 Measure the amount of feces. Note the color, amount, consistency, and odor of feces.

19 Ask the nurse to observe abnormal feces. Then empty the pouch and bedpan into the toilet. Put the pouch in the bag.

20 Remove the gloves, and practice hand hygiene. Put on clean gloves.

21 Fill the basin with warm water. Place the basin on the overbed table on top of the paper towels. Lower the bed rail near you if up.

22 Wash the skin around the stoma. Rinse and pat dry. Use soap or other cleansing agent as directed by the nurse.

23 Apply the skin barrier if it is a separate device.

24 Put a clean ostomy belt on the person (if a belt is worn).

25 Add deodorant to the new pouch.

26 Remove adhesive backing on the pouch.

27 Center the pouch over the stoma. The drain points downward.

28 Press around the skin barrier so the pouch seals to the skin. Apply gentle pressure from the stoma outward.

29 Maintain pressure for 1 to 2 minutes.

30 Connect the belt to the pouch (if a belt is worn).

31 Remove the waterproof pad.

32 Remove the gloves. Decontaminate your hands.

33 Cover the person. Remove the bath blanket.

### POST-PROCEDURE

34 Provide for comfort.

35 Raise or lower bed rails. Follow the care plan.

36 Lower the bed to its lowest position.

37 Place the signal light within reach.

38 Unscreen the person.

39 Clean equipment. Wear gloves for this step.

40 Return equipment to its proper place.

41 Discard the bag according to agency policy. Follow agency policy for soiled linen.

42 Remove the gloves. Practice hand hygiene.

43 Report and record your observations.

Circle the **BEST** answer.

1 Which is *false?*
a A person must have a bowel movement every day.
b Stools are normally brown, soft, and formed.
c Diarrhea occurs when feces move rapidly through the bowels.
d Constipation results when feces move slowly through the colon.

2 The prolonged retention and accumulation of feces in the rectum is called
a Constipation
b Fecal impaction
c Diarrhea
d Anal incontinence

3 Which will *not* promote comfort and safety for bowel elimination?
a Asking visitors to leave the room
b Helping the person to a sitting position
c Offering the bedpan after meals
d Telling the person that you will return very soon

4 Bowel training is aimed at
a Gaining control of bowel movements and developing a regular elimination pattern
b Ostomy control
c Preventing fecal impaction, constipation, and anal incontinence
d Preventing bleeding

5 Which is *not* used for a cleansing enema?
a Soap suds
b Saline
c Oil
d Tap water

6 Which is *false?*
a Enema solutions should be 105° F (40.5° C).
b The Sims' position is used for an enema.
c The enema bag is held 12 inches above the anus.
d The enema solution is given rapidly.

7 In adults, the enema tube is inserted
a 2 inches
b 4 inches
c 6 inches
d 8 inches

8 The oil-retention enema is retained for at least
a 10 to 15 minutes
b 15 to 30 minutes
c 30 to 60 minutes
d 60 to 90 minutes

9 Rectal tubes are left in place no longer than
a 60 minutes
b 30 minutes
c 20 minutes
d 10 minutes

10 Which statement about ostomies is *false?*
a Good skin care around the stoma is essential.
b Deodorants can control odors.
c The person wears a pouch.
d Feces are always liquid.

*Answers to these questions are on p. 818.*

# Nutrition
# and Fluids

## OBJECTIVES

- Define the key terms listed in this chapter
- Explain the purpose and use of the Food Guide Pyramid
- Explain how to use the Dietary Guidelines for Americans
- Describe the functions and major sources of nutrients
- Explain how to use food labels
- Describe factors that affect eating and nutrition
- Describe the special diets and between-meal nourishments
- Identify the signs, symptoms, and precautions relating to regurgitation and aspiration
- Describe fluid requirements and the causes of dehydration
- Explain what to do when the person has special fluid orders
- Explain the purpose of intake and output records
- Identify what is counted as fluid intake
- Explain how to assist with food and fluid needs
- Explain how to assist with calorie counts
- Describe the purpose, methods, and comfort measures for enteral nutrition and IV therapy
- Perform the procedures described in this chapter

## KEY TERMS

**anorexia**　The loss of appetite

**aspiration**　Breathing fluid or an object into the lungs

**calorie**　The amount of energy produced when the body burns food

**Daily Reference Values (DRVs)**　The maximum daily intake values for total fat, saturated fat, cholesterol, sodium, carbohydrate, and dietary fiber

**Daily Value (DV)**　How a serving fits into the daily diet; expressed in a percent (%) based on a daily diet of 2000 calories

**dehydration**　A decrease in the amount of water in body tissues

**dysphagia**　Difficulty *(dys)* swallowing *(phagia)*

**edema**　The swelling of body tissues with water

**enteral nutrition**　Giving nutrients through the gastrointestinal tract *(enteral)*

**flow rate**　The number of drops per minute *(gtt/min)*

**gastrostomy tube**　A tube inserted through a surgically created opening *(stomy)* into the stomach *(gastro)*; stomach tube

**gavage**　Tube feeding

**graduate**　A measuring container for fluid

**intake**　The amount of fluid taken in

**intravenous (IV) therapy**　Giving fluids through a needle or catheter inserted into a vein; IV, IV therapy, and IV infusion

**jejunostomy tube**　A tube inserted into the intestines through a surgically created opening *(stomy)* into the middle part of the small intestine *(jejunum)*

**nasogastric (NG) tube**　A tube inserted through the nose *(naso)* into the stomach *(gastro)*

**nasointestinal tube**　A tube inserted through the nose *(naso)* into the small intestine *(intestinal)*

**nutrient**　A substance that is ingested, digested, absorbed, and used by the body

**nutrition**　The processes involved in the ingestion, digestion, absorption, and use of foods and fluids by the body

**output**　The amount of fluid lost

**percutaneous endoscopic gastrostomy (PEG) tube**　A tube inserted into the stomach *(gastro)* through a stab or puncture wound *(stomy)* made through *(per)* the skin *(cutaneous)*; a lighted instrument *(scope)* allows the doctor to see inside a body cavity or organ *(endo)*

**regurgitation**　The backward flow of food from the stomach into the mouth

Food and water are physical needs. They are necessary for life. The amount and quality of food affect physical and mental well-being. A poor diet and poor eating habits:

- Increase the risk for infection
- Increase the risk for acute and chronic diseases
- Cause chronic illnesses to become worse
- Cause healing problems
- Affect physical and mental function, increasing the risk for accidents and injuries

Eating and drinking provide pleasure. They often are part of social times with family and friends. A friendly, social setting for meals is important. Otherwise, the person may eat poorly.

Many factors affect dietary practices. They include culture, finances, and personal choice. See *Caring About Culture: Mealtime Practices.* Dietary practices also include selecting, preparing, and serving food. The health team considers these factors when planning to meet the person's nutrition needs.

See Box 20-1 for a review of the structure and function of the digestive system.

## BASIC NUTRITION

**Nutrition** is the processes involved in the ingestion, digestion, absorption, and use of foods and fluids by the body. Good nutrition is needed for growth, healing, and body functions. A well-balanced diet and correct calorie intake are needed. A high-fat and high-calorie diet causes weight gain and obesity. Weight loss occurs with a low-calorie diet.

Foods and fluids contain nutrients. A **nutrient** is a substance that is ingested, digested, absorbed, and used by the body. Nutrients are grouped into fats, proteins, carbohydrates, vitamins, minerals, and water.

Fats, proteins, and carbohydrates give the body fuel for energy. The amount of energy provided by a nutrient is measured in calories. A **calorie** is the amount of energy produced when the body burns food.

- 1 gram of fat—9 calories
- 1 gram of protein—4 calories
- 1 gram of carbohydrate—4 calories

---

### BOX 20-1 DIGESTIVE SYSTEM: REVIEW OF BODY STRUCTURE AND FUNCTION

The digestive system breaks down food physically and chemically so it can be absorbed for use by the cells. This process is called *digestion*. The digestive system is also called the *gastrointestinal system (GI system)*. It consists of the *alimentary canal (GI tract)* and the accessory organs of digestion (Fig. 20-1). The alimentary canal extends from the mouth to the anus. Its major parts are the mouth, pharynx, esophagus, stomach, small intestine, and large intestine. The accessory organs of digestion are the teeth, tongue, salivary glands, liver, gallbladder, and pancreas.

Digestion begins in the *mouth (oral cavity)*. The oral cavity receives food and prepares it for digestion. Using chewing motions, the teeth cut, chop, and grind food into smaller particles for digestion and swallowing. The *tongue* aids in chewing and swallowing. *Taste buds* on the tongue contain nerve endings. Taste buds sense sweet, sour, bitter, and salty tastes. *Salivary glands* in the mouth secrete *saliva.* Saliva moistens food particles for easier swallowing and begins the digestion of food. During swallowing, the tongue pushes food into the pharynx.

The *pharynx* (throat) is a muscular tube. Swallowing continues as the pharynx contracts. Contraction of the pharynx pushes food into the *esophagus.* The esophagus is a muscular tube about 10 inches long. It extends from the pharynx to the stomach. Involuntary muscle contrac-

tions called *peristalsis* move food down the esophagus into the stomach.

The *stomach* is a muscular, pouchlike sac in the upper left part of the abdominal cavity. Strong stomach muscles stir and churn food to break it up into even smaller particles. The stomach is lined with a mucous membrane containing glands that secrete *gastric juices.* Food is mixed and churned with the gastric juices to form a semi-liquid substance called *chyme.* Through peristalsis, the chyme is pushed from the stomach into the small intestine.

The *small intestine* is about 20 feet long and has 3 parts. The first part is the duodenum. In the *duodenum,* more digestive juices are added to the chyme. One is called *bile.* Bile is a greenish liquid. It is produced by the *liver* and stored in the *gallbladder.* Juices from the *pancreas* and small intestine are also added to the chyme. The digestive juices chemically break down food so it can be absorbed.

Peristalsis moves the chyme through the two remaining portions of the small intestine: the *jejunum* and the *ileum.* Tiny projections called *villi* line the small intestine. Villi absorb the digested food into the capillaries. Most food absorption takes place in the jejunum and ileum. Chyme eventually enters the large intestine. More fluid is absorbed. The solid waste that remains is eliminated through the anus.

**CARING ABOUT CULTURE**

MEAL TIME PRACTICES

Many cultural groups have their main meal at midday. For example, the *Austrians* do so. They eat light meals in the early evening and at the end of the day. Persons from *Brazil* also eat their main meal at noon. They have a light meal in the evening. A main meal at noon also is common in *Finland, Germany, Greece,* and *Iran.*

Modified from D'Avanzo CE, Geissler EM: *Pocket guide to cultural health assessment,* ed 3, St Louis, 2003, Mosby.

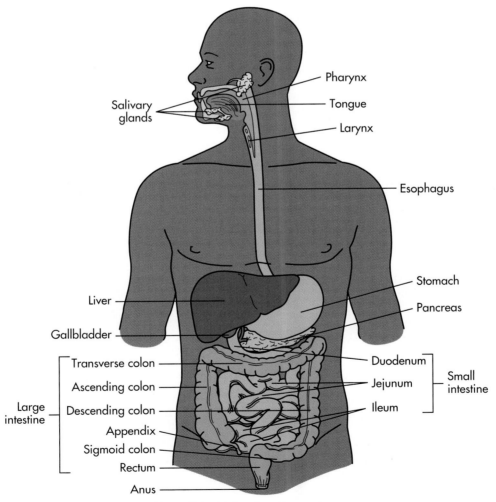

**FIG. 20-1** The digestive system.

## FOOD GUIDE PYRAMID

The *Food Guide Pyramid* promotes wise food choices (Fig. 20-2). It has six food groups:

- Bread, cereal, rice, and pasta
- Vegetables
- Fruits
- Milk, yogurt, and cheese
- Meat, poultry, fish, dry beans, eggs, and nuts
- Fats, oils, and sweets

The pyramid suggests eating more foods at the bottom level (level 1) and lesser amounts at each level moving to the top (level 4). A low-fat diet is the goal. More bread, cereal, rice, and pasta (level 1) and more vegetables and fruits (level 2) are eaten. Food from the milk, yogurt, and cheese group are eaten in moderate amounts. So are foods from the meat, poultry, fish, beans, eggs, and nut group (level 3). Fats, oils, and sweets (level 4) are used sparingly.

Foods from levels 1, 2, and 3 are needed daily. They contain the essential nutrients. No one food or food group contains every nutrient the body needs.

Note the small circles and triangles in the pyramid (see Fig. 20-2). The circles are for fat. The triangles for sugar. All foods have some sugar or fat. The food groups in levels 1 and 2 are low in sugar and fat. They allow the most servings. The result is a low-fat diet. Level 4 foods contain the most fat. Therefore they have the most calories. As you move up the Food Guide Pyramid, fat and calorie amounts increase.

The pyramid is for everyone older than 2 years. Better health is the goal. Many diseases are related to diet and the foods eaten. They include heart disease, high blood pressure, stroke, diabetes, and certain cancers. Follow the Dietary Guidelines for Americans to reduce the risk for such diseases (Box 20-2).

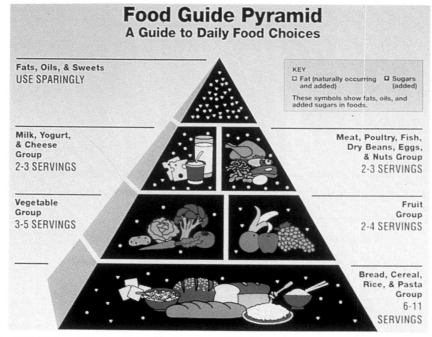

**FIG. 20-2** Food Guide Pyramid. (Courtesy U.S. Dept. of Agriculture, Washington, D.C.)

BOX
20-3 **FOOD GUIDE PYRAMID SERVING SIZES**

**BREAD, CEREALS, RICE, AND PASTA GROUP (6 TO 11 SERVINGS DAILY)**

- 1 slice bread = 1 serving
- 1 ounce ready-to-eat cereal = 1 serving
- ½ cup cooked cereal, rice, or pasta = 1 serving

**VEGETABLE GROUP (3 TO 5 SERVINGS DAILY)**

- 1 cup raw leafy vegetables = 1 serving
- ½ cup other cooked or chopped raw vegetables = 1 serving
- ¾ cup vegetable juice = 1 serving

**FRUIT GROUP (2 TO 4 SERVINGS DAILY)**

- 1 medium apple, orange, or banana = 1 serving
- ½ cup chopped, cooked, or canned fruit = 1 serving
- ¾ cup fruit juice = 1 serving

**MILK, CHEESE, AND YOGURT GROUP (2 TO 3 SERVINGS DAILY)**

- 1 cup milk or yogurt = 1 serving
- ½ to 1 ounce cheese = 1 serving
- 2 ounces process cheese = 1 serving

**MEAT, POULTRY, FISH, DRY BEANS, EGGS, AND NUTS GROUP (2 TO 3 SERVINGS DAILY)**

- 2 to 3 ounces cooked lean meat, poultry, or fish = 1 serving
- ½ cup cooked dry beans = 1 serving
- 1 egg = 1 serving
- 2 tablespoons peanut butter = 1 serving

**FATS, OILS, AND SWEETS GROUP**

- Use sparingly

**BREADS, CEREALS, RICE, AND PASTA GROUP.** This is the base of the pyramid. It allows the most servings—6 to 11 servings a day (Box 20-3). Foods come from grain (wheat, oats, rice, corn, etc.). They provide protein, carbohydrates, iron, thiamin, niacin, and riboflavin. There are small amounts of fats and sugars.

Foods such as pies, cakes, cookies, pastries, donuts, and muffins are made from grains. They are also made with fats and sugars. They are high-fat food choices depending on the amount of fat and sugar added.

**VEGETABLE GROUP.** A person needs 3 to 5 vegetable servings a day (see Box 20-3). Low in fat, they provide fiber, vitamins A and C, carbohydrates, and minerals. A variety of vegetables are eaten—dark green and yellow vegetables, tomatoes, potatoes, and vegetable juices.

Vegetables can become high in fat from food preparation. French fries are very high in fat; a baked or boiled potato is not. Toppings—butter, oil, mayonnaise, salad dressing, sour cream, and sauces—are high in fat. Low-fat toppings, in small amounts, help keep vegetables low in fat.

**FRUIT GROUP.** Fruits contain some sugar and are low in fat. A person needs 2 to 4 fruit servings daily (see Box 20-3). Fruits provide carbohydrates, vitamins A and C, potassium, and other minerals. Fresh fruits and juices are best. Frozen or canned fruits should be unsweetened. Sweetened or syrupy juices are high in sugar and calories.

**MILK, YOGURT, AND CHEESE GROUP.** This group is high in protein, carbohydrates, fat, calcium, and riboflavin. A person needs 2 to 3 servings daily (see Box 20-3). Children and breast-feeding mothers need 3 servings a day.

Skim milk has less fat than whole milk. One cup of skim milk has only a trace of fat (86 calories); 1 cup of whole milk has 8 grams of fat. One cup of whole milk has about 150 calories—72 calories come from fat. Cheese made with skim milk, low or nonfat yogurt, and ice milk rather than ice cream are low in fat.

**MEAT, POULTRY, FISH, DRY BEANS, EGGS, AND NUTS GROUP.** This group is high in protein, fat, iron, and thiamin. It has more fat than the milk, fruit, vegetable, and bread groups. A person needs 2 to 3 servings a day (see Box 20-3).

Meat, poultry, and fish have many calories. Serving size is important. Culture, appetite, personal choice, and the recipe affect serving size. Restaurants offer quarter-pound hamburgers, 12-ounce steaks, 10-ounce lobster tails, and quarters of chickens. *One serving* in this group is 2 to 3 ounces of boned meat, fish, or poultry. A 12-ounce steak is 4 to 6 servings!

This food group is high in fat. Wise food choices lower fat intake and calories. Fish and shellfish are low in fat. Chicken and turkey have less fat than veal, beef, pork, and lamb. Skinless chicken and turkey have even less fat. Veal has less fat than beef. Use lean cuts of beef and pork. Egg yolks have more fat than egg whites. Use low-fat egg substitutes for cooking and baking.

Food preparation is important. Trim fat from meat and poultry. Remove skin from poultry. Roasting, broiling, and baking are better than frying. Gravies and sauces add fat.

Nuts and peanut butter have the most fat in this group. Use them wisely. As shown in Figure 20-3, p. 426, 1 serving of peanut butter (2 tablespoons) equals 1 meat serving (2 to 3 ounces)! Peas and cooked dry beans are very low in fat. Use them often.

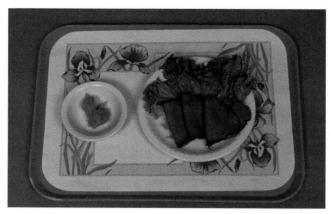

**FIG. 20-3** Two tablespoons of peanut butter (1 serving) equals this 3-ounce portion of beef (1 serving).

**FATS, OILS, AND SWEETS GROUP.** This group is at the top of the pyramid. Fats, oils, and sweets (foods with added sugar) are high in fat with few nutrients. Use them sparingly and as little as possible. This group includes cooking oils, shortening, butter, margarine, salad dressing, soft drinks, sour cream, cream cheese, and frosting. All candy, most desserts (cookies, cake, pie, ice cream), jelly and jam, syrup, and alcohol are included.

You can buy many low-fat foods. Food labels show fat content.

## NUTRIENTS

No food or food group has every essential nutrient. A well-balanced diet has food from levels 1, 2, and 3 of the Food Guide Pyramid. It ensures an adequate intake of essential nutrients:

- *Protein*—is the most important nutrient. It is needed for tissue growth and repair. Sources include meat, fish, poultry, eggs, milk and milk products, cereals, beans, peas, and nuts.
- *Carbohydrates*—provide energy and fiber for bowel elimination. They are found in fruits, vegetables, breads, cereals, and sugar. Carbohydrates break down into sugars during digestion. The sugars are absorbed into the bloodstream. Fiber is not digested. It provides the bulky part of chyme for elimination.

- *Fats*—provide energy. They add flavor to food and help the body use certain vitamins. Sources include meats, lard, butter, shortening, oils, milk, cheese, egg yolks, and nuts. Dietary fat not needed by the body is stored as body fat *(adipose tissue)*.
- *Vitamins*—are needed for certain body functions. They do not provide calories. The body stores vitamins A, D, E, and K. Vitamin C and the B complex vitamins are not stored. They must be ingested daily. The lack of a certain vitamin results in signs and symptoms of an illness. Table 20-1 lists the sources and major functions of common vitamins.
- *Minerals*—are used for many body processes. They are needed for bone and tooth formation, nerve and muscle function, fluid balance, and other body processes. Table 20-2 lists the major functions and dietary sources of common minerals.

## FOOD LABELS

Many foods have labels (Fig. 20-4, p. 428). They are used to plan diets. The food label (Fig. 20-5, p. 428) tells about:

- Serving size
- How the serving fits into the daily diet
- Calories per serving and the number of calories from fat
- The total amount of fat and the amount of saturated fat
- Amount of cholesterol, sodium, and protein
- Total amount of carbohydrates and the amount of dietary fiber and sugars
- Amount of Vitamins A and C, calcium, and iron

How a serving fits into the daily diet is called the **Daily Value (DV).** The DV is expressed in a percent (%). The percent is based on a daily diet of 2000 calories. Some food labels show the maximum daily intake values for total fat, saturated fat, cholesterol, sodium, carbohydrate, and dietary fiber. These are **Daily Reference Values (DRVs).** The DV and DRVs are used as follows:

- No more than 30% of the calories should come from fat.
- Based on a 2000-calorie diet, 65 grams of fat are allowed.
- The food label in Figure 20-5, p. 428, shows that 1 serving has 13 grams of fat, or 20% of the DV.
- The person can have 52 more grams of fat (80%) that day.

| TABLE 20-1 | FUNCTIONS AND SOURCES OF COMMON VITAMINS | |
|---|---|---|
| **Vitamin** | **Major Functions** | **Sources** |
| Vitamin A | Growth; vision; healthy hair, skin, and mucous membranes; resistance to infection | Liver, spinach, green leafy and yellow vegetables, yellow fruits, fish liver oils, egg yolks, butter, cream, whole milk |
| Vitamin $B_1$ (thiamin) | Muscle tone; nerve function; digestion; appetite; normal elimination; carbohydrate use | Pork, fish, poultry, eggs, liver, breads, pastas, cereals, oatmeal, potatoes, peas, beans, soybeans, peanuts |
| Vitamin $B_2$ (riboflavin) | Growth; healthy eyes; protein and carbohydrate metabolism; healthy skin and mucous membranes | Milk and milk products, liver, green leafy vegetables, eggs, breads, cereals |
| Vitamin $B_3$ (niacin) | Protein, fat, and carbohydrate metabolism; nervous system function; appetite; digestive system function | Meat, pork, liver, fish, peanuts, breads and cereals, green vegetables, dairy products |
| Vitamin $B_{12}$ | Formation of red blood cells; protein metabolism; nervous system function | Liver, meats, poultry, fish, eggs, milk, cheese |
| Folic acid | Formation of red blood cells; intestinal function; protein metabolism | Liver, meats, fish, poultry, green leafy vegetables, whole grains |
| Vitamin C (ascorbic acid) | Formation of substances that hold tissues together; healthy blood vessels, skin, gums, bones, and teeth; wound healing; prevention of bleeding; resistance to infection | Citrus fruits, tomatoes, potatoes, cabbage, strawberries, green vegetables, melons |
| Vitamin D | Absorption and metabolism of calcium and phosphorus; healthy bones | Fish liver oils, milk, butter, liver, exposure to sun light |
| Vitamin E | Normal reproduction; formation of red blood cells; muscle function | Vegetable oils, milk, eggs, meats, cereals, green leafy vegetables |
| Vitamin K | Blood clotting | Liver, green leafy vegetables, egg yolks, cheese |

| TABLE 20-2 | FUNCTIONS AND SOURCES OF COMMON MINERALS | |
|---|---|---|
| **Mineral** | **Major Functions** | **Sources** |
| Calcium | Formation of teeth and bones; blood clotting; muscle contraction; heart function; nerve function | Milk and milk products, green leafy vegetables, whole grains, egg yolks, dried peas and beans, nuts |
| Phosphorus | Formation of bones and teeth; use of proteins, fats, and carbohydrates; nerve and muscle function | Meat, fish, poultry, milk and milk products, nuts, egg yolks, dried peas and beans |
| Iron | Allows red blood cells to carry oxygen | Liver, meat, eggs, green leafy vegetables, breads and cereals, dried peas and beans, nuts |
| Iodine | Thyroid gland function; growth; metabolism | Iodized salt, seafood, shellfish |
| Sodium | Fluid balance; nerve and muscle function | Almost all foods |
| Potassium | Nerve function; muscle contraction; heart function | Fruits, vegetables, cereals, meats, dried peas and beans |

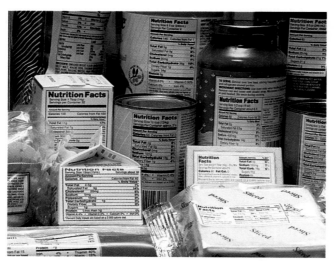

**FIG. 20-4** Most foods have food labels. The labels are required by the Nutrition Labeling and Education Act of 1990.

## FACTORS AFFECTING EATING AND NUTRITION

Many factors affect nutrition and eating habits. Some begin during infancy and continue throughout life. Others develop later.

- *Age.* Age affects nutrition. See Chapter 9. *See Focus on Children: Factors Affecting Eating and Nutrition.*
- *Culture.* Culture influences food choices and food preparation. Frying, baking, smoking, or roasting food and eating raw food are cultural practices. So is the use of sauces and spices. *See Caring About Culture: Food Practices.*
- *Religion.* Selecting, preparing, and eating food often involve religious practices (Box 20-4). A person may follow all, some, or none of the dietary practices of his or her faith. You must respect the person's religious practices.
- *Finances.* People with limited incomes often buy the cheaper carbohydrate foods. Their diets often lack protein and certain vitamins and minerals.

# Nutrition Facts

Serving Size 1 cup (228g)
Servings Per Container 2

**Amount Per Serving**

**Calories** 260     Calories from Fat 120

|  | % Daily Value* |
|---|---|
| **Total Fat** 13g | **20**% |
| Saturated Fat 5g | **25**% |
| *Trans* Fat 2g | |
| **Cholesterol** 30mg | **10**% |
| **Sodium** 660mg | **28**% |
| **Total Carbohydrate** 31mg | **10**% |
| Dietary Fiber 0g | **0**% |
| Sugars 5g | |
| **Protein** 5g | |

| Vitamin A 4% | • | Vitamin C 2% |
|---|---|---|
| Calcium 15% | • | Iron 4% |

\* Percent Daily Values are based on a 2,000 calorie diet. Your Daily Values may be higher or lower depending on your calorie needs:

| | | Calories | 2,000 | 2,500 |
|---|---|---|---|---|
| Total Fat | Less than | | 65g | 80g |
| Sat Fat | Less than | | 20g | 25g |
| Cholesterol | Less than | | 300mg | 300mg |
| Sodium | Less than | | 2,400mg | 2,400mg |
| Total Carbohydrate | | | 300g | 375g |
| Dietary Fiber | | | 25g | 30g |

Calories per gram:
Fat 9    *    Carbohydrate 4    *    Protein 4

**FIG. 20-5** A food label. (From U.S. Food and Drug Administration, July 2003.)

**FOCUS ON CHILDREN**
**FACTORS AFFECTING EATING AND NUTRITION**

Infants are breast-fed or bottle-fed. For bottle-fed babies, the doctor orders the formula to use. Solid foods are introduced at 4 to 6 months. Usually cereal is the first solid food given. Others are added as the infant grows. The nurse tells you what foods the infant can have.

The Food Guide Pyramid applies to children 2 years of age and older. The nurse tells you about the child's needs.

**CARING ABOUT CULTURE**
**FOOD PRACTICES**

Food practices vary among cultural groups. Rice and beans are protein sources in *Mexico*. In the *Philippines*, rice is preferred with every meal. A diet high in sugar and fat is common in *Poland*. Potatoes, rye, and wheat are common. The diet in *China* is high in sodium. The sodium content is from the use of soy sauce and dried and preserved foods.

Eating beef is common in the *United States*. Beef is not eaten in *India*.

Modified from D'Avanzo CE, Geissler EM: *Pocket guide to cultural health assessment,* ed 3, St Louis, 2003, Mosby.

- *Appetite.* Appetite relates to the desire for food. When hungry, a person seeks food. He or she eats until the appetite is satisfied. Aromas and thoughts of food can stimulate the appetite. However, loss of appetite **(anorexia)** can occur. Causes include illness, drugs, anxiety, pain, and depression. Unpleasant sights, thoughts, and smells are other causes.
- *Personal choice.* Food likes and dislikes are personal. They are influenced by food served in the home. Body reactions affect food choices. People usually avoid foods that cause allergic reactions, nausea, vomiting, diarrhea, indigestion, or headaches.
- *Illness.* Appetite usually decreases during illness and recovery from injuries. However, nutritional needs are increased. The body must fight infection, heal tissue, and replace lost blood cells. Nutrients lost through vomiting and diarrhea need replacement. Some diseases and drugs cause a sore mouth. This makes eating painful. Loss of teeth affects chewing, especially protein foods. Illness can affect the ability to prepare and serve meals. Poor nutrition is common in persons needing long-term care. They need good nutrition to correct or prevent health problems. *See Focus on Home Care: Factors Affecting Eating and Nutrition. See Focus on Long-Term Care: Factors Affecting Eating and Nutrition,* p. 430.

## FOCUS ON HOME CARE
### FACTORS AFFECTING EATING AND NUTRITION

You may be assigned to shop for groceries, plan meals, and cook. You need to understand the Food Guide Pyramid, basic nutrition, and food labels. You also need to know the person's food preferences and eating habits. For example, some people have their large meal in the evening, others at noon. Some people eat the same thing for breakfast every day.

Review the foods allowed on the person's diet (p. 431). Consider eating and digestive problems when preparing and serving meals. The nurse and dietitian advise you about what to prepare. A good cookbook is useful for planning and preparing meals.

Plan menus for a full week. Check recipes to make sure that what you need is on hand or on the shopping list. To save money, check newspapers for sales and use coupons. Save all grocery receipts for the person or family member.

Properly store foods. Refrigerate dairy products and most fresh fruits and vegetables right away. Freeze meat, poultry, fish, and frozen foods unless used that day. Dried, packaged, canned, and bottled foods keep well in cabinets. See Chapter 12 for safe food handling.

## BOX 20-4 RELIGION AND DIETARY PRACTICES

**ADVENTIST (SEVENTH DAY ADVENTIST)**
- Coffee, tea, and alcohol are not allowed.
- Beverages with caffeine (colas) are not allowed.
- Some groups have restrictions about beef, pork, lamb, chicken, seafood, and fish.

**BAPTIST**
- Some groups forbid coffee, tea, and alcohol.

**CHRISTIAN SCIENTIST**
- Alcohol and coffee are not allowed.

**CHURCH OF JESUS CHRIST OF LATTER DAY SAINTS (MORMON)**
- Alcohol, coffee, and tea are not allowed.
- Meat is not forbidden, but members are encouraged to eat meat infrequently.

**GREEK ORTHODOX CHURCH**
- Fasting during the Great Lent and before other holy days.
- Meat, fish, and dairy products are not eaten during a fast.

**ISLAM**
- All pork and pork products are forbidden.
- Coffee, tea, and alcohol are not allowed.
- Fasting (no food or fluids) from dawn to sunset during Ramadan.

**JUDAISM (JEWISH FAITH)**
- Foods must be kosher. (Kosher means fit or proper. Food must be prepared according to Jewish law.)
- Meat of kosher animals (cows, goats, and lambs) can be eaten.
- Chickens, ducks, and geese are kosher fowl.
- Kosher fish have scales and fins (tuna, sardines, carp, salmon, herring, whitefish, and so on).
- Pork and shellfish cannot be eaten.
- Milk, milk products, and eggs from kosher animals and fowl are allowed.
- Meat and milk cannot be cooked together.
- Meat and milk products cannot be eaten together.
- Meat and milk products are not prepared or served with the same utensils and dishes. Two sets of utensils and dishes are needed. They are washed and stored separately.
- Fermented grain products (cakes, cookies, noodles, alcohol, and so on) are not consumed during Passover.

**ROMAN CATHOLIC**
- Fasting for 1 hour before receiving Holy Communion.
- Fasting from meat on Ash Wednesday, Good Friday, and all Fridays during Lent.

## FOCUS ON LONG-TERM CARE
### FACTORS AFFECTING EATING AND NUTRITION

OBRA has these requirements for food served in long-term care centers:

- Each person's nutritional and dietary needs are met.
- The person's diet is well-balanced. It is nourishing and tastes good. Food is well seasoned. It is not too salty or too sweet.
- Food is appetizing. It has an appealing aroma and is attractive.
- Hot food is served hot. Cold food is served cold. Food servers keep food at the correct temperature.
- Food is served promptly. Otherwise, hot food cools and cold food warms.
- Food is prepared to meet each person's needs. Some people need food cut, ground, or chopped. Others have special diets ordered by the doctor.
- Each person receives at least three meals a day. A bedtime snack is offered.
- The center provides any special eating equipment and utensils (Fig. 20-6).

Disease or injury can affect the hands, wrists, and arms. Adaptive equipment lets the person eat independently. Make sure the person has needed equipment.

Some centers have areas where the resident can dine with a spouse, family, or friends. They can enjoy holidays, birthdays, anniversaries, and other special events. The dietary department provides the meal, or it is brought by the family.

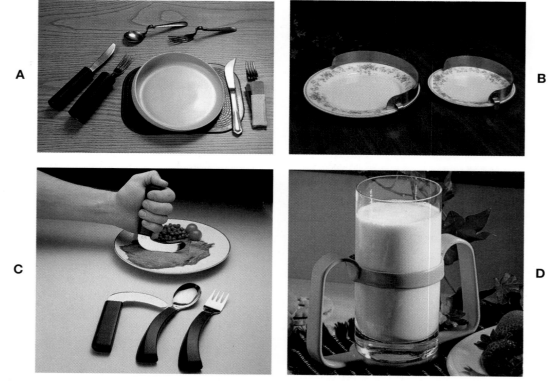

**FIG. 20-6** Eating utensils for persons with special needs. **A,** The curved fork fits over the hand. The rounded plate helps keep food on the plate. Special grips and swivel handles are helpful for some persons. **B,** Plate guards help keep food on the plate. **C,** Knives with rounded blades are rocked back and forth to cut food. The person does not need a fork in one hand and a knife in the other. **D,** Glass or cup holder. (Courtesy Sammons Preston Roylan, An AbilityOne Company, Bolingbrook, Ill.)

# SPECIAL DIETS

Doctors may order special diets for a nutritional deficiency or a disease (Table 20-3). They also order them for weight control or to remove or decrease certain substances in the diet. The doctor, nurses, and dietitian work together to meet the person's nutritional needs. They consider personal choices, religion, culture, food allergies, and eating problems. The nurse and dietitian teach the person and family about the diet.

*Regular diet, general diet,* and *house diet* mean no dietary limits or restrictions. Persons with diabetes or diseases of the heart, kidneys, gallbladder, liver, stomach, or intestines often need special diets. Persons with wounds or pressure ulcers need high-protein diets for healing. Older or disabled persons may have bran added to their food. It provides fiber for bowel elimination. Allergies, excess weight, and other disorders also require special diets.

The sodium-controlled diet is often ordered. So is diabetes meal planning. Persons with difficulty swallowing may need a dysphagia diet.

| TABLE 20-3 SPECIAL DIETS | | |
|---|---|---|
| **Diet** | **Use** | **Foods Allowed** |
| Clear-liquid—foods liquid at body temperature and which leave small amounts of residue; nonirritating and non-gas forming | Postoperatively, acute illness, infection, nausea and vomiting, and in preparation for gastrointestinal exams | Water, tea, and coffee (without milk or cream); carbonated beverages; gelatin; clear fruit juices (apple, grape, cranberry); fat-free clear broth; hard candy, sugar, and Popsicles |
| Full-liquid—foods liquid at room temperature or melt at body temperature | Advance from clear-liquid diet postoperatively; for stomach irritation, fever, nausea, and vomiting; for persons unable to chew, swallow, or digest solid foods | Foods on the clear-liquid diet; custard; eggnog; strained soups; strained fruit and vegetable juices; milk and milk shakes; strained, cooked cereals; plain ice cream and sherbet; pudding; yogurt |
| Mechanical soft—semi-solid foods that are easily digested | Advance from full-liquid diet, chewing problems, gastro-intestinal disorders, and infections | All liquids; eggs (not fried); broiled, baked, or roasted meat, fish, or poultry that is chopped or shredded; mild cheeses (American, Swiss, cheddar, cream, cottage); strained fruit juices; refined bread (no crust) and crackers; cooked cereal; cooked or pureed vegetables; cooked or canned fruit without skin or seeds; pudding; plain cakes and soft cookies without fruit or nuts |
| Fiber- and residue-restricted—food that leaves a small amount of residue in the colon | Diseases of the colon and diarrhea | Coffee, tea, milk, carbonated beverages, strained fruit juices; refined bread and crackers; creamed and refined cereal; rice; cottage and cream cheese; eggs (not fried); plain puddings and cakes; gelatin; custard; sherbet and ice cream; strained vegetable juices; canned or cooked fruit without skin or seeds; potatoes (not fried); strained cooked vegetables; plain pasta; no raw fruits and vegetables |
| High-fiber—foods that increase the amount of residue and fiber in the colon to stimulate peristalsis | Constipation and GI disorders | All fruits and vegetables; whole wheat bread; whole grain cereals; fried foods; whole grain rice; milk, cream, butter, and cheese; meats |

*Continued.*

| TABLE 20-3 | SPECIAL DIETS—CONT'D | |
|---|---|---|
| **Diet** | **Use** | **Foods Allowed** |
| Bland—foods that are mechanically and chemically nonirritating and low in roughage; foods served at moderate temperatures; no strong spices or condiments | Ulcers, gallbladder disorders, and some intestinal disorders; after abdominal surgery | Lean meats; white bread; creamed and refined cereals; cream or cottage cheese; gelatin, plain puddings, cakes, and cookies; eggs (not fried); butter and cream; canned fruits and vegetables without skin and seeds; strained fruit juices; potatoes (not fried); pastas and rice; strained or soft cooked carrots, peas, beets, spinach, squash, and asparagus tips; creamed soups from allowed vegetables; no fried foods |
| High-calorie—calorie intake is increased to about 3000 to 4000; includes 3 full meals and between-meal snacks | Weight gain and some thyroid imbalances | Dietary increases in all foods; large portions of a regular diet with 3 between-meal snacks |
| Calorie-controlled—provides adequate nutrients while controlling calories to promote weight loss and reduction of body fat | Weight reduction | Foods low in fats and carbohydrates and lean meats; avoid butter, cream, rice, gravies, salad oils, noodles, cakes, pastries, carbonated and alcoholic beverages, candy, potato chips, and similar foods |
| High-iron—foods that are high in iron | Anemia; following blood loss for women during the reproductive years | Liver and other organ meats; lean meats; egg yolks; shellfish; dried fruits; dried beans; green leafy vegetables; lima beans; peanut butter; enriched breads and cereals |
| Fat-controlled (low-cholesterol)—foods low in fat and foods prepared without adding fat | Heart disease, gallbladder disease, disorders of fat digestion, liver disease, diseases of the pancreas | Skim milk or buttermilk; cottage cheese (no other cheeses allowed); gelatin; sherbet; fruit; lean meat, poultry, and fish (baked, broiled, or roasted); fat-free broth; soups made with skim milk; margarine; rice, pasta, breads, and cereals; vegetables; potatoes |
| High-protein—aids and promotes tissue healing | For burns, high fever, infection, and some liver diseases | Meat, milk, eggs, cheese, fish, poultry; breads and cereals; green leafy vegetables |
| Sodium-controlled—a certain amount of sodium is allowed | Heart disease, fluid retention, liver disease, and some kidney diseases | Fruits and vegetables and unsalted butter are allowed; adding salt at the table is not allowed; highly salted foods and foods high in sodium are not allowed; the use of salt during cooking may be restricted |
| Diabetes meal planning—the same amount of carbohydrates, protein, and fat are eaten at the same time each day | Diabetes | Determined by nutritional and energy requirements |

## THE SODIUM-CONTROLLED DIET

The average amount of sodium in the daily diet is 3000 to 5000 mg. The body needs no more than 2400 mg. Healthy people excrete excess sodium in the urine.

Heart, liver, and kidney diseases, certain drugs, and some complications of pregnancy cause the body to retain extra sodium. A sodium-controlled diet often is needed. Sodium causes the body to retain water. If there is too much sodium, the body retains more water. Tissues swell with water. There is excess fluid in the blood vessels. The heart has to work harder. That is, the workload of the heart increases. With heart disease, the extra workload can cause serious problems or death. Sodium control decreases the amount of sodium in the body. The body retains less water. Less water in the tissues and blood vessels reduces the heart's workload.

The doctor orders the amount of sodium restriction. Many low-salt or salt-free foods can be bought. Check the food label.

- *2000 mg to 3000 mg sodium diet*—called the *low-salt* or *no-added-salt diet.* Sodium control is mild. All high-sodium foods are omitted (Box 20-5). A small amount of salt is used for cooking. Salt is not added to foods at the table.

- *1000 mg sodium diet*—sodium control is moderate. Food is cooked without salt. Foods high in sodium are omitted. Vegetables high in sodium are restricted in amount. Salt-free products, such as salt-free bread, are used. Diet planning is necessary.

---

### BOX 20-5 HIGH-SODIUM FOODS

**BREAD, CEREAL, RICE, AND PASTA GROUP**

- Saltine crackers
- Baking powder biscuits
- Muffins
- Bisquick
- Pretzels
- Salted crackers
- Quick breads (corn bread, nut bread)
- Pancakes
- Waffles
- Instant cooked cereal
- Processed bran cereals
- Rice
- Noodle mixes
- Corn chips and other salted snacks

**VEGETABLE GROUP**

- Sauerkraut
- Tomato juice
- V-8 juice
- Vegetables in creams or sauces
- Frozen vegetables processed with salt or sodium
- Bloody Mary mixes
- Potato chips
- French fries
- Instant potatoes
- Pickles
- Relishes

**FRUIT GROUP**

- No restrictions

**MILK, YOGURT, AND CHEESE GROUP**

- Buttermilk
- Cheese
- Commercial dips made with sour cream

**MEAT, POULTRY, FISH, DRY BEANS, EGGS, AND NUTS GROUP**

- Bacon
- Ham
- Sausage
- Salt pork
- Hot dogs
- Luncheon meats
- Corned or chopped beef
- Organ meats
- Shellfish
- Sardines
- Herring
- Anchovies
- Caviar
- Kosher meats
- Canned tuna
- Canned salmon
- Mackerel
- Salted nuts or seeds
- Peanut butter

**FATS, OILS, AND SWEETS**

- Salad dressings
- Mayonnaise
- Baked desserts

**OTHER**

- Mineral water
- Club soda
- Canned soups
- Bouillon cubes
- Dried soup mixes
- Olives
- Salted popcorn
- Frozen or canned dinners
- Salt
- Baking powder
- Baking soda
- Celery, onion, garlic, and other seasoning salts
- Meat tenderizers
- Worcestershire sauce
- Soy sauce
- Mustard
- Catsup
- Horseradish
- Sauces: chili, tomato, steak, barbecue

Modified from Lewis SM, Heitkemper MM, Dirksen SR: *Medical-surgical nursing: assessment and management of clinical problems,* ed 5, St Louis, 2000, Mosby.

## DIABETES MEAL PLANNING

Diabetes meal planning is for people with diabetes. Diabetes is a chronic disease from a lack of insulin (Chapter 33). The pancreas produces and secretes insulin. Insulin lets the body use sugar. Without enough insulin, sugar builds up in the bloodstream. It is not used by cells for energy. Diabetes is usually treated with insulin or other drugs, diet, and exercise.

The dietitian and person develop a meal plan. Consistency is key. It involves:

- The person's food preferences—likes and dislikes, eating habits, meal times, culture, and life-style. It may be necessary to limit amounts of food or change how food is prepared.
- Calories needed. The same amount of carbohydrates, protein, and fat are eaten each day.
- Eating meals and snacks at regular times. The person eats at the same time every day.

Meal and snack times also are the same from day to day. Serve the person's meal and snacks on time. The person eats at regular times to maintain a certain blood sugar level.

Always check the tray to see what was eaten. Tell the nurse what the person did and did not eat. If all food was not eaten, a between-meal nourishment is needed (p. 442). The nurse will tell you what to give the person for a snack. It makes up for what was not eaten at the meal. The amount of insulin given also depends on daily food intake. Tell the nurse about changes in the person's eating habits.

## THE DYSPHAGIA DIET

**Dysphagia** means difficulty (*dys*) swallowing (*phagia*). Food thickness is changed to meet the person's needs (Box 20-6). The doctor, speech-language pathologist, occupational therapist, dietitian, and nurse choose the right food thickness.

A *slow swallow* means the person has difficulty getting enough food and fluids for good nutrition and fluid balance. An *unsafe swallow* means that food enters the airway (aspiration). **Aspiration** is breathing fluid or an object into the lungs (p. 446).

You may feed a person with dysphagia. To promote the person's safety, you must:

- Know the signs and symptoms of dysphagia (Box 20-7)
- Position the person's head and neck correctly. Follow the care plan.
- Feed the person according to the care plan.
- Follow aspiration precautions (Box 20-8).
- Report changes in how the person eats.
- Report choking, coughing, or difficulty breathing during or after meals. Also report abnormal breathing or respiratory sounds. Report these observations at once.

---

**BOX 20-6    DYSPHAGIA DIET**

| CONSISTENCY | DESCRIPTION |
|---|---|
| Puree | No lumps; mounds on plate. May be thick like mashed potatoes. |
| Thickened liquid | No lumps, pureed with milk, gravy, or broth to thickness of baby food peaches. Some foods are pureed and thickener added as needed (e.g. many fruits). Does not mound on a plate. May be called creamy or sauce. Stir before serving if the food settles. A spoon is used (baby food consistency). Served in a bowl. |
| Medium thick | The thickness of nectar or V-8 juice (does not hold its shape). Stir right before serving. |
| Extra thick | The thickness of honey. Mounds a bit on a spoon. Drinkable from a cup. Stir before serving. |
| Yogurt-like consistency | The thickness of yogurt; holds its shape. Served with a spoon. |

---

**BOX 20-7    SIGNS AND SYMPTOMS OF DYSPHAGIA**

- The person avoids foods that need chewing.
- Food spills out of the person's mouth while eating.
- Food "pockets" or is "squirreled" in the person's cheeks.
- The person eats slowly, especially solid foods.
- The person complains that food will not go down or the food is stuck.
- The person frequently coughs or chokes before, during, or after swallowing.
- The person regurgitates food after eating (p. 447).
- The person spits out food suddenly and almost violently.
- Food comes up through the person's nose.
- The person is hoarse—especially after eating.
- After swallowing, the person makes gargling sounds while talking or breathing.
- There is excessive drooling of saliva.
- The person complains of frequent heartburn.
- Appetite is decreased.
- There is unexplained weight loss.
- The person has recurrent pneumonia.

# FLUID BALANCE

Water is needed to live. Death can result from too much or too little water. Water is ingested through fluids and foods. Water is lost through urine, feces, and vomit. It is also lost through the skin (perspiration) and the lungs (expiration).

Fluid balance is needed for health. The amount of fluid taken in (**intake**) and the amount of fluid lost (**output**) must be equal. If fluid intake exceeds fluid output, body tissues swell with water. This is called **edema.** Edema is common in people with heart and kidney diseases. **Dehydration** is a decrease in the amount of water in body tissues. Fluid output exceeds intake. Common causes are poor fluid intake, vomiting, diarrhea, bleeding, excess sweating, and increased urine production.

## NORMAL FLUID REQUIREMENTS

An adult needs 1500 ml of water daily to survive. About 2000 to 2500 ml of fluid per day are needed for normal fluid balance. The water requirement increases with hot weather, exercise, fever, illness, and excess fluid losses. *See Focus on Children: Normal Fluid Requirements. See Focus on Older Persons: Normal Fluid Requirements.*

## SPECIAL ORDERS

The doctor may order the amount of fluid a person can have during a 24-hour period. This is done to maintain fluid balance. Found on the care plan, common orders are:

- *Encourage fluids.* The person drinks an increased amount of fluid. The order may be general or state the amount to ingest. Intake records are kept. The person is given a variety of fluids. They are kept within the person's reach. They are served at the correct temperature. Fluids are offered regularly to persons who cannot feed themselves.
- *Restrict fluids.* Fluids are limited to a certain amount. They are offered in small amounts and in small containers. The water pitcher is removed from the room or kept out of sight. Intake records are kept. The person needs frequent oral hygiene. It helps keep mucous membranes of the mouth moist.
- *Nothing by mouth.* The person cannot eat or drink anything. *NPO* is the abbreviation for *non per os.* It means nothing *(non)* by *(per)* mouth *(os).* NPO often is ordered before and after surgery, before some laboratory tests and diagnostic procedures, and in treating certain illnesses. An NPO sign is posted above the bed. The water pitcher and glass are removed. Frequent oral hygiene is needed, but the person must not swallow any fluid. The person is NPO for 6 to 8 hours before surgery and before some laboratory tests and diagnostic procedures.

---

**BOX 20-8    ASPIRATION PRECAUTIONS**

- Help the person with meals and snacks. Follow the care plan.
- Position the person in Fowler's position or upright in a chair for meals and snacks.
- Support the upper back, shoulders, and neck with a pillow. Follow the care plan.
- Observe for signs and symptoms of aspiration during meals and snacks.
- Check the person's mouth after each meal and snack for pocketing. Check inside the cheeks, under the tongue, or on the roof of the mouth. Remove any food present. Report your observations to the nurse.
- Position the person in a chair or in semi-Fowler's position after each meal or snack. The person maintains this position for at least 1 hour after eating. Follow the care plan.
- Provide mouth care after each meal or snack.

---

**FOCUS ON CHILDREN**
**NORMAL FLUID REQUIREMENTS**

Fluid requirements vary with age. Infants and young children have more body water. They need more fluids than adults do. Excess fluid losses cannot be tolerated. They quickly cause death in an infant or child.

---

**FOCUS ON OLDER PERSONS**
**NORMAL FLUID REQUIREMENTS**

The amount of body water decreases with age. Older persons also are at risk for diseases that affect fluid balance. Examples include heart disease, kidney disease, cancer, and diabetes. Some drugs cause the body to lose fluids. Others cause the body to retain water. The older person is at risk for dehydration and edema.

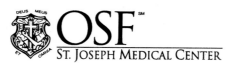

St. Joseph Medical Center

Bloomington, Illinois

## FLUID BALANCE CHART

| | | | |
|---|---|---|---|
| Water Glass | 250cc | Ice Cream | 120cc |
| Styrofoam Cup | 180cc | Ice Chips | 1/2 amt. of |
| Cup (coffee) | 250cc | | cc's in cup |
| Milk Carton | 240cc | | |
| Pop (1 can) | 360cc | Pitcher | |
| Broth-Soup | 175cc | (Yellow) | 1000cc |
| Juice Carton | 120cc | | |
| Juice Glass | 120cc | | |
| Jello | 120cc | | |

DATE _____

| | INTAKE | | | OUTPUT | | | | | |
|---|---|---|---|---|---|---|---|---|---|
| | | | | **URINE** | | **OTHER** | | **CONT. IRRIGATION** | |
| TIME | ORAL | Parenteral | Amt. cc Absbd. | Method Collected | Amt. (cc) | Method Collected | Amt. (cc) | In | Out |
| 2400-0100 | | cc from previous shift | | V | 150 | | | | |
| 0100-0200 | | | | | | Vom. | 150 | | |
| 0200-0300 | | | | | | | | | |
| 0300-0400 | | | | | | | | | |
| 0400-0500 | | | | | | | | | |
| 0500-0600 | 125 | | | V | 200 | | | | |
| 0600-0700 | | | | | | | | | |
| 0700-0800 | | | | | | | | | |
| | 125 | 8 - hour Sub-total | | 8-hr T | 350 | 8-hr T | 150 | | |
| 0800-0900 | 400 | cc from previous shift | | V | 250 | | | | |
| 0900-1000 | 100 | | | | | | | | |
| 1000-1100 | | | | | | | | | |
| 1100-1200 | | | | | | | | | |
| 1200-1300 | 400 | | | V | 250 | | | | |
| 1300-1400 | | | | | | | | | |
| 1400-1500 | 200 | | | | | | | | |
| 1500-1600 | | | | | | | | | |
| | 1100 | 8 - hour Sub-total | | 8-hr T | 500 | 8-hr T | | | |
| 1600-1700 | | cc from previous shift | | V | 270 | | | | |
| 1700-1800 | 350 | | | | | | | | |
| 1800-1900 | 50 | | | | | | | | |
| 1900-2000 | 200 | | | | | | | | |
| 2000-2100 | | | | V | 400 | | | | |
| 2100-2200 | | | | | | | | | |
| 2200-2300 | | | | | | | | | |
| 2300-2400 | | | | | | | | | |
| | 600 | 8 - hour Sub-total | | 8-hr T | 670 | 8-hr T | | | |
| | 1825 | 24 - hour Sub-total | | 24-hr T | 1520 | 24-hr T | 150 | | |

*310'  Marie Mills*

Source Key:

    URINE

V    - Voided
C    - Catheter
INC   - Incontinent
U.C.   - Ureteral Catheter

Source Key:

    OTHER

G.I.T.  - Gastric Intestinal Tube
T.T.   - T. Tube
Vom.  - Vomitus
Liq S.  - Liquid Stool
H.V.   - Hemovac

Form No. MF36722 (Rev. 5/97) **MFI**

**FIG. 20-7** An intake and output record. (Courtesy OSF St. Joseph Medical Center, Bloomington, Ill.)

# INTAKE AND OUTPUT RECORDS

The doctor or nurse may order intake and output (I&O) measurements. I&O records are kept. They are used to evaluate fluid balance and kidney function. They help in evaluating and planning medical treatment. They also are kept when the person has special fluid orders.

All fluids taken by mouth are measured and recorded—water, milk, coffee, tea, juices, soups, and soft drinks. So are foods that melt at room temperature—ice cream, sherbet, custard, pudding, gelatin, and Popsicles. The nurse measures and records IV fluids and tube feedings. Output includes urine, vomitus, diarrhea, and wound drainage.

**MEASURING INTAKE AND OUTPUT.** Intake and output are measured in milliliters (ml) or in cubic centimeters (cc). These metric system measurements are equal in amount—1 ml equals 1 cc. You need to know these amounts.

- 1 ounce equals 30 ml
- A pint is about 500 ml
- A quart is about 1000 ml

You need to know the serving sizes of the bowls, dishes, cups, pitchers, glasses, and other containers. The information may be on the I&O record (Fig. 20-7).

A measuring container for fluid is called a **graduate.** It is used to measure leftover fluids, urine, vomitus, and drainage from suction. Like a measuring cup, the graduate is marked in ounces and in milliliters or cubic centimeters (Fig. 20-8). Plastic urinals and kidney basins often have amounts marked.

An I&O record is kept at the bedside. When intake or output is measured the amount is recorded in the correct column (see Fig. 20-7). Amounts are totaled at the end of the shift. The totals are recorded in the person's chart. They also are shared during the end-of-shift report.

The purpose of measuring I&O and how to help are explained to the person. Some persons measure and record their intake. Family members may help. The urinal, commode, bedpan, or specimen pan is used for voiding. Remind the person not to void in the toilet. Also remind the person not to put toilet tissue into the receptacle.

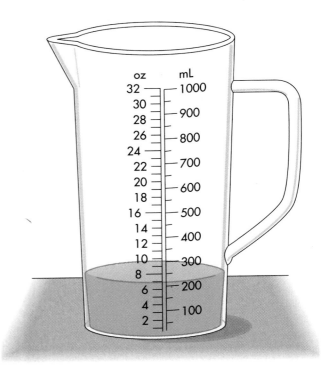

**FIG. 20-8** A graduate marked in ounces and milliliters.

## MEASURING INTAKE AND OUTPUT

*NNAAP*™

### QUALITY OF LIFE

Remember to:
- Knock before entering the person's room
- Address the person by name
- Introduce yourself by name and title

### PRE-PROCEDURE

1 Follow *Delegation Guidelines: Intake and Output*, p. 437. See *Safety Alert: Intake and Output*, p. 437.
2 Explain the procedure to the person.
3 Practice hand hygiene.

4 Collect the following:
  - Intake and output (I&O) record
  - Graduates
  - Gloves

### PROCEDURE

5 Put on gloves.
6 Measure intake as follows:
  a Pour liquid remaining in a container into the graduate.
  b Measure the amount at eye level. Keep the container level.
  c Check the serving amount on the I&O record.
  d Subtract the remaining amount from the full serving amount. Record the amount.
  e Repeat steps 6a through 6d for each liquid.
  f Add the amounts from each liquid together.
  g Record the time and amount on the I&O record.

7 Measure output as follows:
  a Pour the fluid into the graduate used to measure output.
  b Measure the amount at eye level. Keep the container level.
8 Dispose of fluid in the toilet. Avoid splashes.
9 Rinse the graduate. Dispose of rinse into the toilet. Return the graduate to it proper place.
10 Clean and rinse the bedpan, urinal, kidney basin, or other drainage container. Discard the rinse into the toilet. Return the item to its proper place.
11 Remove the gloves. Decontaminate your hands.
12 Record the amount on the I&O record.

### POST-PROCEDURE

13 Report and record your observations.

## MEETING FOOD AND FLUIDS NEEDS

Weakness and illness can affect appetite and ability to eat. So can unpleasant odors, sights, and sounds. An uncomfortable position, the need for oral hygiene, the need to eliminate, and pain also affect appetite.

## PREPARING FOR MEALS

You need to prepare patients and residents for meals. They need to eliminate and have oral care. They need dentures, eyeglasses, and hearing aids in place. If incontinent, they need to be clean and dry. A comfortable position for eating is important.

The setting must be free of unpleasant sights, sounds, and odors. Remove unpleasant equipment from the room.

**DELEGATION GUIDELINES:** *Preparing for Meals*
To prepare a person for a meal, you need this information from the nurse and the care plan:
- How much help the person needs
- Where the person will eat—dining area or room
- What the person uses for elimination—bathroom, commode, bedpan, urinal, or specimen pan
- What type of oral hygiene the person needs
- If the person wear dentures
- How to position the person—in bed or in a chair
- If the person wears eyeglasses or hearing aids
- How the person gets to the dining room—by self or with help
- If the person uses a wheelchair, walker, or cane

**SAFETY ALERT:** *Preparing for Meals*
Before meals, the person needs to eliminate and have oral hygiene. Follow Standard Precautions and the Bloodborne Pathogen Standard. Also follow them when cleaning equipment and the room.

## PREPARING THE PERSON FOR MEALS

### QUALITY OF LIFE

Remember to:
- Knock before entering the person's room
- Address the person by name
- Introduce yourself by name and title

### PRE-PROCEDURE

1 Follow *Delegation Guidelines: Preparing for Meals.* See *Safety Alert: Preparing for Meals.*
2 Explain to the person that it is mealtime.
3 Practice hand hygiene.
4 Collect the following:
- Equipment for oral hygiene
- Bedpan, urinal, or commode and toilet tissue
- Wash basin
- Soap
- Washcloth
- Towel
- Gloves
5 Provide for privacy.

### PROCEDURE

6 Make sure eyeglasses and hearing aids are in place.
7 Assist with oral hygiene. Make sure dentures are in place.
8 Assist with elimination. Make sure the incontinent person is clean and dry.
9 Assist with hand washing.
10 Do the following if the person will eat in bed:
  a Raise the head of the bed to a comfortable position.
  b Clean the overbed table. Adjust it in front of the person.
  c Place the signal light within reach.
  d Unscreen the person.
11 Do the following if the person will sit in a chair:
  a Position the person in a chair or wheelchair.
  b Remove items from the overbed table. Clean the table.
  c Adjust the overbed table in front of the person.
  d Place the signal light within reach.
  e Unscreen the person.
12 Assist the person to the dining area. (This for the person who eats in a dining area.)

### POST-PROCEDURE

13 Return to the room. Knock before entering.
14 Clean and return equipment to its proper place. Wear gloves for this step.
15 Straighten the room. Eliminate unpleasant noise, odors, or equipment.
16 Remove the gloves. Decontaminate your hands.

## SERVING MEAL TRAYS

Food is served in containers that keep foods at the correct temperature. Hot food is kept hot. Cold food is kept cold. You serve meal trays after preparing persons for meals. You can serve trays promptly if they are ready to eat. Prompt serving keeps food at the right temperature.

If a meal tray is not served within 15 minutes, recheck food temperature. To check the temperature, follow agency policy. If not at the right temperature, get another tray. Some agencies allow reheating in a microwave oven.

*See Focus on Long-Term Care: Serving Meal Trays.*

---

**DELEGATION GUIDELINES:** *Serving Meal Trays*

Before serving meal trays, you need this information from the nurse and the care plan:
- What adaptive equipment the person uses
- How much help the person needs opening cartons, cutting food, buttering bread, and so on
- If the person's I&O is measured
- If calorie counts are done (p. 443)

---

**SAFETY ALERT:** *Serving Meal Trays*

Always check food temperature after reheating. Food that is too hot can burn the person.

---

**FOCUS ON LONG-TERM CARE**

SERVING MEAL TRAYS

Nursing centers have special dining programs:
- *Social dining.* Residents eat at a dining room table with 4 to 6 others (Fig. 20-9). Tables have tablecloths or placemats. Food is served as in a restaurant. This program is for persons who are oriented and can feed themselves.
- *Family dining.* Food is served in bowls and on platters. Residents serve themselves like at home.
- *Assistive dining.* The dining room has horseshoe-shaped tables. They are for residents who need help eating. You sit at the center and feed up to 4 people (Fig. 20-10).
- *Low-stimulation dining.* The program prevents distractions during meals. The health team decides on the best place for each person to sit.

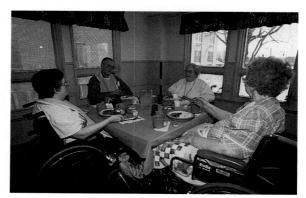

**FIG. 20-9** Residents enjoy a pleasant meal in the dining room.

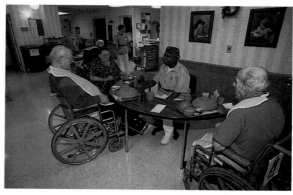

**FIG. 20-10** A horseshoe-shaped table is used for assistive dining. The nursing assistant feeds three residents at one time. Residents are in the company of others.

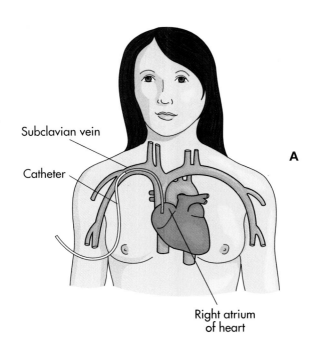

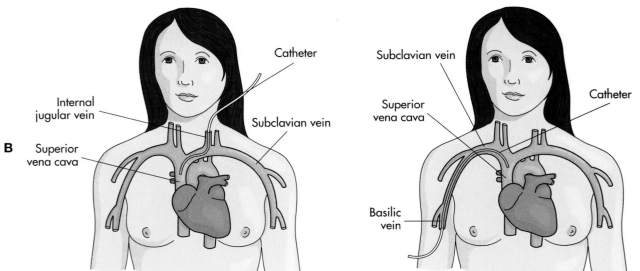

**FIG. 20-23** Central venous sites. **A,** Subclavian vein. The catheter tip is in the right atrium. **B,** Internal jugular vein. The catheter tip is in the superior vena cava. **C,** Basilic vein. This is a peripherally inserted central catheter (PICC).

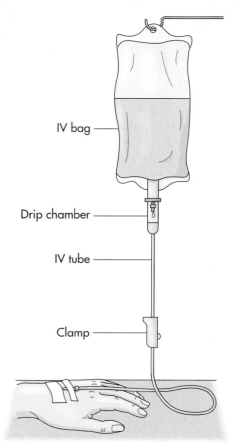

IV bag

Drip chamber

IV tube

Clamp

**FIG. 20-24** Equipment for IV therapy.

**EQUIPMENT.** The basic equipment used in IV therapy is shown in Figure 20-24:
- The solution container is a plastic bag. It is called the *IV bag.*
- A catheter or needle is inserted into a vein (Fig. 20-25). The catheter is a plastic tube. A needle fits over or is inside the catheter for insertion. After insertion, the needle is removed. Butterfly needles also are used.
- The infusion tubing connects the IV bag to the catheter or needle. Fluid drips from the bag into the *drip chamber.* The *clamp* is used to regulate the flow rate.
- The IV bag hangs from the IV pole or ceiling hook. *IV standard* is another name for an IV pole. Portable poles are stored in the supply area. If part of the bed, the pole is stored under the bed frame. It is attached to the head, foot, or side of the bed when needed.

**FLOW RATE.** The doctor orders the amount of fluid to give (infuse) per hour and the amount of time to give it in. With this information, the RN calculates the flow rate. The **flow rate** is the number of drops per minute *(gtt/min).* The abbreviation *gtt* means drops. The Latin word *guttae* means *drops.*

**A**

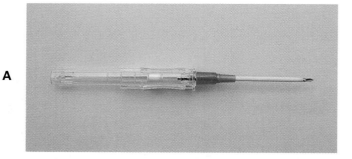

**B**

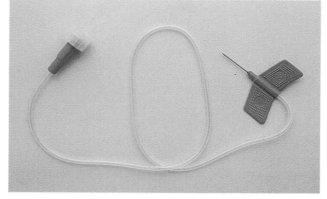

**FIG. 20-25 A,** Intravenous catheter. **B,** Butterfly needle.

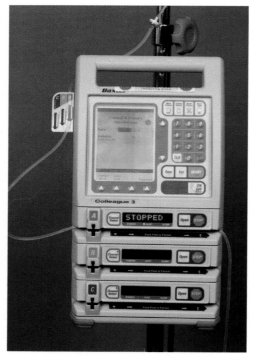

**FIG. 20-26** Electronic IV pump.

The RN sets the clamp for the flow rate. Or an electronic pump is used to control the flow rate (Fig. 20-26). An alarm sounds if something is wrong. Tell the nurse at once if you hear an alarm. *Never change the position of the clamp or adjust any controls on IV pumps.*

You can check the flow rate. The RN tells you the number of drops per minute. To check the flow rate, count the number of drops in 1 full minute (Fig. 20-27). Tell the RN at once if:

- No fluid is dripping
- The rate is too fast
- The rate is too slow

The time tape shows how much fluid to give over a period of time (Fig. 20-28). For example, the doctor orders 1000 ml of fluid over 8 hours. The RN marks the tape in 8 one-hour intervals. To check if fluid is being given on time, compare the fluid line with the time line on the tape. If the fluid line is above or below the time line, the flow rate is too slow or too fast. Tell the RN at once if too much or too little fluid was given.

A rate that is too fast or too slow can be harmful. Changes in flow rate can occur from position changes. Kinked tubes and lying on the tubing also are common problems.

**ASSISTING WITH IV THERAPY.** You help meet the hygiene and activity needs of persons with IVs. *You are never responsible for starting or maintaining IV therapy. Nor do you regulate the flow rate or change IV bags. You never give blood or IV drugs.* However, you assist the RN in providing safe care. Follow the safety measures in Box 20-9, p. 452. Complications can occur from IV therapy. Report any of the signs and symptoms listed in Box 20-10, p. 452, at once.

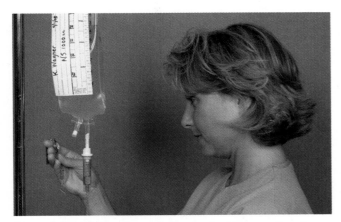

**FIG. 20-27** The flow rate is checked by counting the number of drops per minute.

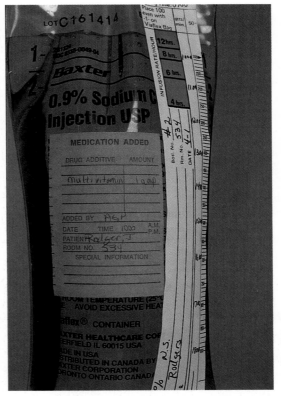

**FIG. 20-28** Time tape applied to an IV bag. (From Elkin MK, Perry AG, Potter PA: *Nursing interventions and clinical skills,* ed 3, St Louis, 2004, Mosby.)

| BOX 20-9 | SAFETY MEASURES FOR IV THERAPY |
| --- | --- |

- Follow Standard Precautions and the Bloodborne Pathogen Standard.
- Do not move the needle or catheter. Needle or catheter position must be maintained. If the needle or catheter is moved, it may come out of the vein. Then fluid flows into tissues (infiltration), or the flow stops.
- Follow the safety measures for restraints (Chapter 11). The nurse may splint or restrain the extremity to prevent movement (Fig. 20-29). This helps prevent the needle or catheter from moving.
- Protect the IV bag, tubing, and needle or catheter when ambulating the person. Portable IV standards are rolled along next to the person (Fig. 20-30).
- Assist the person with turning and repositioning. Move the IV bag to the side of the bed on which the person is lying. Always allow enough slack in the tubing. The needle dislodges from pressure on the tube.
- Tell the nurse at once if bleeding occurs from the insertion site. Follow Standard Precautions and the Bloodborne Pathogen Standard.
- Tell the nurse at once of any signs and symptoms listed in Box 20-10.

| BOX 20-10 | SIGNS AND SYMPTOMS OF IV THERAPY COMPLICATIONS |
| --- | --- |

**LOCAL—AT THE IV SITE**

- Bleeding
- Puffiness or swelling
- Pale or reddened skin
- Complaints of pain at or above the IV site
- Hot or cold skin near the site

**SYSTEMIC—INVOLVING THE WHOLE BODY**

- Fever
- Itching
- Drop in blood pressure
- Pulse rate more than 100 beats per minute
- Irregular pulse
- Cyanosis
- Changes in mental function
- Loss of consciousness
- Difficulty breathing
- Shortness of breath
- Decreasing or no urine output
- Chest pain
- Nausea
- Confusion

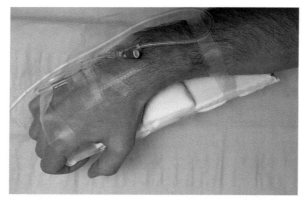

**FIG. 20-29** An armboard prevents movement at an IV site. (From Elkin MK, Perry AG, Potter PA: *Nursing interventions and clinical skills,* ed 2, St Louis, 2000, Mosby.)

## CROSS-TRAINING OPPORTUNITIES

You may be cross-trained as a dietary aide to work in the dietary department. You serve food, prepare trays, and deliver trays to the nursing units. You also distribute and collect menus on the nursing units.

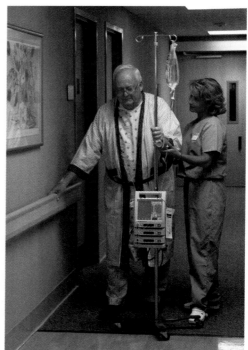

**FIG. 20-30** A person ambulating with an IV.

**Circle the BEST answer.**

**1** Nutrition is
   **a** Fats, proteins, carbohydrates, vitamins, and minerals
   **b** The processes involved in the ingestion, digestion, absorption, and use of food and fluids by the body
   **c** The Food Guide Pyramid
   **d** The balance between calories taken in and used by the body

**2** The Food Guide Pyramid encourages
   **a** A low-fat diet
   **b** A high-fat diet
   **c** A low-fiber diet
   **d** A low-salt diet

**3** How many daily servings of breads, cereals, rice, and pasta are needed?
   **a** 6 to 11
   **b** 3 to 5
   **c** 2 to 4
   **d** 2 to 3

**4** How many daily servings of the meat group are needed?
   **a** 6 to 11
   **b** 3 to 5
   **c** 2 to 4
   **d** 2 to 3

**5** Which food group contains the *most* fat?
   **a** Breads, cereal, rice, and pasta
   **b** Fruits
   **c** Milk, yogurt, and cheese
   **d** Meat, poultry, fish, dry beans, eggs, and nuts

**6** Fats, oils, and sweets
   **a** Are used in moderate amounts
   **b** Are low in calories
   **c** Are used sparingly
   **d** Provide many nutrients

**7** Protein is needed for
   **a** Tissue growth and repair
   **b** Energy and the fiber for bowel elimination
   **c** Body heat and the protection of organs from injury
   **d** Improving the taste of food

**8** Which foods provide th
   **a** Butter and cream
   **b** Tomatoes and potat
   **c** Meats and fish
   **d** Corn and lettuce

**9** Sodium-controlled diets are usually ordered for the following persons *except* those with
   **a** Diabetes
   **b** Heart disease
   **c** Kidney disease
   **d** Liver disease

**10** Mr. Bonner is on a sodium-controlled diet. He wants salt for his chicken. You should
   **a** Bring him the salt
   **b** Tell the nurse
   **c** Remind him that added salt is not allowed on his diet
   **d** Ignore the request

**11** Diabetes meal planning involves the following *except*
   **a** The person's food preferences
   **b** Eating the same amount of carbohydrates, protein, and fat each day
   **c** Eating at regular times
   **d** A high-calorie diet

**12** Adult fluid requirement for normal fluid balance is about
   **a** 1000 to 1500 ml daily
   **b** 1500 to 2000 ml daily
   **c** 2000 to 2500 ml daily
   **d** 2500 to 3000 ml daily

**13** A person is NPO. You should
   **a** Provide a variety of fluids
   **b** Offer fluids in small amounts and small containers
   **c** Remove the water pitcher and glass
   **d** Prevent the person from having oral hygiene

**14** Which are *not* counted as liquid foods?
   **a** Coffee, tea, juices, and soft drinks
   **b** Sauces and melted cheese
   **c** Ice cream and sherbet
   **d** Popsicles and soup

**15** Which action about feeding a person is *incorrect*?
a Ask if he or she wants to pray before eating.
b Use a fork to feed the person.
c Ask the person the order in which to serve foods.
d Engage the person in a pleasant conversation.

**16** To prevent regurgitation after a tubing feeding, the person is positioned in
a Semi-Fowler's position
b Fowler's position
c In the left side-lying position
d In the right side-lying position

**17** A person with a feeding tube is usually
a Allowed a regular diet
b On bedrest
c NPO
d In a coma

**18** You note that the IV flow rate is too slow. You must
a Tell the RN at once
b Adjust the flow rate
c Reposition the person
d Clamp the tubing

**19** A person is bleeding from an IV site. You should
a Remove the IV catheter or needle
b Apply direct pressure
c Call for the RN at once
d Apply a dressing to the site

**20** Which is *not* a sign of IV therapy complications?
a Swelling at the IV site
b Changes in mental function or confusion
c Polyuria
d Changes in blood pressure, pulse, and respirations

*Answers to these questions are on p. 818.*

# Measuring Vital Signs

# OBJECTIVES

- Define the key terms listed in this chapter
- Explain why vital signs are measured
- List the factors affecting vital signs
- Identify the normal ranges for each temperature site
- Know when to use each temperature site
- Identify the pulse sites
- Describe normal respirations
- Describe the factors affecting blood pressure
- Describe the practices followed when measuring blood pressure
- Know the normal vital signs for different age-groups
- Perform the procedures described in this chapter

# KEY TERMS

**apical-radial pulse** Taking the apical and radial pulses at the same time

**blood pressure** The amount of force exerted against the walls of an artery by the blood

**body temperature** The amount of heat in the body that is a balance between the amount of heat produced and the amount lost by the body

**bradycardia** A slow *(brady)* heart rate *(cardia);* less than 60 beats per minute

**diastole** The period of heart muscle relaxation; the period when the heart is at rest

**diastolic pressure** The pressure in the arteries when the heart is at rest

**hypertension** Blood pressure measurements that remain above *(hyper)* a systolic pressure of 140 mm Hg) or a diastolic pressure of 90 mm Hg

**hypotension** When the systolic blood pressure is below *(hypo)* 90 mm Hg and the diastolic pressure is below 60 mm Hg

**pulse** The beat of the heart felt at an artery as a wave of blood passes through the artery

**pulse deficit** The difference between the apical and radial pulse rates

**pulse rate** The number of heartbeats or pulses felt in 1 minute

**respiration** Breathing air into (inhalation) and out of (exhalation) the lungs

**sphygmomanometer** A cuff and measuring device used to measure blood pressure

**stethoscope** An instrument used to listen to the sounds produced by the heart, lungs, and other body organs

**systole** The period of heart muscle contraction; the period when the heart is pumping

**systolic pressure** The amount of force needed to pump blood out of the heart into the arterial circulation

**tachycardia** A rapid *(tachy)* heart rate *(cardia);* more than 100 beats per minute

**vital signs** Temperature, pulse, respirations, and blood pressure

Vital signs reflect the function of three body processes essential for life: regulation of body temperature, breathing, and heart function. The four **vital signs** of body function are:

- Temperature
- Pulse
- Respirations
- Blood pressure

## MEASURING AND REPORTING VITAL SIGNS

A person's vital signs vary within certain limits. They are affected by sleep, activity, eating, weather, noise, exercise, drugs, anger, fear, anxiety, pain, and illness.

Vital signs are measured to detect changes in normal body function. They tell about a person's response to treatment. They often signal life-threatening events. Vital signs are part of assessment in the nursing process. Vital signs are measured:

- During physical exams
- On admission to a health care agency
- As often as required by the person's condition
- Before and after surgery
- Before and after complex procedures or diagnostic tests
- After some care measures, such as ambulation
- After a fall or injury
- When drugs affect the respiratory or circulatory systems
- Whenever there are complaints of pain, dizziness, lightheadedness, fainting, shortness of breath, rapid heart rate, or not feeling well
- As stated on the care plan

Vital signs show even minor changes in a person's condition. Accuracy is essential when you measure, record, and report vital signs. If unsure of your measurements, promptly ask the nurse to take them again.

Unless otherwise ordered, take vital signs with the person lying or sitting. The person is at rest when vital signs are measured. Report the following at once:

- Any vital sign that is changed from a prior measurement
- Vital signs above the normal range
- Vital signs below the normal range

Vital signs are recorded on graphic sheets or entered into the person's computer record. If they are measured often, a flow sheet is used. The doctor or nurse compares current and prior measurements.

## BODY TEMPERATURE

**Body temperature** is the amount of heat in the body. It is a balance between the amount of heat produced and the amount lost by the body. Heat is produced as cells use food for energy. It is lost through the skin, breathing, urine, and feces. Body temperature stays fairly stable. It is lower in the morning and higher in the afternoon and evening. Body temperature is affected by age, weather, exercise, emotions, stress, and illness. Pregnancy and the menstrual cycle are other factors.

Thermometers are used to measure temperature. It is measured using the Fahrenheit (F) and Centigrade or Celsius (C) scale.

### TEMPERATURE SITES

Temperature sites are the mouth, rectum, ear (tympanic membrane), and axilla (underarm). Each site has a normal range (Table 21-1). Oral temperatures are *not* taken if the person:

- Is an infant or a child younger than 6 years
- Is unconscious
- Has had surgery or an injury to the face, neck, nose, or mouth
- Is receiving oxygen
- Breathes through the mouth
- Has a nasogastric tube
- Is delirious, restless, confused, or disoriented
- Is paralyzed on one side of the body
- Has a sore mouth
- Has a convulsive (seizure) disorder

| TABLE 21-1 NORMAL BODY TEMPERATURES | | |
|---|---|---|
| **Site** | **Baseline** | **Normal Range** |
| Rectal | 99.6° F (37.5° C) | 98.6° to 100.6° F (37.0° to 38.1° C) |
| Oral | 98.6° F (37° C) | 97.6° to 99.6° F (36.5 to 37.5° C) |
| Tympanic membrane | 98.6° F (37° C) | 98.6° F (37° C) |
| Axillary | 97.6° F (36.5° C) | 96.6° to 98.6° F (35.9° to 37.0° C) |

Rectal temperatures are taken when the oral route cannot be used. Rectal temperatures are *not* taken if the person has:

- Diarrhea
- A rectal disorder or injury
- Heart disease
- Had rectal surgery
- Confusion or is agitated

The tympanic membrane site has fewer microbes than the mouth or rectum. Therefore the risk of spreading infection is reduced. This site is *not* used if the person has:

- An ear disorder
- Ear drainage

The axillary site is less reliable than the other sites. It is used when the other sites cannot be used.

*See Focus on Children: Temperature Sites. See Focus on Older Persons: Temperature Sites.*

## GLASS THERMOMETERS

The glass thermometer (clinical thermometer) is a hollow glass tube (Fig. 21-1). The tube is filled with a substance—mercury or a mercury-free mixture. When heated, the substance expands and rises in the tube. When cooled, the substance contracts and moves down the tube.

Long- or slender-tip thermometers are used for oral and axillary temperatures. So are thermometers with stubby and pear-shaped tips. Rectal thermometers have stubby tips that are color-coded in red.

Glass thermometers are reusable. However, the following are problems:

- They take a long time to register—3 to 10 minutes depending on the site. Oral temperatures take 2 to 3 minutes. Rectal temperatures take at least 2 minutes. Axillary temperatures take 5 to 10 minutes.
- They break easily. Broken rectal thermometers can injure the rectum and colon.
- The person may bite down and break an oral thermometer. Cuts in the mouth are risks. Swallowed mercury can cause mercury poisoning.

*See Focus on Children: Glass Thermometers.*

---

### ▶ FOCUS ON CHILDREN
**TEMPERATURE SITES**

The oral site is not used for infants and children younger than 6 years. The rectal, axillary, and tympanic membrane sites are used.

---

### ▶ FOCUS ON OLDER PERSONS
**TEMPERATURE SITES**

Older persons have lower body temperatures than younger adults. An oral temperature of 98.6° F may signal fever in an older person.

---

**SAFETY ALERT:** *Temperature Sites*

Rectal temperatures are dangerous for persons with heart disease. The thermometer can stimulate the vagus nerve in the rectum. This nerve also affects the heart. Stimulation of the vagus nerve slows the heart rate. The heart rate can slow to dangerous levels in some persons.

---

### ▶ FOCUS ON CHILDREN
**GLASS THERMOMETERS**

The American Academy of Pediatricians recommends not using mercury-glass thermometers on children. You may care for the child in the home setting. Tell the nurse if there is a mercury-glass thermometer in the home.

---

**SAFETY ALERT:** *Mercury-Glass Thermometers*

If a mercury–glass thermometer breaks, tell the nurse at once. Mercury is a hazardous substance. Do not touch the mercury. Do not let the person do so. The agency must follow special procedures for handling all hazardous materials. See Chapter 10.

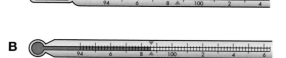
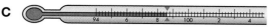

**FIG. 21-1** Types of glass thermometers. **A,** The long or slender tip. **B,** The stubby tip (rectal thermometer). **C,** The pear-shaped tip.

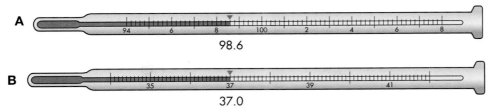

A, A Fahrenheit thermometer. The temperature measurement is 98.6° F.

98.6

B, Centigrade thermometer. The temperature measurement is 37.0° C.

37.0

**FIG. 21-2 A,** A Fahrenheit thermometer. The temperature measurement is 98.6° F. **B,** Centigrade thermometer. The temperature measurement is 37.0° C.

**READING A GLASS THERMOMETER.** Fahrenheit thermometers have long and short lines. Every other long line is marked in an even degree from 94° to 108° F. The short lines mean 0.2 (two tenths) of a degree (Fig. 21-2, *A*).

On a centigrade thermometer, each long line means 1 degree. Degrees range from 34° to 42° C. Each short line means 0.1 (one tenth) of a degree (Fig. 21-2, *B*).

To read a glass thermometer:

- Hold it at the stem (Fig. 21-3). Bring it to eye level.
- Turn it until you can see the numbers and the long and short lines.
- Turn it back and forth slowly until you see the silver or red line.
- Read the nearest degree (long line).
- Read the nearest tenth of a degree (short line)—an even number on a Fahrenheit thermometer.

**USING A GLASS THERMOMETER.** Do the following to prevent infection, promote safety, and obtain an accurate measurement:

- Use only the person's thermometer.
- Use a rectal thermometer only for rectal temperatures.
- Rinse the thermometer under cold, running water if it was soaking in a disinfectant. Dry it from the stem to the bulb end with tissues.
- Check the thermometer for breaks, cracks, and chips. Discard it following agency policy if it is broken, cracked, or chipped.
- Shake down the thermometer so the substance moves down in the tube. Hold it at the stem. Stand away from walls, tables, or other hard surfaces. Flex and snap your wrist until the substance is below the lowest number of the thermometer (94° F or 34° C). See Figure 21-4.

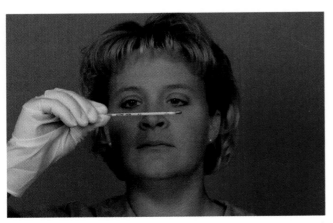

**FIG. 21-3** The thermometer is held at the stem. It is read at eye level.

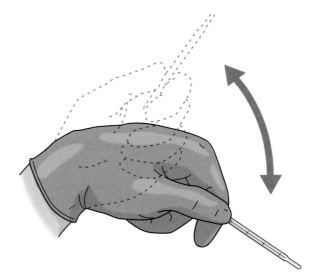

**FIG. 21-4** The wrist is snapped to shake down the thermometer.

- Clean and store the thermometer following agency policy. Wipe it with tissues first to remove mucus, feces, or sweat. Do not use hot water. It causes the mercury or mercury-free mixture to expand so much that the thermometer could break. After cleaning, rinse the thermometer under cold, running water. Then store it in a container with disinfectant solution.
- Use plastic covers following agency policy (Fig. 21-5). To take a temperature, insert the thermometer into a cover. Remove the cover to read the thermometer. Discard the cover after use.
- Practice medical asepsis.
- Follow Standard Precautions and the Bloodborne Pathogen Standard.

**TAKING TEMPERATURES.** Glass thermometers are used for oral, rectal, and axillary temperatures. Special measures are needed for each site.
- *The oral site.* The glass thermometer remains in place 2 to 3 minutes or as required by agency policy.
- *The rectal site.* Lubricate the rectal thermometer for easy insertion and to prevent tissue injury. Hold it in place so it is not lost in the rectum or broken. A glass thermometer remains in the rectum for 2 minutes or as required by agency policy. Privacy is important. The buttocks and anus are exposed. The procedure embarrasses many people.
- *The axillary site.* The axilla must be dry. Do not use this site right after bathing. Hold the glass thermometer in place for 5 to 10 minutes or as required by agency policy.

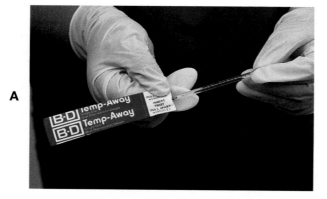

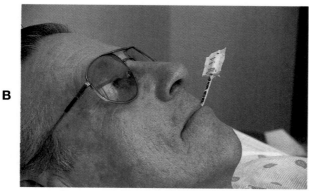

**FIG. 21-5 A,** The thermometer is inserted into a plastic cover. **B,** The person's temperature is taken with the thermometer in a plastic cover.

**DELEGATION GUIDELINES:** *Taking Temperatures*
The nurse may ask you to take temperatures. If so, you need this information from the nurse and the care plan:
- What site to use—oral, rectal, axillary, or tympanic membrane
- What thermometer to use—glass, electronic, or other type
- How long to leave a glass thermometer in place
- When to take temperatures
- Which persons are at risk for elevated temperatures
- What observations to report and record

**SAFETY ALERT:** *Taking Temperatures*
Thermometers are inserted into the mouth, rectum, and axilla. Each area has many microbes. The area may contain blood. Therefore each person has his or her own glass thermometer. This prevents the spread of microbes and infection.
Follow Standard Precautions and the Bloodborne Pathogen Standard when taking temperatures.

## TAKING A TEMPERATURE WITH A GLASS THERMOMETER

NNAAP™

### QUALITY OF LIFE

Remember to:
- Knock before entering the person's room
- Address the person by name
- Introduce yourself by name and title

### PRE-PROCEDURE

1 Follow *Delegation Guidelines: Taking Temperatures.* See *Safety Alerts:*
   - *Temperature Sites*, p. 458
   - *Mercury-Glass Thermometers*, p. 458
   - *Taking Temperatures*
2 Explain the procedure to the person. For an oral temperature, ask the person not to eat, drink, smoke, or chew gum for at least 15 to 20 minutes or as required by agency policy.
3 Collect the following:
   - Oral or rectal thermometer and holder
   - Tissues
   - Plastic covers if used
   - Gloves
   - Toilet tissue (rectal temperature)
   - Water-soluble lubricant (rectal temperature)
   - Towel (axillary temperature)
4 Practice hand hygiene.
5 Identify the person. Check the ID bracelet against the assignment sheet. Call the person by name.
6 Provide for privacy.

### PROCEDURE

7 Put on the gloves.
8 Rinse the thermometer in cold water if it was soaking in a disinfectant. Dry it with tissues.
9 Check for breaks, cracks, or chips.
10 Shake down the thermometer below the lowest number.
11 Insert it into a plastic cover if used.
12 For an *oral temperature:*
   a Ask the person to moisten his or her lips.
   b Place the bulb end of the thermometer under the tongue (Fig. 21-6, p. 462).
   c Ask the person to close the lips around the thermometer to hold it in place.
   d Ask the person not to talk. Remind the person not to bite down on the thermometer.
   e Leave it in place for 2 to 3 minutes or as required by agency policy.
13 For a *rectal temperature:*
   a Position the person in Sims' position.
   b Put a small amount of lubricant on a tissue. Lubricate the bulb end of the thermometer.
   c Fold back top linens to expose the anal area.
   d Raise the upper buttock to expose the anus (Fig. 21-7, p. 462).
   e Insert the thermometer 1 inch into the rectum. Do not force the thermometer. Remember, glass thermometers can break.
   f Hold the thermometer in place for 2 minutes or as required by agency policy. Do not let go of it while it is in the rectum.
14 For an *axillary temperature:*
   a Help the person remove an arm from the gown. Do not expose the person.
   b Dry the axilla with the towel.
   c Place the bulb end of the thermometer in the center of the axilla.
   d Ask the person to place the arm over the chest to hold the thermometer in place (Fig. 21-8, p. 462). Hold it and the arm in place if he or she cannot help.
   e Leave the thermometer in place for 5 to 10 minutes or as required by agency policy.
15 Remove the thermometer.
16 Use tissues to remove the plastic cover. Wipe the thermometer with a tissue if no cover was used. Wipe from the stem to the bulb end.
17 For a *rectal temperature:*
   a Place used toilet tissue on a paper towel or several thicknesses of toilet tissue.
   b Place the thermometer on clean toilet tissue.
   c Wipe the anal area to remove excess lubricant and any feces.
   d Cover the person.
18 For an *axillary temperature:* Help the person put the gown back on.
19 Read the thermometer.
20 Record the person's name and temperature on your note pad or assignment sheet. Write *R* for a rectal temperature. Write *A* for an axillary temperature.
21 Shake down the thermometer.

*Continued.*

## TAKING A TEMPERATURE WITH A GLASS THERMOMETER—CONT'D

*NNAAP™*

### PROCEDURE—CONT'D

22 Clean it according to agency policy.
23 Discard tissue and the paper towel.

24 Remove the gloves. Decontaminate your hands.

### POST-PROCEDURE

25 Provide for comfort.
26 Place the signal light within reach.
27 Unscreen the person.

28 Record the temperature in the proper place. Report any abnormal temperature to the nurse. Note the temperature site.

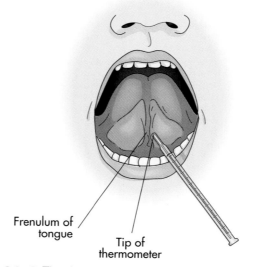

Frenulum of tongue

Tip of thermometer

**FIG. 21-6** The thermometer is placed at the base of the tongue.

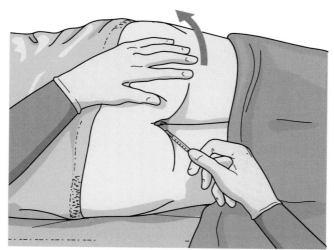

**FIG. 21-7** The rectal temperature is taken with the person in Sims' position. The buttock is raised to expose the anus.

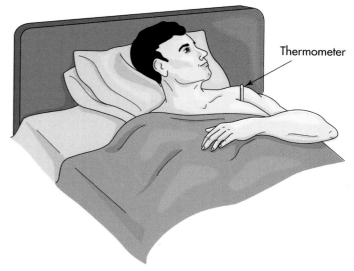

Thermometer

**FIG. 21-8** The thermometer is held in place in the axilla by bringing the person's arm over the chest.

# ELECTRONIC THERMOMETERS

Electronic thermometers are battery-operated (Fig. 21-9). They measure temperature in a few seconds. The temperature is shown on the front of the device. The hand-held unit is kept in a battery charger when not in use.

Electronic thermometers have oral and rectal probes. A disposable cover (sheath) covers the probe. The probe cover is discarded after use. This helps prevent the spread of infection.

**TYMPANIC MEMBRANE THERMOMETERS.** Tympanic membrane thermometers measure temperature at the tympanic membrane in the ear (Fig. 21-10). The covered probe is gently inserted into the ear. The temperature is measured in 1 to 3 seconds.

Tympanic membrane thermometers are comfortable. They are not invasive like rectal thermometers. They are useful for children and confused persons because of their speed and comfort.

*Text continued on p. 466.*

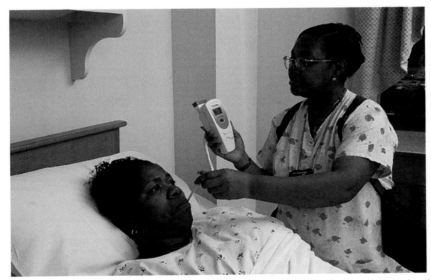

**FIG. 21-9** The covered probe of the electronic thermometer is inserted under the tongue.

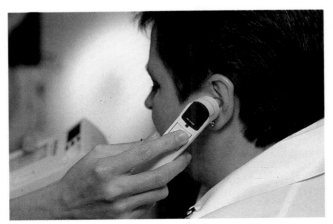

**FIG. 21-10** Tympanic membrane thermometer.

# TAKING A TEMPERATURE WITH AN ELECTRONIC THERMOMETER

## QUALITY OF LIFE

Remember to:
- Knock before entering the person's room
- Address the person by name
- Introduce yourself by name and title

## PRE-PROCEDURE

1 Follow *Delegation Guidelines: Taking Temperatures,* p. 460. See *Safety Alert: Taking Temperatures,* p. 460 *and Safety Alert: Temperature Sites,* p. 458.
2 Explain the procedure to the person. For an oral temperature, ask him or her not to eat, drink, smoke, or chew gum for at least 15 to 20 minutes.
3 Collect the following:
- Thermometer—electronic or tympanic membrane
- Probe (Blue for an oral or axillary temperature. Red for a rectal temperature.)
- Probe covers
- Toilet tissue (rectal temperature)
- Water-soluble lubricant (rectal temperature)
- Gloves
- Towel (axillary temperature)
4 Plug the probe into the thermometer. (This is not done for a tympanic membrane thermometer.)
5 Practice hand hygiene.
6 Identify the person. Check the ID bracelet against the assignment sheet. Call the person by name.

## PROCEDURE

7 Provide for privacy. Position the person for an oral, rectal, axillary, or tympanic membrane temperature.
8 Put on gloves if contact with blood, body fluids, secretions, or excretions is likely.
9 Insert the probe into a probe cover.
10 For an *oral temperature:*
 a Ask the person to open the mouth and raise the tongue.
 b Place the covered probe at the base of the tongue (see Fig. 21-9, p. 463).
 c Ask the person to lower the tongue and close the mouth.
11 For a *rectal temperature:*
 a Place some lubricant on toilet tissue.
 b Lubricate the end of the covered probe.
 c Expose the anal area.
 d Raise the upper buttock.
 e Insert the probe ½ inch into the rectum.
 f Hold the probe in place.
12 For an *axillary temperature:*
 a Help the person remove an arm from the gown. Do not expose the person.
 b Dry the axilla with the towel.
 c Place the covered probe in the axilla.
 d Place the person's arm over the chest.
 e Hold the probe in place.
13 For a *tympanic membrane temperature:*
 a Ask the person to turn his or her head so the ear is in front of you.
 b Pull back on the ear to straighten the ear canal (Fig. 21-11).
 c Insert the covered probe gently.
14 Start the thermometer.
15 Hold the probe in place until you hear a tone or see a flashing or steady light.
16 Read the temperature on the display.
17 Remove the probe. Press the eject button to discard the cover.
18 Record the person's name and temperature on your note pad or assignment sheet. Note the temperature site.
19 Return the probe to the holder.
20 Provide for comfort. Help the person put the gown back on (axillary temperature). For a rectal temperature:
 a Wipe the anal area with tissue to remove lubricant.
 b Cover the person.
 c Discard used toilet tissue.
 d Remove the gloves. Decontaminate your hands.

## TAKING A TEMPERATURE WITH AN ELECTRONIC THERMOMETER—CONT'D

### POST-PROCEDURE

21 Place the signal light within reach.
22 Unscreen the person.
23 Return the thermometer to the charging unit.
24 Decontaminate your hands.

25 Record the temperature in the proper place. Note the temperature site. Report any abnormal temperature.

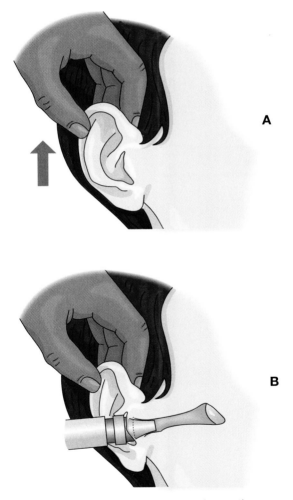

**FIG. 21-11** Using a tympanic membrane thermometer. **A,** The ear is pulled back. **B,** The probe is inserted into the ear canal.

## OTHER THERMOMETERS

Other types of thermometers are used. Follow the manufacturer's instructions.

- *Digital thermometers*—show the temperature on the front of the thermometer (Fig. 21-12). The temperature is measured in about 60 seconds. Some store and recall the last temperature taken. Battery-operated, the device shuts off in about 10 minutes.
- *Disposable oral thermometers*—have small chemical dots (Fig. 21-13). The dots change color when heated. Each dot is heated to a certain temperature before it changes color. These thermometers are used once. They measure temperatures in 45 to 60 seconds.
- *Temperature-sensitive tape*—changes color in response to body heat (Fig. 21-14). The tape is applied to the forehead or abdomen. The measurement takes about 15 seconds.

See *Focus on Children: Other Thermometers.*

---

### FOCUS ON CHILDREN
#### OTHER THERMOMETERS

Pacifier thermometers can be used for children younger than 5 years. They have four parts: a storage cover, a nipple with a sensor, a digital display, and an on-and-off switch. Temperature is measured in about 5 minutes. Follow the manufacturer's instructions for use.

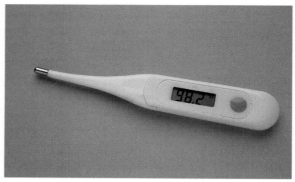

**FIG. 21-12** Digital thermometer.

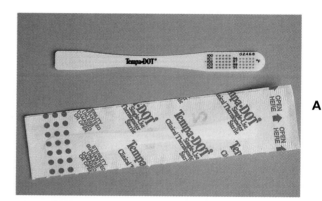

**A**

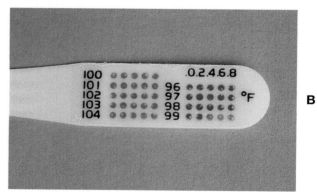

**B**

**FIG. 21-13 A,** Disposable oral thermometer with chemical dots. **B,** The dots change color when heated by the body.

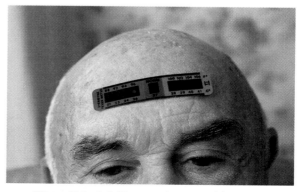

**FIG. 21-14** Temperature-sensitive tape.

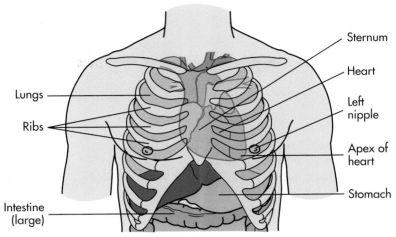

**FIG. 21-15** Location of the heart.

## PULSE

Arteries carry blood from the heart to all body parts (Box 21-1). The **pulse** is the beat of the heart felt at an artery as a wave of blood passes through the artery. A pulse is felt every time the heart beats.

| BOX 21-1 | STRUCTURE AND FUNCTION OF THE HEART AND BLOOD VESSELS |
|---|---|

The heart is a muscle. It pumps blood through the blood vessels to the tissues and cells. The heart lies in the middle to lower part of the chest cavity toward the left side (Fig. 21-15).

The heart has four chambers (see Fig. 7-15, p. 108). Upper chambers receive blood and are called the *atria*. The *right atrium* receives blood from body tissues. The *left atrium* receives blood from the lungs. Lower chambers are called *ventricles*. Ventricles pump blood. The *right ventricle* pumps blood to the lungs for oxygen. The *left ventricle* pumps blood to all parts of the body.

There are two phases of heart action. *Diastole* is the resting phase. Heart chambers fill with blood. *Systole* is the working phase. The heart contracts. Blood is pumped through the blood vessels when the heart contracts.

Blood flows to body tissues and cells through the blood vessels. *Arteries* carry blood away from the heart. Arterial blood is rich in oxygen. The *aorta* is the largest artery. The aorta receives blood directly from the left ventricle. The aorta branches into other arteries that carry blood to all parts of the body (Fig. 21-16). *Veins* return blood to the heart.

See Chapter 7 for more detailed information.

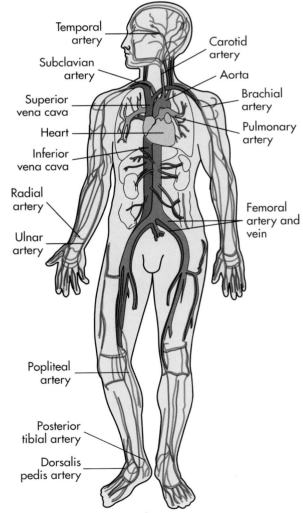

**FIG. 21-16** The arterial system.

## PULSE SITES

The temporal, carotid, brachial, radial, femoral, popliteal, posterior tibial, and dorsalis pedis (pedal) pulses are on each side of the body (Fig. 21-17). Pulses are easy to feel at these sites. The arteries are close to the body's surface and lie over a bone.

The radial site is used most often. It is easy to reach and find. You can take a radial pulse without disturbing or exposing the person. The carotid pulse is taken during CPR and other emergencies (Chapter 40).

The apical pulse is felt over the apex of the heart. The apex is at the tip of the heart, just below the left nipple (p. 472). The apical pulse is taken with a stethoscope.

*See Focus on Children: Pulse Sites.*

**FOCUS ON CHILDREN**
PULSE SITES
The apical site is used for infants and children younger than 2 years. You can use the radial site for children older than 2 years.

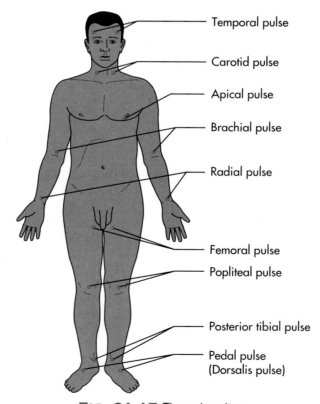

Temporal pulse
Carotid pulse
Apical pulse
Brachial pulse
Radial pulse
Femoral pulse
Popliteal pulse
Posterior tibial pulse
Pedal pulse (Dorsalis pulse)

**FIG. 21-17** The pulse sites.

## USING A STETHOSCOPE

A **stethoscope** is an instrument used to listen to the sounds produced by the heart, lungs, and other body organs (Fig. 21-18). It is used to take apical pulses and blood pressures. The device makes sounds louder for easy hearing.

Follow these rules when using a stethoscope:
- Wipe the earpieces and diaphragm with antiseptic wipes before and after use.
- Warm the diaphragm in your hand (Fig. 21-19).
- Place the earpiece tips in your ears. The bend of the tips points forward. Earpieces should fit snugly to block out noises. They should not cause pain or ear discomfort.
- Place the diaphragm over the artery. Hold it in place as in Figure 21-20.
- Prevent noise. Do not let anything touch the tubing. Ask the person to be silent.

> **SAFETY ALERT: *Stethoscopes***
> Stethoscopes are in contact with many persons and staff. Therefore you must prevent infection. Wipe the earpieces and diaphragm with antiseptic wipes before and after use.

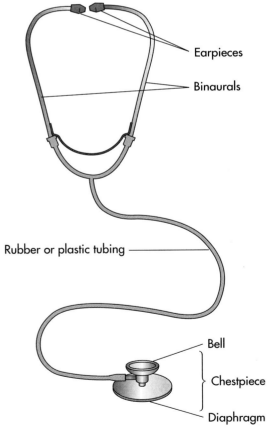

FIG. 21-18 Parts of a stethoscope.

- Earpieces
- Binaurals
- Rubber or plastic tubing
- Bell
- Chestpiece
- Diaphragm

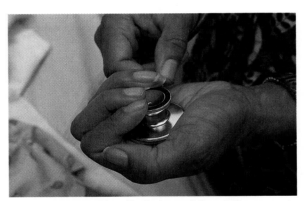

**FIG. 21-19** The diaphragm of the stethoscope is warmed in the palm of the hand.

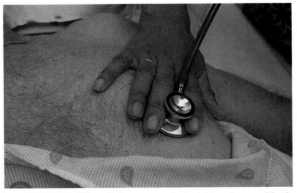

**FIG. 21-20** The stethoscope is held in place with the fingertips of the index and middle fingers.

## PULSE RATE

The **pulse rate** is the number of heartbeats or pulses felt in 1 minute. The rate varies for each age-group (Table 21-2). The pulse rate is affected by many factors. They include elevated body temperature (fever), exercise, fear, anger, anxiety, excitement, heat, position, and pain. These and other factors cause the heart to beat faster. Some drugs also increase the pulse rate. Other drugs slow down the pulse.

The adult pulse rate is between 60 and 100 beats per minute. A rate of less than 60 or more than 100 is considered abnormal. Report abnormal rates to the nurse at once.

- **Tachycardia** is a rapid *(tachy)* heart rate *(cardia)*. The heart rate is more than 100 beats per minute.
- **Bradycardia** is a slow *(brady)* heart rate *(cardia)*. The heart rate is less than 60 beats per minute.

## RHYTHM AND FORCE OF THE PULSE

The rhythm of the pulse should be regular. That is, pulses are felt in a pattern. The same time interval occurs between beats. An irregular pulse occurs when the beats are not evenly spaced or beats are skipped (Fig. 21-21).

Force relates to pulse strength. A forceful pulse is easy to feel. It is described as *strong, full,* or *bounding.* Hard-to-feel pulses are described as *weak, thready,* or *feeble.*

Electronic blood pressure equipment (p. 477) can also count pulses. The pulse rate and blood pressures are shown. Information is not given about pulse rhythm and force. You need to feel the pulse to determine rhythm and force.

| TABLE 21-2 | PULSE RANGES FOR DIFFERENT AGES | |
|---|---|
| Age | Pulse Rates per Minute |
| Birth to 1 year | 80-190 |
| 2 years | 80-160 |
| 6 years | 75-120 |
| 10 years | 70-110 |
| 12 years and older | 60-100 |

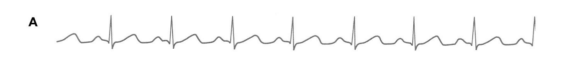

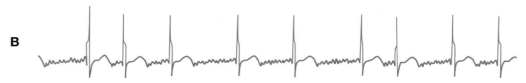

**FIG. 21-21 A,** The electrocardiogram shows a regular pulse. The beats occur at regular intervals. **B,** These beats occur at irregular intervals.

# ◼ TAKING A RADIAL PULSE

The radial pulse is used for routine vital signs. Place the first two or three fingers of one hand against the radial artery. The radial artery is on the thumb side of the wrist (Fig. 21-22). Count the pulse for 30 seconds. Then multiply the number by 2. This gives the number of beats per minute. If the pulse is irregular, count it for 1 minute.

In some agencies, all radial pulses are taken for 1 minute. Follow agency policy.

---

**DELEGATION GUIDELINES:** *Taking Pulses*

Before taking a pulse, you need this information from the nurse and the care plan:

- What pulse to take—radial, apical (p. 472), or apical-radial (p. 473)
- When to take the pulse
- What other vital signs to measure
- How long to count the pulse—30 seconds or 1 minute
- If the nurse has concerns about certain patients or residents
- What observations to report and record:
  —The pulse rate—report a pulse rate less than 60 or more than 100 beats per minute at once
  —If the pulse is regular or irregular
  —Pulse force—strong, full, bounding, weak, thready, or feeble

---

**SAFETY ALERT:** *Taking Pulses*

Do not use your thumb to take a pulse. The thumb has a pulse. You could mistake the pulse in your thumb for the person's pulse. Reporting the wrong pulse rate can harm the person.

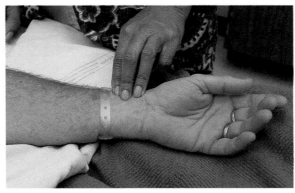

**FIG. 21-22** The middle three fingers are used to take the radial pulse.

---

## TAKING A RADIAL PULSE                                    NNAAP™

### QUALITY OF LIFE

Remember to:
- Knock before entering the person's room
- Address the person by name
- Introduce yourself by name and title

### PRE-PROCEDURE

1 Follow *Delegation Guidelines: Taking Pulses.* See *Safety Alert: Taking Pulses.*
2 Practice hand hygiene.
3 Identify the person. Check the ID bracelet against the assignment sheet. Call the person by name.
4 Explain the procedure to the person.
5 Provide for privacy.

### PROCEDURE

6 Have the person sit or lie down.
7 Locate the radial pulse. Use your first two or three middle fingers (see Fig. 21-22).
8 Note if the pulse is strong or weak, and regular or irregular.
9 Count the pulse for 30 seconds. Multiply the number of beats by 2. Or count the pulse for 1 minute as directed by the nurse or if required by agency policy. (NNAAP™ skills evaluation requires counting the pulse for 1 minute.)
10 Count the pulse for 1 minute if it is irregular.
11 Record the person's name and pulse on your note pad or assignment sheet. Note the strength of the pulse. Note if it was regular or irregular.

### POST-PROCEDURE

12 Provide for comfort.
13 Place the signal light within reach.
14 Unscreen the person.
15 Decontaminate your hands.
16 Report and record the pulse rate and your observations.

## TAKING AN APICAL PULSE

The apical pulse is taken with a stethoscope. This method is used on infants and children up to about 2 years of age. Apical pulses are taken on persons who have heart disease, who have irregular heart rhythms, or who take drugs that affect the heart. The apical pulse is on the left side of the chest slightly below the nipple (Fig. 21-23).

Count the apical pulse for 1 minute. The heartbeat normally sounds like a *lub-dub.* Count each *lub-dub* as one beat. Do not count the *lub* as one beat and the *dub* as another.

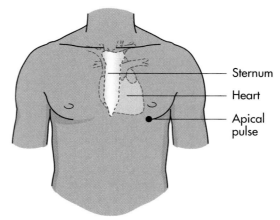

**FIG. 21-23** The apical pulse is located 2 to 3 inches to the left of the sternum (breastbone) and below the left nipple.

## TAKING AN APICAL PULSE

### QUALITY OF LIFE

Remember to:  ▪ Knock before entering the person's room
▪ Address the person by name
▪ Introduce yourself by name and title

### PRE-PROCEDURE

1 Follow *Delegation Guidelines: Taking Pulses,* p. 471. See *Safety Alert: Stethoscopes,* p. 469.
2 Collect a stethoscope and antiseptic wipes.
3 Practice hand hygiene.
4 Identify the person. Check the ID bracelet against the assignment sheet. Call the person by name.
5 Explain the procedure to the person.
6 Provide for privacy.

### PROCEDURE

7 Clean the earpieces and diaphragm with the wipes.
8 Have the person sit or lie down.
9 Expose the nipple area of the left chest. Do not expose a woman's breasts.
10 Warm the diaphragm in your palm.
11 Place the earpieces in your ears.
12 Find the apical pulse. Place the diaphragm 2 to 3 inches to the left of the breastbone and below the left nipple (see Fig. 21-23).
13 Count the pulse for 1 minute. Note if it is regular or irregular.
14 Cover the person. Remove the earpieces.
15 Record the person's name and pulse on your note pad or assignment sheet. Note if the pulse was regular or irregular.

### POST-PROCEDURE

16 Provide for comfort.
17 Place the signal light within reach.
18 Unscreen the person.
19 Clean the earpieces and diaphragm with the wipes.
20 Return the stethoscope to its proper place.
21 Decontaminate your hands.
22 Report and record your observations. Record the pulse rate with *Ap* for apical pulse.

# TAKING AN APICAL-RADIAL PULSE

The apical and radial pulse rates should be equal. Sometimes heart contractions are not strong enough to create pulses in the radial artery. Then the radial pulse rate is less than the apical pulse rate. This may occur in people with heart disease.

To see if the apical and radial rates are equal, two staff members are needed. One takes the radial pulse; the other takes the apical pulse. Taking the apical and radial pulses at the same time is called the **apical-radial pulse**. The **pulse deficit** is the difference between the apical and radial pulse rates. To obtain the pulse deficit, subtract the radial rate from the apical rate. The apical pulse rate is never less than the radial pulse rate.

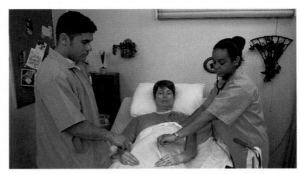

**FIG. 21-24** Taking an apical-radial pulse. One worker takes the apical pulse. The other takes the radial pulse.

## TAKING AN APICAL-RADIAL PULSE

### QUALITY OF LIFE

Remember to:
- Knock before entering the person's room
- Address the person by name
- Introduce yourself by name and title

### PRE-PROCEDURE

1 Follow *Delegation Guidelines: Taking Pulses*, p. 471. See *Safety Alert: Stethoscopes*, p. 469, and *Safety Alert: Taking Pulses*, p. 471.
2 Ask a nurse or a nursing assistant to help you.
3 Collect a stethoscope and antiseptic wipes.
4 Practice hand hygiene.
5 Identify the person. Check the ID bracelet against the assignment sheet. Call the person by name.
6 Explain the procedure to the person.
7 Provide for privacy.

### PROCEDURE

8 Wipe the earpieces and diaphragm with the wipes.
9 Have the person sit or lie down.
10 Warm the diaphragm in your palm.
11 Expose the left nipple area of the chest. Do not expose a woman's breasts.
12 Place the earpieces in your ears.
13 Find the apical pulse. Your helper finds the radial pulse (Fig. 21-24).
14 Give the signal to begin counting.
15 Count the pulse for 1 minute.
16 Give the signal to stop counting.
17 Cover the person. Remove the earpieces.
18 Record the person's name and the apical and radial pulses on your note pad or assignment sheet. Subtract the radial pulse from the apical pulse for the pulse deficit. Note whether the pulse was regular or irregular.

### POST-PROCEDURE

19 Provide for comfort.
20 Place the signal light within reach.
21 Unscreen the person.
22 Clean the earpieces and diaphragm with the wipes.
23 Return the stethoscope to its proper place.
24 Decontaminate your hands.
25 Report and record your observations. Include:
- The apical and radial pulse rates
- The pulse deficit

# RESPIRATIONS

**Respiration** means breathing air into (inhalation) and out of (exhalation) the lungs. Oxygen enters the lungs during inhalation. Carbon dioxide leaves the lungs during exhalation. Each respiration involves one inhalation and one exhalation. The chest rises during inhalation. It falls during exhalation. See Box 21-2 for a review of the respiratory system.

The healthy adult has 12 to 20 respirations per minute. The respiratory rate is affected by the factors that affect temperature and pulse. Heart and respiratory diseases usually increase the respiratory rate.

Respirations are normally quiet, effortless, and regular. Both sides of the chest rise and fall equally. See Chapter 30 for abnormal respiratory patterns.

Count respirations when the person is at rest. Position the person so you can see the chest rise and fall. To a certain extent, a person can control the depth and rate of breathing. People tend to change breathing patterns when they know their respirations are being counted. Therefore the person should not know that you are counting them.

Respirations are counted right after taking a pulse. Keep your fingers or stethoscope over the pulse site. (The person assumes you are taking the pulse.) To count respirations, watch the chest rise and fall. Count them for 30 seconds. Multiply the number by 2 for the number of respirations in 1 minute. If an abnormal pattern is noted, count the respirations for 1 minute. *See Focus on Children: Respirations.*

| TABLE 21-3 | NORMAL RESPIRATORY RATES FOR CHILDREN |
|---|---|
| **Age** | **Respirations per Minute** |
| Newborn | 35 |
| 1 year | 30 |
| 2 years | 25 |
| 4 years | 23 |
| 6 years | 21 |
| 8 years | 20 |
| 10 years | 19 |
| 12 years | 19 |
| 14 years | 18 |
| 16 years | 17 |
| 18 years | 16-18 |

From Hockenberry MJ and others: *Wong's nursing care of infants and children*, ed 7, St Louis, 2003, Mosby.

**DELEGATION GUIDELINES:** *Counting Respirations*

Before counting respirations, you need this information from the nurse and the care plan:

- How long to count respirations—30 seconds or 1 minute
- When to count respirations
- What other vital signs to measure
- What observations to report and record:
  —The respiratory rate
  —Equality and depth of respirations
  —If the respirations were regular or irregular
  —If the person has pain or difficulty in breathing
  —Any respiratory noises
  —Any abnormal respiratory patterns (Chapter 30)

---

**FOCUS ON CHILDREN**
RESPIRATIONS

Infants and children have higher respiratory rates than adults (Table 21-3). Count an infant's respirations for 1 minute.

---

**BOX 21-2 STRUCTURE AND FUNCTION OF THE RESPIRATORY SYSTEM**

Oxygen is needed for life. Every cell needs oxygen. The respiratory system (Fig. 21-25) brings oxygen into the lungs and rids the body of carbon dioxide. *Respiration* is the process of supplying the cells with oxygen and removing carbon dioxide from them. Respiration involves *inhalation* (breathing in) and *exhalation* (breathing out). The terms *inspiration* (breathing in) and *expiration* (breathing out) are also used.

Air enters the body through the *nose*. The air then passes into the *pharynx* (throat), a tube-shaped passageway for both air and food. Air passes from the pharynx into the *larynx* (the voice box). Air passes from the larynx into the *trachea* (the windpipe). The trachea divides at its lower end into the *right bronchus* and *left bronchus*. Each bronchus enters a lung.

On entering the lungs, the bronchi divide many times into smaller branches called *bronchioles*. Eventually the bronchioles further divide. They end in tiny one-celled air sacs called *alveoli*. They are supplied by capillaries.

Oxygen and carbon dioxide are exchanged between the alveoli and capillaries. Blood in the capillaries picks up oxygen from the alveoli. Then the blood returns to the left side of the heart and is pumped to the rest of the body. Alveoli pick up carbon dioxide from the capillaries for exhalation.

Each lung is divided into lobes. The right lung has three lobes; the left lung has two. The lungs are separated from the abdominal cavity by a muscle called the *diaphragm*. A bony framework made up of the ribs, sternum, and vertebrae protects the lungs.

## COUNTING RESPIRATIONS

### PROCEDURE

1 Follow *Delegation Guidelines: Counting Respirations.*
2 Keep your fingers or the stethoscope over the pulse site.
3 Do not tell the person you are counting respirations.
4 Begin counting when the chest rises. Count each rise and fall of the chest as one respiration.
5 Note the following:
   ▪ If respirations are regular
   ▪ If both sides of the chest rise equally
   ▪ The depth of respirations
   ▪ If the person has any pain or difficulty breathing
6 Count respirations for 30 seconds. Multiply the number by 2. (The NNAAP™ skills evaluation requires counting respirations for 1 minute.)
7 Count respirations for 1 minute if they are abnormal or irregular.
8 Record the person's name, respiratory rate, and other observations on your note pad or assignment sheet.

### POST-PROCEDURE

9 Provide for comfort.
10 Place the signal light within reach.
11 Decontaminate your hands.
12 Report and record your observations.

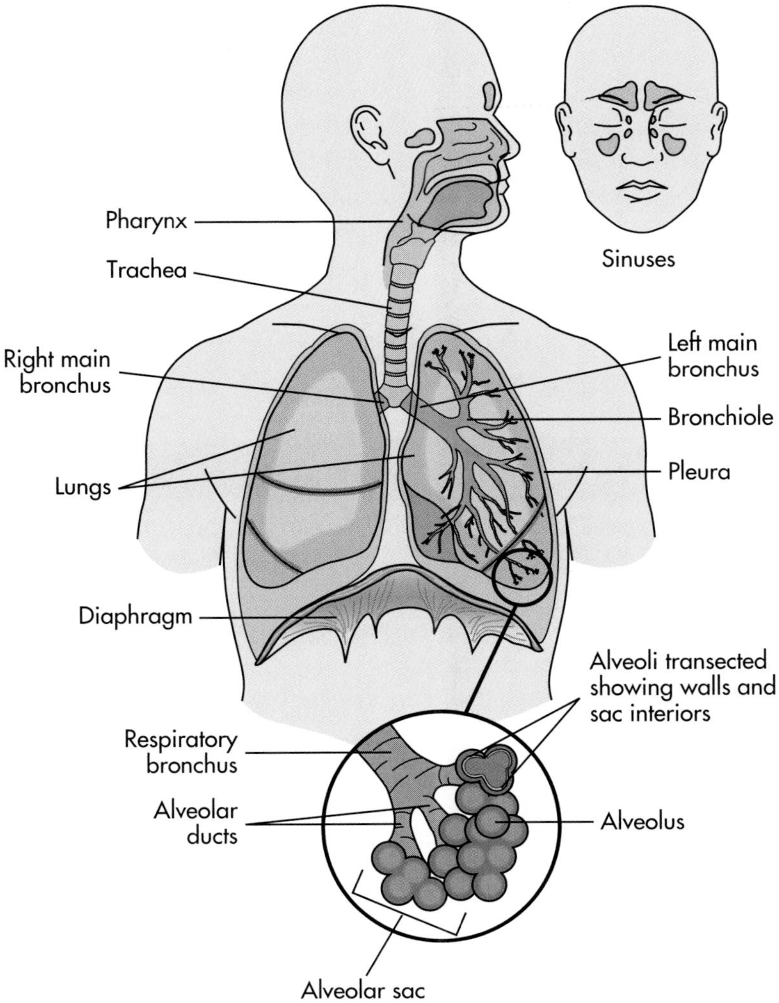

**FIG. 21-25** The respiratory system.

# BLOOD PRESSURE

**Blood pressure** is the amount of force exerted against the walls of an artery by the blood. Blood pressure is controlled by:

- The force of heart contractions
- The amount of blood pumped with each heartbeat
- How easily the blood flows through the blood vessels

The period of heart muscle contraction is called **systole.** The heart is pumping blood. The period of heart muscle relaxation is called **diastole.** The heart is at rest.

Systolic and diastolic pressures are measured. The **systolic pressure** represents the amount of force needed to pump blood out of the heart into the arterial circulation. It is the higher pressure. The **diastolic pressure** reflects the pressure in the arteries when the heart is at rest. It is the lower pressure.

Blood pressure is measured in millimeters (mm) of mercury (Hg). The systolic pressure is recorded over the diastolic pressure. A systolic pressure of 120 mm Hg and a diastolic pressure of 80 mm Hg is written as 120/80 mm Hg.

## NORMAL AND ABNORMAL BLOOD PRESSURES

Blood pressure can change from minute to minute. Factors affecting blood pressure are listed in Box 21-3.

Because it can vary so easily, blood pressure has normal ranges:

- *Systolic pressure*—less than 120 mm Hg
- *Diastolic pressure*—less than 80 mm Hg

Treatment is indicated for measurements that remain above *(hyper)* a systolic pressure of 140 mm Hg or a diastolic pressure of 90 mm Hg. This condition is known as **hypertension.** Report any systolic pressure above 120 mm Hg. A diastolic pressure above 80 mm Hg also is reported. Likewise, systolic pressures below *(hypo)* 90 mm Hg and diastolic pressures below 60 mm Hg are reported. This is called **hypotension.** Some people normally have low blood pressures. However, hypotension may signal a life-threatening problem. *See Focus on Children: Normal and Abnormal Blood Pressures. See Focus on Older Persons: Normal and Abnormal Blood Pressures.*

---

### FOCUS ON CHILDREN
#### NORMAL AND ABNORMAL BLOOD PRESSURES

Infants and children have lower blood pressures than adults. A newborn's blood pressure is usually about 70/55 mm Hg. At 1 year, it increases to 90/55 mm Hg. Blood pressure continues to increase as the child grows older. Adult levels are reached between 14 and 18 years of age.

---

### BOX 21-3 FACTORS AFFECTING BLOOD PRESSURE

- *Age.* Blood pressure increases with age. It is lowest in infancy and childhood. It is highest in adulthood.
- *Gender (male or female).* Women usually have lower blood pressures than men do. Blood pressures rise in women after menopause.
- *Blood volume.* This is the amount of blood in the system. Severe bleeding lowers the blood volume. Therefore the blood pressure lowers. Giving IV fluids rapidly increases the blood volume. The blood pressure rises.
- *Stress.* Stress includes anxiety, fear, and emotions. Blood pressure increases as the body responds to stress.
- *Pain.* Pain generally increases blood pressure. However, severe pain can cause shock. Blood pressure is seriously low in the state of shock (Chapter 40).
- *Exercise.* Blood pressure increases. Do not measure blood pressure right after exercise.
- *Weight.* Blood pressure is higher in overweight persons. It lowers with weight loss.
- *Race.* Black persons generally have higher blood pressures than white persons do.
- *Diet.* A high-sodium diet increases the amount of water in the body. The extra fluid volume increases blood pressure.
- *Drugs.* Drugs can be given to raise or lower blood pressure. Other drugs have the side effects of high or low blood pressure.
- *Position.* Blood pressure is lower when lying down. It is higher in the standing position. Sudden changes in position can cause a sudden drop in blood pressure (orthostatic hypotension). When standing suddenly, the person may have a sudden drop in blood pressure. Dizziness and fainting can occur. See Chapter 22.
- *Smoking.* Blood pressure increases. Nicotine in cigarettes causes blood vessels to narrow. The heart must work harder to pump blood through narrowed vessels.
- *Alcohol.* Excessive alcohol intake can raise blood pressure.

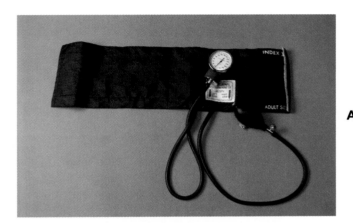

## EQUIPMENT

A stethoscope and a sphygmomanometer are used to measure blood pressure. The **sphygmomanometer** has a cuff and a measuring device. There are three types of sphygmomanometers:

- The *aneroid type* has a round dial and a needle that points to the numbers (Fig. 21-26, *A*).
- The *mercury* type is more accurate than the aneroid type. It has a column of mercury within a calibrated tube (Fig. 21-26, *B*).
- The *electronic* type shows the systolic and diastolic blood pressures on the front of the device (Fig. 21-26, *C*). It also shows the pulse rate. Follow the manufacturer's instructions.

The blood pressure cuff is wrapped around the upper arm. Tubing connects the cuff to the manometer. Another tube connects the cuff to a small, hand-held bulb. A valve on the bulb is turned so the cuff inflates as the bulb is squeezed. The inflated cuff causes pressure over the brachial artery. The valve is turned the other way for cuff deflation. Blood pressure is measured as the cuff is deflated.

Sounds are produced as blood flows through the arteries. The stethoscope is used to listen to the sounds in the brachial artery as the cuff is deflated. Stethoscopes are not needed with electronic manometers. *See Focus on Children: Equipment.*

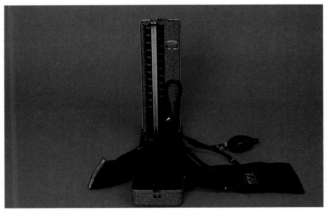

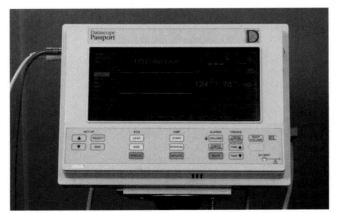

> SAFETY ALERT: *Equipment*
> Mercury is a hazardous substance. Handle mercury manometers carefully. If one breaks, call for the nurse at once. Do not touch the mercury. Do not let the person touch it. The agency must follow special procedures for handling all hazardous substances. See Chapter 10.

**FIG. 21-26** Blood pressure equipment. **A,** Aneroid manometer and cuff. **B,** Mercury manometer and cuff. **C,** Electronic sphygmomanometer.

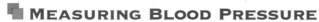

## ◼ MEASURING BLOOD PRESSURE

Blood pressure is normally measured in the brachial artery. Box 21-4 lists the guidelines for measuring blood pressure.

---

**DELEGATION GUIDELINES:** *Measuring Blood Pressure*

Before measuring blood pressure, you need this information from the nurse and the care plan:
- When to measure blood pressure
- If the person has an arm IV infusion, a cast, or dialysis access site
- If the person had breast surgery, what side was the surgery done on
- If the person needs to be lying down, sitting, or standing
- What size cuff to use—regular, pediatric, or extra-large
- What observations to report and record

---

**BOX 21-4** **GUIDELINES FOR MEASURING BLOOD PRESSURE**

- Do not take blood pressure on an arm with an IV infusion, a cast, or a dialysis access site. If a person had breast surgery, do not take blood pressure on that side. Avoid taking blood pressure on an injured arm.
- Let the person rest for 10 to 20 minutes before measuring blood pressure.
- Measure blood pressure with the person sitting or lying. Sometimes the doctor orders blood pressure measured in the standing position.
- Apply the cuff to the bare upper arm. Clothing can affect the measurement.
- Make sure the cuff is snug. Loose cuffs can cause inaccurate readings.
- Use a larger cuff if the person is obese or has a large arm. Ask the nurse what size to use.
- Place the diaphragm of the stethoscope firmly over the brachial artery. The entire diaphragm must have contact with the skin.

- Make sure the room is quiet. Talking, TV, radio, and sounds from the hallway can affect an accurate measurement.
- Have the sphygmomanometer where you can clearly see it.
- Measure the systolic and diastolic pressures. Expect to hear the first blood pressure sound at the point where you felt the radial or brachial pulse. The first sound is the systolic pressure. The point where the sound disappears is the diastolic pressure.
- Take the blood pressure again if you are not sure of an accurate measurement. Wait 30 to 60 seconds before repeating the measurement.
- Tell the nurse at once if you cannot hear the blood pressure.

# MEASURING BLOOD PRESSURE

NNAAP™

## QUALITY OF LIFE

Remember to:
- Knock before entering the person's room
- Address the person by name
- Introduce yourself by name and title

## PRE-PROCEDURE

1 Follow *Delegation Guidelines: Measuring Blood Pressure*. See *Safety Alert: Stethoscopes*, p. 469 *and Safety Alert: Equipment*, p. 477.
2 Collect the following:
- Sphygmomanometer
- Stethoscope
- Antiseptic wipes
3 Practice hand hygiene.
4 Identify the person. Check the ID bracelet against the assignment sheet. Call the person by name.
5 Explain the procedure to the person.
6 Provide for privacy.

## PROCEDURE

7 Wipe the stethoscope earpieces and diaphragm with the wipes.
8 Have the person sit or lie down.
9 Position the person's arm level with the heart. The palm is up.
10 Stand no more than 3 feet away from the manometer. A mercury model is vertical, on a flat surface, and at eye level. The aneroid type is directly in front of you.
11 Expose the upper arm.
12 Squeeze the cuff to expel any remaining air. Close the valve on the bulb.
13 Find the brachial artery at the inner aspect of the elbow.
14 Place the arrow on the cuff over the brachial artery (Fig. 21-27, *A*, p. 480). Wrap the cuff around the upper arm at least 1 inch above the elbow. It is even and snug.
15 *Method 1:*
  a Place the stethoscope earpieces in your ears.
  b Find the radial or brachial artery.
  c Inflate the cuff until you can no longer feel the pulse. Note this point.
  d Inflate the cuff 30 mm Hg beyond the point where you last felt the pulse.
16 *Method 2:*
  a Find the radial or brachial artery.

  b Inflate the cuff until you can no longer feel the pulse. Note this point.
  c Inflate the cuff 30 mm Hg beyond the point where you last felt the pulse.
  d Deflate the cuff slowly. Note the point when you feel the pulse.
  e Wait 30 seconds.
  f Place the stethoscope earpieces in your ears.
  g Inflate the cuff 30 mm Hg beyond the point where you felt the pulse return.
17 Place the diaphragm over the brachial artery (Fig. 21-27, *B*). Do not place it under the cuff.
18 Deflate the cuff at an even rate of 2 to 4 millimeters per second. Turn the valve counterclockwise to deflate the cuff.
19 Note the point where you hear the first sound. This is the systolic reading. It is near the point where the radial pulse or brachial disappeared.
20 Continue to deflate the cuff. Note the point where the sound disappears. This is the diastolic reading.
21 Deflate the cuff completely. Remove it from the person's arm. Remove the stethoscope.
22 Record the person's name and blood pressure on your note pad or assignment sheet.
23 Return the cuff to the case or wall holder.

## POST-PROCEDURE

24 Provide for comfort.
25 Place the signal light within reach.
26 Unscreen the person.
27 Clean the earpieces and diaphragm with the wipes.
28 Return the equipment to its proper place.
29 Decontaminate your hands.
30 Report and record the blood pressure (Fig. 21-28, p. 480).

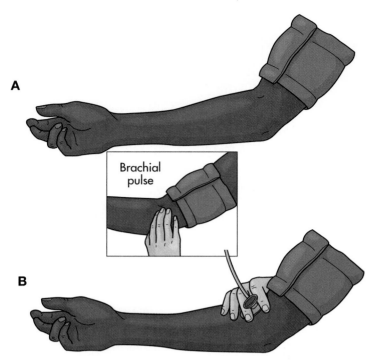

**FIG. 21-27** Measuring blood pressure. **A,** The cuff is over the brachial artery. **B,** The diaphragm of the stethoscope is over the brachial artery.

| Date | Time | Weight | T | P | R | BP | | | | Signatures |
|------|------|--------|------|----|----|--------|--|--|--|------------|
| 10/19 | 0700 | 126 | 98.4 | 72 | 20 | 142/84 | | | | Mary Smith CNA |
| 10/26 | 0715 | 125 | 98.6 | 72 | 18 | 140/84 | | | | Jane Doe CNA |
| 11/2 | 0715 | 126 | 98.6 | 70 | 18 | 144/82 | | | | Mary Smith CNA |
| | | | | | | | | | | |
| | | | | | | | | | | |
| | | | | | | | | | | |
| | | | | | | | | | | |

**FIG. 21-28** Charting sample.

# ■ REVIEW QUESTIONS ■

Circle the **BEST** answer.

1 Which statement is *false?*
  a The vital signs are temperature, pulse, respirations, and blood pressure.
  b Vital signs detect changes in body function.
  c Vital signs change only during illness.
  d Sleep, exercise, drugs, emotions, and noise affect vital signs.

2 Which should you report at once?
  a An oral temperature of 98.4° F
  b A rectal temperature of 101.6° F
  c An axillary temperature of 97.6° F
  d An oral temperature of 99.0° F

3 A rectal temperature is *not* taken when the person
  a Is unconscious
  b Is an infant
  c Has a nasogastric tube
  d Has diarrhea

4 Which gives the *least* accurate measurement of body temperature?
  a Oral site
  b Rectal site
  c Axillary site
  d Tympanic site

5 Which is usually used to take a pulse?
  a The radial pulse
  b The apical-radial pulse
  c The apical pulse
  d The brachial pulse

6 Which is reported to the nurse at once?
  a An adult has a pulse of 120 beats per minute.
  b An infant has a pulse of 130 beats per minute.
  c An adult has a pulse of 80 beats per minute.
  d An adult has a pulse of 64 beats per minute.

7 Which statement about the apical-radial pulse is *true?*
  a It is taken by one person.
  b The radial pulse can be greater than the apical pulse.
  c The apical pulse can be greater than the radial pulse.
  d The apical and radial pulses are always equal.

8 The following describe normal respirations *except*
  a There are 12 to 20 per minute.
  b They are quiet and effortless
  c They are regular with both sides of the chest rising and falling equally
  d The person breathes through the mouth

9 Respirations are usually counted
  a After taking the temperature
  b After taking the pulse
  c Before taking the pulse
  d After taking the blood pressure

10 Which blood pressure is normal for an adult?
  a 88/54 mm Hg
  b 210/100 mm Hg
  c 112/78 mm Hg
  d 152/90 mm Hg

11 When taking a blood pressure, you should do the following *except*
  a Take the blood pressure in the arm with an IV infusion
  b Apply the cuff to a bare upper arm
  c Turn off the TV and radio
  d Locate the brachial artery

12 Which is the systolic blood pressure?
  a The point where the pulse is no longer felt
  b The point where the first sound is heard
  c The point where the last sound is heard
  d The point 30 mm Hg above where the pulse was felt

*Answers to these questions are on p. 818.*

# Exercise and Activity

# OBJECTIVES

- Define the key terms listed in this chapter
- Describe bedrest
- Explain how to prevent the complications of bedrest
- Describe the devices used to support and maintain body alignment
- Explain the purpose of a trapeze
- Describe range-of-motion exercises
- Explain how to help a falling person
- Describe four walking aids
- Perform the procedures described in this chapter

# KEY TERMS

**abduction** Moving a body part away from the midline of the body

**adduction** Moving a body part toward the midline of the body

**ambulation** The act of walking

**atrophy** The decrease in size or a wasting away of tissue

**contracture** The lack of joint mobility caused by abnormal shortening of a muscle

**dorsiflexion** Bending the toes and foot up at the ankle

**extension** Straightening a body part

**external rotation** Turning the joint outward

**flexion** Bending a body part

**footdrop** The foot falls down at the ankle; permanent plantar flexion

**hyperextension** Excessive straightening of a body part

**internal rotation** Turning the joint inward

**orthostatic hypotension** Abnormally low (*hypo*) blood pressure when the person suddenly stands up (*ortho* and *static*); postural hypotension

**plantar flexion** The foot (*plantar*) is bent (*flexion*); bending the foot down at the ankle

**postural hypotension** Orthostatic hypotension

**pronation** Turning the joint downward

**range of motion (ROM)** The movement of a joint to the extent possible without causing pain

**rotation** Turning the joint

**supination** Turning the joint upward

**syncope** A brief loss of consciousness; fainting

---

Being active is important for physical and mental well-being. Most people move about and function without help. Illness, surgery, injury, pain, and aging cause weakness and some activity limits. Some people are in bed for a long time. Some are paralyzed. Some disorders worsen over time. They cause decreases in activity. Examples include arthritis and nervous system and muscular disorders (Chapter 33). Inactivity, whether mild or severe, affects every body system. It also affects mental well-being.

Nurses use the nursing process to promote exercise and activity in all persons to the extent possible. The nursing care plan includes the person's activity level and needed exercises. To help promote exercise and activity, you need to understand:
- Bedrest
- How to prevent complications from bedrest
- How to help with exercise

## BEDREST

The doctor orders bedrest to treat a health problem. Sometimes it is a nursing measure if the person's condition changes. Generally bedrest is ordered to:

- Reduce physical activity
- Reduce pain
- Encourage rest
- Regain strength
- Promote healing

These types of bedrest are common:

- *Bedrest.* Some activities of daily living (ADL) are allowed. Self-feeding, oral hygiene, bathing, shaving, and hair care are often allowed.
- *Strict bedrest.* Everything is done for the person. No ADL are allowed.
- *Bedrest with commode privileges.* The person uses the commode for elimination.
- *Bedrest with bathroom privileges (bedrest with BRP).* The person can use the bathroom for elimination.

The person's care plan and your assignment sheet tell you the activities allowed for each person. Always ask the nurse what bedrest means for each person. Check with the nurse if you have questions about the person's activity limits.

## COMPLICATIONS OF BEDREST

Bedrest and lack of exercise and activity can cause serious complications. Every system is affected. Pressure ulcers, constipation, and fecal impaction can result. Urinary tract infections and renal calculi (kidney stones) can occur. So can blood clots (thrombi) and pneumonia (infection of the lung).

The musculoskeletal system is affected by lack of exercise and activity. A **contracture** is the lack of joint mobility caused by abnormal shortening of a muscle. The contracted muscle is fixed into position, is deformed, and cannot stretch (Fig. 22-1). Common sites are the fingers, wrists, elbows, toes, ankles, knees, and hips. They can also occur in the neck and spine. The person is permanently deformed and disabled. **Atrophy** is the decrease in size or the wasting away of tissue. Tissues shrink in size. Muscle atrophy is a decrease in size or a wasting away of muscle (Fig. 22-2). These complications must be prevented to maintain normal movement.

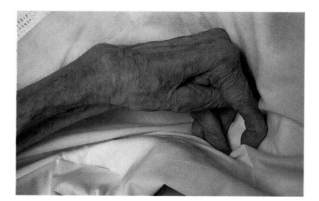

**FIG. 22-1** A contracture.

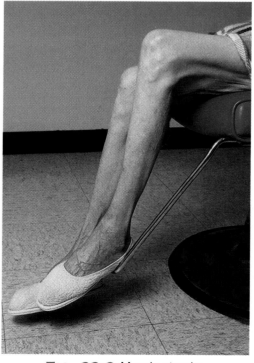

**FIG. 22-2** Muscle atrophy.

Orthostatic hypotension and blood clots (Chapter 27) occur in the cardiovascular system. **Orthostatic hypotension** is abnormally low *(hypo)* blood pressure when the person suddenly stands up *(ortho* and *static)*. When a person moves from lying or sitting to a standing position, the blood pressure drops. The person is dizzy and weak and has spots before the eyes. Syncope can occur. **Syncope** (fainting) is a brief loss of consciousness. (Syncope comes from the Greek word synkoptein. It means to cut short.) Orthostatic hypotension also is called **postural hypotension.** *(Postural* relates to posture or standing.) Box 22-1 lists the measures that prevent orthostatic hypotension. Slowly changing positions is key.

Good nursing care prevents complications from bedrest. Good alignment, range-of-motion exercises, and frequent position changes are important measures. These are part of the care plan.

## POSITIONING

Body alignment and positioning were discussed in Chapter 13. Supportive devices are often used to support and maintain the person in a certain position:

- *Bed boards*—are placed under the mattress. They prevent the mattress from sagging (Fig. 22-3). Usually made of plywood, they are covered with canvas or other material. There are two sections so the head of the bed can be raised. One section is for the head of the bed. The other is for the foot of the bed.
- *Foot boards*—are placed at the foot of mattresses (Fig. 22-4). They prevent plantar flexion that can lead to footdrop. In **plantar flexion,** the foot *(plantar)* is bent *(flexion)*. **Footdrop** is when the foot falls down at the ankle (permanent plantar flexion). The foot board is placed so the soles of the feet are flush against it. The feet are in good alignment as when standing. Foot boards also serve as bed cradles. They prevent pressure ulcers by keeping the top linens off the feet and toes.

| BOX 22-1 | PREVENTING ORTHOSTATIC HYPOTENSION |
|---|---|

- Measure blood pressure, pulse, and respirations with the person supine.
- Position the person in Fowler's position. Raise the head of the bed slowly.
  —Ask the person about weakness, dizziness, or spots before the eyes. Lower the head of the bed if symptoms occur.
  —Measure blood pressure, pulse, and respirations.
  —Keep the person in Fowler's position for a short while. Ask about weakness, dizziness, or spots before the eyes.
- Help the person sit on the side of the bed (Chapter 13).
  —Ask about weakness, dizziness, or spots before the eyes. Help the person to Fowler's position if symptoms occur.
  —Measure blood pressure, pulse, and respirations.
  —Have the person sit on the side of the bed for a short while.
- Help the person stand.
  —Ask about weakness, dizziness, or spots before the eyes. Help the person sit on the side of the bed if any symptoms occur.
  —Measure blood pressure, pulse, and respirations.
- Help the person sit in a chair or walk as directed by the nurse.
  —Ask about weakness, dizziness, or spots before the eyes. If the person is walking, help the person to sit if symptoms occur.
  —Measure blood pressure, pulse, and respirations.
- Report blood pressure, pulse, and respirations to the nurse. Also report other symptoms.

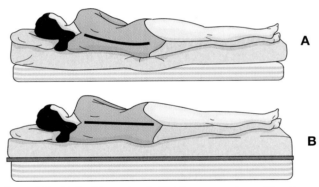

**FIG. 22-3** Bed boards. **A,** Mattress sagging without bed boards. **B,** Bed boards are under mattress. No sagging occurs.

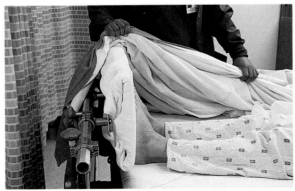

**FIG. 22-4** A foot board. Feet are flush with the board to keep them in normal alignment.

- *Trochanter rolls*—prevent the hips and legs from turning outward (external rotation) (Fig. 22-5). A bath blanket is folded to the desired length and rolled up. The loose end is placed under the person from the hip to the knee. Then the roll is tucked alongside the body. Pillows or sandbags also keep the hips and knees in alignment.
- *Hip abduction wedges*—keep the hips abducted (Fig. 22-6). The wedge is placed between the person's legs. These are common after hip replacement surgery.
- *Hand rolls or hand grips*—prevent contractures of the thumb, fingers, and wrist (Fig. 22-7). Foam rubber sponges, rubber balls, and finger cushions (Fig. 22-8) also are used.
- *Splints*—keep the elbows, wrists, thumbs, fingers, ankles, and knees in normal position. They are usually secured in place with Velcro. Some have foam padding (Fig. 22-9).
- *Bed cradles*—keep the weight of top linens off the feet and toes (Fig. 22-10). The weight of top linens can cause footdrop and pressure ulcers.

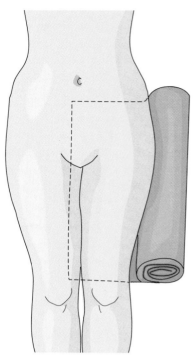

**FIG. 22-5** A trochanter roll is made from a bath blanket. It extends from the hip to the knee.

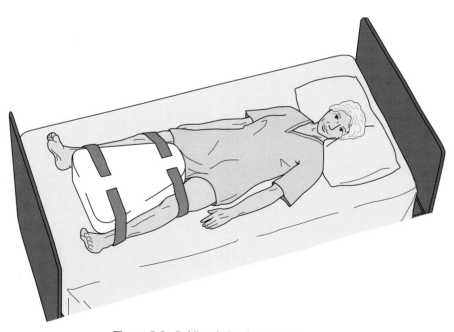

**FIG. 22-6** Hip abduction wedge.

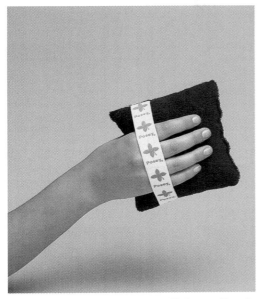

FIG. 22-7 Hand grip. (Courtesy J. T. Posey Co., Arcadia, Calif.)

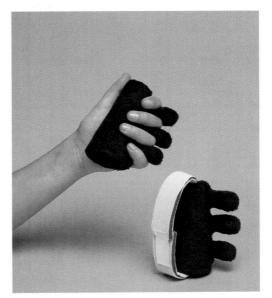

FIG. 22-8 Finger cushion. (Courtesy J. T. Posey Co., Arcadia, Calif.)

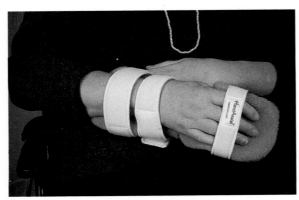

FIG. 22-9 A splint.

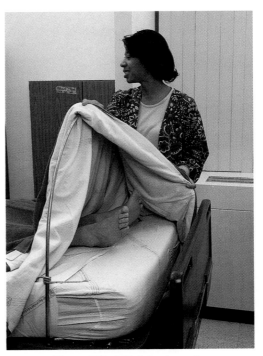

FIG. 22-10 A bed cradle.

## EXERCISE

Exercise helps prevent contractures, muscle atrophy, and other complications of bedrest. Some exercise occurs with ADL and when turning and moving in bed without help. Other exercises are needed for muscles and joints. (See "Range-of-Motion Exercises" and "Ambulation," p. 494.)

A trapeze is used for exercises to strengthen arm muscles. The trapeze hangs from an overbed frame (Fig. 22-11). The person grasps the bar with both hands to lift the trunk off the bed. The trapeze is also used to move up and turn in bed.

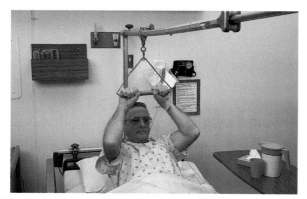

**FIG. 22-11** A trapeze is used to strengthen arm muscles.

## RANGE-OF-MOTION EXERCISES

The movement of a joint to the extent possible without causing pain is the **range of motion (ROM)** of that joint. Range-of-motion exercises involve moving the joints through their complete range of motion (Box 22-2). They are usually done at least 2 times a day.

- *Active* range-of-motion exercises—are done by the person.
- *Passive* range-of-motion exercises—someone moves the joints through their range of motion.
- *Active-assistive* range-of-motion exercises—the person does the exercises with some help.

Bathing, hair care, eating, reaching, and walking all involve joint movements. Persons on bedrest need more frequent range-of-motion exercises. So do those who cannot walk, turn, or transfer themselves because of illness or injury. The doctor or nurse may order range-of-motion exercises.

*See Focus on Children: Range-of-Motion Exercises. See Focus on Long-Term Care: Range-of-Motion Exercises.*

*Text continued on p. 494.*

---

### BOX 22-2   JOINT MOVEMENTS

**Abduction**—moving a body part away from the midline of the body
**Adduction**—moving a body part toward the midline of the body
**Extension**—straightening a body part
**Flexion**—bending a body part
**Hyperextension**—excessive straightening of a body part
**Dorsiflexion**—bending the toes and foot up at the ankle
**Rotation**—turning the joint
**Internal rotation**—turning the joint inward
**External rotation**—turning the joint outward
**Plantar flexion**—bending the foot down at the ankle
**Pronation**—turning the joint downward
**Supination**—turning the joint upward

---

### FOCUS ON CHILDREN
#### RANGE-OF-MOTION EXERCISES

Depending on the child's activity limits, most play activities promote active range-of-motion exercises. For example:
- Kicking a Mylar balloon or foam ball
- Playing "pat-a-cake"
- Having the child clap, kick, jump, or do other motions
- Playing basketball using a wastebasket and a foam ball or wadded paper
- Playing video games for finger and hand movements
- Playing with finger paints, clay, or play dough
- Having tricycle or wheelchair races
- Playing "hide and seek" by hiding a toy in the bed or room

Always check with the nurse for the child's activity limits.

Modified from Wong DL and others: *Whaley & Wong's nursing care of infants and children*, ed 6, St Louis, 1999, Mosby.

**DELEGATION GUIDELINES:** *Range-of-Motion Exercises*

When delegated range-of-motion exercises, you need this information from the nurse and the care plan:

- The kind of range-of-motion exercises ordered—active, passive, active-assistive
- Which joints to exercise
- How often the exercises are done
- How many times to repeat each exercise
- What to report and record:
  —The time the exercises were performed
  —The joints exercised
  —The number of times the exercises were performed on each joint
  —Complaints of pain or signs of stiffness or spasm
  —The degree to which the person took part in the exercises

**SAFETY ALERT:** *Range-of-Motion Exercises*

Range-of-motion exercises can cause injury if not done properly. Muscle strain, joint injury, and pain are possible. Practice the rules in Box 22-3 when performing or assisting with range-of-motion exercises.

Range-of-motion exercises to the neck can cause serious injury if not done properly. Some agencies require that nursing assistants have special training before doing such exercises. Other agencies do not let nursing assistants do them. Know your agency's policy. Perform range-of-motion exercises to the neck only if allowed by your agency and if the nurse instructs you to do so.

---

### FOCUS ON LONG-TERM CARE
#### RANGE-OF-MOTION EXERCISES

OBRA requires an assessment and care planning process to prevent unnecessary loss in a resident's range of motion. Prevention may involve range-of-motion exercises. Sometimes splints and braces are used (p. 503).

OBRA also requires activity programs for residents. Recreational activities promote physical and mental well-being in older persons. Joints and muscles are exercised. Circulation is stimulated. Recreational activities also are social events and are mentally stimulating.

Activities must meet each person's interests and physical, mental, and psychosocial needs. Bingo, movies, dances, exercise groups, shopping trips, museum trips, concerts, and guest speakers are common. Some centers have gardening activities.

The right to personal choice is protected. The person chooses which activities to take part in. Well-being is promoted when the person attends activities of personal choice. The person is not forced to do things that do not interest him or her.

Residents may need help getting to an activity. Some also need help taking part in them. You must assist as needed.

---

**BOX 22-3** | **PERFORMING RANGE-OF-MOTION EXERCISES**

- Exercise only the joints the nurse tells you to exercise.
- Expose only the body part being exercised.
- Use good body mechanics.
- Support the part being exercised.
- Move the joint slowly, smoothly, and gently.
- Do not force a joint beyond its present range of motion or to the point of pain.
- *Perform range-of-motion exercises to the neck only if allowed by agency policy.* In some agencies, only physical or occupational therapists do neck exercises. This is because of the danger of neck injuries.

## PERFORMING RANGE-OF-MOTION EXERCISES

NNAAP™

### QUALITY OF LIFE

Remember to:
- Knock before entering the person's room
- Address the person by name
- Introduce yourself by name and title

### PRE-PROCEDURE

1 Follow *Delegation Guidelines: Range-of-Motion Exercises*, p. 489. See *Safety Alert: Range-of-Motion Exercises*, p. 489.
2 Identify the person. Check the ID bracelet against the assignment sheet. Call the person by name.
3 Explain the procedure to the person.

4 Practice hand hygiene.
5 Obtain a bath blanket.
6 Provide for privacy.
7 Raise the bed for body mechanics. Bed rails are up if used.

### PROCEDURE

8 Lower the bed rail near you if up.
9 Position the person supine.
10 Cover the person with a bath blanket. Fanfold top linens to the foot of the bed.
11 Exercise the neck *if allowed by your agency and if the RN instructs you to do so* (Fig. 22-12):
  a Place your hands over the person's ears to support the head. Support the jaws with your fingers.
  b Flexion—bring the head forward. The chin touches the chest.
  c Extension—straighten the head.
  d Hyperextension—bring the head backward until the chin points up.
  e Rotation—turn the head from side to side.
  f Lateral flexion—move the head to the right and to the left.
  g Repeat flexion, extension, hyperextension, rotation, and lateral flexion 5 times—or the number of times stated on the care plan.
12 Exercise the shoulder (Fig. 22-13, p. 492):
  a Grasp the wrist with one hand. Grasp the elbow with the other hand.
  b Flexion—raise the arm straight in front and over the head.
  c Extension—bring the arm down to the side.
  d Hyperextension—move the arm behind the body. (Do this if the person sits in a straight-backed chair or is standing.)
  e Abduction—move the straight arm away from the side of the body.
  f Adduction—move the straight arm to the side of the body.
  g Internal rotation—bend the elbow. Place it at the same level as the shoulder. Move the forearm down toward the body.
  h External rotation—move the forearm toward the head.

  i Repeat flexion, extension, hyperextension, abduction, adduction, and internal and external rotation 5 times—or the number of times stated on the care plan.
13 Exercise the elbow (Fig. 22-14, p. 492):
  a Grasp the person's wrist with one hand. Grasp the elbow with your other hand.
  b Flexion—bend the arm so the same-side shoulder is touched.
  c Extension—straighten the arm.
  d Repeat flexion and extension 5 times—or the number of times stated on the care plan.
14 Exercise the forearm (Fig. 22-15, p. 492):
  a Pronation—turn the hand so the palm is down.
  b Supination—turn the hand so the palm is up.
  c Repeat pronation and supination 5 times—or the number of times stated on the care plan.
15 Exercise the wrist (Fig. 22-16, p. 492):
  a Hold the wrist with both of your hands.
  b Flexion—bend the hand down.
  c Extension—straighten the hand.
  d Hyperextension—bend the hand back.
  e Radial flexion—turn the hand toward the thumb.
  f Ulnar flexion—turn the hand toward the little finger.
  g Repeat flexion, extension, hyperextension, and radial and ulnar flexion 5 times—or the number of times stated on the care plan.
16 Exercise the thumb (Fig. 22-17, p. 492):
  a Hold the person's hand with one hand. Hold the thumb with your other hand.
  b Abduction—move the thumb out from the inner part of the index finger.
  c Adduction—move the thumb back next to the index finger.
  d Opposition—touch each fingertip with the thumb.

## PERFORMING RANGE-OF-MOTION EXERCISES—CONT'D

NNAAP™

### PROCEDURE—CONT'D

e Flexion—bend the thumb into the hand.

f Extension—move the thumb out to the side of the fingers.

g Repeat abduction, adduction, opposition, flexion, and extension 5 times—or the number of times stated on the care plan.

17 Exercise the fingers (Fig. 22-18, p. 492):

a Abduction—spread the fingers and the thumb apart.

b Adduction—bring the fingers and thumb together.

c Extension—straighten the fingers so the fingers, hand, and arm are straight.

d Flexion—make a fist.

e Repeat abduction, adduction, extension, and flexion 5 times—or the number of times stated on the care plan.

18 Exercise the hip (Fig. 22-19, p. 493):

a Support the leg. Place one hand under the knee. Place your other hand under the ankle.

b Flexion—raise the leg.

c Extension—straighten the leg.

d Abduction—move the leg away from the body.

e Adduction—move the leg toward the other leg.

f Internal rotation—turn the leg inward.

g External rotation—turn the leg outward.

h Repeat flexion, extension, abduction, adduction, and internal and external rotation 5 times—or the number of times stated on the care plan.

19 Exercise the knee (Fig. 22-20, p. 493):

a Support the knee. Place one hand under the knee. Place your other hand under the ankle.

b Flexion—bend the leg.

c Extension—straighten the leg.

d Repeat flexion and extension of the knee 5 times—or the number of times stated on the care plan.

20 Exercise the ankle (Fig. 22-21, p. 493):

a Support the foot and ankle. Place one hand under the foot. Place your other hand under the ankle.

b Dorsiflexion—pull the foot forward. Push down on the heel at the same time.

c Plantar flexion—turn the foot down. Or point the toes.

d Repeat dorsiflexion and plantar flexion 5 times—or the number of times stated on the care plan.

21 Exercise the foot (Fig. 22-22, p. 493):

a Continue to support the foot and ankle.

b Pronation—turn the outside of the foot up and the inside down.

c Supination—turn the inside of the foot up and the outside down.

d Repeat pronation and supination 5 times—or the number of times stated on the care plan.

22 Exercise the toes (Fig. 22-23, p. 493):

a Flexion—curl the toes.

b Extension—straighten the toes.

c Abduction—spread the toes apart.

d Adduction—pull the toes together.

e Repeat flexion, extension, abduction, and adduction 5 times—or the number of times stated on the care plan.

23 Cover the leg. Raise the bed rail if used.

24 Go to the other side. Lower the bed rail near you if up.

25 Repeat steps 12 through 22.

### POST-PROCEDURE

26 Provide for comfort.

27 Cover the person. Remove the bath blanket.

28 Raise or lower bed rails. Follow the care plan.

29 Lower the bed to its lowest level.

30 Place the signal light within reach.

31 Unscreen the person.

32 Return the bath blanket to its proper place.

33 Decontaminate your hands.

34 Report and record your observations.

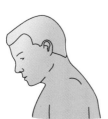
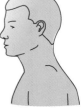
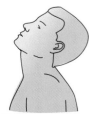

Flexion    Extension    Hyperextension    Rotation    Lateral flexion

**FIG. 22-12** Range-of-motion exercises for the neck.

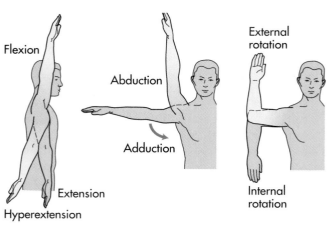

Flexion

Abduction

Adduction

External rotation

Internal rotation

Extension

Hyperextension

**FIG. 22-13** Range-of-motion exercises for the shoulder.

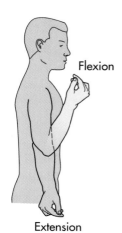

Flexion

Extension

**FIG. 22-14** Range-of-motion exercises for the elbow.

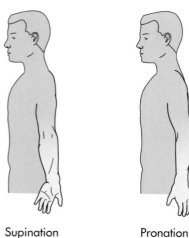

Supination

Pronation

**FIG. 22-15** Range-of-motion exercises for the forearm.

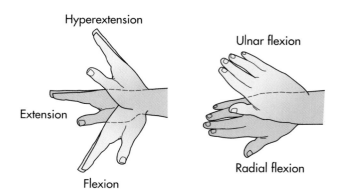

Hyperextension

Extension

Flexion

Ulnar flexion

Radial flexion

**FIG. 22-16** Range-of-motion exercises for the wrist.

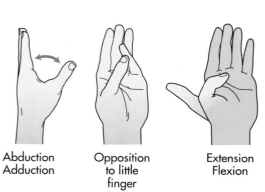

Abduction Adduction

Opposition to little finger

Extension Flexion

**FIG. 22-17** Range-of-motion exercises for the thumb.

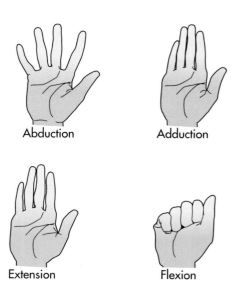

Abduction

Adduction

Extension

Flexion

**FIG. 22-18** Range-of-motion exercises for the fingers.

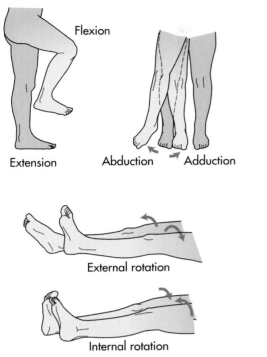

Flexion

Extension    Abduction    Adduction

External rotation

Internal rotation

**FIG. 22-19** Range-of-motion exercises for the hip.

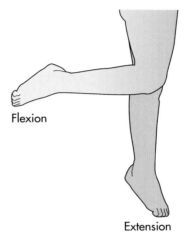

Flexion

Extension

**FIG. 22-20** Range-of-motion exercises for the knee.

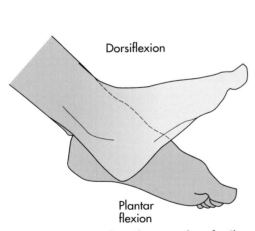

Dorsiflexion

Plantar flexion

**FIG. 22-21** Range-of-motion exercises for the ankle.

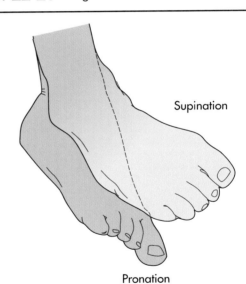

Supination

Pronation

**FIG. 22-22** Range-of-motion exercises for the foot.

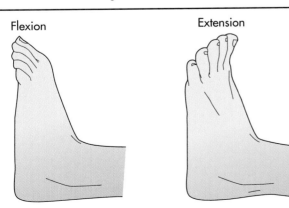

Flexion

Extension

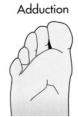

Adduction

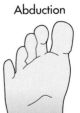

Abduction

**FIG. 22-23** Range-of-motion exercises for the toes.

# AMBULATION

After bedrest, activity increases slowly and in steps. First the person dangles (sits on the side of the bed). Sitting in a bedside chair follows. Next the person walks in the room and then in the hallway. **Ambulation,** the act of walking, is not a problem if complications were prevented. Proper positioning and exercise prevent contractures and muscle atrophy.

Some people are weak and unsteady from bedrest, illness, surgery, or injury. Some persons who use wheelchairs can walk with help. You need to help patients and residents walk according to the care plan. Use a gait (transfer) belt if the person is weak or unsteady. The person also uses hand rails along the wall. Always check the person for orthostatic hypotension (p. 485).

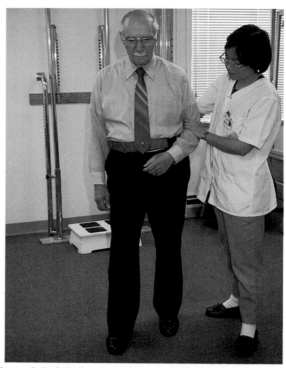

**FIG. 22-24** Assist with ambulation by walking at the person's side. Use a gait belt for the person's safety.

---

**DELEGATION GUIDELINES: *Ambulation***
Before helping with ambulation, you need this information from the nurse and the care plan:
- How much help the person needs
- If the person uses a cane, walker, crutches, or a brace
- Areas of weakness—right arm or leg, left arm or leg
- How far to walk the person
- What observations to report and record
  —How well the person tolerated the activity
  —Complaints of pain or discomfort
  —The distance walked

---

**SAFETY ALERT: *Ambulation***
Practice the safety measures to prevent falls (Chapter 10). Use a gait belt when helping a person with ambulation. Also use it to help the person stand.

---

| Date | Time | |
|------|------|---|
| 8/27 | 1000 | Ambulated 25 feet in the hallway with assist of one and use of a gait belt. Reminded x3 not to shuffle feet. Showed no signs of distress or discomfort. Denies feeling dizzy, lightheaded, or weak. No c/o pain. Assisted to recliner chair and elevated feet after ambulation. BP=132/84 (L) arm sitting. P=76 regular rate and rhythm. R=20 and unlabored. Signal light and water placed within reach. Adam Aims, CNA |

**FIG. 22-25** Charting sample.

# HELPING THE PERSON WALK

NNAAP™

## QUALITY OF LIFE

Remember to:
- Knock before entering the person's room
- Address the person by name
- Introduce yourself by name and title

## PRE-PROCEDURE

1 Follow *Delegation Guidelines: Ambulation.* See *Safety Alert: Ambulation.*
2 Explain the procedure to the person.
3 Practice hand hygiene.
4 Collect the following:
  - Robe and nonskid shoes
  - Paper or sheet to protect bottom linens
  - Gait (transfer) belt
5 Identify the person. Check the ID bracelet against the assignment sheet. Call the person by name.
6 Provide for privacy.

## PROCEDURE

7 Lower the bed to its lowest position. Lock the bed wheels. Lower the bed rail if up.
8 Fanfold top linens to the foot of the bed.
9 Place the paper or sheet under the person's feet. Put the shoes on the person.
10 Help the person dangle. (See procedure: *Helping the Person Sit on the Side of the Bed [Dangle],* p. 255)
11 Help the person put on the robe.
12 Apply the gait belt. (See procedure: *Applying a Transfer Belt,* p. 257.)
13 Help the person stand. (See procedure: *Transferring the Person to a Chair or Wheelchair,* p. 259.) Grasp the gait belt at each side. Or place your arms under the person's arms around to the shoulder blades.
14 Stand at the person's side while he or she gains balance. Hold the belt at the side and back. Or have one arm around the back to support the person.
15 Encourage the person to stand erect with the head up and back straight.
16 Help the person walk. Walk to the side and slightly behind the person. Provide support with the gait belt (Fig. 22-24). Or have one arm around the back to support the person.
17 Encourage the person to walk normally. The heel strikes the floor first. Discourage shuffling, sliding, or walking on tiptoes.
18 Walk the required distance if the person tolerates the activity. Do not rush the person.
19 Help the person return to bed. (See procedure: *Transferring the Person From the Chair or Wheelchair to Bed,* p. 259.)
20 Lower the head of the bed. Help the person to the center of the bed.
21 Remove the shoes. Remove the paper or sheet over the bottom sheet.

## POST-PROCEDURE

22 Provide for comfort. Cover the person.
23 Place the signal light within reach.
24 Raise or lower bed rails. Follow the care plan.
25 Return the robe and shoes to their proper place.
26 Unscreen the person.
27 Decontaminate your hands.
28 Report and record your observations (Fig. 22-25).

# ◼ THE FALLING PERSON

A person may start to fall when standing or walking. The person may be weak, lightheaded, or dizzy. Fainting may occur. Falling may be caused by slipping or sliding on spills, waxed floors, throw rugs, or improper shoes (Chapter 10).

Do not try to prevent the fall. You could injure yourself and the person while twisting and straining to stop the fall. Balance is lost as a person falls. If you try to prevent the fall, you could lose your balance. Thus both you and the person could fall or cause the other person to fall. Head, wrist, arm, hip, and knee injuries could occur.

If a person starts to fall, ease him or her to the floor. This lets you control the direction of the fall. You can also protect the person's head. Do not let the person move or get up before the nurse checks for injuries. Calmly explain that the nurse will check for injuries such as broken bones.

An incident report is completed after all falls. The nurse may ask you to help fill out the report.

## HELPING THE FALLING PERSON

### PROCEDURE

1 Stand with your feet apart. Keep your back straight.
2 Bring the person close to your body as fast as possible. Use the gait belt. Or wrap your arms around the person's waist. You can also hold the person under the arms (Fig. 22-26, *A*).
3 Move your leg so the person's buttocks rest on it (Fig. 22-26, *B*). Move the leg near the person.
4 Lower the person to the floor. The person slides down your leg to the floor (Fig. 22-26, *C*). Bend at your hips and knees as you lower the person.
5 Call a nurse to check the person. Stay with the person.
6 Help the nurse return the person to bed. Get other staff to help if needed.
7 Report the following to the nurse:
   ▪ How the fall occurred
   ▪ How far the person walked
   ▪ How activity was tolerated before the fall
   ▪ Complaints before the fall
   ▪ How much help the person needed while walking
8 Complete an incident report.

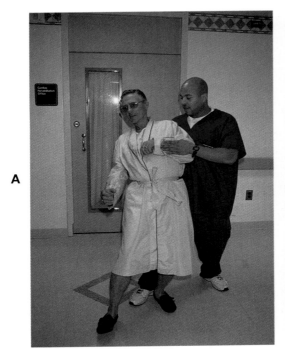

**A**

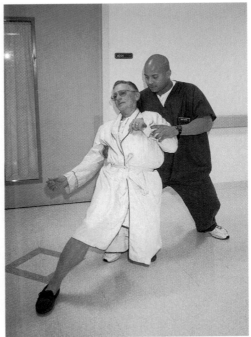

**B**

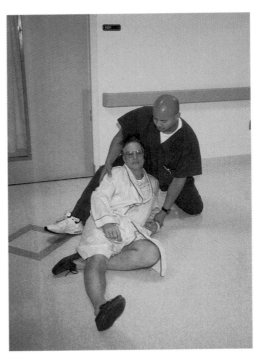

**C**

**FIG. 22-26 A,** The falling person is supported. **B,** The person's buttocks rest on the nursing assistant's leg. **C,** The person is eased to the floor on the nursing assistant's leg.

## WALKING AIDS

Walking aids support the body. The doctor, RN, or physical therapist orders them. The need may be temporary or permanent. The type ordered depends on the person's condition, the amount of support needed, and the type of disability. The physical therapist or RN measures and teaches the person to use the device.

**CRUTCHES.** Crutches are used when the person cannot use one leg or when one or both legs need to gain strength. Some persons with permanent leg weakness can use crutches. They usually use Lofstrand crutches (Fig. 22-27). Axillary crutches extend from the underarm (axilla) to the ground (Fig. 22-28).

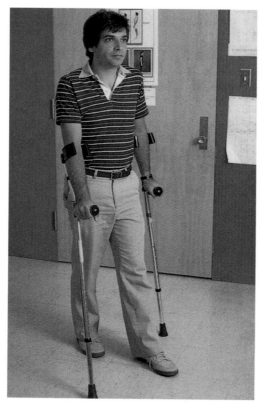

**FIG. 22-27** Lofstrand crutches. (From Elkin MK, Perry AG, Potter PA: *Nursing interventions & clinical skills,* ed 2, St Louis, 2000, Mosby.)

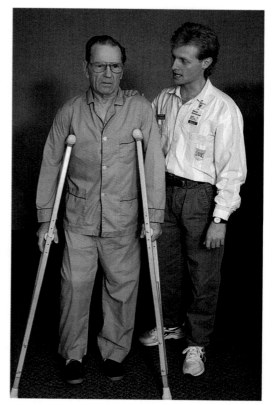

**FIG. 22-28** Axillary crutches. (From Elkin MK, Perry AG, Potter PA: *Nursing interventions & clinical skills,* ed 2, St Louis, 2000, Mosby.)

The person learns to crutch walk, use stairs, and sit and stand. Safety is important. The person on crutches is at risk for falls. Follow these safety measures:

- Check the crutch tips. They must not be worn down, torn, or wet. Replace worn or torn crutch tips. Dry wet tips with a towel or paper towels.
- Check crutches for flaws. Check wooden crutches for cracks and metal crutches for bends.
- Tighten all bolts.
- Street shoes are worn. They must be flat and have nonskid soles.

- Clothes must fit well. Loose clothes may get caught between the crutches and underarms. Loose clothes and long skirts can hang forward and block the person's view of the feet and crutch tips.
- Practice safety rules to prevent falls (Chapter 10).
- Keep crutches within the person's reach. Put them by the person's chair or against a wall.
- Know which crutch gait the person uses:
  —Four-point alternating gait (Fig. 22-29)
  —Three-point alternating gait (Fig. 22-30)
  —Two-point alternating gait (Fig. 22-31, p. 500)
  —Swing-to gait (Fig. 22-32, p. 500)
  —Swing-through gait (Fig. 22-33, p. 500)

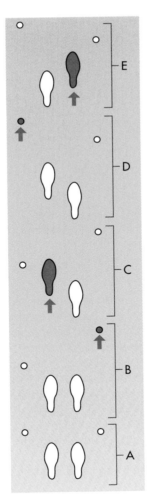

**FIG. 22-29** The four-point alternating gait. The person uses both legs. The right crutch is moved forward and then the left foot. Then the left crutch is moved forward followed by the right foot.

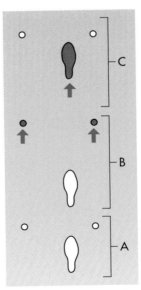

**FIG. 22-30** The three-point alternating gait. One leg is used. Both crutches are moved forward. Then the good foot is moved forward.

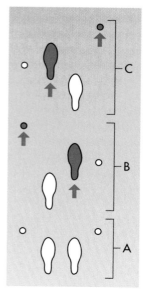

FIG. 22-31 The two-point alternating gait. The person bears some weight on each foot. The left crutch and right foot are moved forward at the same time. Then the right crutch and left foot are moved forward.

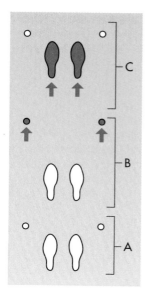

FIG. 22-32 Swing-to gait. The person bears some weight on each leg. Both crutches are moved forward. Then the person lifts both legs and swings to the crutches.

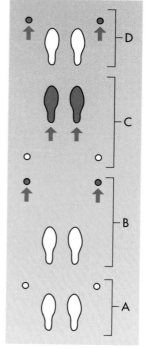

FIG. 22-33 Swing-through gait. The person bears some weight on each leg. Both crutches are moved forward. Then the person lifts both legs and swings through the crutches.

**CANES.** Canes are used for weakness on one side of the body. They help provide balance and support. Single-tip and four-point (quad) canes are common (Fig. 22-34). A cane is held on the *strong side* of the body. (If the left leg is weak, the cane is held in the right hand.) Four-point canes give more support than single-tip canes. However, they are harder to move.

The cane tip is about 6 to 10 inches to the side of the foot. It is about 6 to 10 inches in front of the foot on the strong side. The grip is level with the hip. The person walks as follows:

- *Step A:* The cane is moved forward 6 to 10 inches (Fig. 22-35, A).
- *Step B:* The weak leg (opposite the cane) is moved forward even with the cane (Fig. 22-35, B).
- *Step C:* The strong leg is moved forward and ahead of the cane and the weak leg (Fig. 22-35, C).

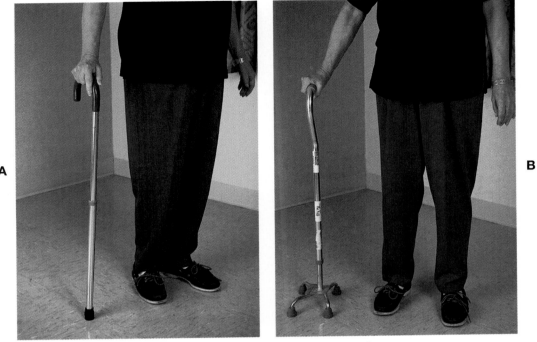

**FIG. 22-34 A,** Single-tip cane. **B,** Four-point cane.

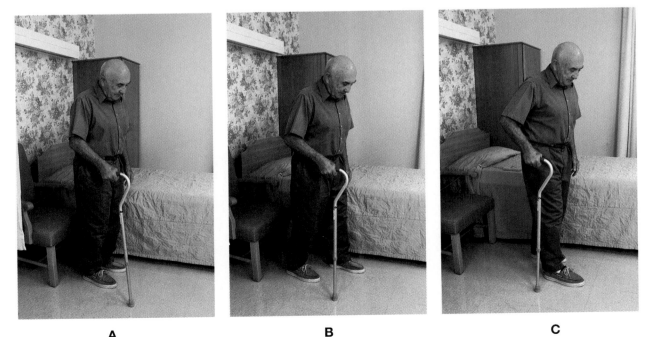

A                    B                    C

**FIG. 22-35** Walking with a cane. **A,** The cane is moved forward about 6 to 10 inches. **B,** The leg opposite the cane (weak leg) is brought forward even with the cane. **C,** The leg on the cane side (strong side) is moved ahead of the cane and the weak leg.

**WALKERS.** A walker is a four-point walking aid (Fig. 22-36). It gives more support than a cane. Many people feel safer and more secure with walkers than with canes. There are many kinds of walkers. The standard walker is picked up and moved about 6 to 8 inches in front of the person. The person then moves the weak leg and foot and then the strong leg and foot up to the walker (Fig. 22-37).

Some people use wheeled walkers. They have wheels on the front legs and rubber tips on the back legs. The person pushes the walker ahead about 6 to 8 inches and then walks up to it. Rubber tips on the back legs prevent the walker from moving while the person is walking or standing. Some have a braking action when weight is applied to the walker's back legs.

Baskets, pouches, and trays attach to the walker (see Fig. 22-36). They are used for needed items. This allows more independence. They also free the hands to grip the walker.

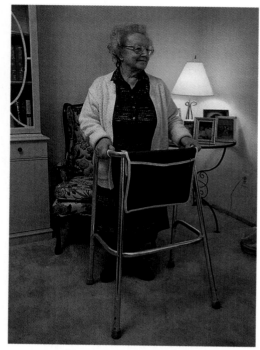

**FIG. 22-36** A walker.

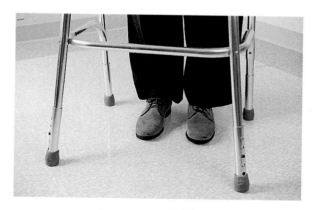

**A**

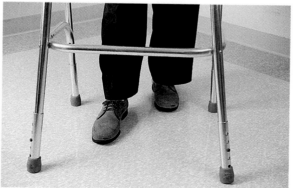

**B**

**FIG. 22-37** Walking with a walker. **A,** The walker is moved about 6 inches in front of the person. **B,** Both feet are moved up to the walker.

**BRACES.** Braces support weak body parts. They also prevent or correct deformities or prevent joint movement. Metal, plastic, or leather is used for braces. A brace is applied over the ankle, knee, or back (Fig. 22-38). An ankle-foot orthosis (AFO) is placed in the shoe (Fig. 22-39). Then the foot is inserted. The device is secured in place with a Velcro strap.

Skin and bony points under braces are kept clean and dry. This prevents skin breakdown. Report redness or signs of skin breakdown at once (Chapter 28). Also report complaints of pain or discomfort. The nurse assesses the skin under braces every shift. The care plan tells you when to apply and remove a brace.

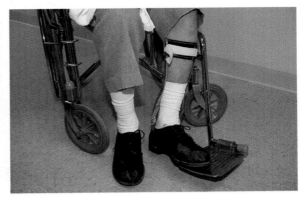

**FIG. 22-38** Leg brace.

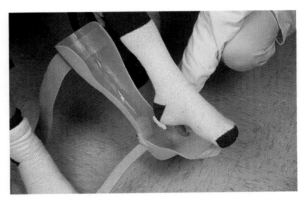

**FIG. 22-39** Ankle-foot orthosis (AFO).

# ■ REVIEW QUESTIONS ■

Circle the **BEST** answer.

1 Ms. Porter is on bedrest. Which is *false?*
   a She has orthostatic hypotension.
   b Bedrest helps reduce pain and promotes healing.
   c Complications of bedrest include pressure ulcers, constipation, and blood clots.
   d Contractures and muscle atrophy can occur.

2 Which helps to prevent plantar flexion?
   a Bed boards
   b A foot board
   c A trochanter roll
   d Hand rolls

3 Which prevents the hip from turning outward?
   a Bed boards
   b A foot board
   c Trochanter roll
   d A leg brace

4 A contracture is
   a The loss of muscle strength from inactivity
   b The lack of joint mobility from shortening of a muscle
   c A decrease in the size of a muscle
   d A blood clot in the muscle

5 A trapeze is used to
   a Prevent footdrop
   b Prevent contractures
   c Strengthen arm muscles
   d Strengthen leg muscles

6 Passive range-of-motion exercises are performed by
   a The person
   b Someone else
   c The person with the help of another
   d The person with the use of a trapeze

7 ROM exercises are ordered for Ms. Porter. You do the following *except*
   a Support the part being exercised
   b Move the joint slowly, smoothly, and gently
   c Force the joint through full range of motion
   d Exercise only the joints indicated by the nurse

8 Flexion involves
   a Bending the body part
   b Straightening the body part
   c Moving the body part toward the body
   d Moving the body part away from the body

9 Which statement about ambulation is *false?*
   a A transfer belt is used if the person is weak or unsteady.
   b The person can shuffle or slide when walking after bedrest.
   c Walking aids may be needed.
   d Crutches, canes, walkers, and braces are common walking aids.

10 You are getting a person ready to crutch walk. You should do the following *except*
   a Check the crutch tips
   b Have the person wear nonskid shoes
   c Get a pair of crutches from physical therapy
   d Tighten the bolts on the crutches

11 A single-tip cane is used
   a At waist level
   b On the strong side
   c On the weak side
   d On either side

Circle **T** if the statement is true and **F** if it is false.

12 T F A single-tip cane and a four-point cane give the same support.
13 T F When using a cane, the feet are moved first.
14 T F Mr. Parker uses a walker. He moves the walker first and then his feet.
15 T F Mr. Parker starts to fall. You should try to prevent the fall.
16 T F A person has a brace. Bony areas need protection from skin breakdown.

*Answers to these questions are on p. 818.*

# Comfort, Rest, and Sleep

# OBJECTIVES

- Define the key terms listed in this chapter
- Explain why comfort, rest, and sleep are important
- List the OBRA room requirements for comfort, rest, and sleep
- Describe four types of pain and the factors that affect pain
- Explain why pain is personal
- List the signs and symptoms of pain
- List the nursing measures that relieve pain
- Explain why meeting basic needs is important for rest
- Identify when rest is needed
- Describe the factors that affect sleep
- Describe the common sleep disorders
- Explain how circadian rhythm affects sleep
- Describe the stages of sleep
- Know the sleep requirements for each age-group
- List the nursing measures that promote rest and sleep

# KEY TERMS

**acute pain**   Pain that is felt suddenly from injury, disease, trauma, or surgery

**chronic pain**   Pain lasting longer than 6 months; it is constant or occurs off and on

**circadian rhythm**   Daily rhythm based on a 24-hour cycle; the day-night cycle or body rhythm

**comfort**   A state of well-being; the person has no physical or emotional pain and is calm and at peace

**discomfort**   Pain

**distraction**   To change the person's center of attention

**enuresis**   Urinary incontinence in bed at night

**guided imagery**   Creating and focusing on an image

**insomnia**   A chronic condition in which the person cannot sleep or stay asleep all night

**NREM sleep**   The phase of sleep when there is *no rapid eye movement;* non-REM sleep

**pain**   To ache, hurt, or be sore; discomfort

**phantom pain**   Pain felt in a body part that is no longer there

**radiating pain**   Pain felt at the site of tissue damage and in nearby areas

**relaxation**   To be free from mental and physical stress

**REM sleep**   The phase of sleep when there is *rapid eye movement*

**rest**   To be calm, at ease, and relaxed; no anxiety and stress

**sleep**   A state of unconsciousness, reduced voluntary muscle activity, and lowered metabolism

■ Comfort, rest, and sleep are needed for well-being. The total person—the physical, emotional, social, and spiritual—is affected by comfort, rest, and sleep problems. Discomfort and pain can be physical or emotional. Whatever the cause, they affect rest and sleep. They also decrease function and quality of life.

Rest and sleep restore energy and well-being. Illness and injury increase the need for rest and sleep. The body needs more energy for healing and repair. When the person is ill or injured, more energy than normal is needed to perform daily functions.

*See Focus on Long-Term Care: Comfort, Rest, and Sleep.*

## COMFORT

**Comfort** is a state of well-being. The person has no physical or emotional pain. He or she is calm and at peace. Age, illness, and activity affect comfort. So do temperature, ventilation, noise, odors, and lighting. Those factors are controlled to meet the person's needs (Chapter 14).

**Pain** or **discomfort** means to ache, hurt, or be sore. It is unpleasant. Comfort and discomfort are subjective. That is, you cannot see, hear, touch, or smell comfort or discomfort. You must rely on what the person says. Report complaints to the nurse. The information is used for the nursing process.

Pain is personal. It differs for each person. What *hurts* to one person may *ache* to another. What one person calls *sore*, another may call *aching*. If a person complains of pain or discomfort, the person *has* pain or discomfort. You must believe the person. You cannot see, hear, feel, or smell the pain.

Pain is a warning from the body. It means there is tissue damage. Pain often causes the person to seek health care.

## TYPES OF PAIN

There are different types of pain. The doctor uses the type of pain when diagnosing. The nurse uses it for the nursing process.

- **Acute pain** is felt suddenly from injury, disease, trauma, or surgery. There is tissue damage. Acute pain lasts a short time, usually less than 6 months. It lessens with healing.
- **Chronic pain** lasts longer than 6 months. Pain is constant or occurs off and on. There is no longer tissue damage. Chronic pain remains long after healing. Arthritis and cancer are common causes.
- **Radiating pain** is felt at the site of tissue damage and in nearby areas. Pain from a heart attack is often felt in the left chest, left jaw, left shoulder, and left arm. Gallbladder disease can cause pain in the right upper abdomen, the back, and the right shoulder (Fig. 23-1).
- **Phantom pain** is felt in a body part that is no longer there. A person with an amputated leg may still sense leg pain (Chapter 33).

### FOCUS ON LONG-TERM CARE
#### COMFORT, REST, AND SLEEP

The following room requirements under OBRA promote quality of life and comfort, rest, and sleep:
- No more than four persons in a room
- Suspended curtain that goes around the bed for privacy
- A bed of proper height and size for the person
- Clean, comfortable mattress
- Linens (sheets, blankets, spreads) that suit weather and climate
- Clean and orderly room
- Odor-free room
- Room temperature between 71° and 81° F
- Acceptable noise level
- Adequate ventilation and room humidity
- Appropriate lighting

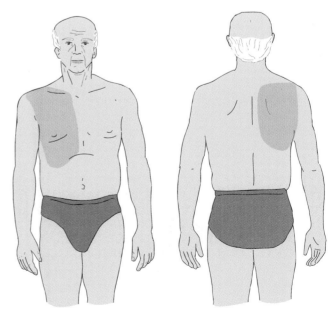

**FIG. 23-1** Gallbladder pain radiates to the right upper abdomen, the back, and the right shoulder.

## FACTORS AFFECTING PAIN

A person may handle pain well one time and poorly the next time. Many factors affect reactions to pain.

**PAST EXPERIENCE.** We learn from past experiences. They help us know what to do or what to expect. Whether it is going to school, driving, taking a test, shopping, having a baby, or caring for children, the past prepares us for similar events at another time. We also learn from the experiences of family and friends.

A person may have had pain before. The severity of pain, its cause, how long it lasted, and if relief occurred all affect the person's current response to pain. Knowing what to expect can help or hinder how the person handles pain.

Some people have not had pain. When it occurs, pain can cause fear and anxiety. They can make pain worse.

**ANXIETY.** Anxiety relates to feelings of fear, dread, worry, and concern. The person is uneasy and tense. The person may feel troubled or threatened. Or the person may sense danger. Something is wrong but the person does not know what or why.

Pain and anxiety are related. Pain can cause anxiety. Anxiety increases how much pain the person feels. Reducing anxiety helps lessen pain. For example, the nurse explains to Mr. Smith that he will have pain after surgery. The nurse also explains that he will receive drugs for pain relief. Mr. Smith knows the cause of the pain. And he knows what to expect. This helps reduce his anxiety and therefore the amount of pain felt.

**REST AND SLEEP.** Rest and sleep restore energy. They reduce body demands, and the body repairs itself. Lack of needed rest and sleep affects thinking and coping with daily life. Sleep and rest needs increase with illness and injury. Pain seems worse when tired or restless. Also, the person tends to focus on pain when tired and unable to rest or sleep.

**ATTENTION.** The more a person thinks about the pain, the worse it seems. Sometimes pain is so severe, it is all the person thinks about. However, even mild pain can seem worse if the person thinks about it all the time.

Pain often seems worse at night. Activity is less, and it is quiet. There are no visitors. The radio or TV is off. Others are asleep. When unable to sleep, the person has time to think about the pain.

**PERSONAL AND FAMILY DUTIES.** Personal and family duties affect pain responses. Often pain is ignored when there are children to care for. Some people go to work with pain. Others deny pain if a serious illness is feared. The illness can interfere with a job, going to school, or caring for children, a partner, or ill parents.

**THE VALUE OR MEANING OF PAIN.** To some people, pain is a sign of weakness. It may mean a serious illness and the need for painful tests and treatments. Therefore pain is ignored or denied. Sometimes pain gives pleasure. The pain of childbirth is one example.

For some persons, pain means not having to work or assume daily routines. Pain is used to avoid certain people or things. The pain is useful. Some people like doting and pampering by others. The person values and wants such attention.

**SUPPORT FROM OTHERS.** Dealing with pain is often easier when family and friends offer comfort and support. The pain of childbirth is easier when a loving father gives support and encouragement. A child bears pain much better when comforted by a caring parent or family member. The use of touch by a valued person is very comforting. Just being nearby also helps.

Some people do not have caring family or friends. They deal with pain alone. Being alone can increase anxiety. The person has more time to think about the pain. Facing pain alone is hard for everyone, especially children and older persons.

**CULTURE.** Culture affects pain responses. In some cultures, the person in pain is *stoic*. To be stoic means to show no reaction to joy, sorrow, pleasure, or pain. Strong verbal and nonverbal reactions to pain are seen in other cultures. *See Caring About Culture: Pain Reactions.*

**AGE.** *See Focus on Children: Factors Affecting Pain. See Focus on Older Persons: Factors Affecting Pain.*

### CARING ABOUT CULTURE
#### PAIN REACTIONS

People of *Mexico* and the *Philippines* may appear stoic in reaction to pain. In the *Philippines*, pain is viewed as the will of God. It is believed that God will give strength to bear the pain.

In *Vietnam*, pain may be severe before pain relief measures are requested. The people of *India* accept pain quietly. They will accept some pain relief measures.

In *China*, showing emotion is a weakness of character. Therefore pain is often suppressed.

From D' Avanzo CE, Geissler EM: *Pocket guide to cultural health assessment*, ed 3, St Louis, 2003, Mosby.

### FOCUS ON CHILDREN
#### FACTORS AFFECTING PAIN

Children may not understand pain. They know it feels bad. They have fewer pain experiences. They do not know what to expect. Also, they do not have many ways to deal with pain. Adults can buy some pain drugs. They know that heat or cold applications help relieve pain. They can distract attention away from the pain with music, working, reading, and hobbies. Children do not know how to relieve their own pain. They rely on adults for help.

Adults must be alert to behaviors and situations that signal a child's pain. Infants cry, fuss, and are restless. Such behaviors also mean hunger and time for a diaper change. Toddlers and preschool children may not have the words to express pain.

### FOCUS ON OLDER PERSONS
#### FACTORS AFFECTING PAIN

Older persons may have decreased pain sensations. They do not feel pain. Or it may not feel severe. The person is at risk for undetected disease or injury. Pain occurs with tissue damage. The pain signals illness or injury. If pain is not felt, the person does not know to seek health care.

Some older persons have many painful health problems. Chronic pain may mask new pain. Older persons may ignore or deny new pain. They may think it relates to a known health problem. Older persons often deny or ignore pain because of what it may mean.

Thinking and reasoning are affected in some older persons. Some cannot verbally communicate pain. Changes in behavior may signal that the person has pain. Nursing staff must be alert for the signs of pain. Always report changes in the person's behavior to the nurse.

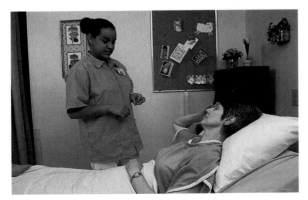

**FIG. 23-2** The person points to the area of pain.

## SIGNS AND SYMPTOMS

You cannot see, hear, feel, or smell the person's pain. You must rely on what the person tells you. Promptly report any information you collect about pain. Use the person's exact words when reporting and recording. The nurse needs the following information to assess the person's pain:

- *Location.* Where is the pain? Ask the person to point to the area of pain (Fig. 23-2). Pain can radiate. Ask the person if the pain is anywhere else and to point to those areas.
- *Onset and duration.* When did the pain start? How long has it lasted?
- *Intensity.* Does the person complain of mild, moderate, or severe pain? Ask the person to rate the pain on a scale of 1 to 10, with 10 as the most severe (Fig. 23-3).
- *Description.* Ask the person to describe the pain. Box 23-1, p. 510, lists some words used to describe pain.
- *Factors causing pain.* These are called *precipitating* factors. To precipitate means to cause. Such factors include moving or turning in bed, coughing or deep breathing, and exercise. Ask what the person was doing before the pain started and when it started.
- *Vital signs.* Measure the person's pulse, respirations, and blood pressure. Increases in these vital signs often occur with acute pain. Vital signs may be normal with chronic pain.
- *Other signs and symptoms.* Does the person have other symptoms—dizziness, nausea, vomiting, weakness, numbness or tingling, or others? Box 23-2, p. 510, lists the signs and symptoms that often occur with pain.

PAIN: Ask patient to rate pain on scale of 1-10

No pain ... Worst pain imaginable

| 0 | 1 | 2 | 3 | 4 | 5 | 6 | 7 | 8 | 9 | 10 |
|---|---|---|---|---|---|---|---|---|---|---|

**FIG. 23-3** Pain rating scale. From deWit SC: *Fundamental concepts and skills for nursing*, Philadelphia, 2001, Saunders.

---

**BOX 23-1 WORDS USED TO DESCRIBE PAIN**

- Aching
- Burning
- Cramping
- Crushing
- Dull
- Gnawing
- Knifelike
- Piercing
- Pressure
- Sharp
- Sore
- Squeezing
- Stabbing
- Throbbing
- Viselike

---

**BOX 23-2 SIGNS AND SYMPTOMS OF PAIN**

**BODY RESPONSES**

- Increased pulse, respirations, and blood pressure
- Nausea
- Pale skin (pallor)
- Sweating (diaphoresis)
- Vomiting

**BEHAVIORS**

- Changes in speech: slow or rapid; loud or quiet
- Crying
- Gasping
- Grimacing
- Groaning
- Grunting
- Holding the affected body part (splinting)
- Irritability
- Maintaining one position; refusing to move
- Moaning
- Quietness
- Restlessness
- Rubbing
- Screaming

---

**BOX 23-3 NURSING MEASURES TO PROMOTE COMFORT AND RELIEVE PAIN**

- Position the person in good alignment. Use pillows for support.
- Keep bed linens tight and wrinkle-free.
- Make sure the person is not lying on drainage tubes.
- Assist with elimination needs.
- Provide blankets for warmth and to prevent chilling.
- Use correct lifting, moving, and turning procedures.
- Wait 30 minutes after pain drugs are given before giving care or starting activities.
- Give a back massage.
- Provide soft music to distract the person.
- Use touch to provide comfort.
- Allow family and friends at the bedside as requested by the person.
- Avoid sudden or jarring movements of the bed or chair.
- Handle the person gently.
- Practice safety measures if the person takes strong pain drugs or sedatives:
  —Keep the bed in the low position.
  —Raise bed rails as directed. Follow the care plan.
  —Check on the person every 10 to 15 minutes.
  —Provide help when the person needs to get up and when he or she is up and about.
- Apply warm or cold applications as directed by the nurse (Chapter 29).
- Provide a calm, quiet, darkened setting.

---

## NURSING MEASURES

The RN uses the nursing process to promote comfort and relieve pain. The care plan may include measures in Box 23-3. See Figure 23-4.

Other measures are often needed. They include distraction, relaxation, and guided imagery. Nurses and physical, occupational, and recreational therapists may assist with these measures. If asked to assist, they tell you what to do.

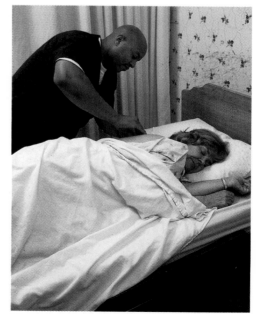

**FIG. 23-4** Measures are implemented to relieve pain. The person is positioned in good alignment with pillows used for comfort. The room is darkened. Blankets provide warmth. A back massage provides touch and promotes relaxation.

**Distraction** means to change the person's center of attention. Attention is moved away from the pain. Music, games, singing, praying, TV, and needlework can distract attention (Fig. 23-5).

**Relaxation** means to be free from mental and physical stress. This state reduces pain and anxiety. The person is taught relaxation methods (Box 23-4). The person is taught to breathe deeply and slowly and to contract and relax muscle groups. A comfortable position is important. So is a quiet room.

**Guided imagery** is creating and focusing on an image (Box 23-5). The person is asked to create a pleasant scene. This is noted on the care plan so all staff members use the same image with the person. A calm, soft voice is used to help the person focus on the image. Soft music, a blanket for warmth, and a darkened room may help. The person is coached to focus on the image and then to practice relaxation exercises.

Doctors often order drugs to control or relieve pain. Nurses give these drugs. Such drugs can cause orthostatic hypotension (Chapter 22). They also can cause drowsiness, dizziness, and coordination problems. Therefore the person is protected from falls and injury. The nurse and care plan alert you to needed safety measures. *See Focus on Children: Nursing Measures.*

---

**BOX 23-4  RELAXATION TAUGHT BY THE NURSE**

"Let's begin by finding as comfortable a position as possible. Arms at your side . . . legs uncrossed. . . . . Move until you feel at ease. . . . . Take a deep breath. Feel your stomach and chest slowly rise. . . .Relax. . . . Now breathe out slowly . . . slowly . . . and relax."

"Count to 4, inhaling on 1 and 2, exhaling on 3 and 4. . . . Continue to breathe slowly. . . . Your body is beginning to relax. . . . Think 'relax'. . . . Feel the parts of your body. . . . Notice any tension in your muscles. . . . Continue to breathe slowly . . . and relax."

"Concentrate on your face . . . your jaws . . . your neck. . . . Notice any tightness. . . . Breathe in warmth and relaxation. . . . Concentrate on any tension in your hands. . . . Notice how they feel. . . . Now make a fist—a tight fist. As you begin to exhale, relax your fist. . . . Good. Notice how your hand feels. . . . Think 'relax'. . . . Your hand feels warm . . . heavy or light. . . . Just relax more . . . and more. Now focus on your forearms. . . . Notice any tension. . . . Relax your arms. . . . Feel your body relaxing. . . . Let the feelings of relaxation spread from your fingers and hands through the muscles of your arms. . . . "

*The nurse then teaches the person to relax other muscle groups throughout the body.*

From Potter PA, Perry AG: *Fundamentals of nursing: concepts, process and practice,* ed 4, St Louis, 1997, Mosby.

---

**BOX 23-5  GUIDED IMAGERY**

"Imagine yourself lying on a cool bed of grass with sounds of rushing water from a nearby stream. It's a balmy day. You turn to see a patch of blue wildflowers in bloom and can smell their fragrance."

From Potter PA, Perry AG: *Fundamentals of nursing: concepts, process and practice,* ed 4, St Louis, 1997, Mosby.

---

**FOCUS ON CHILDREN**
**NURSING MEASURES**

Pacifiers and favorite toys and blankets can comfort infants and young children. So can holding, rocking, touching, and talking or singing to them. Always check with the nurse before picking up and holding a child. Sometimes children are not held for treatment reasons.

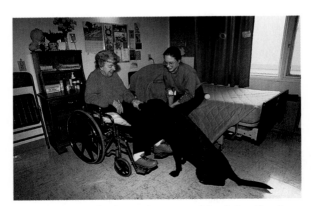

**FIG. 23-5** A comforting pet can provide distraction from pain.

## REST

**Rest** means to be calm, at ease, and relaxed. The person has no anxiety or stress. Rest may involve inactivity. Or the person does things that are calming and relaxing. Examples include reading, music, TV, needlework and prayer. Some people garden, bake, golf, walk, or do woodworking.

You can promote rest by meeting physical needs. Thirst, hunger, and elimination needs can affect rest. So can pain or discomfort. A comfortable position and good alignment are important. A quiet setting promotes rest. So does a clean, dry, and wrinkle-free bed. Some people rest easier in a clean, neat, and uncluttered room.

Meet safety and security needs. The person must feel safe from falling or other injuries. The person is secure with the signal light within reach. Understanding the reasons for care also helps the person feel safe. So does knowing how care is given. That is why you always explain procedures before doing them.

Many people have rituals or routines before resting. These may include going to the bathroom, brushing teeth, and washing the face and hands. Some people pray. Some have a snack or beverage, lock doors, or make sure loved ones are safe at home. The person may want a certain blanket or afghan. Follow routines and rituals whenever possible.

Love and belonging promote rest. Visits or calls from family and friends may relax the person. The person knows that others care and are concerned. Reading cards and letters may also help the person relax and rest (Fig. 23-6).

Self-esteem needs relate to feeling good about oneself. Some people find patient gowns embarrassing. Others fear exposure. Many persons rest better in their own sleepwear. Hygiene and grooming also affect self-esteem. This includes hair care and being clean and odor-free. Hygiene and grooming measures help people feel good about themselves. If esteem needs are met, the person may rest easier.

Some people are refreshed after a 15- or 20-minute rest. Others need more time. Health care routines usually allow time for afternoon rest.

Ill or injured persons need to rest more often. Some rest during or after a procedure. For example, a bath tires Mr. Smith. So does getting dressed. He needs to rest before you make his bed. Some people need a few hours for hygiene and grooming. Others need to rest after meals. Do not push the person beyond his or her limits. Allow rest when needed. Do not rush the person.

Distraction, relaxation, and guided imagery also promote rest. So does a back massage. Plan and organize care to allow uninterrupted rest.

The doctor may order bedrest for a person. Bedrest is presented in Chapter 22.

## SLEEP

**Sleep** is a state of unconsciousness, reduced voluntary muscle activity, and lowered metabolism. An unconscious person is unaware of the environment. He or she cannot respond to people and things in the environment. There are no voluntary arm or leg movements. Metabolism is the burning of food to produce energy for the body. Less energy is needed during sleep. Thus metabolism is reduced during sleep. The sleep state is temporary. People awake from sleep.

Sleep is a basic need. It lets the mind and body rest. The body saves energy. Body functions slow. Vital signs are lower than when awake. Tissue healing and repair occur. Sleep lowers stress, tension, and anxiety. It refreshes and renews the person. The person regains energy and mental alertness. The person thinks and functions better after sleep.

### CIRCADIAN RHYTHM

Sleep is part of circadian rhythm. (*Circa* means *about*. *Dies* means *day*.) **Circadian rhythm** is a daily rhythm based on a 24-hour cycle. It is called the *day-night cycle* or *body rhythm*. It affects functioning. Some people function better in the morning. They are more alert and active. They think and react better. Others do better in the evening.

Circadian rhythm includes a sleep-wake cycle. The person's *biological clock* signals when to sleep and when to wake up. You sleep and wake up at certain times. You may awaken before the alarm clock goes off. That is part of your biological clock. Health care often interferes with a person's circadian rhythm and the sleep-wake cycle. Sleep problems easily occur.

Many people work evening and night shifts. Their bodies must adjust to changes in the sleep-wake cycle.

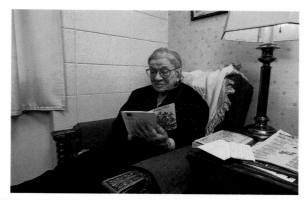

**FIG. 23-6** This nursing center resident reads cards and letters from family and friends.

## BOX 23-6 SLEEP CYCLE

### STAGE 1: NREM SLEEP

- Lightest sleep level
- Lasts a few minutes
- Gradual decrease in vital signs
- Gradual lowering of metabolism
- Person feels drowsy and relaxed
- Person is easily aroused
- Daydreaming feeling after being aroused

### STAGE 2: NREM SLEEP

- Sound sleep
- Relaxation increases
- Still easy to arouse
- Lasts 10 to 20 minutes
- Body functions continue to slow

### STAGE 3: NREM SLEEP

- First stages of deep sleep
- Hard to arouse the person
- Person rarely moves
- Muscles relax completely
- Vital signs decrease
- Lasts 15 to 30 minutes

### STAGE 4: NREM SLEEP

- Deepest stage of sleep
- Hard to arouse the person
- Body rests and is restored
- Vital signs much lower than when awake
- Lasts about 15 to 30 minutes
- Sleepwalking and **enuresis** (urinary incontinence in bed at night) may occur

### REM SLEEP

- Vivid, full-color dreaming
- Usually starts 50 to 90 minutes after sleep has begun
- Rapid eye movements
- Blood pressure, pulse, and respirations may fluctuate
- Voluntary muscles are relaxed
- Mental restoration occurs
- Hard to arouse the person
- Lasts about 20 minutes

Modified from Potter PA, Perry AG: *Fundamentals of nursing,* ed 5, St Louis, 2001, Mosby.

## SLEEP CYCLE

There are two phases of sleep (Box 23-6). **NREM sleep** *(non-REM sleep)* is the phase of sleep where there is *no rapid eye movement.* NREM sleep has 4 stages. Sleep goes from light to deep as the person moves through the four stages.

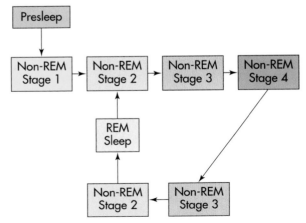

**FIG. 23-7** Adult sleep cycle.

The *rapid eye movement* phase is called **REM sleep.** The person is hard to arouse. Mental restoration occurs. Events and problems of the day are thought to be reviewed. The person prepares for the next day.

There are usually 4 to 6 cycles of NREM and REM sleep during 7 to 8 hours of sleep. Stage 1 of NREM is usually not repeated (Fig. 23-7).

## SLEEP REQUIREMENTS

Sleep needs vary for each age-group. The amount needed decreases with age (Table 23-1, p. 514). Infants need more sleep than toddlers. Toddlers need more than preschool children. School-age children need more than teenagers. Older persons need less sleep than middle-age adults.

## FACTORS AFFECTING SLEEP

Many factors affect the amount and quality of sleep. Quality relates to how well the person slept. It also involves getting needed amounts of NREM and REM sleep.

- *Illness.* Illness increases the need for sleep. However, signs and symptoms of illness can interfere with sleep. They include pain, nausea, vomiting, coughing, difficulty breathing, diarrhea, frequent voiding, and itching. Treatments and therapies can also interfere

| TABLE 23-1 | AVERAGE SLEEP REQUIREMENTS |
| --- | --- |
| Age-Group | Hours per Day |
| Newborns (birth to 4 weeks) | 14 to 18 |
| Infants (4 weeks to 1 year) | 12 to 14 |
| Toddlers (1 to 3 years) | 11 to 12 |
| Preschoolers (3 to 6 years) | 11 to 12 |
| Middle and late childhood (6 to 12 years) | 10 to 11 |
| Adolescents (12 to 18 years) | 8 to 9 |
| Young adults (18 to 40 years) | 7 to 8 |
| Middle-age adults (40 to 65 years) | 7 |
| Older adults (65 years and older) | 5 to 7 |

---

**BOX 23-7  SIGNS AND SYMPTOMS OF SLEEP DISORDERS**

- Hand tremors
- Slowed responses to questions, conversations, or situations
- Reduced word memory; problems finding the right word
- Decreased reasoning and judgment
- Irregular pulse
- Red, puffy eyes
- Dark circles under the eyes
- Moodiness; mood swings
- Disorientation
- Irritability
- Fatigue
- Sleepiness
- Agitation
- Restlessness
- Decreased attention
- Hallucinations (Chapter 34)
- Coordination problems
- Slurred speech

---

with sleep. Often patients and residents are awakened for treatments or drugs. Traction or a cast can cause uncomfortable positions. The emotional effects of illness can affect sleep. These include fear, anxiety, and worry.

- *Nutrition.* Sleep needs increase with weight gain. They decrease with weight loss. Some foods affect sleep. Those with caffeine (chocolate, coffee, tea, colas) prevent sleep. The protein L-tryptophan tends to help sleep. It is found in milk, cheese, and beef.
- *Exercise.* Exercise improves health and fitness. Exercise requires energy. People usually feel good after exercising. Eventually they tire. Being tired helps them sleep well. Exercise before bedtime interferes with sleep. Exercise causes the release of substances into the bloodstream that stimulate the body. Exercise is avoided 2 hours before bedtime.
- *Environment.* People adjust to their usual sleep settings. They get used to such things as the bed, pillows, noises, lighting, and a sleeping partner. Any change in the usual setting can affect the amount and quality of sleep.
- *Drugs and other substances.* Sleeping pills promote sleep. Drugs for anxiety, depression, and pain may cause the person to sleep. However, these drugs and sleeping pills reduce the length of REM sleep. Mental restoration occurs during REM sleep. Behavior problems and sleep deprivation can occur. Alcohol is a drug. It causes drowsiness and sleep. However, it interferes with REM sleep. Those under the influence of alcohol may awaken during sleep. Difficulty returning to sleep is common. Some drugs contain caffeine. Caffeine is a stimulant and prevents sleep. Besides in drugs, caffeine is found in coffee, tea, chocolate, and colas. The side effects of some drugs cause frequent voiding and nightmares.
- *Life-style changes.* Life-style relates to a person's daily routines and way of living. Life-style changes can affect sleep. Travel, vacation, and social events often

affect usual sleep and wake times. Children usually stay up later during school holidays. They may sleep later, too. If work hours change, sleep hours may change. Such changes affect normal sleep-wake cycles and the circadian rhythm.

- *Emotional problems.* Fear, worry, depression, and anxiety affect sleep. Causes include work, personal, or family problems. Loss of a loved one or friend is another cause. Money problems are stressful. People may have problems falling asleep, or they awaken often. Some have problems getting back to sleep.

## SLEEP DISORDERS

Sleep disorders involve repeated sleep problems. The amount and quality of sleep are affected. Sleep disorders affect life-style. Box 23-7 lists the signs and symptoms that occur.

**INSOMNIA.** **Insomnia** is a chronic condition in which the person cannot sleep or stay asleep all night. There are three forms of insomnia:

- Cannot fall asleep
- Cannot stay asleep
- Early awakening and cannot fall back asleep

Emotional problems are common causes of insomnia. The fear of dying during sleep is another cause. Some people are afraid of not waking up. This may occur with heart disease or when told of a terminal illness. The fear of not being able to sleep is another cause. The physical and emotional discomforts of illness can also cause insomnia.

The RN plans measures to promote sleep. However, the emotional or physical problems causing the insomnia also are treated.

**SLEEP DEPRIVATION.** With sleep deprivation, the amount and quality of sleep are decreased. Sleep is interrupted. NREM and REM sleep stages are not completed. Illness, pain, and hospital care are common causes. Patients in intensive care units (ICUs) are at great risk. ICU lights, the many care measures, and equipment sounds interfere with sleep. Factors that affect sleep can also lead to sleep deprivation. The signs and symptoms in Box 23-7 may occur.

**SLEEPWALKING.** The person leaves the bed and walks about. The person is not aware of sleepwalking. He or she has no memory of the event on awakening. Children sleepwalk more than adults. The event may last 3 to 4 minutes or longer.

Stress, fatigue, and some drugs are common causes. Protect the person from injury. Falling is a risk. IVs, catheters, nasogastric tubes, and other tubing can cause injury. The tubes or catheters can be pulled out of the body when the person gets out of bed. Guide sleepwalkers back to bed. They startle easily. Awaken them gently.

## PROMOTING SLEEP

The RN assesses the person's sleep patterns. Report any of the signs and symptoms listed in Box 23-7. Measures are planned to promote sleep (Box 23-8). Follow the care plan. Also report your observations about how the person slept. This helps the nurse evaluate if the person develops a regular sleep pattern. *See Focus on Older Persons: Promoting Sleep. See Focus on Long-Term Care: Promoting Sleep.*

---

### FOCUS ON OLDER PERSONS
#### PROMOTING SLEEP

Older persons have less energy than younger people. They may nap during the day. You need to let the person sleep. Organize the person's care to allow uninterrupted naps.

Some older persons have dementia. Sleep problems are common in some types of dementia. Night wandering is common. Restlessness and confusion increase at night. This increases the risk of falls. It often helps to quietly and calmly direct the person to his or her room. Nighttime wandering in a safe and supervised setting is helpful for some people. The measures listed in Box 23-8 also are tried. Follow the care plan.

---

### FOCUS ON LONG-TERM CARE
#### PROMOTING SLEEP

Many residents have rituals and routines before bedtime. They are allowed if safe. The person may perform hygiene measures in a certain order. Some persons like to check on friends in the center before going to bed. Some have the responsibility of turning off lights at bedtime. A bedtime snack may be important. Some watch TV in bed. Others may read religious writings, pray, or say a rosary before going to sleep.

The person is involved in planning care. The person chooses when to nap or go to bed. The person chooses the measures that promote comfort, rest, and sleep. Follow the care plan and the person's wishes.

---

### BOX 23-8 NURSING MEASURES TO PROMOTE SLEEP

- Organize care for uninterrupted rest.
- Avoid physical activity before bedtime.
- Encourage the person to avoid business or family matters before bedtime.
- Allow a flexible bedtime. Bedtime is when the person is tired, not a certain time.
- Provide a comfortable room temperature.
- Let the person take a warm bath or shower.
- Provide a bedtime snack.
- Avoid caffeine (coffee, tea, colas, chocolate).
- Avoid alcoholic beverages.
- Have the person void before going to bed.
- Make sure incontinent persons are clean and dry. Change a baby's diaper.
- Follow bedtime routines.
- Have the person wear loose-fitting sleepwear.
- Provide for warmth (blankets, socks) for those who tend to be cold.
- Reduce noise.
- Darken the room—close shades, blinds, and the privacy curtain. Shut off or dim lights.
- Dim lights in hallways and the nursing unit.
- Make sure linens are clean, dry, and wrinkle-free.
- Position the person in good alignment and in a comfortable position.
- Support body parts as ordered.
- Give a back massage.
- Provide measures to relieve pain.
- Let the person read. Read to children.
- Let the person listen to music or watch TV.
- Assist with relaxation exercises as ordered.
- Sit and talk with the person.

# ■ REVIEW QUESTIONS ■

Circle the **BEST** answer.

1  These statements are about pain. Which is *false?*
   a  Pain can be seen, heard, smelled, or felt.
   b  Pain is a warning from the body.
   c  Pain is personal. It is different for each person.
   d  Pain is used to make diagnoses.

2  A person has pain in the left chest, the left jaw, and the left shoulder and arm. This is
   a  Acute pain
   b  Chronic pain
   c  Radiating pain
   d  Phantom pain

3  Mr. Smith complains of pain. You should do the following *except*
   a  Ask him to point to where the pain is felt
   b  Ask him when the pain started
   c  Ask him to describe the pain
   d  Ask to look at the pain

4  The nurse gives Mr. Smith a drug for pain. Care is scheduled for this time. You should
   a  Give care before the drug is given
   b  Give care right after the drug is given
   c  Wait 30 minutes to let the drug take effect
   d  Omit the care for the day

5  Mr. Smith was given a drug for pain. To protect him from injury, you should do the following *except*
   a  Keep the bed in the high position
   b  Raise bed rails as directed
   c  Check on him every 10 to 15 minutes
   d  Provide help if he needs to get up

6  Which measure will *not* help relieve pain?
   a  Providing blankets as needed
   b  Keeping the room well lighted
   c  Providing soft music
   d  Giving a back massage

7  Mr. Smith's care plan has these measures. Which will *not* help him rest or sleep?
   a  Having him void before rest or sleep
   b  Helping him to a comfortable position
   c  Helping him walk before rest or sleep
   d  Letting him choose sleepwear

8  Mr. Smith tires easily. His morning care includes a bath, hair care, and getting dressed. His bed is made after he is dressed. When should he rest?
   a  After you complete morning care
   b  After his bath and before hair care
   c  After you make the bed
   d  When he needs to

9  These statements are about sleep. Which is *false?*
   a  Tissue healing and repair occur during sleep.
   b  Voluntary muscle activity increases during sleep.
   c  Sleep refreshes and renews the person.
   d  Sleep lowers stress, tension, and anxiety.

10  Mr. Smith was awake several nights when he first entered the hospital. Which is *false?*
    a  His circadian rhythm may be affected.
    b  NREM and REM sleep are affected.
    c  His biological clock will still tell him when to sleep and wake up.
    d  His functioning may be affected.

11  Mr. Smith is 35 years old. When healthy, he probably needs about
    a  12 to 14 hours of sleep per day
    b  8 to 9 hours of sleep per day
    c  7 to 8 hours of sleep per day
    d  About 6 hours of sleep per day

12  Which will prevent sleep?
    a  Chocolate      c  Milk
    b  Cheese         d  Beef

13  Mr. Smith awakens often during the night. He has problems answering questions and seems moody. His pulse is irregular. His eyes are red and puffy. He is showing signs of
    a  Acute pain
    b  Sleep deprivation
    c  Enuresis
    d  Distraction

14  These measures are part of Mr. Smith's care plan. Which should you question?
    a  Let Mr. Smith choose his bedtime.
    b  Provide hot tea and a cheese sandwich at bedtime.
    c  Position him in good alignment.
    d  Follow his bedtime rituals.

*Answers to these questions are on p. 818.*

# 24

# Admissions, Transfers, and Discharges

# OBJECTIVES

- Define the key terms listed in this chapter
- Describe your role in the admission, transfer, and discharge processes
- Explain how to prepare the room for a new admission
- Measure height and weight
- Explain the reasons for transfers to another nursing unit
- Perform the procedures described in this chapter

# KEY TERMS

**admission** Official entry of a person into an agency

**discharge** Official departure of a person from an agency

**transfer** Moving a person from one room or nursing unit to another

Admission to a hospital or nursing center cause anxiety and fear in patients, residents, and families. They may worry about treatments and surgeries and their outcomes. They may fear serious health problems. The fear of pain is common. People admitted to nursing centers have fears about not going home.

Patients, residents, and their families are in new, strange settings. They worry about where to go, what to do, and what to expect. They worry about meals, finding the bathroom, and how to get help. Strange sights and sounds frighten some people. Similar concerns occur with transfers to other nursing units. Discharge is usually a happy time. However, the person may need home care or long-term care.

Admission, transfer, and discharge are critical events. They involve:
- Privacy and confidentiality
- Reporting and recording
- Understanding and communicating with the person
- Communicating with the health team
- Respect for the person and the person's property
- Being kind, courteous, and respectful
- Promoting comfort and safety

> **SAFETY ALERT:** *Admissions, Transfers, and Discharges*
> The person may develop pain or distress during admission, a transfer, or discharge. If so, call for the nurse at once. Stay with the person. When the nurse arrives, assist as needed.

> **DELEGATION GUIDELINES:** *Admissions, Transfers, and Discharges*
> When admitting, transferring, or discharging a person, you need this information from the nurse:
> - If you need to admit, transfer, or discharge the person
> - The person's method of transportation to or from the agency—car, ambulance, or wheelchair van
> - How the person will move about within the agency—walking, wheelchair, stretcher, or bed
> - Which room and bed to prepare
> - What special equipment and supplies are needed

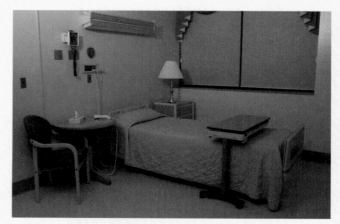

**FIG. 24-1** The room is ready for a new admission.

## ADMISSIONS

Except in emergencies, the admission process starts in the admitting office. **Admission** is the official entry of a person into an agency. Admitting staff or a nurse obtains identifying information for the admission record. This includes the person's full name, age, date of birth, doctor's name, social security number, and religion. The person is given an identification number and an ID bracelet (Chapter 10). A general consent for treatment is signed at this time.

The admitting office tells the nursing unit when there is a new patient or resident. The person's room and bed number are given. Staff from the admitting office brings the person to the nursing unit. In some agencies, the person can walk if able. Most persons require transport by wheelchair or stretcher. *See Focus on Long-Term Care: Admissions.*

### PREPARING THE ROOM

The room must be ready for the new patient or resident. You usually do this. Figure 24-1 shows a room ready for a person to arrive.

*Text continued on p. 522.*

### FOCUS ON LONG-TERM CARE
#### ADMISSIONS

Nursing centers have admission coordinators. They make the person's admission simple and easy. Often admission procedures are done 2 or 3 days before the person enters the center. Identifying information is obtained from the person or family member.

The room assignment is made before the person arrives. Some residents arrive by ambulance or wheelchair van. The attendants take them to their rooms. Some arrive by car. Nurses or nursing assistants take them to their rooms. Some residents want a family member with them. This is a critical and emotional time for the person and family. They do not part until comfortable doing so. Remember, the center is now the person's home.

Persons with dementia and their families may need special help during the admission process. Confusion may increase in the new setting. Fear, agitation, and wanting to leave are common. Family members also are fearful. Many feel guilty about the need for nursing center care. The health team helps the person and family feel safe and welcome.

## PREPARING THE PERSON'S ROOM

### PROCEDURE

1 Follow *Delegation Guidelines: Admissions, Transfers, and Discharges.*
2 Know which room and bed to prepare. Find out if the person will arrive by wheelchair or stretcher.
3 Practice hand hygiene.
4 Collect the following:
   - Admission kit—wash basin, soap, toothpaste, toothbrush, water pitcher, and so on
   - Bedpan and urinal (for a man)
   - Admission form (Fig. 24-2, p. 520)
   - Urine specimen container (if a urine specimen is ordered)
   - Thermometer
   - Sphygmomanometer
   - Stethoscope
   - Gown or pajamas (if needed)
   - Towels and washcloths
   - IV pole (if needed)
   - Other items requested by the nurse

5 If the person is ambulatory or arrives by wheelchair:
   a Open the bed for a hospital patient. Leave the bed closed for a nursing center resident.
   b Lower the bed to its lowest position.
6 If the person arrives by stretcher:
   a Make a surgical bed (Chapter 15)
   b Raise the bed to its highest level.
7 Attach the signal light to the bed linens.
8 Place the thermometer, sphygmomanometer, stethoscope, and admission form on the overbed table.
9 Place the gown or pajamas on the bed.
10 Place the wash basin, soap, toothpaste, toothbrush, and so on in the bedside stand.
11 Place the bedpan, urinal, towels, and washcloths in the bedside stand.
12 Place the water pitcher, glass, and specimen container on the bedside stand or overbed table.
13 Decontaminate your hands.

# ADMISSION NURSING ASSESSMENT

## STATUS UPON ADMISSION

### Admission Notes

Date of admission _____ / _____ / _____    Time _____ a.m. / p.m.

Transported by _____

Accompanied by _____

Age _____ Sex _____ Weight _____ Height: _____ Ft. _____ In.

Vitals: T _____ P _____ (❏ Reg ❏ Irreg) R _____ B/P _____ / _____

Attending physician notified? ❏ No ❏ Yes, date/time _____ / _____ / _____ _____ a.m. / p.m.

Diagnosis: _____ Date last chest x-ray or PPD _____ / _____ / _____

### Allergies

Meds _____

_____

Food _____

_____

Other _____

### Skin Condition

Using the diagrams provided, indicate all body marks such as old/recent scars (surgical and other), bruises, discolorations, abrasions, pressure ulcers, or questionable markings. Indicate size, depth (in cms), color and drainage.

COMMENTS: _____

_____

_____

SPECIAL TREATMENTS & PROCEDURES:

_____

_____

### PAIN

(As described by resident/representative)

**Frequency:**
❏ No pain          ❏ Daily, but not
❏ Less than daily    constant
                   ❏ Constant

**Location:** _____

**Intensity:**
❏ No pain           ❏ Severe pain
❏ Mild pain         ❏ Horrible pain
❏ Distressing pain  ❏ Excruciating
                     pain

Pain on admission:
❏ No  ❏ Yes, describe _____
_____

RIGHT   LEFT

## CURRENT STATUS

### General Skin Condition

Check all that apply.
❏ Reddened  ❏ Pale  ❏ Jaundiced
  ❏ Cyanotic  ❏ Ashen
❏ Dry  ❏ Moist  ❏ Oily  ❏ Warm  ❏ Cold
❏ Edema, site _____

### Physical Status (describe if applicable otherwise indicate NA)

Paralysis/paresis-site, degree _____
Contracture(s)-site, degree _____
Congenital anomalies _____
Prosthesis: _____
Other _____

### Functional Status

**TRANSFERS-ABLE TO TRANSFER**
❏ Independently
❏ 1 person assist
❏ 2 person assist
❏ Total assist

**WEIGHT BEARING-ABLE TO BEAR**
❏ Full weight
❏ Partial weight
❏ Non-weight bearing

**AMBULATION-ABLE TO AMBULATE**
❏ Independently
❏ 1 person assist
❏ 2 person assist
❏ With device
   Type _____
❏ Wheelchair only
❏ Wheelchair/propels self
❏ Bedrest

**SUPPORTIVE DEVICES USED:**
❏ Elastic hose      ❏ Footboard
❏ Bed cradle        ❏ Air mattress
❏ Sheepskin         ❏ Eggcrate
❏ Hand rolls  ❏ Sling  ❏ Trapeze
❏ Other _____

❏ Other _____

### Drug Therapy

| DRUG | DOSE/FREQUENCY | | DRUG | DOSE/FREQUENCY |
|---|---|---|---|---|
| 1 | | 6 | | |
| 2 | | 7 | | |
| 3 | | 8 | | |
| 4 | | 9 | | |
| 5 | | 10 | | |

| NAME–Last | First | Middle | Attending Physician | Record No. | Room/Bed |
|---|---|---|---|---|---|
| | | | | | |

**ADMISSION NURSING ASSESSMENT**
❏ Continued on Reverse

**FIG. 24-2** Admission form. (Courtesy Briggs Corp., Des Moines, Iowa.)

## CURRENT STATUS - CONTINUED

| Hearing | Right | Left | R & L | Vision | Right | Left | R & L | Communication |
|---|---|---|---|---|---|---|---|---|
| Adequate | | | | Adequate | | | | ❑ Clear |
| Adequate w/aid | | | | Adequate w/glasses | | | | ❑ Aphasic  ❑ Dysphasic |
| Poor | | | | Poor | | | | Language(s) Spoken: |
| Deaf | | | | Blind | | | | |

### Oral Assessment / Eating/Nutrition

**Oral Assessment**

Complete oral cavity exam:  ❑ Yes  ❑ No
  If yes, condition _____
_____
Own teeth:  ❑ Yes  ❑ No
  If yes, condition _____
Dentures: Upper  ❑ Comp  ❑ Part
  Lower  ❑ Comp  ❑ Part
Do dentures fit?  ❑ Yes  ❑ No

**Eating/Nutrition**

❑ Dependent  ❑ Independent  ❑ Needs assist
❑ Dysphagic; reason _____
❑ Adaptive equipment (specify) _____
Type/consistency of diet _____
_____

Food likes _____
Food dislikes _____
_____
Bev. preference _____
HS snack preferred:  ❑ Yes  ❑ No

### Sleep Patterns / Bathing/Oral Hyg. / General Grooming

| Sleep Patterns | | Bathing/Oral Hyg. | Indep. | Assist | Dep. | General Grooming | Indep. | Assist | Dep. |
|---|---|---|---|---|---|---|---|---|---|
| Usual bed time _____ a.m./p.m. | | Tub | | | | Shave | | | |
| Usual arising time _____ a.m./p.m. | | Shower | | | | Grooming | | | |
| Usual nap time _____ a.m./p.m. | | Bed bath | | | | Dressing | | | |
| Other _____ | | Oral hygiene | | | | Shampoo | | | |

### Psychosocial Functioning

**FAMILY RELATIONSHIPS:**
  Members visit (frequency) _____
_____
  Closest relationship with _____

**ORIENTED:** ❑ Yes  ❑ No, if No:
**DISORIENTED TO:** ❑ Time  ❑ Place
  ❑ Person
**RESIDENT GIVEN EXPLANATION OF/OR INVOLVED IN PLAN OF CARE?** ❑ Yes  ❑ No
**RESIDENT ORIENTED TO FACILITY?**  ❑ Call light  ❑ Bathroom  ❑ Mealtime  ❑ Activities

**WHICH WORDS BEST DESCRIBE RESIDENT?** ❑ Alert  ❑ Angry  ❑ Fearful
  ❑ Noisy  ❑ Friendly  ❑ Cooperative  ❑ Lethargic  ❑ _____
  ❑ Non-questioning  ❑ Combative
**ANSWERS QUESTIONS:** ❑ Readily  ❑ Reluctantly  ❑ Inappropriately
**MOOD:** ❑ Passive  ❑ Depressed  ❑ Elated  ❑ Quiet  ❑ Secure
  ❑ Questioning  ❑ Talkative  ❑ Homesick  ❑ Wanders mentally
  ❑ Hyperactive  ❑ _____
**COMPREHENSION:** ❑ Slow  ❑ Quick  ❑ Unable to understand
**MOTIVATION:** ❑ Good  ❑ Fair  ❑ Poor
**PERSONAL HABITS:** Smokes?  ❑ Yes  ❑ No  Uses alcohol?  ❑ Yes  ❑ No

### Bowel and Bladder Evaluation

Uses:  ❑ Toilet  ❑ Urinal  ❑ Bedpan  ❑ Bedside commode
**BOWEL HABITS:** Continent?  ❑ Yes  ❑ No  Constipated?  ❑ Yes  ❑ No  Laxative used?  ❑ Yes  ❑ No
  Enemas used?  ❑ Yes  ❑ No  Last bowel movement _____ a.m./p.m.
**BLADDER HABITS:** Continent?  ❑ Yes  ❑ No  Dribbles?  ❑ Yes  ❑ No  Catheter?  ❑ Yes, type _____  ❑ No
  Urine color _____  Consistency _____  Time last voiding _____ a.m./p.m.

### Restorative Programs Indicated / Therapy Indicated

**Restorative Programs Indicated**

Based on the foregoing assessment, check all that apply.

❑ ROM
❑ Splint or brace assistance
❑ Bed mobility training & skill practice
❑ Transfer training & skill practice
❑ Walking training & skill practice

❑ Dressing/grooming training & skill practice
❑ Eating/swallowing training & skill practice
❑ Appliance/prosthesis training & skill practice
❑ Communication training & skill practice
❑ Scheduled toileting
❑ Bladder retraining

Comments: _____
_____

**Therapy Indicated**

❑ Physical
❑ Occupational
❑ Speech
Comments: _____
_____
_____
_____
_____
_____

Completed by:
Signature/Title _____  Date _____

| NAME–Last | First | Middle | Attending Physician | Record No. | Room/Bed |
|---|---|---|---|---|---|
| | | | | | |

**ADMISSION NURSING ASSESSMENT**

**FIG. 24-2, CONT'D.** For legend see opposite page.

## ADMITTING THE PERSON

A nurse usually greets and admits the person. The nurse may ask you to do so if the person has no discomfort or distress. Use the admission record to find out the person's name. To greet the person, call him or her by name. Using your name and title, introduce yourself to the person and family members present (Fig. 24-3). Also make roommate introductions.

During the admission procedure you will:
- Collect some information for the admission form
- Weigh and measure the person
- Obtain a urine specimen if ordered (Chapter 26)
- Orient the person to the room, the nursing unit, and the agency

    *See Focus on Long-Term Care: Admitting the Person.*

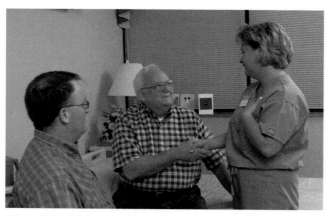

**FIG. 24-3** The nursing assistant introduces herself to the person and family member.

### FOCUS ON LONG-TERM CARE
#### ADMITTING THE PERSON

The person needs to feel comfortable, safe, and secure. Do not rush into admission procedures. Rather, treat the person and family like guests in your home. Offer them coffee, tea, or other beverage. Visit with them. Tell them some of the many good things about the center.

Introduce the person's roommate and residents in nearby rooms. Write down their names for the new resident. Remembering names is hard for many people. This way the person will know others when the family leaves. Other residents can provide comfort and support. They understand, better than anyone else, what entering a nursing center is like.

The center is the person's home. Help make the room as homelike as possible. Also help the person unpack. The person might need help putting clothes away. The person might want to hang pictures or display photos. Show caring and compassion. Help the person feel safe, comfortable, and secure.

When the person is comfortable, complete the admission. A nurse or social worker explains the resident's rights to the person and family. They also get a booklet explaining them.

## ADMITTING THE PERSON

### QUALITY OF LIFE

Remember to:
- Knock before entering the person's room
- Address the person by name
- Introduce yourself by name and title

### PRE-PROCEDURE

1 Follow *Delegation Guidelines: Admissions, Transfers, and Discharges*, p. 518. See *Safety Alert: Admissions, Transfers, and Discharges*, p. 518.

2 Practice hand hygiene.
3 Prepare the room.

### PROCEDURE

4 Greet the person by name. Ask if he or she prefers a certain name.
5 Introduce yourself to the person and others present. Give your name and title. Explain that you assist the nurses in giving care.
6 Introduce the roommate.
7 Provide for privacy. Ask family members or friends to leave the room. Tell them how much time you need and where they can wait comfortably. (Let a family member or friend stay if the person prefers.)
8 Have the person put on a gown or pajamas. Assist as needed. (A nursing center resident can stay dressed if his or her condition permits.)
9 Provide for comfort. The person is in bed or in a chair as directed by the nurse.
10 Measure vital signs (Chapter 21), and measure height and weight. Collect other information for the admission form as requested by the nurse.
11 Complete a clothing and personal belongings list (Chapter 10).
12 Hang clothes in the closet. Put personal items in the drawers and bedside stand.
13 Explain any ordered activity limits.
14 Obtain a urine specimen if ordered. Take the specimen to the storage area or laboratory. Clean equipment, and decontaminate your hands.
15 Orient the person to the area:
  a Give names of the nurses.
  b Identify items in the bedside stand. Explain the purpose of each item.
  c Show how the signal light is used.
  d Show how to use the bed and TV controls.
  e Explain how to make phone calls. Place the phone within reach.
  f Explain visiting hours and policies.
  g Explain where to find the nurses' station, lounge, chapel, dining room, gift shop, and other areas.
  h Explain about newspaper, library, activity, education, religious, and other services.
  i Identify staff—x-ray, laboratory, housekeeping, dietary, physical therapy, and others. Also identify students who are in the agency.
  j Explain when meals and nourishments are served.
16 Fill the water pitcher and glass if oral fluids are allowed.
17 Place the signal light within reach. Place other controls and needed items within reach.
18 Keep the bed in its lowest position.
19 Raise or lower bed rails. Follow the care plan.
20 Unscreen the person.
21 Clean used equipment. Discard used disposable items. Decontaminate your hands.
22 Provide a denture container if needed. Label it with the person's name and room number.
23 Label personal property and personal care equipment for the nursing center resident. Items are labeled with the person's name.

### POST-PROCEDURE

24 Decontaminate your hands.
25 Report and record your observations.

**MEASURING HEIGHT AND WEIGHT.** Height and weight are measured on admission. The person wears only a gown or pajamas. Clothes add weight. Shoes or slippers add weight and height. The person voids before being weighed. A full bladder affects the weight measurement. If a urine specimen is needed, collect it at this time.

Standing, chair, and lift scales are used (Fig. 24-4). Chair and lift scales are used for persons who cannot stand.

Balance the scale at zero before weighing the person. For balance scales, move the weights to zero. A digital scale should read at zero.

The person is weighed daily, weekly, or monthly. This is done to measure weight gain or loss. Weigh the person at the same time of day. Before breakfast is the best time. Food and fluids add weight.

See *Focus on Children: Measuring Height and Weight.*

---

**DELEGATION GUIDELINES:** *Measuring Height and Weight*

Before measuring height and weight, you need this information from the nurse and the care plan:
- When to measure height and weight
- What scale to use
- How to measure height—standing scale or in bed

---

**SAFETY ALERT:** *Measuring Height and Weight*
Follow the manufacturer's instructions when using chair or lift scales. Also follow the agency's procedures. Practice safety measures to prevent falls.

---

**FOCUS ON CHILDREN**
**MEASURING HEIGHT AND WEIGHT**

Birth weight is the baseline for measuring an infant's growth. Weight measurements also are used for the nursing process. To weigh infants, see Chapter 38.

Length is measured in children younger than 2 years. The child lies on a measuring board or on a paper. Two people hold the child still. One holds the head still, and the other extends and holds the legs still. Length is measured from the top of the head to the heels. If using paper, mark the paper at the head and heels. Measure the distance between the two points.

---

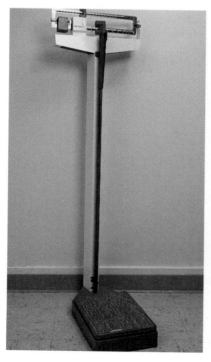
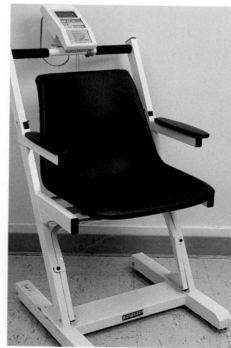
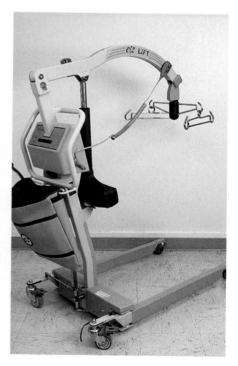

A    B    C

**FIG. 24-4** Types of scales. **A,** Standing scale. **B,** Chair scale. **C,** Lift scale.

## MEASURING HEIGHT AND WEIGHT

*NNAAP™*

### QUALITY OF LIFE

Remember to:
- Knock before entering the person's room
- Address the person by name
- Introduce yourself by name and title

### PRE-PROCEDURE

1 Follow *Delegation Guidelines: Measuring Height and Weight.* See *Safety Alert: Measuring Height and Weight.*
2 Explain the procedure to the person.
3 Ask the person to void.
4 Bring the scale and paper towels to the person's room.
5 Practice hand hygiene.
6 Identify the person. Check the ID bracelet against the assignment sheet. Call the person by name.
7 Provide for privacy.

### PROCEDURE

8 *Balance scale:*
  a Place the paper towels on the scale platform.
  b Raise the height rod.
  c Move the weights to zero (0). The pointer is in the middle.
  d Have the person remove the robe and footwear. Assist as needed.
  e Help the person stand on the scale.
  f Move the weights until the balance pointer is in the middle (Fig. 24-5, p. 526).
  g Record the weight on your note pad or assignment sheet.
  h Ask the person to stand very straight.
  i Lower the height rod until it rests on the person's head (Fig. 24-6, p. 526).
  j Record the height on your note pad or assignment sheet.
9 *Chair scale:*
  a Place both weights on zero (0). Balance the scale following the manufacturer's instructions.
  b Help the person transfer from the wheelchair to the chair scale (see procedure *Transferring the Person to a Chair or Wheelchair,* p. 259).
  c Place the person's feet on the foot platform.

  d Move the weights until the balance pointer is in the middle. Or note the digital display.
  e Record the weight on your notepad or assignment sheet.
10 *Lift scale:*
  a Attach the sling to the lift.
  b Place both weights on zero (0).
  c Level and balance the scale. Follow the manufacturer's instructions.
  d Remove the sling from the scale.
  e Place the person on the sling, and attach it to the lift. Raise the person about 4 inches off the bed (see procedure: *Transferring the Person Using a Mechanical Lift,* p. 267).
  f Move the weights until the balance pointer is in the middle. Or note the digital display.
  g Record the weight on your notepad or assignment sheet.
  h Lower the person to the bed.
  i Remove the sling.
11 Help the person put on a robe and nonskid footwear if he or she will be up. Or help the person back to bed.

### POST-PROCEDURE

12 Provide for comfort.
13 Place the signal light within reach.
14 Raise or lower bed rails. Follow the care plan.
15 Unscreen the person.
16 Discard the paper towels.
17 Return the scale to its proper place.
18 Decontaminate your hands.
19 Report and record the measurements.

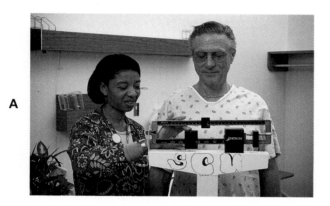

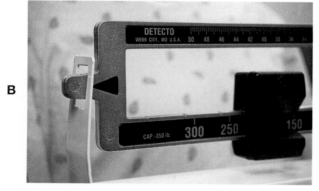

**FIG. 24-5 A,** The person is weighed. **B,** The weight is read when the balance pointer is in the middle.

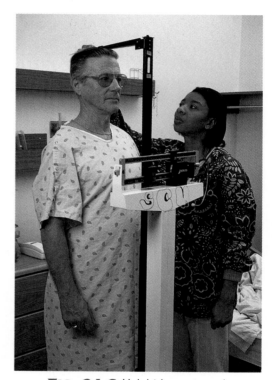

**FIG. 24-6** Height is measured.

## MEASURING HEIGHT—THE PERSON IS IN BED

### QUALITY OF LIFE

Remember to:
- Knock before entering the person's room
- Address the person by name
- Introduce yourself by name and title

### PRE-PROCEDURE

1 Follow *Delegation Guidelines: Measuring Height and Weight*, p. 524. See *Safety Alert: Measuring Height and Weight*, p. 524.
2 Explain the procedure to the person.
3 Practice hand hygiene.
4 Collect a measuring tape and ruler.

5 Ask a co-worker to help you.
6 Identify the person. Check the ID bracelet against the assignment sheet. Call the person by name.
7 Provide for privacy.

### PROCEDURE

8 Position the person supine if this position is allowed.
9 Have your co-worker hold the end of the measuring tape at the person's heel.
10 Pull the measuring tape along the person's body until it extends past the head (Fig. 24-7).

11 Place the ruler flat across the top of the person's head. It extends from the person's head to the measuring tape. Make sure the ruler is level.
12 Record the height on your notepad or assignment sheet.

### POST-PROCEDURE

13 Provide for comfort.
14 Raise or lower bed rails. Follow the care plan.
15 Place the signal light within reach.
16 Unscreen the person.

17 Return equipment to its proper location.
18 Decontaminate your hands.
19 Report and record the height.

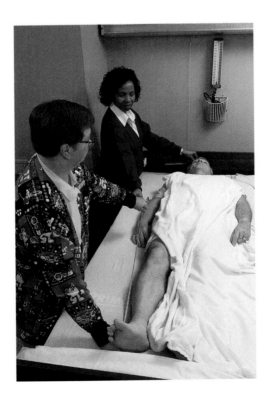

**FIG. 24-7** The person is measured in bed. The tape measure extends from the top of the head to the heel. The ruler is flat across the top of the person's head.

# TRANSFERS

A **transfer** is moving a person from one room or nursing unit to another. Transfers usually relate to a change in condition. Sometimes the person requests a room change. Sometimes roommates do not get along. Changes in care needs are other reasons for transfers.

The doctor, nurse, or social worker explains the reasons for the transfer. The family and business office are notified. You may assist in the transfer. Or you carry out the entire procedure. The person is transported by wheelchair or stretcher. Sometimes the bed is used.

Support and reassurance are needed. The person does not know the staff on the new unit. Use good communication skills. Avoid pat answers such as "It will be OK." Touch can provide comfort at this time. Also introduce the person to the staff and roommate. Wish the person well as you leave him or her.

## TRANSFERRING THE PERSON TO ANOTHER NURSING UNIT

### QUALITY OF LIFE

Remember to:
- Knock before entering the person's room
- Address the person by name
- Introduce yourself by name and title

### PRE-PROCEDURE

1 Follow *Delegation Guidelines: Admissions, Transfers, and Discharges*, p. 518. See *Safety Alert: Admissions, Transfers, and Discharges*, p. 518.
2 Find out where the person is going. Find out if you need to use the bed, a wheelchair, or a stretcher.
3 Explain the procedure to the person.
4 Get a stretcher or wheelchair, a bath blanket, and a utility cart if needed.
5 Practice hand hygiene.
6 Identify the person. Check the ID bracelet against the transfer slip. Call the person by name.

### PROCEDURE

7 Collect the person's belongings and bedside equipment. Place them on the utility cart.
8 Assist the person to the wheelchair or stretcher. Cover the person with a bath blanket.
9 Transport the person to the new room.
10 Introduce the person to the receiving nurse.
11 Help transfer the person to the bed or chair. Help position the person.
12 Bring personal belongings and equipment to the new room. Help put them away.
13 Report the following to the receiving nurse:
  a How the person tolerated the transfer
  b That a nurse will bring the chart, care plan, Kardex, and drugs

### POST-PROCEDURE

14 Return the wheelchair or stretcher and the utility cart to the storage area.
15 Decontaminate your hands.
16 Report and record the following:
- The time of transfer
- Where the person was taken
- How the person was transferred (bed, wheelchair, or stretcher)
- How the person tolerated the transfer
- Who received the person
- Any other observations

17 Strip the bed, and clean the unit. Wear gloves for this step. (The housekeeping staff may do this step.)
18 Decontaminate your hands.
19 Make a closed bed.
20 Decontaminate your hands.

# DISCHARGES

Discharges usually are planned a few days in advance. **Discharge** is the official departure of a person from the agency. The person may be going home, to another hospital, or to a nursing center. Some people may need home care.

The doctor, nurse, dietitian, social worker, and other health team members plan the person's discharge. They teach the person and family about diet, exercise, and drugs. They also teach about procedures and treatments. They arrange for home care, equipment, and special therapies as needed. A doctor's appointment is given.

The nurse tells you when to start the discharge procedure. The doctor must write a discharge order before the person is allowed to leave. The nurse tells you when the person can leave and how to transport him or her. Usually a wheelchair is used. Some agencies let the person walk. Some persons leave by ambulance. Ambulance staff are responsible for the transport.

Use good communication skills when assisting with a discharge. Wish the person and family well as they leave the agency.

A person may want to leave the agency without the doctor's order. Tell the nurse at once if the person expresses the wish or intent to leave. The nurse or social worker handles this matter.

## DISCHARGING THE PERSON

### QUALITY OF LIFE

Remember to:
- Knock before entering the person's room
- Address the person by name
- Introduce yourself by name and title

### PRE-PROCEDURE

1 Follow *Delegation Guidelines: Admissions, Transfers, and Discharges*, p. 518. See *Safety Alert: Admissions, Transfers, and Discharges*, p. 518.
2 Make sure the person can leave. Find out if the person has transportation.
3 Explain the procedure to the person.
4 Practice hand hygiene.
5 Identify the person. Check the ID bracelet against the discharge slip. Call the person by name.

### PROCEDURE

6 Provide for privacy.
7 Help the person dress as needed.
8 Help the person pack. Check all drawers and closets. Make sure all items are collected.
9 Check off the clothing list and the personal belongings list. Give the list to the nurse.
10 Tell the nurse that the person is ready for the final visit. The nurse:
  a Gives prescriptions written by the doctor
  b Provides discharge instructions
  c Gets valuables from the safe
  d Has the person sign the clothing and personal belongings lists
11 Get a wheelchair and a utility cart for the person's belongings. Ask a co-worker to help you.
12 Assist the person into the wheelchair. (See procedure: *Transferring the Person to a Chair or Wheelchair*, p. 259.)
13 Take the person to the exit area. Lock the wheelchair wheels.
14 Help the person out of the wheelchair and into the car.
15 Help put the belongings into the car.

### POST-PROCEDURE

16 Return the wheelchair and cart to the storage area.
17 Decontaminate your hands.
18 Report and record the following:
- The time of discharge
- How the person was transported
- Whom the person was with
- The person's destination
- Any other observations

19 Strip the bed, and clean the unit. Wear gloves for this step. (This may be done by housekeeping staff.)
20 Decontaminate your hands.
21 Make a closed bed.
22 Decontaminate your hands.

# ■ REVIEW QUESTIONS ■

Circle **T** if the statement is true and **F** if it is false.

1   **T F**  Identifying information is obtained when the person arrives on the nursing unit.
2   **T F**  The person is usually transported to the nursing unit by wheelchair or stretcher.
3   **T F**  The bed is opened when preparing the room for a hospital patient.
4   **T F**  The person is greeted by name when he or she arrives on the nursing unit.
5   **T F**  A person complains of pain. You report the pain after completing the admission procedure.
6   **T F**  A urine specimen may be needed on admission.

7   **T F**  You help orient the person to the new setting.
8   **T F**  A robe and slippers are worn when the person is weighed and measured.
9   **T F**  A list is made of clothing and personal belongings during the admission process.
10  **T F**  A person's condition may require a transfer to another nursing unit.
11  **T F**  A doctor's order is required for discharge from the agency.
12  **T F**  You teach the person about diet and drugs.

*Answers to these questions are on p. 818.*

# 25

# Assisting With the Physical Examination

## OBJECTIVES

■ Define the key terms listed in this chapter

■ Explain what to do before, during, and after an examination (exam)

■ Identify the equipment used for an exam

■ Describe how to prepare and drape a person for an exam

■ Explain the rules for assisting with an exam

■ Perform the procedure described in this chapter

## KEY TERMS

**dorsal recumbent position** The supine position with the legs together; horizontal recumbent position

**horizontal recumbent position** The dorsal recumbent position

**knee-chest position** The person kneels and rests the body on the knees and chest; head is turned to one side, arms are above the head or flexed at the elbows, back is straight, and body is flexed about 90 degrees at the hips

**laryngeal mirror** An instrument used to examine the mouth, teeth, and throat

**lithotomy position** The person lies on the back with the hips at the edge of the exam table, knees are flexed, hips are externally rotated, and feet are in stirrups

**nasal speculum** An instrument used to examine the inside of the nose

**ophthalmoscope** A lighted instrument used to examine the internal structures of the eye

**otoscope** A lighted instrument used to examine the external ear and the eardrum (tympanic membrane)

**percussion hammer** An instrument used to tap body parts to test reflexes; reflex hammer

**tuning fork** An instrument vibrated to test hearing

**vaginal speculum** An instrument used to open the vagina so it and the cervix can be examined

Doctors and many RNs perform physical exams. You might be asked to assist them. Exams are done to:

■ Promote health
■ Determine fitness for work
■ Diagnose disease

## YOUR ROLE

What you do depends on agency policies and procedures. It also depends on the examiner's preferences. You may do some or all of the following:

■ Collect linens to drape the person and for the procedure.

■ Collect exam equipment and supplies.
■ Prepare the room.
■ Provide lighting.
■ Transport the person to and from the exam room.
■ Measure vital signs, height, and weight.
■ Position and drape the person.
■ Hand equipment and supplies to the examiner.
■ Label specimen containers.
■ Discard used supplies.
■ Clean equipment.
■ Help the person dress or to a comfortable position after the exam.
■ Follow agency policy for soiled linen.

# EQUIPMENT

Some items needed for an exam are used to give care. You need to know the instruments in Figure 25-1:

- **Laryngeal mirror**—used to examine the mouth, teeth, and throat.
- **Nasal speculum**—used to examine the inside of the nose.
- **Ophthalmoscope**—a lighted instrument used to examine the internal structures of the eye.
- **Otoscope**—a lighted instrument used to examine the external ear and the eardrum (tympanic membrane). Some scopes have parts for examining eyes and ears. They are changed into an ophthalmoscope or otoscope.

- **Percussion hammer**—used to tap body parts to test reflexes. It is also called a *reflex hammer.*
- **Tuning fork**—vibrated to test hearing.
- **Vaginal speculum**—used to open the vagina so it and the cervix can be examined.

Many agencies have exam trays in the supply department. If not, collect the items listed in the procedure: *Preparing the Person for an Examination,* p. 535. Arrange them on a tray or table.

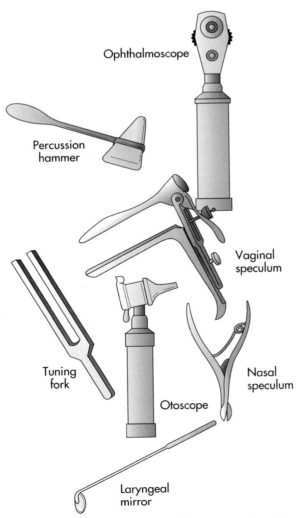

Ophthalmoscope

Percussion hammer

Vaginal speculum

Tuning fork

Otoscope

Nasal speculum

Laryngeal mirror

**FIG. 25-1** Instruments used for a physical exam.

# PREPARING THE PERSON

The physical exam concerns many people. They worry about possible findings. Discomfort, embarrassment, fearing exposure, and not knowing the procedure cause anxiety. You must be sensitive to the person's feelings and concerns. The person is prepared physically and mentally for the exam. The nurse explains its purpose and what to expect. *See Focus on Long-Term Care: Preparing the Person.*

Privacy is protected. The person is screened and the room door closed. All clothes are removed for a complete exam. A patient gown is worn. It reduces the naked feeling and the fear of exposure. So does covering the person with a drape—paper drape, bath blanket, sheet, or drawsheet. Explain that there is little exposure during the exam. Only the part being examined is exposed. *See Focus on Children: Preparing the Person.*

The person voids before the exam. An empty bladder lets the examiner feel the abdominal organs. A full bladder can change the normal position and shape of organs. It also causes discomfort, especially when the abdominal organs are felt. If a urine specimen is needed, obtain it at this time. Explain how to collect the specimen (Chapter 26). Label the container.

Measure height, weight, and vital signs before the exam starts. Record them on the exam form. Then drape and position the person for the exam.

---

**DELEGATION GUIDELINES:** *Preparing the Person*

To prepare a person for an exam, you need this information from the nurse and the care plan:

- When to prepare the person
- Where it will be done—exam room or the person's room
- How to position the person
- What equipment and supplies are needed
- If a urine specimen is needed

---

## FOCUS ON LONG-TERM CARE
### PREPARING THE PERSON

Quality of life is promoted. The resident has the right to personal choice. The doctor or nurse tells the person about the exam. Reasons for it are given. The person is told who will do the exam and when it will be done. The procedure is explained. The exam is done only with the person's consent. The person may want a different examiner. Or the person may want a family member present during the exam and when the results are explained.

---

**SAFETY ALERT:** *Preparing the Person*

Warmth is a major concern during an exam. Protect the person from chilling. Have an extra bath blanket nearby. Also, take measures to prevent drafts.

---

## FOCUS ON CHILDREN
### PREPARING THE PERSON

Babies are undressed for a physical exam. Leave diapers on baby boys to prevent urine sprays. Toddlers, preschool children, and school-age children can wear underpants. They are lowered or removed as needed during the exam.

## PREPARING THE PERSON FOR AN EXAMINATION

### QUALITY OF LIFE

Remember to:
- Knock before entering the person's room
- Address the person by name
- Introduce yourself by name and title

### PRE-PROCEDURE

1 Follow *Delegation Guidelines: Preparing the Person.* See *Safety Alert: Preparing the Person.*
2 Explain the procedure to the person.
3 Practice hand hygiene.
4 Collect the following:
   - Flashlight
   - Sphygmomanometer
   - Stethoscope
   - Thermometer
   - Tongue depressors (blades)
   - Laryngeal mirror
   - Ophthalmoscope
   - Otoscope
   - Nasal speculum
   - Percussion (reflex) hammer
   - Tuning fork
   - Tape measure
   - Gloves
   - Water-soluble lubricant
   - Vaginal speculum
   - Cotton-tipped applicators
   - Specimen containers and labels
   - Disposable bag
   - Kidney basin
   - Towel
   - Bath blanket
   - Tissues
   - Drape (sheet, bath blanket, drawsheet, or paper drape)
   - Paper towels
   - Cotton balls
   - Waterproof bed protector
   - Eye chart (Snellen chart)
   - Slides
   - Gown
   - Alcohol wipes
   - Wastebasket
   - Container for soiled instruments
   - Marking pencils or pens
5 Identify the person. Check the ID bracelet against the assignment sheet. Call the person by name.
6 Provide for privacy.

### PROCEDURE

7 Have the person put on the gown. Tell him or her to remove all clothes. Assist as needed.
8 Ask the person to void. Offer the bedpan, commode, or urinal if necessary. Provide for privacy.
9 Transport the person to the exam room. (This is not done for an exam in the person's room.)
10 Weigh and measure the person (Chapter 24). Record the measurements on the exam form.
11 Help the person onto the exam table. Provide a step stool if necessary. (Omit this step for an exam in the person's room.)
12 Measure vital signs. Record them on the exam form.
13 Raise the bed to its highest level. Raise the far bed rail (if used). (This is not done if an exam table is used.)
14 Position the person as directed (p. 536).
15 Drape the person.
16 Place a bed protector under the buttocks.
17 Raise the bed rail near you (if used).
18 Provide adequate lighting.
19 Put the signal light on for the examiner. Do not leave the person alone.

## POSITIONING AND DRAPING

Sometimes a special position is needed to examine the person. Some positions are uncomfortable and embarrassing. The examiner tells you how to position the person. Before helping the person assume and maintain the position, explain the following:

- Why the position is needed
- How to assume the position
- How the body is draped for warmth and privacy
- How long to expect to stay in the position

The **dorsal recumbent (horizontal recumbent) position** is used to examine the abdomen, chest, and breasts. The person is supine with the legs together. To examine the perineal area, the knees are flexed and hips externally rotated. Drape the person as in Figure 25-2, *A*.

The **lithotomy position** (Fig. 25-2, *B*) is used to examine the vagina. The woman lies on her back. Her hips are at the edge of the exam table. The knees are flexed and the hips externally rotated. The feet are in stirrups. Drape the person as for perineal care (Chapter 16). Some agencies provide socks to cover the feet and calves. Some women cannot assume this position. If so, the examiner tells you how to position the woman.

The **knee-chest position** (Fig. 25-2, *C*) is used to examine the rectum. Sometimes it is used to examine the vagina. The person kneels and rests the body on the knees and chest. The head is turned to one side. The arms are above the head or flexed at the elbows. The back is straight. The body is flexed about 90 degrees at the hips. Apply the drape in a diamond shape to cover the back, buttocks, and thighs. The person can wear socks. *See Focus on Older Persons: Positioning and Draping.*

The *Sims' position* (Fig. 25-2, *D*) is sometimes used to examine the rectum or vagina (Chapter 13). Apply the drape in a diamond shape. The examiner folds back the near corner to expose the rectum or vagina.

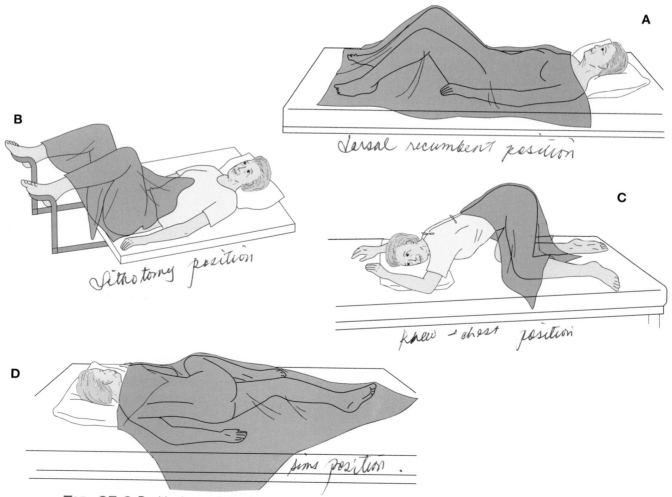

**FIG. 25-2** Positioning and draping for the physical exam. **A,** Dorsal recumbent position. **B,** Lithotomy position. **C,** Knee-chest position. **D,** Sims' position.

# ASSISTING WITH THE EXAMINATION

You may be asked to prepare, position, and drape the person. And you might assist the doctor or RN during the exam. To assist with the exam, follow the rules in Box 25-1. *See Focus on Children: Assisting With the Examination. See Focus on Older Persons: Assisting With the Examination.*

## AFTER THE EXAM

After the exam, the person dresses or returns to bed. Lubricant is used to examine the vagina or rectum. The area is wiped or cleaned before the person dresses or returns to the room. Assist as needed. You also need to:

- Discard disposable items—bed protectors, drapes, tongue blades, cotton balls, and so on.
- Replace supplies so the tray is ready for the next exam.
- Clean reusable items according to agency policy. Return them to the tray or storage area. This includes the otoscope and ophthalmoscope tips, speculum, and stethoscope.
- Cover the exam table with a clean drawsheet or paper.
- Label specimens. Take or send them to the laboratory with a requisition slip.
- Clean and straighten the person's unit or exam room.
- Follow agency policy for soiled linens.

---

### FOCUS ON OLDER PERSONS
#### ASSISTING WITH THE EXAMINATION

Some older persons have dementia. They may resist the examiner's efforts. The person may be agitated and aggressive because of confusion and fear. A person who refuses or resists an exam is not restrained or forced to have it. The exam is tried another time. Sometimes a family member can calm the person. The person's rights are always respected.

---

### FOCUS ON CHILDREN
#### ASSISTING WITH THE EXAMINATION

A parent is present when an infant or child is examined. If the infant or child is uncooperative, the parent may need to hold him or her still during some parts of the procedure. Being kept still may frighten an infant. The child may also fear separation from the parent. Some children have the fear of harm. A calm, comforting manner helps both the child and the parent. The parent may have fears too.

The equipment used is like that for the adult exam. Toys are used to assess development. Vaginal speculums are not used.

---

### FOCUS ON OLDER PERSONS
#### POSITIONING AND DRAPING

The knee-chest position is rarely used for older persons. The side-lying position is used to examine the rectum.

---

### BOX 25-1 RULES FOR ASSISTING WITH THE PHYSICAL EXAMINATION

- Practice hand hygiene before and after the exam.
- Provide for privacy. Close doors. Screen and drape the person. Expose only the body part being examined.
- Position the person as directed by the examiner.
- Place instruments and equipment near the examiner.
- Stay in the room when a female is examined (unless you are a male). When a man examines a female, another female is in the room. This is for the legal protection of the female and the male examiner. A female attendant also adds to the mental comfort of the woman. A female examiner may want a male attendant present when she examines a male. This also is for her legal protection.
- Protect the person from falling.
- Reassure the person throughout the exam.
- Anticipate the examiner's need for equipment and supplies.
- Place paper or paper towels on the floor if the person is asked to stand.
- Follow Standard Precautions and the Bloodborne Pathogen Standard.

## CROSS-TRAINING OPPORTUNITIES

Physical exams often involve laboratory tests and electrocardiograms (ECG or EKG). Doctors use these tests to diagnose disease and evaluate care. You may be cross-trained to assist with or to perform such procedures. They are done by a:

- *Phlebotomist*—draws blood for laboratory study. Phlebotomy means to withdraw blood from a vein. Phlebotomists work in the laboratory. They receive on-the-job training or study at a community college, technical school, or vocational school.
- *EKG or ECG technician*—takes electrocardiograms (Chapter 27). Training occurs on the job. Some community colleges, technical schools, and vocational schools offer EKG courses.

# ■ REVIEW QUESTIONS ■

Circle the **BEST** answer.

**1** The otoscope is used to examine
  **a** Internal structures of the eye
  **b** The external ear and the eardrum
  **c** Reflexes
  **d** The vagina

**2** You are preparing Mrs. Janz for an exam. You should do the following *except*
  **a** Have her void
  **b** Ask her to undress
  **c** Drape her
  **d** Go tell the nurse when she is ready

**3** Which part of Mrs. Janz's exam can you do?
  **a** Test her reflexes
  **b** Inspect her mouth, teeth, and throat
  **c** Measure her height, weight, and vital signs
  **d** Observe her perineum and rectum

**4** Mrs. Janz is supine. Her hips are flexed and externally rotated. Her feet are supported in stirrups. She is in the
  **a** Dorsal recumbent position
  **b** Lithotomy position
  **c** Knee-chest position
  **d** Sims' position

**5** You will assist with Mrs. Janz's exam. Which is *false?*
  **a** Hand hygiene is practiced before and after the exam.
  **b** Instruments are placed near the examiner.
  **c** You leave the room when Mrs. Janz is examined.
  **d** Provide for privacy by screening, closing the door, and proper draping.

*Answers to these questions are on p. 818.*

# Collecting and Testing Specimens

## OBJECTIVES

- Define the key terms listed in this chapter
- Explain why specimens are collected
- Describe the different types of urine specimens
- Explain why urine, stools, and sputum are tested
- Explain the rules for collecting specimens
- Perform the procedures described in this chapter

## KEY TERMS

**acetone** A substance that appears in urine from the rapid breakdown of fat for energy; ketone body or ketone

**glucosuria** Sugar *(glucos)* in the urine *(uria);* glycosuria

**glycosuria** Sugar *(glycos)* in the urine *(uria);* glucosuria

**hematuria** Blood *(hemat)* in the urine *(uria)*

**hemoptysis** Bloody *(hemo)* sputum *(ptysis* means "to spit")

**ketone** Acetone; ketone body

**ketone body** Acetone; ketone

**melena** A black, tarry stool

**sputum** Mucus from the respiratory system that is expectorated (expelled) through the mouth

Specimens *(samples)* are collected and tested to prevent, detect, and treat disease. The doctor orders what specimen to collect and the test needed. Most specimens are tested in the laboratory. All specimens sent to the laboratory require requisition slips. The slip has the person's identifying information and the test ordered. Some tests are done at the bedside. When collecting specimens, follow the rules in Box 26-1.

---

**BOX 26-1 RULES FOR COLLECTING SPECIMENS**

- Follow the rules of medical asepsis.
- Follow Standard Precautions and the Bloodborne Pathogen Standard.
- Use a clean container for each specimen.
- Use the correct container.
- Label the container accurately.
- Do not touch the inside of the container or lid.
- Collect the specimen at the correct time.

- Ask the person not to have a bowel movement when collecting a urine specimen. The specimen must not contain feces.
- Ask the person to put toilet tissue in the toilet or wastebasket. Urine and stool specimens must not contain tissue.
- Place the specimen container in a plastic bag.
- Take the specimen and requisition slip to the laboratory. Or take it to the storage area.

## URINE SPECIMENS

Urine specimens are collected for urine tests. Follow the rules in Box 26-1. *See Focus on Children: Collecting Urine Specimens.*

## ■ THE RANDOM URINE SPECIMEN

The random urine specimen is collected for a urinalysis. No special measures are needed. It is collected at any time. Many people can collect the specimen themselves. Weak and very ill persons need help.

---

**DELEGATION GUIDELINES:** *Urine Specimens*
Before collecting a urine specimen, you need this information from the nurse:
- The type of specimen needed
- What time to collect the specimen
- What special measures are needed
- If you need to test the specimen (p. 548)
- What observations to report and record:
  —Problems obtaining the specimen
  —Color, clarity, and odor of urine
  —Particles in the urine
  —Complaints of pain, burning, urgency, dysuria, or other problems

---

**SAFETY ALERT:** *Urine Specimens*
Microbes can grow in urine. Urine also may contain blood. Follow Standard Precautions and the Bloodborne Pathogen Standard.

---

**FOCUS ON CHILDREN**
**COLLECTING URINE SPECIMENS**
For infants and toddlers who are not toilet-trained, a collection bag is applied to the genital area (p. 548). It is hard for toilet-trained toddlers and young children to void on request and into a collection device. Potty chairs and specimen pans are useful. Remember to use terms the child understands. "Pee pee," "potty," and "tinkle" are examples.

Urine specimens may embarrass older children and teenagers. They do not like clear specimen containers that show urine. Placing the urine specimen container in a paper bag is often helpful.

## COLLECTING A RANDOM URINE SPECIMEN

### QUALITY OF LIFE

Remember to:
- Knock before entering the person's room
- Address the person by name
- Introduce yourself by name and title

### PRE-PROCEDURE

1 Follow *Delegation Guidelines: Urine Specimens.* See *Safety Alert: Urine Specimens.*
2 Explain the procedure to the person.
3 Practice hand hygiene.
4 Collect the following:
   - Voiding receptacle—bedpan and cover, urinal, or specimen pan (Fig. 26-1)

- Specimen container and lid
- Label
- Gloves
- Plastic bag

### PROCEDURE

5 Label the container.
6 Put the container and lid in the bathroom.
7 Identify the person. Check the ID bracelet against the requisition slip. Call the person by name.
8 Provide for privacy.
9 Put on the gloves.
10 Ask the person to void into the receptacle. Remind him or her to put toilet tissue into the wastebasket or toilet. Toilet tissue is not put in the bedpan or specimen pan.

11 Take the receptacle to the bathroom.
12 Pour about 120 ml (4 oz) of urine into the specimen container. Dispose of excess urine.
13 Place the lid on the specimen container. Put the container in the plastic bag.
14 Clean and return the receptacle to its proper place.
15 Assist with hand washing.
16 Practice hand hygiene.

### POST-PROCEDURE

17 Provide for comfort.
18 Place the signal light within reach.
19 Raise or lower bed rails. Follow the care plan.
20 Unscreen the person.

21 Decontaminate your hands.
22 Report and record your observations.
23 Take the specimen and the requisition slip to the storage area or laboratory.

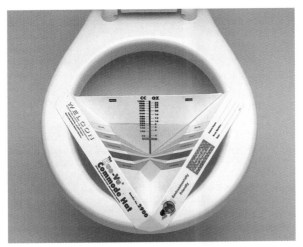

**FIG. 26-1** The specimen pan is placed on the toilet rim. It has a color chart for urine. (Courtesy Welcon, Inc., Forth Worth, Tex.)

# THE MIDSTREAM SPECIMEN

The midstream specimen is also called a *clean-voided specimen* or a *clean-catch specimen*. The perineal area is cleaned before collecting the specimen. This reduces the number of microbes in the urethral area. The person starts to void into a receptacle. Then the person stops the stream of urine, and a sterile specimen container is positioned. The person voids into the container until the specimen is obtained.

Stopping the stream of urine is hard for many people. You may need to position and hold the specimen container in place after the person starts to void.

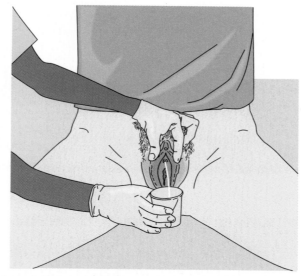

**FIG. 26-2** The labia are separated to collect a midstream specimen.

## COLLECTING A MIDSTREAM SPECIMEN

### QUALITY OF LIFE

Remember to:
- Knock before entering the person's room
- Address the person by name
- Introduce yourself by name and title

### PRE-PROCEDURE

1 Follow *Delegation Guidelines: Urine Specimens*, p. 542. See *Safety Alert: Urine Specimens*, p. 542.
2 Explain the procedure to the person.
3 Practice hand hygiene.
4 Collect the following:
   - Midstream specimen kit (with antiseptic solution)
   - Label
   - Disposable gloves
   - Sterile gloves (if not part of the kit)
   - Voiding receptacle—bedpan, urinal, or commode if needed
   - Plastic bag
   - Supplies for perineal care
5 Label the container.
6 Identify the person. Check the ID bracelet against the requisition slip. Call the person by name.
7 Provide for privacy.

### PROCEDURE

8 Provide perineal care. Remove the gloves, and decontaminate your hands.
9 Open the sterile kit. Use sterile technique (Chapter 12).
10 Put on the sterile gloves.
11 Pour the antiseptic solution over the cotton balls.
12 Open the sterile specimen container. Do not touch the inside of the container or lid. Set the lid down so the inside is up.
13 *For a female*—clean the perineum with cotton balls:
   a Spread the labia with your thumb and index finger. Use your non-dominant hand. (This hand is now contaminated. It must not touch anything sterile.)
   b Clean down the urethral area from front to back. Use a clean cotton ball for each stroke.
   c Keep the labia separated to collect the urine specimen (steps 16 and 17).
14 *For a male*—clean the penis with cotton balls:
   a Hold the penis with your non-dominant hand.
   b Clean the penis starting at the meatus. Use a cotton ball and clean in a circular motion. Start at the center and work outward.
   c Keep holding the penis until the specimen is collected (steps 16 and 17).

15 Ask the person to void into the receptacle.
16 Pass the specimen container into the stream of urine. Keep the labia separated (Fig. 26-2).
17 Collect about 30 to 60 ml of urine (1 to 2 oz).
18 Remove the specimen container before the person stops voiding.
19 Release the labia or penis.
20 Let the person finish voiding into the receptacle.
21 Put the lid on the specimen container. Touch only the outside of the container or lid.
22 Wipe the outside of the container.
23 Place the container in a plastic bag.
24 Provide toilet tissue after the person is done voiding.
25 Take the receptacle to the bathroom.
26 Measure urine if intake and output (I&O) is ordered. Include the amount in the specimen container.
27 Clean the receptacle and other items. Return equipment to its proper place.
28 Remove soiled gloves. Practice hand hygiene.
29 Put on clean gloves.
30 Assist with hand washing
31 Remove the gloves. Decontaminate your hands.

### POST-PROCEDURE

32 Follow steps 17-23 in procedure: *Collecting a Random Urine Specimen*, p. 543.

## THE 24-HOUR URINE SPECIMEN

All urine voided during a 24-hour period is collected for a 24-hour urine specimen. Urine is chilled on ice or refrigerated during this time. This prevents the growth of microbes. A preservative is added to the collection container for some tests.

The person voids to begin the test. Discard this voiding. Save *all* voidings during the next 24 hours. The person and nursing staff must clearly understand the procedure and test period.

---

### COLLECTING A 24-HOUR URINE SPECIMEN

#### QUALITY OF LIFE

Remember to:
- Knock before entering the person's room
- Address the person by name
- Introduce yourself by name and title

#### PRE-PROCEDURE

1 Follow *Delegation Guidelines: Urine Specimens*, p. 542. See *Safety Alert: Urine Specimens*, p. 542.
2 Review the procedure with the nurse.
3 Explain the procedure to the person.
4 Practice hand hygiene.
5 Collect the following:
- Urine container for a 24-hour collection
- Preservative if needed
- Bucket with ice if needed
- Two 24-hour urine specimen labels
- Funnel
- Voiding receptacle—bedpan, urinal, commode, or specimen pan
- Gloves
- Graduate
6 Label the urine container.
7 Identify the person. Check the ID bracelet against the requisition slip. Call the person by name.
8 Arrange equipment in the person's bathroom.
9 Place one label in the bathroom. Place the other near the bed.

#### PROCEDURE

10 Put on the gloves.
11 Offer the bedpan or urinal. Or assist the person to the bathroom or commode.
12 Ask the person to void.
13 Discard the urine, and note the time. This starts the 24-hour collection period.
14 Clean the bedpan, urinal, commode, or specimen pan.
15 Remove the gloves. Practice hand hygiene.
16 Mark the time the test began and the time it ends on the room and bathroom labels. Also mark the urine container.
17 Ask the person to use the bedpan, urinal, commode, or specimen pan when voiding during the next 24 hours. Tell the person to signal after voiding. Remind him or her not to have a bowel movement at the same time and not to put toilet tissue in the receptacle.
18 Put on the gloves.
19 Measure all urine if I&O is ordered.
20 Pour urine into the urine container using the funnel. Do not spill any urine. Restart the test if you spill or discard urine.
21 Clean the receptacle. Remove the gloves, and practice hand hygiene.
22 Add ice to the bucket as needed.
23 Ask the person to void at the end of the 24-hour period. Pour the urine into the urine container. Wear gloves for this step.

#### POST-PROCEDURE

24 Provide for comfort.
25 Place the signal light within reach.
26 Raise or lower bed rails. Follow the care plan.
27 Remove the labels from the room and bathroom.
28 Clean and return equipment to its proper place. Discard disposable items. Wear gloves for this step.
29 Remove the gloves, and practice hand hygiene.
30 Report and record your observations.
31 Take the specimen and requisition slip to the laboratory.

# THE DOUBLE-VOIDED SPECIMEN

*Fresh-fractional urine specimen* is another term for a double-voided specimen. The person voids twice. The first time the bladder is emptied of "stale" urine. "Fresh" urine collects in the bladder after the first voiding. In 30 minutes the person voids again. The second voiding is usually a very small or "fractional" amount of urine.

Fresh-fractional specimens are used to test urine for glucose and ketones (p. 548).

## COLLECTING A DOUBLE-VOIDED SPECIMEN

### QUALITY OF LIFE

Remember to:
- Knock before entering the person's room
- Address the person by name
- Introduce yourself by name and title

### PRE-PROCEDURE

1 Follow *Delegation Guidelines: Urine Specimens*, p. 542. See *Safety Alert: Urine Specimens*, p. 542.
2 Explain the procedure to the person.
3 Practice hand hygiene.
4 Collect the following:
- Voiding receptacle—bedpan, urinal, commode, or specimen pan
- Two specimen containers
- Urine testing equipment
- Gloves

5 Identify the person. Check the ID bracelet against the assignment sheet. Call the person by name.
6 Provide for privacy.

### PROCEDURE

7 Put on the gloves.
8 Ask the person to void into the receptacle. Remind the person not to put toilet tissue in the receptacle.
9 Take the receptacle to the bathroom.
10 Pour some urine into the specimen container.
11 Test the specimen in case you cannot obtain a second specimen (p. 548). Discard the urine.
12 Clean the receptacle, and return the receptacle to its proper place.
13 Remove the gloves. Practice hand hygiene.
14 Assist with hand washing. Wear gloves if needed. Decontaminate your hands after removing gloves.
15 Ask the person to drink an 8-ounce glass of water.
16 Provide for comfort. Raise the bed rails if needed. Place the signal light within reach.
17 Unscreen the person.
18 Decontaminate your hands.
19 Return to the room in 20 to 30 minutes.
20 Repeat steps 6 through 14.

### POST-PROCEDURE

21 Provide for comfort.
22 Raise the bed rails if needed. Follow the care plan.
23 Place the signal light within reach.
24 Unscreen the person.
25 Decontaminate your hands.
26 Report the results of the second test and any other observations.

## COLLECTING A SPECIMEN FROM AN INFANT OR CHILD

Sometimes specimens are needed from infants and children who are not toilet-trained. A collection bag (called a "wee bag") is applied over the urethra. A parent or another staff member assists if the child is upset.

## TESTING URINE

The nurse may ask you to do simple urine tests. You can test for pH, glucose, ketones, and blood using reagent strips. The doctor orders the type and frequency of urine tests.

- *Testing for pH.* Urine pH measures if urine is acidic or alkaline. Changes in normal pH (4.6 to 8.0) occur from illness, foods, and drugs. A routine urine specimen is needed.
- *Testing for glucose and ketones.* In diabetes, the pancreas does not secrete enough insulin (Chapter 33). The body needs insulin to use sugar for energy. If not used, sugar builds up in the blood. Some sugar appears in the urine. **Glucosuria** or **glycosuria** means sugar (*glucos, glycos*) in the urine (*uria*). The diabetic person may also have **acetone (ketone bodies, ketones)** in the urine. These substances appear in urine from the rapid breakdown of fat for energy. The body uses fat for energy if it cannot use sugar. Urine is also tested for ketones. These tests are usually done four times a day—30 minutes before each meal (ac) and at bedtime (HS). The doctor uses the test to make drug and diet decisions. Double-voided specimens are best for these tests.
- *Testing for blood.* Injury and disease can cause blood (*hema*) to appear in the urine (*uria*). This is called **hematuria.** Sometimes blood is seen in the urine. At other times it is unseen (*occult*). A routine urine specimen is needed.

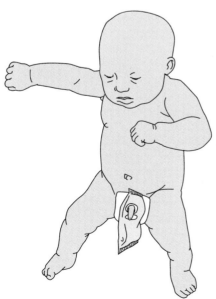

**FIG. 26-3** A collection bag is applied to the perineal area of the infant. Urine collects in the bag for a specimen.

# COLLECTING A URINE SPECIMEN FROM AN INFANT OR CHILD

## QUALITY OF LIFE

Remember to:
- Knock before entering the person's room
- Address the person by name
- Introduce yourself by name and title

## PRE-PROCEDURE

1 Follow *Delegation Guidelines: Urine Specimens*, p. 542. See *Safety Alert: Urine Specimens*, p. 542.
2 Explain the procedure to the child and parents.
3 Practice hand hygiene.
4 Collect the following:
- Collection bag
- Wash basin
- Cotton balls
- Bath towel
- Two diapers
- Specimen container
- Gloves
- Plastic bag
- Scissors

5 Identify the child. Check the ID bracelet against the requisition slip. Call the child by name.
6 Provide for privacy.

## PROCEDURE

7 Put on the gloves.
8 Remove and dispose of the diaper.
9 Clean the perineal area. Use a new cotton ball for each stroke. Rinse and dry the area.
10 Remove the gloves, and practice hand hygiene. Bed rails are up before leaving the bedside.
11 Put on clean gloves.
12 Position the child on the back. Flex the child's knees, and separate the legs.
13 Remove the adhesive backing from the collection bag.
14 Apply the bag to the perineum. Do not cover the anus (Fig. 26-3).
15 Cut a slit in the bottom of a new diaper.
16 Diaper the child.
17 Pull the collection bag through the slit in the diaper.
18 Remove the gloves. Decontaminate your hands.
19 Raise the head of the crib if allowed. This helps urine to collect in the bottom of the bag.
20 Unscreen the child.
21 Decontaminate your hands.
22 Check the child often. Check the bag for urine. (Wear gloves, and provide for privacy.)
23 Provide privacy if the child has voided.
24 Remove the diaper.
25 Remove the collection bag gently.
26 Press the adhesive surfaces of the bag together. Or transfer urine to the specimen container using the drainage tab.
27 Clean the perineal area. Rinse and dry well.
28 Diaper the child.
29 Remove the gloves. Practice hand hygiene.

## POST-PROCEDURE

30 Provide for comfort. Raise the bed rail.
31 Unscreen the child.
32 Label the specimen container. Place it in the plastic bag.
33 Clean and return equipment to its proper place. Discard disposable items. (Wear gloves for this step.)
34 Practice hand hygiene.
35 Report and record your observations.
36 Take the requisition slip and the specimen to the storage area or laboratory.

**USING REAGENT STRIPS.** Reagent strips have sections that change color when they react with urine. To use a reagent strip, dip the strip into urine. Then compare the strip with the color chart on the bottle (Fig. 26-4). The nurse gives you specific instructions for the urine test ordered.

> **SAFETY ALERT:** *Using Reagent Strips*
> When using reagent strips, read and follow the manufacturer's instructions. Otherwise you could get the wrong result. The doctor uses the test results in diagnosing and treating the person. A wrong result could lead to serious harm.

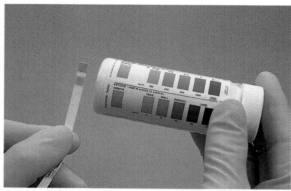

**FIG. 26-4** Reagent strips for sugar and ketones.

## TESTING URINE WITH REAGENT STRIPS

### QUALITY OF LIFE

Remember to:
- Knock before entering the person's room
- Address the person by name
- Introduce yourself by name and title

### PRE-PROCEDURE

1 Follow *Delegation Guidelines: Testing Urine*, p. 548. See *Safety Alert: Testing Urine*, p. 548 and *Safety Alert: Using Reagent Strips.*
2 Explain the procedure to the person.
3 Practice hand hygiene.
4 Identify the person. Check the ID bracelet against the assignment sheet. Call the person by name.

### PROCEDURE

5 Put on the gloves.
6 Collect the following:
   - Urine specimen (routine specimen for ph and occult blood; double-voided specimen for sugar and ketones)
   - Reagent strip as ordered
   - Gloves
7 Remove a strip from the bottle. Put the cap on the bottle at once. It must be on tight.
8 Dip the strip test areas into the urine.
9 Remove the strip after the correct amount of time. See the manufacturer's instructions.
10 Tap the strip gently against the container. This removes excess urine.
11 Wait the required amount of time. See the manufacturer's instructions.
12 Compare the strip with the color chart on the bottle. Read the results.
13 Discard disposable items and the specimen.

### POST-PROCEDURE

14 Clean and return equipment to its proper place.
15 Remove the gloves. Practice hand hygiene.
16 Report and record the results and other observations.

## STRAINING URINE

Stones (*calculi*) can develop in the kidneys, ureters, or bladder. Stones vary in size. Some are pinhead size. Others are as big as an orange. Stones causing severe pain and urinary system damage may require surgical removal. Some stones are passed through urine. Therefore all of the person's urine is strained. Passed stones are sent to the laboratory for examination.

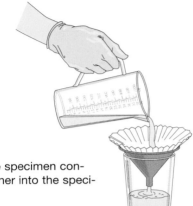

**FIG. 26-5** A strainer is placed in the specimen container. Urine is poured through the strainer into the specimen container.

## STRAINING URINE

### QUALITY OF LIFE

Remember to:
- Knock before entering the person's room
- Address the person by name
- Introduce yourself by name and title

### PRE-PROCEDURE

1 Follow *Delegation Guidelines: Testing Urine*, p. 548. See *Safety Alert: Testing Urine*, p. 548.
2 Explain the procedure to the person. Also explain that the urinal, bedpan, commode, or specimen pan is used for voiding.
3 Practice hand hygiene.
4 Collect the following:
- Strainer or 4 × 4 gauze
- Specimen container
- Bedpan, urinal, commode, or specimen pan
- Two labels stating that all urine is strained
- Gloves
- Plastic bag
5 Identify the person. Check the ID bracelet against the assignment sheet. Call the person by name.
6 Arrange items in the person's bathroom. Place the specimen pan in the toilet.
7 Place one label in the bathroom. Place the other near the bed.

### PROCEDURE

8 Put on the gloves.
9 Offer the bedpan or urinal. Or assist the person to the commode or bathroom.
10 Provide for privacy.
11 Tell the person to signal after voiding.
12 Remove the gloves. Decontaminate your hands.
13 Return when the person signals for you. Knock before entering the room.
14 Decontaminate your hands. Put on gloves.
15 Place the strainer or gauze into the specimen container.
16 Pour urine into the specimen container. Urine passes through the strainer or gauze (Fig. 26-5).
17 Discard the urine.
18 Place the strainer or gauze in the specimen container if any crystals, stones, or particles appear.
19 Provide perineal care if needed.
20 Clean and return equipment to its proper place.
21 Remove soiled gloves. Practice hand hygiene, and put on clean gloves.
22 Assist with hand washing.
23 Remove the gloves. Decontaminate your hands.

### POST-PROCEDURE

24 Provide for comfort.
25 Place the signal light within reach.
26 Raise or lower bed rails. Follow the care plan.
27 Unscreen the person.
28 Label the specimen container. Put it in the plastic bag. (Wear gloves for this step.)
29 Remove the gloves. Decontaminate your hands.
30 Report and record your observations.
31 Take the specimen and requisition slip to the laboratory or storage area.

# STOOL SPECIMENS

When internal bleeding is suspected, feces are checked for blood. Stools are also studied for fat, microbes, worms, and other abnormal contents. The stool specimen must not be contaminated with urine. Some tests require a warm stool. The specimen is taken to the laboratory at once if a warm stool is needed.

*See Focus on Children: Stool Specimens.*

**FOCUS ON CHILDREN**
**STOOL SPECIMENS**

If the child wears a diaper, you can scrape the stool from the diaper.

**DELEGATION GUIDELINES:** *Stool Specimens*
Before collecting a stool specimen, you need this information from the nurse:
- What time to collect the specimen
- What special measures are needed
- If you need to test the specimen
- What observations to report and record:
    —Problems obtaining the specimen
    —Color, amount, consistency, and odor of feces
    —Complaints of pain or discomfort

**SAFETY ALERT:** *Stool Specimens*
Stools contain microbes. And they may contain blood. Follow Standard Precautions and the Bloodborne Pathogen Standard.

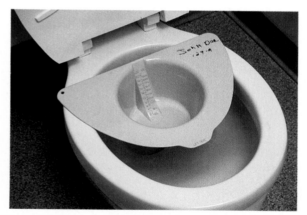

**FIG. 26-6** The specimen pan is placed at the back of the toilet for a stool specimen.

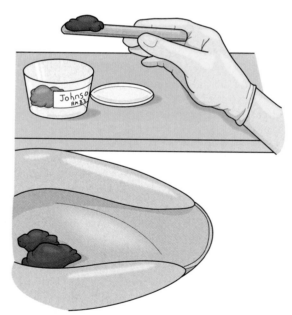

**FIG. 26-7** A tongue blade is used to transfer a small amount of stool from the bedpan to the specimen container.

# COLLECTING A STOOL SPECIMEN

## QUALITY OF LIFE

Remember to:
- Knock before entering the person's room
- Address the person by name
- Introduce yourself by name and title

## PRE-PROCEDURE

1 Follow *Delegation Guidelines: Stool Specimens.* See *Safety Alert: Stool Specimens.*
2 Explain the procedure to the person.
3 Practice hand hygiene.
4 Collect the following:
- Bedpan and cover or commode
- Urinal for voiding
- Specimen pan for the toilet or commode
- Specimen container and lid
- Tongue blade
- Disposable bag
- Gloves
- Toilet tissue
- Laboratory requisition slip
- Plastic bag

## PROCEDURE

5 Label the container.
6 Identify the person. Check the ID bracelet against the requisition slip. Call the person by name.
7 Provide for privacy.
8 Ask the person to void. Provide the bedpan, commode, or urinal for voiding if the person does not use the bathroom. Empty and clean the device.
9 Put the specimen pan on the toilet if the person will use the bathroom. Place it at the back of the toilet (Fig. 26-6).
10 Assist the person onto the bedpan or to the toilet or commode. The person wears a robe and nonskid footwear when up.
11 Ask the person not to put toilet tissue in the bedpan, commode, or specimen pan. Provide a bag for toilet tissue.
12 Place the signal light and toilet tissue within reach. Raise or lower bed rails. Follow the care plan.
13 Decontaminate your hands. Leave the room.

14 Return when the person signals. Knock before entering. Decontaminate your hands.
15 Lower the bed rail near you if up.
16 Put on the gloves. Provide perineal care if needed.
17 Use a tongue blade to take about 2 tablespoons of stool to the specimen container (Fig. 26-7). Take the sample from the middle of a formed stool. If required by agency policy, take stool from 2 different places on the specimen.
18 Put the lid on the specimen container. Do not touch the inside of the lid or container. Place the container in the plastic bag.
19 Wrap the tongue blade in toilet tissue.
20 Discard the tongue blade into the bag.
21 Empty, clean, and disinfect equipment.
22 Remove the gloves. Decontaminate your hands.
23 Return equipment to its proper place.
24 Help the person with hand washing. Wear gloves if necessary.

## POST-PROCEDURE

25 Provide for comfort.
26 Place the signal light within reach.
27 Lower the bed to its lowest position.
28 Raise or lower bed rails. Follow the care plan.
29 Unscreen the person.

30 Take the specimen and requisition slip to the laboratory.
31 Decontaminate your hands.
32 Report and record your observations.

# TESTING STOOLS FOR BLOOD

Blood can appear in stools for many reasons. Ulcers, colon cancer, and hemorrhoids are common causes. Often blood is seen if bleeding is low in the bowels. Stools are black and tarry if there is bleeding in the stomach or upper GI tract. **Melena** is a black, tarry stool.

Sometimes bleeding occurs in very small amounts. Such bleeding is hard to see. Therefore stools are often tested for *occult blood. Occult* means "hidden" or "unseen." The test is often done to screen for colon cancer.

Many factors can affect the test results. One is eating red meat. The person cannot eat red meat for 3 days before the test. Bleeding from hemorrhoids and menstrual periods also affect test results.

**DELEGATION GUIDELINES:** *Testing Stool Specimens*
Before testing a stool specimen, you need this information from the nurse:
- What test is needed
- What equipment to use
- When to test the stool
- Instructions for the test ordered
- If the nurse wants to observe the results of each test
- What observations to report and record:
  —Test results
  —Problems obtaining the specimen
  —Color, amount, consistency, and odor of feces
  —Complaints of pain or discomfort

**SAFETY ALERT:** *Testing Stool Specimens*
You must be accurate when testing stools. Follow the manufacturer's instructions for the test used. Promptly report the results to the nurse.

Stools contain microbes. They may contain blood. Follow Standard Precautions and the Bloodborne Pathogen Standard.

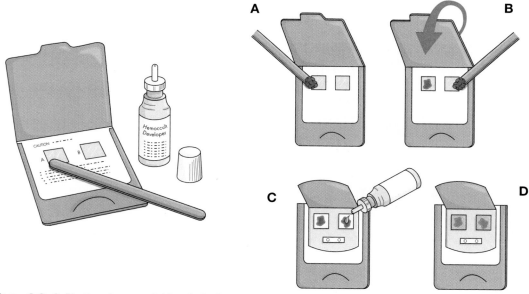

**FIG. 26-8** Testing for occult blood. **A,** Stool is smeared on *box A.* **B,** Stool is smeared on *box B,* and then the flap is closed. **C,** Developer is applied to *boxes A and B.* **D,** Color changes are noted.

## TESTING A STOOL SPECIMEN FOR BLOOD

### QUALITY OF LIFE

Remember to:
- Knock before entering the person's room
- Address the person by name
- Introduce yourself by name and title

### PRE-PROCEDURE

1 Follow *Delegation Guidelines: Testing Stool Specimens.* See *Safety Alert: Testing Stool Specimens.*

2 Explain the procedure to the person.

3 Decontaminate your hands.

### PROCEDURE

4 Collect a stool specimen. (See procedure: *Collecting a Stool Specimen,* p. 553.)

5 Collect the following:
- Paper towels
- Hemoccult test kit
- Tongue blades
- Gloves

6 Put on the gloves.

7 Open the test kit.

8 Use the tongue blade to obtain a small amount of stool.

9 Apply a thin smear of stool on *box A* on the test paper (Fig. 26-8, *A*).

10 Use another tongue blade to obtain stool from another part of the specimen.

11 Apply a thin smear of stool on *box B* on the test paper (Fig. 26-8, *B*).

12 Close the test packet.

13 Turn the test packet to the other side. Open the flap. Apply developer (from the kit) to *boxes A* and *B*. Follow the manufacturer's instructions (Fig. 26-8, *C*).

14 Wait the amount of time noted in the manufacturer's instructions. Time varies from 10 to 60 seconds.

15 Note and record the color changes (Fig. 26-8, *D*).

16 Dispose of the test packet.

17 Wrap the tongue blades with toilet tissue. Then discard them.

18 Dispose of the specimen.

19 Remove the gloves. Decontaminate your hands.

### POST-PROCEDURE

20 Report and record the test results and your observations.

# SPUTUM SPECIMENS

Respiratory disorders cause the lungs, bronchi, and trachea to secrete mucus (Chapter 30). The mucus from the respiratory system is called **sputum** when expectorated *(expelled)* through the mouth. Sputum is not saliva. Saliva ("spit") is a thin, clear liquid. It is produced by the salivary glands in the mouth.

Sputum specimens are studied for blood, microbes, and abnormal cells. The person coughs up sputum from the bronchi and trachea. This is often painful and hard to do. It is easier to collect a specimen in the morning. Secretions collect in the trachea and bronchi during sleep. They are coughed up upon awakening.

The person rinses the mouth with water. Rinsing decreases saliva and removes food particles. Mouthwash is not used. It destroys some of the microbes in the mouth.

The procedure can embarrass the person. Coughing and expectorating sounds can disturb those nearby. Also, sputum is unpleasant to look at. For these reasons, privacy is important. Cover the specimen container, and place it in a bag. Some sputum containers hide the contents.

*See Focus on Children: Sputum Specimens. See Focus on Older Persons: Sputum Specimens.*

---

## FOCUS ON CHILDREN
### SPUTUM SPECIMENS

Breathing treatments and suctioning are often needed to produce a sputum specimen in infants and small children. The RN or respiratory therapist gives the breathing treatment. The nurse suctions the trachea for the specimen. The infant or child is likely to be uncooperative during suctioning. You can assist by holding the child's head and arms still.

---

## FOCUS ON OLDER PERSONS
### SPUTUM SPECIMENS

Older persons may lack the strength to cough up sputum. Coughing is easier after postural drainage. It drains secretions by gravity. Gravity causes fluids to flow down. The person is positioned so a lung part is higher than the airway (Fig. 26-9). The nurse or respiratory therapist does postural drainage.

---

**DELEGATION GUIDELINES:** *Sputum Specimens*

When collecting a sputum specimen is delegated to you, you need this information from the nurse:

- When to collect the specimen
- How much sputum is needed—usually 1 to 2 tablespoons
- If the person uses the bathroom
- If the person can hold the specimen container
- What observations to report and record:
  —The time the specimen was collected
  —The amount of sputum collected
  —How easily the person raised the sputum
  —Sputum color—clear, white, yellow, green, brown, or red
  —Sputum odor—none or foul odor
  —Sputum consistency—thick, watery, or frothy (with bubbles or foam)
  —**Hemoptysis**—bloody *(hemo)* sputum *(ptysis,* meaning "to spit")
  —Any other observations

---

**SAFETY ALERT:** *Sputum Specimens*

Follow Standard Precautions and the Bloodborne Pathogen Standard to prevent contact with mucus. It may contain blood or microbes.

Also follow Airborne Precautions if the person has or may have tuberculosis (TB) (Chapter 33). Protect yourself by wearing a tuberculosis respirator (Chapter 12).

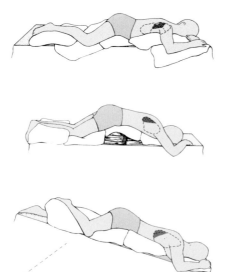

**FIG. 26-9** Some positions for postural drainage. (From Potter PA, Perry AG: *Fundamentals of nursing,* ed 5, St Louis, 2001, Mosby.)

## COLLECTING A SPUTUM SPECIMEN

### QUALITY OF LIFE

Remember to:
- Knock before entering the person's room
- Address the person by name
- Introduce yourself by name and title

### PRE-PROCEDURE

1 Follow *Delegation Guidelines: Sputum Specimens.* See *Safety Alert: Sputum Specimens.*
2 Explain the procedure to the person.
3 Practice hand hygiene.
4 Collect the following:
   - Sputum specimen container and label
   - Laboratory requisition
   - Disposable bag
   - Gloves
   - Tissues
5 Label the container.
6 Identify the person. Check the ID bracelet against the requisition slip. Call the person by name.
7 Provide for privacy. If able, the person goes into the bathroom for the procedure.

### PROCEDURE

8 Ask the person to rinse the mouth out with clear water.
9 Put on the gloves.
10 Have the person hold the container. Only the outside is touched.
11 Ask the person to cover the mouth and nose with tissues when coughing.
12 Ask him or her to take 2 or 3 deep breaths and cough up the sputum.
13 Have the person expectorate directly into the container (Fig. 26-10). Sputum should not touch the outside.
14 Collect 1 to 2 tablespoons of sputum unless told to collect more.
15 Put the lid on the container.
16 Place the container in the bag. Attach the requisition to the bag.
17 Remove the gloves. Decontaminate your hands.

### POST-PROCEDURE

18 Provide for comfort.
19 Place the signal light within reach.
20 Unscreen the person.
21 Decontaminate your hands.
22 Take the bag to the laboratory or storage area.
23 Decontaminate your hands.
24 Report and record your observations.

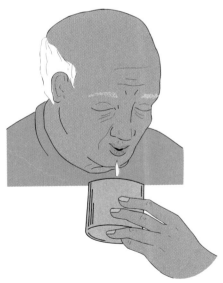

**FIG. 26-10** The person expectorates into the center of the specimen container.

# ■ REVIEW QUESTIONS ■

Circle the **BEST** answer.

1 You are going to collect a random urine specimen. You should do the following *except*
   a Label the container as requested
   b Use the correct container
   c Collect the specimen at the right time
   d Use sterile supplies

2 The perineum is cleaned before collecting a
   a Random specimen
   b Midstream specimen
   c 24-hour urine specimen
   d Double-voided specimen

3 A 24-hour urine specimen involves
   a Collecting all urine voided during a 24-hour period
   b Collecting a random specimen every hour for 24 hours
   c Testing urine for sugar and ketones every day
   d Measuring output every hour for 24 hours

4 Urine is tested for sugar and ketones
   a At bedtime
   b 30 minutes after meals and at bedtime
   c 30 minutes before meals and at bedtime
   d Before breakfast

5 Which specimen is best for sugar and ketone testing?
   a A random specimen
   b A clean-voided specimen
   c A 24-hour specimen
   d A double-voided specimen

6 You need to strain Mr. Powell's urine. Straining urine is done to find
   a Blood
   b Stones
   c Ketones
   d Acetone

7 You note a black, tarry stool. This is called
   a Melena
   b Feces
   c Hemostool
   d Occult blood

8 A stool specimen must be kept warm. After collecting the specimen, you need to
   a Put it in the oven
   b Take it to the storage area
   c Take it to the laboratory
   d Cover it with a towel

9 The best time to collect a sputum specimen is
   a On awakening
   b After meals
   c At bedtime
   d After oral hygiene

10 A sputum specimen is needed. You should ask the person to
   a Use mouthwash
   b Rinse the mouth with clear water
   c Brush the teeth
   d Remove dentures

*Answers to these questions are on p. 818.*

# 27

# The Person Having Surgery

## OBJECTIVES

- Define the key terms listed in this chapter
- Describe the common fears and concerns of surgical patients
- Explain how people are prepared for surgery
- Describe how to prepare a room for the postoperative patient
- List the signs and symptoms to report postoperatively
- Explain how to meet the person's needs after surgery
- Perform the procedures described in this chapter

## KEY TERMS

**anesthesia**  The loss of feeling or sensation produced by a drug

**douche**  The introduction of a fluid into the vagina and the immediate return of the fluid

**elective surgery**  Surgery done by choice to improve the person's life or well-being

**embolus**  A blood clot (*thrombus*) that travels through the vascular system until it lodges in a distant blood vessel

**emergency surgery**  Surgery done immediately to save life or function

**general anesthesia**  The loss of consciousness and all feeling or sensation

**local anesthesia**  The loss of feeling or sensation in a small area

**postoperative**  After surgery

**preoperative**  Before surgery

**regional anesthesia**  The loss of feeling or sensation in a large area of the body

**thrombus**  A blood clot

**urgent surgery**  Surgery needed for the person's health; it is done soon to prevent further damage or disease

---

Surgery is done to remove a diseased body part, remove a tumor, or repair injured tissue. Surgery is also done to make a diagnosis, improve appearance, and relieve symptoms. Restoring function and replacing a body part are other reasons for surgery.

Surgery often requires a hospital stay. Patients are admitted before the surgery. They stay for 2 or more days after the surgery. Same-day surgery (outpatient, one-day, or ambulatory surgery) is common. The person is admitted in the morning and discharged later in the day. Many same-day surgeries are done in clinics or surgical centers that are part of hospitals or doctors' offices.

Surgeries are elective, urgent, or emergency:

- **Elective surgery** is done by choice to improve the person's life or well-being. It is not lifesaving. Joint replacement surgery and cosmetic surgery are examples. The surgery is scheduled in advance.
- **Urgent surgery** is needed for the person's health. It is done soon to prevent further damage or disease. Cancer surgery and coronary artery bypass surgery are examples.
- **Emergency surgery** is done immediately to save life or function. The need is sudden and unexpected. Accidents, stabbings, and bullet wounds often require emergency surgery.

The person is prepared for what happens before, during, and after surgery. This is done by nurses, doctors, and other health team members. You assist as the nurse and care plan direct.

In hospitals, you will care for patients before and after surgery. In nursing centers, many residents are recovering from surgery. Some patients need home care after surgery.

# PSYCHOLOGICAL CARE

Surgery causes many fears and concerns (Box 27-1). The person's deepest and worst fears are often felt. What if you needed surgery tomorrow? Would you fear cancer or losing a body part? Would you worry about pain or death? Who will care for your children and home? Will you have an income to support your family? Imagine having an accident. You wake up hours later. You are told that your right leg was amputated.

Past experiences affect feelings. Some persons have had surgery. Others have not. Family and friends talk about their surgical experiences, which can affect the patient. Most people know about tragic events—surgery on the wrong person or wrong body part, instruments left in the body, death during surgery. Some people do not share their fears and concerns. They may cry, be quiet and withdrawn, or talk about other things. Some pace or are very cheerful.

Mental preparation is important. Respect the person's fears and concerns. Show the person warmth, sensitivity, and caring.

## BOX 27-1 — COMMON FEARS AND CONCERNS OF SURGICAL PATIENTS

**THE FEAR OF . . .**
- Cancer
- Disfigurement and scarring
- Disability
- Pain during surgery
- Waking up during surgery
- Dying during surgery
- Surgery on the wrong body part
- Anesthesia and its effects
- Going to sleep or not waking up after surgery
- Exposure
- Severe pain or discomfort after surgery
- Tubes, needles, and other care equipment
- Complications
- Prolonged recovery
- More surgery or treatments
- Separation from family and friends

**CONCERN ABOUT . . .**
- Caring for children and other family members
- Pets or plants
- The house, lawn, and garden
- Monthly bills, loan payments, mortgages, or rent
- Paying hospital and doctor bills

# PATIENT INFORMATION

The doctor explains the need for surgery to the patient and family. They are told about:
- The surgical procedure, its risks, and possible complications
- The risks from not having surgery
- Who will do the surgery
- When the surgery is scheduled
- How long the surgery will take

Questions from the patient and family are answered. Misunderstandings are cleared up. Instructions about care are given. The doctor and nurse give all information before surgery.

After surgery the doctor talks to the patient and family. The doctor decides what and when to tell them. Often the health team knows the results before the person. Patients and families are anxious to know the results. They may ask you what their reports say. Refer such questions to the nurse. You never tell of any results or diagnosis.

## YOUR ROLE

You can assist in the surgical patient's psychological care. Do the following if you assist in preoperative and postoperative care:
- Listen to the person. He or she may talk about fears and concerns.
- Refer questions about the surgery or its results to the nurse.
- Explain the care you will give. Also explain why the care is needed.
- Follow communication rules (Chapters 4 and 6).
- Use verbal and nonverbal communication (Chapter 6).
- Perform procedures and tasks with skill and ease.
- Report signs (verbal and nonverbal) of fear or anxiety to the nurse.
- Report a request to see a member of the clergy to the nurse.

# PREOPERATIVE CARE

**Preoperative** means before surgery. The preoperative period may be many days or a few minutes. If time permits, the person is prepared mentally and physically for the effects of anesthesia and surgery. The goal is to prevent complications before, during, and after surgery.

## PREOPERATIVE TEACHING

A nurse does the preoperative teaching. The nurse explains what to expect before, during, and after surgery. Teaching includes:

- *Preoperative activities.* This includes tests and their purpose, skin preparation, and personal care. The person learns about the purpose and effects of preoperative drugs.
- *Deep breathing, coughing, and leg exercises.* These are taught and practiced. After surgery, they are done every 1 or 2 hours when the person is awake.
- *The recovery room.* This is where the person wakes up (Fig. 27-1). Recovery room care is explained.
- *Vital signs.* These are taken frequently until stable.
- *Food and fluids.* The person is NPO and has an IV after surgery. The doctor orders food and oral fluids when the person's condition is stable.
- *Turning and repositioning.* These are done every 1 to 2 hours after surgery.
- *Early ambulation.* The person walks as soon as possible after surgery.
- *Pain.* The person is told about the type and amount of pain to expect. Pain relief drugs are explained.
- *Treatments and equipment.* The person may need a urinary catheter, NG tube, oxygen, wound suction, a cast, or traction.
- *Position restrictions.* Some surgeries require certain positions. For example, the hip is abducted after hip replacement surgery (Chapter 33).

    See Focus on Children: Preoperative Teaching.

---

> ### FOCUS ON CHILDREN
> #### PREOPERATIVE TEACHING
> The child and parents are prepared for the surgery. Often play is used to help the child understand what will happen. For example, dolls are used to show the site of surgery. A tour of the operating and recovery rooms also is common. The child and parents meet the nursing staff who will care for the child.

## SPECIAL TESTS

The doctor evaluates the person's circulatory, respiratory, and urinary systems. The person has a chest x-ray, a complete blood count (CBC), and urinalysis. An electrocardiogram (ECG or EKG) detects cardiac (heart) problems (Fig. 27-2). If blood loss is expected, the person's blood is tested to determine blood type. This is called *type and crossmatch.* Other tests depend on the person's condition and the surgery.

The person is prepared for the tests as needed. Test results must be on the chart by the time of surgery.

## NUTRITION AND FLUIDS

A light meal is usually allowed. Then the person is NPO for 6 to 8 hours before surgery. These measures reduce the risk of vomiting and aspiration during anesthesia and after surgery. An NPO sign is placed in the person's room. The water pitcher and glass are removed.

## ELIMINATION

Bowel surgeries may require cleansing enemas. Remember, feces contain microbes. When the intestine is opened, feces can spill into the sterile abdominal cavity. Cleansing enemas prevent this contamination by clearing the colon of feces. Sometimes enemas are given to prevent constipation after surgery. The doctor orders what enema to give and when.

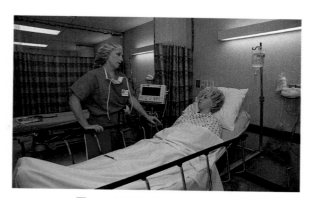

**FIG. 27-1** Recovery room.

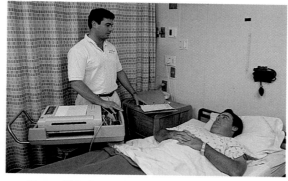

**FIG. 27-2** An electrocardiogram is taken.

Some surgeries require catheters. For pelvic and abdominal surgeries, the bladder must be empty. A full bladder is easily injured during surgery. Catheters also allow accurate output measurements during and after surgery.

If the person does not have a catheter, he or she needs to void before the nurse gives preoperative drugs.

## PERSONAL CARE

Personal care before surgery usually involves:

- *A complete bed bath, shower, or tub bath.* A special soap or cleanser may be ordered. A shampoo is included. The bath and shampoo reduce the number of microbes on the body. This reduces the risk of a wound infection.
- *Removing makeup, nail polish, and artificial nails.* The skin, lips, and nail beds are observed for color and circulation during and after surgery.
- *Hair care.* All hairpins, clips, combs, and other items are removed. So are wigs and hairpieces. Some agencies have the patient wear a surgical cap. A cap keeps hair out of the face and the operative site.
- *Oral hygiene for comfort.* Being NPO causes thirst and a dry mouth. The person must not swallow any water during oral hygiene. *See Focus on Children: Personal Care.*
- *Removing dentures.* Provide denture care. Then store dentures following agency policy. Some people do not like being seen without their dentures. Let them wear their dentures as long as possible. This promotes dignity and self-esteem.
- *Removing other prostheses.* Eyeglasses, contact lenses, artificial eyes, hearing aids, and artificial limbs are examples. Follow agency policy for storage and safekeeping.

---

**FOCUS ON CHILDREN**
**PERSONAL CARE**

Check for loose teeth. Report any loose teeth to the nurse. The nurse notes this on the preoperative checklist and tells the surgery staff. A loose tooth can fall out during anesthesia. The child can aspirate the tooth.

---

## JEWELRY

Jewelry is easily lost or broken during surgery. Transfers to and from the operating room (OR), recovery room, and the person's room also present safety risks. Therefore all jewelry is removed and stored for safekeeping. Record its removal and storage according to agency policy.

The person may want to wear a wedding ring or religious medal. The item is secured in place with gauze and tape according to agency policy. Hand, arm, and breast surgeries can cause swelling of the fingers. Wedding rings are removed for such surgeries.

## SKIN PREPARATION

The skin and hair contain microbes that can enter the body through the surgical incision. Infection is a risk. A *skin prep* removes hair and reduces the number of microbes on the skin.

The incision site and a large area around it are *prepped* (Fig. 27-3, p. 564). This is done right before the surgery. The prep is done in the person's room or in the OR. A hair cream remover is used, or the skin is shaved.

A skin prep kit has a razor, a sponge filled with soap, a basin, and a drape and towel (Fig. 27-4, p. 566). Lather the skin with soap. Then shave in the direction of hair growth (Fig. 27-5, p. 566).

---

**DELEGATION GUIDELINES:** *Skin Preparation*

The nurse may delegate a skin prep to you. When reviewing the procedure with the nurse, you need this information:

- When to do the skin prep
- What site to prep
- What observations to report and record:
  —The area prepared
  —Any cuts, nicks, or scratches
  —Other observations

---

**SAFETY ALERT:** *Skin Preparation*

Any break in the skin is a possible infection site. Be very careful not to cut, scratch, or nick the skin. Follow Standard Precautions and the Bloodborne Pathogen Standard.

*Text continued on p. 567.*

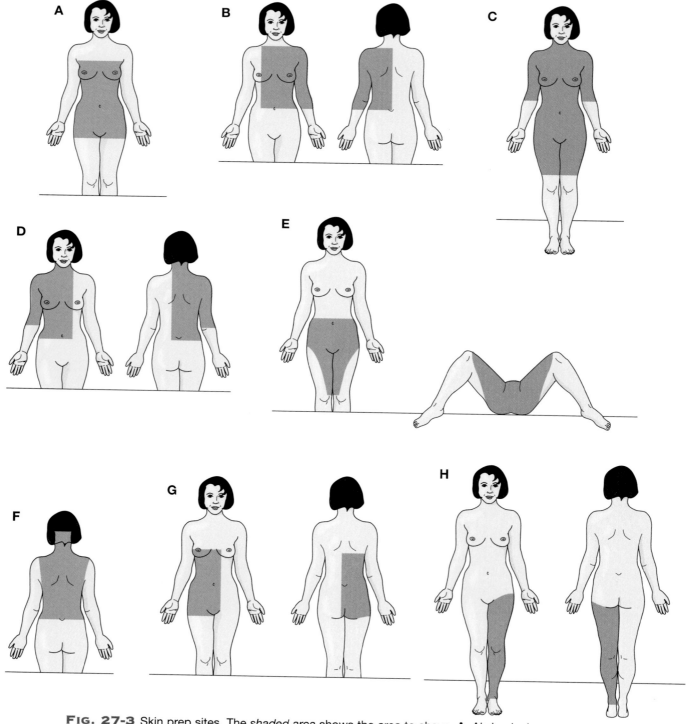

**FIG. 27-3** Skin prep sites. The *shaded area* shows the area to shave. **A,** Abdominal surgery.
**B,** Chest or thoracic surgery. **C,** Open-heart surgery. **D,** Breast surgery. **E,** Perineal surgery. **F,** Cervical spine surgery. **G,** Kidney surgery. **H,** Knee surgery.

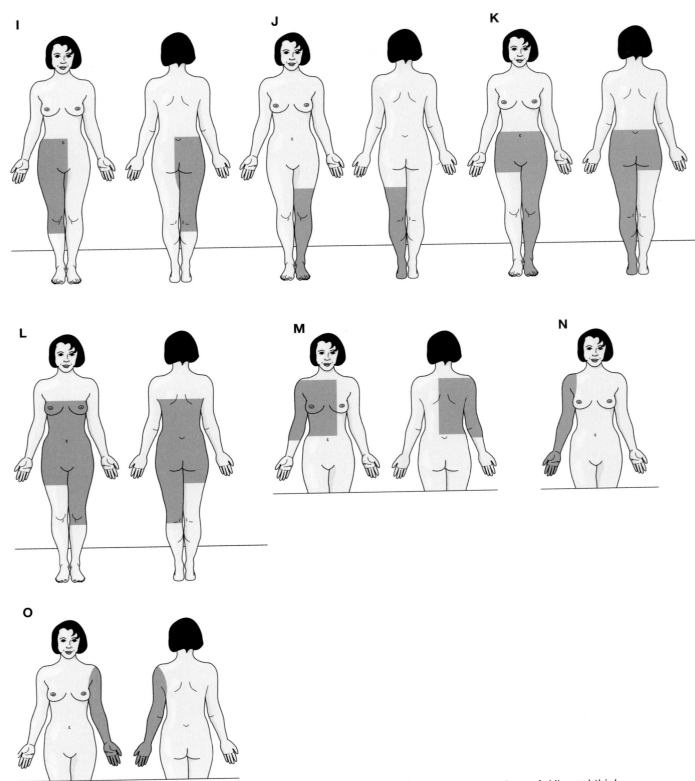

**FIG. 27-3, CONT'D** Skin prep sites. The *shaded area* shows the area to shave. **I,** Hip and thigh surgery. **J,** Lower leg and foot surgery. **K,** Complete lower extremity surgery. **L,** Abdominal and leg surgery. **M,** Upper arm surgery. **N,** Lower arm surgery. **O,** Elbow surgery.

## THE SURGICAL SKIN PREP

### QUALITY OF LIFE

Remember to:
- Knock before entering the person's room
- Address the person by name
- Introduce yourself by name and title

### PRE-PROCEDURE

1 See *Delegation Guidelines: Skin Preparation*, p. 563. See *Safety Alert: Skin Preparation*, p. 563.
2 Explain the procedure to the person.
3 Practice hand hygiene.
4 Collect the following:
- Skin prep kit
- Bath blanket
- Warm water
- Gloves
- Waterproof pad
- Bath towel

5 Identify the person. Check the ID bracelet against the assignment sheet. Call the person by name.
6 Provide for privacy.

### PROCEDURE

7 Make sure you have good lighting.
8 Raise the bed for body mechanics. Lower the bed rail near you (if up).
9 Cover the person with a bath blanket. Fanfold top linens to the foot of the bed.
10 Place the waterproof pad under the area you will shave.
11 Open the skin prep kit.
12 Position the person for the skin prep.
13 Drape him or her with the drape.
14 Add warm water to the basin. Bed rails (if used) are up before you leave the bedside.
15 Put on the gloves.
16 Lather the skin with the sponge.
17 Hold the skin taut. Shave in the direction of hair growth (see Fig. 27-5).
18 Shave outward from the center using short strokes.
19 Rinse the razor often.
20 Make sure the entire area is free of hair. Check for cuts, scratches, or nicks.
21 Rinse the skin thoroughly. Pat dry.
22 Remove the drape and waterproof pad.
23 Remove the gloves. Decontaminate your hands.
24 Return top linens. Remove the bath blanket.

### POST-PROCEDURE

25 Provide for comfort.
26 Raise or lower bed rails. Follow the care plan.
27 Lower the bed to its lowest position.
28 Place the signal light within reach.
29 Unscreen the person.
30 Return equipment to its proper place.
31 Discard supplies. Follow agency policy for soiled linen.
32 Decontaminate your hands.
33 Report and record your observations.

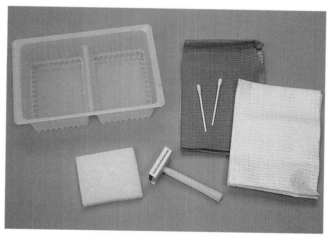

**FIG. 27-4** Skin prep kit.

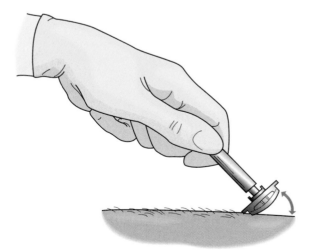

**FIG. 27-5** Shave in the direction of hair growth.

## VAGINAL DOUCHE

A **douche** is the introduction of a fluid into the vagina and the immediate return of the fluid. Doctors order douches to:

- Clean the vagina before surgery
- Relieve pain and inflammation
- Clean the vagina of discharge
- Prevent or remove odor

Drugs, heat, and cold can be applied with a douche. The nurse gives such douches. Some agencies do not allow nursing assistants to give douches.

Douching is not done during menstruation. Nor is it done during late pregnancy or during the first 6 to 8 weeks after childbirth. Douching is not a birth control method. Normally, douching is not needed. Vaginal secretions cleanse the vagina and protect it from infection.

A full bladder can cause discomfort during a douche. Therefore the woman voids before the procedure.

A douche kit has a bag, connecting tubing, and nozzle. Check the nozzle for chips and cracks. Insert the nozzle gently backward and upward (Fig. 27-6). This follows the angle of the vagina when the woman is in the back-lying position.

To give a douche, the genital area is exposed and touched. This area is sexual. Protect the person from sexual abuse. Also protect yourself from being accused

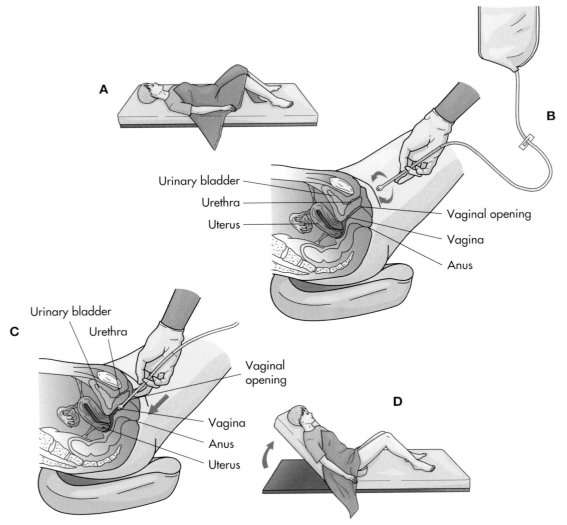

**FIG. 27-6** Giving a douche. **A,** The woman is on her back. **B,** The vulva is cleansed with solution. **C,** The nozzle is inserted 2 to 3 inches into the vagina. Solution flows into the vagina. **D,** The head of the bed is raised to let solution drain from the vagina.

of sexual abuse. Some people do not like being touched. They may interpret the purpose of touch in the wrong way. Culture, religion, and personal values and beliefs affect the meaning of touch. Perform the procedure with skill and in a professional manner:

- Explain the procedure to the person. Get her consent to proceed.
- Protect the right to privacy. Exposure is a form of sexual abuse.
- Be careful what you say. Some words mean different things to different people.
- Be careful what you do. Your nonverbal communication is important.

**DELEGATION GUIDELINES:** *Giving a Douche*
The nurse may ask you to give a douche. Before doing so, make sure the procedure is in your job description and that you have had the necessary training. When reviewing the procedure with the nurse, you need this information:

- When to give the douche
- What solution to use
- How much solution to give
- What the solution temperature should be—usually 100° to 105° F (37.7° to 40.5° C)
- How fast to give the solution—usually 1000 ml over 10 minutes
- What observations to report and record:
  —The time the douche was given
  —The amount, type, and temperature of the solution
  —Amount of discharge
  —Color and odor of returned solution
  —Complaints of pain, burning, or other sensations

**SAFETY ALERT:** *Giving a Douche*
Vaginal secretions may contain blood and microbes. Follow Standard Precautions and the Bloodborne Pathogen Standard.

The nurse tells you what the solution temperature should be—usually 100° to 105° F (37.7° to 40.5° C). If the solution is too hot, you could injure or burn vaginal tissue.

## GIVING A DOUCHE

### QUALITY OF LIFE

Remember to:
- Knock before entering the person's room
- Address the person by name
- Introduce yourself by name and title

### PRE-PROCEDURE

1 Follow *Delegation Guidelines: Giving a Douche.* See *Safety Alert: Giving a Douche.*
2 Explain the procedure to the person.
3 Practice hand hygiene.
4 Collect the following:
   - Douche kit
   - 1000 ml of solution
   - Bath thermometer
   - Bath blanket
   - Bedpan
   - Toilet tissue
   - Waterproof pad
   - Gloves
   - IV pole
   - Water pitcher
   - Equipment for perineal care
5 Identify the person. Check the ID bracelet against the assignment sheet. Call her by name.
6 Provide for privacy.
7 Ask the woman to void. Assist her to the bathroom or commode. Or provide the bedpan. Wear gloves for this step.
8 Remove the gloves. Practice hand hygiene.
9 Raise the bed for body mechanics. Bed rails are up if used.

### PROCEDURE

10 Warm the solution to the temperature directed by the nurse. Follow agency policy for warming the solution and measuring its temperature.
11 Clamp the tubing. Pour the solution into the douche bag.
12 Hang the bag from the IV pole. It should be 12 to 18 inches above the vagina.
13 Cover the person with a bath blanket. Fanfold top linens to the foot of the bed.
14 Position the person supine. Drape her with the bath blanket as for perineal care.
15 Put on gloves.
16 Place the waterproof pad under her buttocks.
17 Give perineal care (see procedure: *Giving Female Perineal Care,* p. 342).
18 Position her on the bedpan.
19 Unclamp the tubing. Let some solution run over the vulva and perineal area.
20 Insert the nozzle 2 to 3 inches into the vagina (see Fig. 27-6). Gently turn the nozzle back and forth during the procedure.
21 Clamp the tubing when the bag is empty. Remove the nozzle.
22 Place the tubing in the douche bag.
23 Raise the head of the bed. This lets solution drain from the vagina into the bedpan.
24 Lower the head of the bed.
25 Remove the bedpan. Dry the perineal area with toilet tissue.
26 Remove the waterproof pad.
27 Take the bedpan into the bathroom. Bed rails are up if used.
28 Clean and return equipment to its proper place.
29 Discard used disposable items.
30 Change damp linen.
31 Remove the gloves. Practice hand hygiene.

### POST-PROCEDURE

32 Provide for comfort.
33 Return top linens. Remove the bath blanket.
34 Lower the bed to its lowest position.
35 Raise or lower bed rails. Follow the care plan.
36 Place the signal light within reach.
37 Unscreen the person.
38 Decontaminate your hands.
39 Report and record your observations.

## THE SURGERY CONSENT

The person's consent is needed before surgery is done. An *operative permit* or *surgical consent* is signed when the person understands the information given by the doctor. The person's spouse or nearest relative may be required to sign the consent. A parent or legal guardian signs for a minor child. The legal guardian signs for a person who is mentally incompetent.

The doctor is responsible for securing written consent. Often this is delegated to an RN. *You do not obtain the person's written consent for surgery.*

## THE PREOPERATIVE CHECKLIST

A preoperative checklist (Fig. 27-7) is placed on the front of the person's chart. When the list is complete, the person is ready for surgery. The nurse may ask you to do some things on the list. Promptly report when you complete each task. Also report any observations. Except for the bed rails, the entire checklist is completed before preoperative drugs are given.

**MARKING THE SURGICAL SITE.** Many agencies mark the surgical site. This is to prevent surgery on the wrong body part. Sometimes the patient marks the body part. This is done as part of the preoperative checklist. It is done before preoperative drugs are given.

## PREOPERATIVE MEDICATION

About 45 minutes to 1 hour before surgery, the preoperative drugs are given. They are given to:
- Help the person relax and feel drowsy
- Reduce respiratory secretions to prevent aspiration
- Prevent nausea and vomiting

The person feels sleepy and lightheaded. Thirst and dry mouth also occur. Falls and accidents are prevented after the drugs are given. Bed rails are raised. The person is not allowed out of bed. Therefore the person voids before the drugs are given. After they are given, the bedpan or urinal is used for voiding.

After the drugs are given, move furniture to make room for the stretcher. Also clean off the overbed table and the bedside stand. This prevents damage to equipment and valuables. Raise the bed to its highest level to transfer the patient from the bed to a stretcher.

## TRANSPORT TO THE OPERATING ROOM

An OR staff member brings a stretcher to the room. The patient is transferred to the stretcher and covered with a bath blanket. The blanket provides warmth and prevents exposure. Falls are prevented. Safety straps are secured and the side rails raised. A pillow is placed under the person's head for comfort.

Identification checks are made. Then the person's chart is given to the OR staff member. The person is transported to the OR. The family may be allowed to go as far as the OR entrance. *See Focus on Children: Transport to the Operating Room.*

## ANESTHESIA

**Anesthesia** is the loss of feeling or sensation produced by a drug. These types of anesthesia are common:
- **General anesthesia** is the loss of consciousness and all feeling or sensation. A drug is given IV, or a gas is inhaled.
- **Regional anesthesia** is the loss of feeling or sensation in a large area of the body. The person is awake. A drug is injected into a body part.
- **Local anesthesia** is the loss of feeling or sensation in a small area. A drug is injected at the site.

Anesthetics are given by specially educated doctors and nurses. An *anesthesiologist* is a doctor who specializes in giving anesthetics. An *anesthetist* is an RN with advanced study giving anesthetics.

---

> ### FOCUS ON CHILDREN
> #### TRANSPORT TO THE OPERATING ROOM
> Some agencies allow a parent to be with the child while anesthesia is given. The parent stays in the OR until the child is asleep.

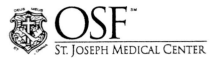

## OSF
ST. JOSEPH MEDICAL CENTER

2200 E. Washington Street, Bloomington, Illinois 61701
Phone (309) 662-3311

## PREOPERATIVE CHECKLIST

DATE OF SURGERY: _____

| CHART PREPARATION | ADEQUATE INITIAL HERE | NOT ADEQUATE INITIAL HERE AND EXPLAIN |
|---|---|---|
| 1. HISTORY AND PHYSICAL ON CHART    HT. _____ WT. _____ | | |
| 2. SURGICAL CONSENT ON CHART, SIGNED | | |
| 3. CONSENT FOR ADM BLOOD/BLOOD PROD. | | |
| 4. PREGNANCY TEST OBTAINED WHEN INDICATED | | |
| 5. URINALYSIS REPORT ON CHART | | |
| 6. BLOOD WORK    TYPE _____ | | |
| 7. TYPE AND CROSSMATCH | | |
| 8. CHEST X-RAY REPORT ON CHART | | |
| 9. EKG REPORT ON CHART   READ _____ | | |
| 10. KNOWN ALLERGIES AND SENSITIVITIES NOTED ON CHART | | |
| 11. KNOWN EXPOSURE AND/OR ALLERGY TO **LATEX** NOTED ON CHART | | |

| PATIENT PREPARATION | ADEQUATE INITIAL HERE | NOT ADEQUATE INITIAL HERE AND EXPLAIN |
|---|---|---|
| 12. FAMILY NOTIFIED OF SURGERY   NAME _____  DATE/TIME _____ | | |
| 13. PATIENT IDENTIFICATION ON WRIST | | |
| 14. ALL PROSTHESES REMOVED (INCLUDING DENTURES, WIGS, HAIRPINS, CONTACT LENSES, COSMETICS, NAIL POLISH, ARTIFICIAL EYES, LIMBS, ETC.) | | |
| 15. ALL JEWELRY REMOVED | | |
| 16. CLOTHING REMOVED EXCEPT HOSPITAL GOWN WITH TIES | | |
| 17. SURGICAL PREP DONE | | |
| 18. TIME OF LAST MEAL OR FLUIDS _____ TIME | | |
| 19. PRE-OP TPR AND BP:  T_____ P_____ R_____ BP_____ | | |
| 20. VOIDED TIME _____ OR FOLEY | | |
| 21. PRE-OP IV AND/OR ANTIBIOTIC:    TIME: | | |

| | DRUG | DOSAGE | ROUTE |
|---|---|---|---|
| PREOPERATIVE MEDICATION GIVEN, | | | |

TIME _____ GIVEN BY _____

☐ SIDE RAILS UP

READY FOR O.R.    DATE _____ TIME _____ SIGNATURE _____

PATIENT IDENTIFIED BY TRANSPORTER AND STAFF NURSE    TIME _____

FLOOR NURSE SIGNATURE _____  OR TRANSPORTER SIGNATURE _____  OR NURSE SIGNATURE _____

| IDENTIFICATION OF INITIALS | | | |
|---|---|---|---|
| INITIALS | SIGNATURE | INITIALS | SIGNATURE |
| | | | |
| | | | |
| | | | |

**FIG. 27-7** Preoperative checklist. (Courtesy OSF St. Joseph Medical Center, Bloomington, Ill.)

# POSTOPERATIVE CARE

After surgery (**postoperative**), the person is taken to the recovery room (RR). This is often called the postanesthesia room (PAR) or postanesthesia care unit (PACU). The recovery room is near the OR. There the person recovers from anesthesia. This takes 1 to 2 hours. The person is watched very closely. Vital signs are taken and observations are made often. The person returns to his or her room when:

- Vital signs are stable.
- Respiratory function is good.
- The person can respond and call for needed help.

The doctor gives the transfer order when appropriate.

## PREPARING THE PERSON'S ROOM

The room must be ready for the person. This is done after the person is taken to the OR. You can do the following:

- Make a surgical bed
- Place equipment and supplies in the room:
  —Thermometer
  —Stethoscope
  —Sphygmomanometer
  —Kidney basin
  —Tissues
  —Waterproof bed protector
  —Vital signs flow sheet
  —I&O record
  —IV pole
  —Other items as directed by the nurse
- Raise the bed to its highest position
- Lower bed rails
- Move furniture out of the way for the stretcher

## RETURN FROM THE RECOVERY ROOM

The recovery staff calls the nursing unit when the person is ready for transfer. The transport is done by the recovery room nurses. A nurse meets the person in the room. Then the person is transferred from the stretcher to bed. Assist as needed. Also help position the person.

Vital signs are taken and observations made. They are compared with those taken in the recovery room. The nurse checks dressings for bleeding. Catheter, IV, and other tube placements and functions are checked. Bed rails are raised. The signal light is placed within the person's reach. Necessary care and treatments are given. Then the family can see the person.

# MEASUREMENTS AND OBSERVATIONS

Your role in postoperative care depends on the person's condition. Often you will measure vital signs and observe the person's condition. Vital signs are usually measured:

- Every 15 minutes the first hour
- Every 30 minutes for 1 to 2 hours
- Every hour for 4 hours
- Then every 4 hours

The nurse tells you how often to check the person. This is an important function. Be alert for the signs and symptoms in Box 27-2. Report them to the nurse at once.

---

**BOX 27-2 POSTOPERATIVE OBSERVATIONS**

- Choking
- Bleeding from the incision, drainage tubes, or suction tubes
- A drop or rise in blood pressure
- A pulse more than 100 or less than 60 beats per minute
- A weak or irregular pulse
- A rise or drop in body temperature
- Hypoxia (Chapter 30)
- The need for upper airway suctioning—rapid respirations, difficulty breathing, moist-sounding respirations or gurgling, restlessness, cyanosis (Chapter 30)
- Shallow, slow breathing
- Rapid, gasping, or difficult respirations
- Weak cough
- Complaints of thirst
- Restlessness
- Cold, moist, clammy, or pale skin
- Cyanosis (bluish color) of the lips or nails
- Increased drainage on or under dressings
- Drainage on bed linens (including bottom linens and pillowcases)
- Complaints of pain or nausea
- Vomiting
- Confusion or disorientation
- The amount, character, and time of the first voiding after surgery
- Intake and output
- IV flow rate
- The appearance of drainage from a urinary catheter, NG tube, or wound suction
- Any other observation that signals a change in condition

## POSITIONING

The person is positioned for comfort and to prevent complications. The type of surgery affects positioning. Position restrictions may be ordered. The person is usually positioned for easy and comfortable breathing. Also, stress on the incision is prevented. When the person is supine, the head of the bed is usually raised slightly. The person's head may be turned to the side. This prevents aspiration if vomiting occurs.

Repositioning is done every 1 to 2 hours to prevent respiratory and circulatory complications. Turning may be painful. Provide support. Use smooth, gentle motions. Pillows and other positioning devices are used as the nurse directs (Chapters 13 and 22).

The nurse tells you when to reposition the person and the positions allowed. Usually you assist the nurse. Sometimes you turn and reposition the person yourself. This occurs when the person's condition is stable and care is simple. *See Focus on Older Persons: Positioning.*

## COUGHING AND DEEP BREATHING

Respiratory complications are prevented. One major complication is *pneumonia.* It is an inflammation and infection in the lung. Another is *atelectasis,* the collapse of a portion of the lung. Coughing and deep-breathing exercises and incentive spirometry help prevent these complications (Chapter 30). *See Focus on Older Persons: Coughing and Deep Breathing.*

## STIMULATING CIRCULATION

Circulation must be stimulated. This is important for blood flow in the legs. If blood flow is sluggish, blood clots may form. They can form in the deep leg veins (Fig. 27-8, *A*). A blood clot (**thrombus**) can break loose and travel through the bloodstream. It then becomes an embolus. An **embolus** is a blood clot that travels through the vascular system until it lodges in a distant vessel (Fig. 27-8, *B*). An embolus from a vein lodges in the lungs (pulmonary embolus). A pulmonary embolus can cause severe respiratory problems and death. *See Focus on Older Persons: Stimulating Circulation.*

---

**FOCUS ON OLDER PERSONS**
POSITIONING

Many older persons have stiff and painful joints. Sore muscles, bones, and joints occur from being on the operating room table. Turn and reposition older persons slowly and gently.

---

**FOCUS ON OLDER PERSONS**
COUGHING AND DEEP BREATHING

Older person are at risk for respiratory complications. Respiratory muscles are weaker. Lung tissue is less elastic. The person has less strength for coughing. Coughing, deep breathing, and incentive spirometry are very important.

---

**FOCUS ON OLDER PERSONS**
STIMULATING CIRCULATION

Older persons are at risk for thrombi and emboli. Blood is pumped through the body with less force. Circulation is already sluggish.

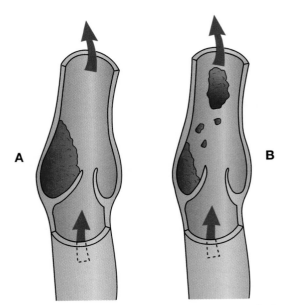

**FIG. 27-8 A,** A blood clot is attached to the wall of a vein. The *arrows* show the direction of blood flow. **B,** Part of the thrombus breaks off and becomes an embolus. The embolus will travel in the bloodstream until it lodges in a distant vessel.

**LEG EXERCISES.** Leg exercises increase venous blood flow and help prevent thrombi. If the person has had leg surgery, a doctor's order is needed for the exercises.

The nurse tells you when to do the exercises. They are done at least every 1 or 2 hours while the person is awake. Assist if the person is weak. These exercises are done 5 times:

- Making circles with the toes. This rotates the ankles.
- Dorsiflexing and plantar flexing the feet (Chapter 22).
- Flexing and extending one knee and then the other (Fig. 27-9).
- Raising and lowering a leg off the bed (Fig. 27-10). Repeat with the other leg.

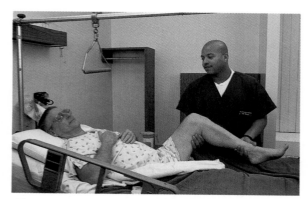

**FIG. 27-9** The knee is flexed and then extended.

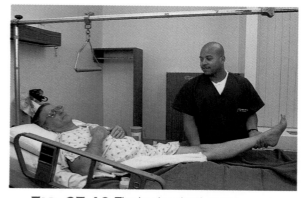

**FIG. 27-10** The leg is raised and lowered.

**ELASTIC STOCKINGS.** Elastic stockings help prevent thrombi. The elastic exerts pressure on the veins. The pressure promotes venous blood flow to the heart. The stockings also are called *anti-embolism* or *anti-embolic (AE) stockings.* They are ordered for persons at risk for thrombi:

- Postoperative patients
- Persons with heart and circulatory disorders
- Persons on bedrest
- Pregnant women

Stockings come in thigh-high or knee-high lengths. The nurse measures the person for the correct size. They are applied before the person gets out of bed. Otherwise the person's legs can swell from sitting or standing. Stockings are hard to put on when the legs are swollen. They are removed every 8 hours for 30 minutes or according to the care plan. The person lies in bed while they are off. This prevents the legs from swelling.

The person usually has two pairs of stockings. One pair is washed while the other pair is worn. Wash the stockings by hand with a mild soap. Hang them to dry.

---

**DELEGATION GUIDELINES:** *Elastic Stockings*
Before you apply elastic stockings, you need this information from the nurse and the care plan:

- What size to use—small, medium, or large
- What length to use—thigh-high or knee-high
- When to remove and reapply them
- What observations to report and record:
  —When you applied the stockings
  —Skin color and temperature
  —Leg and foot swelling
  —Signs of skin breakdown
  —Complaints of pain, tingling, or numbness
  —When you removed the stockings and for how long
  —When you reapplied the stockings
  —When you washed the stockings

---

**SAFETY ALERT:** *Elastic Stockings*
Stockings should not have twists, creases, or wrinkles after you apply them. Twists can affect circulation. Creases and wrinkles can cause skin breakdown.

## APPLYING ELASTIC STOCKINGS

NNAAP™

### QUALITY OF LIFE

Remember to:
- Knock before entering the person's room
- Address the person by name
- Introduce yourself by name and title

### PRE-PROCEDURE

1 Follow *Delegation Guidelines: Elastic Stockings.* See *Safety Alert: Elastic Stockings.*
2 Explain the procedure to the person.
3 Practice hand hygiene.
4 Obtain elastic stockings in the correct size and length.
5 Identify the person. Check the ID bracelet against the assignment sheet. Call the person by name.
6 Provide for privacy.
7 Raise the bed for body mechanics. Bed rails are up if used.

### PROCEDURE

8 Lower the bed rail near you if up.
9 Position the person supine.
10 Expose the legs. Fanfold top linens toward the thighs.
11 Turn the stocking inside out down to the heel (Fig. 27-11, *A*).
12 Slip the foot of the stocking over the toes, foot, and heel (Fig. 27-11, *B*).
13 Grasp the stocking top. Slip it over the foot and heel. Pull it up the leg. It turns right side out as it is pulled up. The stocking is even and snug (Fig. 27-11, *C*).
14 Remove twists, creases, or wrinkles.
15 Repeat steps 11 through 14 for the other leg.

### POST-PROCEDURE

16 Cover the person.
17 Provide for comfort.
18 Lower the bed.
19 Raise or lower bed rails. Follow the care plan.
20 Place the signal light within reach.
21 Unscreen the person.
22 Decontaminate your hands.
23 Report and record your observations.

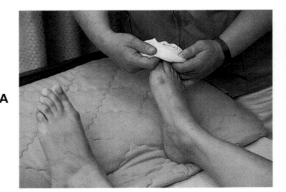
A

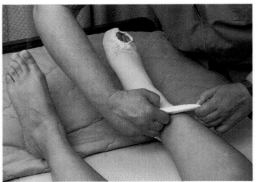
B

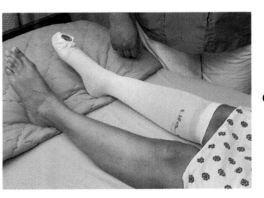
C

**FIG. 27-11** Applying elastic stockings. **A,** The stocking is turned inside out down to the heel. **B,** The stocking is slipped over the toes, foot, and heel. **C,** The stocking turns right side out as it is pulled up over the leg.

**ELASTIC BANDAGES.** Elastic bandages have the same purposes as elastic stockings. They also provide support and reduce swelling from injuries. Sometimes they are used to hold dressings in place. They are applied to arms and legs. The nurse gives you directions about the area to bandage. When applying bandages:

- Use the correct size. Use the proper length and width to bandage the extremity.
- Position the part in good alignment.
- Face the person during the procedure.
- Start at the lower (*distal*) part of the extremity. Work upward to the top (*proximal*) part.
- Expose fingers or toes if possible. This allows circulation checks.
- Apply the bandage with firm, even pressure.
- Check the color and temperature of the extremity every hour.
- Reapply a loose or wrinkled bandage.
- Replace a moist or soiled bandage.

**DELEGATION GUIDELINES:** *Elastic Bandages*
Before applying an elastic bandage, you need this information from the nurse and the care plan:
- Where to apply the bandage
- What width and length to use
- When to remove the bandage and for how long
- What to do if the bandage is wet or soiled
- What observations to report and record:
  —When you applied the bandage
  —Skin color and temperature
  —Swelling of the part
  —Signs of skin breakdown
  —Complaints of pain, itching, tingling, or numbness
  —When you removed the bandage and for how long
  —When you reapplied the bandage

**SAFETY ALERT:** *Elastic Bandages*
Elastic bandages must be firm and snug. However, they must not be tight. A tight bandage can affect circulation.

Some agencies do not let nursing assistants apply elastic bandages. Know your agency's policy.

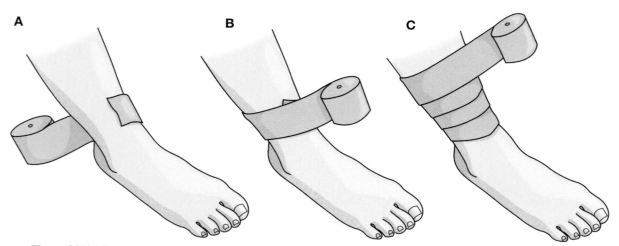

**FIG. 27-12** Applying an elastic bandage. **A,** The roll of the bandage is up. The loose end is at the bottom. **B,** The bandage is applied to the smallest part with two circular turns. **C,** The bandage is applied with spiral turns in an upward direction.

## APPLYING ELASTIC BANDAGES

### QUALITY OF LIFE

Remember to:
- Knock before entering the person's room
- Address the person by name
- Introduce yourself by name and title

### PRE-PROCEDURE

1 Follow *Delegation Guidelines: Elastic Bandages*. See *Safety Alert: Elastic Bandages*.
2 Explain the procedure to the person.
3 Practice hand hygiene.
4 Collect the following:
  - Elastic bandage as directed by the nurse
  - Tape or metal clips (unless the bandage has Velcro)

5 Identify the person. Check the ID bracelet against the assignment sheet. Call the person by name.
6 Provide for privacy.
7 Raise the bed for body mechanics. Bed rails are up if used.

### PROCEDURE

8 Lower the bed rail near you if up.
9 Help the person to a comfortable position. Expose the part you will bandage.
10 Make sure the area is clean and dry.
11 Hold the bandage so the roll is up. The loose end is on the bottom (Fig. 27-12, *A*).
12 Apply the bandage to the smallest part of the wrist, foot, ankle, or knee.
13 Make two circular turns around the part (Fig. 27-12, *B*).

14 Make overlapping spiral turns in an upward direction. Each turn overlaps about ⅔ of the previous turn (Fig. 27-12, *C*).
15 Apply the bandage smoothly with firm, even pressure. It is not tight.
16 Secure the bandage in place with Velcro, tape, or clips. The clips are not under the body part.
17 Check the fingers or toes for coldness or cyanosis (bluish color). Ask about pain, itching, numbness, or tingling. Remove the bandage if any are noted. Report your observations to the nurse.

### POST-PROCEDURE

18 Provide for comfort.
19 Place the signal light within reach.
20 Lower the bed.
21 Raise or lower bed rails. Follow the care plan.

22 Unscreen the person.
23 Decontaminate your hands.
24 Report and record your observations.

**SEQUENTIAL COMPRESSION DEVICES.** A sequential compression device (SCD) is a sleeve that wraps around the leg (Fig. 27-13). Made of cloth or plastic, it is secured in place with Velcro. The device is attached to a pump. The pump inflates the device with air. This promotes venous blood flow to the heart by causing pressure on the veins. Then the pump deflates the device. After deflation, the device is inflated again. The inflation and deflation sequence is repeated as ordered by the doctor.

## EARLY AMBULATION

Early ambulation prevents circulatory complications such as thrombi. It also prevents pneumonia, atelectasis, constipation, and urinary tract infections.

The person usually walks the day of surgery. The person dangles first. Blood pressure and pulse are measured. If they are stable, the person is assisted out of bed. The person does not walk very far, just in the room. Distance increases as the person gains strength.

The nurse tells you when the person can walk. Usually you assist the nurse the first time.

## WOUND HEALING

The incision needs protection. Healing is promoted and infection prevented. Sterile dressing changes are done by the doctor or nurse. Your agency may let you do simple dressing changes. See Chapter 28 for wound care.

## NUTRITION AND FLUIDS

The person returns from the OR with an IV. Continued IV therapy depends on the type of surgery and the person's condition. Anesthesia can cause nausea and vomiting. Diet progresses from NPO to clear liquids, to full liquids, to a regular diet. The doctor orders the diet. Frequent oral hygiene is important when the person is NPO.

Some patients have nasogastric tubes (Chapter 20). Often the NG tube is attached to suction to keep the stomach empty. The person is NPO and has an IV.

## ELIMINATION

Anesthesia, the surgery, and being NPO affect normal bowel and urinary elimination. Pain relief drugs can cause constipation. Measures to promote elimination are practiced as directed by the nurse (Chapters 18 and 19).

Intake and output are measured. The person must void within 8 hours after surgery. Report the time and amount of the first voiding. If the person does not void within 8 hours, a catheterization is usually ordered. Some patients have catheters after surgery. See Chapter 18 for care of the person with a catheter.

Fluid intake and a regular diet are needed for bowel elimination. Suppositories or enemas may be ordered for constipation. Rectal tubes may be ordered for flatulence.

## COMFORT AND REST

Pain is common after surgery. The degree of pain depends on the extent of surgery, incision site, and if drainage tubes, casts, or other devices are present. Positioning during surgery can cause muscle strains and discomfort. The doctor orders drugs for pain relief. The nurse uses the nursing process to promote comfort and rest. Many of the measures listed in Chapter 23 are part of the person's care plan.

## PERSONAL HYGIENE

Personal hygiene is important for physical and mental well-being. Wound drainage and skin prep solutions can irritate the skin and cause discomfort. NPO causes a dry mouth and breath odors. Moist, clammy skin from blood pressure changes or elevated body temperatures also causes discomfort. Frequent oral hygiene, hair care, and a complete bed bath the day after surgery help refresh and renew the person. The gown is changed whenever it is wet or soiled.

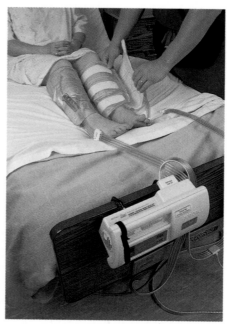

**FIG. 27-13** Sequential compression device. (From deWit SC: *Fundamental concepts and skills for nursing*, Philadelphia, 2001, Saunders.)

**Circle the BEST answer.**

**1** Which is *true* of elective surgery?
  a It is done immediately.
  b The need is sudden and unexpected.
  c It is scheduled for a later date.
  d General anesthesia is always used.

**2** Mr. Long said he was afraid of surgery. What should you do?
  a Call his clergyman.
  b Listen and use touch.
  c Change the subject.
  d Tell his family.

**3** You can assist in Mr. Long's preoperative care by explaining
  a The reason for the surgery
  b The procedures you are doing
  c The risks and possible complications of surgery
  d What to expect during and after surgery

**4** Preoperatively, Mr. Long is
  a NPO
  b Allowed only water
  c Given a regular breakfast
  d Given a tube feeding

**5** Cleansing enemas are given preoperatively to
  a Clean the colon of feces
  b Prevent bleeding
  c Relieve flatus
  d Prevent pain

**6** A skin prep is done preoperatively to
  a Completely bathe the body
  b Sterilize the skin
  c Reduce the amount of hair and microbes on the skin
  d Destroy non-pathogens and pathogens

**7** When doing a skin prep
  a Shave in the direction opposite of hair growth
  b Shave toward the center of the specific area
  c Do not cut, scratch, or nick the skin
  d Use an electric razor

**8** Preoperative medication was given. Mr. Long
  a Must stay in bed
  b Can use the bathroom
  c Can use the commode to void
  d Can have sips of water

**9** General anesthesia
  a Is a specially educated nurse
  b Is the loss of consciousness and feeling or sensation
  c Is a specially educated doctor
  d Is the loss of sensation or feeling in a body part

**10** Coughing and deep breathing after surgery prevent
  a Bleeding
  b A pulmonary embolus
  c Respiratory complications
  d Pain and discomfort

**11** Leg exercises are ordered for Mr. Long. Which is *false*?
  a They stimulate circulation.
  b They prevent thrombi.
  c They are done 5 times every 1 or 2 hours.
  d They are done only for leg surgery.

**12** Postoperatively, Mr. Long's position is changed
  a Every 2 hours
  b Every 3 hours
  c Every 4 hours
  d Every shift

**13** Mr. Long wears elastic stockings to
  a Prevent blood clots
  b Hold dressings in place
  c Reduce swelling after injury
  d Prevent atelectasis

**14** When applying an elastic bandage
  a The part is in good alignment
  b Cover the fingers or toes if possible
  c Apply it from the largest to smallest part of the extremity
  d Apply it from the upper to the lower part of the extremity

Circle **T** if the statement is true and **F** if it is false.

15  **T F** Hair is kept out of the face for surgery by using pins, clips, or combs.

16  **T F** Nail polish is removed before surgery.

17  **T F** Women can wear makeup to surgery.

18  **T F** Pajamas are worn to the operating room.

19  **T F** Contact lenses are removed before surgery.

20  **T F** A surgical bed is made for the person's return from the recovery room.

21  **T F** A drop in a person's blood pressure is reported to the nurse at once.

22  **T F** The person walks the first time 2 days after surgery.

23  **T F** Intake and output are measured after surgery.

24  **T F** A surgical patient should void within 8 hours after surgery.

*Answers to these questions are on p. 818.*

# Wound Care

## OBJECTIVES

- Define the key terms listed in this chapter
- Describe the different types of wounds
- Describe skin tears, pressure ulcers, and circulatory ulcers and how to prevent them
- Identify the pressure points in each body position
- Describe the process, types, and complications of wound healing
- Describe what to observe about wounds and wound drainage
- Explain how to secure dressings
- Explain the rules for applying dressings
- Explain the purpose of binders and how to apply them
- Describe how to meet the basic needs of persons with wounds
- Perform the procedure described in this chapter

## KEY TERMS

**abrasion** A partial-thickness wound caused by the scraping away or rubbing of the skin

**arterial ulcer** An open wound on the lower legs and feet caused by poor arterial blood flow

**bedsore** A pressure ulcer, pressure sore, or decubitus ulcer

**chronic wound** A wound that does not heal easily

**circulatory ulcer** An open wound on the lower legs and feet caused by decreased blood flow through the arteries or veins; vascular ulcer

**clean-contaminated wound** Occurs from the surgical entry of the reproductive, urinary, respiratory, or gastrointestinal system

**clean wound** A wound that is not infected; microbes have not entered the wound

**closed wound** Tissues are injured but the skin is not broken

**contaminated wound** A wound with a high risk of infection

**contusion** A closed wound caused by a blow to the body; a bruise

**decubitus ulcer** A pressure ulcer, pressure sore, or bedsore

**dehiscence** The separation of wound layers

**dirty wound** An infected wound

**epidermal stripping** Removing the epidermis (outer skin layer) as tape is removed from the skin

**evisceration** The separation of the wound along with the protrusion of abdominal organs

**full-thickness wound** The dermis, epidermis, and subcutaneous tissue are penetrated; muscle and bone may be involved

**gangrene** A condition in which there is death of tissue

**hematoma** A collection of blood under the skin and tissues

**hemorrhage** The excessive loss of blood in a short time

**incision** An open wound with clean, straight edges; usually intentionally made with a sharp instrument

**infected wound** A wound containing large amounts of microbes and that shows signs of infection; a dirty wound

**intentional wound** A wound created for therapy

**laceration** An open wound with torn tissues and jagged edges

**open wound** The skin or mucous membrane is broken

**partial-thickness wound** The dermis and epidermis of the skin are broken

**penetrating wound** An open wound in which the skin and underlying tissues are pierced

**pressure sore** A bedsore, decubitus ulcer, or pressure ulcer

**pressure ulcer** Any injury caused by unrelieved pressure; decubitus ulcer, bedsore, or pressure sore

**puncture wound** An open wound made by a sharp object; entry of the skin and underlying tissues may be intentional or unintentional

**purulent drainage** Thick green, yellow, or brown drainage

**sanguineous drainage** Bloody drainage *(sanguis)*

**serosanguineous drainage** Thin, watery drainage *(sero)* that is blood-tinged *(sanguineous)*

**serous drainage** Clear, watery fluid *(serum)*

**shock** Results when organs and tissues do not get enough blood

**skin tear** A break or rip in the skin; the epidermis separates from the underlying tissues

**stasis ulcer** An open wound on the lower legs and feet caused by poor blood return through the veins; venous ulcer

**trauma** An accident or violent act that injures the skin, mucous membranes, bones, and internal organs

**unintentional wound** A wound resulting from trauma

**vascular ulcer** A circulatory ulcer

**venous ulcer** A stasis ulcer

**wound** A break in the skin or mucous membrane

---

A **wound** is a break in the skin or mucous membrane. Wounds result from many causes:

- Surgical incisions
- **Trauma**—an accident or violent act that injures the skin, mucous membranes, bones, and internal organs. Examples: falls, vehicle crashes, gun shots, stabbings, human and animal bites, burns, and frostbite
- Pressure ulcers from poor skin care and immobility (p. 585)
- Circulatory ulcers from decreased blood flow through the arteries or veins (p. 591)

The wound is a portal of entry for microbes. Thus infection is a major threat. Wound care involves preventing infection and further injury to the wound and nearby tissues. Blood loss and pain also are prevented.

Your role in wound care depends on state law, your job description, and the person's condition. Whatever your role, you need to know the types of wounds, how wounds heal, and how to promote wound healing. A review of surgical asepsis will help you understand this chapter (Chapter 12).

## TYPES OF WOUNDS

Types of wounds are described in Box 28-1, p. 585. Wounds also are described by their cause:

- **Abrasion**—a partial-thickness wound caused by the scraping away or rubbing of the skin
- **Contusion**—a closed wound caused by a blow to the body (a bruise)
- **Incision**—an open wound with clean, straight edges; usually intentionally made with a sharp instrument
- **Laceration**—an open wound with torn tissues and jagged edges
- **Penetrating wound**—an open wound in which the skin and underlying tissues are pierced
- **Puncture wound**—an open wound made by a sharp object; entry of the skin and underlying tissues may be intentional or unintentional

*See Focus on Older Persons: Types of Wounds.*

---

> ### FOCUS ON OLDER PERSONS
> #### TYPES OF WOUNDS
>
> Older persons have thin and fragile skin. They are at risk for skin tears. A **skin tear** is a break or rip in the skin. The epidermis (top skin layer) separates from the underlying tissues. The hands, arms, and lower legs are common sites for skin tears.
>
> Skin tears are caused by friction, shearing (Chapter 13), pulling, or pressure on the skin. Bumping a hand, arm, or leg on any hard surface can cause a skin tear. Beds, bed rails, chairs, wheelchair footplates, and tables are dangers. So is holding the person's arm or leg too tight. Be careful when moving, repositioning, or transferring the person. Bathing, dressing, and other tasks can cause skin tears. So can pulling buttons and zippers across fragile skin. Your jewelry (rings, bracelets, watches) also can cause skin tears.
>
> Skin tears are painful. They are a portal of entry for microbes. Wound complications can develop. Tell the nurse at once if you cause or find a skin tear.
>
> To prevent skin tears:
> - Keep your fingernails short and smoothly filed.
> - Keep the person's fingernails short and filed smoothly. Report long and tough toenails to the nurse.
> - Do not wear rings with large or raised stones. Do not wear bracelets.
> - Dress the person in soft clothing with long sleeves and long pants.
> - Follow the care plan and safety rules to lift, move, position, transfer, bathe, and dress the person.
> - Prevent shearing and friction.
> - Use a lift sheet to lift and turn the person in bed.
> - Provide good lighting. It helps prevent the person from bumping into furniture, walls, and equipment.

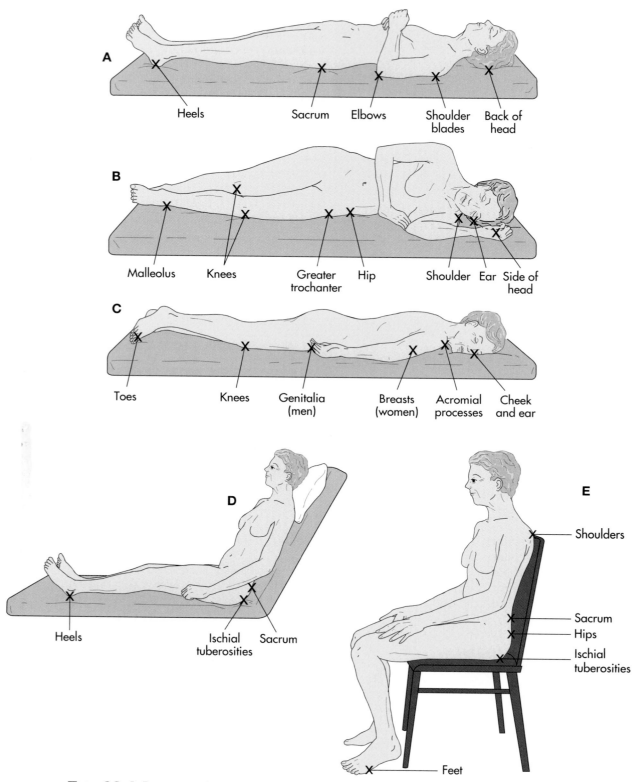

**FIG. 28-1** Pressure points. **A,** Supine position. **B,** Lateral position. **C,** Prone position. **D,** Fowler's position. **E,** Sitting position.

**TYPES OF WOUNDS**

**INTENTIONAL AND UNINTENTIONAL WOUNDS**

- **Intentional wound**—is created for therapy. Surgical incisions are examples. So are venipunctures for starting IVs and for drawing blood specimens.
- **Unintentional wound**—results from trauma. See p. 583.

**OPEN AND CLOSED WOUNDS**

- **Open wound**—when the skin or mucous membrane is broken. Intentional and most unintentional wounds are open.
- **Closed wound**—tissues are injured but the skin is not broken. Bruises, twists, and sprains are examples.

**CLEAN AND DIRTY WOUNDS**

- **Clean wound**—is not infected. Microbes have not entered the wound. Closed wounds are usually clean. So are intentional wounds created under surgically aseptic conditions. The reproductive, urinary, respiratory, and gastrointestinal systems are not entered.
- **Clean-contaminated wound**—occurs from the surgical entry of the reproductive, urinary, respiratory, or gastrointestinal system. These systems are not sterile and contain normal flora.

- **Contaminated wound**—has a high risk of infection. Unintentional wounds are generally contaminated. Wound contamination also occurs from breaks in surgical asepsis and spillage of intestinal contents. Tissues may show signs of inflammation.
- **Infected wound (dirty wound)**—contains large amounts of microbes and shows signs of infection. Examples include old wounds, surgical incisions into infected areas, and traumatic injuries that rupture the bowel.
- **Chronic wound**—does not heal easily. Pressure ulcers and circulatory ulcers are examples.

**PARTIAL- AND FULL-THICKNESS WOUNDS (DESCRIBE WOUND DEPTH)**

- **Partial-thickness wound**—the dermis and epidermis of the skin are broken.
- **Full-thickness wound**—the dermis, epidermis, and subcutaneous tissue are penetrated. Muscle and bone may be involved.

## PRESSURE ULCERS

A **pressure ulcer (decubitus ulcer, bedsore, pressure sore)** is any injury caused by unrelieved pressure. It usually occurs over a bony prominence. *Prominence* means to stick out. A *bony prominence* is an area where the bone sticks out or projects out from the flat surface of the body. The shoulder blades, elbows, hips, sacrum, knees, ankles, heels, and toes are bony prominences (Fig. 28-1). *See Focus on Older Persons: Pressure Ulcers.*

## CAUSES

Pressure, friction, and shearing are common causes of skin breakdown and pressure ulcers. Other factors include breaks in the skin, poor circulation to an area, moisture, dry skin, and irritation by urine and feces.

Pressure occurs when the skin over a bony area is squeezed between hard surfaces. The bone is one hard surface. The other is usually the mattress or chair seat. Squeezing or pressure prevents blood flow to the skin and underlying tissues. Lack of blood flow means oxygen and nutrients cannot get to the cells. Therefore involved skin and tissues die (Fig. 28-2).

**FOCUS ON OLDER PERSONS**
PRESSURE ULCERS

Older and disabled persons are at great risk for pressure ulcers. Their skin is easily injured. Causes include age-related skin changes, chronic disease, and general debility.

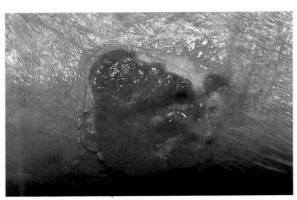

**FIG. 28-2** A pressure ulcer.

Friction scrapes the skin. An open area, the scrape is a portal of entry for microbes. The open area needs to heal. A good blood supply is needed. Infection is prevented so healing occurs. A poor blood supply or an infection can lead to a pressure ulcer.

Shearing is when the skin sticks to a surface (usually the bed or chair) while deeper tissues move downward (Chapter 13). This occurs when the person slides down in the bed or chair. Blood vessels and tissues are damaged. Blood flow to the area is reduced.

## PERSONS AT RISK

Persons at risk for pressure ulcers are those who:
- Are confined to bed or chair
- Need some or total help in moving
- Have loss of bowel or bladder control
- Have poor nutrition
- Have poor fluid balance
- Have altered mental awareness
- Have problems sensing pain or pressure
- Have circulatory problems
- Are older
- Are obese or very thin

  See Focus on Children: Persons at Risk.

## SIGNS OF PRESSURE ULCERS

The first sign of a pressure ulcer is pale skin or a reddened area. Color changes may be hard to notice in persons with dark skin. The person may complain of pain, burning, or tingling in the area. Some do not feel anything unusual. Box 28-2 describes pressure ulcer stages.

## SITES

Pressure ulcers usually occur over bony areas. The bony areas are called *pressure points*. This is because they bear the weight of the body in a certain position (see Fig. 28-1). Pressure from body weight can reduce the blood supply to the area.

In obese people, pressure ulcers can occur in areas where skin is in contact with skin. Common sites are between abdominal folds, the legs, and the buttocks and under the breasts. Friction occurs in these areas.

Persons who spend a lot of time in bed are at risk for pressure ulcers on the ears. This is from pressure of the ear on the mattress when in the side-lying position.

---

### FOCUS ON CHILDREN
#### PERSONS AT RISK

Infants and children also are at risk for pressure ulcers. Poor mobility, lack of bowel and bladder control (incontinence), poor nutrition, and infection are risk factors. Pressure, friction, and shearing are causes. Epidermal stripping is another cause. **Epidermal stripping** is removing the epidermis (outer skin layer) as tape is removed from the skin. Newborns are at risk because of having fragile skin.

---

| BOX 28-2 | STAGES OF PRESSURE ULCERS |
|---|---|
| Stage 1 | The skin is red. The color does not return to normal when the skin is relieved of pressure (Fig. 28-3, *A*). The skin is intact. |
| Stage 2 | The skin cracks, blisters, or peels (Fig. 28-3, *B*). There may be a shallow crater. |
| Stage 3 | The skin is gone. Underlying tissues are exposed (Fig. 28-3, *C*). The exposed tissue is damaged. There may be drainage from the area. |
| Stage 4 | Muscle and bone are exposed and damaged (Fig. 28-3, *D*). Drainage is likely. |

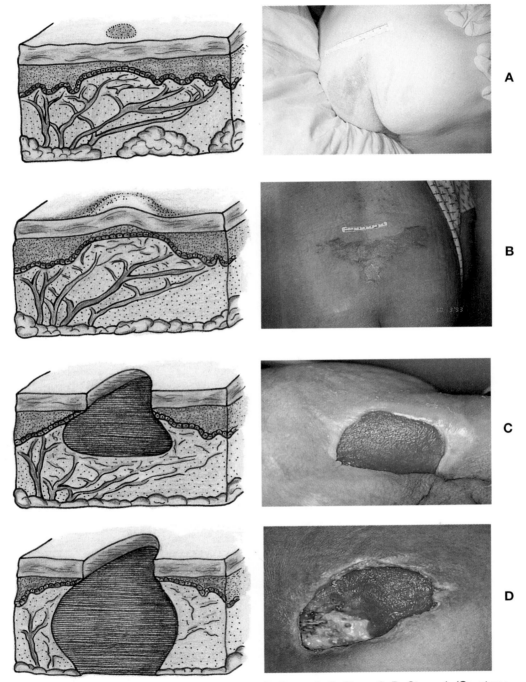

**FIG. 28-3** Stages of pressure ulcers. **A,** Stage 1. **B,** Stage 2. **C,** Stage 3. **D,** Stage 4. (Courtesy Laurel Wiersema-Bryant, RN, MSN, Clinical Nurse Specialist, Barnes-Jewish Hospital, St. Louis.)

## PREVENTION AND TREATMENT

Preventing pressure ulcers is much easier than trying to heal them. Good nursing care, cleanliness, and skin care are essential. The measures in Box 28-3 help prevent skin breakdown and pressure ulcers. Follow the person's care plan.

The person at risk for pressure ulcers is placed on a surface that reduces or relieves pressure. Such surfaces include foam, air, alternating air, gel, or water mattresses. The health team decides on the best surface for the person.

The doctor orders wound care products, drugs, treatments, and special equipment to promote healing. The nurse and care plan tell you what to do. These protective devices are often used to prevent and treat pressure ulcers and skin breakdown:

---

### BOX 28-3 MEASURES TO PREVENT PRESSURE ULCERS

- Follow the repositioning schedule in the person's care plan. The person is repositioned at least every 2 hours. Some persons are repositioned every 15 minutes.
- Position the person according to the care plan. Use pillows for support as instructed by the nurse. The 30-degree lateral position is recommended (Fig. 28-4).
- Prevent shearing and friction during lifting and moving procedures.
- Prevent shearing. Do not raise the head of the bed more than 30 degrees. Follow the care plan.
- Prevent friction by applying a thin layer of cornstarch to the bottom sheets.
- Provide good skin care. The skin must be clean and dry after bathing. The skin is free of moisture from urine, stools, perspiration, and wound drainage.
- Minimize skin exposure to moisture. Check incontinent persons (those without bowel or bladder control) often. Also check persons who perspire heavily and those with wound drainage. Change linens and clothing as needed, and provide good skin care.
- Check with the nurse before using soap. Soap can dry and irritate the skin.

- Apply a moisturizer to dry areas such as the hands, elbows, legs, ankles, and heels. The nurse tells you what to use and the areas that need attention.
- Give a back massage when repositioning the person. *Do not massage bony areas.*
- Keep linens clean, dry, and free of wrinkles.
- Apply powder where skin touches skin.
- Do not irritate the skin. Avoid scrubbing or vigorous rubbing when bathing or drying the person.
- Do not massage over pressure points. *Never rub or massage reddened areas.*
- Use pillows and blankets to prevent skin from being in contact with skin. They also reduce moisture and friction.
- Keep the heels off the bed. Use pillows or other devices as the nurse directs. Place the pillows or devices under the lower legs from midcalf to the ankles.
- Use protective devices as the nurse and care plan direct.
- Remind persons sitting in chairs to shift their positions every 15 minutes. This decreases pressure on bony points.
- Report any signs of skin breakdown or pressure ulcers at once.

---

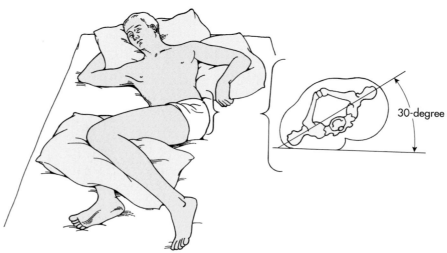

**FIG. 28-4** The 30-degree lateral position. Pillows are placed under the head, shoulder, and leg. This position inclines (lifts up) the hip to avoid pressure on the hip. The person does not lie on the hip as in the side-lying position. (From Bryant RA and others: Pressure ulcers. In Bryant RA, editor: *Acute and chronic wounds: nursing management,* St Louis, 1992, Mosby.)

- *Bed cradle.* A bed cradle (Anderson frame) is a metal frame placed on the bed and over the person. Top linens are brought over the cradle to prevent pressure on the legs and feet (Fig. 28-5). Top linens are tucked in at the bottom of the mattress and mitered. They are also tucked under mattress sides. This protects the person from air drafts and chilling. *See Focus on Home Care: Bed Cradles.*
- *Elbow protectors.* These devices are made of foam rubber or sheepskin. They fit the shape of the elbow (Fig. 28-7). Some have straps to secure them in place. Friction is prevented between the bed and the elbow.
- *Heel elevators.* Pillows or special cushions are used to raise the heels off the bed (Fig. 28-8). Special braces and splints also are used to keep pressure off the heels.

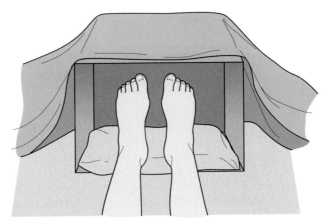

FIG. 28-6 A box serves as a bed cradle. It keeps top linens off the feet.

> ### FOCUS ON HOME CARE
> #### BED CRADLES
> A cardboard box is useful as a bed cradle (Fig. 28-6). The nurse tells you how to line the box to prevent pressure on the heels.

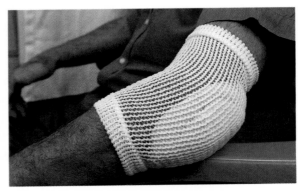

FIG. 28-7 Elbow protector.

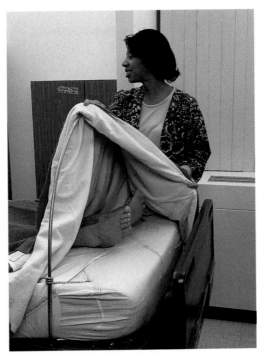

FIG. 28-5 A bed cradle. Linens are brought over the top of the cradle.

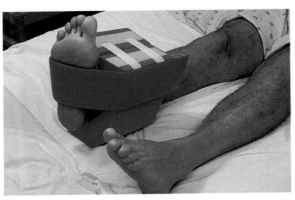

FIG. 28-8 Heel elevator.

- *Flotation pads.* Flotation pads or cushions (Fig. 28-9) are like waterbeds. They are used for chairs and wheelchairs. They are made of a gel-like substance. The outer case is heavy plastic. The pad is placed in a pillowcase or special cover. The cover protects the skin.
- *Eggcrate-like mattress.* This is a foam pad that looks like an egg carton (Fig. 28-10). Peaks in the mattress distribute the person's weight more evenly. It is placed on top of the regular mattress. The eggcrate-like mattress is put in a special cover. The cover protects against moisture and soiling. Only a bottom sheet is used to cover the eggcrate-like mattress and cover. No other bottoms linens are used.
- *Special beds.* Some beds have air flowing through the mattresses (Fig. 28-11). The *person floats* on the mattress. Body weight is distributed evenly. There is little pressure on bony parts. Other beds allow repositioning without moving the person. The person is turned to the prone or supine position or tilted various degrees. Alignment does not change. Pressure points change as the position changes. There is little friction. Some beds constantly rotate from side to side. They are useful for persons with spinal cord injuries.
- *Other equipment.* Trochanter rolls and footboards also are used (Chapter 22).

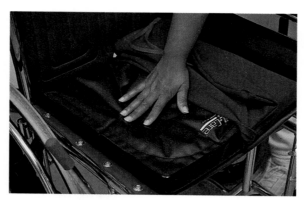

**FIG. 28-9** Flotation pad.

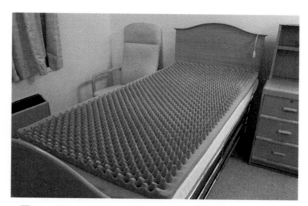

**FIG. 28-10** Eggcrate-like mattress on the bed.

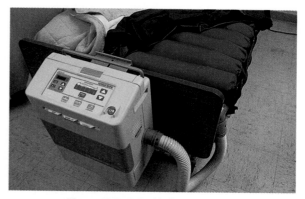

**FIG. 28-11** Air flotation bed.

# CIRCULATORY ULCERS

Some people have diseases that affect blood flow to and from the legs and feet. Such poor circulation can lead to pain, open wounds, and swelling of tissues (*edema*). Infection and gangrene can result from the open wound and poor circulation. **Gangrene** is a condition in which there is death of tissue (Chapter 33).

The doctor orders drugs and treatments as needed. The RN uses the nursing process to meet the person's needs (Box 28-4). Preventing skin breakdown on the legs and feet is very important.

**Circulatory ulcers (vascular ulcers)** are open wounds on the lower legs and feet caused by decreased blood flow through arteries or veins. Persons with diseases affecting the blood vessels are at risk. These wounds are painful and hard to heal.

## STASIS ULCERS

**Stasis ulcers (venous ulcers)** are open wounds on the lower legs and feet caused by poor blood return through the veins (Fig. 28-12). Valves in the leg veins do not close well. Therefore the veins do not pump blood back to the heart normally. Blood and fluid collect in the legs and feet. Small veins in the skin can rupture. Remember, hemoglobin gives blood its red color. When veins rupture, hemoglobin enters the tissues. This causes the skin to turn brown. The skin is dry, leathery, and hard. Itching is common.

The heels and inner aspect of the ankles are common sites for stasis ulcers. They can occur from skin injury. Scratching is a common cause. Or the ulcers occur spontaneously.

---

| BOX 28-4 | MEASURES TO PREVENT CIRCULATORY ULCERS |
|---|---|

- Remind the person not to sit with the legs crossed.
- Position the person according to the care plan.
- Do not use elastic or rubber band–type of garters to hold socks or hose in place.
- Do not dress the person in tight clothes.
- Keep the feet clean and dry. Clean and dry between the toes.
- Do not scrub or rub the skin during bathing and drying.
- Keep linens clean, dry, and wrinkle-free.
- Avoid injury to the legs and feet.
- Make sure shoes fit well.
- Keep pressure off the heels and other bony areas. Use pillows or other devices as the nurse and care plan direct.
- Check the person's legs and feet. Report skin breaks or changes in skin color.
- Do not massage over pressure points. *Never rub or massage reddened areas.*
- Follow the care plan for walking and exercise.

---

Stasis ulcers are painful and make walking difficult. They weep fluid. Infection is a risk. Healing is slow.

**RISK FACTORS.** Risk factors for stasis ulcers include:
- History of blood clots
- History of varicose veins
- Decreased mobility
- Obesity
- Leg or foot injury
- Advanced age
- Surgery on the bones and joints
- Inflammation of a vein

**PREVENTION AND TREATMENT.** Preventing skin breakdown is important. Follow the person's care plan (see Box 28-4). Stasis ulcers are hard to heal. The doctor may order elastic stockings or elastic bandages (Chapter 27). Professional foot care is important.

## ARTERIAL ULCERS

**Arterial ulcers** are open wounds on the lower legs and feet caused by poor arterial blood flow. The leg and foot may feel cold and look blue or shiny. The ulcer is often painful at rest. Pain is usually worse at night.

These ulcers are caused by diseases or injuries that decrease arterial blood flow to the legs and feet. High blood pressure and diabetes are common causes. So are narrowed arteries from aging. Smoking is another risk factor.

Arterial ulcers are found between the toes, on top of the toes, and on the outer side of the ankle. The heels are common sites for persons on bedrest. These ulcers can occur on pressure sites from shoes that fit poorly.

The doctor treats the disease causing the ulcer. Drugs, wound care, and a walking and exercise program are ordered. Professional foot care is important. Follow the care plan (see Box 28-4) and prevent further injury.

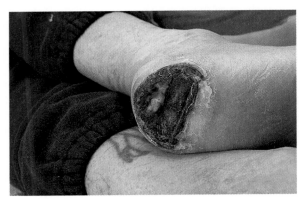

**FIG. 28-12** Stasis ulcer.

# WOUND HEALING

The healing process has three phases:
- *Inflammatory phase* (3 days). Bleeding stops. A scab forms over the wound. The scab protects against microbes entering the wound. Blood supply to the wound increases. The blood brings nutrients and healing substances. Because blood supply increases, signs and symptoms of inflammation appear. They are redness, swelling, heat or warmth, and pain. Loss of function may occur.
- *Proliferative phase* (day 3 to day 21). *Proliferate* means to multiply rapidly. Tissue cells multiply to repair the wound.
- *Maturation phase* (day 21 to 2 years). The scar gains strength. The red, raised scar becomes thin and pale.

## TYPES OF WOUND HEALING

Healing occurs through primary intention, secondary intention, or tertiary intention. With *primary intention (first intention, primary closure)*, the wound is closed by bringing the wound edges together. Sutures (stitches), staples, clips, special glue, or adhesive strips hold the wound edges together.

*Secondary intention (second intention)* is used for contaminated and infected wounds. Wounds are cleaned and dead tissue removed. Wound edges are not brought together. The wound gaps. Healing occurs naturally. However, healing takes longer and leaves a larger scar. The threat of infection is great.

*Tertiary intention (third intention, delayed intention)* involves leaving a wound open and closing it later. It combines secondary and primary intention. Infection and poor circulation are common reasons for tertiary intention.

## COMPLICATIONS OF WOUND HEALING

Many factors affect healing and increase the risk of complications. The type of wound is one factor. Other factors include the person's age, general health, nutrition, and life-style.

Good circulation is important. Age, smoking, circulatory disease, and diabetes all affect circulation. Certain drugs (Coumadin and heparin) prolong bleeding.

Good nutrition is needed. Protein is needed for tissue growth and repair.

Infection is a risk for persons with immune system changes and for those taking antibiotics. Antibiotics kill pathogens. Specific antibiotics kill specific pathogens. In doing so, an environment may be created that allows other pathogens to grow and multiply.

**HEMORRHAGE AND SHOCK. Hemorrhage** is the excessive loss of blood in a short time (Chapter 40). If bleeding is not stopped, death results. Hemorrhage may be internal or external. Internal hemorrhage cannot be seen. Bleeding occurs inside the body into tissues and body cavities. A hematoma may form. A **hematoma** is a collection of blood under the skin and tissues. The area is swollen and is reddish blue in color. Shock, vomiting blood, coughing up blood, and loss of consciousness are signs of internal hemorrhage.

You can see external bleeding. Common signs are bloody drainage and dressings soaked with blood. Gravity causes fluid to flow down. Blood can flow down and collect under the part. Check under the body part for pooling of blood. As with internal hemorrhage, shock can occur.

**Shock** results when organs and tissues do not get enough blood (Chapter 40). Blood pressure falls, the pulse is rapid and weak, and respirations are rapid. The skin is cold, moist, and pale. The person is restless and may complain of thirst. Confusion and loss of consciousness occur as shock worsens.

Hemorrhage and shock are emergencies. Alert the nurse at once. Assist as requested.

> **SAFETY ALERT:** *Hemorrhage and Shock*
> Follow Standard Precautions and the Bloodborne Pathogen Standard when in contact with blood. Gloves, gowns, masks, and eye protection are necessary when blood splashes and splatters are likely.

**INFECTION.** Wound contamination can occur during or after the injury. Trauma often causes contaminated wounds. Surgical wounds can be contaminated during or after surgery. An infected wound appears inflamed (reddened) and has drainage (p. 594). The wound is painful and tender. The person has a fever.

**DEHISCENCE. Dehiscence** is the separation of wound layers (Fig. 28-13). Separation may involve the

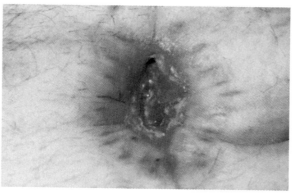

**FIG. 28-13** Wound dehiscence. (Courtesy Morison M: *A colour guide to the nursing management of wounds*, London, 1992, Wolfe Medical Publishers.)

skin layer or underlying tissues. Abdominal wounds are commonly affected. Coughing, vomiting, and abdominal distention place stress on the wound. The person often describes the sensation of the wound "popping open."

**EVISCERATION.** **Evisceration** is the separation of the wound along with the protrusion of abdominal organs (Fig. 28-14). Causes are the same as for dehiscence.

Dehiscence and evisceration are surgical emergencies. The wound is covered with large sterile dressings saturated with sterile saline. You must tell the nurse at once and help prepare the person for surgery.

## WOUND APPEARANCE

Doctors and nurses observe the wound and its drainage. They observe for healing and complications. You need to make certain observations when assisting with wound care (Box 28-5). Report and record your observations according to agency policy. *See Focus on Home Care: Wound Appearance.*

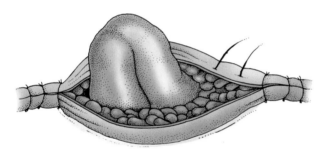

**FIG. 28-14** Wound evisceration. (From Ignatavicius DD, Workman ML: *Medical-surgical nursing: critical thinking for collaborative care,* ed 4, Philadelphia, 2002, Saunders.)

### FOCUS ON HOME CARE
#### WOUND APPEARANCE

The RN may ask you to take photos of wounds. The photos help the RN assess and evaluate the wound. Before taking a photo, make sure the person has signed a consent for photography. (The RN obtains the consent.) If using a Polaroid camera, write the person's name, the date, and time on the back of the photo. For regular film or a digital camera, note the frame number, the person's name, and the date and time in the person's record.

The photo does not replace making accurate observations. See Box 28-5.

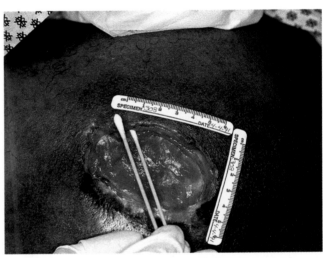

**FIG. 28-15** The size and depth of this pressure ulcer are measured. (From Potter PA, Perry AG: *Fundamentals of nursing,* ed 5, St Louis, 2001, Mosby.)

---

### BOX 28-5 WOUND OBSERVATION

- Wound location
  —Multiple wounds may exist from surgery or trauma.
- Wound size and depth (measure in centimeters)
  —Size: Measure from top to bottom and side to side (Fig. 28-15).
  —Depth: (1) Insert a sterile swab inside the deepest part of the wound. (2) Remove the swab and measure the distance on the swab. *Measure depth only when the wound is open and with the nurse's supervision.*
  —Use a disposable ruler. For a nondisposable ruler, clean the ruler following agency policy.
- Wound appearance
  —Is the wound red and swollen?
  —Is the area around the wound warm to touch?

  —Are sutures, staples, or clips intact or broken?
  —Are wound edges closed or separated?
  —Did the wound break open?
- Drainage (p. 594)
  —Is the drainage serous, sanguineous, serosanguineous, or purulent?
  —What is the amount of drainage?
- Odor
  —Does the wound or drainage have an odor?
- Surrounding skin
  —Is surrounding skin intact?
  —What is the color of surrounding skin?
  —Are surrounding tissues swollen?

# WOUND DRAINAGE

During injury and the inflammatory phase of wound healing, fluid and cells escape from the tissues. The amount of drainage may be small or large. This depends on wound size and location. Bleeding and infection also affect the amount and kind of drainage. Wound drainage is observed and measured.

- **Serous drainage**—clear, watery fluid (Fig. 28-16, *A*). The fluid in a blister is serous. *Serous* comes from the word *serum*. Serum is the clear, thin, fluid portion of the blood. Serum does not contain blood cells or platelets.
- **Sanguineous drainage**—bloody drainage (Fig. 28-16, *B*). The Latin word *sanguis* means blood. The amount and color of sanguineous drainage is important. Hemorrhage is suspected when large amounts are present. Bright drainage means fresh bleeding. Older bleeding is darker.
- **Serosanguineous drainage**— thin, watery drainage *(sero)* that is blood-tinged *(sanguineous)* (Fig. 28-16, *C*).
- **Purulent drainage**—thick green, yellow, or brown drainage (Fig. 28-16, *D*).

Drainage must leave the wound for healing. If drainage is trapped inside the wound, underlying tissues swell. The wound may heal at the skin level, but underlying tissues do not close. Infection and other complications can occur.

When large amounts of drainage are expected, the doctor inserts a drain. A *Penrose drain* is a rubber tube that drains onto a dressing (Fig. 28-17). It opens onto the dressing. Therefore it is an open drain. Microbes can enter the drain and wound.

Closed drainage systems prevent microbes from entering the wound. A drain is placed in the wound and attached to suction. The Hemovac (Fig. 28-18) and Jackson-Pratt (Fig. 28-19) systems are examples. Other systems are used depending on wound type, size, and location.

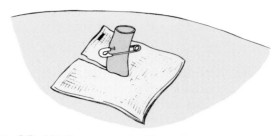

**FIG. 28-17** Penrose drain. The safety pin prevents the drain from slipping into the wound. (From Potter PA, Perry AG: *Fundamentals of nursing*, ed 5, St Louis, 2001, Mosby.)

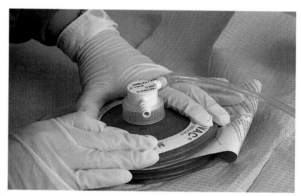

**FIG. 28-18** Hemovac. Drains are sutured to the wound and connected to the reservoir. (From Potter PA, Perry AG: *Fundamentals of nursing*, ed 5, St Louis, 2001, Mosby.)

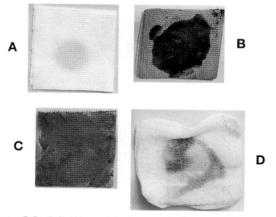

**FIG. 28-16** Wound drainage. **A,** Serous drainage. **B,** Sanguineous drainage. **C,** Serosanguineous drainage. **D,** Purulent drainage. (From Potter PA, Perry AG: *Fundamentals of nursing*, ed 5, St Louis, 2001, Mosby.)

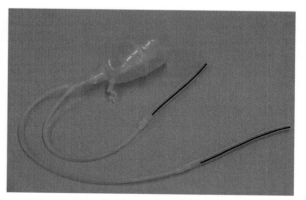

**FIG. 28-19** The Jackson-Pratt drainage system. (From Elkin MK, Perry AG, Potter PA: *Nursing interventions & clinical skills*, ed 2, St Louis, 2000, Mosby.)

Drainage is measured in three ways:

- Noting the number and size of dressings with drainage. What is the amount and kind of drainage? Are dressings saturated? Is drainage on just part of the dressing? If so, which part? Is drainage through some or all layers?
- Weighing dressings before applying them to the wound. The weight of each new dressing is noted. Dressings are weighed after removal. The dry dressing weight is subtracted from the wet dressing weight. (Wet dressings weigh more.)
- Measuring the amount of drainage in the collection container if closed drainage is used.

## DRESSINGS

Wound dressings have many functions:

- They protect wounds from injury and microbes.
- They absorb drainage.
- They remove dead tissue.
- They promote comfort.
- They cover unsightly wounds.
- They provide a moist environment for wound healing.
- When bleeding is a problem, pressure dressings help control bleeding.

Dressing type and size depend on many factors. These include the type of wound, its size and location, and amount of drainage. Infection is a factor. The dressing's function and the frequency of dressing changes are other factors. The doctor and nurse choose the best type of dressing for each wound.

## TYPES OF DRESSINGS

Dressings are described by the material used and application method. There are many dressing products. The following are common:

- *Gauze.* It comes in squares, rectangles, pads, and rolls (Fig. 28-20). Gauze dressings absorb moisture.
- *Nonadherent gauze.* It is a gauze dressing with a non-stick surface. It does not stick to the wound. It removes easily without injuring tissue.
- *Transparent adhesive film.* Air can reach the wound but fluids and bacteria cannot. The wound is kept moist. Drainage is not absorbed. The transparent film allows wound observation.

Some dressings contain special agents to promote wound healing. If you assist with the dressing change, the nurse explains its use to you.

Dressing application methods involve dry and wet dressings:

- *Dry-to-dry dressing (dry dressing).* A dry gauze dressing is placed over the wound. More dressings are placed on top of the first dressing as needed. Drainage is absorbed by the dressing and is removed with the dressing. A dry dressing can stick to the wound. The dressing is removed carefully to prevent tissue injury and discomfort.
- *Wet-to-dry dressing.* A gauze dressing saturated with a solution is applied over the wound. More dressings are applied as needed. They also are moistened with solution. The solution softens dead tissue in the wound. The dead tissue is absorbed by the dressing and is removed with the dressing. The dressings are removed when dry.
- *Wet-to-wet dressing.* Gauze dressings saturated with solution are placed in the wound. The dressing is kept moist.

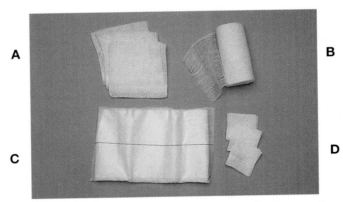

**FIG. 28-20** Gauze dressings. **A,** 4 × 4. **B,** Gauze roll. **C,** Abdominal pad (ABD). **D,** 2 × 2.

## SECURING DRESSINGS

Dressings must be secured over wounds. Microbes can enter the wound and drainage can escape if the dressing is dislodged. Tape and Montgomery ties are used to secure dressings. Binders also hold dressings in place.

**TAPE.** Adhesive, paper, plastic, and elastic tapes are common. Adhesive tape sticks well to the skin. However, the adhesive remaining on the skin is hard to remove. It can irritate the skin. An abrasion occurs if skin is removed with tape. Many people are allergic to adhesive tape. Paper and plastic tapes usually do not cause allergic reactions. Elastic tape allows movement of the body part.

Tape is applied to secure the top, middle, and bottom of the dressing (Fig. 28-21). The tape extends several inches beyond each side of the dressing. *The tape must not circle the entire body part. If swelling occurs, circulation to the part is impaired.*

**MONTGOMERY TIES.** Montgomery ties (Fig. 28-22) are used for large dressings and frequent dressing changes. A Montgomery tie has an adhesive strip and a cloth tie. When the dressing is in place, the adhesive strips are placed on both sides of the dressing. Then the cloth ties are secured over the dressing. Two or three Montgomery ties may be needed on each side. The ties are undone for the dressing change. The adhesive strips are not removed unless soiled.

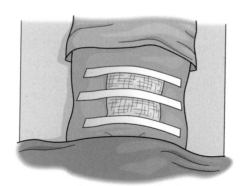

**FIG. 28-21** Tape is applied at the top, middle, and bottom of the dressing. The tape extends several inches beyond both sides of the dressing.

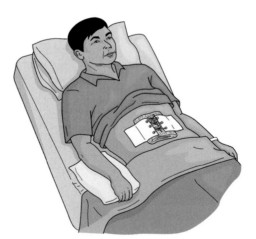

**FIG. 28-22** Montgomery ties.

# APPLYING DRESSINGS

The doctor usually does the first dressing change after surgery. The nurse follows the doctor's order for dressing changes. The nurse may ask you to assist with dressing changes. Some agencies let you apply simple, dry, nonsterile dressings to simple wounds. Box 28-6 lists the rules for applying dressings.

*See Focus on Children: Applying Dressings. See Focus on Older Persons: Applying Dressings. See Focus on Home Care: Applying Dressings.*

---

**DELEGATION GUIDELINES:** *Applying Dressings*

When applying a dressing is delegated to you, make sure that:

- Your state allows you to perform the procedure
- The procedure is in your job description
- You have the necessary education and training
- You review the procedure with the nurse
- A nurse is available to answer questions and to supervise you

If the above conditions are met, you need this information from the nurse:

- When to change the dressing
- When the person received a drug for pain relief; how long it needs to take effect
- How to secure the dressing—tape or Montgomery ties
- What kind of tape to use—adhesive, paper, plastic, or elastic
- What observations to report and record:
  - —A red or swollen wound
  - —An area around the wound that is warm to touch
  - —If wound edges are closed or separated
  - —A wound that has broken open
  - —Drainage appearance: clear, bloody, or watery and blood-tinged; thick and green, yellow, or brown
  - —The amount of drainage
  - —Wound or drainage odor
  - —Intactness and color of surrounding tissues
  - —Swelling of surrounding tissues

---

**SAFETY ALERT:** *Applying Dressings*

Contact with blood, body fluids, secretions, or excretions is likely. Follow Standard Precautions and the Bloodborne Pathogen Standard. Wear personal protective equipment as needed.

---

**BOX 28-6 RULES FOR APPLYING DRY, NONSTERILE DRESSINGS**

- Allow pain drugs time to take effect. The dressing change may cause discomfort. The nurse gives the drug and tells you how long to wait.
- Meet fluid and elimination needs before you begin.
- Collect needed equipment and supplies before you begin.
- Control your nonverbal communication. Wound odors, appearance, and drainage may be unpleasant. Do not communicate your thoughts and reactions to the person.
- Remove soiled dressings so the person cannot see the soiled side. The drainage and its odor may upset the person.
- Do not force the person to look at the wound. A wound can affect body image and self-esteem. The nurse helps the person deal with the wound.
- Remove tape by pulling it toward the wound.
- Remove dressings gently. They may stick to the wound, drain, or surrounding skin.
- Observe the wound, and report your observations. See *Delegation Guidelines: Applying Dressings.*

---

**FOCUS ON CHILDREN**
**APPLYING DRESSINGS**

Children are often afraid of dressing changes. Tape removal is often painful. Wound appearance can be frightening. A calm, cooperative child helps prevent contamination of the sterile field. A parent or caregiver holds the child so the wound can be reached with ease. The child is often comforted by holding or playing with a favorite toy.

---

**FOCUS ON OLDER PERSONS**
**APPLYING DRESSINGS**

Older persons have thin, fragile skin. Skin tears must be prevented. Extreme care is necessary when removing tape.

---

**FOCUS ON HOME CARE**
**APPLYING DRESSINGS**

Gather needed supplies before leaving the agency. The RN may ask you to call him or her after removing the old dressings. During the call, report your observations. Then the RN tells you how to proceed.

# APPLYING A DRY, NONSTERILE DRESSING

## QUALITY OF LIFE

Remember to:
- Knock before entering the person's room
- Address the person by name
- Introduce yourself by name and title

## PRE-PROCEDURE

1 Follow *Delegation Guidelines: Applying Dressings,* p. 597. See *Safety Alert: Applying Dressings,* p. 597.
2 Explain to the person what you are going to do.
3 Allow time for pain relief drugs to take effect.
4 Provide for fluid and elimination needs.
5 Practice hand hygiene.
6 Collect needed supplies and equipment:
   - Gloves
   - Personal protective equipment as needed
   - Tape or Montgomery ties
   - Dressings as directed by the nurse
   - Adhesive remover
   - Scissors
   - Plastic bag
   - Bath blanket
7 Identify the person. Check the ID bracelet against the assignment sheet. Call the person by name.
8 Provide for privacy.
9 Arrange your work area. You should not have to reach over or turn your back on the work area.
10 Raise the bed for body mechanics. Bed rails are up if used.

## PROCEDURE

11 Lower the bed rail near you if up.
12 Help the person to a comfortable position.
13 Cover the person with a bath blanket. Fanfold top linens to the foot of the bed.
14 Expose the affected body part.
15 Make a cuff on the plastic bag. Place it within reach.
16 Put on a gown and mask if needed.
17 Put on the gloves.
18 Undo Montgomery ties or remove tape:
   a Montgomery ties: fold ties away from the wound.
   b Tape: hold the skin down. Gently pull the tape toward the wound.
19 Remove adhesive from the skin if necessary. Wet a 4 × 4 gauze dressing with the adhesive remover. Clean away from the wound.
20 Remove gauze dressings. Start with the top dressing. The soiled side is away from the person's sight. Put dressings in the bag. They must not touch the outside of the bag.
21 Remove the dressing directly over the wound very gently. It may stick to the wound or drain.
22 Observe the wound, drain site, and wound drainage (see Box 28-5).
23 Remove the gloves, and put them into the bag. Decontaminate your hands.
24 Put on clean gloves.
25 Open the dressings.
26 Cut the length of tape needed.
27 Apply dressings as directed by the nurse.
28 Secure the dressings in place. Use tape or Montgomery ties.
29 Remove your gloves, and put them in the bag. Decontaminate your hands.

## POST-PROCEDURE

30 Provide for comfort.
31 Cover the person. Remove the bath blanket.
32 Place the signal light within reach.
33 Lower the bed to its lowest position.
34 Raise or lower bed rails. Follow the care plan.
35 Unscreen the person.
36 Discard supplies into the bag. Tie the bag closed. Discard the bag according to agency policy.
37 Clean your work surface. Follow the Bloodborne Pathogen Standard.
38 Decontaminate your hands.
39 Report and record your observations.

# BINDERS

Binders are applied to the abdomen, chest, or perineal areas. They promote healing by:

- Supporting wounds
- Holding dressings in place
- Promoting circulation—swelling is prevented or reduced
- Promoting comfort
- Preventing injury

Box 28-7 lists the rules for applying these binders:

- *Straight abdominal binder*—provides abdominal support and holds dressings in place (Fig. 28-23). It is applied with the person supine. The top part is at the person's waist. The lower part is over the hips. The binder is secured in place with pins, hooks, or Velcro.
- *Breast binder*—supports the breasts after breast surgery (Fig. 28-24). It also applies pressure to the breasts after childbirth in the non-breastfeeding mother. Pressure from the binder helps dry up the milk in the breasts. The binder also promotes comfort and supports swollen breasts after childbirth. The woman is supine when it is applied. The binder is pulled snugly across the chest and secured in place.
- *T-binders*—secure dressings in place after rectal and perineal surgeries. The single T-binder is for women (Fig. 28-25, *A*). The double T-binder is for men (Fig. 28-25, *B*). If perineal dressings are large, women may need double T-binders. The waistbands are brought around the waist and pinned at the front. The tails are brought between the legs and up to the waistband. They are pinned in place at the waistband.

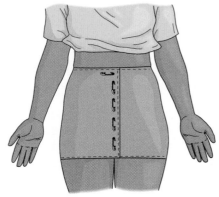

**FIG. 28-23** Straight abdominal binder.

> **SAFETY ALERT: *Binders***
> Binders must be applied properly. Otherwise, severe discomfort, skin irritation, and circulatory and respiratory complications can occur. The binder's effectiveness and the person's safety depend on correct application.

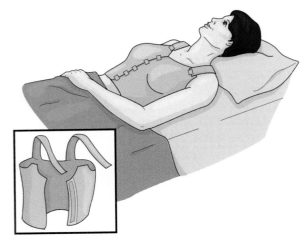

**FIG. 28-24** Breast binder.

> | BOX 28-7 | RULES FOR APPLYING BINDERS |
> | --- | --- |
>
> - Apply the binder so there is firm, even pressure over the area.
> - Apply the binder so it is snug. It must not interfere with breathing or circulation.
> - Position the person in good alignment.
> - Reapply the binder if it is loose, wrinkled, or out of position or causes discomfort.
> - Secure pins so they point away from the wound.
> - Change binders that are moist or soiled. This prevents the growth of microbes.

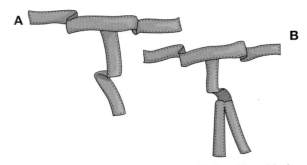

**FIG. 28-25 A,** Single T-binder. **B,** Double T-binder.

# HEAT AND COLD APPLICATIONS

Heat and cold applications are often ordered for wound care (Chapter 29). Doctors order them to promote healing, promote comfort, and reduce tissue swelling.

# MEETING BASIC NEEDS

The wound can affect the person's basic needs. However, it is only one aspect of the person's care. Remember, the *person* has the wound.

The person is recovering from surgery or trauma. The wound causes pain and discomfort. The wound and the pain may affect breathing and moving. Turning, repositioning, and walking may be painful. Handle the person gently. Allow pain drugs to take effect before giving care.

Good nutrition is needed for healing. However, pain and discomfort can affect appetite. So can odors from wound drainage. Remove soiled dressings promptly from the room. Use room deodorizers as directed. Also keep drainage containers out of the person's sight. Tell the nurse if the person has a taste for certain foods or drinks.

Infection is always a threat. Follow Standard Precautions and the Bloodborne Pathogen Standard. Carefully observe the wound (see Box 28-5). Also observe for signs and symptoms of infection.

Delayed healing is a risk for persons who are older or obese or have poor nutrition. Poor circulation and diabetes also affect healing. These conditions are risk factors for infection.

Many fears affect safety and security needs. The person fears scarring, disfigurement, delayed healing, and infection. Fears about the wound "popping open" are common. Medical bills are other concerns. Continued hospital care, home care, or long-term care may be needed.

Victims of violence have many other concerns. Future attacks, finding and convicting the attacker, and fear for family members are common concerns. Victims of domestic, child, and elder abuse often hide the source of their injuries.

The wound may be large or small. Others can see wounds on the face, arms, or legs. Clothing can hide some wounds. Wound drainage may have odors. Some wounds are large and disfiguring. They can affect sexual performance or feelings of sexual attractiveness. Amputation of a finger, hand, arm, toe, foot, or leg can affect function, everyday activities, and job. Eye injuries can affect vision. Abdominal trauma and surgery can affect eating and elimination.

Whatever the wound site or size, it affects function and body image. Love, belonging and self-esteem needs are affected. You must be sensitive to the person's feelings. The person may be sad and tearful or angry and hostile. Adjustment may be hard and rehabilitation necessary. Be gentle and kind, give thoughtful care, and practice good communication. Other health team members—social workers, psychiatrists, and the clergy—may be involved in the person's care.

# ■ REVIEW QUESTIONS ■

Circle the **BEST** answer.

1 Sally Jones fell off her bike. She has a laceration on her right leg. Which is *false?*
 a She has an open wound.
 b She has an infected wound.
 c She has a contaminated wound.
 d She has an unintentional wound.

2 A person had rectal surgery. The person has a
 a Clean wound
 b Dirty wound
 c Clean-contaminated wound
 d Contaminated wound

3 The skin and underlying tissues are pierced. This is
 a A penetrating wound
 b An incision
 c A contusion
 d An abrasion

4 Which can cause skin tears?
 a Keeping your nails trim and smooth
 b Dressing the person in soft clothing
 c Wearing rings
 d Handling the person gently

5 Which can cause pressure ulcers?
 a Repositioning the person every 2 hours
 b Scrubbing and rubbing the skin
 c Applying lotion to dry areas
 d Keeping linens clean, dry, and wrinkle-free

6 Which are *not* used to treat pressure ulcers?
 a Special beds
 b Waterbeds and flotation pads
 c Plastic drawsheets and waterproof pads
 d Heel elevators and elbow protectors

7 A person has a stasis ulcer. Which measure should you question?
 a Use elastic garters to hold socks in place.
 b Do not cut or trim toenails.
 c Avoid injury to the person's legs.
 d Apply elastic stockings.

8 Which is *not* a common site for arterial ulcers?
 a Between the toes
 b On top of the toes
 c On the outer side of the ankle
 d Behind the knee

9 A wound appears red and swollen. The area around it is warm to touch. These are signs of
 a The inflammatory phase of wound healing
 b The proliferative phase of wound healing
 c Healing by primary intention
 d Healing by secondary intention

10 A wound is separating. This is called
 a Dehiscence
 b Tertiary intention
 c Evisceration
 d Hematoma

11 Clear, watery drainage from a wound is called
 a Purulent drainage
 b Serous drainage
 c Sero-purulent drainage
 d Serosanguineous drainage

12 You note large amounts of sanguineous drainage in a Hemovac. Which is *true?*
 a The person is bleeding.
 b You need to tell the doctor.
 c The person has an infection.
 d The person has a Penrose drain.

13 A dressing does the following *except*
 a Protect the wound from injury
 b Absorb drainage
 c Provide moisture for wound healing
 d Support the wound and reduce swelling

14 To secure a dressing, apply tape
 a Around the entire part
 b To the top and bottom of the dressing
 c To the top, middle, and bottom of the dressing
 d As the person prefers

15 An abdominal binder is used to
 a Prevent blood clots
 b Prevent wound infection
 c Provide support and hold dressings in place
 d Decrease circulation and swelling

*Answers to these questions are on p. 819.*

# Heat and Cold Applications

## OBJECTIVES

- Define the key terms listed in this chapter
- Identify the purposes, effects, and complications of heat and cold applications
- Identify the persons at risk for complications from heat and cold applications
- Explain the differences between moist and dry heat and cold applications
- Describe the rules for applying heat and cold
- Explain how cooling and warming blankets are used
- Perform the procedures described in this chapter

## KEY TERMS

**compress**  A soft pad applied over a body area
**constrict**  To narrow
**cyanosis**  Bluish skin color
**dilate**  To expand or open wider
**hyperthermia**  A body temperature *(thermia)* that is much higher *(hyper)* than the person's normal range

**hypothermia**  A very low *(hypo)* body temperature *(thermia)*
**pack**  A treatment that involves wrapping a body part with a wet or dry application

Doctors order heat and cold applications to promote healing and comfort. They also reduce tissue swelling. Heat and cold have opposite effects on body function. Severe injuries and changes in body function can occur. The risks are great. You must understand the purposes, effects, and complications of heat and cold applications.

In some agencies, only nurses apply heat and cold. Other agencies let nursing assistants do so. Before you perform these procedures, make sure that:
- Your state allows you to perform the procedure
- The procedure is in your job description
- You have the necessary training
- You know how to use the equipment
- You review the procedure with a nurse
- A nurse is available to answer questions and to supervise you

## HEAT APPLICATIONS

Heat applications can be applied to almost any body part. They are often used for musculoskeletal injuries or problems (sprains, arthritis). Heat:
- Relieves pain
- Relaxes muscles

- Promotes healing
- Reduces tissue swelling
- Decreases joint stiffness

When heat is applied to the skin, blood vessels in the area dilate. **Dilate** means to expand or open wider (Fig. 29-1). Blood flow increases. Tissues have more oxygen and nutrients for healing. Excess fluid is removed from the area faster. The skin is red and warm.

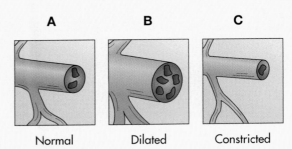

A        B        C

Normal        Dilated        Constricted

**FIG. 29-1  A,** Blood vessel under normal conditions. **B,** Dilated blood vessel. **C,** Constricted blood vessel.

## COMPLICATIONS

High temperatures can cause burns. Pain, excessive redness, and blisters are danger signs. Report these signs at once. Also observe for pale skin. When heat is applied too long, blood vessels **constrict** (narrow) (see Fig. 29-1, C). Blood flow decreases. Tissues receive less blood. Tissue damage occurs, and the skin is pale.

Fair-skinned people are at great risk for complications. Their fragile skin is easily burned. Persons with problems sensing heat or pain are also at risk. Nervous system damage, loss of consciousness, and circulatory disorders affect sensation. So do confusion and some drugs.

Persons with metal implants are at risk. Metal conducts heat. Deep tissues can be burned. Pacemakers and joint replacements are made of metal. Do not apply heat in the implant area.

Heat is not applied to a pregnant woman's abdomen. The heat can affect fetal growth.

*See Focus on Children: Complications From Heat Applications. See Focus on Older Persons: Complications From Heat Applications.*

> ### FOCUS ON CHILDREN
> #### COMPLICATIONS FROM HEAT APPLICATIONS
> Infants and young children have fragile skin. They are at risk for burns. They need careful observation. Always respond when they cry. Crying is a way to communicate pain.

> ### FOCUS ON OLDER PERSONS
> #### COMPLICATIONS FROM HEAT APPLICATIONS
> Older persons have thin and fragile skin. Burns are a risk. Changes from aging and health problems increase the risk for burns. They include circulatory and nervous system changes. Some drugs affect the ability to sense pain. Confused persons and those with dementia may not recognize pain. Look for behavior changes. They can signal pain.

## MOIST AND DRY APPLICATIONS

With a *moist heat application,* water is in contact with the skin. Water conducts heat. Moist heat has greater and faster effects than dry heat. Heat penetrates deeper with a moist application. To prevent injury, moist heat applications have lower (cooler) temperatures than dry heat applications.

With *dry heat applications,* water is not in contact with the skin. Dry heat has advantages:
- A dry heat application stays at the desired temperature longer.
- Dry heat does not penetrate as deeply as moist heat.

Because water is not used, dry heat needs higher (hotter) temperatures to achieve the desired effect. Therefore burns are still a risk.

> ### DELEGATION GUIDELINES: *Applying Heat and Cold*
> If your agency allows you to apply heat and cold, you need this information from the nurse and the care plan:
> - The type of application—hot compress or pack, commercial compress, hot soak, sitz bath, aquathermia pad; ice bag, ice collar, ice glove, cold pack, or cold compress
> - How to cover the application
> - The application site
> - What temperature to use
> - How long to leave the application in place
> - What observations to report and record:
>   —Complaints of pain, numbness, or burning
>   —Excessive redness
>   —Blisters
>   —Pale, white, or gray skin
>   —Cyanosis (bluish skin color)
>   —Shivering
>   —Time, site, and length of the application
> - What observations to report at once

> ### SAFETY ALERT: *Applying Heat and Cold*
> Protect the person from injury during heat and cold applications. Practice the rules in Box 29-1 to prevent burns and other complications.

## BOX 29-1  RULES FOR APPLYING HEAT AND COLD

- Know how to use the equipment.
- Measure the temperature of moist applications. Use a bath thermometer. Or follow agency policy for measuring temperature.
- Follow agency policies for safe temperature ranges. See Table 29-1 for guidelines.
- Do not apply *very hot* (above 106° to 115° F [41.1° to 46.1° C]) applications. Tissue damage can occur. A nurse applies *very hot* applications.
- Ask the nurse what the temperature of the application should be:
  —Heat: cooler temperatures are needed for persons at risk.
  —Cold: warmer temperatures are needed for persons at risk.
- Know the precise site of the application. Ask the nurse to show you the site.
- Cover dry heat or cold applications before applying them. Use a flannel cover, towel, or pillowcase. Follow agency policy.
- Observe the skin every 5 minutes for signs of complications. See *Delegation Guidelines: Applying Heat and Cold.*
- Do not let the person change the temperature of the application.
- Ask the nurse how long to leave the application in place. Carefully watch the time. Heat and cold are applied for no longer than 15 to 20 minutes.
- Follow the rules of electrical safety when using electrical appliances to apply heat.
- Provide for privacy. Properly drape and screen the person. Expose only the body part where you will apply heat or cold.
- Place the signal light within the person's reach.

## TABLE 29-1  HEAT AND COLD TEMPERATURE RANGES

| Temperature | Fahrenheit Range | Centigrade Range |
|---|---|---|
| Very hot | 106° to 115° F | 41.1° to 46.1° C |
| Hot | 98° to 106° F | 36.6° to 41.1° C |
| Warm | 93° to 98° F | 33.8° to 36.6° C |
| Tepid | 80° to 93° F | 26.6° to 33.8° C |
| Cool | 65° to 80° F | 18.3° to 26.6° C |
| Cold | 50° to 65° F | 10.0° to 18.3° C |

Modified from Perry AG, Potter PA: *Clinical nursing skills and techniques,* ed 5, St Louis, 2002, Mosby.

## HOT COMPRESSES

Hot compresses are moist heat applications. A **compress** is a soft pad applied over a body area. It is usually made of cloth. The application usually is left in place for 20 minutes. Sometimes an aquathermia pad (p. 612) is applied over the compress. It maintains the temperature of the compress.

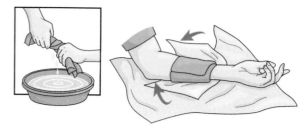

**FIG. 29-2** A hot compress is covered with plastic and a bath towel. These keep the compress warm.

## APPLYING HOT COMPRESSES

### QUALITY OF LIFE

Remember to:
- Knock before entering the person's room
- Address the person by name
- Introduce yourself by name and title

### PRE-PROCEDURE

1 Follow *Delegation Guidelines: Applying Heat and Cold*, p. 604. See *Safety Alert: Applying Heat and Cold*, p. 604.
2 Explain the procedure to the person.
3 Practice hand hygiene.
4 Collect the following:
- Basin
- Bath thermometer
- Small towel, washcloth, or gauze squares
- Plastic wrap or aquathermia pad
- Ties, tape, or rolled gauze
- Bath towel
- Waterproof pad
5 Identify the person. Check the ID bracelet against the assignment sheet. Call the person by name.
6 Provide for privacy.

### PROCEDURE

7 Place the waterproof pad under the body part.
8 Fill the basin ½ to ⅔ full with hot water as directed by the nurse. Measure water temperature.
9 Place the compress in the water.
10 Wring out the compress.
11 Apply the compress to the area. Note the time.
12 Cover the compress quickly. Use one of the following as directed by the nurse:
  a Apply plastic wrap and then a bath towel (Fig. 29-2). Secure the towel in place with ties, tape, or rolled gauze.
  b Apply an aquathermia pad (p. 612).
13 Place the signal light within reach.
14 Raise or lower bed rails. Follow the care plan.
15 Check the area every 5 minutes. Check for redness and complaints of pain, discomfort, or numbness. Remove the compress if any occur. Tell the nurse at once.
16 Change the compress if cooling occurs.
17 Remove the compress after 20 minutes or as directed by the nurse. Pat dry the area. (If the bed rail is up, lower it for this step.)

### POST-PROCEDURE

18 Provide for comfort.
19 Unscreen the person.
20 Raise or lower bed rails. Follow the care plan.
21 Place the signal light within reach.
22 Clean equipment. Discard disposable items. (Wear gloves for this step.)
23 Follow agency policy for soiled linen.
24 Decontaminate your hands.
25 Report and record your observations.

## HOT SOAKS

For a hot soak, a body part is put into water. This usually is used for smaller parts—a hand, lower arm, foot, or lower leg (Fig. 29-3). A tub is used for larger areas. Comfort and body alignment are maintained during the hot soak.

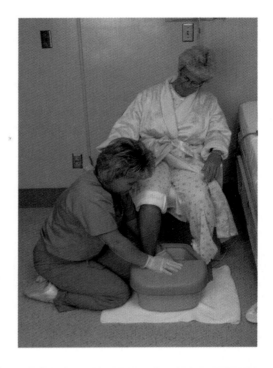

FIG. 29-3 A hot soak. This device has a bubbling action.

## THE HOT SOAK

### QUALITY OF LIFE

Remember to:
- Knock before entering the person's room
- Address the person by name
- Introduce yourself by name and title

### PRE-PROCEDURE

1 Follow *Delegation Guidelines: Applying Heat and Cold*, p. 604. See *Safety Alert: Applying Heat and Cold*, p. 604.
2 Explain the procedure to the person.
3 Practice hand hygiene.
4 Collect the following:
 - Water basin or an arm or foot bath
 - Bath thermometer
 - Bath blanket
 - Waterproof pads
5 Identify the person. Check the ID bracelet against the assignment sheet. Call the person by name.
6 Provide for privacy.

### PROCEDURE

7 Position the person for the procedure. Place the signal light within reach.
8 Place a waterproof pad under the area.
9 Fill the container ½ full with hot water as directed by the nurse. Measure water temperature.
10 Expose the area. Avoid unnecessary exposure.
11 Place the part into the water. Pad the edge of the container with a towel. Note the time.
12 Cover the person with a bath blanket for extra warmth.
13 Check the area every 5 minutes. Check for redness and complaints of pain, numbness, or discomfort. Discontinue the soak if any of these occur. Wrap the part in a towel, and tell the nurse at once.
14 Check water temperature every 5 minutes. Change water as necessary. Wrap the part in a towel while changing the water.
15 Remove the part from the water in 15 to 20 minutes. Pat dry.

### POST-PROCEDURE

16 Follow steps 18 through 25 in procedure: *Applying Hot Compresses*.

## ■ THE SITZ BATH

The sitz bath involves immersing the perineal and rectal areas into warm or hot water. The sitz bath usually lasts 20 minutes. (*Sitz* means *seat* in German.) Sitz baths are common after rectal or female pelvic surgery, for hemorrhoids, and after childbirth. They are used to:

- Clean perineal and anal wounds
- Promote healing
- Relieve pain and soreness
- Increase circulation
- Stimulate voiding

The disposable plastic sitz bath fits onto the toilet seat (Fig. 29-4). A sitz tub is a built-in fixture with a deep seat (Fig. 29-5).

> **SAFETY ALERT:** *Sitz Baths*
> Blood flow increases to the perineum and rectum. Therefore less blood flows to other body parts. The person may become weak or feel faint. Drowsiness can occur from the bath's relaxing effect. Observe for signs of weakness, faintness, or fatigue. Also protect the person from injury. Check the person often. Keep the signal light within reach, and prevent chills and burns.

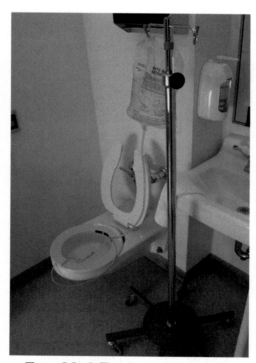

**FIG. 29-4** The disposable sitz bath.

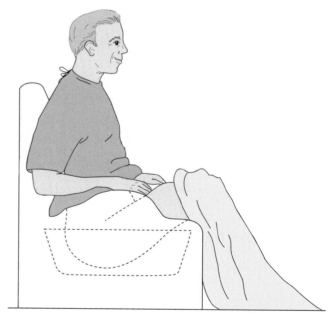

**FIG. 29-5** The built-in sitz bath.

## ASSISTING THE PERSON TO TAKE A SITZ BATH

### QUALITY OF LIFE

Remember to:   • Knock before entering the person's room
              • Address the person by name
              • Introduce yourself by name and title

### PRE-PROCEDURE

1 Follow *Delegation Guidelines: Applying Heat and Cold*, p. 604. See *Safety Alert: Applying Heat and Cold*, p. 604, and *Safety Alert: Sitz Baths.*
2 Explain the procedure to the person.
3 Practice hand hygiene.
4 Collect the following:
   • Disposable sitz bath if used
   • Wheelchair if the built-in sitz bath is used
   • Bath thermometer

• Two bath blankets, bath towels, and a clean gown
• Footstool if the person is short
• Disinfectant solution
• Utility gloves
5 Identify the person. Check the ID bracelet against the assignment sheet. Call the person by name.
6 Provide for privacy.

### PROCEDURE

7 Do one of the following:
   **a** Place the disposable sitz bath on the toilet seat.
   **b** Transport the person by wheelchair to the sitz bathroom.
8 Fill the sitz bath ⅔ full with water as directed by the nurse. Measure water temperature.
9 Pad the metal part of the sitz bath with towels. Pad the part in contact with the person.
10 Secure the gown above the waist.
11 Help the person sit in the sitz bath.
12 Place a bath blanket around the shoulders. Place another over the legs for warmth.
13 Provide a footstool if the edge of the sitz bath causes pressure under the knees.

14 Place the signal light within reach. Provide for comfort.
15 Stay with a person who is weak or unsteady.
16 Check the person every 5 minutes for complaints of weakness, faintness, and drowsiness. Check for a rapid pulse. If any occur, call for the nurse. Assist the person back to bed.
17 Help the person out of the sitz bath after 20 minutes or as directed by the nurse.
18 Assist the person with drying and dressing.
19 Assist the person back to bed.

### POST-PROCEDURE

20 Provide for comfort.
21 Unscreen the person.
22 Place the signal light within reach.
23 Raise or lower bed rails. Follow the care plan.
24 Clean the sitz bath with disinfectant solution. Wear utility gloves.

25 Clean and return reusable items to their proper place. Follow agency policy for soiled linen. Wear gloves for this step.
26 Decontaminate your hands.
27 Report and record your observations.

## HOT PACKS

A **pack** is a treatment that involves wrapping a body part with a wet or dry application. The application can be hot or cold. There are single-use (disposable) or reusable packs. Some can be used for heat or cold. The manufacturer's instructions tell you how to activate the heat or cold (Fig. 29-6). For example, some hot packs are put in boiling water for a few minutes. Or they are warmed in a microwave oven. For other types, you strike, knead, or squeeze the package to activate the heat.

Reusable packs are cleaned after use. They are wiped with alcohol or washed with soap and water. Follow agency policy and the manufacturer's instructions.

**SAFETY ALERT:** *Commercial Hot Packs*
Read warning labels and follow the manufacturer's instructions to safely use a commercial hot pack.

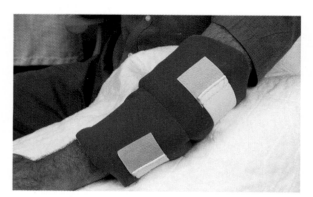

**FIG. 29-7** Hot pack secured with Velcro.

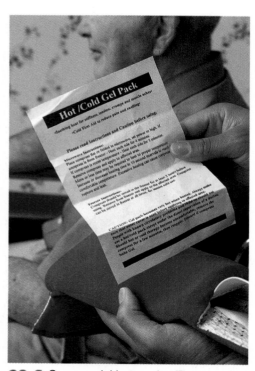

**FIG. 29-6** Commercial hot packs. The manufacturer's instructions tell how to activate the heat.

## APPLYING A HOT PACK

### QUALITY OF LIFE

Remember to:
- Knock before entering the person's room
- Address the person by name
- Introduce yourself by name and title

### PRE-PROCEDURE

1 Follow *Delegation Guidelines: Applying Heat and Cold*, p. 604. See *Safety Alert: Applying Heat and Cold*, p. 604, and *Safety Alert: Commercial Hot Packs*.
2 Explain the procedure to the person.
3 Practice hand hygiene.
4 Collect the following:
   - Commercial pack
   - Towel
   - Pack cover
   - Ties, tape, or rolled gauze (if needed)
   - Waterproof pad
5 Heat the pack. Follow the manufacturer's instructions.
6 Put the pack in the cover.
7 Identify the person. Check the ID bracelet against the assignment sheet. Call the person by name.
8 Provide for privacy.

### PROCEDURE

9 Place the waterproof pad under the body part.
10 Apply the pack quickly. Note the time.
11 Secure the pack in place with ties, tape, or rolled gauze. Some packs are secured with Velcro straps (Fig. 29-7).
12 Place the signal light within reach.
13 Raise or lower bed rails. Follow the care plan.
14 Check the area every 5 minutes. Check for redness and complaints of pain, discomfort, or numbness. Remove the pack if any occur. Tell the nurse at once.
15 Change the pack if cooling occurs.
16 Remove the pack after 20 minutes or as directed by the nurse. Pat the area dry. (If the bed rail is up, lower it for this step.)

### POST-PROCEDURE

17 Follow steps 18 through 25 in procedure: *Applying Hot Compresses*, p. 606.
18 Clean a reusable pack. Follow agency policy and the manufacturer's instructions.

## THE AQUATHERMIA PAD

The aquathermia pad (Aqua-K, K-Pad) is an electric device used for dry heat. Tubes inside the pad are filled with distilled water. Heated water flows to the pad through a hose (Fig. 29-8). Another hose returns water to the heating unit. The water is reheated and returned back into the pad.

Keep the heating unit level with the pad and connecting hoses. Water must flow freely. Hoses must not have kinks and bubbles. The temperature is set at 105° F (40.5° C) with a key. Then the key is removed. This prevents anyone from changing the temperature. The temperature often is set in the supply department. The key is kept there.

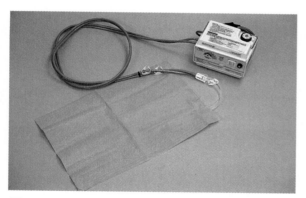

**FIG. 29-8** The aquathermia pad and heating unit.

---

**SAFETY ALERT: *The Aquathermia Pad***

When using an aquathermia pad, practice these safety measures:

- Follow electrical safety precautions (Chapter 10).
- Check the device for damage or other flaws.
- Follow the manufacturer's instructions.
- Place the heating unit on an even, uncluttered surface. This prevents it from being knocked over or knocked off of the surface.
- Use a flannel cover to insulate the pad. It absorbs perspiration at the application site. (Some agencies use a towel or pillowcase.)
- Secure the pad in place with ties, tape, or rolled gauze. Do not use pins. They can puncture the pad and cause leaks.
- Do not place the pad under the person or under a body part. This prevents the escape of heat. Burns can result if heat cannot escape.
- *See Focus on Home Care: The Aquathermia Pad.*

---

### FOCUS ON HOME CARE
#### THE AQUATHERMIA PAD

Many people have heating pads with electric coils made of wire. The coils present fire hazards if they break. Always make sure the heating pad is in good repair.

The temperature is easily adjusted. Burns are a great risk. Check the temperature often. Make sure the person has not changed it.

Some devices serve as heating pads and cold applications. They are filled with a special fluid. The pad is kept in the freezer until needed. For a heating pad, heat it following the manufacturer's instructions.

## APPLYING AN AQUATHERMIA PAD

### QUALITY OF LIFE

Remember to:
- Knock before entering the person's room
- Address the person by name
- Introduce yourself by name and title

### PRE-PROCEDURE

1 Follow *Delegation Guidelines: Applying Heat and Cold*, p. 604. See *Safety Alert: Applying Heat and Cold*, p. 604, and *Safety Alert: The Aquathermia Pad.*
2 Explain the procedure to the person.
3 Practice hand hygiene.
4 Collect the following:
   - Aquathermia pad and heating unit
   - Distilled water
   - Flannel cover, pillowcase, or towel
   - Ties, tape, or rolled gauze
5 Identify the person. Check the ID bracelet against the assignment sheet. Call the person by name.
6 Provide for privacy.

### PROCEDURE

7 Fill the heating unit to the fill line with distilled water.
8 Remove bubbles. Place the pad and tubing below the heating unit. Tilt the heating unit from side to side.
9 Set the temperature as the nurse directs (usually 105° F [40.5° C]). Remove the key. (Give the key to the nurse after the procedure.)
10 Place the pad in the cover.
11 Plug in the unit. Let water warm to the desired temperature.
12 Set the heating unit on the bedside stand. Keep the pad and connecting hoses level with the unit. Hoses must not have kinks.
13 Apply the pad to the part. Note the time.
14 Secure the pad in place with ties, tape, or rolled gauze. Do not use pins.
15 Unscreen the person. Place the signal light within reach.
16 Raise or lower bed rails. Follow the care plan.
17 Check the person every 5 minutes. Check the skin for redness, swelling, and blisters. Ask about pain, discomfort, or decreased sensation. Remove the pad if any occur. Tell the nurse at once.
18 Remove the pad at the specified time. (If bed rails are up, lower the near one for this step.)

### POST-PROCEDURE

19 Follow steps 18 through 25 in procedure: *Applying Hot Compresses*, p. 606.

# COLD APPLICATIONS

Cold applications are often used to treat sprains and fractures. They reduce pain, prevent swelling, and decrease circulation and bleeding. Cold cools the body when fever is present.

Cold has the opposite effect of heat. When cold is applied to the skin, blood vessels constrict (see Fig. 29-1, C, p. 603). Blood flow decreases. Less oxygen and nutrients are carried to the tissues. Cold applications are useful right after injury. Decreased blood flow reduces the amount of bleeding. Less fluid collects in the tissues. Cold has a numbing effect on the skin. This helps reduce or relieve pain in the part.

## COMPLICATIONS

Complications include pain, burns and blisters, and **cyanosis** (bluish skin color). Burns and blisters occur from intense cold. They also occur when dry cold is in direct contact with the skin. When cold is applied for a long time, blood vessels dilate. Blood flow increases. The prolonged application of cold has the same effects as heat applications.

Fair-skinned persons have fragile skin. They are at great risk for complications. So are persons with mental or sensory impairments. *See Focus on Children: Complications From Cold Applications. See Focus on Older Persons: Complications From Cold Applications.*

## MOIST AND DRY APPLICATIONS

Cold applications are moist or dry:
- Dry cold—ice bag, ice collar, and ice glove
- Moist cold—cold compresses
- Moist or dry—cold packs

Moist cold applications penetrate deeper than dry ones. Therefore moist applications are not as cold as dry applications. Prevent injuries from cold applications (see Box 29-1, p. 605).

## ICE BAGS, ICE COLLARS, ICE GLOVES, AND DRY COLD PACKS

Ice bags, ice collars, and ice gloves are dry cold applications. The device is filled with crushed ice. Then it is placed in a cover.

Commercial cold packs are reusable or single-use (disposable). Single-use cold packs are discarded after use. To activate the cold, follow the manufacturer's instructions. You will need to strike, knead, or squeeze the pack. Reusable cold packs are kept in the freezer. They are cleaned after use (see "Hot Packs," p. 610).

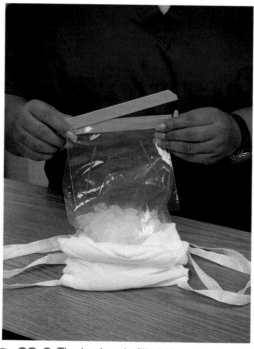

**FIG. 29-9** The ice bag is filled ½ to ⅔ full with ice.

---

> ### FOCUS ON CHILDREN
> #### COMPLICATIONS FROM COLD APPLICATIONS
> Infants and children are at risk for complications from cold applications. Check them often.

> ### FOCUS ON OLDER PERSONS
> #### COMPLICATIONS FROM COLD APPLICATIONS
> Older persons are at risk for complications from cold applications. Check them often.

Some devices have an outer covering. It allows direct application to the skin. If not, place the device in a cover. If the cover becomes moist, remove it and apply a dry one.

*See Focus on Home Care: Ice Bags, Ice Collars, Ice Gloves, and Dry Cold Packs.*

> **FOCUS ON HOME CARE**
> ICE BAGS, ICE COLLARS, ICE GLOVES, AND DRY COLD PACKS
>
> Disposable ice packs are common in home settings. A bag of frozen peas or corn can serve as an ice bag. So can plastic bags. Fill the bag with ice. Then close it securely to prevent leaks. Wrap the pack, bag of peas or corn, or plastic bag in a towel, dishcloth, or pillowcase.

> **SAFETY ALERT:** *Commercial Cold Packs*
> Follow the manufacturer's instructions to safely use a commercial cold pack.

## APPLYING AN ICE BAG, ICE COLLAR, ICE GLOVE, OR DRY COLD PACK

### QUALITY OF LIFE

Remember to:
- Knock before entering the person's room
- Address the person by name
- Introduce yourself by name and title

### PRE-PROCEDURE

1 Follow *Delegation Guidelines: Applying Heat and Cold*, p. 604. See *Safety Alert: Applying Heat and Cold*, p. 604 and *Safety Alert: Commercial Cold Packs*.
2 Explain the procedure to the person.
3 Practice hand hygiene.
4 Collect the following:
   - Cold pack or ice bag, collar, or glove
   - Crushed ice
   - Flannel cover, towel, or pillowcase
   - Paper towels
5 Apply an ice bag, collar, or glove:
   a Fill it with water. Put in the stopper. Turn the device upside down to check for leaks.
   b Empty the device.

c Fill the device $\frac{1}{2}$ to $\frac{2}{3}$ full with crushed ice or ice chips (Fig. 29-9).
d Remove excess air. Bend, twist, or squeeze the device. Or press it against a firm surface.
e Place the cap or stopper on securely.
f Dry the device with the paper towels.
g Place the device in the cover.
6 Apply a cold pack:
   a Squeeze, knead, or strike the cold pack as directed by the manufacturer. This releases cold.
   b Place the pack in the cover.
7 Identify the person. Check the ID bracelet against the assignment sheet. Call the person by name.
8 Provide for privacy.

### PROCEDURE

9 Apply the device. Secure it in place with ties, tape, or rolled gauze. Note the time.
10 Place the signal light within reach. Raise or lower bed rails. Follow the care plan.
11 Check the skin every 5 minutes. Check for blisters; pale, white, or gray skin; cyanosis; and shiv-

ering. Ask about numbness, pain, or burning. Remove the device if any occur. Tell the nurse at once.
12 Remove the device after 20 minutes or as directed by the nurse.

### POST-PROCEDURE

13 Follow steps 18 through 25 in procedure: *Applying Hot Compresses*, p. 606.

14 Clean a reusable cold pack. Follow agency policy and the manufacturer's instructions.

## COLD COMPRESSES

Applying a cold compress is like applying a hot compress. The cold compress is a moist application. Moist cold compresses are left in place no longer than 20 minutes.

---

## APPLYING COLD COMPRESSES

### QUALITY OF LIFE

Remember to:
- Knock before entering the person's room
- Address the person by name
- Introduce yourself by name and title

### PRE-PROCEDURE

1 Follow *Delegation Guidelines: Applying Heat and Cold*, p. 604. See *Safety Alert: Applying Heat and Cold*, p. 604.
2 Explain the procedure to the person.
3 Practice hand hygiene.
4 Collect the following:
 - Large basin with ice
 - Small basin with cold water
 - Gauze squares, washcloths, or small towels
 - Waterproof pad
 - Bath towel
5 Identify the person. Check the ID bracelet against the assignment sheet. Call the person by name.
6 Provide for privacy.

### PROCEDURE

7 Place the waterproof pad under the affected body part. Expose the area.
8 Place the small basin with cold water into the large basin with ice.
9 Place the compresses into the cold water.
10 Wring out a compress.
11 Apply the compress to the part. Note the time.
12 Check the area every 5 minutes. Check for blisters; pale, white, or gray skin; cyanosis; or shivering. Ask about numbness, pain, or burning. Remove the compress if any occur. Tell the nurse at once.
13 Change the compress when it warms. Usually compresses are changed every 5 minutes.
14 Remove the compress after 20 minutes or as directed by the nurse.
15 Pat dry the area.

### POST-PROCEDURE

16 Follow steps 18 through 25 in procedure: *Applying Hot Compresses*, p. 606.

# COOLING AND WARMING BLANKETS

**Hyperthermia** is a body temperature (*thermia*) that is much higher (*hyper*) than the person's normal range. With hyperthermia, body temperature is usually greater than 103° F (39.4° C). It is often called *heat stroke* when caused by hot weather. Other causes include illness, dehydration, and not being able to perspire. Lowering the person's body temperature is necessary. Otherwise death can occur. The doctor orders ice packs applied to the head, neck, underarms, and groin. Sometimes cooling blankets are used alone or with ice packs.

A cooling blanket is an electric device. Made of rubber or plastic, the device has tubes filled with fluid. The fluid flows through the tubes. The blanket is placed on the bed and covered with a sheet. The blanket is turned on the cool setting and allowed to cool. The person lies on the blanket. The person's vital signs are measured often. Rapid and excess cooling are prevented.

**Hypothermia** is a very low (*hypo*) body temperature (*thermia*). Body temperature is less than 95° F (35° C). Cold weather is a common cause. The person is warmed to prevent death. Treatment may include a warming blanket. A warming blanket is like a cooling blanket except warm settings are used. Vital signs are checked often to prevent rapid or excess warming.

When used for cooling, the device is called a *hypothermia blanket*. When used for warming, it is called a *hyperthermia blanket*. The device has warm and cool settings.

*See Focus on Children: Cooling and Warming Blankets.*

> ### FOCUS ON CHILDREN
> #### COOLING AND WARMING BLANKETS
> Rapid temperature changes can occur in infants and children. Observe them closely. Measure temperature as the nurse directs. Always report the measurement at once. Also report any changes in vital signs or in the child's condition.

# ■ REVIEW QUESTIONS ■

Circle the **BEST** answer.

1 Local heat has these effects *except*
   a Pain relief
   b Muscle relaxation
   c Healing
   d Decreased blood flow

2 The greatest threat from heat applications is
   a Infection
   b Burns
   c Chilling
   d Pressure ulcers

3 Who has the greatest risk of complications from local heat applications?
   a A 10-year-old boy
   b A teenager
   c A 40-year-old woman
   d An older person

4 These statements are about moist heat applications. Which is *false*?
   a Water is in contact with the skin.
   b The effects of moist heat are less than with a dry heat application.
   c Moist heat penetrates deeper than dry heat.
   d A moist heat application has a lower temperature than a dry heat application.

5 A hot application is usually between
   a 80° and 93° F
   b 93° and 98° F
   c 98° and 106° F
   d 106° and 115° F

6 These statements are about sitz baths. Which is *false*?
   a The perineal and rectal areas are immersed in warm or hot water.
   b The sitz bath lasts 25 to 30 minutes.
   c They clean the perineum, relieve pain, increase circulation, or stimulate voiding.
   d Weakness and fainting can occur.

7 Mrs. Parks is using an aquathermia pad. Which is *false*?
   a It is a dry heat application.
   b The temperature is usually set at 105° F.
   c Electrical safety precautions are practiced.
   d Pins secure the pad in place.

8 Cold applications
   a Reduce pain, prevent swelling, and decrease circulation
   b Dilate blood vessels
   c Prevent the spread of microbes
   d Prevent infection

9 Which is *not* a complication of cold applications?
   a Pain
   b Burns and blisters
   c Cyanosis
   d Infection

10 Before applying an ice bag
   a Place the bag in a freezer
   b Measure the temperature of the bag
   c Place the bag in a cover
   d Provide perineal care

11 Moist cold compresses are left in place no longer than
   a 20 minutes
   b 30 minutes
   c 45 minutes
   d 60 minutes

12 A cooling blanket is used for
   a Hypothermia
   b Hyperthermia
   c Cyanosis
   d Shivering

*Answers to these questions are on p. 819.*

# Oxygen Needs

# OBJECTIVES

- Define the key terms listed in this chapter
- Describe the factors affecting oxygen needs
- Identify the signs and symptoms of hypoxia and altered respiratory function
- Describe the tests used to diagnose respiratory problems
- Explain the measures that promote oxygenation
- Describe the oxygen devices
- Explain how to safely assist with oxygen therapy
- Explain how to assist in the care of persons with artificial airways
- Describe the safety measures for suctioning
- Explain how to assist in the care of persons on mechanical ventilation
- Explain how to assist in the care of persons with chest tubes
- Perform the procedures described in this chapter

# KEY TERMS

**allergy** A sensitivity to a substance that causes the body to react with signs and symptoms

**apnea** The lack or absence *(a)* of breathing *(pnea)*

**Biot's respirations** Rapid and deep respirations followed by 10 to 30 seconds of apnea

**bradypnea** Slow *(brady)* breathing *(pnea)*; respirations are fewer than 12 per minute

**Cheyne-Stokes respirations** Respirations gradually increase in rate and depth and then become shallow and slow; breathing may stop *(apnea)* for 10 to 20 seconds

**dyspnea** Difficult, labored, or painful *(dys)* breathing *(pnea)*

**hemoptysis** Bloody *(hemo)* sputum *(ptysis* means "to spit")

**hemothorax** Blood *(hemo)* in the pleural space *(thorax)*

**hyperventilation** Respirations are rapid *(hyper)* and deeper than normal

**hypoventilation** Respirations are slow *(hypo)*, shallow, and sometimes irregular

**hypoxemia** A reduced amount *(hypo)* of oxygen *(ox)* in the blood *(emia)*

**hypoxia** Cells do not have enough *(hypo)* oxygen *(oxia)*

**intubation** Inserting an artificial airway

**Kussmaul respirations** Very deep and rapid respirations

**mechanical ventilation** Using a machine to move air into and out of the lungs

**orthopnea** Breathing *(pnea)* deeply and comfortably only when sitting *(ortho)*

**orthopneic position** Sitting up *(ortho)* and leaning over a table to breathe

**oxygen concentration** The amount (percent) of hemoglobin containing oxygen

**pleural effusion** The escape and collection of fluid *(effusion)* in the pleural space

**pneumothorax** Air *(pneumo)* in the pleural space *(thorax)*

**pollutant** A harmful chemical or substance in the air or water

**respiratory arrest** When breathing stops

**respiratory depression** Slow, weak respirations at a rate of fewer than 12 per minute

**suction** The process of withdrawing or sucking up fluid *(secretions)*

**tachypnea** Rapid *(tachy)* breathing *(pnea)*; respirations are 24 or more per minute

Oxygen ($O_2$) is a gas. It has no taste, odor, or color. It is a basic need required for life. Death occurs within minutes if breathing stops. Serious illnesses occur without enough oxygen. Illness, surgery, and injuries affect the amount of oxygen in the blood and cells.

You assist in the care of persons with oxygen needs. You must give safe and effective care. See Box 30-1 for a review of the respiratory system.

## FACTORS AFFECTING OXYGEN NEEDS

The respiratory and cardiovascular systems must function properly for cells to get enough oxygen. Any disease, injury, or surgery involving these systems affects the intake and use of oxygen. Body systems depend on each other. Altered function of any system (for example, the nervous, musculoskeletal, or urinary system) affects oxygen needs. Oxygen needs are affected by:

- *Respiratory system status.* Structures must be intact and function. An open (*patent*) airway is needed. Alveoli must exchange $O_2$ and $CO_2$.
- *Cardiovascular system function.* Blood must flow to and from the heart. Narrowed vessels affect blood flow. Capillaries and cells must exchange $O_2$ and $CO_2$.
- *Red blood cell count.* Red blood cells (RBCs) contain hemoglobin. Hemoglobin picks up oxygen in the lungs and carries it to the cells. The bone marrow must produce enough RBCs. Poor diet, chemotherapy, and leukemia affect bone marrow function. Blood loss also reduces the number of RBCs.

- *Nervous system function.* Nervous system diseases and injuries can affect respiratory muscles. Breathing may be difficult or impossible. Brain damage affects respiratory rate, rhythm, and depth. Narcotics and depressant drugs affect the brain. They slow respirations. $O_2$ and $CO_2$ blood levels also affect brain function. Respirations increase when $O_2$ is lacking. The body tries to bring in more oxygen. Respirations also increase when $CO_2$ increases. The body tries to get rid of $CO_2$.
- *Aging.* Respiratory muscles weaken. Lung tissue is less elastic. Strength for coughing decreases. The person must cough and remove secretions from the upper airway. Otherwise, *pneumonia* (inflammation of the lung) can develop. Older persons are at risk for respiratory complications after surgery.
- *Exercise.* $O_2$ needs increase with exercise. Normally, respiratory rate and depth increase to bring enough $O_2$ into the lungs. Persons with heart and respiratory diseases may have enough oxygen at rest. However, even slight activity can increase $O_2$ needs. Their bodies may not be able to bring in $O_2$ and carry it to cells.
- *Fever.* $O_2$ needs increase. Respiratory rate and depth increase to meet the body's needs.
- *Pain.* $O_2$ needs increase. Respirations increase to meet this need. However, chest and abdominal injuries and surgeries often involve respiratory muscles. It hurts to breathe in and out.
- *Drugs.* Some drugs depress the respiratory center in the brain. **Respiratory depression** means slow, weak respirations at a rate of fewer than 12 per minute. Respirations are too shallow to bring enough $O_2$ into the lungs. **Respiratory arrest** is when breathing stops. Narcotics (morphine, Demerol, and others) can have these effects. (Narcotic comes from the Greek word *narkoun*. It means "stupor" or "to be numb.") In safe amounts, these drugs relieve severe pain.

---

**BOX 30-1  THE RESPIRATORY SYSTEM: STRUCTURE AND FUNCTION**

Oxygen is needed for life. Every cell needs oxygen. The respiratory system (Fig. 30-1, p. 622) brings oxygen into the lungs. It rids the body of carbon dioxide. The process of supplying the cells with oxygen and removing carbon dioxide from them is called *respiration*. Respiration involves *inhalation* (breathing in) and *exhalation* (breathing out). The terms *inspiration* (breathing in) and *expiration* (breathing out) are also used.

Air enters the body through the *nose*. Then air passes into the *pharynx* (throat), a tube-shaped passageway for air and food. Air passes from the pharynx into the *larynx* (the voice box). Air passes from the larynx into the *trachea* (the windpipe).

The trachea divides at its lower end into the *right bronchus* and *left bronchus*. Each bronchus enters a lung.

On entering the lungs, the bronchi further divide many times into smaller branches called *bronchioles*. The bronchioles subdivide and end in tiny one-cell air sacs called *alveoli*. They are supplied by capillaries.

Oxygen and carbon dioxide are exchanged between the alveoli and capillaries. Blood in the capillaries picks up oxygen from the alveoli. The blood returns to the left side of the heart and is pumped to the rest of the body. Alveoli pick up carbon dioxide from the capillaries for exhalation.

Each lung is divided into lobes. The right lung has three lobes; the left lung has two. The lungs are separated from the abdominal cavity by a muscle called the *diaphragm*. A bony framework consisting of the ribs, sternum, and vertebrae protects the lungs.

Substance abusers are at risk for respiratory depression and respiratory arrest. They can overdose on drugs.

- *Smoking.* Smoking causes lung cancer and chronic obstructive pulmonary disease (COPD). It is a risk factor for coronary artery disease.

- *Allergies.* An **allergy** is a sensitivity to a substance that causes the body to react with signs and symptoms. Runny nose, wheezing, and congestion are common. Mucous membranes in the upper airway swell. With severe swelling, the airway closes. Shock and death are risks. Pollens, dust, foods, drugs, and cigarette smoke often cause allergies. Chronic bronchitis and asthma are risks.

- *Pollutant exposure.* A **pollutant** is a harmful chemical or substance in the air or water. Examples are dust, fumes, toxins, asbestos, coal dust, and sawdust. They damage the lungs. Pollutant exposure occurs in home, work, and public settings.

- *Nutrition.* Good nutrition is needed to produce red blood cells. The body needs iron and vitamins (vitamin $B_{12}$, vitamin C, and folic acid) to produce RBCs.

- *Alcohol.* Alcohol depresses the brain. Excessive amounts reduce the cough reflex and increase the risk of aspiration. Obstructed airway and pneumonia are risks from aspiration.

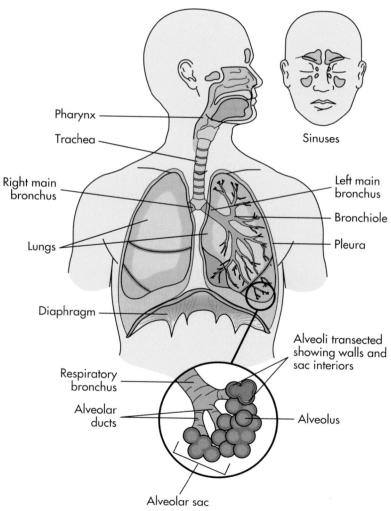

**FIG. 30-1** The respiratory system.

# ALTERED RESPIRATORY FUNCTION

Respiratory system function involves three processes. Respiratory function is altered if even one process is affected.

- Air moves into and out of the lungs.
- $O_2$ and $CO_2$ are exchanged at the alveoli.
- The blood carries $O_2$ to the cells and removes $CO_2$ from them.

## HYPOXIA

**Hypoxia** means that cells do not have enough *(hypo)* oxygen *(oxia)*. Cells do not receive enough oxygen. They cannot function properly. Anything that affects respiratory function can cause hypoxia. The brain is very sensitive to inadequate $O_2$. Restlessness is an early sign. So are dizziness and disorientation. Report the signs and symptoms in Box 30-2 to the nurse at once.

Hypoxia is life-threatening. All organs need oxygen to function. Oxygen is given. The cause of the hypoxia is treated.

## ABNORMAL RESPIRATIONS

Adults normally have 12 to 20 respirations per minute. Infants and children have faster rates. Normal respirations are quiet, effortless, and regular. Both sides of the chest rise and fall equally. The following breathing patterns are abnormal (Fig. 30-2):

- **Tachypnea**—rapid *(tachy)* breathing *(pnea)*. Respirations are 24 or more per minute. Fever, exercise, pain, pregnancy, airway obstruction, and hypoxemia are common causes. **Hypoxemia** is a reduced amount *(hypo)* of oxygen *(ox)* in the blood *(emia)*.
- **Bradypnea**—slow *(brady)* breathing *(pnea)*. Respirations are fewer than 12 per minute. Drug overdose and central nervous system disorders are common causes.

| BOX 30-2 | SIGNS AND SYMPTOMS OF HYPOXIA |
|---|---|

- Restlessness
- Dizziness
- Disorientation
- Confusion
- Behavior and personality changes
- Problems concentrating and following directions
- Apprehension
- Anxiety
- Fatigue
- Agitation
- Increased pulse rate
- Increased rate and depth of respirations
- Sitting position, often leaning forward
- Cyanosis (bluish color to the skin, lips, mucous membranes, and nail beds)
- Dyspnea

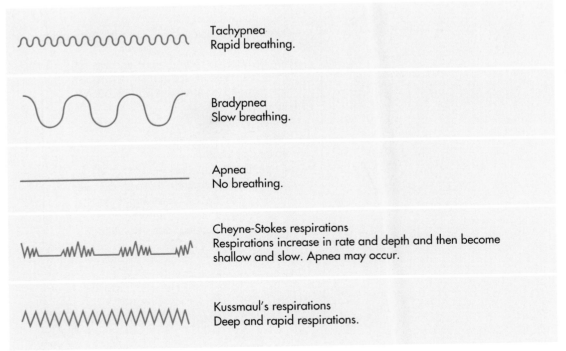

**FIG. 30-2** Some breathing patterns. (Modified from Phipps WJ and others: *Medical-surgical nursing: health and illness perspectives,* ed 7, St Louis, 2003, Mosby.)

- **Apnea**—lack or absence *(a)* of breathing *(pnea)*. It occurs in cardiac arrest and respiratory arrest. Sleep apnea and periodic apnea of newborns are other types of apnea.
- **Hypoventilation**—respirations are slow *(hypo)*, shallow, and sometimes irregular. Lung disorders affecting the alveoli are common causes. Pneumonia is an example. Other causes include obesity, airway obstruction, and drug side effects. Nervous system and musculoskeletal disorders affecting the respiratory muscles are other causes.
- **Hyperventilation**—respirations are rapid *(hyper)* and deeper than normal. Its many causes include asthma, emphysema, infection, fever, nervous system disorders, hypoxia, anxiety, pain, and some drugs.
- **Dyspnea**—difficult, labored, or painful *(dys)* breathing *(pnea)*. Heart disease, exercise, and anxiety are common causes.
- **Cheyne-Stokes respirations**—respirations gradually increase in rate and depth. Then they become shallow and slow. Breathing may stop (apnea) for 10 to 20 seconds. Drug overdose, heart failure, renal failure, and brain disorders are common causes. Cheyne-Stokes is common when death is near.
- **Orthopnea**—breathing *(pnea)* deeply and comfortably only when sitting *(ortho)*. Common causes include emphysema, asthma, pneumonia, angina pectoris, and other heart and respiratory disorders.
- **Biot's respirations**—rapid and deep respirations followed by 10 to 30 seconds of apnea. They occur with nervous system disorders.
- **Kussmaul respirations**—very deep and rapid respirations. They signal diabetic coma.

## ASSISTING WITH ASSESSMENT AND DIAGNOSTIC TESTS

Altered respiratory function may be an acute or chronic problem. Report your observations promptly and accurately (Box 30-3). Quick action is needed to meet the person's oxygen needs. Measures are taken to correct the problem and prevent it from getting worse.

The doctor uses these tests to find the cause of the problem:

- *Chest x-ray (CXR)*. An x-ray is taken of the chest. Lung changes are studied. All clothing and jewelry from the waist to the neck are removed. An x-ray gown is worn.
- *Lung scan*. The lungs are scanned to see what areas are not getting air or blood. The person inhales radioactive gas. *Radioactive* means to give off radiation.

---

| BOX 30-3 | SIGNS AND SYMPTOMS OF ALTERED RESPIRATORY FUNCTION |

- Signs and symptoms of hypoxia (see Box 30-2)
- Any abnormal breathing pattern (p. 623)
- Complaints of shortness of breath or being "winded" or "short-winded"
- Cough (note frequency and time of day):
  —Dry and hacking
  —Harsh and barking
  —Productive (produces sputum) or nonproductive
- Sputum
  —Color: clear, white, yellow, green, brown, or red
  —Odor: none or foul odor
  —Consistency: thick, watery, or frothy (with bubbles or foam)
  —**Hemoptysis:** bloody *(hemo)* sputum *(ptysis* means "to spit"); note if sputum is bright red, dark red, blood-tinged, or streaked with blood
- Noisy respirations
  —Wheezing
  —Wet-sounding respirations
  —Crowing sounds
- Chest pain (note location)
  —Constant or intermittent (comes and goes)
  —Person's description (stabbing, knife-like, aching)
  —What makes it worse (movement, coughing, yawning, sneezing, sighing, deep breathing)
- Cyanosis
  —Skin
  —Mucous membranes
  —Lips
  —Nail beds
- Changes in vital signs
- Body position
  —Sitting upright
  —Leaning forward or hunched over a table

A radioisotope is injected into a vein. A *radioisotope* is a substance that gives off radiation. Lung tissue getting air and blood flow "take up" the substance. A scanner senses areas with the substance. All clothing and jewelry from the waist to the neck are removed. An x-ray gown is worn.

- *Bronchoscopy.* A scope *(scopy)* is passed into the trachea and bronchi *(broncho)*. Airway structures are checked for bleeding and tumors. Tissue samples *(biopsy)* are taken. Or mucus plugs and foreign objects are removed. The person is NPO for 6 to 8 hours before the procedure. This reduces the risk of vomiting and aspiration. An anesthetic is given. After the procedure, the person is NPO and watched carefully until the gag and swallow reflexes return. This usually takes about 2 hours. The nurse directs preoperative and postoperative care.

- *Thoracentesis.* The pleura *(thora)* is punctured. Air or fluid is removed *(centesis)* from it. The doctor inserts a needle through the chest wall into the pleural sac. Injury or disease can cause it to fill with air, blood, or fluid. Sometimes fluid is removed for laboratory study. Anti-cancer drugs can be injected into the pleural sac. This takes a few minutes. Vital signs are taken. Then a local anesthetic is given. The person sits up and leans forward. He or she is asked not to talk, cough, or move suddenly (Fig. 30-3). Afterward a dressing is applied to the puncture site. Vital signs are taken. A chest x-ray is taken to detect lung damage. The person is observed for shortness of breath, dyspnea, cough, sputum, chest pain, cyanosis, vital sign changes, and other respiratory signs and symptoms.

- *Pulmonary function tests.* These tests measure the amount of air moving into and out of the lungs *(volume)*. They also measure how much air the lungs can hold *(capacity)*. The person takes as deep a breath as possible. Using a mouthpiece, the person blows into a machine (Fig. 30-4). The tests help assess the risk for lung diseases or postoperative lung complications. They also measure the progress of lung diseases and its treatment. Fatigue is common after the tests. The person needs to rest.

- *Arterial blood gases (ABGs).* A radial or femoral artery is punctured to obtain arterial blood. Laboratory tests measure the amount of oxygen in the blood. Hemorrhage from the artery must be prevented. Pressure is applied to the artery for at least 5 minutes after the procedure. Pressure is applied longer if there are blood-clotting problems. The procedure is done by a specially trained nurse, respiratory therapist, or laboratory technician.

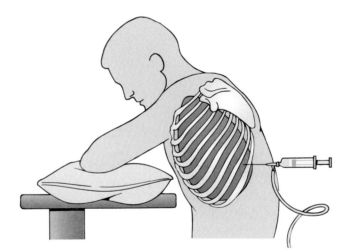

**FIG. 30-3** The person is positioned for a thoracentesis. (From Pagana KD, Pagana TJ: *Mosby's manual of diagnostic and laboratory tests*, ed 2, St Louis, 2002, Mosby.)

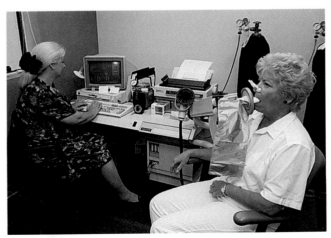

**FIG. 30-4** Pulmonary function testing.

**PULSE OXIMETRY.** Pulse oximetry measures *(metry)* oxygen *(oxi)* concentration in arterial blood. **Oxygen concentration** is the amount (percent) of hemoglobin containing oxygen. The normal range is 95% to 100%. For example, if 97% of all the hemoglobin (100%) carries $O_2$, tissues get enough oxygen. If only 90% contains $O_2$, tissues do not get enough. Measurements are used to prevent and treat hypoxia.

A sensor attaches to a finger, toe, earlobe, nose, or forehead (Fig. 30-5). Light beams on one side of the sensor pass through the tissues. A detector on the other side measures the amount of light passing through the tissues. Using this information, the oximeter measures the $O_2$ concentration. The value and pulse rate are shown. Oximeter alarms sound if:

- $O_2$ concentration is low
- The pulse is too fast or slow
- Other problems occur

A good sensor site is needed. Swollen sites are avoided. So are sites with skin breaks. Finger and toe sites are avoided if circulation is poor.

Bright light, nail polish, fake nails, and movements affect measurements. Place a towel over the sensor to block bright light. Remove nail polish, or use another site. Do not use a finger site if the person has fake nails.

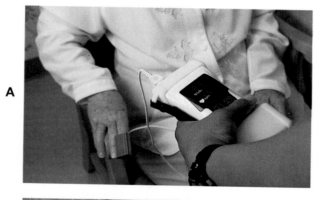

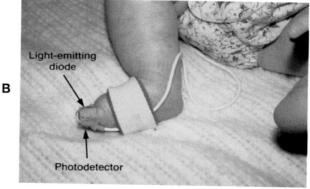

Light-emitting diode

Photodetector

**FIG. 30-5 A,** Pulse oximetry sensor is attached to a finger. **B,** The sensor is attached to an infant's great toe. **(B** from Hockenberry MJ and others: *Wong's nursing care of infants and children,* ed 7, St Louis, 2003, Mosby.)

Movements from shivering, seizures, or tremors affect finger sensors. The earlobe is a better site when there are such problems. Blood pressure cuffs affect blood flow. If using a finger site, do not measure blood pressure on that side.

Report and record measurements accurately. Use $SpO_2$ when recording the oxygen concentration value:
S = saturation
p = pulse
$O_2$ = oxygen

*See Focus on Children: Pulse Oximetry. See Focus on Older Persons: Pulse Oximetry. See Focus on Home Care: Pulse Oximetry.*

---

**DELEGATION GUIDELINES:** *Pulse Oximetry*
When assisting with pulse oximetry, you need this information from the nurse and care plan:
- What site to use
- How to use the equipment
- What sensor to use
- What type of tape to use
- The alarm limits for $SpO_2$ and pulse rate:
  —Tell the nurse at once if the $SpO_2$ goes below the alarm limit (usually 95%)
  —Tell the nurse at once if the pulse goes above or below the alarm limit
- When to do the measurement
- If the apical or radial site is used for the pulse
- How often to check the sensor site (usually every 2 hours)
- What observations to report and record:
  —The date and time
  —The $SpO_2$ and display pulse rate
  —Apical or radial pulse rate
  —What the person was doing at the time
  —Oxygen flow rate (p. 635) and the device used (p. 634)
  —Reason for the measurement: routine or change in condition
  —Other observations

---

**SAFETY ALERT:** *Pulse Oximetry*
The person's condition can change rapidly. Pulse oximetry does not lessen the need for good observations. Observe for signs and symptoms of hypoxia.

---

**COLLECTING SPUTUM SPECIMENS.** Respiratory disorders cause the lungs, bronchi, and trachea to secrete mucus. Mucus from the respiratory system is called *sputum* when expectorated *(expelled)* through the mouth. Sputum specimens are studied for blood, microbes, and abnormal cells. See Chapter 26.

► **FOCUS ON CHILDREN**
PULSE OXIMETRY

The sensor is attached to the sole of a foot, palm of the hand, finger, toe, or earlobe (see Fig. 30-5, *B*). If the child moves a lot, the earlobe is a better site.

► **FOCUS ON HOME CARE**
PULSE OXIMETRY

Oxygen concentration is often measured with vital signs. The pulse oximeter is portable. It must be accurate. After applying the sensor, check the person's pulse (radial or apical). Compare it with the displayed pulse. The pulse rates should be the same.

► **FOCUS ON OLDER PERSONS**
PULSE OXIMETRY

Older persons often have poor circulation from aging or vascular disease. Blood flow to the toe or finger may be poor. Use the ear, nose, and forehead sites.

# USING A PULSE OXIMETER

## QUALITY OF LIFE

Remember to:
- Knock before entering the person's room
- Address the person by name
- Introduce yourself by name and title

### PRE-PROCEDURE

1 Follow *Delegation Guidelines: Pulse Oximetry.* See *Safety Alert: Pulse Oximetry.*
2 Explain the procedure to the person.
3 Practice hand hygiene.
4 Collect the following:
 - Oximeter and sensor
 - Nail polish remover
 - Cotton balls
 - $SpO_2$ flow sheet
 - Tape
 - Towel
5 Identify the person. Check the ID bracelet against your assignment sheet. Call the person by name.
6 Provide for privacy.

### PROCEDURE

7 Provide for comfort.
8 Remove nail polish from the fingernail or toenail. Use nail polish remover and a cotton ball.
9 Dry the site with a towel.
10 Clip or tape the sensor to the site.
11 Turn on the oximeter.
12 Set the high and low alarm limits for $SpO_2$ and pulse rate. Turn on audio and visual alarms.
13 Check the person's pulse (apical or radial) with the pulse on the display. The pulses should be equal. Tell the nurse if the pulses are not equal.
14 Read the $SpO_2$ on the display. Note the value on the flow sheet and your assignment sheet.
15 Leave the sensor in place for continuous monitoring. Otherwise, turn off the device and remove the sensor.

### POST-PROCEDURE

16 Provide for comfort.
17 Place the signal light within the person's reach.
18 Raise or lower bed rails. Follow the care plan.
19 Unscreen the person.
20 Return the device to its proper place unless monitoring is continuous.
21 Decontaminate your hands.
22 Report and record the $SpO_2$, the pulse rate, and your other observations.

## PROMOTING OXYGENATION

To get enough oxygen, air must move deep into the lungs. Air must reach the alveoli where $O_2$ and $CO_2$ are exchanged. Disease and injury can prevent air from reaching the alveoli. Pain and immobility interfere with deep breathing and coughing. So do narcotics. Therefore secretions collect in the airway and lungs. They interfere with air movement and lung function. Secretions also provide a place for microbes to grow and multiply. Infection is a threat.

Oxygen needs must be met. The following measures are common in care plans.

### POSITIONING

Breathing is usually easier in semi-Fowler's and Fowler's position. Persons with difficulty breathing often prefer sitting up and leaning over a table to breathe. This is called the **orthopneic position.** (*Ortho* means sitting or standing. *Pnea* means breathing.) Place a pillow on the table to increase the person's comfort (Fig. 30-6).

Frequent position changes are needed. Unless the doctor limits positioning, the person must not lie on one side for a long time. Secretions pool. The lungs cannot expand on that side. Position changes are needed at least every 2 hours. Follow the care plan.

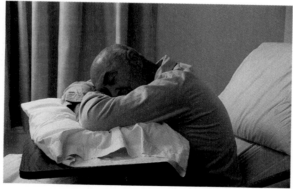

**FIG. 30-6** The person is in the orthopneic position. A pillow is on the overbed table for the person's comfort.

## COUGHING AND DEEP BREATHING

Coughing removes mucus. Deep breathing moves air into most parts of the lungs. Coughing and deep-breathing exercises help persons with respiratory problems. They are done after surgery and during bedrest. The exercises are painful after surgery or injury. Breaking an incision open while coughing is a fear.

Coughing and deep breathing help prevent pneumonia and atelectasis. *Atelectasis* is the collapse of a portion of the lung. It occurs when mucus collects in the airway. Air cannot get to a part of the lung. The lung collapses. Atelectasis is a risk after surgery. Bedrest, lung diseases, and paralysis are other risk factors.

Some doctors order coughing and deep breathing every 1 or 2 hours while the person is awake. Others want them done 4 times a day.

*See Focus on Children: Coughing and Deep Breathing.*

---

**DELEGATION GUIDELINES:** *Coughing and Deep Breathing*

When delegated coughing and deep-breathing exercises, you need this information from the nurse and the care plan:

- When to do them
- How many deep breaths and coughs the person needs to do
- What observations to report and record:
  —The number of times the person coughed and deep-breathed
  —How the person tolerated the procedure

---

> **FOCUS ON CHILDREN**
> **COUGHING AND DEEP BREATHING**
>
> Party favors are useful for helping children deep breathe. They include paper blowouts, horns, whistles, pinwheels, and others. They are fun and colorful.

## ASSISTING WITH COUGHING AND DEEP-BREATHING EXERCISES

### QUALITY OF LIFE

Remember to:
- Knock before entering the person's room
- Address the person by name
- Introduce yourself by name and title

### PRE-PROCEDURE

1 Follow *Delegation Guidelines: Coughing and Deep Breathing.*
2 Explain the procedure to the person.
3 Practice hand hygiene.
4 Identify the person. Check the ID bracelet against the assignment sheet. Call the person by name.
5 Provide for privacy.

### PROCEDURE

6 Help the person to a comfortable sitting position: dangling, semi-Fowler's, or Fowler's.
7 Have the person deep breathe:
  a Have the person place the hands over the rib cage (Fig. 30-7).
  b Ask the person to exhale. Explain that the ribs should move as far down as possible.
  c Have the person take a deep breath. It should be as deep as possible. Remind the person to inhale through the nose.
  d Ask the person to hold the breath for 3 seconds.
  e Ask the person to exhale slowly through pursed lips (Fig. 30-8, p. 630). The person should exhale until the ribs move as far down as possible.
  f Repeat this step 4 more times.
8 Ask the person to cough:
  a Have the person interlace the fingers over the incision (Fig. 30-9, *A*, p. 630). The person can also hold a pillow or folded towel over the incision (Fig. 30-9, *B*, p. 630).
  b Have the person take in a deep breath as in step 7.
  c Ask the person to cough strongly twice with the mouth open.

### POST-PROCEDURE

9 Provide for comfort.
10 Raise or lower bed rails. Follow the care plan.
11 Place the signal light within reach.
12 Unscreen the person.
13 Decontaminate your hands.
14 Report and record your observations (Fig. 30-10, p. 630).

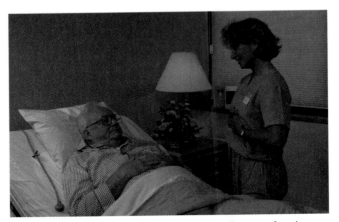

**FIG. 30-7** The hands are over the rib cage for deep breathing.

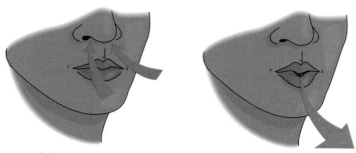

**FIG. 30-8** The person inhales through the nose and exhales through pursed lips during the deep-breathing exercise.

A

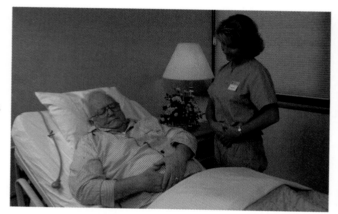
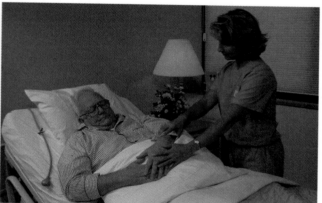

B

**FIG. 30-9** The person supports an incision for the coughing exercise. **A,** Fingers are interlaced over the incision. **B,** A pillow is held over the incision.

| Date | Time | |
|------|------|---|
| 3/27 | 1000 | Assisted resident with coughing and deep breathing exercises. 5 deep breaths and coughs performed. Resident tolerated procedure well. States, "It is getting easier every day." Left sitting up in chair after procedure per resident request. Tray table with water and signal light within reach. Jean Hein, CNA |

**FIG. 30-10** Charting sample.

## INCENTIVE SPIROMETRY

*Incentive* means to encourage. A *spirometer* is a machine that measures the amount (volume) of air inhaled. With incentive spirometry the person is encouraged to inhale until reaching a preset volume of air. Balls or bars in the machine let the person see air movement when inhaling (Fig. 30-11).

Incentive spirometry also is called *sustained maximal inspiration (SMI)*. *Sustained* means constant. *Maximal* means the most or the greatest. And *inspiration* relates to breathing in. SMI means inhaling as deeply as possible and holding that breath for a certain time. The breath is usually held for at least 3 seconds.

The goal is to improve lung function. Atelectasis is prevented or treated. Like yawning or sighing, breathing is long, slow, and deep. This moves air deep into the lungs. Secretions loosen. $O_2$ and $CO_2$ exchange occurs between the alveoli and capillaries.

The device is used as follows:
- The spirometer is placed upright.
- The person exhales normally.
- He or she seals the lips around a mouthpiece.
- A slow, deep breath is taken until the balls rise to the desired height.
- The breath is held for 3 to 6 seconds to keep the balls floating.
- The person removes the mouthpiece and exhales slowly. The person may cough at this time.
- After some normal breaths, the device is used again.

The nurse and care plan tell you the following:
- How often the person needs incentive spirometry
- How many breaths the person needs to take
- The desired height of the floating balls

Follow agency policy for cleaning and replacing disposable mouthpieces.

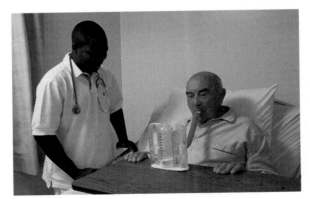

**FIG. 30-11** The person uses a spirometer.

# ASSISTING WITH OXYGEN THERAPY

Disease, injury, and surgery often interfere with breathing. The amount of $O_2$ in the blood may be less than normal (hypoxemia). If so, the doctor orders oxygen therapy.

Oxygen is treated as a drug. The doctor orders the amount of oxygen to give, the device to use, and when to give it. Some people need oxygen constantly. Others need it for symptom relief—chest pain or shortness of breath. Oxygen helps relieve chest pain. Persons with respiratory diseases may have enough oxygen at rest. With mild exercise or activity, they become short of breath. Oxygen helps to relieve the shortness of breath.

*You do not give oxygen.* The nurse and respiratory therapist start and maintain oxygen therapy. You assist the nurse in providing safe care.

## OXYGEN SOURCES

Oxygen is supplied as follows:

- *Wall outlet.* $O_2$ is piped into each person's unit (Fig. 30-12).
- *Oxygen tank.* The oxygen tank is placed at the bedside. Small tanks are used during emergencies and transfers. They also are used by persons who walk or use wheelchairs (Fig. 30-13). A gauge tells how much oxygen is left (Fig. 30-14). Tell the nurse if the tank is low.

- *Oxygen concentrator.* The machine removes oxygen from the air (Fig. 30-15). A power source is needed. If not portable, the person stays near the machine. A portable oxygen tank is needed for power failures and mobility.
- *Liquid oxygen system.* A portable unit is filled from a stationary unit (Fig. 30-16). The portable unit has enough oxygen for about 8 hours of use. A dial shows the amount of oxygen in the unit. Tell the nurse if the unit is low. The portable unit can be worn over the shoulder. This allows the person to be mobile.

*See Focus on Home Care: Oxygen Sources.*

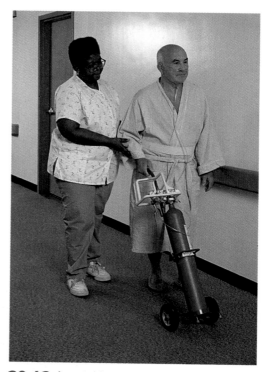

**FIG. 30-13** A portable oxygen tank is used when walking.

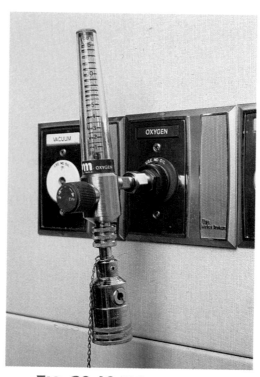

**FIG. 30-12** Wall oxygen outlet.

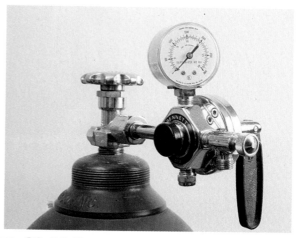

**FIG. 30-14** The gauge shows the amount of oxygen in the tank.

**SAFETY ALERT:** *Liquid Oxygen Systems*
Liquid oxygen is very cold. If touched, it can freeze the skin. Never tamper with the equipment. Doing so is unsafe and could damage the equipment. Follow agency procedures and the manufacturer's instructions when working with liquid oxygen.

> ## FOCUS ON HOME CARE
> ### OXYGEN SOURCES
>
> Oxygen tanks, oxygen concentrators, and liquid oxygen systems are used in home care. The type ordered depends on the person's needs. It is maintained by a medical supply company. Keep the company's name and phone number near the phone.
>
> The patient and family must practice safety measures where oxygen is used and stored. This includes measures to prevent fires (Box 30-4). Keep a fire extinguisher in the room.

> ## BOX 30-4 SAFETY RULES FOR FIRE AND USING OXYGEN
>
> - Place "No Smoking" signs in the room and on the room door.
> - Remove smoking materials from the room—cigarettes, cigars, pipes, matches, and lighters.
> - Remove materials from the room that ignite easily—alcohol, nail polish remover, oils, greases.
> - Keep oxygen sources and oxygen tubing away from heat sources and open flames. These include candles, stoves, heating ducts, radiators, heating pipes, space heaters, and kerosene heaters and lamps.
> - Turn off electrical items before unplugging them.
> - Use electrical items that are in good repair—shaver, radio, TV, and others.
> - Use only electrical items with three-prong plugs.
> - Do not use materials that cause static electricity (wool and synthetic fabrics).
> - Turn off the oxygen if a fire occurs. Get the person and family out of the home. Call the fire department.

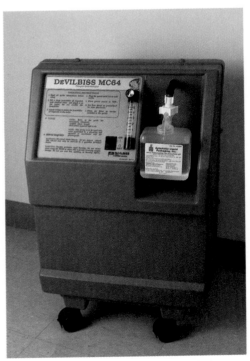

**FIG. 30-15** Oxygen concentrator.

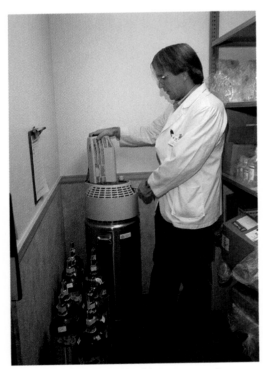

**FIG. 30-16** Liquid oxygen system.

## OXYGEN DEVICES

The doctor orders the device used to give oxygen. These devices are common:

- *Nasal cannula* (Fig. 30-17). The prongs are inserted into the nostrils. A band goes over the ears and under the chin to keep the device in place. A cannula allows eating and drinking. Tight prongs can irritate the nose. Pressure on the ears and cheekbones is possible.

- *Simple face mask* (Fig. 30-18). Covers the nose and mouth. The mask has small holes in the sides. $CO_2$ escapes when exhaling.

- *Partial-rebreather mask* (Fig. 30-19). A bag is added to the simple face mask. The bag is for exhaled air. When breathing in, the person inhales oxygen and some exhaled air. Some room air also is inhaled. The bag should not totally deflate when inhaling.

- *Non-rebreather face mask* (Fig. 30-20). Prevents exhaled air and room air from entering the bag. Exhaled air leaves through holes in the mask. When inhaling, only oxygen from the bag is inhaled. The bag must not totally collapse during inhalation.

- *Venturi mask* (Fig. 30-21). Precise amounts of oxygen are given. Color-coded adaptors show the amount of oxygen given.

Talking and eating are hard to do with a mask. Listen carefully. Moisture can build up under masks. Keep the face clean and dry. This helps prevent irritation from the mask. Masks are removed for eating. Usually oxygen is given by cannula during meals.

*See Focus on Children: Oxygen Devices.*

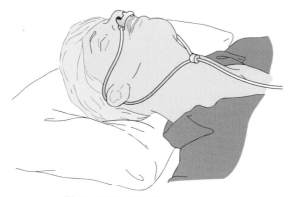

**FIG. 30-17** Nasal cannula.

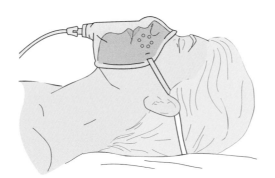

**FIG. 30-18** Simple face mask.

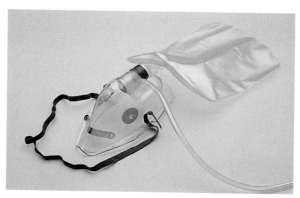

**FIG. 30-20** Non-rebreather mask.

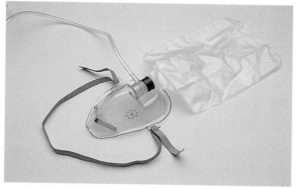

**FIG. 30-19** Partial-rebreather mask.

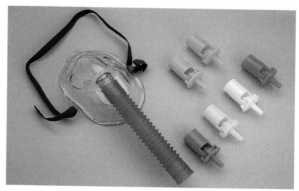

**FIG. 30-21** Venturi mask.

## OXYGEN FLOW RATES

The *flow rate* is the amount of oxygen given. It is measured in liters per minute (L/min). The doctor orders 2 to 15 liters of $O_2$ per minute. The nurse or respiratory therapist sets the flow rate (Fig. 30-23).

The nurse and care plan tell you the person's flow rate. When giving care and checking the person, always check the flow rate. Tell the nurse at once if it is too high or too low. A nurse or respiratory therapist will adjust the flow rate. Some states and agencies let nursing assistants adjust $O_2$ flow rates. Know your agency's policy.

A
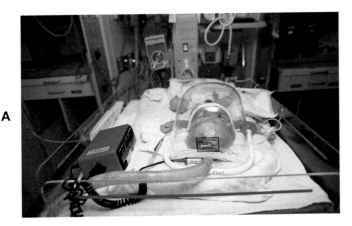

B
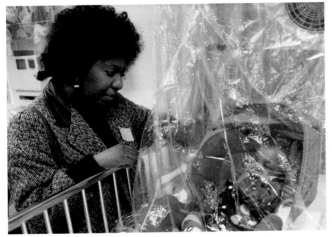

**FIG. 30-22 A,** Oxygen hood. **B,** Mist tent. (From Hockenberry MJ and others: *Wong's nursing care of infants and children,* ed 7, St Louis, 2003, Mosby.)

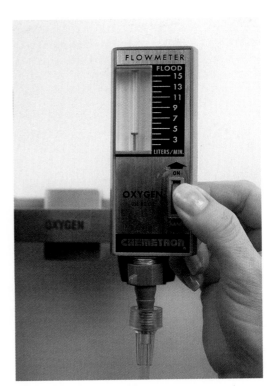

**FIG. 30-23** The flowmeter is used to set the oxygen flow rate.

# OXYGEN ADMINISTRATION SET-UP

Oxygen is a dry gas. If not humidified (made moist), oxygen dries the airway's mucous membranes. Distilled water is added to the humidifier to create water vapor (Fig. 30-24). Oxygen picks up water vapor as it flows into the system. Bubbling in the humidifier means water vapor is being produced. Low flow rates (1 to 2 L/min) by cannula usually do not need humidification.

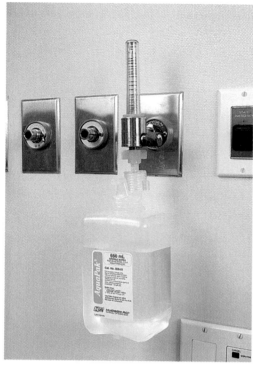

**FIG. 30-24** Oxygen administration system with humidifier.

> **DELEGATION GUIDELINES:** *Oxygen Administration Set-Up*
>
> If setting up oxygen is delegated to you, you need this information from the nurse:
> - The person's name and room and bed number
> - What oxygen device was ordered
> - If humidification was ordered

> **SAFETY ALERT:** *Oxygen Administration Set-Up*
>
> You do not give oxygen. Tell the nurse when the oxygen administration system is set up. The nurse turns on the oxygen, sets the flow rate, and applies the oxygen device.

## SETTING UP FOR OXYGEN ADMINISTRATION

### QUALITY OF LIFE

Remember to:
- Knock before entering the person's room
- Address the person by name
- Introduce yourself by name and title

### PRE-PROCEDURE

1 Follow *Delegation Guidelines: Oxygen Administration Set-Up.* See *Safety Alert: Oxygen Administration Set-Up.*
2 Practice hand hygiene.
3 Collect the following:
- Oxygen device with connecting tubing
- Flowmeter
- Humidifier (if ordered)
- Distilled water (if using a humidifier)
4 Identify the person. Check the ID bracelet against the assignment sheet. Call the person by name.
5 Explain to the person what you are going to do.

## SETTING UP FOR OXYGEN ADMINISTRATION—CONT'D

### PROCEDURE

6 Make sure the flowmeter is in the *OFF* position.
7 Attach the flowmeter to the wall outlet or to the tank.
8 Fill the humidifier with distilled water.
9 Attach the humidifier to the bottom of the flowmeter.

10 Attach the oxygen device and connecting tubing to the humidifier. *Do not set the flowmeter. Do not apply the oxygen device on the person.*

### POST-PROCEDURE

11 Discard packaging.
12 Make sure the cap is securely on the distilled water. Store it according to agency policy.
13 Provide for comfort.
14 Place the signal light within reach.

15 Decontaminate your hands.
16 Tell the nurse when you are done. *The nurse will:*
  - *Turn on the oxygen and set the flow rate*
  - *Apply the oxygen device on the person*

## OXYGEN SAFETY

You assist the nurse with oxygen therapy. You do not give oxygen. You do not adjust the flow rate unless allowed by your state and agency. However, you must give safe care. Follow the rules in Box 30-5. Also follow the rules in Box 30-4.

---

**BOX 30-5  SAFETY RULES FOR OXYGEN THERAPY**

- Never remove the oxygen device.
- Make sure the oxygen device is secure but not tight.
- Check for signs of irritation from the device. Check behind the ears, under the nose (cannula), and around the face (mask). Also check the cheekbones.
- Keep the face clean and dry when a face mask is used.
- Never shut off oxygen flow.
- Do not adjust the flow rate unless allowed by your state and agency.
- Tell the nurse at once if the flow rate is too high or too low.
- Tell the nurse at once if the humidifier is not bubbling.
- Secure connecting tubing in place. Tape or pin it to the person's garment following agency policy.
- Make sure there are no kinks in the tubing.
- Make sure the person does not lie on any part of the tubing.
- Report signs and symptoms of hypoxia, respiratory distress, or abnormal breathing patterns to the nurse at once (see Boxes 30-2 and 30-3).
- Give oral hygiene as directed. Follow the care plan.
- Make sure the oxygen device is clean and free of mucus.
- Maintain an adequate water level in the humidifier.

# ARTIFICIAL AIRWAYS

Artificial airways keep the airway patent (open). They are needed:
- When disease, injury, secretions, or aspiration obstructs the airway
- By some persons who are semiconscious or unconscious
- When the person is recovering from anesthesia
- For mechanical ventilation (p. 642)

**Intubation** means inserting an artificial airway. Artificial airways are usually plastic and disposable. They come in adult, pediatric, and infant sizes. These airways are common:
- *Oropharyngeal airway*—inserted through the mouth and into the pharynx (Fig. 30-25, *A*). A nurse or respiratory therapist inserts the airway.
- *Nasopharyngeal airway*—inserted through a nostril and into the pharynx (Fig. 30-25, *B*). A nurse or respiratory therapist inserts the airway.
- *Endotracheal (ET) tube*—inserted through the mouth or nose and into the trachea (Fig. 30-25, *C*). A doctor inserts it using a lighted scope. Some RNs and respiratory therapists are trained to insert ET tubes. A cuff is inflated to keep the airway in place.

- *Tracheostomy tube*—inserted through a surgically created opening *(ostomy)* into the trachea *(tracheo)* (Fig. 30-25, *D*). Some have cuffs. The cuff is inflated to keep the tube in place. Doctors perform tracheostomies.

Vital signs are checked often. Observe for hypoxia and other signs and symptoms. If an airway comes out or is dislodged, tell the nurse at once. The person needs frequent oral hygiene. Follow the care plan for oral hygiene.

Gagging and choking feelings are common. Imagine something in your mouth, nose, or throat. Comfort and reassure the person. Remind the person that the airway helps breathing. Use touch to show you care.

Persons with ET tubes cannot speak. Some tracheostomy tubes allow the person to speak. Paper and pencils, Magic Slates, communication boards, and hand signals are ways to communicate. Follow the care plan.

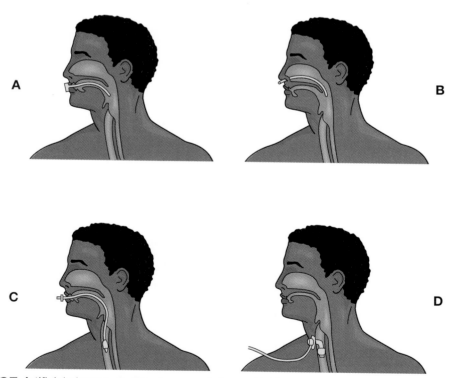

**FIG. 30-25** Artificial airways. **A,** Oropharyngeal airway. **B,** Nasopharyngeal airway. **C,** Endotracheal tube. **D,** Tracheostomy tube.

## TRACHEOSTOMIES

Tracheostomies are temporary for mechanical ventilation (p. 642). They are permanent when airway structures are surgically removed. Cancer, severe airway trauma, or brain damage may require a permanent tracheostomy. *See Focus on Children: Tracheostomies.*

A tracheostomy tube is plastic or metal. It has three parts (Fig. 30-26):

- The *obturator* has a round end. It is used to insert the outer cannula (tube). Then it is removed. (The obturator is placed within easy reach in case the tracheostomy tube falls out and needs to be reinserted. It is taped to the wall or bedside stand.)
- The *inner cannula* is inserted and locked in place. It is removed for cleaning and mucus removal. This keeps the airway patent.
- The *outer cannula* is secured in place with ties around the neck or a Velcro collar. The outer cannula is not removed.

Some plastic tracheostomy tubes do not have inner cannulas. These are used for persons who are suctioned often. With frequent suctioning, mucus does not stick to the cannula.

The cuffed tracheostomy tube is used for mechanical ventilation. It provides a seal between the cannula and the trachea (see Fig. 30-25, *D*). The cuff prevents air from leaking around the tube. It also prevents aspiration. A nurse or respiratory therapist inflates and deflates the cuff.

The tube must not come out (extubation). If not secure, it could come out with coughing or if pulled on. A loose tube moves up and down. It can damage the trachea.

The tube must remain patent (open). If able, the person coughs up secretions. Otherwise suctioning is needed (p. 640). *Call for the nurse if you note signs and symptoms of hypoxia or respiratory distress. Also call the nurse if the outer cannula comes out.*

Nothing must enter the stoma. Otherwise the person can aspirate. These safety measures are needed:

- Dressings do not have loose gauze or lint.
- The stoma or tube is covered when outdoors. The person wears a stoma cover, scarf, or shirt or blouse that buttons at the neck. The cover prevents dust, insects, and other small particles from entering the stoma.
- The stoma is not covered with plastic, leather, or similar materials. They prevent air from entering the stoma. The person cannot breathe.
- Tub baths are taken. If showers are taken, a shower guard is worn. A hand-held nozzle is used to direct water away from the stoma.
- The person is assisted with shampooing. Water must not enter the stoma.
- The stoma is covered when shaving.
- Swimming is not allowed. Water will enter the tube or stoma.
- Medical-alert jewelry is worn. The person carries a medical-alert ID card.

---

### FOCUS ON CHILDREN
#### TRACHEOSTOMIES

Some children have congenital defects. (*Congenitus* is a Latin word that means "to be born with.") Congenital defects are present at birth. Tracheostomies are needed for some congenital defects affecting the neck and airway.

Some infections cause airway structures to swell. This obstructs airflow. So does foreign body aspiration. These situations can require emergency tracheostomies.

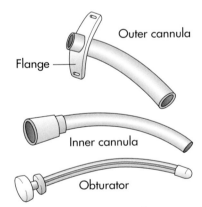

**FIG. 30-26** Parts of a tracheostomy tube.

**TRACHEOSTOMY CARE.** Tracheostomy care involves:
- Cleaning the inner cannula to remove mucus and keep the airway patent
- Cleaning the stoma to prevent infection and skin breakdown
- Applying clean ties or a Velcro collar to prevent infection

You can assist the nurse with tracheostomy care. It is done daily or every 8 to 12 hours. Excess secretions, soiled ties or collar, or soiled or moist dressings are other reasons for this care.

*See Focus on Children: Tracheostomy Care.*

---

**SAFETY ALERT:** *Tracheostomy Care*
When the ties are removed, you must hold the outer cannula in place. The ties or collar must be secure but not tight. For an adult, a finger should slide under the ties or collar (Fig. 30-27, *B*).

Mucus may contain microbes or blood. Follow Standard Precautions and the Bloodborne Pathogen Standard.

---

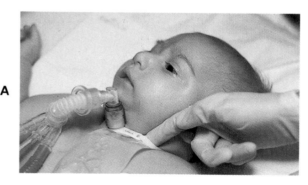

**A**

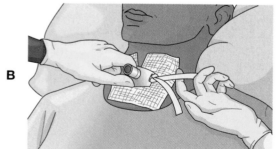

**B**

**FIG. 30-27 A,** For children, only a fingertip is inserted under the ties. **B,** For an adult, a finger is inserted under the ties. (**A** from Hockenberry MJ and others: *Wong's nursing care of infants and children*, ed 7, St Louis, 2003, Mosby.)

---

**FOCUS ON CHILDREN**
TRACHEOSTOMY CARE
The ties must be secure but not tight. Only a fingertip should slide under the ties (Fig. 30-27, *A*). Ties are too loose if you can slide your whole finger under them.
Help the nurse by holding the child still. Position the child's head as the nurse directs.

---

## SUCTIONING THE AIRWAY

Secretions can collect in the upper airway. Retained secretions:
- Obstruct airflow into and out of the airway
- Provide an environment for microbes
- Interfere with $O_2$ and $CO_2$ exchange

Hypoxia can occur. Usually coughing removes secretions. Some persons cannot cough, or the cough is too weak to remove secretions. They need suctioning.

**Suction** is the process of withdrawing or sucking up fluid (*secretions*). A tube connects to a suction source (wall outlet or suction machine) at one end and to a suction catheter at the other end. The catheter is inserted into the airway. Secretions are withdrawn through the catheter.

### SUCTIONING ROUTES
The nose, mouth, and pharynx make up the upper airway. The trachea and bronchi are the lower parts of the airway.
- *Oropharyngeal* route. The mouth (*oro*) and pharynx (*pharyngeal*) are suctioned. A suction catheter is passed through the mouth and into the pharynx. The Yankauer suction catheter is often used for thick secretions (Fig. 30-28). It is larger and stiffer than other suction catheters.
- *Nasopharyngeal* route. The nose (*naso*) and pharynx (*pharyngeal*) are suctioned. The suction catheter is passed through the nose and into the pharynx.
- *Lower airway* suctioning. This is done through an ET or a tracheostomy tube (p. 638).

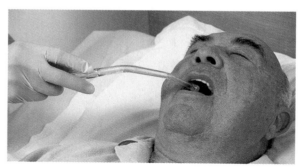

**FIG. 30-28** The Yankauer suction catheter.

The lungs are hyperventilated before suctioning the lower airway. *Hyperventilate* means to give extra *(hyper)* breaths *(ventilate)*. An Ambu bag is used (Fig. 30-29). It is attached to an oxygen source. Then the oxygen delivery device is removed from the ET or tracheostomy tube. The Ambu bag is attached to the ET or tracheostomy tube. To give a breath, the bag is squeezed with both hands. The nurse or respiratory therapist gives 3 to 5 breaths.

Oxygen is treated like a drug. You do not give drugs. Therefore you need to check if your state and agency allow you to use an Ambu bag attached to an oxygen source.

*See Focus on Children: Suctioning.*

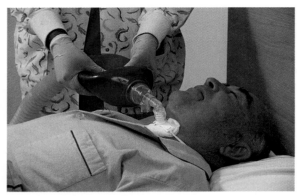

**FIG. 30-29** Using an Ambu bag. Two hands are used to squeeze the bag.

---

**SAFETY ALERT:** *Suctioning*

If not done correctly, suctioning can cause serious harm. Suctioning removes oxygen from the airway. The person does not get oxygen during suctioning. Hypoxia and life-threatening problems can occur. They arise from the respiratory, cardiovascular, and nervous systems. Cardiac arrest can occur. Infection and airway injury are possible.

You can assist the nurse with suctioning. Follow the principles and safety measures in Box 30-6.

Always keep needed suction equipment and supplies at the bedside. When suctioning is needed, you do not have time to collect supplies from the supply area.

Mucus may contain microbes or blood. Follow Standard Precautions and the Bloodborne Pathogen Standard.

---

### ► FOCUS ON CHILDREN
#### SUCTIONING

Suctioning may frighten children. They need clear explanations about the procedure. As with other care, you may need to hold the child still. To do so, control the child's head and arm movements.

---

### BOX 30-6   PRINCIPLES AND SAFETY MEASURES FOR SUCTIONING

- Review the procedure with the nurse. Know what the nurse expects you to do.
- Report coughing and signs and symptoms of respiratory distress to the nurse. They signal the need for suctioning. Suctioning is done as needed *(prn)*—not on a schedule.
- Sterile technique is used. This helps prevent microbes from entering the airway.
- The nurse tells you the catheter size needed. If too large, it can injure the airway.
- Suction is not applied while inserting the catheter. When suction is applied, air is sucked out of the airway.
- The catheter is inserted smoothly. This helps prevent injury to the mucous membranes.
- A suction cycle involves inserting the catheter, suctioning, and removing the catheter. A suction cycle takes no more than 10 to 15 seconds. For infants and children, the suction cycle is limited to 5 seconds. (Hold your breath during the suction cycle. This helps you experience what the person feels during suctioning.)
- The catheter is cleared with water or saline between suction cycles.
- The nurse waits 20 to 30 seconds between each suction cycle. Some agencies require waiting 60 seconds.
- The suction catheter is passed (inserted) no more than 3 times. Injury and hypoxia are risks each time the suction catheter is passed.
- Check the person's pulse, respirations, and pulse oximeter measurement before, during, and after the procedure. Also observe the person's level of consciousness. Tell the nurse at once if any of these occur:
  —A drop in pulse rate or a pulse rate less than 60 beats per minute
  —Irregular cardiac rhythms
  —A drop or rise in blood pressure
  —Respiratory distress
  —A drop in the $SpO_2$ (p. 626)

# MECHANICAL VENTILATION

Weak muscle effort, airway obstruction, and damaged lung tissue cause hypoxia. Nervous system diseases and injuries can affect the respiratory center in the brain. Nerve damage interferes with messages between the lungs and the brain. Drug overdose depresses the brain. With severe problems, the person cannot breathe. Or normal blood oxygen levels are not maintained. Often mechanical ventilation is needed.

**Mechanical ventilation** is using a machine to move air into and out of the lungs (Fig. 30-30). Oxygen enters the lungs, and carbon dioxide leaves them. An ET or tracheostomy tube is needed for mechanical ventilation.

Alarms sound when something is wrong. One alarm means the person is disconnected from the ventilator. The nurse shows you how to reconnect the ET or tracheostomy tube. *When any alarm sounds, first check to see if the person's tube is attached to the ventilator. If not, attach it to the ventilator.* Then tell the nurse at once about the alarm. Do not reset alarms.

Persons needing mechanical ventilation are very ill. Other problems and injuries are common. Some persons are confused or disoriented or cannot think clearly. The machine and fear of dying frighten many. Some are relieved to get enough oxygen. Many fear needing the machine for life. Mechanical ventilation can be painful for those with chest injuries or chest surgery. Tubes and hoses restrict movement. This causes more discomfort.

The nurse may ask you to assist with the person's care. See Box 30-7.

*See Focus on Long-Term Care: Mechanical Ventilation. See Focus on Home Care: Mechanical Ventilation.*

---

### FOCUS ON LONG-TERM CARE
#### MECHANICAL VENTILATION

Some persons need mechanical ventilation for a few hours or days. Others need it for a longer time. They may require long-term or subacute care. Often the person needs weaning from the ventilator. That is, the person needs to breathe without the machine. The respiratory therapist and RN plan the weaning process. The process may take many weeks.

---

### FOCUS ON HOME CARE
#### MECHANICAL VENTILATION

Home care is an option for some ventilator-dependent persons. The RN teaches you how to care for the person. Family members learn how to assist with the person's care. Make sure that you can reach an RN by phone when in the person's home. Make sure delegated tasks are allowed by your state and agency.

---

## BOX 30-7 CARE OF PERSONS ON MECHANICAL VENTILATION

- Keep the signal light within reach.
- Make sure hoses and connecting tubing have slack. They must not pull on the artificial airway. Answer signal lights promptly. The person depends on others for basic needs.
- Explain who you are and what you are going to do. Do this whenever you enter the room.
- Give the day, date, and time every time you give care.
- Report signs of respiratory distress or discomfort at once.
- Do not change settings on the machine or reset alarms.
- Follow the care plan for communication. The person cannot talk. Use agreed-upon hand or eye signals for "yes" and "no." Everyone must use the same signals. Otherwise, communication does not occur. Some persons can use paper and pencils, Magic Slates, communication boards, and hand signals.
- Ask questions that have simple answers. It may be hard to write long responses.
- Watch what you say and do. This includes when you are near and away from the person and family. They pay close attention to your verbal and nonverbal communication. Do not say or do anything that could upset the person.
- Use touch to comfort and reassure the person. Also tell the person about the weather, pleasant news events, and gifts and cards.
- Meet the person's basic needs. Follow the care plan.
- Tell the person when you are leaving the room and when you will return.

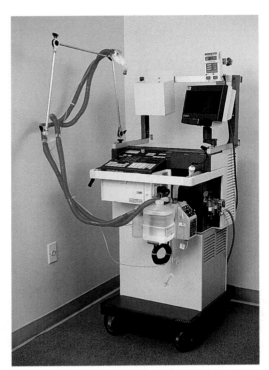

**FIG. 30-30** A mechanical ventilator.

## CHEST TUBES

Air, blood, or fluid can collect in the pleural space (sac or cavity). This occurs when the chest is entered because of injury or surgery.

- **Pneumothorax** is air *(pneumo)* in the pleural space *(thorax)*.
- **Hemothorax** is blood *(hemo)* in the pleural space *(thorax)*.
- **Pleural effusion** is the escape and collection of fluid *(effusion)* in the pleural space.

Pressure occurs when air, blood, or fluid collects in the pleural space. The pressure collapses the lung. Air cannot reach affected alveoli. $O_2$ and $CO_2$ are not exchanged. Respiratory distress and hypoxia result. Pressure on the heart threatens life. It affects the heart's ability to pump.

The doctor inserts chest tubes to remove the air, fluid, or blood (Fig. 30-31). The sterile procedure is done in surgery, in the emergency room, or at the bedside. A nurse assists.

Chest tubes attach to a drainage system (Fig. 30-32, p. 644). The system must be airtight. Air must not enter the pleural space. Water-seal drainage keeps the system airtight. The bottles in Figure 30-33, p. 644, show how the system works:

- A chest tube attaches to connecting tubing.
- Connecting tubing attaches to a tube in the drainage container.
- The tube in the drainage container extends under water. The water prevents air from entering the chest tube and then the pleural space.

See Box 30-8, p. 644, for care of the person with chest tubes.

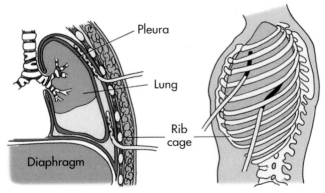

**FIG. 30-31** Chest tubes inserted into the pleural space. (From Elkin MK, Perry AG: Potter PA: *Nursing interventions & clinical skills,* ed 3, St Louis, 2004, Mosby.)

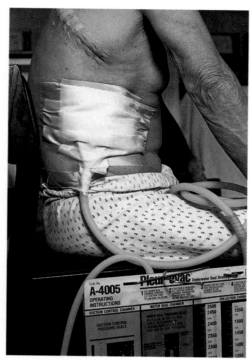

**FIG. 30-32** Chest tubes attached to a disposable water-seal drainage system. (From Elkin MK, Perry AG: Potter PA: *Nursing interventions & clinical skills,* ed 3, St Louis, 2004, Mosby.)

# CARDIOPULMONARY RESUSCITATION

Persons with respiratory injuries and problems are at risk for respiratory and cardiac arrest. See Chapter 40.

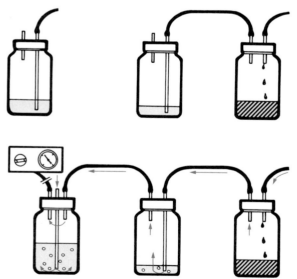

**FIG. 30-33** Water-seal drainage system. (From Potter PA, Perry AG: *Fundamentals of nursing,* ed 5, St Louis, 2001, Mosby.)

| BOX 30-8 | CARE OF THE PERSON WITH CHEST TUBES |
|---|---|

- Keep the drainage system below the chest.
- Measure vital signs as directed. Report vital sign changes at once.
- Report signs and symptoms of hypoxia and respiratory distress at once. Also report complaints of pain or difficulty breathing.
- Keep connecting tubing coiled on the bed. Allow enough slack so the chest tubes are not dislodged when the person moves. If tubing hangs in loops, drainage collects in the loop.
- Prevent tubing kinks. Kinks obstruct the chest tube. Air, blood, or fluid collects in the pleural space.
- Observe chest drainage. Report any change in chest drainage at once. This includes increases in drainage or the appearance of bright red drainage.
- Record chest drainage according to agency policy.
- Turn and position the person as directed. Be careful and gentle to prevent chest tubes from dislodging.
- Assist the person with coughing and deep breathing as directed.
- Assist with incentive spirometry as directed.
- Note bubbling in the drainage system. Tell the nurse at once if bubbling increases, decreases, or stops.
- Tell the nurse at once if any part of the system is loose or disconnected.
- Keep sterile petrolatum gauze at the bedside. It is needed if a chest tube comes out.
- Call for help at once if a chest tube comes out. Cover the insertion site with sterile petrolatum gauze. Stay with the person. Follow the nurse's directions.

# ■ REVIEW QUESTIONS ■

Circle the **BEST** answer.

1 Alcohol and narcotics affect oxygen needs because they
   a Depress the brain
   b Are pollutants
   c Cause allergies
   d Cause a pneumothorax

2 Hypoxia is
   a Not enough oxygen in the blood
   b The amount of hemoglobin that contains oxygen
   c Not enough oxygen in the cells
   d The lack of carbon dioxide

3 An early sign of hypoxia is
   a Cyanosis
   b Increased pulse and respiratory rates
   c Restlessness
   d Dyspnea

4 A person can breathe deeply and comfortably only while sitting. This is called
   a Biot's respirations
   b Orthopnea
   c Bradypnea
   d Kussmaul respirations

5 The person needs to rest after
   a A chest x-ray
   b A lung scan
   c Arterial blood gases
   d Pulmonary function tests

6 A person's $SpO_2$ is 98%. Which is *true?*
   a The pulse oximeter is wrong.
   b The pulse is 98 beats per minute.
   c The measurement is within normal range.
   d The person needs suctioning.

7 Which is *not* a site for a pulse oximetry sensor?
   a Toe
   b Finger
   c Ear lobe
   d Upper arm

8 You are assisting with coughing and deep breathing. Which is *false?*
   a The person inhales through pursed lips.
   b The person sits in a comfortable sitting position.
   c The person inhales deeply through the nose.
   d The person holds a pillow over an incision.

9 Which is useful for deep breathing?
   a Pulse oximeter
   b Incentive spirometry
   c Chest tubes
   d Partial-rebreather mask

10 When assisting with oxygen therapy, you can
   a Turn the oxygen on and off
   b Start the oxygen
   c Decide what device to use
   d Keep connecting tubing secure and free of kinks

11 A person has a tracheostomy. Which is *false?*
   a The inner cannula is removed for cleaning.
   b The outer cannula is removed for cleaning.
   c The outer cannula must be secured in place.
   d The person must be protected from aspiration.

12 A person has a tracheostomy. The person can do the following *except*
   a Shampoo
   b Shave
   c Shower with a hand-held nozzle
   d Swim

13 A person has a tracheostomy. The nurse removes the ties. You must
   a Remove the inner cannula
   b Clean the flange and stoma
   c Remove the dressing
   d Hold the outer cannula in place

14 These statements are about suctioning. Which is *true?*
   a Suction is applied while inserting the catheter.
   b Suctioning is done every 2 hours.
   c A suction cycle is no more than 10 to 15 seconds.
   d The catheter is inserted 4 or more times.

15 Suctioning requires
   a Mechanical ventilation
   b Sterile technique
   c An artificial airway
   d Chest tubes

**16** Which is used to hyperventilate the lungs?
  a Incentive spirometer
  b Pulse oximeter
  c Ambu bag
  d Partial-rebreather mask

**17** Mr. Long requires mechanical ventilation. Which is *false?*
  a He has an ET or a tracheostomy tube.
  b The signal light is always within his reach.
  c Touch provides comfort and reassurance.
  d You can reset alarms on the ventilator.

**18** An alarm sounds on Mr. Long's ventilator. What should you do *first?*
  a Reset the alarm.
  b Check to see if his airway is attached to the ventilator.
  c Call the nurse at once.
  d Ask him what is wrong.

**19** A person has a pneumothorax. This is
  a Fluid in the pleural space
  b Blood in the pleural space
  c Air in the pleural space
  d Secretions in the pleural space

**20** Chest tubes are attached to water-seal drainage. You should do the following *except*
  a Tell the nurse if bubbling increases, decreases, or stops
  b Make sure the tubing is not kinked
  c Keep the drainage system below the person's chest
  d Hang tubing in loops

*Answers to these questions are on p. 819.*

# Rehabilitation and Restorative Care

## OBJECTIVES

- Define the key terms listed in this chapter
- Describe how rehabilitation involves the whole person
- Identify the complications to prevent
- Identify the common reactions to rehabilitation
- Describe how rehabilitation can help a person work
- List the common rehabilitation services
- Explain your role in rehabilitation and restorative care
- Explain how to promote quality of life

## KEY TERMS

**activities of daily living (ADL)** The activities usually done during a normal day in a person's life

**disability** Any lost, absent, or impaired physical or mental function

**prosthesis** An artificial replacement for a missing body part

**rehabilitation** The process of restoring the person to the highest possible level of physical, psychological, social, and economic function

**restorative aide** A nursing assistant with special training in restorative nursing and rehabilitation skills

**restorative nursing care** Care that helps persons regain their health, strength, and independence

Disease, injury, and surgery can affect body function. So can birth injuries and birth defects (Chapter 36). Often more than one function is lost. Losses are temporary or permanent. Eating, bathing, dressing, and walking are hard or seem impossible. Some persons cannot work. Others cannot care for children or family.

A **disability** is any lost, absent, or impaired physical or mental function. Causes are acute or chronic (Box 31-1):

- An *acute problem* has a short course. Recovery is complete. A fracture is an acute problem.
- A *chronic problem* has a long course. The problem is controlled—not cured—with treatment. Arthritis is a chronic health problem.

Disabilities are short-term or long-term. The person may depend totally or in part on others for basic needs. The degree of disability affects how much function is possible.

**Rehabilitation** is the process of restoring the person to the highest possible level of physical, psychological, social, and economic function. The focus is on improving abilities. For some persons the goal is to return to work. For others, self-care is the goal. Sometimes improved function is not possible. Then the goal is to prevent further loss of function. This helps the person maintain the best possible quality of life.

Some persons are weak. Many cannot perform activities of daily living. **Restorative nursing care** is care that helps persons regain their health, strength, and independence. Some people have more progressive illnesses. They become more and more disabled. Rehabilitation and restorative nursing programs do the following:

- Help maintain the highest level of function
- Prevent unnecessary decline in function

*See Focus on Long-Term Care: Rehabilitation and Restorative Care.*

# RESTORATIVE NURSING

Restorative nursing helps persons regain their health, strength, and independence. It may involve measures that promote:
- Self-care
- Elimination
- Positioning
- Mobility
- Communication
- Cognitive function

Many persons need restorative nursing and rehabilitation. Often it is hard to separate them. In many agencies, they mean the same thing. Both focus on the whole person.

## RESTORATIVE AIDES

Some agencies have restorative aides. A **restorative aide** is a nursing assistant with special training in restorative nursing and rehabilitation skills. These aides assist the nursing and health teams as needed.

There is no required training for restorative aides. The agency decides on their roles and functions. Then needed training is provided. Some schools offer courses for restorative aides.

Usually nursing assistants are promoted to restorative aide positions. Those chosen have excellent work ethics, job performance, and skills.

# REHABILITATION AND THE WHOLE PERSON

An illness or injury has physical, psychological, and social effects. So does a disability. Suppose an illness left you paralyzed from the waist down? Answer these questions:
- Would you be angry, afraid, or depressed?
- How would you move about?
- How would you care for yourself?
- How would you care for your family?
- How would you shop, go to church, or visit friends?
- What job could you do?
- How would you support yourself?

The person with a disability needs to adjust physically, psychologically, socially, and economically. Abilities—what the person can do—are stressed. Complications are prevented. They can lead to further disability.

*See Focus on Children: The Whole Person. See Focus on Older Persons: The Whole Person.*

---

**BOX 31-1  COMMON HEALTH PROBLEMS REQUIRING REHABILITATION**

- Alcoholism
- Amputation
- Brain tumor
- Burns
- Cerebral palsy
- Chronic obstructive pulmonary disease
- Head injury
- Myocardial infarction (heart attack)
- Parkinson's disease
- Spinal cord injury
- Spinal cord tumor
- Stroke
- Substance abuse

---

**FOCUS ON LONG-TERM CARE**
**REHABILITATION AND RESTORATIVE CARE**

Some nursing center residents have physical disabilities. Causes include strokes, fractures, amputations, or other injuries. They need to regain function or adjust to a long-term disability. Often these residents return home.

Other residents have progressive illnesses. They become more and more disabled. The goals are to help them maintain their highest level of function and to prevent unnecessary decline in function.

---

**FOCUS ON CHILDREN**
**THE WHOLE PERSON**

Disabilities occur from birth defects or from illness, injury, or surgery. They can affect normal growth and development (Chapter 8). For normal growth and development the child needs hand skills, mobility, communication, play, and relationships with parents, family, and peers. A disability can affect one or more of these factors.

---

**FOCUS ON OLDER PERSONS**
**THE WHOLE PERSON**

Rehabilitation often takes longer in older persons than in other age-groups. Changes from aging affect healing, mobility, vision, hearing, and other functions (Chapter 9). Chronic health problems can slow recovery. Older persons also are at risk for injuries. Long or fast-paced rehabilitation programs are hard for them. Their programs usually are slower-paced.

## PHYSICAL ASPECTS

Rehabilitation begins when the person seeks health care. It starts with preventing complications. They can occur from bedrest, prolonged illness, or recovery from surgery or injury. Bowel and bladder problems are prevented. So are contractures and pressure ulcers. Good alignment, turning and repositioning, range-of-motion exercises, and supportive devices are needed (Chapters 13 and 22). Good skin care also prevents pressure ulcers (Chapters 16 and 28).

Bladder training may be needed (Chapter 18). The method depends on the person's problems, abilities, and needs. Some need bowel training (Chapter 19). The goals are to gain control of bowel movements and have regular elimination. Fecal impaction, constipation, and fecal incontinence are prevented. Follow the care plan and the nurse's instructions.

Self-care is a major goal. **Activities of daily living (ADL)** are the activities usually done during a normal day in a person's life. ADL include bathing, oral hygiene, dressing, eating, elimination, and moving about. The health team evaluates the person's ability to perform ADL. They also consider the need for self-help devices.

Sometimes the hands, wrists, and arms are affected. Self-help devices are often needed. Equipment is changed, made, or bought to meet the person's needs. Eating devices include glass holders, plate guards, and silverware with curved handles or cuffs (Chapter 20). Some devices attach to splints (Fig. 31-1). Some persons cannot perform back-and-forth brushing motions for oral hygiene. Electric toothbrushes are helpful. Longer handles attach to combs, brushes, and sponges (Fig. 31-2). There are self-help devices for cooking, dressing, writing, and other tasks (Fig. 31-3).

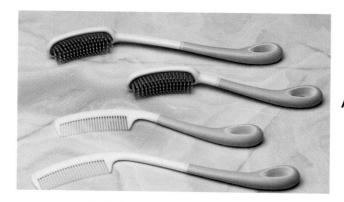

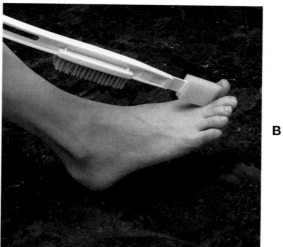

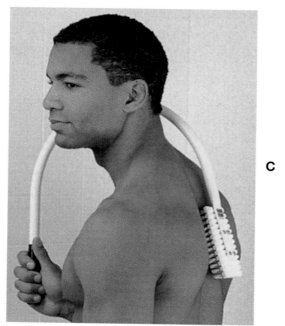

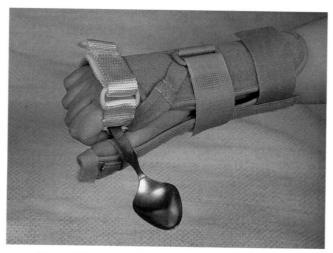

**FIG. 31-1** Eating device attached to a splint.

**FIG. 31-2 A,** Long-handled combs and brushes for hair care. **B,** Long-handled brush for bathing. **C,** Brush with a curved handle. (**A** and **B** courtesy North Coast Medical Inc., Morgan Hill, Calif.; **C** courtesy Sammons Preston Roylan, An AbilityOne Company, Bolingbrook, Ill.)

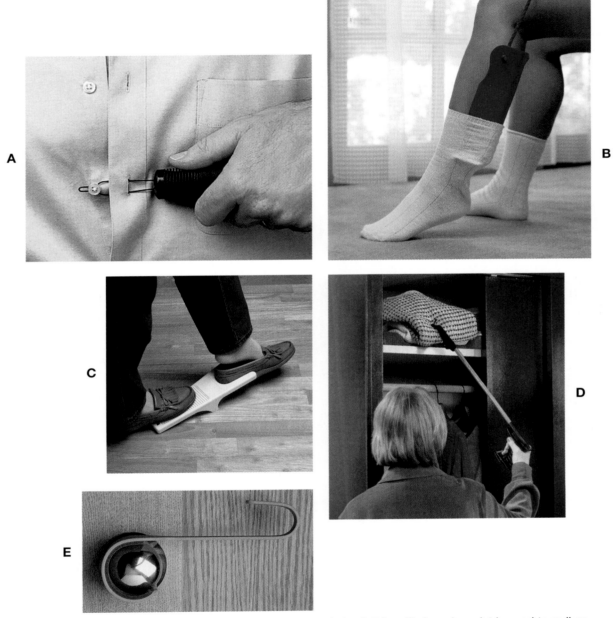

**FIG. 31-3 A,** A button hook is used to button and zip clothing. **B,** A sock assist is used to pull on socks and stockings. **C,** A shoe remover is used to take off shoes. **D,** Reachers are helpful to remove items from high shelves. **E,** A doorknob turner increases leverage to help turn the knob. (**A, B, C,** and **E** courtesy North Coast Medical Inc., Morgan Hill, Calif.; **D** courtesy Sammons Preston Roylan, An AbilityOne Company, Bolingbrook, Ill.)

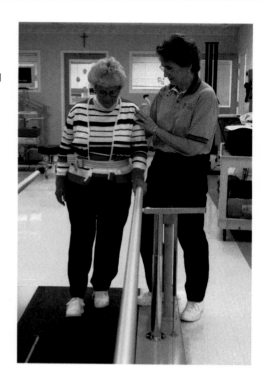

FIG. 31-4 The person is assisted with walking in physical therapy.

FIG. 31-5 The person uses a transfer board.
A, The person transfers from the wheelchair to bed.
B, The person transfers from the wheelchair to the bathtub.

**A**

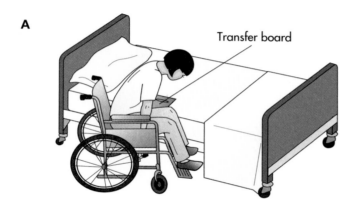

Transfer board

**B**

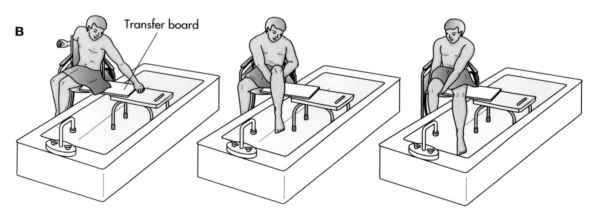

Transfer board

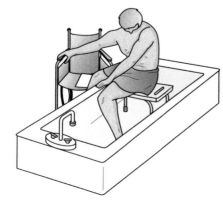

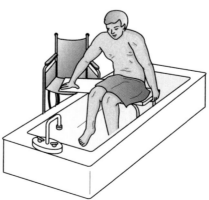

The person may need crutches or a walker, cane, or brace. Physical therapy is common after musculoskeletal and nervous system diseases, injuries, and surgeries (Fig. 31-4). Some people need wheelchairs. If possible, they learn wheelchair transfers. Such transfers include to and from the bed, toilet, bathtub, sofa, and chair and in and out of cars (Figs. 31-5 and 31-6).

A **prosthesis** is an artificial replacement for a missing body part. The person learns how to use an artificial arm or leg (Chapter 33). Eye and breast prostheses are other examples. The goal is for the prosthesis to be like the missing body part in function and appearance.

Difficulty swallowing (*dysphagia*) may occur after a stroke. The person may need a dysphagia diet (Chapter 20). When possible, exercises are taught to improve swallowing. Some persons cannot swallow. They need enteral nutrition (Chapter 20). Difficulty speaking (*aphasia*) may occur from a stroke (Chapter 33). Speech therapy and communication devices (Chapter 6) are helpful.

Some persons need mechanical ventilation (Chapter 30). Some are weaned from the ventilator. Others must learn to live with life-long mechanical ventilation.

*See Focus on Long-Term Care: Physical Aspects.*

> ### FOCUS ON LONG-TERM CARE
> #### PHYSICAL ASPECTS
> Some nursing centers have special rehabilitation programs:
> - Cardiac rehabilitation—for heart disorders (Chapter 33).
> - Neurological rehabilitation—for nervous system disorders (Chapter 33).
> - Respiratory rehabilitation—for respiratory system disorders (Chapters 30 and 33).
> - Rehabilitation of complex medical and surgical conditions—such as postoperative wound care (Chapter 28) and unstable diabetes (Chapter 33).
>
> Persons in rehabilitation programs usually return home after a short stay. Some need home care or assisted-living housing. Others require long-term care.

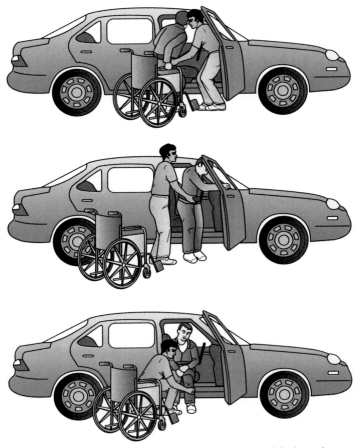

**FIG. 31-6** The person transfers from the wheelchair to the car.

## PSYCHOLOGICAL AND SOCIAL ASPECTS

A disability can affect function and appearance. Self-esteem and relationships may suffer. The person may feel unwhole, useless, unattractive, unclean, or undesirable. The person may deny the disability. The person may expect therapy to correct the problem. He or she may be depressed, angry, and hostile.

Successful rehabilitation depends on the person's attitude. The person must accept his or her limits and be motivated. The focus is on abilities and strengths. Despair and frustration are common. Progress may be slow. Learning a new task is a reminder of the disability. Old fears and emotions may recur.

Remind persons of their progress. They need help accepting disabilities and limits. Give support, reassurance, and encouragement. Meeting psychological and social needs is part of the care plan. Spiritual support helps some persons.

## ECONOMIC ASPECTS

Some persons cannot return to their jobs. The person is assessed for work skills, past work history, interests, and talents. A job skill may be restored or a new one learned. The goal is for the person to become gainfully employed. Assistance is often given in finding a job.

## THE REHABILITATION TEAM

Rehabilitation is a team effort. The person is the key member of the team. The family, doctor, nursing team, and other health team members assist the person in setting goals and planning (Chapter 1). All help the person regain function and independence.

The team meets often to discuss the person's progress. Changes in the rehabilitation plan are made as needed. The person and family attend the meetings when possible. Families are key members of the team. They provide support and encouragement. Often they help with care when the person returns home.

### YOUR ROLE

Every part of your job focuses on promoting the person's independence. Preventing decline in function also is a goal. The many procedures, care measures, and rules in this book apply. Safety, communication, legal, and ethical aspects apply. So do the measures in Box 31-2.

---

**BOX 31-2  ASSISTING WITH REHABILITATION AND RESTORATIVE CARE**

- Follow the nurse's instructions carefully.
- Follow the person's care plan.
- Follow the person's daily routine.
- Provide for safety (Chapter 10).
- Protect the person's rights. Privacy and personal choice are very important.
- Report early signs and symptoms of complications. They include pressure ulcers, contractures, and bowel and bladder problems.
- Keep the person in good alignment at all times (Chapter 13).
- Use safe transfer methods (Chapter 13).
- Practice measures to prevent pressure ulcers (Chapter 28).
- Turn and reposition the person as directed.
- Perform range-of-motion exercises as instructed.
- Apply assistive devices as ordered.
- Do not pity the person or give sympathy.
- Encourage the person to perform ADL to the extent possible.

- Allow time for the person to complete tasks. Do not rush the person.
- Give praise when even a little progress is made.
- Provide emotional support and reassurance.
- Try to understand and appreciate the person's situation, feelings, and concerns.
- Provide for spiritual needs.
- Practice the methods developed by the rehabilitation team when assisting the person.
- Practice the task that the person must do. This helps you guide and direct the person.
- Know how to apply the person's self-help devices.
- Know how to use and operate special equipment used by the person.
- Stress what the person can do. Focus on abilities and strengths—not disabilities and weaknesses.
- Remember that muscles will atrophy if not used.
- Have a hopeful outlook.

# REHABILITATION SERVICES

Some persons need extended hospital care. Some need subacute or long-term care. Others receive outpatient care. Home care agencies and day care centers often provide needed services.

Some people are transferred to rehabilitation centers. There are centers for persons who are blind, deaf, mentally retarded, or physically disabled or who have speech problems. There are centers for persons who are mentally ill.

*See Focus on Children: Rehabilitation Services. See Focus on Home Care: Rehabilitation Services. See Focus on Long-Term Care: Rehabilitation Services.*

# QUALITY OF LIFE

Successful rehabilitation and restorative care improve the person's quality of life. A hopeful and winning outlook is helpful. Often the process is slow and frustrating. Promoting quality of life helps the person's at-

---

## FOCUS ON CHILDREN
### REHABILITATION SERVICES

Federal laws require that schools provide needed therapies. In-school therapy is required to meet the child's learning needs.

---

## FOCUS ON HOME CARE
### REHABILITATION SERVICES

The rehabilitation team assesses the person's home setting (Box 31-3, p. 656). Changes in the home are made as needed. Some persons require personal attendants 24 hours a day.

---

## FOCUS ON LONG-TERM CARE
### REHABILITATION SERVICES

OBRA requires that nursing centers provide services required by the person's comprehensive care plan. If a person requires physical therapy, it must be provided. If occupational therapy is required, it must be provided. The same holds for speech and other therapies. All services require a doctor's order.

---

titude. The more the person can do alone, the better his or her quality of life. To promote quality of life:

- *Protect the right to privacy.* The person relearns old or practices new skills in private. No one needs to watch. They do not need to see mistakes, falls, spills, or clumsiness. Nor do they need to see anger or tears. Privacy protects dignity and promotes self-respect.
- *Encourage personal choice.* This gives the person control. Not being able to control body movements or functions is very frustrating. Persons are allowed and encouraged to control their lives to the extent possible. Persons who are sad and depressed may not want to make choices. Encourage them to do so. It can help them feel in control of those things that affect them. Personal choice is important in planning care.
- *Protect the right to be free from abuse and mistreatment.* Sometimes improvement is not seen for weeks. Learning to use a self-help device takes time. Learning to speak after a stroke can take a long time. So can learning how to dress when there is paralysis. What seems simple is often very hard for the person. Repeated explanations and demonstrations may have no or little results. You may become upset and short-tempered. Or other staff or the family may have such behaviors. Protect the person from physical and mental abuse and mistreatment. No one can shout, scream, or yell at the person. Nor can they call the person names. They cannot hit or strike the person. Unkind remarks are not allowed. Report signs of abuse or mistreatment to the nurse.
- *Learn to deal with your anger and frustration.* The person does not choose loss of function. If the process upsets you, think how the person must feel. Discuss your feelings with the nurse. The nurse can suggest ways to help you control or express your feelings. Perhaps you can assist other persons for a while.
- *Encourage activities.* Encourage the person to join in group activities. There may be concern about how others view the disability. Provide support and reassurance. Remind the person that others have disabilities. They can give support and understanding. Allow personal choice. The person should do what interests him or her. The person usually chooses activities that he or she can do.
- *Provide a safe setting.* It must meet the person's needs. Needed changes are made. The overbed table and bedside stand are moved to the person's strong side. The person may need a special chair. If unable to use the signal light, another way is needed to communicate with the staff. The rehabilitation team suggests these and other changes. They explain the need and purpose to the person and family.
- *Show patience, understanding, and sensitivity.* Progress may be slow and hard to see. The person may be upset and discouraged. Give support, encouragement, and praise when needed. Stress the person's abilities and strengths. Do not give pity or sympathy.

## BOX 31-3 HOME ASSESSMENT

### OUTDOORS

- Where is parking? How far is the parking area to the door?
- Where is the motor vehicle parked?
- Where is the mailbox?
- How wide are the doors?
- Can the person turn a key?
- Can the person open and close doors?
- Are ramps needed?
- Are handrails needed?
- Are entrances lighted?
- Does the person have access to private or public transportation?
- Can the person drive a motor vehicle?
- How wide and high are ramps and sidewalks?

### INDOORS

- Are there floor obstructions?
- Are there steps in the home? Where are they? How many are there?
- How is furniture arranged?
- Can the person use the furniture?
- Where are phones?
- Can the person open and close windows?
- How are floors covered (wall-to-wall carpeting, tile, hardwood floors, throw rugs)?
- Can the person use a wheelchair throughout the home?
- Where is the fuse or circuit-breaker box?
- Can the person control the heat?
- Are walkways, doors, and halls wide enough for wheelchair use?
- Does the building have an elevator?

### KITCHEN

- Can the person access the stove, sink, cupboards, storage areas, work space, refrigerator, and other appliances?
- How high is the sink and countertop?
- Is there an opening under the sink for wheelchair access?
- Can the person turn faucets on and off?
- Can the person use the microwave?
- Can the person reach stove knobs?
- Can the person reach appliances?

### BATHROOM

- How high are the sink, toilet, shower, and tub?
- Can the person reach the faucets?
- Can the person turn the faucets on and off?

### BATHROOM—CONT'D

- Is there space for a wheelchair and other assistive devices?
- Can the person get into and out of the tub or shower?
- Are there grab bars by the toilet, shower, and tub?

### BEDROOM

- How high is the person's bed?
- Can the person access the closet? Can the person reach rods and shelves?
- Can the person transfer into and out of bed safely? Is there space around the bed for the person to move?
- How is furniture arranged? Does it allow for a wheelchair or assistive devices?

### SAFETY

- Is the house number clearly visible and readable during an emergency?
- Are deadbolts and locks secure? Can the person use them?
- Can the person see and talk to a visitor at the door without being seen?
- Are steps, porch, and front door lighted?
- Are the steps, porch, and front door protected from rain, sleet, and snow?
- Is there a nonslip doormat?
- Can the person use the phone?
- Are emergency phone numbers clearly posted?
- Can the person control water temperature?
- Do electrical outlets have childproof covers?
- Where are the smoke detectors? Are they working?
- Are rooms and hallways well-lighted?
- Can the person turn indoor and outdoor lighting on and off?
- Can the person exit the home in an emergency?
- Is oxygen used? Are safety measures for oxygen use in place?
- Can the person access the phone, TV, radio, and lights while in bed?
- Are space heaters used? Are safety measures in place?
- Does the person have good judgment for cooking and stove use?
- Is there a safe play area for children?
- Can the person safely dispose of blood, body fluids, secretions, and excretions?
- Is there a pest-free method of trash storage?

Modified from Hoeman SP: *Rehabilitation nursing: process, application, and outcomes*, ed 3, St Louis, 2002, Mosby.

# ■ REVIEW QUESTIONS ■

Circle the **BEST** answer.

1 Rehabilitation and restorative care focus on
   a What the person cannot do
   b What the person can do
   c The whole person
   d The person's rights

2 Mr. Olson's rehabilitation begins with preventing
   a Angry feelings
   b Contractures and pressure ulcers
   c Illness and injury
   d Loss of self-esteem

3 Mr. Olson has weakness on his right side. ADL are
   a Done by him to the extent possible
   b Done by you
   c Postponed until he can use his right side
   d Supervised by a therapist

4 Persons with disabilities are likely to feel the following *except*
   a Undesirable
   b Angry and hostile
   c Depressed
   d Relief

5 Which statement about disabled persons is *false?*
   a They can never work again.
   b They may need to learn a new job skill.
   c They are evaluated for work abilities.
   d They receive help in finding a job.

6 Which statement is *false?*
   a Sympathy and pity help the person adjust to the disability.
   b You should know how to apply self-help devices.
   c You should know how to use equipment used in the person's care.
   d You need to convey hopefulness to the person.

7 Mr. Olson is learning to use a walker. He asks to have music played. You should
   a Tell him music is not allowed
   b Choose some music
   c Ask him to choose some music
   d Ask a therapist to choose some music

8 Mr. Olson's right side is weak. The signal light is on his right side. You move it to the left side. You have promoted his quality of life by
   a Protecting him from abuse and mistreatment
   b Allowing personal choice
   c Providing for his safety
   d Taking part in his activities

Circle **T** if the statement is true and **F** if it is false.

9 T F A person's speech therapy should be done in private.
10 T F You tell Mr. Olson that he cannot have dessert until he does his exercises. This is abuse and mistreatment.
11 T F Rehabilitation programs for older persons are usually slower-paced than those for younger persons.
12 T F Only the doctor and physical therapist make up the rehabilitation team.
13 T F Nursing assistants and restorative aides are involved in the person's rehabilitation program.
14 T F You need to stress the person's abilities and strengths.

*Answers to these questions are on p. 819.*

# Hearing and Vision Problems

## OBJECTIVES

- Define the key terms listed in this chapter
- Explain otitis media and Meniere's disease
- Describe the effects of hearing loss and vision loss
- Describe how to communicate with the hearing-impaired person
- Explain how to communicate with the speech-impaired person
- Explain the purpose of a hearing aid
- Describe how to care for a hearing aid
- Explain the differences between glaucoma and cataracts
- Describe how to protect an artificial eye from loss or damage
- Explain how to assist a blind person
- Perform the procedure described in this chapter

## KEY TERMS

**braille** A writing system that uses raised dots for each letter of the alphabet; the first 10 letters also represent 0 through 9

**cerumen** Earwax

**deafness** Hearing loss in which it is impossible for the person to understand speech through hearing alone

**hearing loss** Difficulty hearing normal conversations

**tinnitus** Ringing in the ears

**vertigo** Dizziness

Sight and hearing allow communication, learning, and moving about. They are important for self-care, work, and many other activities. They also have a role in safety and security needs. For example, you see dark clouds and hear tornado warning sirens. You know to seek shelter.

Many people have some degree of hearing or vision loss. Common causes include birth defects, accidents, infections, diseases, and aging.

damage the tympanic membrane (eardrum) or the ossicles (see Fig. 32-1). These structures are needed for hearing. Permanent hearing loss can occur.

Fluid builds up in the ear. Pain (earache) and hearing loss occur. So do fever and ringing in the ears (**tinnitus**). The doctor orders antibiotics. *See Focus on Children: Otitis Media.*

## EAR DISORDERS

The ear functions in hearing and balance. Middle ear infections, Meniere's disease, and hearing loss are presented here. To review the structures and functions of the ear, see Box 32-1, p. 660.

### OTITIS MEDIA

Otitis media is infection (*itis*) of the middle (*media*) ear (*ot*). It is acute or chronic. Chronic otitis media can

### FOCUS ON CHILDREN
#### OTITIS MEDIA

Otitis media is common in infants and children. It is most common between 6 months and 3 years of age. Infants cannot tell you about pain. For earaches, they pull at their ears or roll their heads. They may be irritable, cry a lot, sleep poorly, and have diarrhea. Fever, vomiting, and loss of appetite often occur.

The ear is a sense organ (Fig. 32-1). It functions in hearing and balance. It is divided into the *external ear*, *middle ear*, and *inner ear*.

The external ear (outer part) is called the *pinna* or *auricle*. Sound waves are guided through the external ear into the *auditory canal*. Glands in the auditory canal secrete a waxy substance called *cerumen*. The auditory canal extends about 1 inch to the *eardrum*. The eardrum *(tympanic membrane)* separates the external and middle ear.

The middle ear is a small space. It contains the *eustachian tube* and three small bones called *ossicles*. The eustachian tube connects the middle ear and the throat. Air enters the eustachian tube so that there is equal pressure on both sides of the eardrum. The ossicles amplify sound received from the eardrum. They transmit the sound to the inner ear. The three ossicles are:

- The *malleus*, which looks like a hammer
- The *incus*, which resembles an anvil
- The *stapes*, which is shaped like a stirrup

The inner ear consists of the *semicircular canals* and the *cochlea*. The cochlea looks like a snail shell. It contains fluid. The fluid carries sound waves from the middle ear to the *auditory nerve*. The auditory nerve then carries the message to the brain.

The three semicircular canals are involved with balance. They sense the head's position and changes in position and send messages to the brain.

## MENIERE'S DISEASE

Meniere's disease is a chronic disease of the inner ear. The increased fluid causes pressure in the middle ear. Tinnitus, hearing loss, and vertigo occur. **Vertigo** means dizziness. Whirling and spinning sensations are felt. Severe dizziness causes nausea and vomiting. Attacks last a few minutes to many hours.

Drugs, fluid restriction, and a low-salt diet decrease fluid in the ear. Safety is needed during vertigo. The person must lie down. Falls are prevented. Bed rails are used according to the care plan. The head is kept still. The person avoids turning the head. To talk to the person, stand directly in front of him or her. When movement is necessary, the person moves slowly. Sudden movements are avoided. So are bright or glaring lights. Assist with walking. The person should not walk alone in case vertigo occurs.

## HEARING LOSS

**Hearing** loss means difficulty hearing normal conversations. Losses range from mild to severe. Deafness is the most severe form. **Deafness** is hearing loss in which it is impossible for the person to understand speech through hearing alone.

Hearing loss occurs in all age-groups. Men are at higher risk for hearing loss than are women. Whites are at greater risk than are blacks. Common causes are:

- Age-related changes in the inner ear. It is harder to hear high-pitched sounds.
- Noise. Exposure to a very loud sound just once can cause hearing loss. Or it can occur over a long time.

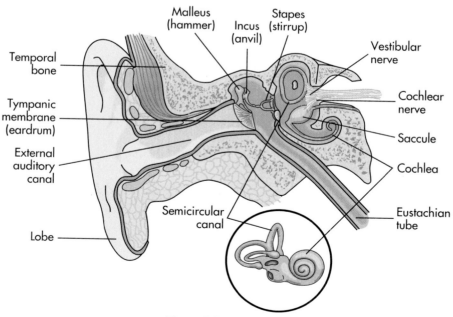

**FIG. 32-1** The ear.

Loud music from stereos and headphones, traffic, airplanes, power tools, and industrial machines are some examples of harmful noise.

- Infections
- Heart conditions
- Stroke
- Head injuries
- Tumors
- Drugs (some antibiotics and too much aspirin are examples)
- Heredity
- Birth defects

Temporary hearing loss can occur from earwax (**cerumen**). It blocks the ear canal. Hearing improves after earwax is removed. It is removed by a doctor or nurse.

---

**SAFETY ALERT:** *Hearing Loss*
Do not try to remove ear wax. This is done by a doctor or a nurse. Do not insert anything, including cotton swabs, into the ear.

---

Clear speech, responding to others, safety, and awareness of surroundings require hearing. Many people deny hearing problems. They relate hearing loss to aging. *See Focus on Older Persons: Hearing Loss. See Focus on Children: Hearing Loss.*

**EFFECTS ON THE PERSON.** A person may not notice gradual hearing loss. Others may see changes in the person's behavior or attitude. They may not relate hearing loss to the changes. Symptoms of hearing loss in children and adults include:

- Speaking too loudly
- Leaning forward to hear
- Turning and cupping the better ear toward the speaker
- Answering questions or responding inappropriately
- Asking for words to be repeated

Psychological and social effects are less obvious. People may give wrong answers or responses. Therefore they tend to shun social events to avoid embarrassment. Often they feel lonely, bored, and left out. Only parts of conversations are heard. They may become suspicious. They think others are talking about them or are talking softly on purpose. Some control conversations to avoid responding or being labeled "senile" because of poor answers. Straining and working to hear can cause fatigue, frustration, and irritability.

Hearing is needed for speech. How you pronounce words and voice volume depend on how you hear yourself. Hearing loss may result in slurred speech. Words may be pronounced wrong. Some have monotone speech or drop word endings. It may be hard to understand what the person says. Do not assume or pretend that you understand what the person says. Otherwise serious problems can result. Follow the guidelines in Box 32-2.

**COMMUNICATION.** Hearing-impaired persons may wear hearing aids or read lips. They watch facial expressions, gestures, and body language. Follow the measures in Box 32-3, p. 662, to help the person hear or lip-read (speech-read). Some people learn sign language (Figs. 32-2, p. 662, and 32-3, p. 663).

Some people have *hearing assistance* dogs (hearing guide dogs). The dog alerts the person to sounds. Examples include phones, doorbells, smoke detectors, alarm clocks, sirens, and oncoming cars.

*Text continued on p. 664.*

---

**FOCUS ON OLDER PERSONS**
HEARING LOSS

According to the National Institute on Aging, one third (33%) of Americans between the ages of 65 and 74 years have hearing loss. More than one half (50%) of persons age 85 years and older have hearing loss.

---

**FOCUS ON CHILDREN**
HEARING LOSS

Ear infection is the most common cause of hearing loss in children. Birth defects, illness, and injury are other causes. Infants with hearing loss often fail to start talking. Lack of attention and failing grades are early signs of hearing loss in children.

---

**BOX 32-2 COMMUNICATING WITH THE SPEECH-IMPAIRED PERSON**

- Listen, and give the person your full attention.
- Ask the person questions to which you know the answer. This helps you learn how the person speaks.
- Determine the subject being discussed. This helps you understand main points.
- Ask the person to repeat or rephrase statements if necessary.
- Repeat what the person has said. Ask if your understanding is correct.
- Ask the person to write down key words or the message.
- Watch the person's lip movements.
- Watch facial expressions, gestures, and body language for clues about what is being said.

**BOX 32-3** **COMMUNICATING WITH THE HEARING-IMPAIRED PERSON**

- Gain attention. Alert the person to your presence. Raise an arm or hand, or lightly touch the person's arm. Do not startle or approach the person from behind.
- Position yourself at the person's level. If the person is sitting, you sit. If the person is standing, you stand.
- Face the person when speaking. Do not turn or walk away while you are talking. Do not talk to the person from the doorway or another room.
- Make sure the person is wearing his or her hearing aid. Make sure it is turned on and working.
- Stand or sit in good light. Shadows and glares affect the person's ability to see your face clearly.

- Make sure the person is wearing needed eyeglasses or contact lenses. This helps the person see your face for speech-reading.
- Speak clearly, distinctly, and slowly.
- Speak in a normal tone of voice. Do not shout.
- Adjust the pitch of your voice as needed. Ask the person if he or she can hear you better:
  —If the person does not wear a hearing aid, lower the pitch if you are a female. Women's voices are higher-pitched and are harder to hear than lower-pitched male voices.
  —If the person wears a hearing aid, raise the pitch slightly.

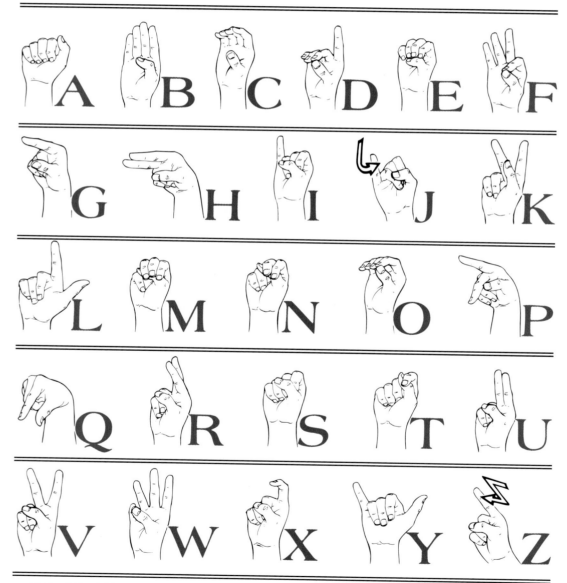

**FIG. 32-2** Manual alphabet. (Courtesy National Association of the Deaf, Silver Spring, Md.)

**BOX 32-3 COMMUNICATING WITH THE HEARING-IMPAIRED PERSON—CONT'D**

- Do not cover your mouth, smoke, eat, or chew gum while talking. Mouth movements are affected.
- Keep your hands away from your face. The person must be able to clearly see your face.
- Stand or sit on the side of the better ear.
- State the topic of conversation first.
- Tell the person when you are changing the subject. State the new subject of conversation.
- Use short sentences and simple words.
- Use gestures and facial expressions to give useful clues.
- Write out important names and words.

- Say things in another way if the person does not seem to understand.
- Keep conversations and discussions short. This avoids tiring the person.
- Repeat and rephrase statements as needed.
- Be alert to the messages sent by your facial expressions, gestures, and body language.
- Reduce or eliminate background noises. For example, turn off radios, stereos, televisions, air conditioners, and fans.

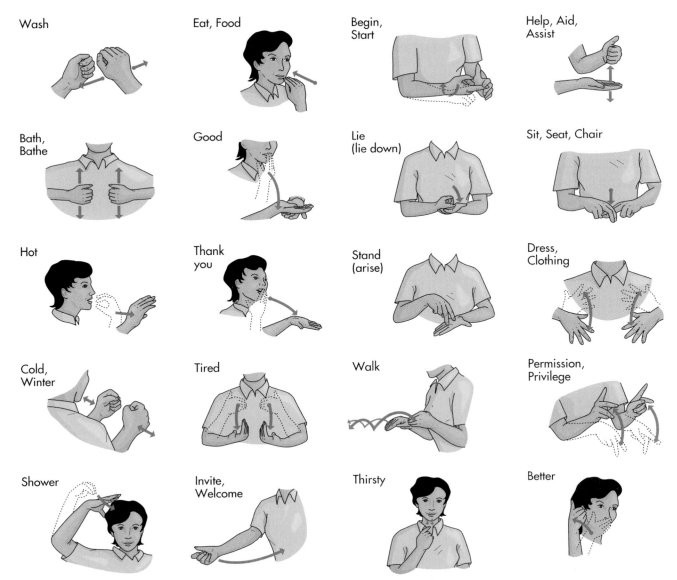

**FIG. 32-3** Sign language examples.

**HEARING AIDS.** A *hearing aid* makes sounds louder (Fig. 32-4). It does not correct or cure the hearing problem. Hearing ability does not improve. The person hears better because the device makes sounds louder. Background noise and speech are louder. The measures in Box 32-3 apply.

Sometimes hearing aids do not seem to work properly. Try these simple measures:

- Check if the hearing aid is *on*. It has an *on* and *off* switch.
- Check the battery position.
- Insert a new battery if needed.
- Clean the earmold if necessary.

Hearing aids are costly. Handle and care for them properly. Report lost or damaged hearing aids to the nurse at once. *Check with the nurse before washing a hearing aid. Also follow the manufacturer's instructions.* Remove the battery at night. When not in use, turn the hearing aid off.

# EYE DISORDERS

Vision loss occur at all ages. Problems range from mild vision loss to complete blindness. Vision loss is sudden or gradual in onset. One or both eyes are affected. See Box 32-4 for a review of the structures and functions of the eye.

## GLAUCOMA

Fluid pressure within the eye increases. This damages the optic nerve. Vision loss with eventual blindness occurs. Onset is gradual or sudden. Peripheral vision is lost. The person sees through a tunnel (Fig. 32-6). Blurred vision, halos around lights, and sensitivity to glares occur.

| BOX 32-4 | STRUCTURES AND FUNCTIONS OF THE EYE |
| --- | --- |

Receptors for vision are in the eyes. The eye is a delicate organ that is easily injured. Bones of the skull, eyelids and eyelashes, and tears protect the eyes from injury. Eye structures are shown in Figure 32-5. The eye has three layers:

- The *sclera*, the white of the eye, is the outer layer. It is made of tough connective tissue.
- The *choroid* is the second layer. Blood vessels, the *ciliary muscle*, and the *iris* make up the choroid. The iris gives the eye its color. The opening in the middle of the iris is the *pupil*. Pupil size varies with the amount of light entering the eye. The pupil constricts (narrows) in bright light and dilates (widens) in dim or dark places.
- The *retina* is the inner layer of the eye. Receptors for vision and the nerve fibers of the optic nerve are in the retina.

Light enters the eye through the *cornea*. The cornea is the transparent part of the outer layer that lies over the eye. Light rays pass to the *lens*, which lies behind the pupil. The light is then reflected to the retina and carried to the brain by the optic nerve.

The *aqueous chamber* separates the cornea from the lens. The chamber is filled with a fluid called *aqueous humor*. The fluid helps the cornea keep its shape and position. The *vitreous body* is behind the lens. The vitreous body is a gelatin-like substance that supports the retina and maintains the eye's shape.

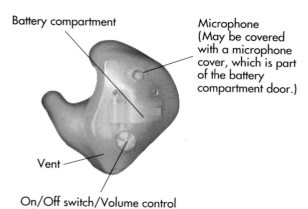

Battery compartment

Microphone (May be covered with a microphone cover, which is part of the battery compartment door.)

Vent

On/Off switch/Volume control

**FIG. 32-4** A hearing aid. (Courtesy Siemens Hearing Instruments, Piscataway, NJ.)

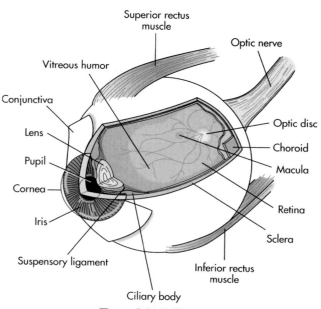

Superior rectus muscle

Optic nerve

Vitreous humor

Conjunctiva

Lens

Pupil

Cornea

Iris

Suspensory ligament

Ciliary body

Optic disc

Choroid

Macula

Retina

Sclera

Inferior rectus muscle

**FIG. 32-5** The eye.

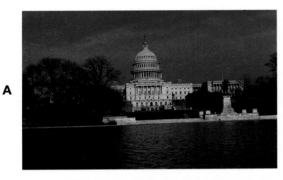

A

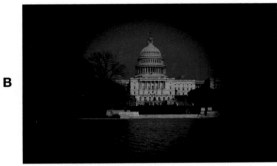

B

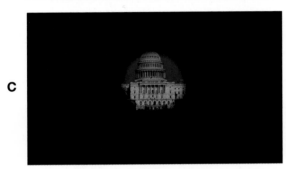

C

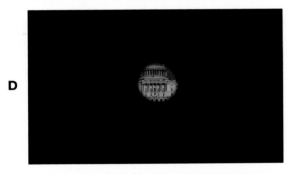

D

E

**FIG. 32-6 A,** Normal vision. **B,** Peripheral (tunnel) vision. **C, D,** and **E,** Vision loss continues, with eventual blindness.

Glaucoma is a major cause of vision loss. Persons older than 40 years are at risk. African-Americans and Asian-Americans are at greater risk than are white Americans. Other risk factors include a family history of the disease, diabetes, and past eye injuries or surgeries.

Treatment involves drug therapy and possibly surgery. The goal is to prevent further damage to the optic nerve. Prior damage cannot be reversed.

## CATARACT

The lens of the eye becomes cloudy (*opaque*). Light cannot enter the eye (Fig. 32-7). Cataract comes from the Greek word that means *waterfall*. Trying to see is like looking through a waterfall. Vision blurs and dims. Print and colors look faded. The person is sensitive to light and glares. A cataract can occur in one or both eyes. Aging is the most common cause.

Surgery is the only treatment. The lens is removed. A plastic lens is put into the eye. Vision returns to near normal. Postoperative care includes the following:

- Keep the eye shield in place as directed. Some doctors allow the shield off during the day if eyeglasses are worn. The shield is worn for sleep, including naps.
- Remind the person not to rub or press the affected eye.
- Do not bump the eye.
- Do not shower or shampoo the person without a doctor's order.
- Report eye drainage or complaints of pain at once.

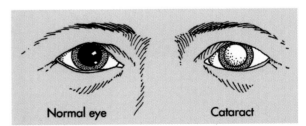

Normal eye          Cataract

**FIG. 32-7** One eye is normal. The other has a cataract. (From Phipps WJ and others: *Medical-surgical nursing: concepts and clinical practice,* ed 5, St Louis, 1995, Mosby.)

## CORRECTIVE LENSES

Eyeglasses and contact lenses can correct many vision problems. Some people wear glasses for reading or seeing at a distance. Others wear them for all activities. Contact lenses are usually worn while awake.

**EYEGLASSES.** Lenses are hardened glass or plastic. Clean them daily and as needed. Wash glass lenses with warm water. Dry them with soft tissue. Plastic lenses scratch easily. Use special cleaning solutions, tissues, and cloths.

**CONTACT LENSES.** Contact lenses fit on the eye. They are easily lost. There are hard and soft contacts. Depending on the type, contacts can be worn for 12 to 24 hours, 1 week, or longer. To remove and clean them, follow the manufacturer's instructions and agency procedures.

Report redness or eye drainage from the eyes at once. Also report complaints of eye pain or blurred vision.

---

**DELEGATION GUIDELINES:** *Eyeglasses*
When you need to clean eyeglasses, find out if a special cleaning solution is needed. Then follow the manufacturer's instructions.

---

**SAFETY ALERT:** *Eyeglasses*
Glasses are costly. Protect them from breakage or other damage. When not worn, put them in their case. Place the case in the bedside stand or in the drawer in the overbed table.

---

## CARING FOR EYEGLASSES

### QUALITY OF LIFE

Remember to:
- Knock before entering the person's room
- Address the person by name
- Introduce yourself by name and title

### PRE-PROCEDURE

1 Follow *Delegation Guidelines: Eyeglasses.* See *Safety Alert: Eyeglasses.*
2 Explain the procedure to the person.
3 Practice hand hygiene.
4 Collect the following:
   - Eyeglass case
   - Cleaning solution or warm water
   - Tissues or cloth

### PROCEDURE

5 Remove the glasses:
   a Hold the frames in front of the ear on both sides (Fig. 32-8, *A*).
   b Lift the frames from the ears. Bring the glasses down away from the face (Fig. 32-8, *B*).
6 Clean the glass with the cleaning solution or warm water. Dry the lenses with tissues.
7 Open the eyeglass case.
8 Fold the glasses. Put them in the case. Do not touch the clean lenses.
9 Place the glass case in the top drawer of the bedside stand or in the drawer of the overbed table. Or put the glasses back on the person as follows:
   a Unfold the glasses.
   b Hold the frames at each side. Place them over the ears.
   c Adjust the glasses so the nosepiece rests on the nose.
   d Return the glass case to the drawer in the bedside stand.
10 Decontaminate your hands.

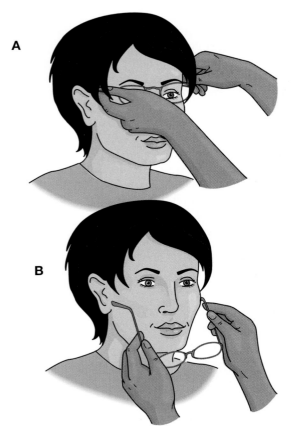

FIG. 32-8 **A,** To remove eyeglasses, hold the frames in front of the ear on both sides. **B,** Lift the frames from the ears. Bring the glasses down away from the face.

## ARTIFICIAL EYES

Removal of an eyeball is sometimes done because of injury or disease. The person is fitted with an ocular (eye) prosthesis (Fig. 32-9). It matches the other eye in color and shape. The person cannot see out of the artificial eye. The other eye may have normal or impaired vision.

Some prostheses are permanent implants. Others are removable. If the prosthesis is removable, the person is taught to remove, clean, and insert it.

The prosthesis is the person's property. Protect it from loss or damage. Follow these measures if the eye is not inserted after removal:

- Wash the eye with mild soap and warm water. Rinse well.
- Line a container with a soft cloth or 4 × 4 gauze. This prevents scratches and damage to the eye.
- Fill the container with water or a saline (salt) solution.
- Place the eye in the container. Close the container.
- Label the container with the person's name and room number.
- Place the labeled container in the bedside stand.
- Wash the eye socket with warm water or saline. Use a washcloth or gauze square. Remove excess moisture with a gauze square.
- Wash the eyelid with mild soap and warm water. Clean from the inner to outer aspect of the eye (Chapter 16). Dry the eyelid.

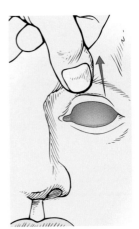
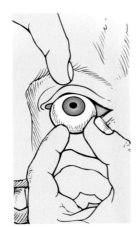
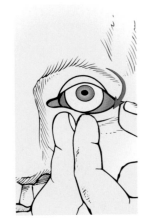

FIG. 32-9 An ocular prosthesis is inserted. (From Lewis SM, Heitkemper MM, Dirksen SR: *Medical-surgical nursing: assessment and management of clinical problems,* ed 5, St Louis, 2000, Mosby.)

## BLINDNESS

Birth defects, accidents, and eye diseases are among the many causes of blindness. It is also a complication of some diseases. The level of blindness varies. Some people are totally blind. Others sense some light but have no usable vision. Still others have some usable vision but cannot read newsprint. The legally blind person sees at 20 feet what a person with normal vision sees at 200 feet.

Loss of sight is serious. Adjustments are hard and long. Special education and training are needed. Moving about, daily activities, reading braille, and using a guide dog (seeing-eye dog) all require training.

**Braille** is a writing system that uses raised dots. Dots are arranged for each letter of the alphabet. The first 10 letters also represent 0 through 9 (Fig. 32-10). Braille is read with the fingers (Fig. 32-11). Many books, magazines, and newspapers are in braille.

Braille is hard to learn, especially for many older people. There are many audio books. They are found in bookstores and libraries.

Blind persons learn to move about using a white cane with a red tip or using a guide dog. Both are used worldwide by persons who are blind. The guide dog sees for the person. The dog is aware of danger and guides the person through traffic.

Treat the blind person with respect and dignity—not with pity. Most blind people adjust well and lead independent lives. Some were blind for a long time; others for a short time. Follow the practices in Box 32-5. *See Focus on Home Care: Blindness.*

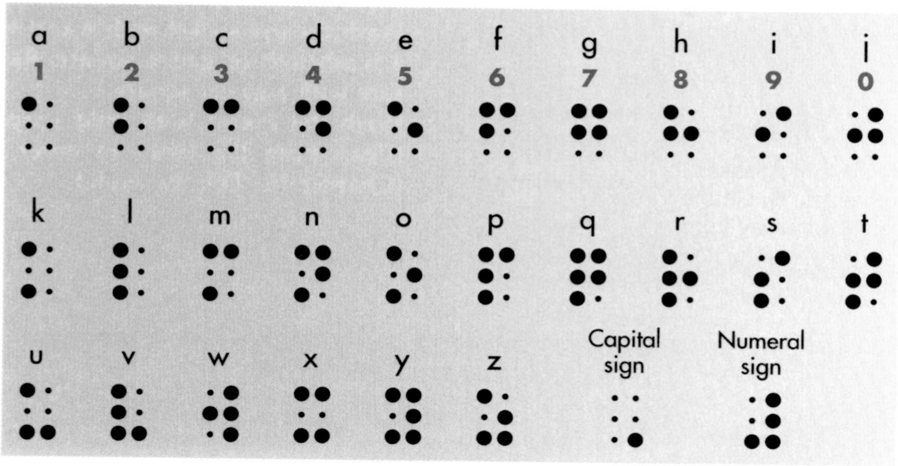

**FIG. 32-10** Braille.

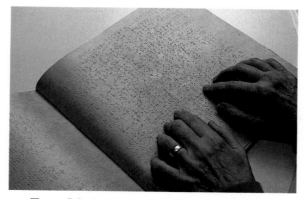

**FIG. 32-11** Braille is read with the fingers.

### FOCUS ON HOME CARE

**BLINDNESS**

The practices in Box 32-5 apply in the home setting. A safe setting is important. Outdoor walks and stairs must be free of toys, ice, and snow. Furniture, closets, drawers, shelves, and other items are arranged to meet the person's needs. Always replace items where you found them. Do not rearrange the person's belongings.

## BOX 32-5 CARING FOR THE BLIND PERSON

- Ask the person how much he or she can see. Do not assume the person is totally blind or that the person has some vision.
- Provide lighting as the person prefers. Tell the person when the lights are on or off.
- Adjust blinds and shades to prevent glares. Sunny days and bright, snowy days cause glares.
- Face the person when speaking. Speak slowly and clearly.
- Use a normal tone of voice. Do not shout or speak loudly. Blindness does not mean the person has hearing loss.
- Identify yourself. Give your name, title, and reason for being there. Do not touch the person until you have indicated your presence.
- Identify others. Explain where each person is located and what the person is doing.
- Address the person by name. This tells the person that you are directing a comment or question to him or her.
- Do not avoid using the words "see," "look," or "read."
- Orient the person to the room. Describe the layout. Also describe the location and purpose of furniture and equipment.
- Let the person move about. Let him or her touch and find furniture and equipment.
- Do not leave the person in the middle of a room. Make sure the person can reach a wall or furniture.
- Do not rearrange furniture and equipment.
- Keep doors open or shut. Never leave them partly open.
- Give step-by-step explanations of procedures as you perform them. Indicate when the procedure is over.
- Offer assistance. Simply say "May I help you?" Respect the person's answer.
- Tell the person when you are leaving the room.
- Assist the person in walking. Walk slightly ahead of him or her (Fig. 32-12). Tell the person which arm is offered. Never push, pull, or guide the person in front of you. Walk at a normal pace.
- Tell the person when you are coming to a curb or steps. State if the steps are up or down.
- Inform the person of doors, turns, furniture, and other obstructions when assisting with ambulation.
- Give specific directions. Say "right behind you," "on your left," or "in front of you." Avoid phrases like "over here" or "over there."
- Keep hallways and walkways free of carts, equipment, toys, and other items.
- Assist in food selection. Read menus to the person.
- Avoid plates, napkins, placemats, and tablecloths with patterns and designs. These items should be solid colors and provide contrast. For example, place a white plate on a dark placemat or tablecloth.
- Explain the location of food and beverages. Use the face of a clock (Chapter 20). Or guide the person's hand to each item on the tray.
- Cut meat, open containers, butter bread, and perform other similar activities if needed.
- Keep the signal light within the person's reach.
- Provide a radio, compact disks or audiotapes, audio books, television, and braille books.
- Let the person perform self-care if able.

**FIG. 32-12** The blind person walks slightly behind the nursing assistant. She touches the assistant's arm lightly.

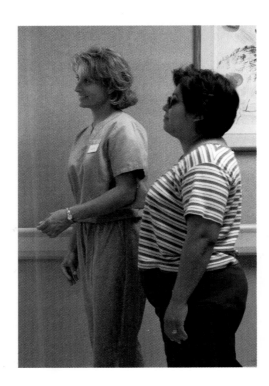

# ■ REVIEW QUESTIONS ■

Circle the **BEST** answer.

1 Mr. Percy has Meniere's disease. Which is *true?*
   a He has a middle ear infection.
   b Vertigo is a symptom.
   c Hearing aids will correct the problem.
   d He may have a speech problem.

2 Mr. Percy's care includes preventing
   a Infection
   b Falls
   c Pain
   d Deafness

3 Mr. Young has a hearing loss. He may do the following *except*
   a Avoid social events
   b Become suspicious
   c Control conversations
   d Lie down because of dizziness

4 Which is *not* an obvious effect of hearing loss?
   a Loneliness and boredom
   b Speaking too loudly
   c Asking to repeat things
   d Answering questions poorly

5 You are talking to Mr. Young. You should do the following *except*
   a Speak clearly, distinctly, and slowly
   b Sit or stand where there is good light
   c Shout
   d Stand or sit on the side of the better ear

6 You are talking to Mr. Young. You can do the following *except*
   a State the topic
   b Chew gum
   c Use short sentences and simple words
   d Write out important names and words

7 A person has a speech problem. You should do the following *except*
   a Pretend to understand so the person is not embarrassed
   b Have the person write key words
   c Ask the person to repeat or rephrase statements when necessary
   d Watch lip movements

8 Mr. Young has a hearing aid. The hearing aid
   a Corrects the hearing problem
   b Makes sounds louder
   c Makes speech clearer
   d Lowers background noise

9 Mr. Young's hearing aid does not seem to be working. First, you should
   a See if it is turned on
   b Wash it with soap and water
   c Have it repaired
   d Remove the batteries

10 Mr. Percy has a cataract. Which is *true?*
   a Surgery is the only treatment.
   b There is no cure.
   c He will become blind.
   d There is pressure in the eye.

11 Mr. Percy is not wearing his eyeglasses. They should be
   a Soaked in a cleansing solution
   b Kept within his reach
   c Put in the case and in the bedside stand
   d Placed on the overbed table

12 Braille involves
   a A white cane with a red tip for walking
   b Raised dots arranged for letters of the alphabet
   c An artificial eye
   d Audio books

13 Mrs. Hart is blind. You should do the following *except*
   a Identify yourself
   b Move equipment and furniture to provide variety
   c Explain procedures step by step
   d Have her walk behind you

14 You can provide for Mrs. Hart's safety by the following *except*
   a Keeping doors open or closed
   b Informing her of steps and curbs
   c Having her stand in the middle of the room
   d Turning on lights

*Answers to these questions are on p. 819.*

# Common Health Problems

# OBJECTIVES

- Define the key terms listed in this chapter
- Describe how cancer is treated
- Describe arthritis and the care required
- Explain how to care for persons in casts, in traction, and with hip pinnings
- Describe the care required for osteoporosis
- Describe the effects of amputation
- Describe signs and symptoms of stroke and the care required
- Describe the care needs of persons with Parkinson's disease and multiple sclerosis
- Identify the causes of head and spinal cord injuries and the care required
- Describe common respiratory disorders and the care required
- Identify the signs, symptoms, and treatment of hypertension
- List the risk factors for coronary artery disease
- Describe the care required by persons with heart disease
- Describe the care required by persons with urinary system disorders
- Identify the signs, symptoms, and complications of diabetes
- Explain the care required by persons with digestive problems
- Describe the signs and symptoms of communicable diseases and the care required

# KEY TERMS

**amputation** The removal of all or part of an extremity

**aphasia** The inability *(a)* to speak *(phasia)*

**arthritis** Joint *(arthr)* inflammation *(itis)*

**arthroplasty** The surgical replacement *(plasty)* of a joint *(arthro)*

**benign tumor** A tumor that grows slowly and within a local area

**cancer** Malignant tumor

**closed fracture** The bone is broken but the skin is intact; simple fracture

**compound fracture** Open fracture

**expressive aphasia** Difficulty expressing or sending out thoughts

**expressive-receptive aphasia** Difficulty expressing or sending out thoughts and difficulty receiving information

**fracture** A broken bone

**gangrene** A condition in which there is death of tissue

**hemiplegia** Paralysis on one side of the body

**hyperglycemia** High *(hyper)* sugar *(glyc)* in the blood *(emia)*

**hypoglycemia** Low *(hypo)* sugar *(glyc)* in the blood *(emia)*

**malignant tumor** A tumor that grows fast and invades other tissues; cancer

**metastasis** The spread of cancer to other body parts

**open fracture** The broken bone has come through the skin; compound fracture

**paraplegia** Paralysis from the waist down

**quadriplegia** Paralysis from the neck down

**receptive aphasia** Difficulty receiving information

**simple fracture** Closed fracture

**stomatitis** Inflammation *(itis)* of the mouth *(stomat)*

**tumor** A new growth of abnormal cells; tumors are benign or malignant

**ureterostomy** The surgical creation of an artificial opening *(stomy)* between the ureter *(uretero)* and the abdomen

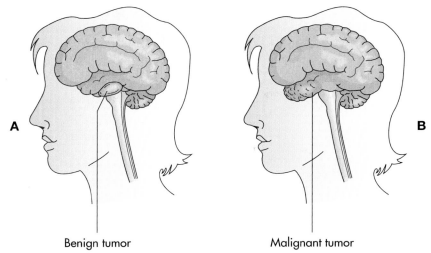

A    Benign tumor

B    Malignant tumor

FIG. 33-1 **A,** Benign tumors grow within a local area. **B,** Malignant tumors invade other tissues.

Understanding common health problems gives meaning to the required care. Refer to Chapter 7 while you study this chapter.

# CANCER

Cells reproduce for tissue growth and repair. Cells divide in an orderly way. Sometimes cell division and growth are out of control. A mass or clump of cells develops. This new growth of abnormal cells is called a **tumor.** Tumors are benign or malignant (Fig. 33-1):

- A **benign tumor** grows slowly and within a local area. It does not spread to other body parts. It usually does not cause death.
- A **malignant tumor (cancer)** grows fast. It invades other tissues (Fig. 33-2).

**Metastasis** is the spread of cancer to other body parts (Fig. 33-3, p. 674). Cancer cells break off the tumor and travel to other body parts. New tumors grow in other body parts. This occurs if the cancer is not treated and controlled.

Cancer can occur almost anywhere. The most common sites are the skin, lung, colon, rectum, breast, prostate, uterus, and urinary tract. Cancer is the second leading cause of death in the United States. It occurs in all ages.

Exact causes are unknown. The National Cancer Institute cites these risk factors:

- Tobacco—smoking tobacco, chewing tobacco and snuff, and secondhand smoke.
- Exposure to radiation—sun, sunlamps, tanning booths, x-ray procedures.
- Alcohol.
- Diet—high-fat diet, being seriously overweight.
- Chemicals and other substances—metals, pesticides, asbestos, and others.
- Diethylstilbestrol—a synthetic form of estrogen used between the early 1940s and 1971. It was given during pregnancy to prevent certain problems.
- Close relatives with certain types of cancer—melanoma and cancers of the breast, ovary, prostate, and colon.

If detected early, cancer can be treated and controlled (Box 33-1, p. 674). Treatment depends on the type of tumor, its site and size, and if it has spread. One or more of the following treatments are used.

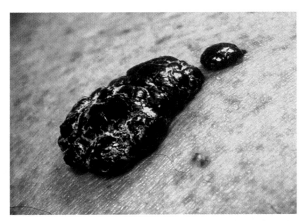

FIG. 33-2 Malignant tumor on the skin. (From Belcher AE: *Cancer nursing,* St Louis, 1992, Mosby.)

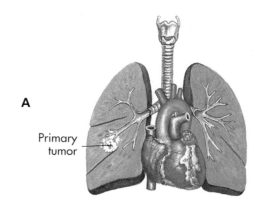

**A**

Primary
tumor

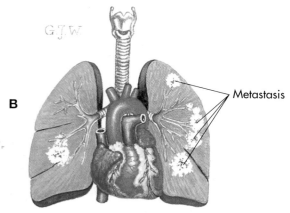

**B**

Metastasis

**FIG. 33-3 A,** Tumor in the lung. **B,** Tumor has metastasized to the other lung. (Modified from Belcher AE: *Cancer nursing*, St Louis, 1992, Mosby.)

| BOX 33-1 | SOME SIGNS AND SYMPTOMS OF CANCER |
| --- | --- |

- Thickening or lump in the breast or any other part of the body
- Obvious change in a wart or mole
- A sore that does not heal
- Nagging cough or hoarseness
- Changes in bowel or bladder habits
- Indigestion or difficulty swallowing
- Unexplained changes in weight
- Unusual bleeding or discharge

Modified from National Cancer Institute: *What you need to know about cancer: an overview*, NIH Publication No. 00-1566, modified September 16, 2002.

## SURGERY

Surgery removes tumors. It is done to cure or control cancer. It also relieves pain from advanced cancer. Some surgeries are very disfiguring. Self-esteem and body image are affected.

## RADIATION THERAPY

Radiation therapy also is called *radiotherapy.* It kills cells. X-ray beams are aimed at the tumor. Cancer cells and normal cells receive radiation. Both are destroyed. Radiation therapy:

- Destroys certain tumors.
- Shrinks a tumor before surgery.
- Destroys cancer cells that may remain in an area after surgery.
- Controls tumor growth to prevent or relieve pain.

Side effects depend on the body part treated. Burns, skin breakdown, and hair loss can occur at the treatment site. The doctor may order special skin care measures. Fatigue is common. Extra rest is needed. Discomfort, nausea and vomiting, diarrhea, and loss of appetite (*anorexia*) are other side effects.

## CHEMOTHERAPY

*Chemotherapy* involves drugs that kill cells. It is used to:

- Shrink a tumor before surgery.
- Kill cells that break off the tumor when given after surgery. The goal is to prevent metastasis.
- Relieve symptoms caused by the cancer.

Chemotherapy affects normal cells and cancer cells. Side effects depend on the drug used:

- Gastrointestinal irritation. Poor appetite, nausea, vomiting, and diarrhea result. **Stomatitis,** an inflammation (*itis*) of the mouth (*stomat),* may occur.
- Hair loss (*alopecia).*
- Decreased production of blood cells. Bleeding and infection are risks. The person may feel weak and tired.

## HORMONE THERAPY

Hormone therapy prevents cancer cells from getting or using hormones needed for their growth. Drugs are given that prevent the production of certain hormones. Organs or glands that produce a certain hormone are removed. For example, a breast cancer might need estrogen for growth. Then the ovaries are removed.

Side effects of hormone therapy include fatigue, fluid retention, weight gain, hot flashes, nausea and vomiting, appetite changes, and blood clots. Fertility is affected in men and women. Men also may experience impotence and loss of sexual desire.

## BIOLOGICAL THERAPY

Biological therapy (*immunotherapy)* helps the immune system. It helps the body fight cancer. It also protects the body from cancer treatment side effects.

Side effects include flu-like symptoms—chills, fever, muscle aches, weakness, loss of appetite, nausea, vomiting, and diarrhea. Bleeding, bruising, and swelling may occur. So can skin rashes.

## THE PERSON'S NEEDS

Persons with cancer have many needs. They include:

- Pain relief or control
- Rest and exercise
- Fluids and nutrition
- Preventing skin breakdown
- Preventing bowel problems (Constipation occurs from pain relief drugs. Diarrhea occurs from radiation therapy, chemotherapy, or biological therapy.)
- Dealing with treatment side effects
- Psychological and social needs
- Spiritual needs
- Sexual needs

Psychological and social needs are great. Anger, fear, and depression are common. Some surgeries are disfiguring. The person may feel unwhole, unattractive, or unclean. The person and family need support.

Talk to the person. Do not avoid the person because you are uncomfortable. Use touch and listening to show that you care. Often the person needs to talk and have someone listen. Being there when needed is important. You may not have to say anything. Just listen.

Spiritual needs are important. A spiritual leader may provide comfort. To many people, spiritual needs are just as important as physical needs.

Persons dying of cancer are often referred to hospice programs (Chapters 1 and 41). Support is given to the person and family.

*See Focus on Children: Cancer.*

## MUSCULOSKELETAL DISORDERS

Musculoskeletal disorders affect movement. Injury and age-related changes are common causes.

### ARTHRITIS

**Arthritis** means joint *(arth)* inflammation *(itis)*. It is the most common joint disease. Pain and decreased mobility occur in the affected joints. There are two basic types of arthritis.

**OSTEOARTHRITIS (DEGENERATIVE JOINT DISEASE).** This occurs with aging. Joint injury and obesity are other causes. Finger and thumb joints are often affected (Fig. 33-4). The disease also occurs in the hips, knees, and spine. These joints bear the body's weight.

Signs and symptoms are joint stiffness, pain, swelling, and tenderness. Joint stiffness occurs with rest and lack of motion. Pain occurs with weight-bearing and joint motion. Severe pain affects rest, sleep, and mobility. Cold weather and dampness seem to increase symptoms.

There is no cure. Treatment involves:

- *Pain relief.* Drugs decrease swelling and relieve pain. Heat applications and warm baths or showers relieve pain and stiffness. So does water therapy in a heated pool. Sometimes cold applications are used to relieve pain or numb the area.
- *Exercise.* Exercise decreases pain, increases flexibility, and improves blood flow. It helps with weight control and promotes fitness. Mental well-being improves. The person is taught what exercises to do.

---

### FOCUS ON CHILDREN
#### CANCER

Leukemia is the most common type of cancer in children. White blood cells *(leuk)* in the blood *(emia)* increase in number. Other common sites are the brain, bones, lymph nodes, nervous system, muscles, and kidneys. Warning signs of cancer in children include:

- A mass or swelling
- Paleness and fatigue
- Easy bruising
- Limping
- Bone pain
- Recurrent or persistent fever
- Morning headaches, often with vomiting
- White dot or reflex in the eye
- Weight loss

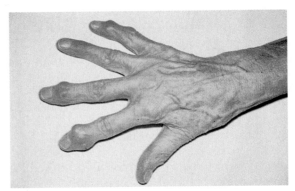

**FIG. 33-4** Bony growths called *Heberden nodes* occur in the finger joints. (From Kamal A, Brocklehurst JC: *A color atlas of geriatric medicine*, ed 2, St Louis, 1991, Mosby.)

- *Rest and joint care.* Regular rest protects the joints from overuse. Relaxation methods are helpful. Canes and walkers provide support. Splints support weak joints and keep them in alignment.
- *Weight control.* Weight loss is stressed for persons who are obese. It reduces stress on weight-bearing joints. It also helps prevent further injury.
- *Healthy life-style.* Arthritis support programs can help the person develop a good outlook. Abilities and strengths are stressed. The focus also is on fitness, exercise, rest, managing stress, and good nutrition.

The person's care plan includes measures to prevent falls. Help is given with activities of daily living (ADL) as needed. Elevated toilet seats are helpful when hip and knee motion is limited. Some people need joint replacement surgery.

**RHEUMATOID ARTHRITIS.** Rheumatoid arthritis (RA) is an inflammatory disease. It causes joint pain, swelling, and stiffness. More common in women, the onset is usually during middle age. It also occurs during the 20s and 30s.

RA occurs on both sides of the body. For example, if the right wrist is involved, so is the left wrist. The wrist and finger joints closest to the hand are commonly affected (Fig. 33-5). Neck, shoulders, elbows, hips, knees, ankles, and feet joints can be affected. Joints are tender, warm, and swollen. Fatigue and fever are common. The person may not feel well. RA symptoms can last for many years. Other body parts may be affected.

RA varies from person to person. Some people have flare-ups and then feel better. In others, the disease is active most of the time.

Treatment goals are to relieve pain, reduce inflammation, and slow down or stop joint damage. Improved well-being and function are other goals. The person's care plan may include:
- Rest balanced with exercise. More rest is needed when RA is active. More exercise is needed when it is not.
- Good body alignment.
- Positioning to prevent contractures and deformities. Bed boards, a bed cradle, trochanter rolls, and pillows are used.
- 8 to 10 hours of sleep each night. Morning and afternoon rest periods are needed.
- An exercise program. It includes range-of-motion exercises.
- Walking aids and self-help device as needed.
- Splints to support affected joints. They also reduce pain and swelling.
- Safety measures to prevent falls.
- Measures to reduce stress.

Drugs are ordered for pain relief and to reduce inflammation. Heat or local cold applications may be ordered. Some persons need joint replacement surgery.

Emotional support is needed. A good outlook is important. Persons need to stay as active as possible. The

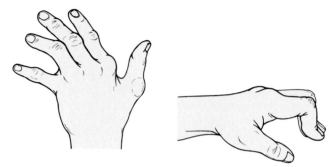

**FIG. 33-5** Deformities caused by rheumatoid arthritis. (From Lewis SM, Heitkemper MM, Dirksen SR: *Medical-surgical nursing: assessment and management of clinical problems*, ed 5, St Louis, 2000, Mosby.)

> **FOCUS ON CHILDREN**
> **RHEUMATOID ARTHRITIS**
> When RA occurs in children, it is called *juvenile rheumatoid arthritis (JRA)*. Signs and symptoms include swollen, painful, stiff joints; fever and rash; and swollen lymph nodes. JRA can affect growth and development. Eye inflammation is another complication.

more they can do for themselves, the better off they are. Give encouragement and praise. Listen when the person needs to talk.

*See Focus on Children: Rheumatoid Arthritis.*

**TOTAL JOINT REPLACEMENT.** **Arthroplasty** is the surgical replacement (*plasty*) of a joint (*arthro*). Ankle, knee, hip, shoulder, wrist, finger, and toe joints can be replaced. The diseased joint is removed. It is replaced with a prosthesis (Fig. 33-6). The surgery relieves pain and restores joint motion.

## OSTEOPOROSIS

With osteoporosis, the bone (*osteo*) becomes porous and brittle (*porosis*). Bones are fragile and break easily. Spine, hip, and wrist fractures are common.

Older persons are at risk. So are women after menopause. The ovaries do not produce estrogen after menopause. The lack of estrogen causes bone changes. So do low levels of dietary calcium.

Persons who are white or of Southeast Asian descent are at greater risk than other ethnic groups. A family history of the disease is a risk factor. So are tobacco use, alcoholism, lack of exercise, bedrest, and immobility. Exercise and activity are needed for bone strength. For bone to form properly, it must bear weight. If not, calcium is absorbed. The bone becomes porous and brittle.

Back pain, gradual loss of height, and stooped posture occur. Fractures are a major threat. Sometimes bones are so brittle that slight activity can cause a fracture. Turning in bed, getting up from a chair, or coughing can cause a fracture. Fractures are great risks from falls and accidents.

Prevention is important. The diet must contain enough calcium and vitamin D. Often doctors order calcium and vitamin supplements. Estrogen is ordered for some women. Exercise should include weight bearing (walking, jogging, stair climbing, and so on) and strength training (lifting weights). Smoking and alcohol are avoided. Caffeine is limited. Good posture is important. Some people wear back braces or corsets. Others need walking aids. Protect the person from falls and accidents (Chapter 10). Turn and reposition the person gently.

## FRACTURES

A **fracture** is a broken bone. Tissues around the fracture (muscles, blood vessels, nerves, and tendons) are injured. Fractures are open or closed (Fig. 33-7):

- **Closed fracture (simple fracture).** The bone is broken but the skin is intact.
- **Open fracture (compound fracture).** The broken bone has come through the skin.

Falls and accidents are causes. Bone tumors, metastatic cancer, and osteoporosis are other causes. Signs and symptoms of a fracture are:

- Pain and tenderness
- Swelling
- Limited movement
- Loss of function
- Deformity (the part is in an abnormal position)
- Bruising and skin color changes at the fracture site
- Bleeding (internal or external)

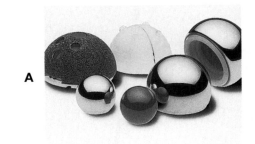
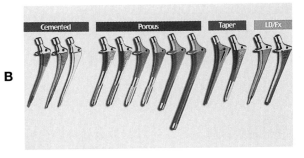
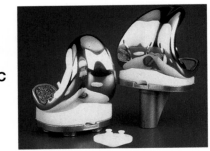

**FIG. 33-6 A,** Hip replacement prosthesis. **B,** Hip replacement prosthesis stems. **C,** Knee replacement prosthesis. (Courtesy Zimmer, Inc., a Bristol-Meyers Squibb Company, Warsaw, Ind.)

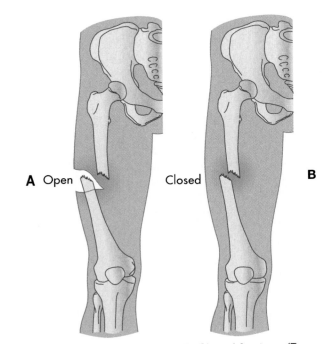

**FIG. 33-7 A,** Open fracture. **B,** Closed fracture. (From Thibodeau GA, Patton KT: *The human body in health & disease,* ed 3, St Louis, 2002, Mosby.)

For healing, bone ends are brought into normal position. This is called *reduction*:

- *Closed reduction* involves moving the bone back into place. The skin is not opened.
- *Open reduction* involves surgery. The bone is exposed and brought back into alignment. Nails, rods, pins, screws, plates, or wires keep the bone in place (Fig. 33-8).

After reduction, movement of the bone ends is prevented. This is done with a cast or traction. Other devices—splints, walking boots, external fixation devices—also are used (Fig. 33-9). *See Focus on Children: Fractures.*

**CAST CARE.** Casts are made of plaster of paris, plastic, or fiberglass (Fig. 33-10). Before casting, the part is covered with stockinette. This protects the skin. Moistened cast rolls are wrapped around the part. Plastic and fiberglass casts dry quickly. A plaster of paris cast dries in 24 to 48 hours. It is odorless, white, and shiny when dry. When wet, it is gray and cool and has a musty smell. The nurse may ask you to assist with care (Box 33-2).

*Text continued on p. 683.*

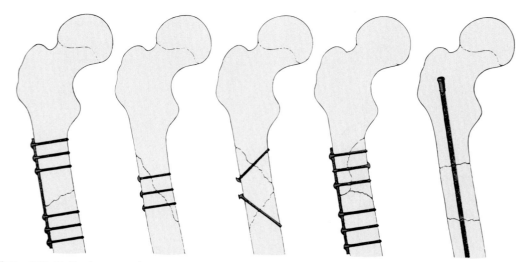

**FIG. 33-8** Devices used to reduce a fracture. (From Beare PG, Meyers JL: *Adult health nursing,* ed 3, St Louis, 1998, Mosby.)

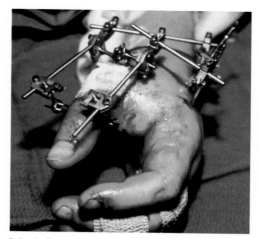

**FIG. 33-9** External fixation device. (From Lewis SM, Heitkemper MM, Dirksen SR: *Medical-surgical nursing: assessment and management of clinical problems,* ed 5, St Louis, 2000, Mosby.)

> ### FOCUS ON CHILDREN
> #### FRACTURES
> Falls and accidents involving motor vehicles, bicycles, skate boards, and roller blades are common causes of fractures in children. Fractures in infants may be a sign of child abuse.

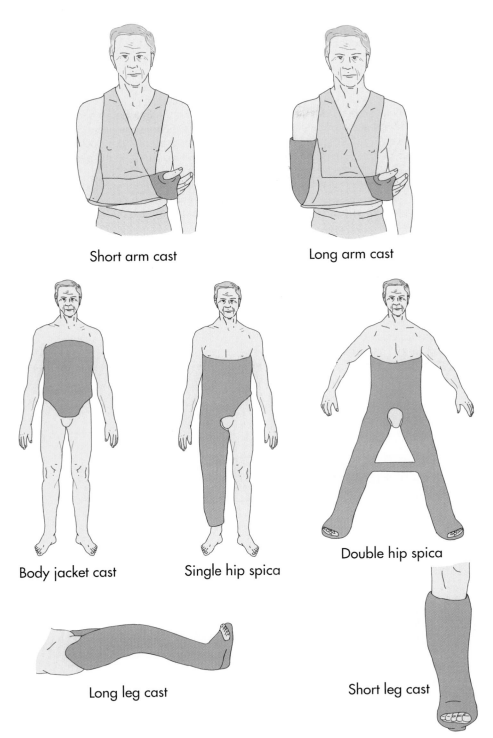

Short arm cast

Long arm cast

Body jacket cast

Single hip spica

Double hip spica

Long leg cast

Short leg cast

**FIG. 33-10** Common casts.

## BOX 33-2 RULES FOR CAST CARE

- Do not cover the cast with blankets, plastic, or other material. A plaster cast gives off heat as it dries. Covers prevent the escape of heat. Burns can occur if the heat cannot escape.
- Turn the person every 2 hours. All cast surfaces are exposed to the air at one time or another. Turning promotes even drying.
- Do not place a wet cast on a hard surface. It flattens the cast. The cast must keep its shape. Use pillows to support the entire length of the cast (Fig. 33-11).
- Support a wet cast with your palms when turning and positioning the person (Fig. 33-12). Fingertips can dent the cast. The dents can cause pressure areas that can lead to skin breakdown.
- Protect the person from rough cast edges. Petaling involves covering the cast edges with tape (Fig. 33-13).
- Keep the cast dry. A wet cast loses its shape. Some casts are near the perineal area. The nurse may apply a waterproof material around the perineal area after the cast dries.
- Do not let the person insert anything into the cast. Itching under the cast causes an intense desire to scratch. Items used for scratching (pencils, coat hangers, knitting needles, back scratchers) can open the skin. An infection can develop. Scratching items can wrinkle the stock-

inette or be lost into the cast. Both can cause pressure and lead to skin breakdown.
- Elevate a casted arm or leg on pillows. This reduces swelling.
- Have enough help when turning and repositioning the person. Plaster casts are heavy and awkward. Balance is lost easily.
- Position the person as directed.
- Report these signs and symptoms at once:
  —Pain: pressure ulcer, poor circulation, or nerve damage
  —Swelling and a tight cast: reduced blood flow to the part
  —Pale skin: reduced blood flow to the part
  —Cyanosis: reduced blood flow to the part
  —Odor: infection
  —Inability to move the fingers or toes: pressure on a nerve
  —Numbness: pressure on a nerve or reduced blood flow to the part
  —Temperature changes: cool skin means poor circulation; hot skin means inflammation
  —Drainage on or under the cast: infection
  —Chills, fever, nausea, and vomiting: infection

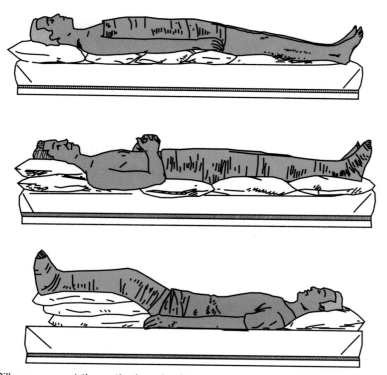

**FIG. 33-11** Pillows support the entire length of the wet cast. (From Harkness GA, Dincher JR: *Medical-surgical nursing: total patient care,* ed 10, St Louis, 1999, Mosby.)

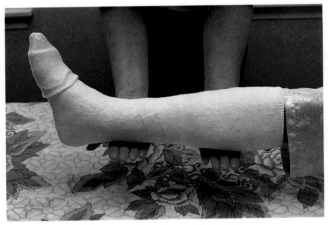

**FIG. 33-12** The cast is supported with the palms during lifting.

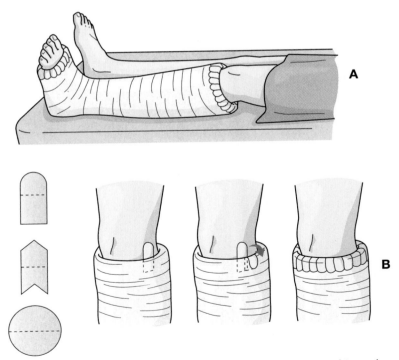

**FIG. 33-13 A,** The edges of the cast are petaled. **B,** Pieces of tape are used to make petals. The petal is placed inside the cast and then brought over the edge.

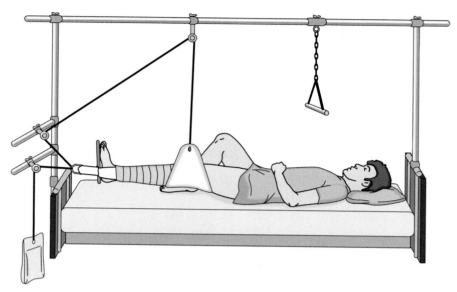

**FIG. 33-14** Traction set-up. Note the weights, pulleys, and ropes. (From Phipps WJ and others: *Medical-surgical nursing: health and illness perspectives,* ed 7, St Louis, 2003, Mosby.)

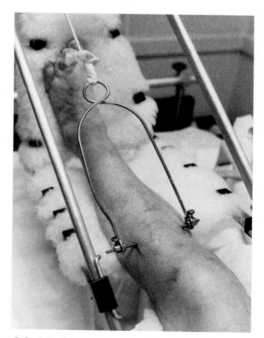

**FIG. 33-15** Skeletal traction is attached to the bone. (From Christensen BL, Kockrow EO: *Adult health nursing,* ed 4, St Louis, 2003, Mosby.)

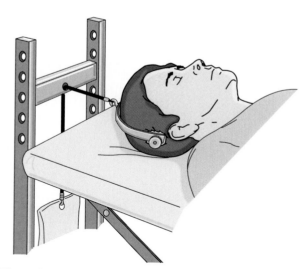

**FIG. 33-16** Tongs are inserted into the skull for cervical spine traction. (From Phipps WJ and others: *Medical-surgical nursing: health and illness perspectives,* ed 7, St Louis, 2003, Mosby.)

**TRACTION.** Traction reduces and immobilizes fractures. A steady pull from two directions keeps the bone in place. Traction is also used for muscle spasms, to correct or prevent deformities, and to relieve pressure on a nerve. Weights, ropes, and pulleys are used (Fig. 33-14). Traction is applied to the neck, arms, legs, or pelvis.

*Skin traction* is applied to the skin. Tape, a boot, or a splint is used. Weights are attached to the device (see Fig. 33-14). *Skeletal traction* is applied directly to the bone. Wires or pins are inserted through the bone (Fig. 33-15). For cervical traction, tongs are applied to the skull (Fig. 33-16). Weights are attached to the device.

The nurse may ask you to assist with the person's care (Box 33-3).

**HIP FRACTURES.** Fractured hips are common in older persons (Fig. 33-17). Older women are at risk. Healing is slower in older people. Slow healing and other health problems affect the person's condition and care. Postoperative problems present life-threatening risks. They include pneumonia, atelectasis, urinary tract infections, and thrombi in the leg veins. Pressure ulcers, constipation, and confusion are other risks.

The fracture is fixed in position with a pin, nail, plate, screw, or prosthesis (Fig. 33-18, p. 684). Some persons need rehabilitation after surgery. Box 33-4, p. 684, describes the care required. *See Focus on Home Care: Hip Fractures. See Focus on Long-Term Care: Hip Fractures.*

---

**BOX 33-3  CARING FOR PERSONS IN TRACTION**

- Keep the person in good body alignment.
- Do not remove the traction.
- Keep weights off the floor. Weights must hang freely from the traction setup (Fig. 33-14).
- Do not add or remove weights from the traction setup.
- Perform range-of-motion exercises for the uninvolved body parts as directed.
- Position the person as directed. Usually only the back-lying position is allowed. Sometimes slight turning is allowed.
- Provide the fracture pan for elimination.
- Give skin care as directed.
- Put bottom linens on the bed from the top down. The person uses the trapeze to raise the body off the bed.
- Check pin, nail, wire, or tong sites for redness, drainage, or odors. Report any observations to the nurse at once.
- Observe for the signs and symptoms listed under cast care (Box 33-2). Report these observations to the nurse at once.

---

**FOCUS ON LONG-TERM CARE**
**HIP FRACTURES**

Older persons often require rehabilitation after a hip fracture. If home care is not possible, the person requires subacute or long-term care. The person usually returns home after successful rehabilitation. Adduction, internal rotation, and severe hip flexion are avoided.

---

**FOCUS ON HOME CARE**
**HIP FRACTURES**

The prosthesis can dislocate (move out of place) with adduction, internal rotation (turning inward), and severe hip flexion. The person avoids the following for 6 to 8 weeks after surgery:

- Lying on the affected side
- Sitting in low seats
- Sitting with the legs crossed
- Bending from the waist
- Bending to put on shoes and socks or stockings

An occupational therapist helps the person learn self-care activities. Assistive devices are used for dressing (Chapter 31). A raised toilet seat is needed for elimination. A shower chair is needed for bathing. The person uses a pillow or abductor splint between the legs when in bed.

A physical therapist helps the person learn muscle-strengthening exercises. A walker is usually needed for ambulation.

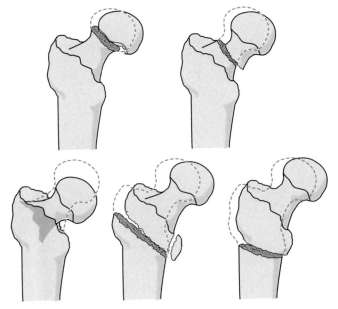

**FIG. 33-17** Hip fractures. (From Phipps WJ and others: *Medical-surgical nursing: health and illness perspectives,* ed 7, St Louis, 2003, Mosby.)

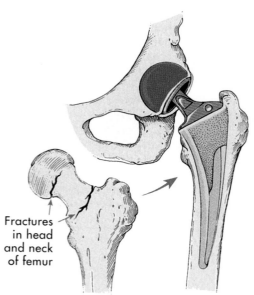

**FIG. 33-18** Hip fracture repaired with a prosthesis. (Modified from Christensen BL, Kockrow EO: *Adult health nursing,* ed 4, St Louis, 2003, Mosby.)

Fractures in head and neck of femur

---

**BOX 33-4   CARE OF THE PERSON WITH A HIP FRACTURE**

- Give good skin care. Skin breakdown can occur rapidly.
- Encourage incentive spirometry and coughing and deep-breathing exercises as directed. See Chapter 30.
- Turn and reposition the person as directed. Turning and positioning depend on the type of fracture and the surgery performed. Usually the person is not positioned on the operative side.
- Keep the operated leg abducted at all times. The leg is abducted when the person is supine, being turned, or in a side-lying position. Use pillows (Fig. 33-19) or abductor splints as directed (Chapter 22).
- Prevent external rotation of the hip (turning outward). Use trochanter rolls, pillows, sandbags, or abductor splints as directed.
- Perform range-of-motion exercises as directed (Chapter 22). Do not exercise the affected leg.
- Provide a straight-back chair with armrests. The person needs a high, firm seat. A low, soft chair is not used.
- Place the chair on the unaffected side.
- Assist the nurse in transferring the person.
- Do not let the person stand on the operated leg unless allowed by the doctor.
- Support and elevate the leg as directed when the person is in the chair.
- Apply elastic stockings as directed (Chapter 27).
- Remind the person not to cross his or her legs.

---

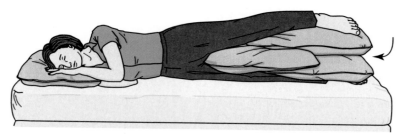

**FIG. 33-19** Pillows are used to keep the hip in abduction. (From Phipps WJ and others: *Medical-surgical nursing: health and illness perspectives,* ed 7, St Louis, 2003, Mosby.)

## LOSS OF A LIMB

An **amputation** is the removal of all or part of an extremity. Severe injuries, tumors, severe infection, and circulatory disorders are common causes. So is gangrene.

**Gangrene** is a condition in which there is death of tissue. Causes include infection, injuries, and circulatory disorders. These conditions affect blood flow. The tissues do not get enough oxygen and nutrients. Poisonous substances and waste products build up in the tissues. Tissue death results. Tissues become black, cold, and shriveled (Fig. 33-20). Surgery is needed to remove dead tissue. If untreated, gangrene spreads through the body. It can cause death.

Much support is needed. The amputation affects the person's life. Appearance, daily activities, moving about, and work are some areas affected.

The person is fitted with a prosthesis—an artificial replacement for a missing body part (Fig. 33-21). The stump is conditioned so the prosthesis fits. This involves shrinking and shaping the stump into a cone shape (Fig. 33-22). The person learns exercises to strengthen other limbs. Occupational and physical therapists help the person use the prosthesis.

The person may feel that the limb is still there. Or the person may complain of pain in the amputated part. This is called *phantom limb pain.* This is a normal reaction. It may occur for a short time after surgery. Some persons have phantom limb pain for many years.

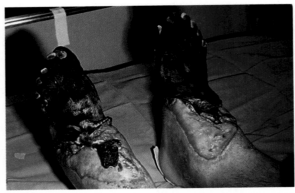

**FIG. 33-20** Gangrene. (Courtesy Cameron Bangs, MD. From Auerbach PS: *Wilderness medicine: management of wilderness and environmental emergencies,* ed 3, St Louis, 1995, Mosby.)

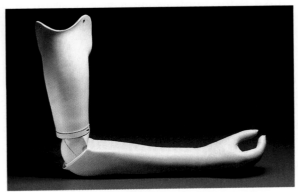

**FIG. 33-21** Arm prosthesis. (Courtesy Motion Control, Subsidiary of Fillauer, Salt Lake City, Utah.)

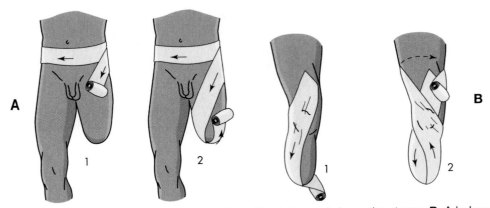

**FIG. 33-22 A,** A midthigh amputation is bandaged to shrink and shape the stump. **B,** A below-the-knee amputation is bandaged to shrink and shape the stump. (From Phipps WJ and others: *Medical-surgical nursing: health and illness perspectives,* ed 7, St Louis, 2003, Mosby.)

# NERVOUS SYSTEM DISORDERS

Nervous system disorders can affect mental and physical functions. They can affect the ability to speak, understand, feel, see, hear, touch, think, control bowels and bladder, or move.

## STROKE

Stroke is a disease affecting the blood vessels that supply blood to the brain. It also is called a *cerebrovascular accident (CVA)*. The main causes are:
- *A ruptured blood vessel.* Bleeding occurs in the brain.
- *Blood clots.* A blood clot blocks blood flow to the brain.

Brain cells in the area affected do not get oxygen and nutrients. Brain cells die. Brain damage occurs. Functions controlled by that part of the brain are lost or impaired.

Stroke is the third leading cause of death in the United States. It is the leading cause of disability in adults. See Box 33-5 for warning signs. The person needs emergency care.

Sometimes warning signs last a few minutes. This is called a *transient ischemic attack (TIA)*. (*Transient* means temporary or short term. *Ischemic* means to hold back [ischein] blood [hemic].) Blood supply to the brain is interrupted for a short time. Sometimes a TIA occurs before a stroke. Medical care is needed.

Stroke occurs in all age-groups. Risk factors are:
- Age—older persons are at greater risk than younger persons
- Gender—men are at higher risk than women
- African-American descent—this ethnic group is at greater risk than other ethnic groups
- Hypertension (high blood pressure)
- A family history of stroke
- Cardiovascular disease
- Smoking
- Diabetes
- High blood cholesterol
- Inactivity
- Obesity
- Excessive alcohol use
- Drug abuse

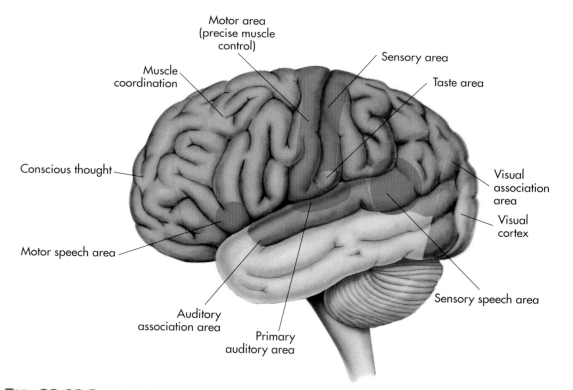

**FIG. 33-23** Functions lost from a stroke depend on the area of brain damage. (From Thibodeau GA, Patton KT: *The human body in health & disease,* ed 3, St Louis, 2002, Mosby.)

Stroke can occur suddenly. Warning signs may occur (see Box 33-5). The person may have nausea, vomiting, and memory loss. Unconsciousness, noisy breathing, high blood pressure, slow pulse, redness of the face, and seizures may occur. So can paralysis on one side of the body **(hemiplegia)**. The person may lose bowel and bladder control and the ability to speak. **Aphasia** is the inability *(a)* to speak *(phasia)*.

If the person survives, some brain damage is likely. Functions lost depend on the area of brain damage (Fig. 33-23). The effects of a stroke include:
- Loss of face, hand, arm, leg, or body control
- Hemiplegia
- Changing emotions (crying easily or mood swings, sometimes for no reason)
- Difficulty swallowing (dysphagia)
- Dimmed vision
- Aphasia
- Slow or slurred speech
- Changes in sight, touch, movement, and thought
- Impaired memory
- Urinary frequency, urgency, or incontinence
- Depression
- Frustration

Behavior changes occur. The person may forget about or ignore the weaker side. This is called *neglect*. It is from loss of vision or movement and feeling on that side. Sometimes thinking is affected. The person may not recognize or know how to use common items. ADL and other tasks are hard to do. The person may forget what to do and how to do it. If the person does know, the body may not respond.

Rehabilitation starts at once. The person may depend in part or totally on others for care. The health team helps the person regain the highest possible level of function (Box 33-6).

**APHASIA.** There are two basic types of aphasia. **Expressive aphasia** is difficulty expressing or sending out thoughts. Thinking is clear. There are problems speaking, spelling, counting, gesturing, or writing. The person thinks one thing but says another. For example, the person thinks about food but asks for a book. People are called the wrong names even when names are known. Some people produce sounds and no words. The person may cry or swear for no reason.

**Receptive aphasia** relates to difficulty receiving information. The person has trouble understanding what is said or read. People and common objects are not recognized. The person may not know how to use a fork, toilet, cup, TV, phone, or other items.

With *receptive* aphasia, messages are not interpreted. With *expressive* aphasia, messages are not sent. Some people have both types. This is called **expressive-receptive aphasia.**

The person has many emotional needs. Frustration, depression, and anger are common. Communication is needed to function and relate to others. The person wants to communicate but cannot. You need to be patient and kind.

*See Focus on Home Care: Stroke. See Focus on Long-Term Care: Stroke.*

---

| BOX 33-6 | CARE OF THE PERSON WITH A STROKE |
|---|---|

- The lateral position prevents aspiration.
- Coughing and deep breathing are encouraged.
- The bed is kept in semi-Fowler's position.
- Turning and repositioning are done at least every 2 hours.
- Food and fluid needs are met.
- Elastic stockings prevent thrombi (blood clots) in the legs.
- Range-of-motion exercises prevent contractures.
- A catheter is inserted, or a bladder training program is started.
- A bowel training program may be needed.
- Safety precautions are practiced. Use bed rails according to the care plan.
- Keep the signal light within reach. It is on the person's unaffected side. If unable to use the signal light, check the person often.
- The person does as much self-care as possible. Assist as needed.
- Communication methods are established. Magic Slates, pencil and paper, a picture board, or other methods are used. Limit questions to those that have "yes" or "no" answers. Speak slowly. Allow the person time to respond (Chapter 6).
- Good skin care prevents pressure ulcers.
- Speech, physical, and occupational therapies are ordered.
- Assistive devices are used as needed (Chapter 31).
- Support, encouragement, and praise are given.

---

### FOCUS ON HOME CARE
#### STROKE

Many stroke survivors return home. A partner or family members assist with the person's care. Home care is often needed. The care measures in Box 33-6 continue in the home. The nurse and therapists also recommend changes in the home setting to help the person function.

---

### FOCUS ON LONG-TERM CARE
#### STROKE

Some stroke survivors need subacute or long-term care. Some persons return home after rehabilitation. Long-term care is often permanent for those who totally depend on others for care. Many measures listed in Box 33-6 are part of the person's care.

## PARKINSON'S DISEASE

Parkinson's disease is a slow, progressive disorder with no cure. Degeneration of a part of the brain occurs. Persons older than 50 years are at risk. Signs and symptoms become worse over time (Fig. 33-24). They include:

- *Tremors*—often start in one finger and spread to the whole arm. Pill-rolling movements (rubbing of the thumb and index finger) may occur.
- *Stiff muscles*—in the arms, legs, neck, and trunk.
- *Slow movement*—the person has a slow, shuffling gait.
- *Stooped posture and impaired balance*—it is hard to walk. Falls are a risk.
- *Mask-like expression*—the person cannot blink and smile. A fixed stare is common.

Other signs and symptoms develop over time. They include swallowing and chewing problems, constipation, and bladder problems. Sleep problems and depression can occur. So can memory loss, slow thinking, and emotional changes (fear and insecurity). Speech changes occur. They include slurred, monotone, and soft speech. Some people talk too fast or repeat what they say.

The doctor orders drugs for Parkinson's disease. Exercise and physical therapy are ordered to improve strength, posture, balance, and mobility. Therapy is needed for speech and swallowing problems. The person may need help with eating and self-care. Normal elimination is a goal. Safety measures prevent injury. The person is treated with dignity and respect.

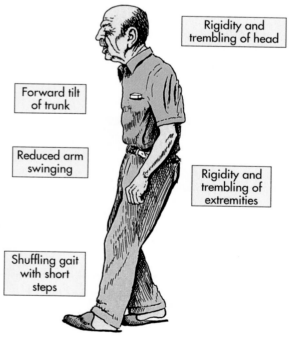

Rigidity and trembling of head

Forward tilt of trunk

Reduced arm swinging

Rigidity and trembling of extremities

Shuffling gait with short steps

**FIG. 33-24** Signs of Parkinson's disease. (From Thibodeau GA, Patton KT: *The human body in health & disease*, ed 3, St Louis, 2002, Mosby.)

## MULTIPLE SCLEROSIS

Multiple sclerosis (MS) is a chronic disease. *Multiple* means many. *Sclerosis* means hardening or scarring. The myelin (which covers nerve fibers) in the brain and spinal cord is destroyed. Nerve impulses are not sent to and from the brain in a normal manner. Functions are impaired or lost. There is no cure.

Symptoms usually start between the ages of 20 and 40 years. Women are affected more often than are men. Whites are at greater risk than other groups.

MS can present as follows:

- *Benign form.* Little or no symptom progress after the first attack.
- *Relapsing-remitting.* The person has a series of attacks. Then symptoms lessen or disappear (remission). At some point, there are flare-ups (relapses). With each flare-up, more symptoms can occur.
- *Primary progressive.* The person's condition gradually declines. There are no remissions.
- *Secondary progressive.* The person has flare-ups and remissions. After many years, the person's condition declines.
- *Progressive-relapsing.* The person's condition gradually declines. Acute attacks occur. They leave new symptoms and more damage.
- *Malignant MS.* Decline is rapid. Severe disability or death occurs shortly after onset.

Symptoms depend on the damaged area. Vision problems may occur. Muscle weakness and balance problems affect standing and walking. Paralysis can occur. Tremors, numbness and tingling, loss of feeling, speech problems, dizziness, and poor coordination are common. Problems with concentration, attention, memory, judgment, and behavior may occur. Fatigue increases such problems. Bowel, bladder, and sexual function problems occur. Respiratory muscle weakness is common. So are anger and depression.

Persons with MS are kept active as long as possible. They need to do as much self-care as possible. The care plan reflects the person's changing needs. Skin care, hygiene, and range-of-motion exercises are important. So are turning, positioning, coughing, and deep breathing. Injuries are prevented. So are complications from bedrest. Bowel and bladder elimination is promoted. *See Focus on Home Care: Multiple Sclerosis.*

### FOCUS ON HOME CARE
#### MULTIPLE SCLEROSIS

The person may need help with housekeeping to avoid fatigue. As mobility decreases, the person depends more on others. Occupational and physical therapists are often involved in the person's care. The National Multiple Sclerosis Society can provide resources for the person and family.

## HEAD INJURIES

Injuries can involve the scalp, skull, and brain tissue. Some injuries are minor. They cause temporary loss of consciousness. Others are more serious. Brain tissue is bruised or torn. Bleeding can occur in the brain or nearby structures. Permanent brain damage or death may result.

Causes include falls, accidents, and sports injuries. Often there are other injuries. Spinal cord injuries are likely. If the person survives, some permanent damage is likely. Paralysis, mental retardation, and personality changes may be permanent. The same is true for speech, breathing, bowel, and bladder problems.

Rehabilitation is required. Nursing care depends on the person's needs and remaining abilities. *See Focus on Children: Head Injuries.*

## SPINAL CORD INJURIES

Spinal cord injuries can permanently damage the nervous system. Common causes are stab or bullet wounds, accidents, falls, and sports injuries. Cervical traction is often needed (see Fig. 33-16). The person in cervical traction has a special bed. It keeps the spine straight at all times.

Problems depend on the level of injury. The higher the level of injury, the more functions lost (Fig. 33-25). With lumbar injuries, leg function is lost. Injuries at the thoracic level cause loss of muscle function below the chest. Injuries at the lumbar or thoracic levels cause paraplegia. **Paraplegia** is paralysis from the waist down. Cervical injuries cause loss of function to the arms, chest, and below the chest. **Quadriplegia** is paralysis from the neck down.

If the person survives, rehabilitation is necessary. Care measures are listed in Box 33-7, p. 690. Emotional needs require attention. Reactions to paralysis and loss of function are often severe.

*See Focus on Long-Term Care: Spinal Cord Injuries, p. 690. See Focus on Home Care: Spinal Cord Injuries, p. 690.*

### FOCUS ON CHILDREN
#### HEAD INJURIES

Birth injuries are a major cause of head trauma in newborns. As children grow older, motor vehicle accidents, wheel-related sports (bikes, scooters, skates, skateboards), and falls are the major causes of traumatic brain injury (TBI).

Falls are a great danger for infants and toddlers. Falling down stairs and from windows are common accidents. See Chapter 10 for safety practices to prevent falls.

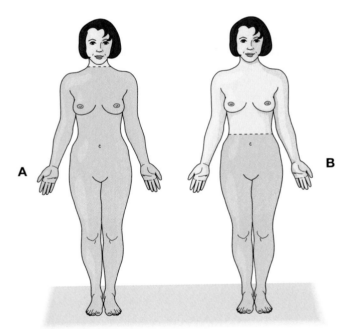

**FIG. 33-25** The *shaded areas* show the areas of paralysis. **A,** Quadriplegia. **B,** Paraplegia.

- Prevent falls. Follow the care plan for safety measures and bed rail use.
- Keep the bed in the low position.
- Keep the signal light within reach. If unable to use the signal light, check the person often.
- Prevent burns. Check bath water, heat applications, and food for proper temperature.
- Turn and reposition at least every 2 hours.
- Prevent pressure ulcers. Follow the care plan.
- Maintain good alignment at all times. Use supportive devices according to the care plan.
- Follow bowel and bladder training programs.
- Maintain muscle function, and prevent contractures. Assist with range-of-motion and other exercises as directed.
- Assist with food and fluids as needed. Provide self-help devices as ordered.
- Give emotional and psychological support.
- Follow the person's rehabilitation plan.

**FOCUS ON LONG-TERM CARE**
**SPINAL CORD INJURIES**

Some rehabilitation centers focus on spinal cord injuries. The person learns to function at the highest possible level. He or she learns to use self-help, assistive, and other devices. The person needs the care listed in Box 33-7.

**FOCUS ON HOME CARE**
**SPINAL CORD INJURIES**

Rehabilitation continues when the person goes home. The RN, physical therapist, and occupational therapist suggest changes in the home to meet the person's needs. Ramps for wheelchair use usually are needed. So are changes in the kitchen, bathroom, and bedroom. For example, the refrigerator door may need to open from the other side. Shelves may need rearranging. A raised toilet seat, grab bars by the toilet and tub, bathtub seats, and transfer boards may help the person. The person may need a hospital bed, trapeze, and bedside commode. Furniture in all rooms is arranged for wheelchair access.

The person may need help with activities of daily living and housekeeping. Follow the nurse's directions and the care plan.

# RESPIRATORY DISORDERS

The respiratory system brings oxygen ($O_2$) into the lungs and removes carbon dioxide ($CO_2$) from the body. Respiratory disorders interfere with this function and threaten life.

## CHRONIC OBSTRUCTIVE PULMONARY DISEASE

Three disorders are grouped under chronic obstructive pulmonary disease (COPD). They are chronic bronchitis, emphysema, and asthma. These disorders interfere with the exchange of $O_2$ and $CO_2$ in the lungs. They obstruct airflow.

**CHRONIC BRONCHITIS.** Chronic bronchitis occurs after repeated episodes of bronchitis. Bronchitis means inflammation (*itis*) of the bronchi (*bronch*). Smoking is the major cause. Infection, air pollution, and industrial dusts are other causes.

*Smoker's cough* in the morning is often the first symptom. At first the cough is dry. Over time, the person coughs up mucus. Mucus may contain pus. The cough becomes more frequent. The person has difficulty breathing and tires easily. Mucus and inflamed breathing passages obstruct airflow into the lungs. The body cannot get normal amounts of oxygen.

The person must stop smoking. Oxygen therapy and breathing exercises are often ordered. Respiratory tract infections are prevented. If one occurs, prompt treatment is needed.

**EMPHYSEMA.** In emphysema, the alveoli enlarge. They become less elastic. They do not expand and shrink normally with breathing in and out. As a result, some air is trapped in the alveoli when exhaling. Trapped air is not exhaled. Over time, more alveoli are involved. Therefore more air is trapped. $O_2$ and $CO_2$ exchange cannot occur in affected alveoli.

Smoking is the most common cause. The person has shortness of breath and a cough. At first, shortness of breath occurs with exertion. Over time, it occurs at rest. Sputum may contain pus. As more air is trapped in the lungs, the person develops a *barrel chest* (Fig. 33-26). Breathing is easier when the person sits upright and slightly forward (Chapter 30).

The person must stop smoking. Respiratory therapy, breathing exercises, oxygen, and drug therapy are ordered.

**ASTHMA.** The airway narrows with asthma. Dyspnea results. Asthma is triggered by allergies and emotional stress. Smoking, respiratory infections, exertion, and cold air are other triggers. Symptoms are mild to severe. Wheezing and coughing are common.

Sudden attacks *(asthma attacks)* can occur. There is shortness of breath, wheezing, coughing, rapid pulse, sweating, and cyanosis. The person gasps for air and is very frightened. Fear makes the attack worse.

Asthma is treated with drugs. Severe attacks may require emergency room treatment. The person and family are taught how to prevent asthma attacks. Repeated attacks can damage the respiratory system.

## PNEUMONIA

Pneumonia is an inflammation and infection of lung tissue. Affected tissues fill with fluid. $O_2$ and $CO_2$ exchange is affected.

Bacteria, viruses, aspiration, and immobility are causes. The person is very ill. Fever, chills, painful cough, chest pain on breathing, and a rapid pulse occur. Cyanosis may be present. Sputum is thick and green, yellowish, or rust colored. The color depends on the cause.

Drugs are ordered for infection and pain. Fluid intake is increased because of fever. Fluids also thin mucous secretions. Thin secretions are easier to cough up. IV fluids and oxygen may be needed. The person needs plenty of rest. The semi-Fowler's position eases breathing. Standard Precautions are followed. Transmission-Based Precautions are used depending on the cause. Mouth care is important. Frequent linen changes are needed because of fever. *See Focus on Children: Pneumonia. See Focus on Older Persons: Pneumonia.*

> ### FOCUS ON CHILDREN
> #### PNEUMONIA
> Pneumonia occurs in children of all ages. It is more common in infants and toddlers.

> ### FOCUS ON OLDER PERSONS
> #### PNEUMONIA
> Changes from aging, diseases, and decreased mobility increase the risk of pneumonia in older persons. Decreased mobility after surgery also is a risk factor. Drugs and other diseases can mask signs and symptoms of pneumonia. Pneumonia can lead to death.
>
> Aspiration pneumonia is common in older persons. Dysphagia, decreased cough and gag reflexes, and nervous system disorders are risk factors. So are substances that depress the brain—narcotics, sedatives, alcohol, and drugs for general anesthesia.

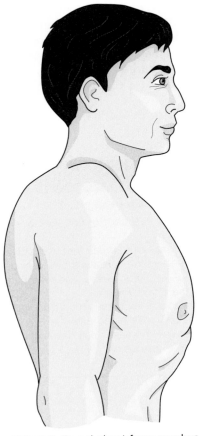

**FIG. 33-26** Barrel chest from emphysema.

## TUBERCULOSIS

Tuberculosis (TB) is a bacterial infection. It affects the lungs. It also can occur in the kidneys and bones. If TB is untreated, death can occur. TB drug therapy was introduced in the 1940s. The number of cases declined after that. The number began to increase in the late 1980s.

TB is spread by airborne droplets with coughing, sneezing, speaking, and singing (Chapter 12). Nearby persons can inhale the bacteria. Those who have close, frequent contact with an infected person are at risk. TB is more likely to occur in close, crowded areas. Age, poor nutrition, and HIV infection are other risk factors.

An active infection may not occur for many years. Chest x-ray and TB testing can detect the disease. Signs and symptoms are tiredness, loss of appetite, weight loss, fever, and night sweats. Coughing occurs. The cough is more frequent over time. Sputum production also increases. Chest pain occurs.

Drugs for TB are given. The mouth and nose are covered with tissues when coughing or sneezing. Tissues are flushed down the toilet. Or they are placed in a paper bag and burned. In health care agencies, tissues are placed in a biohazard bag. Hand washing after contact with sputum is essential. Standard Precautions and Airborne Precautions are practiced.

# CARDIOVASCULAR DISORDERS

Cardiovascular disorders are the leading causes of death in the United States. Problems occur in the heart or blood vessels.

## HYPERTENSION

With hypertension *(high blood pressure)*, the resting blood pressure is too high. The systolic pressure is 140 mm Hg or higher. Or the diastolic pressure is 90 mm Hg or higher. Such measurements must occur two or more times. *Prehypertension* occurs when the systolic pressure is between 120 and 139 mm Hg or the diastolic pressure is between 80 and 89 mm Hg. See Box 33-8 for risk factors.

Narrowed blood vessels are a common cause. When vessels narrow, the heart pumps with more force to move blood through the vessels. Kidney disorders, head injuries, some pregnancy problems, and adrenal gland tumors are other causes.

Hypertension can damage other organs. It can lead to stroke, heart attack, heart failure, kidney failure, and blindness.

Usually hypertension is found when blood pressure is measured. Signs and symptoms develop over time. Headache, blurred vision, dizziness, and nosebleeds occur.

Certain drugs can lower blood pressure. A healthy diet, a healthy weight, and regular exercise are needed. No smoking is allowed. Alcohol and caffeine are limited. Managing stress and sleeping well also lower blood pressure.

---

**BOX 33-8   RISK FACTORS FOR HYPERTENSION**

**FACTORS YOU CANNOT CHANGE**

- Age—45 years or older for men; 55 years or older for women
- Gender—younger men are at greater risk than younger women; the risk increases for women after menopause
- Race—African-Americans are at greater risk than whites
- Family history—tends to run in families

**FACTORS YOU CAN CHANGE**

- Being overweight—related to diet, lack of exercise, and atherosclerosis
- Stress—increased sympathetic nervous system activity
- Tobacco use—nicotine narrows blood vessels
- High-salt diet—sodium causes fluid retention; increased fluid raises the blood volume
- Excessive alcohol—increases chemical substances in the body that increase blood pressure
- Lack of exercise—increases risk of being overweight
- Atherosclerosis—arteries narrow because of fatty buildup in the vessels

## CORONARY ARTERY DISEASE

The coronary arteries are in the heart. They supply the heart with blood. In coronary artery disease (CAD), the coronary arteries narrow. One or all are affected. Therefore the heart muscle gets less blood. The most common cause is atherosclerosis (Fig. 33-27). Fatty material collects on the arterial walls. The narrowed arteries block blood flow. Blockage may be total or partial. Permanent damage occurs in the part of the heart receiving its blood supply from the blocked artery.

CAD is the leading cause of death in the United States. The major complications of CAD are angina pectoris and myocardial infarction (heart attack). Treatment involves reducing risk factors. Some risk factors cannot be controlled:

- Gender—men are at greater risk than women
- Age—CAD is more common in older persons
- Family history
- Race—African-Americans are at greater risk than whites, Hispanics, or Asian-Americans
  Other factors can be controlled:
- Being overweight
- Smoking
- Lack of exercise
- High blood cholesterol
- Hypertension
- Diabetes
- Stress

**ANGINA PECTORIS.** Angina *(pain)* pectoris *(chest)* means chest pain. The chest pain is from reduced blood flow to a part of the heart muscle (myocardium). It is commonly called *angina*. It occurs when the heart needs more oxygen. Normally blood flow to the heart increases when the need for oxygen increases. Exertion, a heavy meal, stress, and excitement increase the heart's need for oxygen. In CAD, narrowed vessels prevent increased blood flow.

Chest pain is described as a tightness or pressure. Some complain of discomfort in the chest (Fig. 33-28). Pain in the jaw, neck, and down one or both arms is common. The person may be pale, feel faint, and perspire. Dyspnea is common. The person stops activity to rest. Rest often relieves symptoms in 3 to 15 minutes. Rest reduces the heart's need for oxygen. Therefore normal blood flow is achieved. Heart damage is prevented.

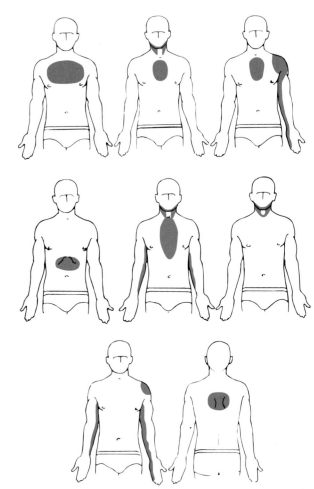

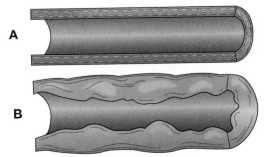

**FIG. 33-27 A,** Normal artery. **B,** Fatty deposits collect on the artery walls in atherosclerosis.

**FIG. 33-28** *Shaded areas* show where the pain of angina is located. (From Phipps WJ and others: *Medical-surgical nursing: concepts and clinical practice,* ed 5, St Louis, 1995, Mosby.)

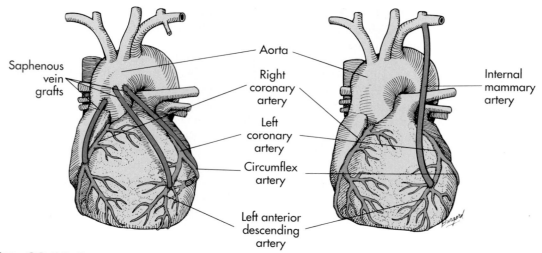

**FIG. 33-29** Coronary artery bypass surgery. (From Phipps WJ and others: *Medical-surgical nursing: concepts and clinical practice,* ed 5, St Louis, 1995, Mosby.)

Besides rest, a *nitroglycerin* tablet is taken when an angina attack occurs. It is placed under the tongue. There it dissolves and is rapidly absorbed into the bloodstream. Tablets are kept with the person at all times. The person takes a tablet and then tells the nurse.

Things that cause angina are avoided. These include overexertion, heavy meals and overeating, and emotional stress. The person needs to stay indoors during cold weather or during hot, humid weather. Exercise programs are helpful. They are supervised by the doctor.

Surgery can open or bypass the diseased part of the artery (Fig. 33-29). Increased blood flow to the heart is the goal. Angina pectoris often leads to heart attack. Chest pain that is not relieved by rest and nitroglycerin may signal a heart attack. The person needs emergency care.

**MYOCARDIAL INFARCTION.** *Myocardial* refers to the heart muscle. *Infarction* means tissue death. With myocardial infarction (MI), part of the heart muscle dies. This is from lack of blood flow to the heart muscle.

Common terms for MI are *heart attack, coronary, coronary thrombosis,* and *coronary occlusion.* Blood flow to the heart muscle is suddenly blocked. A thrombus (blood clot) blocks blood flow through an artery with atherosclerosis. The area of damage may be small or large (Fig. 33-30). Sudden cardiac death *(cardiac arrest)* can occur (Chapter 40).

Signs and symptoms are listed in Box 33-9. MI is an emergency. Efforts are made to:
- Relieve pain
- Stabilize vital signs
- Give oxygen
- Calm the person
- Prevent life-threatening problems

> ### ▶ FOCUS ON HOME CARE
> #### MYOCARDIAL INFARCTION
> Cardiac rehabilitation continues. The person may go to a fitness center or health club for exercise. Many hospitals have fitness centers. Some persons go to indoor malls for walking. Normal activities are increased slowly. The person returns to work with the doctor's approval.

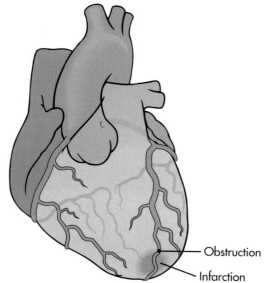

**FIG. 33-30** Myocardial infarction. (From Lewis SM, Heitkemper MM, Dirksen SR: *Medical-surgical nursing: assessment and management of clinical problems,* ed 5, St Louis, 2000, Mosby.)

Activity is increased slowly. Drugs and measures to prevent problems are continued. Cardiac rehabilitation is planned. It involves exercise and teaching about drugs, diet, sex, and life-style changes. The goal is to prevent another heart attack. The person may need surgery to open or bypass the diseased artery. *See Focus on Home Care: Myocardial Infarction.*

## HEART FAILURE

Heart failure or congestive heart failure (CHF) occurs when the heart cannot pump blood normally. Blood backs up. Tissue congestion occurs.

- *Left-sided failure.* The left side of the heart cannot pump blood normally. Blood backs up into the lungs. Respiratory congestion occurs. The person has dyspnea, increased sputum, cough, and gurgling sounds in the lungs. Also, the rest of the body does not get enough blood. Signs and symptoms occur from effects on the organs. Poor blood flow to the brain causes confusion, dizziness, and fainting. The kidneys produce less urine. The skin is pale. Blood pressure falls. A very severe form of left-sided failure is *pulmonary edema* (fluid in the lungs). It is an emergency. Death can occur.
- *Right-sided failure.* The right side of the heart cannot pump blood normally. Blood backs up into the venous system. Feet and ankles swell. Neck veins bulge. Liver congestion affects liver function. The abdomen becomes congested with fluid. The right side of the heart pumps less blood to the lungs. Normal blood flow does not occur from the lungs to the left side of the heart. The left side has less blood to pump to the body. As with left-sided heart failure, organs receive less blood. The signs and symptoms described for left-sided failure occur.

A damaged or weakened heart usually causes heart failure. MI and hypertension are common causes. So are damaged heart valves.

Drugs strengthen the heart. They also reduce the amount of fluid in the body. A sodium-controlled diet is ordered. Oxygen is given. Semi-Fowler's or Fowler's position is preferred for breathing. If acutely ill, the person needs hospital care.

You may assist with these aspects of the person's care:
- Maintaining bedrest or a limited activity program
- Measuring intake and output
- Measuring weight daily
- Assisting with pulse oximetry
- Restricting fluids as ordered
- Preventing skin breakdown and pressure ulcers
- Performing range-of-motion exercises
- Assisting with transfers or ambulation
- Assisting with self-care activities
- Maintaining good body alignment
- Applying elastic stockings

*See Focus on Children: Heart Failure. See Focus on Older Persons: Heart Failure.*

---

**BOX 33-9    SIGNS AND SYMPTOMS OF MYOCARDIAL INFARCTION**

- Sudden, severe chest pain
- Pain is usually on the left side
- Pain is described as crushing, stabbing, or squeezing; some describe pain in terms of someone sitting on the chest
- Pain may radiate to the neck and jaw, and down the arm or to other sites
- Pain is more severe and lasts longer than angina pectoris
- Pain is not relieved by rest and nitroglycerin
- Indigestion
- Dyspnea
- Nausea
- Dizziness
- Perspiration
- Pallor
- Cyanosis
- Cold and clammy skin
- Low blood pressure
- Weak and irregular pulse
- Fear and apprehension
- A feeling of doom

---

**FOCUS ON CHILDREN**
**HEART FAILURE**

Congenital heart defects can cause heart failure in children. (*Congenital* comes from the Latin word *congenitus.* It means to be born with.)

---

**FOCUS ON OLDER PERSONS**
**HEART FAILURE**

Many older persons suffer from heart failure. They may need home care or long-term care.

Older persons are at risk for skin breakdown. Tissue swelling, poor circulation, and fragile skin combine to increase the risk of pressure ulcers. Good skin care and regular position changes are needed.

# URINARY SYSTEM DISORDERS

The kidneys, ureters, bladder, and urethra are the major urinary system structures. Disorders can occur in these structures.

## URINARY TRACT INFECTIONS

Urinary tract infections (UTIs) are common. Infection in one area can involve the entire system. Microbes can enter the system through the urethra. Catheterization, urological exams, intercourse, poor perineal hygiene, and poor fluid intake are common causes. UTI is a common nosocomial infection (Chapter 12).

Women are at high risk. Microbes can easily enter the short female urethra. Prostate gland secretions help protect men from UTIs. *See Focus on Older Persons: Urinary Tract Infections.*

**CYSTITIS.** Cystitis is a bladder *(cyst)* infection *(itis)*. It is caused by bacteria. The following are common:
- Urinary frequency
- Oliguria—scant *(olig)* urine *(uria)*
- Urgency
- Dysuria—difficult or painful *(dys)* urination *(uria)*
- Pain or burning on urination
- Foul-smelling urine
- Hematuria—blood *(hemat)* in the urine *(uria)*
- Pyuria—pus *(py)* in the urine *(uria)*
- Fever

Antibiotics are ordered. Fluids are encouraged—usually 2000 ml per day. If untreated, cystitis can lead to pyelonephritis.

**PYELONEPHRITIS.** Pyelonephritis is inflammation *(itis)* of the kidney *(nephr)* pelvis *(pyelo)*. Infection is the most common cause. Cloudy urine may contain pus, mucus, and blood. Chills, fever, back pain, and nausea and vomiting occur. So do the signs and symptoms of cystitis. Treatment involves antibiotics and fluids.

## URINARY DIVERSIONS

Sometimes the urinary bladder is surgically removed. Cancer and bladder injuries are common reasons. When the bladder is removed, a new pathway is needed for urine to exit the body. The new pathway is called a *urinary diversion.*

Often an ostomy is involved. A **ureterostomy** is the surgical creation of an artificial opening *(stomy)* between the ureter *(uretero)* and the abdomen (Fig. 33-31). The nurse provides stoma care in the early postoperative period. You may care for persons with long-standing ureterostomies.

The person wears a ureterostomy pouch over the stoma (Fig. 33-32). Urine drains through the stoma into the pouch. The pouch is replaced anytime it leaks. Leakage can cause skin irritation, breakdown, and infection. Follow Standard Precautions and the Bloodborne Pathogen Standard when giving stoma care or emptying the pouch.

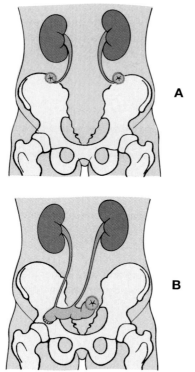

**FIG. 33-31** Ureterostomies. **A,** Both ureters are brought through the skin onto the abdomen. The person has two stomas. **B,** The ileal conduit. A small section of the intestine (ileum) is removed. One end is sutured closed. The other end is brought through the skin onto the abdomen to form a stoma. The ureters are attached to the resected ileum. (From Beare PG, Meyers JL: *Adult health nursing,* ed 3, St Louis, 1998, Mosby.)

---

### FOCUS ON OLDER PERSONS
#### URINARY TRACT INFECTION

An enlarged prostate increases the risk of a UTI in older men. Incomplete bladder emptying, perineal soiling from fecal incontinence, and poor nutrition increase the risk of UTI in older men and women.

## RENAL CALCULI

Renal calculi are kidney *(renal)* stones *(calculi)*. White men between the ages of 20 and 40 years are at risk. Bedrest, immobility, and poor fluid intake are risk factors. Stones vary in size. Signs and symptoms include:

- Severe, cramping pain in the back and side just below the ribs
- Pain in the abdomen, thigh, and urethra
- Nausea and vomiting
- Fever and chills
- Dysuria—difficult or painful *(dys)* urination *(uria)*
- Urinary frequency
- Urinary urgency
- Oliguria—scant *(olig)* urine *(uria)*
- Hematuria—blood *(hemat)* in the urine *(uria)*
- Foul-smelling urine

Drugs are given for pain relief. The person needs to drink about 2000 to 3000 ml of fluid a day. Increased fluids help stones pass through the urine. All urine is strained (Chapter 26). Surgical removal of the stone may be necessary. Some dietary changes can prevent stones.

## RENAL FAILURE

In renal failure (kidney failure), the kidneys do not function or are severely impaired. Waste products are not removed from the blood. The body retains fluid. Heart failure and hypertension easily result. Renal failure may be acute or chronic. The person is very ill.

**ACUTE RENAL FAILURE.** Acute renal failure is sudden. There is severe decreased blood flow to the kidneys. Causes include severe bleeding, myocardial infarction (heart attack), heart failure, burns, infection, and severe allergic reactions. Hospital care is needed.

At first, *oliguria* (scant amount of urine) occurs. Urine output is less than 400 ml in 24 hours. This phase lasts a few days to 2 weeks. Then diuresis occurs. *Diuresis* means the process *(esis)* of passing *(di)* urine *(ur)*. Large amounts of urine are produced—1000 to 5000 ml a day. Kidney function improves and returns to normal during the recovery phase. This can take from 1 month to 1 year. Some persons develop chronic renal failure.

Every system is affected by the buildup of waste products in the blood. Death can occur.

Treatment involves drugs, restricted fluids, and diet therapy. The diet is high in carbohydrates. It is low in protein and potassium. The care plan will likely include:

- Measuring and recording urine output every hour. Report an output of less than 30 ml per hour to the nurse at once.
- Measuring and recording intake and output every shift
- Restricting fluid intake
- Measuring weight daily
- Turning and repositioning at least every 2 hours
- Measures to prevent pressure ulcers
- Frequent oral hygiene
- Measures to prevent infection
- Coughing and deep-breathing exercises
- Measures to meet emotional needs

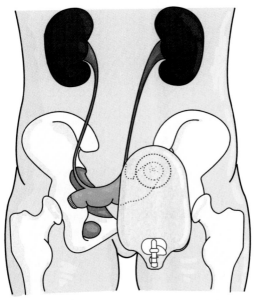

**FIG. 33-32** Ureterostomy pouch.

> **BOX 33-10** SIGNS AND SYMPTOMS OF CHRONIC RENAL FAILURE
>
> - Yellow, tan, or dusky skin
> - Dry, itchy skin
> - Thin, brittle skin
> - Bruises
> - Bad breath (*halitosis*)
> - Inflammation of the mouth (*stomatitis*)
> - Nausea and vomiting
> - Loss of appetite
> - Weight loss
> - Diarrhea or constipation
> - Decreased urine output
> - Bleeding tendencies
> - Susceptibility to infection
> - Hypertension
> - Congestive heart failure
> - Gastric ulcers
> - GI bleeding
> - Irregular pulse
> - Abnormal breathing patterns
> - Burning sensation in the legs and feet
> - Muscle twitching
> - Leg cramps at night
> - Fatigue
> - Sleep disorders
> - Headache
> - Convulsions
> - Confusion
> - Coma

> **BOX 33-11** CARE OF THE PERSON IN CHRONIC RENAL FAILURE
>
> - A diet low in protein, potassium, and sodium
> - Fluid restriction
> - Measuring blood pressure in the supine, sitting, and standing positions
> - Measuring weight daily
> - Measuring and recording intake and output
> - Turning and repositioning
> - Measures to prevent pressure ulcers
> - Range-of-motion exercises
> - Measures to prevent itching (bath oils, lotions, creams)
> - Measures to prevent injury and bleeding
> - Frequent oral hygiene
> - Measures to prevent infection
> - Measures to prevent diarrhea or constipation
> - Measures to meet emotional needs
> - Measures to promote rest

**CHRONIC RENAL FAILURE.** The kidneys cannot meet the body's needs. Nephrons of the kidney are destroyed over many years. Hypertension and diabetes are common causes. Infections, urinary tract obstructions, and tumors are other causes.

Signs and symptoms appear when 80% to 90% of kidney function is lost (Box 33-10). Every body system is affected as waste products build up in the blood.

Treatment includes fluid restriction, diet therapy, drugs, and dialysis. *Dialysis* is the process of removing waste products from the blood. It requires specially trained nurses. Some persons have kidney transplants.

Nursing measures are listed in Box 33-11.

# THE ENDOCRINE SYSTEM

The endocrine system is made up of glands. The endocrine glands secrete hormones that affect other organs and glands. Diabetes is the most common endocrine disorder.

## DIABETES

In this disorder the body cannot produce or use insulin properly. Insulin is needed for sugar use. Insulin is secreted by the pancreas. Sugar builds up in the blood. Cells do not have enough sugar for energy. They cannot perform their functions. There are three types of diabetes:

- *Type 1*—occurs most often in children and young adults. The pancreas produces little or no insulin. Onset is rapid. There is increased thirst and urination, constant hunger, weight loss, blurred vision, and extreme fatigue.
- *Type 2*—occurs in adults. Persons older than 40 years are at risk. Obesity and hypertension are risk factors. The pancreas secretes insulin. However, the body cannot use it well. Onset is slow. The person has fatigue, nausea, frequent urination, increased thirst, weight loss, and blurred vision. Infections are frequent. Wounds heal slowly.
- *Gestational diabetes*—develops during pregnancy. (Gestation comes from *gestare*. It means to bear.) It usually goes away after the baby is born. However, the woman is at risk for type 2 diabetes later in life.

Diabetes must be controlled. Otherwise complications occur. These include blindness, renal failure, nerve damage, hypertension, and circulatory disorders. Circulatory disorders can lead to stroke, heart attack, and slow wound healing. Foot and leg wounds are very serious. Infection and gangrene can occur. Sometimes amputation is needed.

Risk factors include a family history of the disease. For type 1, whites are at greater risk than nonwhites. Type 2 is more common in older and overweight persons. These ethnic groups are at risk for type 2:

- African-Americans
- Native Americans
- Asian-Americans and Pacific Islander–Americans
- Hispanics

Type 1 is treated with daily insulin therapy, healthy eating (Chapter 20), and exercise. Type 2 is treated with healthy eating and exercise. Many persons with type 2 take oral drugs. Some need insulin. Overweight persons need to lose weight.

Both types require blood glucose monitoring. Good foot care is needed. Corns, blisters, and calluses can lead to an infection and amputation.

The person's blood sugar level can fall too low or go too high:

- **Hypoglycemia** means low *(hypo)* sugar *(glyc)* in the blood *(emia)*.
- **Hyperglycemia** means high *(hyper)* sugar *(glyc)* in the blood *(emia)*.

See Table 33-1 for their causes, signs, and symptoms. Both can lead to death if not corrected. You must call for the nurse at once. *See Focus on Children: Diabetes.*

> ### FOCUS ON CHILDREN
> #### DIABETES
> You may prepare meals for the child with diabetes. Follow the child's diet carefully. Also prepare snacks for the child to take to school. The snack is needed in case the child's blood sugar level drops.

| TABLE 33-1 HYPOGLYCEMIA AND HYPERGLYCEMIA | Causes | Signs and Symptoms |
|---|---|---|
| Hypoglycemia (low blood sugar) | Too much insulin or diabetic drugs<br>Omitting a meal<br>Delayed meal<br>Eating too little food<br>Increased exercise<br>Vomiting | Hunger<br>Weakness<br>Trembling; shakiness<br>Sweating<br>Headache<br>Dizziness<br>Faintness<br>Rapid pulse<br>Low blood pressure<br>Rapid, shallow respirations<br>Confusion<br>Changes in vision<br>Cold, clammy skin<br>Convulsions<br>Unconsciousness |
| Hyperglycemia (high blood sugar) | Undiagnosed diabetes<br>Not enough insulin or diabetic drugs<br>Eating too much food<br>Too little exercise<br>Physical or emotional stress | Weakness<br>Drowsiness<br>Thirst<br>Hunger<br>Frequent urination<br>Leg cramps<br>Flushed face<br>Sweet breath odor<br>Slow, deep, and labored respirations<br>Rapid, weak pulse<br>Low blood pressure<br>Dry skin<br>Blurred vision<br>Headache<br>Nausea and vomiting<br>Convulsions<br>Coma |

## DIGESTIVE DISORDERS

The digestive system breaks down food so the body can absorb it. Solid wastes are eliminated. Diarrhea, constipation, flatulence, and fecal incontinence are discussed in Chapter 19. So is care of persons with colostomies and ileostomies.

### DIVERTICULAR DISEASE

Many people have small pouches in their colons. The pouches bulge outward through weak spots in the colon (Fig. 33-33). Each pouch is called a *diverticulum*. (*Diverticulare* means to turn inside out.) The condition of having these pouches is called *diverticulosis*. (*Osis* means condition of.) The pouches can become infected or inflamed. This is called *diverticulitis*. (*Itis* means inflammation.)

Age is a risk factor. About half of all Americans between 60 and 80 years of age have diverticulosis. It occurs in almost every person older than 80 years. A low-fiber diet and constipation also are risk factors.

When feces enter the pouches, the pouches can become inflamed and infected. The person has abdominal pain and tenderness on the lower left side of the abdomen. Fever, nausea and vomiting, chills, cramping, and constipation are likely. Bloating, rectal bleeding, frequent urination, and pain while urinating can occur.

A ruptured pouch is a rare complication. Feces spill out into the abdomen. This leads to a severe, life-threatening infection. A pouch also can cause a blockage in the intestine (intestinal obstruction). Feces and gas cannot move past the blocked part. These problems require surgery.

The doctor orders needed dietary changes. Sometimes antibiotics are ordered. Surgery is needed for severe disease, obstruction, and ruptured pouches. The diseased part of the bowel is removed. Sometimes a colostomy is necessary (Chapter 19).

### VOMITING

Vomiting means expelling stomach contents through the mouth. It signals illness or injury. It can be life-threatening. Aspirated vomitus can obstruct the airway. Vomiting large amounts of blood can lead to shock. These measures are needed:

- Follow Standard Precautions and the Bloodborne Pathogen Standard.
- Turn the person's head well to one side. This prevents aspiration.
- Place a kidney basin under the person's chin.
- Move vomitus away from the person.
- Provide oral hygiene. This helps remove the bitter taste of vomitus.
- Eliminate odors.
- Change linens as necessary.
- Observe vomitus for color, odor, and undigested food. If it looks like coffee grounds, it contains digested blood. This signals bleeding. Report your observations.
- Measure, report, and record the amount of vomitus. Note the amount on the I&O record.
- Save a specimen for laboratory study.
- Dispose of vomitus after the nurse observes it.

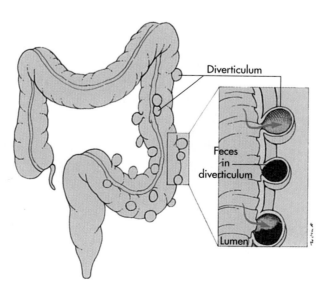

**FIG. 33-33** Diverticulosis. (From Christensen BL, Kockrow EO: *Adult health nursing*, ed 4, St Louis, 2003, Mosby.)

# COMMUNICABLE DISEASES

Communicable diseases are contagious or infectious diseases. They can be transmitted from one person to another in these ways:

- *Direct*—from the infected person
- *Indirect*—from dressings, linens, or surfaces
- *Airborne*—through sneezing or coughing
- *Vehicle*—through ingesting contaminated food, water, drugs, blood, or fluids
- *Vector*—from animals, fleas, and ticks

Table 33-2 outlines common communicable childhood diseases. Standard Precautions and Transmission-Based Precautions are followed for all communicable diseases.

## HEPATITIS

Hepatitis is an inflammation of the liver. It can be mild or cause death. Signs and symptoms are listed in Box 33-12. Treatment involves rest, a healthy diet, fluids, and no alcohol. Recovery takes about 8 weeks.

| BOX 33-12 | SIGNS AND SYMPTOMS OF HEPATITIS |
| --- | --- |

- Loss of appetite
- Weakness, fatigue, exhaustion
- Nausea and vomiting
- Fever
- Skin rash
- Dark urine
- Yellowish color to the skin and whites of the eyes (*jaundice*)
- Itching
- Light-colored stools
- Diarrhea or constipation
- Headache
- Chills
- Abdominal pain or discomfort
- Muscle aches
- Weight loss

| TABLE 33-2 | COMMON COMMUNICABLE CHILDHOOD DISEASES | |
| --- | --- | --- |
| **Disease** | **Transmission** | **Signs and Symptoms** |
| Chickenpox (*varicella*) | Direct contact and airborne contact with respiratory secretions; direct contact with skin lesions | Fever, rash, and skin lesions |
| Diphtheria | Direct or indirect contact with respiratory secretions and skin lesions from the person or a carrier | Sore throat, fever, nasal discharge, enlarged lymph glands in the neck, cough, hoarseness, patches (*lesions*) on the tonsils, pharynx, larynx, nasal membranes, and skin |
| Measles (*rubeola*) | Direct or indirect contact with nasal secretions | Fever, cough, rash, inflammation of the mucous membranes of the nose, nasal discharge; bronchitis |
| Mumps | Direct contact with saliva droplets | Fever, headache, swollen salivary glands, earache |
| Whooping cough (*pertussis*) | Airborne or direct contact with droplets from the respiratory tract | Fever, sneezing, severe cough at night, coughs are short and rapid followed by a "whoop" or crowing sound with inhalation |
| Poliomyelitis | Airborne or direct contact with respiratory secretions; direct contact with feces | Fever, sore throat, headache, nausea and vomiting, loss of appetite, abdominal pain, neck and spinal stiffness, paralysis |
| German measles (*rubella*) | Airborne or direct contact with secretions from the nose and pharynx | Fever, headache, loss of appetite, nasal inflammation, sore throat, cough, rash |
| Scarlet fever | Airborne or direct contact with nasal and pharyngeal secretions | Fever, chills, headache, vomiting, abdominal pain, red and swollen tonsils and pharynx, rash |

Protect yourself and others. Follow Standard Precautions and the Bloodborne Pathogen Standard. Transmission-Based Precautions are ordered as necessary (Chapter 12). Assist the person with hygiene and hand washing as needed.

There are five major types of hepatitis.

**HEPATITIS A.** This type is spread by the fecal-oral route. The virus is ingested when eating or drinking contaminated food or water. It is also ingested when eating or drinking from a contaminated vessel. Causes include poor sanitation, crowded living conditions, poor nutrition, and poor hygiene. Anal sex and IV drug abuse also are causes.

Persons with fecal incontinence, confusion, or dementia can cause contamination. Carefully look for contaminated items and areas.

Handle bedpans, feces, and rectal thermometers carefully. Good hand washing is needed by everyone, including the person. Assist with hand washing after bowel movements.

**HEPATITIS B.** The hepatitis B virus (HBV) is the cause. It is present in the blood and body fluids (saliva, semen, vaginal secretions) of infected persons. It is spread by:
- Contaminated blood products
- IV drug use
- Sexual contact, especially anal sex
  (For the HBV vaccine, see Chapter 12.)

**HEPATITIS C.** This type is spread by blood contaminated with the virus. A person may have the virus but no symptoms. Serious liver disease and damage may show up years later. Even without symptoms, the person can transmit the disease. The virus is spread by:
- Blood contaminated with the virus
- IV drug use
- Inhaling cocaine through contaminated straws
- Contaminated needles used for tattooing and body piercing
- High-risk sexual activity

**HEPATITIS D AND HEPATITIS E.** Hepatitis D occurs in persons infected with the hepatitis B virus (HBV). It is spread the same way as HBV. Hepatitis E occurs in countries with contaminated water supplies. It is spread by the fecal-oral route. *See Focus on Children: Hepatitis.*

> ### FOCUS ON CHILDREN
> #### HEPATITIS
> Hepatitis A is more common in preschool and school-age children. Poor hygiene after defecation leads to contaminated eating and drinking vessels. Also, young children often put their hands into their mouths.

# ACQUIRED IMMUNODEFICIENCY SYNDROME

Acquired immunodeficiency syndrome (AIDS) is caused by a virus. The virus is called the *human immunodeficiency virus (HIV).* It attacks the immune system. The person's ability to fight other diseases is affected. Many new drugs help reduce complications and prolong life. AIDS has no vaccine and no cure at present. It is a life-threatening disease.

The virus is spread through certain body fluids—blood, semen, vaginal secretions, and breast milk. HIV is not spread by saliva, tears, sweat, sneezing, coughing, insects, or casual contact. The virus is transmitted mainly by:
- Unprotected anal, vaginal, or oral sex with an infected person ("Unprotected" is without a new latex or polyurethane condom.)
- Needle and syringe sharing among IV drug users
- HIV-infected mothers before or during childbirth
- HIV-infected mothers through breast-feeding

The virus enters the bloodstream through the rectum, vagina, penis, mouth, or skin breaks. Small breaks in the vagina or rectum may occur when the penis, finger, or other objects are inserted. Gum disease can cause breaks in the gums. The virus can enter the bloodstream through these mucous membrane breaks (mouth, vagina, rectum). Babies can become infected during pregnancy, shortly after birth, or from breast-feeding.

The virus is carried in the contaminated blood left in needles or syringes. When the devices are shared, contaminated blood enters the bloodstream. Needle-sticks pose a threat to the health team.

> ### BOX 33-13 SIGNS AND SYMPTOMS OF AIDS
> - Loss of appetite
> - Weight loss
> - Fever
> - Headache
> - Night sweats
> - Diarrhea
> - Painful or difficulty swallowing
> - Tiredness, extreme or constant
> - Skin rashes
> - Swollen glands in the neck, underarms, and groin
> - Cough
> - Shortness of breath
> - Sores or white patches in the mouth or on the tongue
> - Purple blotches or bumps on the skin that look like bruises but do not disappear
> - Blurred vision
> - Confusion
> - Forgetfulness
> - Dementia (Chapter 35)

The virus is very fragile. It cannot live outside the body. HIV is not spread by casual, everyday contact. Such contact includes using public telephones, restrooms, swimming pools, hot tubs, or water fountains. Other forms of casual contact include talking to, hugging, or dancing with an infected person. HIV is not transmitted by food prepared by the infected person.

Box 33-13 lists the signs and symptoms of AIDS. Some persons infected with HIV are symptom-free for 8 to 10 years. However, they carry the virus. They can spread it to others.

Persons with AIDS develop other diseases. Their immune system is damaged. They cannot fight other diseases. The person is at risk for pneumonia, TB, Kaposi sarcoma (a cancer), and nervous system damage. Memory loss, loss of coordination, paralysis, mental health disorders, and dementia signal nervous system damage.

You may care for persons with AIDS or those who are HIV carriers (Box 33-14). You may have contact with the person's blood and body fluids. Mouth-to-mouth contact is possible during CPR. Protect yourself and others from the virus. Follow Standard Precautions and the Bloodborne Pathogen Standard. *These precautions apply when caring for all persons.* A person may have the HIV virus but no symptoms. In some persons, HIV is not yet diagnosed. *See Focus on Older Persons: AIDS.*

## SEXUALLY TRANSMITTED DISEASES

Sexually transmitted diseases (STDs) are spread by oral, vaginal, or anal sex (Table 33-3, p. 704). At least one partner must have an STD. Some people do not have signs and symptoms or are not aware of an infection. Others know but do not seek treatment because of embarrassment.

STDs often occur in the genital and rectal areas. They also occur in the ears, mouth, nipples, throat, tongue, eyes, and nose. Using condoms helps prevent the spread of STDs, especially HIV and AIDS. Some STDs are also spread through skin breaks, by contact with infected body fluids (blood, semen, saliva), or by contaminated blood or needles.

Standard Precautions and the Bloodborne Pathogen Standard are followed.

---

| BOX 33-14 | CARING FOR THE PERSON WITH AIDS |
|---|---|

- Practice Standard Precautions.
- Follow the Bloodborne Pathogen Standard.
- Provide daily hygiene. Avoid irritating soaps.
- Provide oral hygiene before meals and at bedtime. A toothbrush with soft bristles is best.
- Provide oral fluids as ordered.
- Measure and record intake and output.
- Measure weight daily.
- Encourage deep-breathing and coughing exercises as ordered.
- Prevent pressure ulcers.
- Assist with range-of-motion exercises and ambulation as ordered.
- Encourage self-care as able. The person may need assistive devices (walker, commode, eating devices).
- Encourage the person to be as active as possible.
- Change linens and garments as often as needed when fever is present.
- Be a good listener. Provide emotional support.

---

> ## FOCUS ON OLDER PERSONS
> ### AIDS

Persons age 50 years and older are at risk. The Centers for Disease Control and Prevention (CDC) reported that through December 2000, there were 84,044 cases of AIDS in persons age 50 years and older. They get and spread HIV through sexual contact and IV drug use. However, they do not consider themselves to be at risk. They tend to be less informed about the disease. And they tend not to practice safe sex. A blood transfusion between 1978 and 1985 increases the risk of HIV.

Aging and other diseases can mask the signs and symptoms of AIDS. Older persons are less likely to be tested for HIV/AIDS. Often the person dies without the disease being diagnosed. You must follow Standard Precautions and the Bloodborne Pathogen Standard.

| TABLE 33-3 | SEXUALLY TRANSMTTED DISEASES | |
|---|---|---|
| **Disease** | **Signs and Symptoms** | **Treatment** |
| Herpes | Painful, blister-like sores on or near the genitals, mouth, or anus (Fig. 33-34) The sores may have a watery discharge Pain, itching, burning, and tingling in the affected area Vaginal discharge Pain during urination or intercourse Fever Swollen glands | No known cure Anti-viral drugs |
| Genital warts | *Male*—Warts appear on the penis, anus, genitalia, or throat *Female*—Warts appear near the vagina, cervix, labia, or throat | Application of special ointment that causes the warts to dry up and fall off Surgical removal may be necessary if the ointment is not effective |
| HIV/AIDS | See p. 702. | See p. 702. |
| Gonorrhea | Burning and pain on urination Urinary frequency and urgency Genital discharge (vagina, urethra, rectum) | Antibiotic drugs |
| Chlamydia | May not show symptoms Discharge from the penis or vagina Burning or pain on urination Testicular pain or swelling Vaginal bleeding Rectal inflammation and/or discharge Pain during intercourse Diarrhea Nausea Abdominal pain Fever | Antibiotic drugs |
| Pubic lice | Intense itching | Over-the-counter or prescription lice treatment Washing or dry-cleaning all exposed clothing, bedding, and towels |
| Trichomoniasis (occurs in women; men are carriers) | No symptoms Frothy, thick, foul-smelling, yellow vaginal discharge Genital itching and irritation Burning and pain on urination Genital swelling | Metronidazole |
| Syphilis | *Stage 1*—10 to 90 days after exposure Painless sores (*chancres*) on penis, in the vagina, or on genitalia; the chancre may also be on the lips or inside of mouth, or anywhere else on the body *Stage 2*—About 3 to 6 weeks after the sores General fatigue, loss of appetite, nausea, fever, headache, rash, swollen glands, sore throat, bone and joint pain, hair loss, lesions on the lips and genitalia Symptoms may come and go for many years *Stage 3*—3 to 15 years after infection Central nervous system damage (including paralysis), heart damage, blindness, liver damage, mental health problems, death | Penicillin and other antibiotic drugs |

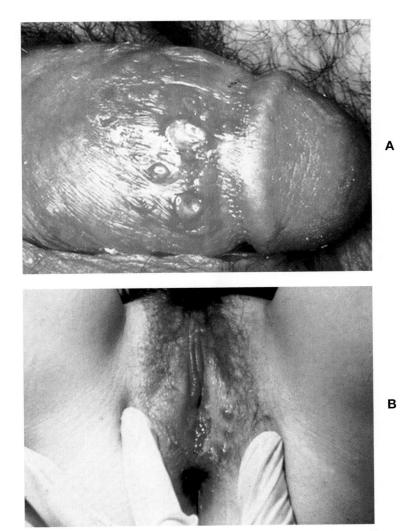

**FIG. 33-34** Herpes. **A,** Sores on the penis. **B,** Sores on the female perineum. (Courtesy United States Public Health Service, Washington, DC.)

Circle the **BEST** answer.

**1** Which is *not* a warning sign of cancer?
  **a** Painful, swollen joints
  **b** A sore that does not heal
  **c** Unusual bleeding or discharge
  **d** Nagging cough or hoarseness

**2** Joan Martin has arthritis. Care includes the following *except*
  **a** Preventing contractures
  **b** Range-of-motion exercises
  **c** A cast or traction
  **d** Assisting with ADL

**3** A cast needs to dry. Which is *false?*
  **a** The cast is covered with blankets or plastic.
  **b** The person is turned so the cast dries evenly.
  **c** The entire cast is supported with pillows.
  **d** The cast is supported by the palms when lifted.

**4** A person has an arm cast. The following are reported at once *except*
  **a** Pain, numbness, or inability to move the fingers
  **b** Chills, fever, or nausea and vomiting
  **c** Odor, cyanosis, or temperature changes of the skin
  **d** Pulse rate of 75 and output of 900 ml during your shift

**5** A person is in traction. You should do the following *except*
  **a** Perform range-of-motion exercises as directed
  **b** Keep the weights off the floor
  **c** Remove the weights if the person is uncomfortable
  **d** Give skin care at frequent intervals

**6** After a hip pinning, the operated leg is
  **a** Abducted at all times
  **b** Adducted at all times
  **c** Externally rotated at all times
  **d** Flexed at all times

**7** Joan Martin has osteoporosis. She is at risk for
  **a** Fractures
  **b** An amputation
  **c** Phantom limb pain
  **d** Paralysis

**8** A person had a stroke. The care plan includes the following. Which should you question?
  **a** Semi-Fowler's position
  **b** Range-of-motion exercises every 2 hours
  **c** Turn, reposition, and skin care every 2 hours
  **d** Bed in the highest horizontal position

**9** Receptive aphasia means that the person has trouble
  **a** Talking
  **b** Writing
  **c** Understanding messages
  **d** Using gestures

**10** A person has Parkinson's disease. Which is *false?*
  **a** Part of the brain is affected.
  **b** Mental function is affected first.
  **c** Stiff muscles, slow movements, and a shuffling gait occur.
  **d** The person is protected from injury.

**11** A person has multiple sclerosis. Which is *false?*
  **a** Nerve impulses are sent to and from the brain in a normal manner.
  **b** Symptoms begin in young adulthood.
  **c** There is no cure.
  **d** Over time, the person depends on others for care.

**12** Persons with head or spinal cord injuries require
  **a** Rehabilitation
  **b** Speech therapy
  **c** Long-term care
  **d** Psychiatric care

**13** A person has emphysema. Which is *false?*
  **a** The person has dyspnea only with activity.
  **b** Smoking is the most common cause.
  **c** Breathing is usually easier sitting upright and slightly forward.
  **d** Sputum may contain pus.

**14** Which is *not* a complication of hypertension?
  **a** Stroke
  **b** Heart attack
  **c** Renal failure
  **d** Parkinson's disease

15 A person has hypertension. Treatment will likely include the following *except*
  a No smoking and regular exercise
  b A high-sodium diet
  c A low-calorie diet if the person is obese
  d Drugs to lower the blood pressure

16 A person has angina pectoris. Which is *true?*
  a Damage to the heart muscle occurs.
  b The pain is described as crushing, stabbing, or squeezing.
  c The pain is relieved with rest and nitroglycerin.
  d The pain is always on the left side of the chest.

17 A person is having a myocardial infarction. Which is *false?*
  a The person is having a heart attack.
  b This is an emergency.
  c The person may have a cardiac arrest.
  d The person does not have enough blood to supply the body with needed oxygen.

18 A person has heart failure. These measures are ordered. Which should you question?
  a Encourage fluids
  b Measure intake and output
  c Measure weight daily
  d Perform range-of-motion exercises

19 A person has cystitis. This is
  a A kidney infection
  b Kidney stones
  c A urinary diversion
  d A bladder infection

20 The person with a urinary diversion
  a Wears a pouch
  b Needs dialysis
  c Has urine strained
  d Has urine tested before meals and at bedtime

21 A person has chronic renal failure. Care includes the following *except*
  a A diet low in protein, potassium, and sodium
  b Measuring urinary output every hour
  c Measures to prevent pressure ulcers
  d Measuring weight daily

22 Which is *not* a sign of diabetes?
  a Increased urine production
  b Weight gain
  c Hunger
  d Increased thirst

23 Joan Martin has diabetes. She needs the following *except*
  a Exercise
  b Good foot care
  c A sodium-controlled diet
  d Healthy eating

24 Vomiting is dangerous because of
  a Aspiration
  b Diverticular disease
  c Fluid loss
  d Stroke

25 AIDS and hepatitis require
  a Airborne Precautions
  b Droplet Precautions
  c Standard Precautions
  d Contact Precautions

26 AIDS is spread by contact with infected
  a Blood
  b Urine
  c Tears
  d Saliva

27 These statements are about HIV and AIDS. Which is *false?*
  a Standard Precautions and the Blood Pathogen Standard are followed.
  b The person may have nervous system damage.
  c The person is at risk for infection.
  d The person always shows some signs and symptoms.

28 Which statement is *false?*
  a STDs are usually spread by sexual contact.
  b STDs can affect the genital area and other parts of the body.
  c Signs and symptoms of STDs are always obvious.
  d Some STDs result in death.

*Answers to these questions are on p. 819.*

# 34

# Mental Health Problems

# OBJECTIVES

- Define the key terms listed in this chapter
- Explain the difference between mental health and mental illness
- List the causes of mental illness
- Explain how personality develops
- Describe three anxiety disorders
- Explain the defense mechanisms used to relieve anxiety
- Describe common phobias
- Explain schizophrenia
- Describe bipolar disorder and depression
- Describe three personality disorders
- Describe substance abuse
- Explain two types of eating disorders
- Describe the care required by persons with mental health disorders

# KEY TERMS

**affect** Feelings and emotions

**anxiety** A vague, uneasy feeling in response to stress

**compulsion** Repeating an act over and over again

**conscious** Awareness of the environment and experiences; the person knows what is happening and can control thoughts and behaviors

**defense mechanism** An unconscious reaction that blocks unpleasant or threatening feelings

**delusion** A false belief

**delusion of grandeur** An exaggerated belief about one's importance, wealth, power, or talents

**delusion of persecution** A false belief that one is being mistreated, abused, or harassed

**ego** The part of the personality dealing with reality; deals with thoughts, feelings, reasoning, good sense, and problem solving

**emotional illness** Mental illness, mental disorder, psychiatric disorder

**hallucination** Seeing, hearing, or feeling something that is not real

**id** The part of the personality at the unconscious level; concerned with pleasure

**mental** Relating to the mind; something that exists in the mind or is done by the mind

**mental disorder** Mental illness, emotional illness, psychiatric disorder

**mental health** The person copes with and adjusts to everyday stresses in ways accepted by society

**mental illness** A disturbance in the ability to cope or adjust to stress; behavior and function are impaired; mental disorder, emotional illness, psychiatric disorder

**obsession** A recurrent, unwanted thought or idea

**panic** An intense and sudden feeling of fear, anxiety, terror, or dread

**paranoia** A disorder (para) of the mind (noia); false beliefs (delusions) and suspicion about a person or situation

**personality** The set of attitudes, values, behaviors, and traits of a person

**phobia** Fear, panic, or dread

**psychiatric disorder** Mental illness, mental disorder, emotional illness

**psychosis** A state of severe mental impairment

**stress** The response or change in the body caused by any emotional, physical, social, or economic factor

**stressor** Any factor that causes stress

**subconscious** Memory, past experiences, and thoughts of which the person is not aware; they are easily recalled

**superego** The part of the personality concerned with right and wrong

**unconscious** Experiences and feelings that cannot be recalled

The whole person has physical, social, psychological, and spiritual parts. Each part affects the other. A physical problem has social, mental, and spiritual effects. Likewise, mental health problems affect the person physically, socially, and spiritually. A social problem can have physical, mental health, and spiritual effects.

## BASIC CONCEPTS

Physical illnesses range from mild to severe. The common cold is at one extreme. The person has chills, fever, and respiratory congestion. At the other extreme is a life-threatening illness. Mental illness has the same extremes.

### MENTAL HEALTH

**Mental** relates to the mind. It is something that exists in the mind or is done by the mind. Therefore mental health involves the mind. Mental health and mental illness involve stress:

- **Stress**—is the response or change in the body caused by any emotional, physical, social, or economic factor.
- **Mental health**—means that the person copes with and adjusts to everyday stresses in ways accepted by society.
- **Mental illness**—is a disturbance in the ability to cope with or adjust to stress. Behavior and function are impaired. **Mental disorder, emotional illness,** and **psychiatric disorder** also mean mental illness.

    Causes of mental health disorders include:
- Not being able to cope or adjust to stress
- Chemical imbalances
- Genetics
- Drug or substance abuse
- Social and cultural factors

### PERSONALITY

**Personality** is the set of attitudes, values, behaviors, and traits of a person. Personality starts to develop at birth. It is affected by many factors. They include genes, culture, environment, parenting, and social experiences.

Maslow's theory of basic needs (Chapter 6) affects personality development. Lower-level needs must be met before higher-level needs. Physical needs are met before safety and security, love and belonging, self-esteem, and self-actualization needs. A child who grows up hungry, neglected, cold, or abused will not feel safe and secure. Higher-level needs cannot be met. Unmet needs at any age affect personality development.

Growth and development tasks (Chapter 8) also affect personality development. There is a sequence, order, and pattern to growth and development. Certain tasks must be accomplished at each stage. Each stage lays the foundation for the next stage.

Freud's theory of personality development involves the id, ego, and superego. It involves three levels of awareness:

- **Conscious**—awareness of the environment and experiences. The person knows what is happening. He or she can control thoughts and behavior.
- **Subconscious**—memory, past experiences, and thoughts of which the person is not aware. They are easily recalled.
- **Unconscious**—experiences and feelings that cannot be recalled.

The **id** part of the personality is at the unconscious level. The id is concerned with pleasure. The need for pleasure must be satisfied almost right away. The id deals with hunger, comfort, sex, and warmth. People are not aware that they behave and act in ways to satisfy the id.

The **ego** deals with reality, with what is happening in the person's world. Thoughts, feelings, reasoning, good sense, and problem solving occur in the ego. The ego decides what to do and when.

The **superego** is concerned with right and wrong. Morals and values are in the superego. The superego judges what the ego thinks and does. It is like a parent helping a child look at behaviors.

## ANXIETY DISORDERS

**Anxiety** is a vague, uneasy feeling in response to stress. The person may not know why or the cause. The person senses danger or harm—real or imagined. The person acts to relieve the unpleasant feeling. Often anxiety occurs when needs are not met.

Some anxiety is normal. Persons with mental health problems have higher levels of anxiety. Signs and symptoms depend on the degree of anxiety (Box 34-1).

Anxiety level depends on the stressor. A **stressor** is any factor that causes stress. It can be physical, emotional, social, or economic. Past experiences affect how a person reacts. So does the number of stressors. A stressor may produce mild anxiety. Anxiety may be higher at another time.

Coping and defense mechanisms are used to relieve anxiety. Some are healthy. Others are not. Coping mechanisms include eating, drinking, smoking, exercising, fighting, and talking about the problem. Some people play music, go for a walk, take a hot bath, or want to be alone.

**Defense mechanisms** are unconscious reactions that block unpleasant or threatening feelings (Box 34-2). Used by everyone, defense mechanisms protect the ego. Some use of defense mechanisms is normal. With mental health problems, they are used poorly.

## BOX 34-1 SIGNS AND SYMPTOMS OF ANXIETY

- A "lump" in the throat
- "Butterflies" in the stomach
- Rapid pulse
- Rapid respirations
- Increased blood pressure
- Rapid speech
- Voice changes
- Dry mouth
- Sweating
- Nausea
- Diarrhea
- Urinary frequency and urgency
- Poor attention span
- Difficulty following directions
- Difficulty sleeping
- Loss of appetite

## PANIC DISORDER

Panic is the highest level of anxiety. **Panic** is an intense and sudden feeling of fear, anxiety, terror, or dread. Onset is sudden with no obvious reason. The person cannot function. Signs and symptoms of anxiety are severe. *Panic attacks* can last for a few minutes or for hours. They can occur often.

## PHOBIAS

**Phobia** means fear, panic, or dread. The person has an intense fear of an object, situation, or activity. Common phobias are fear of:

- Being in an open, crowded, or public place (agoraphobia—*agora* means marketplace)
- Being in pain or seeing others in pain (algophobia—*algo* means pain)
- Water (aquaphobia—*aqua* means water)
- Being in or being trapped in an enclosed or narrow space (claustrophobia—*claustro* means closing)
- The slightest uncleanliness (mysophobia—*myso* means anything that is disgusting)
- Night or darkness (nyctophobia—*nycto* means night or darkness)
- Fire (pyrophobia—*pryo* means fire)
- Strangers (xenophobia—*xeno* means strange)

The person avoids what is feared. When faced with the fear, the person has high anxiety and cannot function.

## BOX 34-2 DEFENSE MECHANISMS

**Compensation.** *Compensate* means to make up for, replace, or substitute. The person makes up for or substitutes a strength for a weakness.
EXAMPLE: A boy is not good in sports. But he learns to play music.

**Conversion.** *Convert* means to change. An emotion is shown or changed into a physical symptom.
EXAMPLE: A girl does not want to read out loud in school. She complains of a headache.

**Denial.** *Deny* means refusing to accept or believe something that is true. The person refuses to face or accept unpleasant or threatening things.
EXAMPLE: A man had a heart attack. He continues to smoke after being told to quit.

**Displacement.** *Displace* means to move or take the place of. An individual moves behaviors or emotions from one person, place, or thing to a safe person, place, or thing.
EXAMPLE: You are angry with your boss. You yell at a friend.

**Identification.** *Identify* means to relate or recognize. A person assumes the ideas, behaviors, and traits of another person.
EXAMPLE: A neighbor is a high school cheerleader. A little girl practices cheerleading in her back yard.

**Projection.** *Project* means to blame another. An individual blames another person or object for unacceptable behaviors, emotions, ideas, or wishes.

EXAMPLE: A girl fails a test. She blames a friend for not helping her study.

**Rationalization.** *Rational* means sensible, reasonable, or logical. An acceptable reason or excuse is given for one's behavior or actions. The real reason is not given.
EXAMPLE: A man is often late for work. He did not get a raise. He says that the boss does not like him.

**Reaction formation.** A person acts in a way opposite to what he or she truly feels.
EXAMPLE: A man does not like his boss. He buys the boss an expensive birthday gift.

**Regression.** *Regress* means to move back or to retreat. The person retreats or moves back to an earlier time or condition.
EXAMPLE: A 3-year-old wants a baby bottle when a new baby comes into the family.

**Repression.** *Repress* means to hold down or keep back. The person keeps unpleasant or painful thoughts or experiences from the conscious mind. They cannot be recalled or remembered.
EXAMPLE: A child was sexually abused. Now 33 years old, she has no memory of the event.

## OBSESSIVE-COMPULSIVE DISORDER

An **obsession** is a recurrent, unwanted thought or idea. **Compulsion** is repeating an act over and over again (a ritual). The act may not make sense, but the person has much anxiety if the act is not done.

Common rituals are hand washing, constant checking to make sure the oven or iron is off, cleaning, and counting to a certain number. Some persons with obsessive-compulsive disorder (OCD) also have depression, eating disorders, substance abuse, and other anxiety disorders.

## SCHIZOPHRENIA

*Schizophrenia* means split *(schizo)* mind *(phrenia)*. It is a severe, chronic, disabling brain disease. It involves:

- **Psychosis**—a state of severe mental impairment. The person does not view the real or unreal correctly.
- **Delusion**—a false belief. For example, a person believes he is God. Or a person believes she is a movie star.
- **Hallucination**—seeing, hearing, or feeling something that is not real. A person may see animals, insects, or people that are not real.
- **Paranoia**—a disorder *(para)* of the mind *(noia)*. The person has false beliefs (delusions). He or she is suspicious about a person or situation. For example, a woman believes her food is poisoned.
- **Delusion of grandeur**—an exaggerated belief about one's importance, wealth, power, or talents. For example, a man believes he is Superman. Or a woman believes she is the Queen of England.
- **Delusion of persecution**—the false belief that one is being mistreated, abused, or harassed. For example, a person believes that someone is "out to get" him or her.

The person with schizophrenia has a severe mental impairment *(psychosis)*. Thinking and behavior are disturbed. The person has false beliefs *(delusions)*. He or she also has hallucinations. That is, the person sees, hears, or feels things that are not real. The person has problems relating to others. He or she may be paranoid. That is, the person is suspicious about a person or situation. Responses are inappropriate. Communication is disturbed. The person may ramble or repeat what another says. Sometimes speech cannot be understood. The person may withdraw. That is, the person lacks interest in others. He or she is not involved with people or society. The person may sit for hours alone without moving, speaking, or responding.

Some persons *regress*. To regress means to retreat or move back to an earlier time or condition. For example, a 5-year-old wets the bed when there is a new baby. This is normal. Healthy adults do not act like infants or children. However, regression often occurs in schizophrenia.

## AFFECTIVE DISORDERS

**Affect** relates to feelings and emotions. Affective disorders involve feelings, emotions, and moods.

### BIPOLAR DISORDER

*Bipolar* means two *(bi)* poles or ends *(polar)*. The person with bipolar disorder has severe extremes in mood, energy, and ability to function. There are emotional lows *(depression)* and emotional highs *(mania)*. The disorder also is called manic-depressive illness. The person may:

- Be more depressed than manic
- Be more manic than depressed
- Alternate between depression and mania

The disorder tends to run in families. See Box 34-3 for the signs and symptoms of mania and depression. They can range from mild to severe. Bipolar disorder can damage relationships and affect school or work performance. Some people are suicidal.

### MAJOR DEPRESSION

Depression involves the body, mood, and thoughts. Symptoms (see Box 34-3) affect work, study, sleep, eating, and other activities. The person is very sad. He or she loses interest in daily activities.

Depression may occur just once. It may be caused by a stressful event such as death of a partner, parent, or child. Divorce and loss of job are other stressful events. For some people, episodes of depression occur throughout life.

*See Focus on Older Persons: Depression.*

---

**FOCUS ON OLDER PERSONS**

**DEPRESSION**

Depression is common in older persons. They have many losses—death of family and friends, loss of health, loss of body functions, loss of independence. Loneliness and the side effects of some drugs also are causes. See Box 34-4 for the signs and symptoms of depression in older persons.

Depression in older persons is often overlooked or a wrong diagnosis is made. Often the person is thought to have a cognitive disorder (Chapter 35). Therefore the depression often is untreated.

---

**BOX 34-3  SIGNS AND SYMPTOMS OF BIPOLAR DISORDER**

**MANIA**

Increased energy, activity, and restlessness
Excessively "high," overly good mood
Extreme irritability
Racing thoughts and talking very fast
Jumping from one idea to another
Easily distracted; problems concentrating
Little sleep needed
Unrealistic beliefs in one's abilities and powers
Poor judgment
Spending sprees
A lasting period of behavior that is different from usual
Increased sexual drive
Abuse of drugs (particularly cocaine, alcohol, and sleeping pills)
Aggressive behavior
Denial that anything is wrong

**DEPRESSION**

Lasting sad, anxious, or empty mood
Feelings of hopelessness
Feelings of guilt, worthlessness, or helplessness
Loss of interest or pleasure in activities once enjoyed
Loss of interest in sex
Decreased energy; a feeling of fatigue or being "slowed down"
Problems concentrating, remembering, or making decisions
Restlessness or irritability
Sleeping too much, or unable to sleep
Change in appetite
Unintended weight loss or gain
Chronic pain or other symptoms not caused by physical illness or injury
Thoughts of death or suicide
Suicide attempts

Modified from *Bipolar Disorder,* National Institute of Mental Health, NIH Pub No 02-3679, 2001.

---

**BOX 34-4  SIGNS AND SYMPTOMS OF DEPRESSION IN OLDER PERSONS**

- Fatigue
- Lack of interest
- Inability to experience pleasure
- Feelings of uselessness
- Feelings of hopelessness
- Feelings of helplessness
- Decreased sexual interest
- Increased dependency
- Anxiety
- Slow or unreliable memory
- Paranoia
- Agitation
- Focus on the past
- Thoughts of death
- Thoughts of suicide
- Difficulty completing activities of daily living
- Changes in sleep patterns
- Lower energy level
- Poor grooming
- Withdrawal from people and interests
- Muscle aches
- Abdominal pain
- Nausea and vomiting
- Dry mouth
- Headaches

Modified from Lueckenotte AG: *Gerontologic nursing,* ed 2, St Louis, 2000, Mosby.

## PERSONALITY DISORDERS

Personality disorders involve rigid and maladaptive behaviors. To *adapt* means to change or adjust. *Mal* means bad, wrong, or ill. *Maladaptive* means to change or adjust in the wrong way. Because of their behaviors, those with personality disorders cannot function well in society. Personality disorders include:

- *Abusive personality.* The person copes with anxiety by abusing others. Behavior may be violent.
- *Paranoid personality.* The person is very suspicious. There is distrust of others.
- *Antisocial personality.* The person has poor judgment. He or she lacks responsibility and is hostile. The person is not loyal to any person or group. Morals and ethics are lacking. Others are blamed for actions and behaviors. The rights of others do not matter. The person has no guilt. He or she does not learn from experiences or punishment. The person is often in trouble with the police.

## SUBSTANCE ABUSE

Substance abuse occurs when a person overuses or depends on drugs or alcohol. Dependence may be emotional, psychological, or physical. According to the Substance Abuse and Mental Health Services Administration, almost 17 million Americans age 12 years or older abused or were dependent on alcohol or illegal drugs in 2001.

Substance abuse affects school and work performance, relationships, health, appearance, and behavior. Money is needed to buy drugs. Therefore money problems are common. Some people steal money or items to sell for drug money.

Legal and illegal drugs are abused. Legal drugs are approved for use in the United States. Doctors prescribe them. Illegal drugs are not approved for use. They are obtained through illegal means.

Commonly abused drugs are listed in Box 34-5. These drugs affect the nervous system. Some depress the nervous system. Others stimulate it. All affect the mind and thinking.

# EATING DISORDERS

Eating disorders involve disturbances in eating behaviors. The two common eating disorders are anorexia nervosa and bulimia nervosa.

# ANOREXIA NERVOSA

*Anorexia* means no (*a*) appetite (*orexis*). *Nervosa* relates to *nerves* or *emotions.* Anorexia nervosa occurs when a person has an intense fear of weight gain and obesity. It occurs mainly in teenage girls and young women.

The person believes she is fat despite being dangerously thin (Fig. 34-1). Poor eating habits include:
- Avoiding food and meals
- Choosing a few foods and eating them in small amounts
- Weighing and measuring food

Intense exercise and vomiting are common. Some people abuse laxatives and enemas to rid the body of food. Laxatives are drugs that rid the intestines of feces through defecation.

Diuretic abuse also may occur. These drugs cause the kidneys to produce large amounts of urine. Extra fluid in the body is lost, causing weight loss.

The person has a poor self-image and may avoid people. Sleep problems and depression may occur. The person may not have monthly menstrual periods. Serious health problems can result. Death is a risk from cardiac arrest or suicide.

| BOX 34-5 | COMMONLY ABUSED SUBSTANCES |
|---|---|

Alcohol
Ativan
Cocaine—Big C, Blow, Coke, Flake, Lady, Nose Candy, Snow, Rock
Codeine
Ecstasy—E, Fantasy, XTC, Adam, Clarity, Lover's Speed
Hallucinogens—LSD, PCP
Hashish
Heroin
Inhalants—glue, paint, solvents
Librium
Marijuana
Methadone
Methamphetamine—Meth, Speed, Ice, Chalk, Crank, Fire, Glass, Crystal
Morphine
OxyContin—Oxy, OC, Oxycotton, Killer
Serax
Valium
Xanax

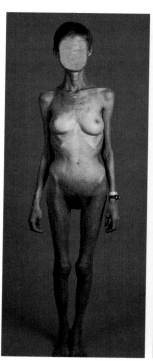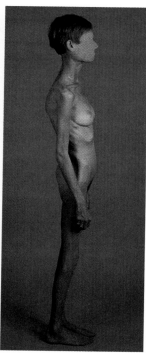

**FIG. 34-1** A person with anorexia nervosa. (Courtesy George D. Comerci, MD, Tucson, Arizona. In Jarvis C: *Physical examination and health assessment,* ed 4, Philadelphia, 2004, WB Saunders.)

## BULIMIA NERVOSA

*Bulimia* comes from the Greek words for ox *(bous)* and hunger *(limos).* It occurs mainly in teenage girls and young women.

Binge eating occurs. That is, the person eats a large amount of food. Then the body is purged (rid) of the food eaten to prevent weight gain. Vomiting, laxatives, enemas, diuretics, fasting, and intense exercise are some methods used.

## CARE AND TREATMENT

Treatment of mental health problems involves having the person explore his or her thoughts and feelings. This is done through psychotherapy and group, occupational, art, and family therapies. Often drugs are ordered.

The RN uses the nursing process to meet the person's needs. The needs of the total person must be met. This includes physical, safety and security, and emotional needs.

Communication is important. Be alert to nonverbal communication. This includes the person's nonverbal communication and your own.

Circle the **BEST** answer.

**1** Stress is
  **a** The way a person copes with and adjusts to everyday living
  **b** A response or change in the body caused by some factor
  **c** A mental or emotional disorder
  **d** A thought or idea

**2** Personality is
  **a** The id and the ego
  **b** A person's attitudes, values, behaviors, and traits
  **c** How a person copes with stress
  **d** A false thought or idea

**3** Experiences in the subconscious
  **a** Can be recalled
  **b** Cannot be recalled
  **c** The person is aware of
  **d** The person can project to others

**4** Which is concerned with right and wrong?
  **a** The id
  **b** The ego
  **c** The superego
  **d** The conscious

**5** Defense mechanisms are used to
  **a** Blame others
  **b** Make excuses for behavior
  **c** Return to an earlier time
  **d** Block unpleasant feelings

**6** These statements are about defense mechanisms. Which is *false*?
  **a** Mentally healthy persons use them.
  **b** They protect the ego.
  **c** They relieve anxiety.
  **d** They prevent mental illness.

**7** A phobia is
  **a** A serious mental health problem
  **b** A false belief
  **c** An intense fear of something
  **d** Feelings and emotions

**8** Mr. Porter cleans and cleans his room. This behavior is
  **a** A Delusion
  **b** A Hallucination
  **c** A Compulsion
  **d** An Obsession

**9** Ms. Mills believes that she is married to a rock singer. This is called a
  **a** Fantasy
  **b** Delusion of grandeur
  **c** Delusion of persecution
  **d** Hallucination

**10** Mr. Walker believes that someone is trying to kill him. This belief is called a
  **a** Fantasy
  **b** Delusion of grandeur
  **c** Delusion of persecution
  **d** Hallucination

**11** Bipolar disorder means that the person
  **a** Is very suspicious
  **b** Has anxiety
  **c** Is very unhappy and feels unwanted
  **d** Has severe mood swings

**12** A person with an abusive personality may
  **a** Abuse drugs or alcohol
  **b** Have an eating disorder
  **c** Have bulimia
  **d** Have violent behavior

*Answers to these questions are on p. 819.*

# 35

# Confusion and Dementia

## OBJECTIVES

- Define the key terms listed in this chapter
- Describe confusion and its causes
- List the measures that help confused persons
- Explain the difference between delirium, depression, and dementia
- Describe Alzheimer's disease (AD)
- Describe the signs, symptoms, and behaviors of AD
- Explain the care required by persons with AD and other dementias
- Describe the effects of AD on the family

## KEY TERMS

**delirium**   A state of temporary but acute mental confusion

**delusion**   A false belief

**dementia**   The loss of cognitive and social function caused by changes in the brain

**hallucination**   Seeing, hearing, or feeling something that is not real

**pseudodementia**   False *(pseudo)* dementia

**sundowning**   Signs, symptoms, and behaviors of AD increase during hours of darkness

Changes in the brain and nervous system occur with aging (Box 35-1). Certain diseases affect the brain. Changes in the brain can affect cognitive function. (*Cognitive* relates to knowledge.) Quality of life is affected. Cognitive functioning involves:

- Memory
- Thinking
- Reasoning
- Ability to understand
- Judgment
- Behavior

Acute confusion (*delirium*) occurs suddenly. It is usually temporary. Causes include infection, illness, injury, drugs, and surgery. Treatment is aimed at the cause.

Confusion caused by physical changes cannot be cured. Some measures help improve function (Box 35-2). You must meet the person's physical and safety needs.

## CONFUSION

Confusion has many causes. Diseases, infections, hearing and vision loss, and drug side effects are some causes. So is brain injury. With aging, there is reduced blood supply to the brain. Brain cells are lost. Personality and mental changes can result. Memory and the ability to make good judgments are lost. A person may not know people, the time, or the place. Some people gradually lose the ability to perform daily activities. Behavior changes are common. The person may be angry, restless, depressed, and irritable.

---

**BOX 35-1   CHANGES IN THE NERVOUS SYSTEM FROM AGING**

- Brain cells are lost.
- Nerve conduction slows.
- Response and reaction times are slower.
- Reflexes are slower.
- Vision and hearing decrease.
- Taste and smell decrease.
- Touch and sensitivity to pain decrease.
- Blood flow to the brain is reduced.
- Sleep patterns change.
- Memory is shorter.
- Forgetfulness occurs.
- Dizziness can occur.

## BOX 35-2 CARING FOR THE CONFUSED PERSON

- Follow the person's care plan.
- Provide for safety.
- Face the person. Speak clearly and slowly.
- Call the person by name every time you are in contact with him or her.
- State your name. Show your name tag.
- Give the date and time each morning. Repeat as needed during the day or evening.
- Explain what you are going to do and why.
- Give clear, simple directions and answers to questions.
- Ask clear and simple questions. Give the person time to respond.
- Keep calendars and clocks with large numbers in the person's room and in nursing areas (Fig. 35-1). Remind the person of holidays, birthdays, and special events.
- Have the person wear eyeglasses and hearing aids as needed.
- Use touch to communicate (Chapter 6).
- Place familiar objects and pictures within the person's view.

- Provide newspapers, magazines, TV, and radio. Read to the person if appropriate.
- Discuss current events with the person.
- Maintain the day-night cycle. Open curtains, shades, and drapes during the day. Close them at night. Use a night-light at night. The person wears regular clothes during the day—not sleepwear.
- Provide a calm, relaxed, and peaceful setting. Prevent loud noises, rushing, and congested hallways and dining rooms.
- Follow the person's routine. Meals, bathing, exercise, TV, and other activities have a schedule. This promotes a sense of order and what to expect.
- Break tasks into small steps when helping the person.
- Do not rearrange furniture or the person's belongings.
- Encourage the person to take part in self-care.
- Be consistent.

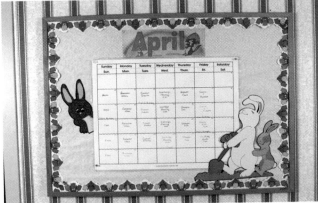

**FIG. 35-1** A large calendar can help confused persons.

## DEMENTIA

**Dementia** is the loss of cognitive function and social function. It is caused by changes in the brain. (*De* means from. *Mentia* means mind.) Alzheimer's disease (AD) is the most common type of dementia. Other types and causes are listed in Box 35-3.

Dementia is not a normal part of aging. Most older people do not have dementia. Some early warning signs include:
- Recent memory loss that affects job skills
- Problems with common tasks (for example, dressing, cooking, driving)

## BOX 35-3 TYPES AND CAUSES OF DEMENTIA

- Alzheimer's disease—see p. 720
- Alcohol-related dementia and Korsakoff disease—alcohol has a toxic effect on brain cells
- AIDS-related dementia—Chapter 33
- Brain tumors—Chapter 33
- Cerebrovascular disease—diseased blood vessels *(vascular)* in the brain *(cerebro)*
- Delirium—a temporary state of acute confusion
- Depression— see p. 720 and Chapter 34
- Drugs—some drugs affect how the brain functions
- Huntington's disease—a nervous system disease
- Infection—Chapter 12
- Multi-infarct dementia—many *(multi)* strokes leave areas of damage *(infarct)*
- Multiple sclerosis—Chapter 33
- Parkinson's disease—Chapter 33
- Stroke—Chapter 33
- Syphilis—Chapter 33
- Trauma and head injury—Chapter 33

- Problems with language; forgetting simple words
- Getting lost in familiar places
- Misplacing things and putting things in odd places (for example, putting a watch in the oven)
- Personality changes
- Poor or decreased judgment (for example, going outdoors in the snow without shoes)
- Loss of interest in life

The person needs to see a doctor. The doctor orders many tests. Treatment depends on the cause and problem. Some dementias can be reversed. When the cause is removed, so are the signs and symptoms. Treatable causes include:

- Drugs
- Alcohol
- Delirium
- Depression
- Tumors
- Heart, lung, and blood vessel problems
- Head injuries
- Infection
- Vision and hearing problems

Permanent dementias result from changes in the brain. They have no cure. Function declines over time. Parkinson's disease causes changes in the brain. So does cardiovascular disease. Multi-infarct dementia (MID) is caused by many (*multi*) strokes. The stroke leaves an area of damage called an *infarct*. AD is the most common type of permanent dementia.

**Pseudodementia** means false (*pseudo*) dementia. The person has the signs and symptoms of dementia. However, there are no changes in the brain. This can occur with delirium and depression. Both can be treated. A correct diagnosis is very important.

## DELIRIUM AND DEPRESSION

Delirium and depression can be mistaken for dementia. They occur alone or with dementia. Or the person with dementia suffers from delirium and depression.

**DELIRIUM.** **Delirium** is a state of temporary but acute mental confusion. Onset is sudden. It is common in older persons with acute or chronic illnesses. Infections, heart and lung diseases, and poor nutrition are common causes. So are hormone disorders. Hypoglycemia is also a cause (Chapter 33). Alcohol and many drugs can cause delirium. Delirium has a short course. It can last for a few hours to as long as 1 month.

Delirium signals physical illness in older persons and in persons with dementia. It is an emergency. The cause must be found and treated. Signs and symptoms of delirium include:

- Anxiety
- Disorientation
- Tremors
- Hallucinations (p. 722)
- Delusions (p. 722)
- Attention problems
- Decline in level of consciousness
- Memory problems

**DEPRESSION.** Depression is the most common mental health problem in older persons. It is often overlooked. A correct diagnosis is needed for proper treatment. Otherwise the person and family have unnecessary emotional, physical, social, and financial discomfort.

Depression, aging, and some drug side effects have similar signs and symptoms. They include:

- Sadness
- Inactivity
- Difficulty thinking
- Problems concentrating
- Feelings of despair
- Problems sleeping
- Changes in appetite
- Fatigue
- Agitation
- Withdrawal

## ALZHEIMER'S DISEASE

Alzheimer's disease (AD) is a brain disease. Brain cells that control intellectual and social function are damaged. These functions are affected:

- Memory
- Thinking
- Reasoning
- Judgment
- Language
- Behavior
- Mood
- Personality

The person has problems with work and everyday functions. Problems with family and social relationships occur. There is a steady decline in memory and mental function.

The disease is gradual in onset. It progresses over 3 to 20 years. It gets worse and worse. AD occurs in both men and women. Women live longer than men do. Therefore more women have AD. Some people in their 40s and 50s have AD. However, it usually occurs after the age of 65. It is often diagnosed around the age of 80. The cause is unknown. A family history of AD and Down syndrome (Chapter 36) are risk factors. Close relatives of persons with Down syndrome also may be at risk.

## SIGNS OF AD

The classic sign of AD is *gradual loss of short-term memory.* Other early signs include:
- Problems finding or speaking the right word
- Not recognizing objects
- Forgetting how to use simple, everyday things (like a pencil)
- Forgetting to turn off the stove, close windows, or lock doors
- Mood and personality changes
- Agitation
- Poor judgment (may cause odd behavior)

AD affects the ability to perform complex and simple tasks. Problems with complex tasks appear first. The person has problems using the phone, driving, managing money, planning meals, and working. Over time, problems occur with simple tasks. These include bathing, dressing, eating, using the toilet, and walking. See Box 35-4 for other signs of AD.

## STAGES OF AD

AD is often described in terms of three stages (Box 35-5, p. 722). Sometimes it is described as having seven stages:
- No cognitive decline
- Very mild cognitive decline
- Mild cognitive decline
- Moderate cognitive decline
- Moderately severe cognitive decline
- Severe cognitive decline
- Very severe cognitive decline

Signs and symptoms become more severe with each stage. The disease ends in death.

## BEHAVIORS

The following behaviors are common with AD.

**WANDERING.** Persons with AD are not oriented to person, time, and place. They may wander away and not find their way back. Wandering may be by foot, car, bicycle, or other means. They may be with you one moment and gone the next.

Judgment is poor. They cannot tell what is safe or dangerous. Life-threatening accidents are great risks. They can walk into traffic or into a nearby river, lake, ocean, or forest. If not properly dressed, heat or cold exposure is a risk.

Wandering may have no cause. Or the person may be looking for something or someone—the bathroom, the bedroom, a child, or a partner. Pain, drug side effects, stress, restlessness, and anxiety are possible causes. Sometimes finding the cause prevents wandering.

For persons living at home, the Alzheimer's Association has a Safe Return program. The program is nationwide. It serves to identify and safely return persons who wander or become lost. A small fee is charged. A family member completes a form and provides a picture. These are entered into a national database. The person receives an ID (wallet card, bracelet or necklace, clothing labels). Anyone finding a person can call the Safe Return number on the ID. Safe Return then calls the family member or caregiver. Some persons are reported missing. Safe Return can provide the person's information and photo to the police.

---

**BOX 35-4  OTHER SIGNS AND SYMPTOMS OF AD**

- Forgets recent events
- Forgets simple directions
- Forgets conversations
- Forgets appointments
- Forgets names (including family members)
- Forgets the names of everyday things (clock, radio, TV, and so on)
- Forgets words
- Substitutes unusual words and names for what is forgotten
- Loses train of thought
- Speaks in a native language
- Curses or swears
- Misplaces things
- Puts things in odd places
- Has problems writing checks or balancing checkbooks
- Gives away large amounts of money
- Does not recognize or understand numbers
- Has problems following conversations
- Has problems reading

- Has problems writing
- Becomes lost in familiar settings
- Forgets where he or she is
- Does not know how to get back home
- Wanders from home
- Cannot tell or understand time
- Cannot tell or understand dates
- Cannot solve everyday problems (iron is left on, stove burners left on, food burning on the stove, and so on)
- Cannot perform everyday tasks (dressing, bathing, brushing teeth, and so on)
- Distrusts others
- Is stubborn
- Withdraws socially
- Is restless
- Becomes suspicious
- Becomes fearful
- Does not want to do things
- Sleeps more than usual

---

**BOX 35-5  STAGES OF ALZHEIMER'S DISEASE**

**STAGE 1: MILD**

- Memory loss—forgetfulness; forgets recent events
- Problems finding words, finishing thoughts, following directions, and remembering names
- Poor judgment; bad decisions (including when driving)
- Disoriented to time and place
- Lack of spontaneity—less outgoing or interested in things
- Blames others for mistakes, forgetfulness, and other problems
- Moodiness
- Problems performing everyday tasks

**STAGE 2: MODERATE**

- Restlessness—increases during the evening hours
- Sleep problems
- Memory loss increases—may not know family and friends
- Dulled senses—cannot tell the difference between hot and cold; cannot recognize dangers
- Fecal and urinary incontinence
- Needs help with activities of daily living (ADL)—bathing, feeding, and dressing self; afraid of bathing; will not change clothes
- Loses impulse control—foul language, poor table manners, sexual aggression; rudeness

- Movement and gait problems—walks slowly, has a shuffling gait
- Communication problems—cannot follow directions; problems with reading, writing, and math; speaks in short sentences or single words; statements may not make sense
- Repeats motions and statements—moves things back and forth constantly; says the same thing over and over again
- Agitation—behavior may be violent

**STAGE 3: SEVERE**

- Seizures (Chapter 40)
- Cannot speak—may groan, grunt, or scream
- Does not recognize self or family members
- Depends totally on others for all activities of daily living
- Disoriented to person, time, and place
- Totally incontinent of urine and feces
- Cannot swallow—choking and aspiration are risks
- Sleep problems increase
- Becomes bed bound—cannot sit or walk
- Coma
- Death

---

**SUNDOWNING.** With **sundowning,** signs, symptoms, and behaviors of AD increase during hours of darkness. It occurs in the late afternoon and evening hours. As daylight ends and darkness starts, confusion and restlessness increase. So do anxiety, agitation, and other symptoms. Behavior is worse after the sun goes down. It may continue throughout the night.

Sundowning may relate to being tired or hungry. Poor light and shadows may cause the person to see things that are not there. Persons with AD may be afraid of the dark.

**HALLUCINATIONS.** A **hallucination** is seeing, hearing, or feeling something that is not real. Senses are dulled. Affected persons see animals, insects, or people that are not present. Some hear voices. They may feel bugs crawling or feel that they are being touched.

Sometimes the problem is caused by impaired vision or hearing. The person needs to wear eyeglasses and hearing aids as prescribed.

**DELUSIONS.** **Delusions** are false beliefs. People with AD may think they are some other person. Some believe they are in jail, are being killed, or are being attacked. A person may believe that the caregiver is someone else. Many other false beliefs can occur.

**CATASTROPHIC REACTIONS.** These are extreme responses. The person reacts as if there is a disaster or tragedy. The person may scream, cry, or be agitated or combative. These reactions are common from too many stimuli. Eating, music or TV playing, and being asked questions all at once can overwhelm the person.

**AGITATION AND RESTLESSNESS.** The person may pace, hit, or yell. Common causes are pain or discomfort, anxiety, lack of sleep, and too many or too few stimuli. Hunger and the need to eliminate also are causes. A calm, quiet setting helps calm the person. So does meeting basic needs.

Caregivers can cause these behaviors. A caregiver may rush the person or be impatient. Or mixed verbal and nonverbal messages are sent. Caregivers always need to look at how their behaviors affect other persons.

**AGGRESSION AND COMBATIVENESS.** These behaviors include hitting, pinching, grabbing, biting, or swearing. They may result from agitation and restlessness. They frighten others.

Sometimes these behaviors are part of the individual's personality. Or pain, fatigue, too much stimulation, caregiver stress, and feeling lost or abandoned are causes. The behaviors can occur during care measures (bathing, dressing) that upset or frighten the person. See Chapter 6 for dealing with the angry person. See Chapter 10 for workplace violence. Also follow the person's care plan.

**SCREAMING.** Persons with AD have communication problems. At first, it is hard to find the right words. As AD progresses, the person speaks in short sentences or in words. Often speech is not understandable.

The person screams to communicate. It is common in persons who are very confused and have poor communication skills. The person may scream a word or a name. Or the person just makes screaming sounds.

Possible causes include hearing and vision problems, pain or discomfort, fear, and fatigue. Too much or not enough stimulation is another cause. The person may react to a caregiver or family member by screaming.

Sometimes these measures are helpful:
- Providing a calm, quiet setting
- Playing soft music
- Having the person wear hearing aids and eyeglasses
- Having a family member or favorite caregiver comfort and calm the person
- Using touch to calm the person

**ABNORMAL SEXUAL BEHAVIORS.** Sexual behaviors are labeled abnormal because of how and when they occur. Persons with AD are not oriented to person, time, and place. Sexual behaviors may involve the wrong person, the wrong place, and the wrong time. They also cannot control behavior. Healthy persons do not undress or expose themselves in front of others. They do not masturbate or engage in sexual pleasures in public. They know their sexual partners. Persons with AD often mistake someone else for a sexual partner. The person kisses and hugs the other person.

Some behaviors are not sexual. Touching, scratching, and rubbing the genitals can signal infection, pain, or discomfort in the urinary or reproductive system. Poor hygiene is another cause. So is being wet or soiled from urine or feces.

The nurse encourages the person's sexual partner to show affection. Their normal practices are encouraged. Examples include hand holding, hugging, kissing, and touching. When a person masturbates in public, lead the person to his or her room. Provide for privacy and safety. Good hygiene prevents itching. Clean the person quickly and thoroughly after elimination. Do not let the person stay wet or soiled.

The RN assesses the person for urinary or reproductive system problems. The doctor is contacted as necessary.

**REPETITIVE BEHAVIORS.** *Repetitive* means to repeat over and over again. Persons with AD repeat the same motions over and over again. For example, the person folds the same napkin over and over. Or the person says the same words over and over. Or the same question is asked. Such behaviors do not harm the person. However, they can annoy caregivers and the family.

Harmless acts are allowed. Music, picture books, exercise, and movies are distracting. Taking the person for a walk can help. Such measures also help when words or questions are repeated.

## CARE OF THE PERSON WITH AD AND OTHER DEMENTIAS

Usually the person is cared for at home until symptoms are severe. Adult day care may help. Often nursing center care is required. Sometimes hospital care is needed for other illnesses. You may care for persons with AD or other dementias in any of these settings. The person and family need your support and understanding.

People with AD do not choose to be forgetful, incontinent, agitated, or rude. Nor do they choose to have other behaviors, signs, and symptoms of the disease. They cannot control what is happening to them. The disease causes the behaviors. *The disease is responsible, not the person.*

Currently AD has no cure. Symptoms worsen over many years. The rate varies from person to person. Over time, persons with AD depend on others for care. Safety, hygiene, nutrition and fluids, elimination, and activity needs must be met. So must comfort and sleep needs. The person's care plan will include many of the measures listed in Box 35-6, p. 724.

Comfort and safety are important. Good skin care and alignment prevent skin breakdown and contractures. You must take special care to treat these persons with dignity and respect. They have the same rights as persons who are alert and active. Talk to them in a calm voice. Always explain what you are going to do. Massage, soothing touch, music, and aromatherapy are comforting and relaxing. The person may need hospice care as death nears (Chapter 41).

The person can have other health problems and injuries. However, the person may not know there is pain, fever, constipation, incontinence, or other signs and symptoms. Carefully observe the person. Report any change in the person's usual behavior to the nurse.

Infection is a major risk. The person cannot fully tend to self-care. Infection can occur from poor hygiene. This includes poor skin care, oral hygiene, and perineal care after bowel and bladder elimination. Inactivity and immobility can cause pneumonia and pressure ulcers.

The person needs to feel useful, worthwhile, and active. This promotes self-esteem. Therapists work with
*Text continued on p. 726.*

## BOX 35-6 CARE OF PERSONS WITH AD AND OTHER DEMENTIAS

### ENVIRONMENT

- Follow established routines.
- Avoid changing rooms or roommates.
- Place picture signs on rooms, bathrooms, dining rooms, and other areas (Fig. 35-2).
- Keep personal items where the person can see them.
- Stay within the person's sight to the extent possible.
- Place memory aids (large clocks, calendars) where the person can see them.
- Keep noise levels low.
- Play music and show movies from the person's past.
- Select tasks and activities specific to the person's cognitive abilities and interests.

### COMMUNICATION

- Approach the person in a calm, quiet manner.
- Approach the person from the front. Do not approach the person from the side or the back. This can startle the person.
- Call the person by name.
- Identify other people by their names. Avoid pronouns (he, she, them, and so on).
- Follow the rules of communication (Chapters 4 and 6).
- Practice measures to promote communication (Chapter 6).
- Use gestures or cues. Point to objects.
- Speak in a calm, gentle voice.
- Speak slowly. Use simple words and sentences.
- Let the person speak. Do not interrupt or rush the person.
- Give the person time to respond.
- Do not criticize, correct, or argue with the person.
- Present one idea, question, or instruction at a time.
- Ask simple questions having simple answers. Do not ask complex questions.
- Do not present the person with many choices.
- Provide simple explanations of all procedures and activities.
- Give consistent responses.

### SAFETY

- Remove harmful, sharp, and breakable objects from the area. This includes knives, scissors, glass, dishes, razors, and tools.
- Provide plastic eating and drinking utensils. This helps prevent breakage and cuts.
- Place safety plugs in electrical outlets.
- Keep cords and electrical equipment out of reach.
- Remove electrical appliances from the bathroom. Examples include hair dryers, curling irons, make-up mirrors, and electric shavers.
- Store personal care items (shampoo, deodorant, lotion, and so on) in a safe place.
- Keep childproof caps on medicine containers and household cleaners.
- Store household cleaners and drugs in locked storage areas.

- Store dangerous equipment and tools in a safe place.
- Remove knobs from stoves, or place childproof covers on the knobs.
- Remove dangerous appliances and power tools from the home.
- Remove firearms from the home.
- Store car keys in a safe place.
- Supervise the person who smokes.
- Store cigarettes, cigars, pipes, matches and other smoking materials in a safe place.
- Practice safety measures to prevent falls (Chapter 10).
- Practice safety measures to prevent fires (Chapter 10).
- Practice safety measures to prevent burns (Chapter 10).
- Practice safety measures to prevent poisoning (Chapter 10).
- Keep all doors to kitchens, utility rooms, and housekeeping closets locked.

### WANDERING

- Follow agency policy for locking doors and windows. In home settings, locks are often placed at the top and bottom of doors (Fig. 35-3). The person is not likely to look for a lock in such places.
- Keep door alarms and electronic doors turned on. The alarm goes off when the door is opened.
- Follow agency policy for fire exits. Everyone must be able to leave the building if there is a fire.
- Make sure the person wears an ID bracelet or Safe Return ID at all times.
- Exercise the person as ordered. Adequate exercise often reduces wandering.
- Involve the person in activities—folding napkins, dusting a table, sorting socks, rolling yarn, sweeping, sanding blocks of wood, or watering plants.
- Do not use restraints. Restraints require a doctor's order. They also tend to increase confusion and disorientation.
- Do not argue with the person who wants to leave. The person does not understand what you are saying.
- Go with the person who insists on going outside. Make sure he or she is properly dressed. Guide the person inside after a few minutes (Fig. 35-4, p. 726).
- Let the person wander in enclosed areas. Many nursing centers have enclosed areas where residents can walk about (Fig. 35-5, p. 726). They provide a safe place for the person to wander.

### SUNDOWNING

- Complete treatments and activities early in the day.
- Provide a calm, quiet setting late in the day.
- Do not restrain the person.
- Encourage exercise and activity early in the day.
- Meet nutrition needs. Hunger can increase restlessness.
- Promote elimination. The need to eliminate can increase restlessness.

## BOX 35-6  CARE OF PERSONS WITH AD AND OTHER DEMENTIAS—CONT'D

### SUNDOWNING—CONT'D

- Do not try to reason with the person. He or she cannot understand what you are saying.
- Do not ask the person to tell you what is bothering him or her. Communication is impaired. The person does not understand what you are asking. He or she cannot think or speak clearly.

### HALLUCINATIONS AND DELUSIONS

- Make sure the person wears eyeglasses and hearing aids as needed. Follow the care plan.
- Do not argue with the person. He or she does not understand what you are saying.
- Reassure the person. Tell him or her that you will provide protection from harm.
- Distract the person with some item or activity. Taking the person for a walk may be helpful.
- Use touch to calm and reassure the person.
- Eliminate noises that the person could misinterpret. TV, radio, stereos, furnaces, air conditioners, and other things could affect the person.
- Check lighting. Make sure there are no glares, shadows, or reflections.
- Cover or remove mirrors. The person could misinterpret his or her reflection.

### SLEEP

- Follow bedtime rituals.
- Use night-lights so the person can see. They help prevent accidents and disorientation.
- Limit caffeine during the day.
- Discourage naps during the day.
- Encourage exercise during the day.
- Reduce noises.

### BASIC NEEDS

- Meet food and fluid needs (Chapter 20). Provide finger foods. Cut food and pour liquids as needed.
- Provide good skin care (Chapter 16). Keep the person's skin free of urine and feces.

- Promote urinary and bowel elimination (Chapters 18 and 19).
- Provide incontinence care as needed (Chapters 18 and 19).
- Promote exercise and activity during the day (Chapter 22). This helps reduce wandering and sundowning behaviors. The person may also sleep better.
- Reduce intake of coffee, tea, and cola drinks. These contain caffeine. Caffeine is a stimulant. It can increase restlessness, confusion, and agitation.
- Provide a quiet, restful setting (Chapter 23). Soft music is better than loud TV programs.
- Play music during care activities such as bathing and during meals.
- Promote personal hygiene (Chapter 16). Do not force the person into a shower or tub. People with AD are often afraid of bathing. Try bathing the person when he or she is calm. Use the person's preferred bathing method (tub bath, shower, bed bath). Provide privacy, and keep the person warm. Do not rush the person.
- Provide oral hygiene (Chapter 16).
- Choose clothing that is comfortable and simple to put on. Front-opening garments are easy to put on. Pullover tops are harder to put on. And the person may become frightened when his or her head is inside the pullover top.
- Select clothing that closes with Velcro. Such items are easy to put on and take off. Buttons, zippers, snaps, and other closures can frustrate the person.
- Offer simple clothing choices (Fig. 35-6, p. 726). Let the person choose between two shirts or two blouses, two pants or two slacks, and so on.
- Lay clothing out in the order it will be put on. Hand the person one clothing item at a time. Tell or show the person what to do. Do not rush him or her.
- Have equipment ready for any procedure. This reduces the amount of time the person is involved in care measures.
- Observe for signs and symptoms of health problems (Chapters 5 and 33).
- Prevent infection (Chapter 12).

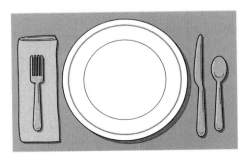

FIG. 35-2 Signs give cues to persons with dementia.

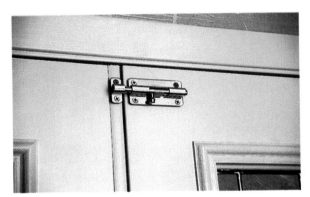

FIG. 35-3 A slide lock is at the top of the door.

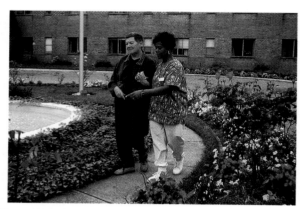

**FIG. 35-4** Walk outside with the person who wanders. Then guide the person back inside after a few minutes.

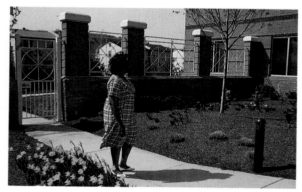

**FIG. 35-5** An enclosed garden allows persons with AD to wander in a safe setting.

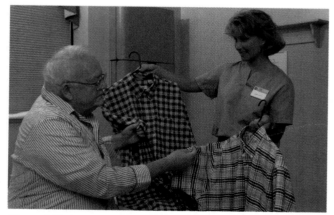

**FIG. 35-6** The person with AD is offered simple clothing choices.

one person, a small group, or a large group. Therapies and activities focus on the person's strengths and past successes. For example:

- A woman used to cook. She helps clean fruit.
- A man was a good dancer. Activities are planned so he can dance.
- A man likes to clean. He helps with dusting.

Supervised activities meet the person's needs and cognitive abilities. The person's interests are considered. Activities are based on what the person enjoys and can do. Some people like crafts, exercise, gardening, and listening and moving to music. Others like sing-alongs, reminiscing, and board games. Some like to string beads, fold towels, or roll dough. Massage, range-of-motion exercises, and touch are also important therapies.

*See Focus on Long-Term Care: Caring for Persons With AD and Other Dementias.*

## THE FAMILY

The person may live at home or with a partner, children, or other family members. The family gives care. Or someone stays with the person. Health care is sought when the family cannot deal with the situation or meet the person's needs. Home health care may help for a while. Adult day care is an option (Chapter 9). Long-term care is needed when:

- Family members cannot meet the person's needs
- The person no longer knows the caregiver
- Family members have health problems
- Money problems occur
- The person's behaviors present dangers to self or others

Diagnostic tests, doctor's visits, drugs, and home care are costly. So is long-term care. The person's medical care can drain family finances.

The family has special needs. Caring for the person at home or in a nursing center is stressful. There are physical, emotional, social, and financial stresses. Adult children are in the *sandwich generation.* They are caught between their own children who need attention and an ill parent who needs care. Caring for two families is stressful. Often adult children have jobs too.

Caregivers can suffer from anger, anxiety, depression, and sleeplessness. Some cannot concentrate or are irritable. They can develop health problems. They need to take care of their own health. A healthy diet, exercise, and plenty of rest are needed. Asking for help is important. The caregiver needs to feel free to ask family and friends for help.

Caregivers need much support and encouragement. Many join AD support groups. The groups are sponsored by hospitals, nursing centers, and the Alzheimer's Association. The Alzheimer's Association has chapters in cities and towns across the country. Support groups offer encouragement and advice.

## FOCUS ON LONG-TERM CARE
### CARING FOR PERSONS WITH AD AND OTHER DEMENTIAS

Many nursing centers have special care units for persons with AD and other dementias. Some units are secured. This means that entrances and exits are locked. Persons in these units have a safe setting to move about it. They cannot wander away. Some persons have aggressive behaviors that disrupt or threaten others. They may need a secured unit.

At some point, the secured unit is no longer needed for safe care. For example, the person's condition progresses from stage 2 to stage 3. The person cannot sit or walk. Wandering is not a concern. The person is transferred to another unit.

Quality of life is important for all persons with confusion and dementia. Nursing center residents have rights under OBRA. They may not know or be able to exercise their rights. However, the family knows the person's rights. They want those rights protected. They want respect and dignity for the loved one.

The person has the right to privacy and confidentiality. Protect the person from exposure. Only those involved in the person's care are present for care and procedures. The person is allowed to visit in private. Space is provided for a private visit. Protect confidentiality. Do not share information about the person's care and condition with others.

Personal choice is important. If able, simple choices are encouraged. For example, a person chooses to wear a dress or slacks. Watching or not watching TV may be a simple choice. The family makes choices if the person cannot. They choose bath times, menus, clothing, activities, and other care.

The person has the right to keep and use personal items. Some items provide comfort. A pillow, blanket, afghan, or sweater may have meaning to the person. The person may not know why or even recognize the item. Still, it is important. Personal items are kept safe. Protect the person's property from loss or damage.

These persons must be kept free from abuse, mistreatment, and neglect. Caring for persons with confusion and dementia is often very frustrating. Some behaviors are hard to deal with. Family and staff can become short-tempered and angry. Protect the person from abuse (Chapter 2). Report any signs of abuse to the nurse at once. Be patient and calm when caring for these persons. Talk with the nurse if you are becoming upset. Sometimes an assignment change is needed for a while.

All persons have the right to be free from restraints. Restraints require a doctor's order. They are used only if it is the best way to protect the person. They are not used for staff convenience. Restraints can make confusion and demented behaviors worse. The nurse tells you when to use restraints.

Activity and a safe setting promote quality of life (see Box 35-6). Safe, calm, and quiet activities are needed. The recreational therapist and other health team members will find activities that are best for each person. These are part of the person's care plan.

---

People in similar situations share their feelings, anger, frustration, guilt, and other emotions. They also share coping and caregiving ideas.

The family often feels helpless. No matter what is done, the person only gets worse. Much time, money, energy, and emotion are needed to care for the person. Anger and resentment may result. Guilt feelings are common. The family also knows that the person did not choose the disease. They know that the person does not choose to have its signs, symptoms, and behaviors. Sometimes behaviors are embarrassing. The family may be upset and angry that the loved one cannot show love or affection.

The family is an important part of the health team. They help plan the person's care whenever possible. They need to learn how to bathe, feed, dress, and give oral hygiene to the person. They also need to learn how to provide a safe setting. The RN and support group will help the family learn to give necessary care. *See Focus on Home Care: The Family.*

## FOCUS ON HOME CARE
### THE FAMILY

Home care is an option for many families. They may need someone to prepare the person's meals. Help is often needed with bathing and elimination. Someone needs to supervise the person while family members work, do errands, or have time to themselves. The amount and kind of care depend on the person's needs and the family's ability to provide care.

## VALIDATION THERAPY

Validation therapy may be part of the person's care plan. The therapy is based on the following principles:

- All behavior has meaning.
- Development occurs in a sequence, order, and pattern. Certain tasks must be completed during a stage of development. A stage cannot be skipped. Each stage is the basis for the next stage.
- If a person does not successfully complete a stage of development, unresolved issues and emotions may surface later in life.
- A person may return to the past to resolve such issues and emotions.
- Caregivers need to listen and provide empathy.
- Attempts are not made to correct the person's thoughts or bring the person back to reality. For example:
  —While going from room to room, Mrs. Bell calls for her babies. In reality, her babies died shortly after birth. The caregiver does not tell Mrs. Bell that her babies died after they were born. Instead, the caregiver says: "Tell me about your babies."

—Mrs. Brown sits all day on a bench by the window. She says that she is at the train station waiting to meet her husband. In reality, her husband was killed during World War II. Buried in England, he never returned home. The caregiver does not remind Mrs. Brown of what happened. Instead, the caregiver encourages Mrs. Brown to talk about her husband.

—Mr. Garcia was 3 years old when his father died. He holds a ball constantly. He is very upset when anyone tries to remove it from his hand. He calls for his father and repeats "play ball, play ball." The caregiver does not remind Mr. Garcia that he is 80 years old and that his father died many years ago. Instead, the caregiver says, "Tell me about playing ball."

The health team decides if validation therapy might help a person. If so, it will be part of the person's care plan. Proper use of validation therapy requires special training. If the therapy is used in your agency, you will receive the training needed to use it correctly.

# ■ REVIEW QUESTIONS ■

Circle the **BEST** answer.

1 Cognitive function relates to the following *except*
   a Memory loss and personality
   b Thinking and reasoning
   c Ability to understand
   d Judgment and behavior

2 A person is confused after surgery. The confusion is likely to be
   a Permanent
   b Temporary
   c Caused by an infection
   d Caused by a brain injury

3 The confused person is
   a Restrained in bed at night
   b Given many tasks to keep busy
   c Easily distracted
   d Never a danger to self or others

4 Joe Dunn has delusions. A delusion is
   a A false belief
   b An illness caused by changes in the brain
   c Seeing, hearing, or feeling something that is not real
   d Alzheimer's disease

5 Joe Dunn has AD. Which is *true?*
   a AD occurs only in older persons.
   b Diet and drugs can control the disease.
   c AD and delirium are the same.
   d AD ends in death.

6 The following are common in persons with AD *except*
   a Memory loss, poor judgment, and sleep disturbances
   b Loss of impulse control and the ability to communicate
   c Wandering, delusions, and hallucinations
   d Paralysis, dyspnea, and pain

7 Sundowning means that
   a The person becomes sleepy when the sun sets
   b Behaviors become worse in the late afternoon and evening hours
   c Behavior improves at night
   d The person is in the third stage of the disease

8 Joe Dunn is screaming. You know that this is
   a An agitated reaction
   b His way of communicating
   c Caused by a delusion
   d A repetitive behavior

9 AD support groups do the following *except*
   a Provide care
   b Offer encouragement and care ideas
   c Provide support for the family
   d Promote the sharing of feelings and frustrations

10 Joe Dunn tends to wander. You should do the following *except*
   a Make sure doors alarms are turned on
   b Make sure he wears an ID bracelet
   c Help him with exercise as ordered
   d Tell him where to wander safely

11 Safety is important for Joe Dunn. Which is *false?*
   a Safety plugs are placed in electrical outlets.
   b Cleaners and drugs are kept locked up.
   c He can keep smoking materials.
   d Sharp and breakable objects are removed from his environment.

12 You are caring for Joe Dunn. Which is *false?*
   a You can reason with him.
   b Touch can calm and reassure him.
   c A calm, quiet setting is important.
   d Help is needed with ADL.

*Answers to these questions are on p. 820.*

# Developmental Disabilities

## OBJECTIVES

- Define the key terms listed in this chapter
- Identify the areas of function limited by a developmental disability
- Explain how a developmental disability affects the child and family across the life span
- Explain when developmental disabilities occur
- Describe the causes of developmental disabilities
- Explain how the various developmental disabilities affect a person's function

## KEY TERMS

**convulsion**  A seizure

**developmental disability**  A disability occurring before 22 years of age

**diplegia**  Similar body parts are affected on both sides of the body

**seizure**  The violent and sudden contractions or tremors of muscle groups; convulsion

**spastic**  Uncontrolled contractions of skeletal muscles

Many diseases, illnesses, and injuries causing disability occur in adulthood. However, some infants have congenital defects. (*Congenital* means present at birth.) The defects result in disabilities. Childhood illnesses and injuries also can result in disabilities.

A disability occurring before 22 years of age is called a **developmental disability.** It can be a physical, cognitive, psychological, sensory, or speech disability. It is severe and permanent. Function is limited in three or more life skills:

- Self-care
- Understanding and expressing language
- Learning
- Mobility
- Self-direction
- Capacity for independent living
- Economic self-sufficiency (supporting oneself financially)

Developmentally disabled children become adults. They are not children forever. They need lifelong assistance, support, and special services. Both the child and parents grow older. Often it is harder to care for an older child or adult. It may be hard to lift or move the person. A parent may become ill, injured, or disabled or die. Yet the disabled person still needs care.

Some children are severely disabled. They need long-term care in centers for those who are developmentally disabled. Some nursing centers admit developmentally disabled adults. OBRA requires that centers provide age-appropriate activities for them. Staff must have special training to meet their care needs.

Developmental disabilities are caused before, during, and after birth. These conditions are common:

- Mental retardation
- Down syndrome
- Cerebral palsy
- Autism
- Epilepsy
- Spina bifida

## MENTAL RETARDATION

Mental retardation involves low intellectual function. Adaptive behavior is impaired. (*Intellectual function* relates to learning, thinking, and reasoning. *Adapt* means to change or adjust.) The Arc of the United States is a national organization focused on mental retardation. According to the Arc, mental retardation involves:

- *An IQ score below 70 to 75.* The person learns at a slower rate than normal. The ability to learn is less than normal.
- *Limits in two or more adaptive skill areas.* The skills are needed to live, work, and play. They involve communication, self-care, home living, social skills, and leisure. They also involve health and safety, self-direction, basic academics, community use, and work. Activities of daily living are hard for the person. Understanding the behavior of others is limited. So is the ability to respond in socially correct ways.
- *The condition being present before 18 years of age.*

Brain development is impaired. It can occur before birth, during birth, or before the age of 18 years. Causes are listed in Box 36-1.

Mental retardation ranges from mild to severe. Some persons are mildly affected. They are slow to learn in school. As adults, they can function in society with some support. For example, help is needed finding a job. Support is not needed every day. Some persons need much support every day at home or at work. Still others need constant support in all areas.

The Arc believes that children with mental retardation should live in a family. They should learn and play with children with and without disabilities. As adults, they should control their lives to the greatest extent possible. They should speak, make choices, and act for themselves. They should live in a home and have friends. They should do meaningful work and enjoy adult activities.

The Arc recognizes the sexuality of persons with mental retardation. They have physical, emotional, and social needs and desires. Reproductive organs develop. Remember, adaptive skills vary from moderate to severe. Some have life partners. Others marry and have children. Some persons can control their sexual

urges. Others cannot. The type and location of their sexual responses may be inappropriate. Also, some adults sexually abuse persons with mental retardation. The Arc believes that persons with mental retardation:

- Have the right to privacy
- Have the right to love and be loved
- Have the right to develop friendships and emotional relationships
- Should learn about sex, sexual abuse, safe sex, and other sex and sexuality issues

## DOWN SYNDROME

Down syndrome (DS) is named for the doctor who identified the syndrome. DS is often caused by an extra 21st chromosome. At fertilization, a male sex cell (sperm) unites with a female sex cell (ovum). Each sex cell has 23 chromosomes. When they unite, the cell has 46 chromosomes. In DS, an extra chromosome is present. The person has 47 chromosomes. Thus DS occurs at fertilization.

DS causes some level of mental retardation. It is usually moderate to severe. The child also has certain features caused by the extra chromosome (Fig. 36-1):

- Small head
- Oval-shaped eyes that slant upward
- Flat face
- Short, wide neck
- Large tongue
- Wide, flat nose
- Small ears
- Short stature
- Short, wide hands with stubby fingers
- Low muscle tone

---

### BOX 36-1 CAUSES OF MENTAL RETARDATION

**GENETIC CONDITIONS**

Abnormal genes from one or both parents
Down syndrome
Fragile X syndrome

**DURING PREGNANCY**

Alcohol use (fetal alcohol syndrome)
Drug use
Poor nutrition
German measles (rubella)
Diabetes
HIV infection
Lack of oxygen to the brain

**DURING BIRTH**

Head injury
Prematurity
Low birth weight
Lack of oxygen to the brain

**AFTER BIRTH**

Childhood diseases (whooping cough, chicken pox, measles)
Head injuries
Near drowning
Mercury poisoning
Lead poisoning
Poor nutrition
Child abuse (including shaken baby syndrome)

---

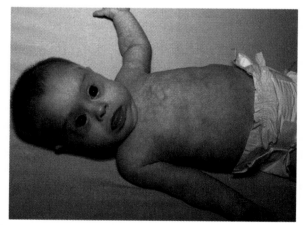

**FIG. 36-1** An infant with Down syndrome. (From Hockenberry MJ and others: *Wong's nursing care of infants and children*, ed 7, St Louis, 2003, Mosby.)

Many children with DS have heart defects. They tend to have vision and hearing problems. They are at risk for ear infections, respiratory infections, and thyroid gland problems. Leukemia also is a risk. After age 35 years, persons with DS are at risk for Alzheimer's disease.

Persons with DS need speech, language, physical, and occupational therapies. Most learn self-care skills. They also need health and sex education. Weight gain and constipation often are problems. They need a well-balanced diet and regular exercise.

# CEREBRAL PALSY

Cerebral palsy (CP) is a term applied to a group of disorders involving muscle weakness or poor muscle control *(palsy)*. The defect is in the motor region of the brain *(cerebral)*. Abnormal movements, posture, and coordination result. The defect results from brain damage. It occurs before, during, or within a few months after birth. Lack of oxygen to the brain is the usual cause. Congenital brain defects (faulty brain development) are other causes. There is no cure.

Infants at risk include those who:
- Are premature
- Have low birth weight
- Do not cry in the first 5 minutes after birth
- Need mechanical ventilation
- Have bleeding in the brain
- Have heart, kidney, or spinal cord defects
- Have blood problems
- Have seizures
- Have fetal alcohol syndrome

Brain damage in infancy and early childhood also can result in CP. Lack of oxygen to the brain can occur from:
- Choking (Chapter 40)
- Poisoning
- Near drowning
- Head injuries from accidents, falls, or child abuse (including shaken baby syndrome)
- Meningitis (inflammation of the covering around the brain and spinal cord)
- Encephalitis (inflammation of the brain)

Body movements and body parts are affected. These types are the most common:
- *Spastic cerebral palsy. Spastic* comes from *spastikos.* It means to draw in. **Spastic** means uncontrolled contractions of skeletal muscles. Muscles contract or shorten. They are stiff and cannot relax. One or both sides of the body may be involved. Posture, balance, and movement are affected. The arms may be affected. If so, there are problems with eating, writing, dressing, and other activities of daily living.

- *Athetoid cerebral palsy.* The person cannot control movements. *Athetoid* comes from *athetos.* It means not fixed. The person has constant, slow, weaving or writhing motions. These occur in the trunk, arms, hands, legs, and feet. Sometimes the tongue, face, and neck muscles are involved. Drooling and grimacing result.

Certain terms describe the body parts involved:
- *Hemiplegia.* The arm and leg on one side are affected.
- *Diplegia. Di* means twice. **Diplegia** means that similar body parts are affected on both sides of the body. Both arms or both legs are paralyzed. The legs are commonly involved.
- *Quadriplegia.* Both arms and both legs are paralyzed. So are the trunk and neck muscles.

The person with CP can have many other impairments. They include:
- Mental retardation
- Learning disabilities
- Hearing impairments
- Speech impairments
- Vision impairments
- Drooling
- Bladder and bowel control problems
- Seizures
- Difficulty swallowing
- Attention deficit hyperactivity disorder (short attention span, poor concentration, increased activity)
- Breathing problems from poor posture
- Pressure ulcers from immobility

Care needs depend on the degree of brain damage. The goal is for the person to be as independent as possible. Physical, occupational, and speech therapy can help. Some need eyeglasses and hearing aids. Surgery and drugs can help some muscle problems.

# AUTISM

Autism begins in early childhood—between 18 months and 3 years. (*Autos* means self.) It is a brain disorder with no cure. Social skills, verbal and nonverbal communication skills, behavior, and play are impaired. It is hard for the child to relate to people. Boys are affected more than girls are.

Children are mildly to severely affected. The following are common:
- Slow language development
- Talks later than other children
- Repeats words or phrases
- Does not start or maintain conversations
- Uses gestures
- Repeats body movements (hand flapping, hand twisting, rocking)
- Short attention span

- Spends time alone
- Little or no eye contact
- Over-reacts to touch
- Does not like to cuddle
- Little reaction to pain
- Frequent tantrums for no apparent reason
- Strong attachment to a single item, idea, activity, or person
- Needs routines
- Does not like change
- Does not fear danger
- Does not respond to others
- May act deaf
- Does not respond to his or her name
- Very active or very quiet
- Aggressive or violent behavior
- May injure self

With therapy, the person can learn to change or control behaviors. Many therapies are used. They include:

- Behavior modification
- Speech and language therapy
- Music therapy
- Auditory training
- Sensory therapies
- Physical therapy
- Occupational therapy
- Drug therapy
- Diet therapy
- Communication therapy
- Recreation therapy

The person needs to develop social and work skills. Children with autism become adults. Some adults work and live independently. Others need support and help from family and community services. Some live in group homes or residential care centers.

Persons with autism may have other disorders. Mental retardation and epilepsy are common.

## EPILEPSY

The Epilepsy Foundation of America describes epilepsy as a chronic condition produced by temporary changes in the brain's electrical function. These changes occur from time to time. They involve bursts of electrical energy that cause seizures. The seizures affect awareness, movement, or sensation. (Epilepsy comes from *epilepsia*. It means seizure.)

A **seizure** (or **convulsion**) involves violent and sudden contractions or tremors of muscle groups. Movements are uncontrolled. The person may lose consciousness. Seizures can occur in one part of the brain. They are *partial seizures*. Some seizures involve the whole brain. They are *generalized seizures*.

A single seizure does not mean epilepsy. In epilepsy, seizures recur. The person has a permanent brain injury or defect. Known causes include:

- Brain injury before, during, or after birth
- Lack of oxygen before, during, or after birth
- Problems with brain development before birth
- The mother having an injury or infection during pregnancy
- Head trauma (accidents, gun shot wounds, sports injuries, falls, blows to the head)
- Chemical imbalance
- Poor nutrition
- Brain tumor
- Childhood fevers
- Poison—such as lead and alcohol
- Infection—such as meningitis and encephalitis
- Stroke

Children and young adults are commonly affected. However, epilepsy can develop at any time during the person's life. It can occur with any problem affecting the brain. Such problems include:

- Cerebral palsy
- Mental retardation
- Autism
- Alzheimer's disease
- Stroke
- Tumor
- Traumatic brain injury

There is no cure at this time. Doctors order drugs to prevent seizures. The drugs control seizures in many people. For other persons, drug therapy does not work.

When controlled, epilepsy usually does not affect learning and activities of daily living. Activity and job limits occur in severe cases. For example, a person has seizures at any time. The person may not be allowed to drive. This may limit job choices. Also, the person is at risk for accidents and injuries. Safety measures are needed. They are needed for the home, workplace, transportation, and recreation.

These persons have an increased risk of death. They have higher rates of suicide and sudden unexplained death syndrome. They also have higher rates of accidental death, especially drowning.

See Chapter 40 for the emergency care of persons having seizures.

## SPINA BIFIDA

Spina bifida is a defect of the spinal column. (*Spina* means backbone. *Bifid* means split in two parts.) The defect occurs during the first month of pregnancy. Hydrocephalus often occurs with spina bifida (p. 736).

Bones of the spinal column are called *vertebrae.* They protect the spinal cord. In spina bifida, vertebrae do not form properly. This leaves a split in the vertebrae. The split leaves the spinal cord unprotected. Only a membrane covers the spinal cord. The spinal cord contains nerves. The nerves send messages to and from the brain. If the spinal cord is unprotected, nerve damage occurs. Affected body parts do not function properly. Paralysis may occur. Bowel and bladder problems are common. Infection is a threat.

Spina bifida can occur anywhere in the spine. The lower back is the most common site. Types of spina bifida include:

- *Spina bifida occulta. Occult* means hidden. The vertebrae are closed. A defect occurs in the vertebrae closure. In other words, the defect is hidden. The spinal cord and nerves are normal. The person has a dimple or tuft of hair on the back (Fig. 36-2). Often there are no symptoms. Foot weakness and bowel and bladder problems can occur.
- *Spina bifida cystica. Cystica* means pouch or sac. Part of the spinal column is in the pouch or sac. A membrane or a thin layer of skin covers the sac. It looks like a large blister. The pouch is easily injured. Infection is a threat. There are two types of spina bifida cystica (Fig. 36-3):
  —*Meningocele. Meningo* comes from *meninx.* It means membrane. *Cele* means hernia or swelling. Meninges are the connective tissue that covers and protects the brain and spinal cord. Cerebrospinal fluid also protects the brain and spinal cord. The sac contains meninges and cerebrospinal fluid (see Fig. 36-3, *A* and Fig. 36-4). The sac does not contain nerve tissue. The spinal cord and nerves are usually normal. Nerve damage usually does not occur. Surgery corrects the defect.
  —*Myelomeningocele* (or *meningomyelocele*). *Myelo* means spinal cord. The pouch contains nerves, spinal cord, meninges, and cerebrospinal fluid (see Fig. 36-3, *B*). Nerve damage occurs. Loss of function occurs below the level of damage. Leg paralysis and lack of sensation are common problems. So is the lack of bowel and bladder control. The defect is closed with surgery. Some children walk with braces or crutches. Others use wheelchairs.

Some children have learning problems. They may have problems with attention, language, reading, and math. They are at high risk for obesity, GI disorders, and mobility problems. Skin breakdown, depression, and social and sexual issues are other risks.

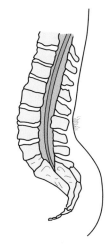

**FIG. 36-2** Spina bifida occulta.

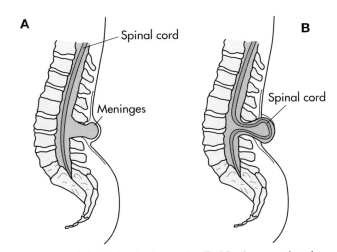

**FIG. 36-3 A,** Meningocele. **B,** Meningomyelocele.

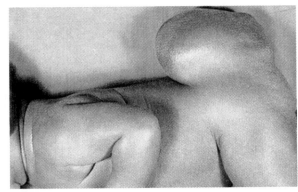

**FIG. 36-4** Meningocele. (From Zitelli BJ, Davis HW: *Atlas of pediatric physical diagnosis,* St Louis, 1987, Gower Medical Publishing.)

# HYDROCEPHALUS

With hydrocephalus, cerebrospinal fluid collects in and around the brain. (*Hydro* means water. *Cephalo* means head.) The head enlarges (Fig. 36-5). Pressure inside the head increases. Mental retardation and neurological damage occur without treatment.

A shunt is placed in the brain. It allows cerebrospinal fluid to drain. The shunt is a long, flexible tube. It goes from the brain to a body cavity (Fig. 36-6). Fluid drains from the brain through the tube. Usually it drains into the abdomen or a heart chamber. The shunt must remain open *(patent)*. If blocked, the cerebrospinal fluid cannot drain from the brain.

The person can have many problems. Vision problems, seizures, and learning disabilities can occur.

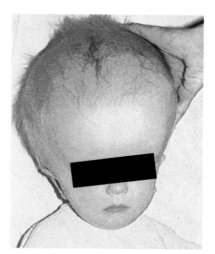

**FIG. 36-5** Hydrocephalus. (From Hart CA, Broadhead RL: *Color atlas of pediatric infectious diseases,* London, 1992, Mosby-Wolfe.)

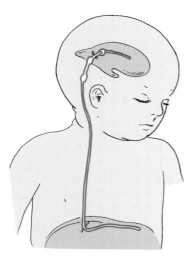

**FIG. 36-6** A shunt drains fluid from the brain. (From Hockenberry MJ and others: *Wong's nursing care of infants and children,* ed 7, St Louis, 2003, Mosby.)

# ■ REVIEW QUESTIONS ■

Circle the **BEST** answer.

1 All developmental disabilities occur
  a At birth
  b From trauma
  c During pregnancy
  d Before 22 years of age

2 These statements are about developmental disabilities. Which is *true?*
  a Self-care, learning, and mobility are always affected.
  b The disability is severe and permanent.
  c Physical and intellectual impairment occur together.
  d The person cannot hold a job.

3 The person with mental retardation
  a Has delayed development of sexual organs
  b Does not have the skills to live, work, and play
  c Requires care in a special setting
  d Learns at a slower rate than normal

4 Mental retardation
  a Is always severe
  b Can occur before, during, or after birth
  c Is caused by an extra chromosome
  d Affects the motor region of the brain

5 Down syndrome occurs
  a At fertilization
  b During the first month of pregnancy
  a Any time before, during, or after birth
  d From trauma

6 The person with Down syndrome always has some degree of
  a Cerebral palsy
  b Autism
  c Impaired mobility
  d Mental retardation

7 Cerebral palsy is usually caused by
  a An extra chromosome
  b High fever
  c Lack of oxygen to the brain
  d Infection during pregnancy

8 The person with spastic type of cerebral palsy has problems with
  a Learning
  b Drooling
  c Posture, balance, and movement
  d Weaving motions of the trunk, arms, and legs

9 Autism begins
  a At fertilization
  b During pregnancy
  c At birth
  d In early childhood

10 The person with autism has
  a Impaired movement
  b Problems relating to people
  c Diplegia
  d Mental retardation

11 The person with epilepsy has
  a Seizures
  b Diplegia
  c Athetoid movements
  d Spastic movements

12 Which is used to control epilepsy
  a Physical therapy
  b Occupational therapy
  c Drugs
  d A shunt

13 Spina bifida involves
  a Nerve damage
  b A defect in the spinal column
  c Seizures
  d Mental retardation

14 Which is common in spina bifida?
  a Short attention span
  b Hearing and vision problems
  c Seizures
  d Bowel and bladder problems

15 Hydrocephalus often occurs with
  a Down syndrome
  b Mental retardation
  c Spina bifida
  d Autism

*Answers to these questions are on p. 820.*

# Sexuality

## OBJECTIVES

- Define the key terms listed in this chapter
- Describe sex and sexuality
- Explain why sexuality is important throughout life
- Describe five types of sexual relationships
- Explain how injury, illness, and aging can affect sexuality
- Explain how the nursing team can promote sexuality
- Describe how to deal with sexually aggressive persons

## KEY TERMS

**bisexual**  A person who is attracted to both sexes

**erectile dysfunction**  Impotence

**heterosexual**  A person who is attracted to members of the other sex

**homosexual**  A person who is attracted to members of the same sex

**impotence**  The inability of the male to have an erection; erectile dysfunction

**menopause**  When menstruation stops

**sex**  Physical activities involving the reproductive organs; done for pleasure or to have children

**sexuality**  The physical, psychological, social, cultural, and spiritual factors that affect a person's feelings and attitudes about his or her sex

**transsexual**  A person who believes that he or she is a member of the other sex

**transvestite**  A person who becomes sexually excited by dressing in the clothes of the other sex

---

Sexuality involves the whole person. Patients and residents, young and old, are total persons. Total persons have sexuality.

## SEX AND SEXUALITY

**Sex** is the physical activities involving the reproductive organs (Box 37-1, p. 740). It is done for pleasure or to have children. **Sexuality** is the physical, psychological, social, cultural, and spiritual factors that affect a person's feelings and attitudes about his or her sex. Sexuality involves the personality and body. It affects how a person behaves, thinks, dresses, and responds to others.

Sexuality develops when a baby's sex is known. It is shown in names, colors, and toys. Blue is for boys and pink for girls. Dolls are for girls. Trains are for boys. By age 2 years, children know their own sex. Three-year-olds know the sex of other children. They learn male and female roles from adults (Fig. 37-4, p. 741). Children learn that boys and girls each behave in certain ways.

As children grow older, interest increases about the body and how it works. Teens are more aware of sex and the body. Their bodies respond to stimulation. They engage in sexual behaviors. They kiss, embrace, pet, or have intercourse. Pregnancy and sexually transmitted diseases (Chapter 33) are great risks.

Sex has more meaning as young adults mature. Attitudes and feelings are important. Partners are selected. They decide about sex before marriage and birth control.

Sexuality is important throughout life. Attitudes and sex needs change with aging. They are affected by life events. These include divorce, death of a partner, injury, and illness.

*Text continued on p. 742.*

## BOX 37-1 REVIEW OF THE STRUCTURE AND FUNCTION OF THE REPRODUCTIVE SYSTEM

### THE MALE REPRODUCTIVE SYSTEM

The male reproductive system is shown in Figure 37-1. The *testes (testicles)* are the male sex glands *(gonads)*. Male sex cells *(sperm cells)* are produced in the testes. So is *testosterone,* the male hormone. This hormone is needed for reproductive organ function and for male secondary sex characteristics (Chapter 8). The testes are suspended between the thighs in a sac called the *scrotum.*

Sperm travel from the testis to the *epididymis.* The epididymis is a coiled tube on top and to the side of the testis. From the epididymis, sperm travel through a tube called the *vas deferens.* Each vas deferens joins a *seminal vesicle.* The two seminal vesicles store sperm and produce *semen.* Semen is a fluid that carries sperm. The ducts of the seminal vesicles join to form the *ejaculatory duct.* The ejaculatory duct passes through the prostate gland.

The *prostate gland,* shaped like a donut, lies below the bladder. The gland secretes fluid into the semen. As the ejaculatory ducts leave the prostate, they join the *urethra.* It also runs through the prostate. The urethra is the outlet for urine and semen. The penis contains the urethra.

The *penis* is outside the body and has *erectile* tissue. With sexual arousal, blood fills the erectile tissue. The penis becomes enlarged, hard, and erect. The erect penis can enter the female vagina. The semen, which contains sperm, is released into the vagina.

### THE FEMALE REPRODUCTIVE SYSTEM

The female reproductive system is shown in Figure 37-2. The female gonads are two almond-shaped glands called *ovaries.* An ovary is on each side of the uterus in the abdominal cavity.

The ovaries contain eggs (*ova*). Ova are female sex cells. One egg (*ovum*) is released monthly during the woman's reproductive years. Release of an ovum is called *ovulation.*

The ovaries also secrete the female hormones *estrogen* and *progesterone.* These hormones are needed for reproductive system function and the development of female secondary sex characteristics (Chapter 8).

When an ovum is released from an ovary, it travels through a *fallopian tube.* There are two fallopian tubes, one on each side. The tubes are attached at one end to the uterus. The ovum travels through a fallopian tube to the uterus.

The *uterus* is a hollow, muscular organ shaped like a pear. It is in the center of the pelvic cavity behind the bladder and in front of the rectum. The main part of the uterus is the *fundus.* The neck or narrow section of the uterus is the *cervix.* Tissue lining the uterus is called the *endometrium.* The endometrium has many blood vessels. If sex cells from the male and female unite into one cell, that cell implants into the endometrium. There it grows into a baby. The uterus serves as a place for the unborn baby to grow and receive nourishment.

The cervix projects into a muscular canal called the *vagina.* The vagina opens to the outside of the body. It is just behind the urethra. The vagina receives the penis during sexual intercourse and is part of the birth canal. Glands in the vaginal wall keep it moistened with secretions.

The female's external genitalia are called the *vulva* (Fig. 37-3). The *mons pubis* is covered with hair in the adult female. The *labia majora* and *labia minora* are two folds of tissue on each side of the vaginal opening. The *clitoris* is a small organ composed of erectile tissue. The clitoris becomes enlarged and hard when sexually stimulated.

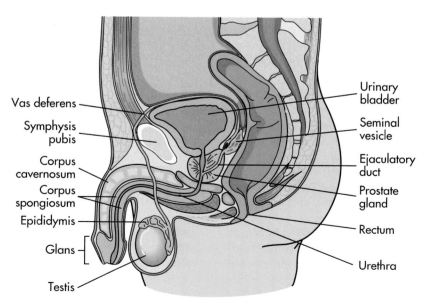

**FIG. 37-1** Male reproductive system.

## BOX 37-1   REVIEW OF THE STRUCTURE AND FUNCTION OF THE REPRODUCTIVE SYSTEM—CONT'D

### MENSTRUATION

The endometrium is rich in blood to nourish the cell that grows into an unborn baby *(fetus)*. If pregnancy does not occur, the endometrium breaks up. It leaves the body through the vagina. This process is called *menstruation.* Menstruation occurs about every 28 days. This is also called the *menstrual cycle.*

Day 1 of the cycle starts with menstruation. Blood flows from the uterus through the vaginal opening. Menstrual flow lasts 3 to 7 days. Ovulation occurs during the next phase. An ovum matures in the ovary and is released. This usually occurs on or about day 14 of the cycle.

Meanwhile, estrogen and progesterone (female hormones) are secreted by the ovaries. These hormones cause the endometrium to thicken for pregnancy. If pregnancy does not occur, the hormones decrease in amount. This causes blood supply to the endometrium to decrease. The endometrium breaks up. It is discharged through the vagina. Another menstrual cycle begins.

### FERTILIZATION

To reproduce, a male sex cell *(sperm)* must unite with a female sex cell *(ovum)*. The uniting of the sperm and ovum into one cell is called *fertilization.* A sperm has 23 chromosomes. An ovum has 23 chromosomes. When the two cells unite, the fertilized cell has 46 chromosomes.

During intercourse, millions of sperm are deposited in the vagina. Sperm travel up the cervix, through the uterus, and into the fallopian tubes. If a sperm and an ovum unite in a fallopian tube, fertilization occurs. Pregnancy occurs. The fertilized cell travels down the fallopian tube to the uterus. After a short time, the fertilized cell implants in the thick endometrium and grows during pregnancy.

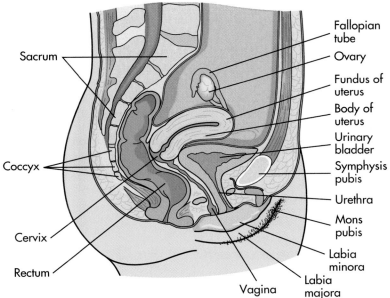

**FIG. 37-2** Female reproductive system.

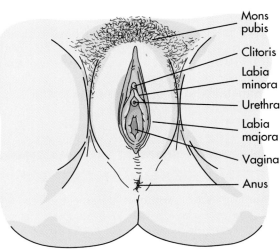

**FIG. 37-3** External female genitalia.

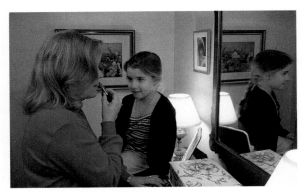

**FIG. 37-4** This little girl is learning female sex roles from her mother.

# SEXUAL RELATIONSHIPS

A **heterosexual** is attracted to members of the other sex. Men are attracted to women. Women are attracted to men. Sexual behavior is male-female.

A **homosexual** is attracted to members of the same sex. Men are attracted to men. Women are attracted to women. *Gay* refers to homosexuality. Homosexual men are called *gay men. Lesbian* refers to a female homosexual. Before the 1960s and 1970s, many gay persons were secret about their sexual orientation. Now many gay persons openly express their sexual preference and relationships.

**Bisexuals** are attracted to both sexes. Some have same-gender and male-female behaviors. They often marry and have children. They may seek a same-gender relationship or experience outside of marriage.

**Transsexuals** believe that they are members of the other sex. A male believes he is a female in a man's body. A female believes she is a male in a woman's body. They often feel "trapped" in the wrong body. Most have always had these feelings. As children they usually behave like the other sex. Many seek psychiatric treatment. Some have sex-change operations.

**Transvestites** become sexually excited by dressing in clothes of the other sex. Most are men. Often they marry and are heterosexual. They dress as men most of the time. They usually dress as women in private. Some dress completely as women. Others focus on bras and panties. The sex partner may not know about the practice. Some partners take part in transvestite activities. Some transvestites have same-gender friends with similar interests.

# INJURY, ILLNESS, AND SURGERY

Injury, illness, and surgery can affect sexual function. The person may feel unclean, unwhole, unattractive, or mutilated. Attitudes may change. The person may feel unfit for closeness and love. Therefore some sexual problems are psychological. Time and understanding are helpful. So is a caring partner. Some need counseling.

**Impotence (erectile dysfunction)** is the inability of the male to have an erection. Diabetes, spinal cord injuries, and multiple sclerosis are causes. So are prostate problems and alcoholism. Heart and circulatory disorders, drugs, and drug abuse are other causes. Some drugs for high blood pressure cause impotence. So do other drugs. Some drugs treat impotence.

Heart disease and stroke can affect sexual ability. So can chronic obstructive pulmonary disease and nervous system disorders. Reproductive system surgeries have physical and psychological effects. Prostate or testes removal affects erections. Removal of the uterus, ovaries, or a breast affects women.

Changes in sexual function greatly impact the person. Fear, anger, worry, and depression are common. They are seen in the person's behavior and comments. The person's feelings are normal and expected. Follow the care plan. It helps the person deal with his or her feelings.

# AGE-RELATED CHANGES

Reproductive organs change with aging. In men, the hormone *testosterone* decreases. It affects strength, sperm production, and reproductive tissues. These changes affect sexual activity. An erection takes longer. The phase between erection and orgasm is also longer. Orgasm is less forceful than when younger. Erections are lost quickly. The time between erections is also longer. Older men may need the penis stimulated for arousal.

Fatigue, overeating, and drinking too much affect erections. Some men fear performance problems. They may avoid closeness.

**Menopause** is when menstruation stops. The woman can no longer have children. This occurs between 45 and 55 years of age. Female hormones (*estrogen* and *progesterone*) decrease. The uterus, vagina, and genitalia shrink (*atrophy*). Vaginal walls thin. There is vaginal dryness. These make intercourse uncomfortable or painful. Arousal takes longer. The time between excitement and orgasm is longer. Orgasm is less intense. The pre-excitement state returns more quickly.

Frequency of sex decreases for many older persons. Reasons relate to weakness, fatigue, and pain. Reduced mobility, aging, and chronic illness are factors.

Some people do not have intercourse. This does not mean loss of sexual needs or desires. Often needs are expressed in other ways. They hold hands, touch, caress, and embrace. These bring closeness and intimacy.

Sexual partners are lost through death and divorce. Or a partner needs hospital or nursing center care. These situations occur in adults of all ages. *See Focus on Older Persons: Age-Related Changes.*

# MEETING SEXUAL NEEDS

The nursing team promotes the meeting of sexual needs. The measures in Box 37-2 may be part of the person's care plan. *See Focus on Long-Term Care: Meeting Sexual Needs.*

## FOCUS ON OLDER PERSONS
### AGE-RELATED CHANGES

Love, affection, and intimacy are needed throughout life. Older persons have many losses. Children leave home. Friends and family die. People retire. Health problems occur. Strength decreases. Appearances change. It helps to feel close to another person. Older persons love, fall in love, hold hands, embrace, and have sex.

## FOCUS ON LONG-TERM CARE
### MEETING SEXUAL NEEDS

Married couples in nursing centers can share the same room. This is an OBRA requirement. The couple has lived together for a long time. Long-term care is no reason to keep them apart. They can share the same bed if their conditions permit. A double, queen-size, or king-size bed is provided by the couple or the center.

Single persons may develop relationships. They are allowed time together, not kept apart (Fig. 37-5).

## BOX 37-2 PROMOTING SEXUALITY

- Let the person practice grooming routines. Assist as needed. For women, this includes applying makeup, nail polish, lotion, and cologne. Many women shave their legs and underarms and pluck eyebrows. Men may use after-shave lotion and cologne. Hair care is important to men and women.
- Let the person choose clothing. Hospital gowns embarrass both men and women. Street clothes are worn if the person's condition permits.
- Protect the right to privacy. Do not expose the person. Drape and screen the person.
- Accept the person's sexual relationships. The person may not share your sexual attitudes, values, or practices. The person may have a homosexual, premarital, or extramarital relationship. Do not judge or gossip about relationships.
- Allow privacy. You can usually tell when people want to be alone. If the person has a private room, close the door for privacy. Some agencies have *Do Not Disturb* signs for doors. Let the person and partner know how much time they have alone. For example, remind them about meal times, drugs, and treatments. Tell other staff members that the person wants time alone.
- Knock before you enter any room. This is a simple courtesy that shows respect for privacy.
- Consider the person's roommate. Privacy curtains provide little privacy. Arrange for privacy when the roommate is out of the room. Sometimes roommates offer to leave for a while. If the roommate cannot leave, the nurse finds other private areas.
- Allow privacy for masturbation. It is a normal form of sexual expression and release. Close the privacy curtain and the door. Knock before you enter any room. This saves you and the person embarrassment. Sometimes confused persons masturbate in public areas. Lead the person to a private area. Or distract him or her with an activity.

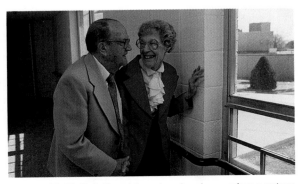

**FIG. 37-5** Relationships develop in nursing centers.

# THE SEXUALLY AGGRESSIVE PERSON

Some persons want the health team to meet their sexual needs. They flirt or make sexual advances or comments. Some expose themselves, masturbate, or touch staff. This can anger or embarrass the staff member. These reactions are normal. Often there are reasons for the person's behavior. Understanding this helps you deal with the matter.

Sexually aggressive behaviors have many causes. They include:

- Nervous system disorders including confusion, disorientation, and dementia
- Drug side effects
- Fever
- Poor vision

The person may confuse someone with his or her partner. Or the person cannot control behavior. The cause is changes in mental function. The healthy person controls sexual urges. Changes in the brain make control difficult. Sexual behavior in these cases is usually innocent.

Sometimes touch serves to gain attention. For example, Mr. Olson had a stroke. He cannot speak or move his right side. Your buttocks are near him. To get your attention, he touches your buttocks. His behavior is not sexual.

Sometimes masturbation is a sexually aggressive behavior. Some persons touch and fondle the genitals for sexual pleasure. However, urinary or reproductive system disorders can cause genital soreness or itching. So can poor hygiene and being wet or soiled from urine or feces. Touching genitals could signal a health problem.

Sometimes the purpose of touch is sexual. For example, a man wants to prove that he is attractive and can perform sexually. He acts sexually. You must be professional about the matter:

- Ask the person not to touch you. State the places where you were touched.
- Tell the person that you will not do what he or she wants.
- Tell the person what behaviors make you uncomfortable. Politely ask the person not to act that way.
- Allow privacy if the person is becoming aroused. Provide for safety. Raise bed rails if ordered for the person, place the signal light within reach, and so on (Chapter 10). Tell the person when you will return.
- Discuss the matter with the nurse. The nurse can help you understand the behavior.

The care plan has measures to deal with sexually aggressive behaviors. They are based on the cause of the behavior. Many agencies have classes to help staff deal with such behavior.

## PROTECTING THE PERSON

The person must be protected from unwanted sexual comments and advances. This is sexual abuse (Chapter 2). Tell the nurse right away. A staff member, patient, resident, family member, or visitor cannot sexually abuse another person.

# SEXUALLY TRANSMITTED DISEASES

Some diseases are spread by sexual contact. They are discussed in Chapter 33.

Circle the **BEST** answer.

1  Sex involves
   a  The organs of reproduction
   b  Attitudes and feelings
   c  Cultural and spiritual factors
   d  Masturbation

2  Sexuality is important to
   a  Small children
   b  Teenagers and young adults
   c  Middle-age adults
   d  Persons of all ages

3  Impotence is
   a  When menstruation stops
   b  A reaction to disfigurement
   c  Not being able to achieve an erection
   d  No sexual activity

4  Reproductive organs change with aging.
   a  True
   b  False

5  Mr. and Mrs. Green live in a nursing center. Which will *not* promote their sexuality?
   a  Allowing their normal grooming routines
   b  Having them wear hospital gowns
   c  Allowing them privacy
   d  Accepting their relationship

6  Two nursing center residents are holding hands. Nursing staff should keep them apart.
   a  True
   b  False

7  Mr. and Mrs. Green want some time alone. The nursing team can do the following *except*
   a  Close the room door
   b  Put a *Do Not Disturb* sign on the door
   c  Tell other staff that Mr. and Mrs. Green want some time alone
   d  Close the privacy curtain so no one can hear them

8  Mr. Cole is masturbating in the dining room. You should do the following *except*
   a  Cover him and take him quietly to his room
   b  Scold him
   c  Provide privacy
   d  Tell the nurse

9  Mr. and Mrs. Green should each have a room.
   a  True
   b  False

10 A person makes sexual advances to you. You should do the following *except*
   a  Discuss the matter with the nurse
   b  Do what the person asks
   c  Explain that the behaviors make you uncomfortable
   d  Ask the person not to touch you

*Answers to these questions are on p. 820.*

# Caring for Mothers and Newborns

# OBJECTIVES

- Define the key terms listed in this chapter
- Describe how to meet an infant's safety and security needs
- Identify the signs and symptoms of illness in infants
- Explain how to help mothers with breast-feeding
- Describe three forms of baby formulas
- Explain how to bottle-feed babies
- Explain how to burp a baby
- Describe how to give cord care
- Describe the purposes of circumcision, needed observations, and the required care
- Explain how to bathe infants
- Explain why infants are weighed
- Describe the care needed by mothers after childbirth
- Perform the procedures described in this chapter

# KEY TERMS

**circumcision** The surgical removal of foreskin from the penis

**episiotomy** Incision *(otomy)* into the perineum

**lochia** The vaginal discharge that occurs after childbirth

**postpartum** After *(post)* childbirth *(partum)*

**umbilical cord** The structure that carries blood, oxygen, and nutrients from the mother to the fetus

Mothers and newborns usually have short hospital stays. Some need home care after discharge. Common reasons for home care include:

- Complications in the mother before or after childbirth
- Help with other young children in the home
- Multiple births (twins, triplets, and so on)
- Help with meals and housekeeping

Babies are helpless. They depend on others for their basic needs. Babies have physical, safety and security, and love and belonging needs. A review of growth and development will help you care for babies (Chapter 8).

# INFANT SAFETY AND SECURITY

Babies cannot protect themselves. They need to feel safe and secure. They feel secure when warm and when wrapped and held snugly. Babies cry to communicate. They cry when wet, hungry, hot or cold, tired, uncomfortable, or in pain. To promote safety and security, respond to their cries and feed them when hungry. See Chapter 10 for infant safety measures. Also follow the measures in Box 38-1, p. 748.

Nursery equipment must be safe and in good repair. Use the guidelines in Box 38-2, p. 749 to check nursery equipment in an agency or home setting.

# SIGNS AND SYMPTOMS OF ILLNESS

Babies can become ill quickly. Signs and symptoms may be sudden. You must be very alert. Report any of the signs and symptoms in Box 38-3, p. 750, to the nurse at once.

Tell the nurse when a sign or symptom began. You may need to measure the child's temperature, pulse, and respirations (Chapter 21). The nurse tells you what temperature site to use—tympanic, rectal, or axillary. Apical pulses are taken on infants and young children.

*Text continued on p. 750.*

## BOX 38-1  INFANT SAFETY

- Follow the safety measures listed in Chapter 10.
- Keep the baby warm. Check windows for drafts. Close windows securely.
- Keep your fingernails short. Do not wear fake nails. Long nails can scratch the baby.
- Do not wear rings or bracelets. Jewelry can scratch the baby.
- Use both hands to lift a newborn. Use one hand to support the head and upper back. Use your other hand to support the legs. Do not lift a newborn by the arms.
- Hold the baby securely. Use the cradle hold, football hold, or shoulder hold (Fig. 38-1).
- Support the baby's head and neck when lifting or holding the baby. Neck support is necessary for the first 3 months after birth.
- Handle the baby with gentle, smooth movements. Avoid sudden or jerking movements. Do not startle the baby.
- Hold and cuddle infants. It is comforting and helps them learn to feel love and security.
- Talk, sing, or play with the baby often. Talk to the baby during the bath, dressing, and diapering.
- Respond to the baby's crying. Babies cry when hungry, uncomfortable, wet, frightened, or tired or when they want attention. They communicate by crying. Responding to their cries helps them feel safe and secure.
- Tighten all nuts, bolts, and screws on cribs, highchairs, and other infant furniture. Do this periodically.
- Check mattress hooks to make sure none are bent or broken.
- Keep one hand on the baby at all times. This includes when he or she is on a changing table. Otherwise the baby can roll off the changing table and strangle on the safety straps. (see Chapter 10).
- Make sure the crib is within hearing distance of the caregivers.
- Do not put a pillow, quilts, or soft toys in the crib. They can cause suffocation.
- Do not lay an infant on soft bedding products. This includes fluffy, plush products such as sheepskin, quilts, comforters, pillows, and toys. These soft products can cover the baby's nose and mouth and cause suffocation.
- Do not place infants on an adult's or child's bed, waterbed, or bunk bed. The following are risks:
  —Death from entrapment. The baby can get trapped between the bed and the wall; between the bed and another object; or between the bed frame, headboard, or footboard.
  —Death from suffocation in soft bedding. This includes pillows, quilts, and comforters.
  —Death from suffocation after falling onto piles of clothing, plastic bags, pillows, cushions, or other soft materials.
- Lay babies on their backs for sleep. *Do not lay babies on their stomachs for sleep. This can interfere with chest expansion and breathing. The baby can suffocate.* Infants can lie on their sides and stomachs when awake.
- Keep pins and small objects out of the baby's reach.
- Do not shake powders directly over the baby. The powder can get into the baby's eyes and lungs. Shake some on your hand away from the baby.

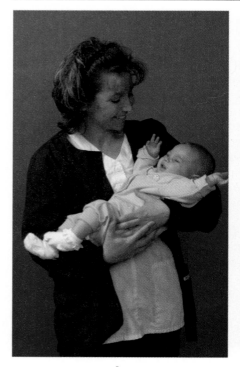 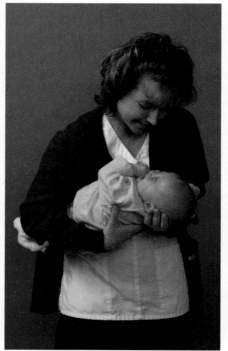 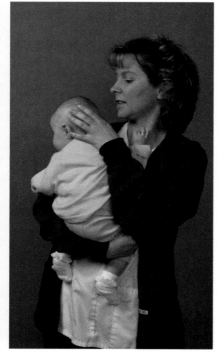

**A**                **B**                **C**

**FIG. 38-1** Holding a baby. **A,** The cradle hold. **B,** The football hold. **C,** The shoulder hold.

## BOX 38-2 SAFETY GUIDE FOR NEW AND USED NURSERY EQUIPMENT

### CRIBS

- Slats are spaced no more than 2⅜ inches (60 mm) apart.
- No slats are missing or cracked.
- The mattress fits snugly—less than a 2-finger width between the edge of mattress and crib side.
- The mattress support is securely attached to the head and footboards.
- Corner posts are no higher than 1/16-inch (1.5 mm) to prevent entanglement of clothing or other objects worn by the child.
- There are no cutouts in the headboard and footboard to allow head entrapment.
- Drop-side latches cannot be easily released by the baby.
- Drop-side latches securely hold the side rails in the raised position.
- All screws or bolts that secure parts of the crib are present and tight.

### CRIB TOYS

- Strings or cords do not dangle into the crib.
- A crib gym or mobile has a label warning to remove the device from the crib when the child can push on the hands and knees or reaches 5 months of age, whichever comes first.
- Toy parts are too large to be a choking hazard.

### GATES AND ENCLOSURES

- Gate openings are too small to entrap a child's head or neck.
- The gate has a pressure bar or other fastener that will resist forces exerted by a child.

### HIGHCHAIRS

- The highchair has crotch strap that must be used when restraining a child in a highchair.
- The highchair has restraining straps that are independent of the tray.
- The tray locks securely.
- Buckles on straps are easy to fasten and unfasten.
- The highchair has a wide, stable base.
- Caps or plugs on tubing are firmly attached and cannot be pulled off and choke a child.
- A folding highchair has an effective locking device to keep the chair from collapsing.

### PLAYPENS

- Playpens or travel cribs have top rails that automatically lock when lifted into the normal use position.
- The playpen does not have a rotating hinge in the center of the top rails.
- A drop-side mesh playpen or mesh crib has a label about never leaving a side in the down position.
- Playpen mesh has small weave (less than ¼-inch openings).
- The mesh has no tears, holes, or loose threads.
- The mesh is securely attached to the top rail and floorplate.
- A wooden playpen has slats spaced no more than 2⅜ inches (60 mm) apart.

### RATTLES, SQUEEZE TOYS, AND TEETHERS

- Rattles, squeeze toys, and teethers have handles too large to lodge in the baby's throat.
- Rattles do not have ball-shaped ends.
- Squeeze toys do not contain a squeaker that could detach and choke a baby.

### TOY CHESTS

- The toy chest has no latch to entrap the child within the chest.
- The toy chest has a spring-loaded lid support that will not require periodic adjustment. It will support the lid in any position to prevent lid slam.
- The chest has ventilation holes or spaces in the front and sides or under the lid in case the child gets caught inside.

### WALKERS

- The walker has safety features to help prevent a fall down stairs.

### BACK CARRIERS

- Leg openings are small enough to prevent the child from slipping out.
- Leg openings are large enough to prevent chafing.
- The folding mechanism has frame joints.
- There is a padded covering over the metal frame near the baby's face.

### BASSINETS AND CRADLES

- The item has a sturdy bottom and a wide base for stability.
- The item has smooth surfaces—no protruding staples or other hardware that could injure the baby.
- Legs have strong, effective locks to prevent folding while in use.
- The mattress is firm and fits snugly.
- Wood or metal cradles have slats spaced to more than 2⅜ inches (60 mm) apart.

### CARRIER SEATS

- The item has a wide, sturdy base for stability.
- The item has nonskid feet to prevent slipping.
- Supporting devices lock securely.
- The seat has a crotch and waist strap.
- The buckle or strap is easy to use.

From the U.S. Consumer Product Safety Commission: *The safe nursery,* CPSC 202, Washington DC.

*Continued*

**BOX 38-2** SAFETY GUIDE FOR NEW AND USED NURSERY EQUIPMENT—CONT'D

**CHANGING TABLES**

- The table has safety straps to prevent falls. (*Note:* Remember to keep one hand on a baby at all times.)
- The table has drawers or shelves that are easy to reach without leaving the baby unattended.

**HOOK-ON CHAIRS**

- The chair has a restraining strap.
- The chair has a clamp that locks onto the table for added security.
- Caps or plugs on tubing are firmly attached and cannot be pulled off and choke a child.
- The hook-on chair has a warning never to place the chair where the child can push off with the feet.

**PACIFIERS**

- The item has no ribbons, strings, cords, or yarn attached.
- The shield is large and firm enough so it cannot fit into the child's mouth.

- The guard or shield has ventilation holes so the baby can breath if the shield does get into the mouth.
- The pacifier nipple has no holes or tears that might cause it to break off in the baby's mouth.

**STROLLERS AND CARRIAGES**

- There is a wide base to prevent tipping.
- The seat belt and crotch strap securely attach to the frame.
- The seat buckle is easy to use.
- Brakes securely lock the wheels.
- The shopping basket is low on the back and located directly over or in front of the rear wheels.
- When used in the carriage position, the leg openings can be closed.

**BOX 38-3** SIGNS AND SYMPTOMS OF ILLNESS IN BABIES

- The baby has jaundice—a yellowish color to the skin and whites of the eyes.
- The baby looks sick.
- The baby has redness or drainage around the cord stump or circumcision.
- The baby has a high temperature (Chapter 21).
- The baby is limp and slow to respond.
- The baby cries all the time or does not stop crying.
- The baby is flushed, pale, or perspiring.
- The baby has noisy, rapid, difficult, or slow respirations.
- The baby is coughing or sneezing.
- The baby has reddened or irritated eyes.
- The baby turns his or her head to one side or puts a hand to one ear (signs of an earache).
- The baby screams for a long time.
- The baby is feeding poorly or has skipped feedings.
- The baby has vomited most of the feeding or vomits between feedings.
- The baby has hard, formed stools or watery stools.
- Stools are light-colored.
- The baby has a rash.

# HELPING MOTHERS BREAST-FEED

Many mothers breast-feed their babies. Breast-fed babies usually nurse every 2 or 3 hours (8 to 12 times a day). They are fed on demand. That is, they are fed when hungry, not on a schedule. Babies nurse for a short time the first few days (5 to 10 minutes at each breast). Eventually, nursing time takes 10 to 20 minutes at each breast.

Nurses help new mothers learn to breast-feed. They also teach breast care. Mothers and babies learn how to nurse in a very short time. Tell the nurse if the mother or baby is having problems breast-feeding.

Mothers may need help getting ready to breast-feed. They may need help with hand washing and positioning. Assist as needed. Make sure the signal light is within reach before you leave the room. Also provide for privacy. Follow the measures in Box 38-4 to help with breast-feeding. *See Focus on Home Care: Helping Mothers Breast-Feed*, p. 752.

## BOX 38-4 HELPING WITH BREAST-FEEDING

- Practice hand hygiene and Standard Precautions. Remember, HIV can be transmitted through breast milk (Chapter 33).
- Help the mother wash her hands. She needs clean hands before handling her breasts.
- Help the mother to a comfortable position. The cradle position, side-lying position, and football hold are the basic positions for breast-feeding (Fig. 38-2).
- Change the baby's diaper if necessary. Bring the baby to the mother.
- Make sure the mother holds the baby close to her breast.
- Have the mother use her nipple to stroke the baby's cheek or lower lip. This stimulates the *rooting reflex.* The baby turns his or her head toward the breast and starts to suck.
- Have the mother keep breast tissue away from the baby's nose with her thumb (Fig. 38-3, p. 752).
- Give her a baby blanket to cover the baby and her breast. This promotes privacy.
- Encourage nursing from both breasts at each feeding. If the baby finished the last feeding at the right breast, the baby starts the next feeding at the right breast. The mother can use a pin on her bra strap as a reminder of which breast to start with.
- Remind her how to remove the baby from the breast. To break the suction between the baby and the breast, she can insert a finger into a corner of the baby's mouth (Fig. 38-4, p. 752).
- Help the mother burp the baby if necessary (p. 755). The baby is burped after nursing at one breast. Then the baby is burped after nursing at the other breast.
- Remind the mother to air-dry her nipples after a feeding.
- Change the baby's diaper after the feeding.
- Lay the baby in the crib if he or she has fallen asleep. *Remember to lay the baby on his or her back. Do not lay the baby on his or her stomach.*
- Encourage the mother to wear a nursing bra day and night. The bra supports the breasts and promotes comfort.
- Encourage the mother to place nursing pads in the bra. The pads absorb leaking milk.
- Have the mother apply cream (if prescribed) to her nipples after each feeding. The cream prevents nipples from drying and cracking. Remind her to wash her breasts with water before a feeding to remove the cream.
- Help the mother straighten clothing after the feeding if necessary.
- Remind the mother to wash her breasts with a clean washcloth and warm water. Soap is not used. It can cause the nipples to dry and crack. Nipples are air-dried after washing to prevent cracking and soreness.

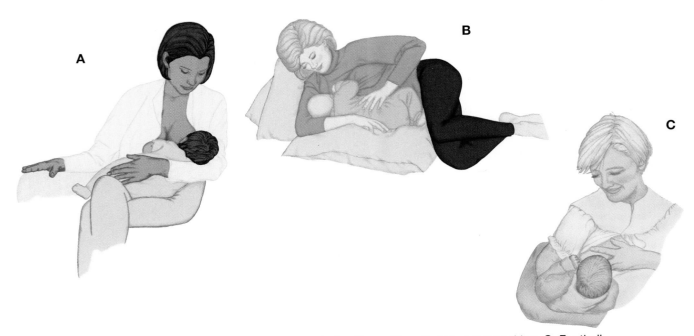

**FIG. 38-2** Basic breast-feeding positions. **A,** Cradle position. **B,** Side-lying position. **C,** Football hold. (From James SR, Ashwill JW, Droske SC: *Nursing care of children: principles and practice,* ed 2, Philadelphia, 2002, WB Saunders.)

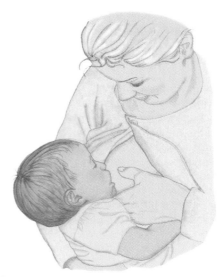

**FIG. 38-3** The mother supports her breast with one hand. The thumb is on top of the breast to keep breast tissue away from the baby's nose. (From James SR, Ashwill JW, Droske SC: *Nursing care of children: principles and practice,* ed 2, Philadelphia, 2002, WB Saunders.)

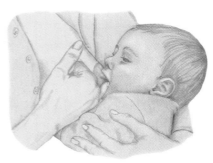

**FIG. 38-4** The mother inserts a finger into the corner of the baby's mouth to remove the baby from the breast. (From James SR, Ashwill JW, Droske SC: *Nursing care of children: principles and practice,* ed 2, Philadelphia, 2002, WB Saunders.)

## FOCUS ON HOME CARE
### HELPING MOTHERS BREAST-FEED

When the mother is nursing, stay within hearing distance in case she needs help.

The nursing mother needs good nutrition. Remember the following when planning meals or grocery shopping:

- Calorie intake may increase. The nurse tells you what the mother's calorie intake needs to be.
- The mother should have 3 servings a day from the milk, yogurt, and cheese group. She can drink whole, 2%, or skim milk. The nurse tells you if more servings are needed.
- Include foods high in calcium in the diet.
- The mother should avoid spicy and gas-forming foods. They can cause cramping and diarrhea in the infant. She should avoid onions, garlic, spices, cabbage, brussels sprouts, asparagus, and beans.
- Chocolate, cola beverages, coffee, and tea contain caffeine. They are used in moderation. Caffeine can cause the baby to be fussy or gassy.

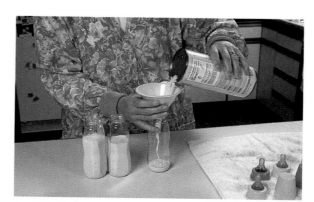

**FIG. 38-5** Ready-to-feed formula is poured from the can into the bottle. A funnel is used to prevent spilling.

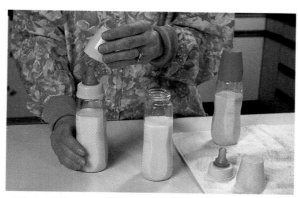

**FIG. 38-6** Bottles are capped for storage in the refrigerator.

# ⬛ BOTTLE-FEEDING BABIES

Formula is given to babies who are not breast-fed. The doctor prescribes the formula. It provides the essential nutrients needed by the infant.

Formula comes in three forms:

- *Ready-to-feed.* It is ready to use. It is poured from the can into the baby bottle (Fig. 38-5). The can may have more than one feeding. Refrigerate the can after opening it. Use its contents within 24 hours.
- *Powdered.* Container directions tell how much powder and water to use.
- *Liquid concentrate.* Container directions tell you how much liquid and water to use.

Bottles are prepared one at a time or in batches for the whole day. Follow the container directions carefully. Measure exact amounts. Extra bottles are capped (Fig. 38-6) and stored in the refrigerator. These bottles are used within 24 hours.

Protect the baby from infection. Wash formula containers before opening them. Also, baby bottles, caps, and nipples must be as clean as possible. Disposable equipment is used in hospitals. Reusable equipment may be used in homes. Reusable bottle-feeding equipment is carefully washed in hot, soapy water or in a dishwasher. Complete rinsing is needed to remove all soap. Some bottles have plastic liners that are discarded after one use.

> **SAFETY ALERT:** *Cleaning Baby Bottles*
> Baby bottles, caps, and nipples must be thoroughly rinsed to remove all soap. Otherwise, the baby takes in soap with the feeding. This can cause serious stomach and intestinal irritation.

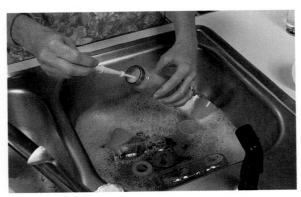

**FIG. 38-7** A bottle brush is used to clean inside a baby bottle.

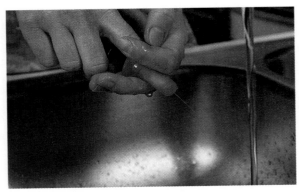

**FIG. 38-8** Water is squeezed through the nipple during washing and rinsing.

## CLEANING BABY BOTTLES

### PRE-PROCEDURE

1 See *Safety Alert: Cleaning Baby Bottles.*
2 Practice hand hygiene.
3 Collect the following:
  - Bottles, nipples, and caps
  - Funnel
  - Can opener
  - Bottle brush
  - Dishwashing soap
  - Other items used to prepare formula
  - Towel

### PROCEDURE

4 Wash the bottles, nipples, caps, funnel, and can opener in hot, soapy water. Wash other items used to prepare formula.
5 Clean inside baby bottles with the bottle brush (Fig. 38-7).
6 Squeeze hot, soapy water through the nipples (Fig. 38-8). This removes formula.
7 Rinse all items thoroughly in hot water. Squeeze hot water through the nipples to remove soap.
8 Lay a clean towel on the counter.
9 Stand bottles upside down to drain. Place nipples, caps, and other items on the towel. Let the items dry.

# FEEDING THE BABY

Bottle-fed babies want to be fed every 3 to 4 hours. The amount of formula taken increases as they grow older. The nurse or the mother tells you how much formula a baby needs at each feeding. Babies usually take as much formula as they need. The baby stops sucking and turns away from the bottle when satisfied.

Babies are not given cold formula out of the refrigerator. A bottle is warmed before the feeding. Warm the bottle in a container of lukewarm water. Or hold it under warm running tap water. The formula should feel warm. Test the temperature by sprinkling a few drops on the inside of your wrist (Fig. 38-9). The guidelines in Box 38-5 will help you bottle-feed babies.

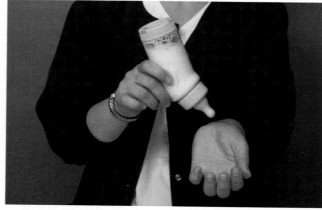

**FIG. 38-9** Formula should feel warm on the inside of your wrist.

**SAFETY ALERT:** *Feeding the Baby*
Do not set the bottle out to warm at room temperature. This takes too long and allows the growth of microbes. Do not heat formula in microwave ovens. The formula can heat unevenly and burn the baby's mouth.

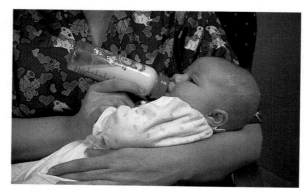

**FIG. 38-10** The bottle is tilted so that formula fills the bottle neck and nipple.

**BOX 38-5** **BOTTLE-FEEDING BABIES**

- Warm a refrigerated bottle so the formula feels warm to the inside of your wrist.
- Assume a comfortable position for the feeding.
- Hold the baby close to you. Relax and snuggle the baby.
- Stroke the baby's cheek or lip with the nipple. The baby's head will turn to the nipple.
- Tilt the bottle so that the neck of the bottle and the nipple are always full (Fig. 38-10). Otherwise some air is in the neck or nipple. The baby sucks air into the stomach. The air causes cramping and discomfort.
- Do not prop the bottle and lay the baby down for the feeding (Fig. 38-11).
- Burp the baby when he or she has taken half the formula. Also burp the baby at the end of the feeding.
- Do not leave the baby alone with a bottle.
- Do not force the baby to finish the bottle.
- Discard remaining formula. Do not save or reheat it for another feeding.
- Wash the bottle, cap, and nipple after the feeding (see procedure: *Cleaning Baby Bottles*, p. 753).

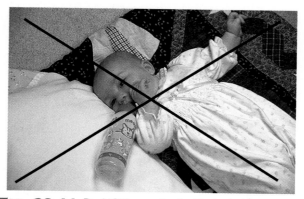

**FIG. 38-11** Do NOT prop the bottle to feed the baby.

# BURPING THE BABY

Babies take in air during feedings. Air in the stomach and intestines causes cramping and discomfort. This can lead to vomiting. Burping helps get rid of the air. Most babies burp mid-way through and after a feeding.

Burping a baby also is called *bubbling*. Figure 38-12 shows two burping positions. You can hold the infant over your shoulder. First place a clean diaper or towel over your shoulder. This protects your clothing if the baby "spits up." Or you can support the baby in a sitting position on your lap. Hold the towel or diaper in front of the baby. To burp the baby, gently pat or rub the baby's back with circular motions. Do this for 2 or 3 minutes. *Remember to support the infant's head and neck for the first 3 months after birth.*

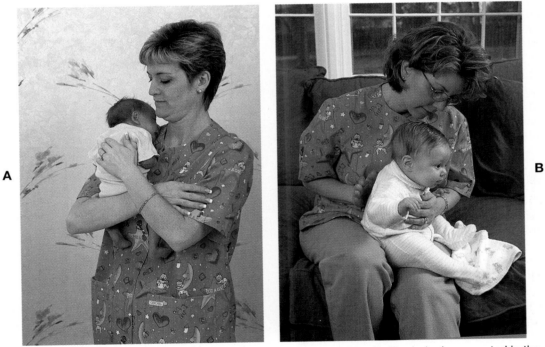

**FIG. 38-12** Burping a baby. **A,** The baby is held over the shoulder. **B,** The baby is supported in the sitting position.

## DIAPERING

Babies should wet at least 6 to 8 times a day. Newborns usually have a bowel movement with every feeding. As they grow older, an elimination pattern develops. Some babies have 1, 2, or 3 stools a day.

Stools are usually soft and unformed. Hard, formed stools signal constipation. Report this to the nurse at once. Watery stools mean diarrhea. Diarrhea is very serious in infants. Their fluid balance is upset quickly (Chapter 20). Tell the nurse at once if you suspect diarrhea.

Diapers are changed when wet or soiled. Cloth and disposable diapers are available. Cloth diapers are reused. No diaper pins are needed if they have Velcro fasteners. The danger of sticking the baby or yourself with a diaper pin is avoided. To properly care for cloth diapers:

- Rinse a soiled cloth diaper in the toilet.
- Store soiled diapers in a diaper pail.
- Wash them daily or every 2 days.
- Wash them separately from other laundry items.
- Wash them in hot water. Use a baby laundry detergent.
- Put them through the wash cycle a second time without detergent. This helps remove all soap.
- Hang them outside to dry if possible. This gives them a fresh, clean smell. Otherwise, dry them in the dryer.

Disposable diapers are secured with Velcro or tape strips. Fold soiled diapers so the soiled area is on the inside. Then discard the diaper in the trash container. Do not flush it down the toilet. Using disposable diapers is more costly than using cloth ones.

Changing diapers often helps prevent diaper rash. Moisture, feces, and urine irritate the baby's skin. When changing diapers, make sure the baby is clean and dry before applying a clean diaper. If a diaper rash develops, tell the nurse at once. The nurse will tell you what to do.

**DELEGATION GUIDELINES:** *Diapering a Baby*
Before changing a baby's diaper, you need this information from the nurse and the care plan:
- The size and type of diaper to use (cloth or disposable)
- If you need to give cord care (p. 758) or circumcision care (p. 759)
- What lotion or cream to use
- What observations to report and record:
  —Color, amount, consistency, and odor of stools
  —Condition of the baby's skin and genital area
  —Redness or irritation of the skin or genital area
  —Blood or discharge on the diaper

**SAFETY ALERT:** *Diapering a Baby*
You must keep the baby safe during diapering. The baby may squirm, wiggle, or kick and cry. You must prevent falls:
- Gather all needed supplies before you begin.
- Place the baby on a firm surface. If the baby is on a table, make sure it is sturdy.
- Always keep one hand on a baby who is on a table.
- Never look away from the baby.

If diaper pins are used for cloth diapers, the pins must point away from the abdomen. If it opens, a pin pointing toward the abdomen can pierce the skin and damage internal organs.

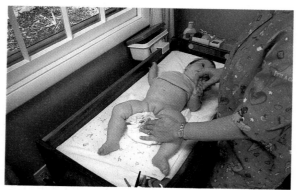

**FIG. 38-13** The front of the diaper is used to clean the genital area.

## DIAPERING A BABY

### PRE-PROCEDURE

1 Follow *Delegation Guidelines: Diapering a Baby*. See *Safety Alert: Diapering a Baby*.
2 Practice hand hygiene.
3 Collect the following:
  - Gloves
  - Clean diaper
  - Waterproof changing pad
  - Washcloth
  - Disposable wipes or cotton balls
  - Basin of warm water
  - Baby soap
  - Baby lotion or cream
4 Place the changing pad under the baby.

### PROCEDURE

5 Put on the gloves.
6 Unfasten the dirty diaper. Place diaper pins out of the baby's reach.
7 Wipe the genital area with the front of the diaper (Fig. 38-13). Wipe from the front to the back.
8 Fold the diaper so urine and feces are inside. Set the diaper aside.
9 Clean the genital area from front to back. Use a wet washcloth, disposable wipes, or cotton balls. Wash with mild soap and water for a large amount of feces or if the baby has a rash. Rinse thoroughly, and pat the area dry.
10 Give cord care (p. 758) and clean the circumcision (p. 759) at this time.
11 Apply cream or lotion to the genital area and buttocks. Do not use too much. Caking can occur.
12 Raise the baby's legs. Slide a clean diaper under the buttocks.
13 Fold a cloth diaper so extra thickness is in the front for a boy (Fig. 38-14, *A*). For girls, fold the diaper so the extra thickness is at the back (Fig. 38-14, *B*).
14 Bring the diaper between the baby's legs.
15 Make sure the diaper is snug around the hips and abdomen. It is loose near the penis if the circumcision has not healed. It is below the umbilicus if the cord stump has not healed.
16 Secure the diaper in place. Use the tape strips or Velcro on disposable diapers (Fig. 38-15, *A*, p. 758). Make sure the tabs stick in place. Use baby pins or Velcro for cloth diapers. Pins point away from the abdomen (Fig. 38-15, *B*, p. 758).
17 Apply plastic pants if cloth diapers are worn. Do not use plastic pants with disposable diapers. They already have waterproof protection.
18 Put the baby in the crib, infant seat, or other safe location.

### POST-PROCEDURE

19 Rinse feces from the cloth diaper in the toilet.
20 Store used cloth diapers in a covered pail. Put a disposable diaper in the trash.
21 Remove the gloves. Practice hand hygiene.
22 Report and record your observations.

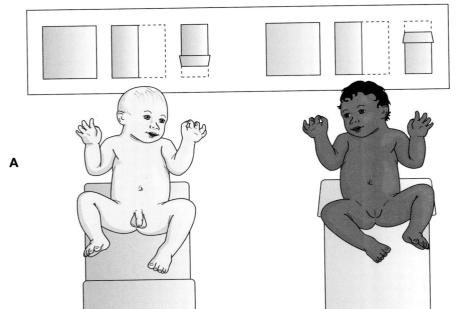

A

B

**FIG. 38-14 A,** A cloth diaper is folded in front for boys. **B,** The diaper has a fold in the back for girls.

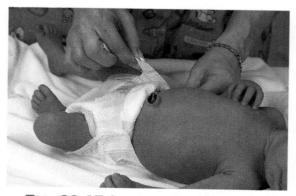

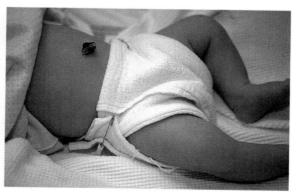

**A**

**B**

**FIG. 38-15** Securing a diaper. **A,** A disposable diaper secured in place with tape strips. **B,** Diaper pins secure a cloth diaper. Pins point away from the abdomen. NOTE: The diapers in **A** and **B** are below the cord.

# CARE OF THE UMBILICAL CORD

The **umbilical cord** connects the mother and the fetus (unborn baby). It carries blood, oxygen, and nutrients from the mother to the fetus (Fig. 38-16). The cord is not needed after birth. Shortly after delivery, the doctor clamps and cuts the cord. A cord stump is left on the baby. The stump dries up and falls off in 2 to 3 weeks. Slight bleeding can occur when the cord comes off.

The cord provides a place for microbes to grow. You need to keep it clean and dry. Cord care is done at each diaper change. Cord care is continued for 1 or 2 days after the cord comes off. It involves the following:

- Keep the stump clean and dry. Do not get the stump wet.
- Wipe the base of the stump with alcohol (Fig. 38-17). Use an alcohol wipe or a cotton ball moistened with alcohol. The alcohol promotes drying.
- Keep the diaper below the cord as in Figure 38-15. This prevents the diaper from irritating the stump. It also keeps the cord from becoming wet from urine.
- Give sponge baths until the cord falls off. Then the baby can have a tub bath.
- Do not pull the cord off—even if looks ready to fall off.
- Report the following to the nurse:
  —Swelling, redness, odor, or drainage from the stump
  —Bleeding from the cord or navel area

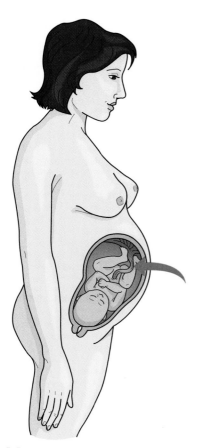

**FIG. 38-16** The umbilical cord connects the mother and fetus.

# CIRCUMCISION

Boys are born with foreskin on the penis. The surgical removal of foreskin from the penis is called a **circumcision** (Chapter 18). The procedure allows good hygiene. It is thought to prevent urinary tract infections in infants and cancer of the penis. It is usually done before the baby leaves the hospital. Circumcision is a religious ceremony in the Jewish faith.

The penis will look red, swollen, and sore. However, the circumcision should not interfere with voiding. Carefully observe for signs of bleeding and infection. There should be no odor or drainage. Also check the diaper for bleeding. The area should heal in 10 to 14 days.

Circumcision care involves the following:

- Clean the penis at each diaper change. This is very important after a bowel movement.
- Use mild soap and water, plain water, or commercial wipes as the nurse directs.
- Apply a petrolatum gauze dressing or petroleum jelly to the penis as the nurse directs. This protects the penis from urine and feces. It also prevents the penis from sticking to the diaper. Use a cotton swab to apply the petroleum jelly (Fig. 38-18).
- Apply the diaper loosely. This prevents the diaper from irritating the penis.

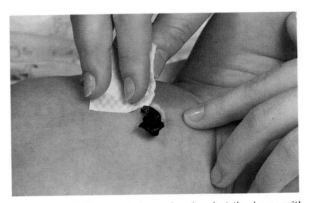

**FIG. 38-17** The cord stump is wiped at the base with alcohol.

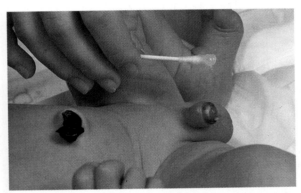

**FIG. 38-18** Petroleum jelly is applied to the circumcised penis.

# BATHING AN INFANT

A bath is important for cleanliness. Though babies do not get very dirty, they need good skin care. Baths comfort and relax babies. They also provide a wonderful time to hold, touch, and talk to babies. Stimulation is important for development. Being touched and held helps babies learn safety, security, and love and belonging.

Planning is an important part of the bath. You cannot leave the baby alone if you forget something. Gather needed equipment, supplies, and the baby's clothes before you start the bath. Everything you need must be within your reach.

There are two bath procedures for babies. Sponge baths are given until the cord stump falls off and the umbilicus and circumcision heal. *The cord must not get wet.* The tub bath is given after the cord site and circumcision heal (Fig. 38-19).

*See Focus on Home Care: Bathing an Infant.*

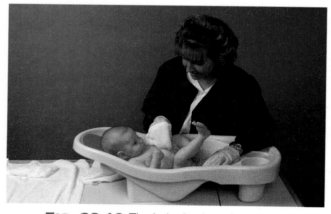

**FIG. 38-19** The baby is given a tub bath.

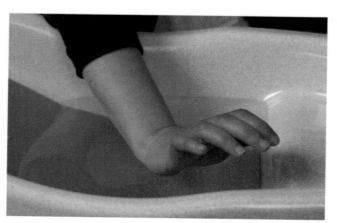

**FIG. 38-20** The inside of the wrist is used to test bath water temperature.

**DELEGATION GUIDELINES:** *Bathing an Infant*
Before bathing an infant, you need this information from the nurse and the care plan:
- What type of bath to give—sponge bath or tub bath
- What water temperature to use—usually 100° to 105° F (37.7° to 40.5° C)
- When to bathe the infant
- If you should apply lotion after the bath
- What observations to report and record

**SAFETY ALERT:** *Bathing an Infant*
To protect an infant during a bath, follow these safety measures:
- Turn up the thermostat and close windows and doors about 20 minutes before the bath. Room temperature should be 75° to 80° F for the bath. The room may be too warm for you. Remove a sweater or lab coat or roll up your sleeves before starting the bath.
- Measure bath water temperature with a bath thermometer. The nurse tells you what temperature to use (usually 100° to 105° F [37.7° to 40.5° C]). Or test water temperature with the inside of your wrist (Fig. 38-20). The water should feel warm and comfortable to your wrist. Babies have delicate skin and are easily burned.
- Never leave the baby alone on a table or in the bathtub.
- Always keep one hand on the baby if you must look away for a moment.
- Hold the baby securely during the bath. Babies are very slippery when they are wet. A wet, squirming baby is hard to hold.

**FOCUS ON HOME CARE**
**BATHING AN INFANT**
Bath time is part of the baby's daily routine. Some mothers bathe their babies in the morning. Others do so in the evening. Evening baths have important advantages:
- The bath is comforting and relaxing. This helps some babies sleep longer at night.
- Working fathers are usually home in the evening. The evening bath lets them be involved.

Sometimes fathers bathe babies so mothers can rest or tend to other children. Follow the family's routine when working in the home.

## GIVING A BABY A SPONGE BATH

### PRE-PROCEDURE

1 Follow *Delegation Guidelines: Bathing an Infant*. See *Safety Alert: Bathing an Infant*.
2 Practice hand hygiene.
3 Place the following items in your work area:
   - Bath basin
   - Bath thermometer
   - Bath towel
   - Two hand towels
   - Receiving blanket
   - Washcloth
   - Clean diaper
   - Clean clothing for the baby
   - Cotton balls
   - Baby soap
   - Baby shampoo
   - Baby lotion
   - Gloves

### PROCEDURE

4 Fill the bath basin with warm water. Water temperature should be 100° to 105° F (37.7° to 40.5° C). Measure water temperature with the bath thermometer or use the inside of your wrist. The water should feel warm and comfortable on your wrist.
5 Provide for privacy.
6 Identify the baby according to agency policy.
7 Put on gloves.
8 Undress the baby. Leave the diaper on.
9 Wash the baby's eyelids (Fig. 38-21, p. 762):
   a Dip a cotton ball into the water.
   b Squeeze out excess water.
   c Wash one eyelid from the inner part to the outer part.
   d Repeat this step for the other eye with a new cotton ball.
10 Moisten the washcloth and make a mitt (Chapter 16). Clean the outside of the ear and then behind the ear. Repeat this step for the other ear. Be gentle.
11 Rinse and squeeze out the washcloth. Make a mitt with the washcloth.
12 Wash the baby's face (Fig. 38-22, p. 762). Clean inside the nostrils with the washcloth. *Do not use cotton swabs to clean inside the nose.* Pat the face dry.
13 Pick up the baby. Hold the baby over the bath basin using the football hold. Support the baby's head and neck with your wrist and hand.

14 Wash the baby's head (Fig. 38-23, p. 762):
   a Squeeze a small amount of water from the washcloth onto the baby's head.
   b Apply a small amount of baby shampoo to the head.
   c Wash the head with circular motions.
   d Rinse the head by squeezing water from a washcloth over the baby's head. Rinse thoroughly. Do not get soap in the baby's eyes.
   e Use a small hand towel to dry the head.
15 Lay the baby on the table.
16 Remove the diaper.
17 Wash the front of the body. Use a soapy washcloth. Or apply soap to your hands and wash the baby with your hands. Do not get the cord wet. Rinse thoroughly. Pat dry. Be sure to wash and dry all creases and folds.
18 Turn the baby to the prone position. Repeat step 17 for the back and buttocks.
19 Give cord care. Clean the circumcision.
20 Apply baby lotion to the baby's body as directed by the nurse.
21 Put a clean diaper and clean clothes on the baby.
22 Wrap the baby in the receiving blanket. Put the baby in the crib or other safe area.

### POST-PROCEDURE

23 Clean and return equipment and supplies to the proper place. Do this step when the baby is settled.
24 Remove the gloves. Practice hand hygiene.
25 Report and record your observations.

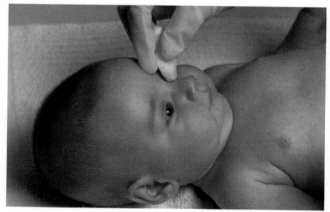

**FIG. 38-21** Wash the baby's eyelids with cotton balls. The eyelids are cleaned from the inner to the outer part.

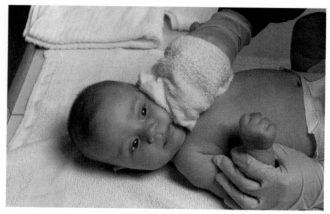

**FIG. 38-22** The baby's face is washed with a mitted washcloth.

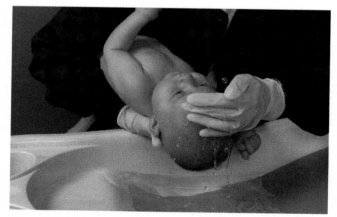

**FIG. 38-23** The baby's head is washed over the bath basin.

## GIVING A BABY A TUB BATH

### PROCEDURE

1 Follow steps 1 through 16 in procedure: *Giving a Baby a Sponge Bath*, p. 761.
2 Hold the baby as in Figure 38-24:
   a Place one hand under the baby's shoulders. Your thumb should be over the baby's shoulder. Your fingers should be under the arm.
   b Support the buttocks with your other hand. Slide your hand under the thighs. Hold the far thigh with your other hand.
3 Lower the baby into the water feet first.
4 Wash the front of the baby's body. Wash all folds and creases. Rinse thoroughly.
5 Reverse your hold. Use your other hand to hold the baby.
6 Wash the baby's back. Rinse thoroughly.
7 Reverse your hold again. Hold the baby with your other hand.
8 Wash the genital area.
9 Lift the baby out of the water and onto a towel.
10 Wrap the baby in the towel. Also cover the baby's head.
11 Pat the baby dry. Dry all folds and creases.
12 Follow steps 20 through 25 in procedure: *Giving a Baby a Sponge Bath*, p. 761.

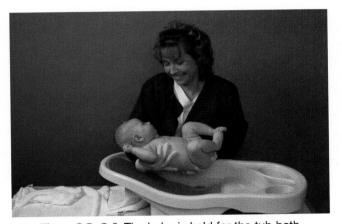

**FIG. 38-24** The baby is held for the tub bath.

## NAIL CARE

The baby's fingernails and toenails are kept short. Otherwise, the baby can scratch himself or herself and others. Nails are best cut when the baby is sleeping. The baby is quiet and will not squirm or fuss. Use nail clippers, or file nails with an emery board. If using nail clippers, clip nails straight across as for an adult (Chapter 17).

# ■ WEIGHING INFANTS

The infant's birth weight is the baseline for measuring growth. The RN uses weight measurements in the assessment step of the nursing process. They also are used to evaluate the amount of breast milk taken during breast-feeding. The baby is weighed before and after breast-feeding. The difference in the weights is the amount of milk taken in during breast-feeding. It tells the nurse if the baby is getting enough milk.

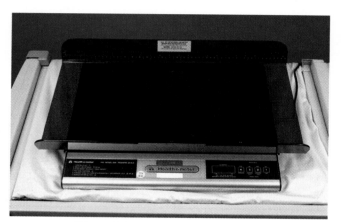

**FIG. 38-25** Digital infant scale.

**DELEGATION GUIDELINES:** *Weighing an Infant*
If weighing an infant is delegated to you, you need this information from the nurse and the care plan:
- When to weigh the baby
- If the baby is breast-fed or bottle-fed—breast-fed babies wear the same diaper, clothes, and blanket for each weight measurement

**SAFETY ALERT:** *Weighing an Infant*
You must meet the baby's safety needs. Protect the baby from chills. Keep the room warm and free of drafts. Also protect the baby from falling. Always keep a hand over the baby when taking the weight measurement. Remember to keep one hand on the baby if you need to look away.

## WEIGHING AN INFANT

### PRE-PROCEDURE

1 Follow *Delegation Guidelines: Weighing an Infant.* See *Safety Alert: Weighing an Infant.*
2 Practice hand hygiene.
3 Collect the following:
- Baby scale (Fig. 38-25)
- Paper for the scale
- Items for diaper changing (see procedure: *Diapering a Baby*, p. 757)
- Gloves

### PROCEDURE

4 Identify the baby following agency policy.
5 Place the paper on the scale. Adjust the scale to zero (0).
6 Put on the gloves.
7 Undress the baby, and remove the diaper. Clean the genital area.
8 Lay the baby on the scale. Keep one hand over the baby to prevent falling.
9 Read the digital display or move the pointer until the scale is balanced.
10 Note the measurement.
11 Diaper and dress the baby. Lay the baby in the crib.
12 Remove and discard the gloves. Practice hand hygiene.

### POST-PROCEDURE

13 Return the scale to its proper place.
14 Decontaminate your hands.
15 Report and record your observations.

## CARE OF THE MOTHER

**Postpartum** means after *(post)* childbirth *(partum).* The postpartum period starts with birth of the baby. It ends 6 weeks later. The mother's body returns to its normal state during this time. The mother adjusts physically and emotionally to childbirth.

The uterus returns almost to its pre-pregnant size. This is called *involution of the uterus.* If the mother does not breast-feed, she can expect a menstrual period within 3 to 8 weeks. Breast-feeding is not an effective method of birth control. Without birth control measures, the mother can get pregnant again.

A vaginal discharge occurs after childbirth. It is called **lochia.** (Lochia comes from the Greek word *lochos,* which means *childbirth.)* Lochia consists of blood and other matter left in the uterus from childbirth. The lochia changes color and decreases in amount during the postpartum period:

- *Lochia rubra*—is dark or bright red *(rubra)* discharge. Mainly blood, it is seen during the first 3 to 4 days.
- *Lochia serosa*—is pinkish brown *(serosa)* drainage. It lasts until about 10 days after birth.
- *Lochia alba*—is whitish *(alba)* drainage. It continues for 2 to 6 weeks after birth.

Lochia increases with breast-feeding and activity. When she stands after lying or sitting, the mother may feel a gush of lochia. She wears a sanitary napkin to absorb the lochia. Normally, lochia smells like menstrual flow. Foul-smelling lochia signals infections.

Good perineal care is important. Sanitary pads are changed often. When wiping after elimination, the mother wipes from front to back. Sanitary napkins are applied and removed from front to back. Good hand washing is essential after perineal care, changing sanitary napkins, and elimination. Standard Precautions and the Bloodborne Pathogen Standard are followed.

Some mothers have episiotomies. An **episiotomy** is an incision *(otomy)* into the perineum. *(Episeion* means *pubic region.)* The doctor performs this procedure during childbirth. It increases the size of the vaginal opening for the baby. The incision is sutured after delivery. The doctor may order sitz baths for comfort and hygiene (Chapter 29). Like other incisions, complications can develop. These include infection and wound separation *(dehiscence).* Tell the nurse at once if the mother complains of pain, discomfort, or a discharge.

Some mothers deliver by *cesarean section (C-section).* The doctor makes an incision into the abdominal wall. The baby is delivered through the incision. This is done when:
- The baby must be delivered to save the baby's or mother's life
- The baby is too large to pass through the birth canal
- The mother has a vaginal infection that could be transmitted to the baby
- A normal vaginal delivery will be difficult for the baby or mother

The C-section incision needs to heal. See Chapter 28 for wound healing and wound care.

The mother has emotional reactions after childbirth. Hormone changes, life-style changes, and lack of sleep can cause mood swings. So can frequent visits and telephone calls from family and friends. Some interfere or offer advice and opinions about parenting. The mother can help herself by resting when the baby sleeps. She needs time for herself and her partner. She may feel better after pampering herself with a shower, washing and styling her hair, and getting dressed. These can be done while the baby sleeps.

Complications can occur during pregnancy, labor, and delivery. They also can occur in the postpartum period. Report any sign or symptom listed in Box 38-6 to the nurse at once.

---

**BOX 38-6  SIGNS AND SYMPTOMS OF POSTPARTUM COMPLICATIONS**

- Fever of 100.4° F or higher
- Abdominal or perineal pain
- Foul-smelling vaginal discharge
- Bleeding from an episiotomy or C-section incision
- Redness, swelling, or drainage from an episiotomy or C-section incision
- Saturating a sanitary napkin within 1 hour of application
- Red lochia after lochia has changed color to pinkish brown or white
- Burning on urination
- Leg pain, tenderness, or swelling
- Sadness or feelings of depression
- Breast pain, tenderness, or swelling

# ■ REVIEW QUESTIONS ■

Circle the **BEST** answer.

1  A baby's head and neck is supported for the first
   a  7 to 10 days
   b  Month
   c  3 months
   d  6 months

2  Zach is a newborn. When holding him you should do the following *except*
   a  Hold him securely
   b  Cuddle him
   c  Sing and talk to him
   d  Hold him on his stomach

3  Which is *false?*
   a  Zach's crib should be within hearing distance of caregivers.
   b  Zach needs a pillow for sleep.
   c  Zach is positioned on his back for sleep.
   d  Crib rails are up at all times.

4  Report the following to the nurse *except*
   a  Zach looks flushed and is perspiring
   b  Zach has watery stools
   c  Zach's eyes are red and irritated
   d  Zach spits up a small amount when burped

5  Zach is breast-fed. The mother should do the following *except*
   a  Wash her hands
   b  Hold Zach close to her breast
   c  Stimulate the rooting reflex
   d  Clean her breasts with soap and water

6  A breast-fed baby is burped
   a  Every 5 minutes
   b  After nursing from one breast
   c  After nursing from both breasts
   d  After half the formula is taken

7  Zach is going to be bottle-fed. You do the shopping. Which formula should you buy?
   a  The one that is on sale
   b  The ready-to-feed type
   c  The one ordered by the doctor
   d  The powdered form

8  You are to warm Zach's bottle. Which is *true?*
   a  The bottle is warmed in the microwave.
   b  The formula is warmed at room temperature.
   c  The formula should feel warm on the inside of your wrist.
   d  The formula is warmed in a pan for 5 minutes.

9  When bottle-feeding Zach, you should
   a  Burp him every 5 minutes
   b  Save remaining formula for the next feeding
   c  Tilt the bottle so that formula fills the neck of the bottle and the nipple
   d  Leave him alone with the bottle

10  Zach's cord has not yet healed. His diaper should be
    a  Loose over the cord
    b  Snug over the cord
    c  Below the cord
    d  Disposable

11  Zach's cord stump is cleaned with
    a  Soap and water
    b  Baby shampoo
    c  Plain water
    d  Alcohol

12  Zach's cord and the circumcision are cleaned
    a  Once a day
    b  When he has a bowel movement
    c  Three times a day
    d  At every diaper change

13  Bath water for Zach should be
    a  85° to 90° F
    b  90° to 95° F
    c  95° to 100° F
    d  100° to 105° F

14  Which should you use to wash Zach's nose?
    a  A mitted washcloth
    b  Alcohol wipes
    c  A cotton swab
    d  Cotton balls

15  A mother has a red vaginal discharge the first few days after childbirth. This
    a  Is a menstrual period
    b  Signals a postpartum complication
    c  Is lochia rubra
    d  Is from her episiotomy

# ■ REVIEW QUESTIONS ■

**16** A cesarean delivery involves
  **a** A vaginal incision
  **b** A perineal incision
  **c** An abdominal incision
  **d** A normal delivery through the birth canal

Circle **T** if the statement is true and **F** if it is false.

**17** **T F** Zach's diapers are changed whenever he is wet.

**18** **T F** Zach's cord and circumcision have not healed. He should have a sponge bath.

**19** **T F** Cotton swabs are used to clean Zach's ears.

**20** **T F** Zach is being breast-fed. He is weighed with his diaper on.

*Answers to these questions are on p. 820.*

# Assisted Living

# OBJECTIVES

- Define the key terms listed in this chapter
- Identify the purpose of and services provided by assisted living facilities
- Identify the person's rights
- Identify the types of assisted living facilities and the living areas offered
- Describe the physical and environmental requirements of assisted living facilities
- Describe the requirements for assisted living facility staff
- Describe the requirements for persons who want to live in assisted living facilities
- Explain the purpose of a service plan
- Explain how to assist with housekeeping and laundry
- Explain how to assist with food handling, preparation, and storage
- Explain how to assist with medications
- Identify the reasons for transferring, discharging, or evicting a person

# KEY TERMS

**medication reminder**  Reminding the person to take drugs, observing them being taken as prescribed, and charting that they were taken

**service plan**  A written plan listing the services needed by the person and who provides them

---

Many older people do not need nursing center care. However, they cannot or do not want to live alone. Many need some help with self-care. Some have physical or cognitive problems and disabilities. Still others need help taking drugs. Others do not want to live alone.

Assisted living settings offer quality of life with independence and companionship. An *assisted living residence* provides housing, support services, and health care to persons needing help with activities of daily living. Some needs are scheduled, such as taking drugs at certain times. Others are unscheduled—elimination, transfers, getting a snack, or taking a walk.

**SAFETY ALERT:** *Assisted Living*
Residents have the same diseases and illnesses as persons at home, in hospitals, and in nursing centers. They are at risk for infections. This includes sexually transmitted and other communicable diseases (Chapter 33). Follow Standard Precautions and the Bloodborne Pathogen Standard when contact with blood, body fluids, secretions, excretions, or potentially contaminated items and surfaces is likely.

## PURPOSE

People are living longer, and there are more older people than before. Divorce rates are high. Some remarry; others do not. Today's older persons had some birth control options. Many had small families. And the United States is a mobile society. Children grow-up and move far away from their families. For these reasons, many older persons live alone without family nearby. When help is needed, often there is no one to assist them.

According to the American Association of Retired Persons (AARP), most assisted living residents need help taking drugs and with bathing, dressing, elimination, and eating. Almost half are cognitively impaired. This means that they have problems with thinking, reasoning, and judgment. Some residents use wheelchairs or motorized scooters.

A homelike setting is provided. Residents have a secure setting and 24-hour supervision. They are given three meals a day. There are laundry, housekeeping, and transportation services. Social and recreational services are offered. So are some health services. Services are added or reduced as the person's needs change.

Some assisted living facilities are part of nursing centers or retirement communities. Others are separate facilities. Most states have laws, rules, and regulations that control assisted living facilities. Residents' rights are part of such laws (Box 39-1). Also, licensure is usually required.

## LIVING AREAS

Living areas vary. A small apartment has a bedroom, bathroom, living area, kitchen, and laundry area (Figs. 39-1 and 39-2). Some people just want a bedroom and bathroom. Others share a bedroom and bathroom with a roommate. Box 39-2 lists the requirements and features of assisted living units. Box 39-3 lists environmental requirements.

## ALZHEIMER'S CARE UNITS

Some residents have Alzheimer's disease or other dementias (Chapter 35). State requirements must be met. They relate to care, the setting, staffing, activities, safety, and the family's role in meeting the person's needs.

---

### BOX 39-1 RESIDENT'S RIGHTS (ASSISTED LIVING)

Assisted facility residents have the right to:

- Be treated with dignity, respect, consideration, and fairness
- Keep and use personal items
- Have personal items kept safe and secure
- Help develop a service plan
- Choose activities, schedules, and daily routines
- Choose a doctor, pharmacy, or other service provider
- Receive the services stated in the service plan
- Review and change the service plan at any time
- Refuse services and to be advised of the consequences of refusing
- Be fully informed in advance about care and treatment and of any changes in that care or treatment that may affect his or her well-being
- Privacy and dignity, especially during personal care or services
- Take part in or refuse to take part in social, recreational, rehabilitative, religious, political, or community activities
- Interact with people inside and outside of the facility
- Send and receive mail unopened
- Make and receive private phone calls
- Visit with others in private
- Arrange for medical and personal care
- Leave the building at any time and not be locked into any room, building, or on facility premises during the day or night
- 24-hour access to the building and its common areas

- Share a unit with a life partner if both partners consent and if both partners are facility residents
- Contact an ombudsman (Chapter 9)
- Freely criticize the facility, file grievances, or make complaints to appropriate agencies
- Be free of chemical and physical restraints
- Be free of abuse or neglect
- Refuse to perform work for the facility
- Perform work for the facility if it consents and if the agreed upon work arrangement (including pay rate) is part of the service plan
- Confidentiality of the medical record
- Access and copy personal files maintained by the facility
- Be transferred, discharged, or evicted by the facility according to the admission contract
- Manage and control personal funds or to be given an accounting of personal funds entrusted to the facility
- Be free from financial abuse
- Privacy in financial and personal affairs
- Be informed, in writing, of fee changes according to the admission agreement
- Be encouraged and assisted in the exercise of these rights as a resident and as a citizen
- Complete an advance directive
- Refuse to take part in research
- Request to relocate or refuse to relocate within the facility
- Organize resident councils

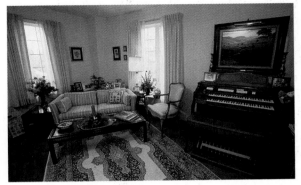

**FIG. 39-1** A living area in an assisted living apartment.

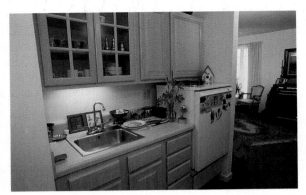

**FIG. 39-2** A kitchen in an assisted living apartment.

## BOX 39-2  REQUIREMENT AND FEATURES OF ASSISTED LIVING UNITS

- A door that locks; the person keeps a key
- A telephone jack
- An emergency communication system
- A window or door that provides natural light
- Lighted common areas
- A window or door that allows safe exit in an emergency
- A mailbox for each person
- A bathroom that provides privacy:
  - A sink in the bathroom or in the next room (sink is not used for food preparation)
  - A bathtub or shower that has a shower curtain and nonslip surfaces
  - Ventilation or a window that opens
- Grab bars for the toilet and bathtub or shower
- Other assistive devices needed for safety and identified in the service plan
- Smoke detectors
- A bed (frame and mattress) that is clean and in good repair
- Adequate general and task lighting
- An easy chair
- A table and chair for meals
- Adjustable window covers that provide privacy
- A dresser or storage space for clothing and personal items
- Food preparation appliances—sink, stove, refrigerator with freezer, and storage for food and cooking items

## BOX 39-3  ENVIRONMENTAL REQUIREMENTS

- The facility is clean, safe, orderly, odor-free, and in good repair.
- The facility is free of insects and rodents.
- Garbage is stored in covered containers lined with plastic bags. Bags are removed from the facility at least once a week.
- Hot water temperatures are between 95° F and 120° F in areas used by residents.
- The hot and cold water supply meets hygiene needs.
- Common bathrooms have toilet paper, soap, and cloth towels, paper towels, or a dryer.
- Clean linens are handled, transported, and stored to prevent contamination.
- Soiled linen and clothing are stored in closed containers away from food, kitchen, and dining areas.
- Oxygen containers are stored according to the manufacturer's instructions.
- Cleaning solutions, insecticides, and other hazardous substances are stored in their original containers. They are in locked cabinets in rooms separate from food, dining areas, and drugs.
- Pets or animals are controlled to protect residents and maintain sanitation.
- Employees have access to a first aid kit.

Persons with Alzheimer's disease have poor judgment. They cannot follow directions. And they tend to wander. A safe setting is needed. They need supervision and help leaving the building in an emergency (p. 775).

The person needs a comfortable routine and schedule. Activities provide stimulation and promote the person's highest level of function. The activities must be things the person once enjoyed doing and can still do to a limited and safe extent.

Staff must have training about Alzheimer's disease. Many states require ongoing or annual training about Alzheimer's disease and related dementias.

## STAFF REQUIREMENTS

Staff requirements vary from state to state. Some require nursing assistant training and competency evaluation. Others require training in the following areas:
- The needs and goals of assisted living residents
- Promoting dignity, independence, and resident rights
- Using service plans
- Ethics and confidentiality of records and information
- Hygiene and infection control
- Nutrition and menu planning
- Food preparation, service, and storage
- Housekeeping and sanitation
- Preventing and reporting abuse and neglect
- Incident reports
- Fire and disaster procedures
- Assisting with drugs
- Early signs of illness and the need for health care
- Safety measures
- Communication skills
- Special needs of persons with Alzheimer's disease and other dementias
- CPR and first aid

Criminal background checks may be required. The facility cannot employ a person with a criminal record.

## RESIDENT REQUIREMENTS

Assisted living is for persons needing some help with activities of daily living (ADL). Some persons are paralyzed or chronically ill. However, they do not need help with complex medical problems. If nursing services are needed, home health care is arranged.

Mobility is often a requirement. The person walks or is mobile with a wheelchair or motor scooter. The person must be able to leave the building in an emergency. Stable health is another requirement. Only limited health care or treatment is needed.

Assisted living is not for people who have greater care needs or require skilled nursing services.

### SERVICE PLAN

A **service plan** is a written plan listing the services needed by the person and who provides them. It also addresses how much help is needed. The plan relates to ADL, activities and social services, dietary needs, taking drugs, and special needs. Health services are included.

For example, a person needs help getting dressed. The service plan states that you will assist the person. The service plan also states that a nurse will replace the person's catheter. The person needs physical therapy after a hip fracture. The service plan states a physical therapist will visit. And the person needs help taking drugs. A family member will assist the person.

The plan is reviewed yearly and when the person's condition, wants, or service needs change.

## SERVICES

Help is given with ADL. Meals, housekeeping, and laundry services are provided. There is a 24-hour emergency communication system. It is used for an emergency or to call for help.

Social, educational, and religious services are common. So are transportation, shopping, banking, and money management services.

### MEALS

Three meals a day and snacks are provided. The time between the evening meal and breakfast usually is no more than 14 hours. It can be longer if there is a nutritious evening snack. Special dietary needs are met. Also, the week's menu is posted for residents to review.

Residents are encouraged to eat in the dining room with other persons. They can eat in their rooms if they want to. Special eating utensils are provided as needed. So is help with eating, opening cartons, buttering bread, cutting meat, and so on (Chapter 20).

## HOUSEKEEPING

Housekeeping measures help prevent infection. They also keep living units neat and clean:
- Dust furniture at least weekly.
- Vacuum floors at least weekly and as needed.
- Wipe up spills right away.
- Use a dust mop or broom to sweep. Use a dustpan to collect dust and crumbs.
- Sweep daily or more often as needed.
- Make sure toilets are flushed after each use.
- Rinse the sink after washing, shaving, or oral hygiene.
- Clean the tub or shower after each use.
- Remove and dispose of hair from the sink, tub, or shower.
- Hang towels to dry. Or place them in a hamper.
- Clean the bathroom surfaces every day. Use a disinfectant or water and detergent to clean all surfaces. They include:
  —The toilet bowl, seat, and outside areas of the toilet
  —The floor
  —The sides, walls, and curtain or door of the tub or shower
  —Towel racks and toilet tissue, toothbrush, and soap holders
  —The sink and mirror
  —Windowsills
- Mop or vacuum the bathroom floor every day.
- Empty bathroom wastebaskets every day.
- Put out clean towels and washcloths every day.
- Wash bath mats, the wastebasket, and laundry hamper every week.
- Replace toilet and facial tissue as needed.
- Open bathroom windows for a short time, and use air fresheners.

## FOOD HANDLING, PREPARATION, AND STORAGE

Certain measures are needed when handling, preparing, and storing food. They protect against infection:
- Handle meat and poultry safely. Follow the safe handling instructions on food labels (Fig. 39-3).
- Cook meats and poultry adequately.
- Protect leftover foods. Place leftover food in small containers. Cover containers with lids, foil, or plastic wrap. Date and refrigerate containers as soon as possible.
- Use leftover food within 2 or 3 days.
- Wash eating and cooking items. Use liquid detergent and hot water. Wash glasses and cups first. Follow with silverware, plates, bowls, and then pots and pans. Rinse items well with hot water.
- Place washed eating and cooking items in a drainer to dry. Air-drying is more aseptic than towel drying.
- Rinse dishes before loading them into a dishwasher. Use dishwasher soap.
- Do not wash pots and pans and cast iron, wood, and some plastic items in a dishwasher.

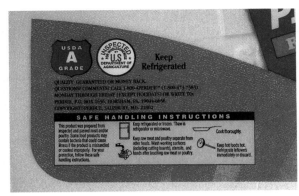

**FIG. 39-3** Safe handling instructions for meat and poultry. They are required by the U.S. Department of Agriculture.

- Clean kitchen appliances, counters, tables, and other surfaces after each meal. Use a clean sponge or dishcloth. Moisten it with water and detergent.
- Remove grease spills and splashes. Use a liquid surface cleaner.
- Clean sinks with scouring powder.
- Dispose of garbage, leftovers, and other soiled supplies after each meal. A garbage disposal is best for food and liquid garbage. Do not put bones in the garbage disposal.
- Recycle paper, boxes, cans, and plastic containers according to facility policy.
- Empty garbage at least once a day.

## LAUNDRY

Laundry services include providing clean bed linens. Residents can use a washing machine, dryer, iron, and ironing board. When assisting with laundry, follow these guidelines:
- Wear gloves when handling soiled laundry (see *Safety Alert: Assisted Living*, p. 769).
- Follow the person's preferences.
- Follow care label directions.
- Sort items by color and fabric. Separate white, colored, and dark items. Separate sturdy and delicate fabrics.
- Empty pockets.
- Fasten buttons, zippers, snaps, hooks, and other closures.
- Wash heavily soiled items separately.
- Follow detergent directions.
- Select the correct wash cycle and water temperature. Follow care label directions and the person's preferences.
- Select the correct drying temperature and cycle. Follow care label directions and the person's preferences.
- Fold, hang, or iron clothes as the person prefers.

## NURSING SERVICES

Some facilities provide limited nursing services. The nurse assesses each person and monitors health. The nurse supervises tasks delegated to caregivers. The nurse also gives medications to persons who cannot manage their own drugs.

## MEDICATION ASSISTANCE

Drugs must be taken as prescribed. The five rights of drug administration are:

- The right drug
- The right dose (amount)
- The right route (by mouth, injection, applied to the skin, inhalation, vaginally, or rectally)
- The right time
- The right person

Your role in assisting with drugs depends on your state's laws, agency policy, and your training and education. It may involve one or more of the following. *Remember, you do not give drugs (Chapter 2).*

- Reminding the person it is time to take a drug
- Reading the drug label to the person
- Opening containers for persons who cannot do so
- Checking the dosage against the drug label
- Providing water, juice, milk, crackers, applesauce, or other food and fluids as needed
- Making sure the person takes the right drug, the right amount, at the right time, and in the right way
- Charting that the person took or refused to take the drug
- Storing drugs

Residents manage and take their own drugs if able. This is called *self-directed medication management.* The person knows drugs by name, color, or shape. The person knows what drugs to take, the correct doses, and when and how to take them. The person can question changes in the usual drug routine. For example, the person comments that a pill is not broken in half. Or the person says that a pill looks different. Report comments or questions to the nurse.

Pill organizers are often used (Fig. 39-4). They have sections for days and times. The person, a family member or legal representative, or a nurse prepares the organizer for the week. The person then takes the drugs on the right day and at the right time.

Some people need medication reminders. A **medication reminder** means reminding the person to take drugs, observing them being taken as prescribed, and charting that they were taken.

**MEDICATION RECORD.** A medication record is kept for each person needing help with drugs. The record includes:

- The person's name
- Drug name, dose, directions, and route of administration
- Date and time to take the drug
- Date and time help was given
- Signature or initials of the person assisting

**DRUG ERRORS.** Report any drug error to the RN. Also complete an incident report. An error means one or more of the following:

- Taking another person's drugs
- Taking the wrong drug
- Taking the wrong dose
- Taking a drug at the wrong time
- Taking a drug by the wrong route
- Not taking a drug when ordered

**STORING DRUGS.** Drugs are kept in a secure place. This prevents someone else from taking them. If the facility stores the drugs, they are kept in a locked container, cabinet, or area.

Some persons manage and store their own drugs. If the room is shared, each person's ability to safely have drugs is assessed. If safety is a factor, drugs are kept in a locked container.

All drugs must have the original pharmacy label. They are stored as directed on the label. For example, some drugs are refrigerated. Others are kept away from light. The label also has an expiration date. Expired or discontinued drugs are disposed of following facility procedures.

## ACTIVITIES AND RECREATION

Residents are urged to take part in activity and recreational programs. Social, physical, and community activities promote well-being and independence. An activities director plans, organizes, and conducts the activity program. These activities are put on a weekly or monthly calendar. It also tells about community events and activities.

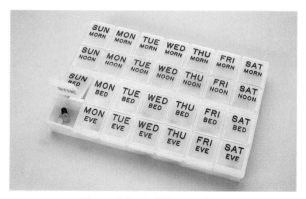

**FIG. 39-4** Pill organizer.

## SPECIAL SERVICES AND SAFETY NEEDS

Sometimes emergencies occur. Some people need help getting out of bed or transferring to a wheelchair. Then they can leave the building with little or no help.

Other people cannot walk or use a wheelchair or motor scooter. They need attendants. If an attendant is needed, the facility and the person agree on how and who will meet the person's needs. An attendant is needed 24 hours a day.

## TRANSFER, DISCHARGE, AND EVICTION

Residents can be transferred, discharged, or evicted. The facility must tell the person about the action as required by state law. Reasons for such action are:

- The facility can no longer meet the person's health needs. The person is a threat to the health and safety of self or others. Or the facility cannot provide needed care.
- The person fails to pay for services.
- The person fails to comply with facility policies or rules.
- The person wants to transfer.
- The facility closes.

Circle the **BEST** answer.

**1** Assisted living provides the following *except*
  a  Nursing care
  b  Housing
  c  Help with activities of daily living
  d  Support services

**2** These statements are about assisted living. Which is *false?*
  a  Each person has a private apartment.
  b  Some have Alzheimer's care units.
  c  24-hour security is provided.
  d  Three meals a day are provided.

**3** Assisted living staff must
  a  Complete a nursing assistant training and competency evaluation program
  b  Meet state requirements
  c  Assist with drugs
  d  Provide transportation

**4** Assisted living facilities often require the following *except*
  a  That persons be mobile
  b  That persons have stable health
  c  That persons require only limited care
  d  That persons speak English

**5** A service plan
  a  Describes nursing care needs
  b  Describes the services needed and who provides them
  c  Lists the drugs the person needs to take
  d  Lists service fees and charges

**6** Assisted living residents are encouraged to eat
  a  In their rooms
  b  In the dining room
  c  At home
  d  At community events

**7** You assist with housekeeping. Which is *false?*
  a  Dusting and vacuuming are done at least weekly.
  b  Spills are wiped up right away.
  c  Bathroom surfaces are cleaned daily.
  d  Spills and splashes are wiped up after meals.

**8** You assist with food. Which is *false?*
  a  Safe handling instructions are followed.
  b  Leftover food is used in 3 to 5 days.
  c  Garbage is emptied at least once a day.
  d  Pots and pans are washed by hand.

**9** You assist with laundry. Which is *true?*
  a  Care label directions are followed.
  b  Clothes are washed in hot water.
  c  Clothes are ironed.
  d  All white fabrics are washed together.

**10** Usually assisted living staff are allowed to
  a  Give drugs
  b  Give medication reminders
  c  Refill drugs
  d  Prepare pill organizers

**11** Drugs are kept
  a  In the person's closet
  b  In the person's drawer
  c  In a locked container, cabinet, or area
  d  By the family

**12** Which of these violates an assisted living resident's rights?
  a  Covering the person during personal care
  b  Giving the person unopened mail
  c  Keeping information confidential
  d  Choosing activities for the person

**13** A person wants to attend a concert. Which statement is *true?*
  a  The concert must be approved by the facility.
  b  The person must return by 10 PM.
  c  An attendant must go with the person.
  d  The facility must respect the person's choice.

**14** The facility cannot provide a person with all needed services. Which is *true?*
  a  The facility must hire more staff.
  b  The family must provide the needed care.
  c  The facility can ask the person to transfer.
  d  The person's service plan needs to change.

*Answers to these questions are on p. 820.*

# Basic
# Emergency Care

## OBJECTIVES

- Define the key terms listed in this chapter
- Describe the general rules of emergency care
- Identify the signs of cardiac arrest and obstructed airway
- Describe the signs, symptoms, and emergency care for hemorrhage
- Identify the signs, symptoms, and emergency care for shock
- Describe the types of seizures and how to care for a person during a seizure
- Describe the causes, types, and emergency care for burns
- Identify the common causes and emergency care for fainting
- Describe the signs, symptoms, and emergency care for stroke
- Perform the procedures described in this chapter

## KEY TERMS

**anaphylaxis** A life-threatening sensitivity to an antigen

**cardiac arrest** The heart and breathing stop suddenly and without warning

**convulsion** A seizure

**fainting** The sudden loss of consciousness from an inadequate blood supply to the brain

**first aid** Emergency care given to an ill or injured person before medical help arrives

**hemorrhage** The excessive loss of blood in a short time

**respiratory arrest** Breathing stops but heart action continues for several minutes

**seizure** Violent and sudden contractions or tremors of muscle groups; convulsion

**shock** Results when organs and tissues do not get enough blood

Emergencies can occur anywhere. Sometimes you can save a life if you know what to do. You are encouraged to take a first aid course and a basic life support (BLS) course. These courses prepare you to give emergency care.

*The basic life support procedures in this chapter are given as information. They do not replace certification training. You need a basic life support course for health care providers.*

(paramedics, emergency medical technicians) rush to the scene. They treat, stabilize, and transport persons with life-threatening problems. Their ambulances have emergency drugs, equipment, and supplies. They communicate with doctors in hospital emergency rooms. The doctors tell them what to do. To activate the EMS system, dial 911. Or call the local fire or police department or the telephone operator.

Each emergency is different. However, the rules in Box 40-1 apply to any emergency. *See Focus on Long-Term Care: Emergency Care.*

## EMERGENCY CARE

**First aid** is the emergency care given to an ill or injured person before medical help arrives. Its goals are to:
- Prevent death
- Prevent injuries from becoming worse

In an emergency, the Emergency Medical Services (EMS) system is activated. Emergency personnel

> **SAFETY ALERT:** *Emergency Care*
> During emergencies, contact with blood, body fluids, excretions, and secretions is likely. Follow Standard Precautions and the Bloodborne Pathogen Standard to the extent possible.

# BASIC LIFE SUPPORT

When the heart and breathing stop, the person is clinically dead. Blood and oxygen are not circulated through the body. Brain damage and other organ damage occur within minutes. Basic life support (BLS) procedures support breathing and circulation. These lifesaving measures require speed, skill, and efficiency.

*The discussion and procedures that follow assume that the person does not have injuries from trauma. If injuries are present, special measures are needed to position the person and open the airway. Such measures are learned during a BLS certification course.*

## FOCUS ON LONG-TERM CARE
### EMERGENCY CARE

In nursing centers, a nurse decides when to activate the EMS system. The nurse tells you how to help. If a person has stopped breathing or is in cardiac arrest, the nurse may start cardiopulmonary resuscitation (CPR) (p. 780). Some centers allow nursing assistants to start CPR. Others do not. Know your center's policy about CPR.

Death is expected in persons suffering from terminal illnesses. Usually these persons are not resuscitated (Chapter 41). This information is in the care plan.

# CARDIAC ARREST

The heart and breathing can stop suddenly and without warning. This is a state of **cardiac arrest.** Permanent brain damage occurs unless breathing and circulation are restored.

Cardiac arrest is a sudden, unexpected, and dramatic event. It can occur while driving, shoveling snow, playing golf or tennis, watching TV, eating, and sleeping. Cardiac arrest can occur anywhere and at any time. Common causes include heart disease, drowning, electrical shock, severe injury, foreign-body airway obstruction (FBAO), and drug overdose. These causes lead to an abnormal heart rhythm called *ventricular fibrillation.* The heart cannot pump blood. A normal rhythm must be restored (p. 796). Otherwise the person will die.

# RESPIRATORY ARREST

**Respiratory arrest** is when breathing stops but heart action continues for several minutes. If breathing is not restored, cardiac arrest occurs. Causes of respiratory arrest include:

- Drowning
- Stroke
- Foreign-body airway obstruction (FBAO)
- Drug overdose
- Electric shock (including lightning strikes)
- Smoke inhalation
- Suffocation
- Heart attack
- Coma
- Other injuries

## BOX 40-1   GENERAL RULES OF EMERGENCY CARE

- Know your limits. Do not do more than you are able. Do not perform an unfamiliar procedure. Do what you can under the circumstances.
- Stay calm. This helps the person feel more secure.
- Know where to find emergency supplies.
- Follow Standard Precautions and the Bloodborne Pathogen Standard to the extent possible.
- Check for life-threatening problems. Check for breathing, a pulse, and bleeding.
- Keep the person lying down or as you found him or her. Moving the person could make an injury worse.
- Perform necessary emergency measures.
- Call for help, or have someone activate the EMS system. *Do not hang up until the operator has hung up.* Give the operator the following information:
  —Your location: street address and city, cross streets or roads, and landmarks
  —Telephone number you are calling from

  —What happened (for example, heart attack, accident, fire)—police, fire equipment, and ambulances may be needed
  —How many people need help
  —Condition of victims, obvious injuries, and life-threatening situations
  —What aid is being given
- Do not remove clothes unless you have to. If you must remove clothing, tear or cut garments along the seams.
- Keep the person warm. Cover the person with a blanket, coats, or sweaters.
- Reassure the conscious person. Explain what is happening and that help was called.
- Do not give the person food or fluids.
- Keep bystanders away. They invade privacy and tend to stare, give advice, and comment about the person's condition. The person may think the situation is worse than it really is.

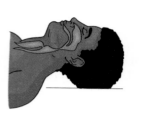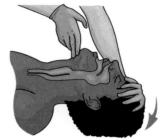

**FIG. 40-1** The head-tilt/chin-lift maneuver opens the airway. One hand is on the person's forehead. Pressure is applied to tilt the head back. The chin is lifted with the fingers of the other hand.

## CHAIN OF SURVIVAL

The American Heart Association's (AHA's) basic life support courses teach the adult Chain of Survival. These actions are taken for heart attack, cardiac arrest, stroke, and FBAO (choking). They also apply to other life-threatening problems. They are done as soon as possible. Any delay reduces the person's chance of surviving.

Chain of Survival actions are:
- *Early access to the emergency response system.* This means activating the EMS system. Hospitals and nursing centers call special codes for life-threatening emergencies.
- *Early CPR.*
- *Early defibrillation.* See p. 796.
- *Early advanced care.* This is given by EMS staff, doctors, and nurses. They give drugs and perform life-saving measures.

*See Focus on Children: Chain of Survival.*

## CARDIOPULMONARY RESUSCITATION FOR ADULTS

Cardiopulmonary resuscitation (CPR) must be started at once when a person is in cardiac arrest. It provides oxygen to the brain and heart until advanced emergency care is given. There are three major signs of cardiac arrest:
- No response
- No breathing
- No pulse

The person's skin is cool, pale, and gray. The person is not coughing or moving.

CPR has three basic parts (the ABCs of CPR):
- Airway
- Breathing
- Circulation

**AIRWAY.** The respiratory passages (airway) must be open to restore breathing. The airway is often obstructed (blocked) during cardiac arrest. The person's tongue falls toward the back of the throat and blocks the airway. The *head-tilt/chin-lift maneuver* opens the airway (Fig. 40-1):
- Position the person supine on a hard, flat surface.
- Kneel or stand at the person's side.
- Place the palm of one hand on the forehead.
- Tilt the head back by pushing down on the forehead with your palm.
- Place the fingers of the other hand under the bony part of the chin.
- Lift the chin as you tilt the head backward with your other hand.

When the airway is open, check for vomitus, loose dentures, or other objects. These can obstruct the airway during rescue breathing. Remove dentures and wipe vomitus away with your index and middle fingers. Wear gloves, or cover your fingers with a cloth. Although you must not waste time, try to protect dentures from loss or damage.

**BREATHING.** Air is not inhaled when breathing stops. The person must get oxygen. If not, permanent brain damage and organ damage occur. The person is given *rescue breathing.*

Before you start rescue breathing, check for adequate breathing (Fig. 40-2). It should take no more than 10 seconds to do the following:
- Maintain an open airway.
- Place your ear over the person's mouth and nose.
- Observe the person's chest.
- *Look* to see if the chest rises and falls.
- *Listen* for the escape of air.
- *Feel* for the flow of air on your cheek.

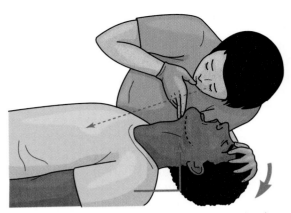

**FIG. 40-2** Determining adequate breathing. *Look* to see if the chest rises and falls. *Listen* for the escape of air. *Feel* for the flow of air on your cheek.

Rescue breathing involves inflating the person's lungs. *Mouth-to-mouth* breathing (Fig. 40-3) involves placing your mouth over the person's mouth. Contact with the person's blood, body fluids, secretions, or excretions is likely. To give mouth-to-mouth breathing:

- Keep the airway open.
- Pinch the person's nostrils shut. Use your thumb and index finger. Use the hand on the forehead. Shutting the nostrils prevents air from escaping through the nose.
- Take a deep breath.
- Place your mouth tightly over the person's mouth.
- Blow air into the person's mouth slowly. You should see the chest rise as the lungs fill with air. You should also hear air escape when the person exhales.
- Remove your mouth from the person's mouth. Then take in a quick, deep breath.

*Mouth-to-barrier device* breathing is used in the workplace. A barrier device is placed over the person's mouth and nose. It prevents contact with the person's mouth and blood, body fluids, secretions, or excretions (Fig. 40-4). The seal must be tight.

The Ambu bag (Chapter 30) is another barrier device. It is used to give oxygen during rescue breathing.

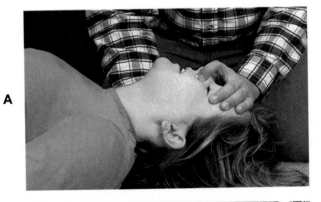

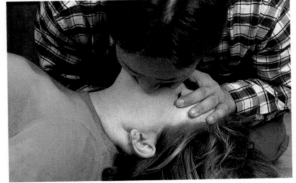

**FIG. 40-3** Mouth-to-mouth rescue breathing. **A,** The person's airway is opened. The nostrils are pinched shut. **B,** The person's mouth is sealed by the rescuer's mouth.

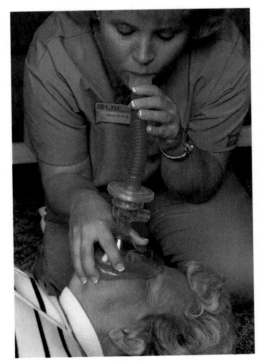

**FIG. 40-4** Barrier device.

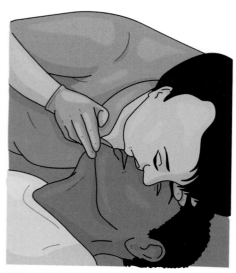

**FIG. 40-5** Mouth-to-nose breathing.

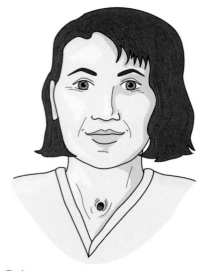

**FIG. 40-6** A stoma in the neck. The person breathes in and out of the stoma.

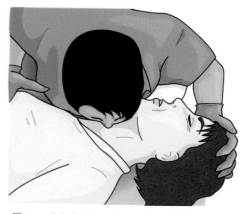

**FIG. 40-7** Mouth-to-stoma breathing.

Mouth-to-mouth breathing is not always possible. The *mouth-to-nose* breathing is used when:

- You cannot ventilate through the person's mouth
- You cannot open the mouth
- You cannot make a tight seal for mouth-to-mouth breathing
- The mouth is severely injured
- Rescuing a drowning victim

The mouth is closed for mouth-to-nose breathing. The head-tilt/chin-lift method opens the airway. Pressure is placed on the chin to close the mouth. To give a breath, place your mouth over the person's nose and blow air into the nose (Fig. 40-5). After giving a breath, remove your mouth from the person's nose.

Some people breathe through openings *(stomas)* in their necks (Fig. 40-6). To give *mouth-to-stoma* breathing, seal your mouth around the stoma and blow air into the stoma (Fig. 40-7). Before giving mouth-to-mouth or mouth-to-nose breathing, always check to see if a person has a stoma. Other rescue breathing methods are not effective if the person has a stoma.

When you start CPR, give 2 breaths first. Allow exhalation after each breath. Then give breaths at a rate of 10 to 12 breaths per minute. During CPR, 2 breaths are given after every 15 chest compressions.

**CIRCULATION.** The brain and other organs must receive blood. Otherwise, permanent damage results. In cardiac arrest, the heart has stopped beating. Blood must be pumped through the body some other way. Chest compressions force blood through the circulatory system.

Before starting chest compressions, check for a pulse. Use the carotid artery on the side near you. To find the carotid pulse, place two fingers on the person's trachea (windpipe). Then slide your fingertips down off the trachea to the groove of the neck (Fig. 40-8). While checking for a pulse, also look for signs of circulation. See if the person has started breathing or is coughing or moving.

The heart lies between the sternum (breastbone) and the spinal column. When pressure is applied to the sternum, the sternum is depressed. This compresses the heart between the sternum and spinal column (Fig. 40-9). For effective chest compressions, the person must be supine and on a hard, flat surface. And, proper hand position is needed (Fig. 40-10):

- Use 2 or 3 fingers to find the lower part of the person's rib cage on the side near you. Use the hand closest to the person's feet.
- Move your fingers up along the rib cage to the notch at the center of the chest. The notch is where the ribs and sternum meet.
- Place the heel of your other hand on the lower half of the sternum by your index finger.
- Remove your fingers from the notch.

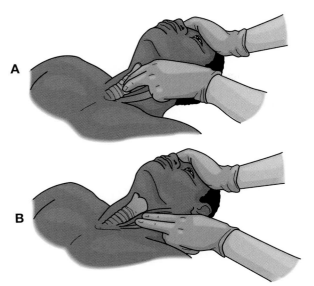

**FIG. 40-8** Locating the carotid pulse. **A,** Two fingers are placed on the trachea. **B,** The fingers are moved down into the groove of the neck to the carotid pulse.

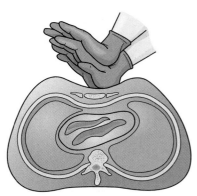

**FIG. 40-9** The heart lies between the sternum and spinal column. The heart is compressed when pressure is applied to the sternum.

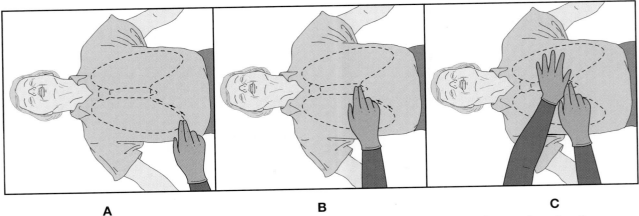

**A**  **B**  **C**

**FIG. 40-10** Proper hand position for CPR. **A,** Find the rib cage. **B,** Move your fingers along the rib cage to the notch. **C,** Place the heel of your hand next to your index finger.

- Place your other hand on the hand that is on the sternum.
- Extend or interlace your fingers. Keep them off the chest.

You must be positioned properly for chest compressions. Your arms are straight. Your shoulders are directly over your hands (Fig. 40-11). Exert firm downward pressure to depress the sternum about 1½ to 2 inches in the adult. Then release pressure without removing your hands from the chest. Give compressions in a regular rhythm at a rate of 100 per minute.

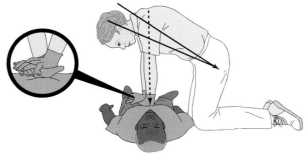

**FIG. 40-11** To give chest compressions, the arms are straight and shoulders are over the hands.

**PERFORMING ADULT CPR.** CPR is done only for cardiac arrest. You must determine if cardiac arrest or fainting has occurred. *CPR is done when the person does not respond, is not breathing, and has no pulse.*

CPR is done alone or with another person. *Never practice CPR on another person.* Serious damage can be done. Mannequins are used to learn CPR.

## ADULT CPR—ONE RESCUER

### PROCEDURE

1 Check if the person is responding. Tap or gently shake the person, call the person by name, and shout "Are you OK?"
2 Call for help. Activate the EMS system or the agency's emergency response system.
3 Position the person supine. Logroll the person so there is no twisting of the spine. The person must be on a hard, flat surface. Place the person's arms alongside the body.
4 Open the airway. Use the head-tilt/chin-lift method.
5 Check for breathing. *Look* to see if the chest rises and falls. *Listen* for the escape of air. *Feel* for the flow of air on your cheek.
6 Give 2 slow breaths if the person is not breathing or is not breathing adequately. Each breath takes 2 seconds. Let the person's chest deflate between breaths.
7 Check for a carotid pulse and for breathing, coughing, and moving. This should take 5 to 10 seconds. Use your other hand to keep the airway open with the head-tilt/chin-lift method. Start chest compressions if there are no signs of circulation.
8 Give chest compressions at a rate of 100 per minute. Give 15 compressions and then 2 slow breaths.
  a Establish a rhythm, and count out loud. (Try: "1 and, 2 and, 3 and, 4 and, 5 and, 6 and, 7 and, 8 and, 9 and, 10 and, 11 and, 12 and, 13 and, 14 and, 15.")
  b Open the airway, and give 2 slow breaths.
  c Repeat this step until 4 cycles of 15 compressions and 2 breaths are given.
9 Check for a carotid pulse. Also check for breathing, coughing, and moving.
10 Continue CPR if the person has no signs of circulation. Begin with chest compressions. Continue the cycle of 15 compressions and 2 breaths. Check for circulation every few minutes.
11 Do the following if the person has signs of circulation.
  a Check for breathing.
  b Position the person in the recovery position (p. 796) if the person is breathing.
  c Monitor breathing and circulation.
12 Do the following if the person has signs of circulation but breathing is absent.
  a Give 1 rescue breath every 5 seconds. This is at a rate of 10 to 12 breaths per minute.
  b Monitor circulation.

# ADULT CPR—TWO RESCUERS

## PROCEDURE

1 Check if the person is responding. Tap or gently shake the person, call the person by name, and shout "Are you OK?" One rescuer activates the EMS system or the agency's emergency response system.

2 Open the airway, and check for breathing. Use the head-tilt/chin-lift method.

3 Give 2 slow rescue breaths if the person is not breathing or if breathing is inadequate. Let the lungs deflate between breaths.

4 Check for a pulse using the carotid artery. Also check for breathing, coughing, and moving.

5 Perform two-person CPR (Fig. 40-12) if there are no signs of circulation:
   a One rescuer gives chest compressions at a rate of 100 per minute. Count out loud in a rhythm.

(Try: "1 and, 2 and, 3 and, 4 and, 5 and, 6 and, 7 and, 8 and, 9 and, 10 and, 11 and, 12 and, 13 and, 14 and, 15.")
   b The other rescuer gives 2 slow breaths after every 15 compressions. Pause for the breaths. Continue chest compressions after the breaths.

6 One rescuer does the following after 4 cycles of 15 compressions and 2 breaths:
   a Gives 2 slow breaths.
   b Checks for circulation—carotid pulse, breathing, coughing, and moving.

7 Continue with 15 compressions and 2 slow breaths if the person has no signs of circulation. Start with chest compressions.

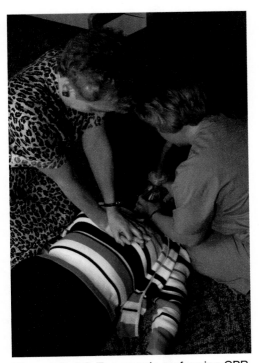

**FIG. 40-12** Two people performing CPR.

# CPR FOR INFANTS AND CHILDREN

Cardiac arrest caused by heart disease is rare in children. More common causes involve diseases and injuries that lead to respiratory arrest or circulatory failure (p. 780).

CPR for infants (younger than 1 year) and young children (1 to 8 years) differs from adult CPR. If a child is not responding:

- And you are alone:
  —Shout for help
  —Perform CPR for 1 minute
  —Activate the EMS system
- And someone is with you:
  —Have the person activate the EMS system
  —Perform two-rescuer CPR

The head-tilt/chin-lift method is used to open the airway in infants and children. The jaw-thrust method is used if head or neck injury is suspected. Remember, accidents and injuries are major causes of cardiac arrest in infants and children. To use the jaw-thrust method (Fig. 40-13):

- Place 1 or more fingers under each side of the lower jaw at the angle of the jaw.
- Lift the jaw forward. Do not tilt the head.
  Infant and child CPR also differs from adult CPR in these ways:
- You will kneel at the child's side near the head.
- Suspect injuries. To turn the child onto his or her back, use the logrolling method (Chapter 13). With logrolling, you turn the person as a unit. Keep the head, neck, and spine straight.
- To perform rescue breathing on an infant, you will cover the infant's nose and mouth with your mouth (Fig. 40-14).
- The brachial pulse is used to check circulation in infants (Chapter 21). For children, the carotid pulse is used.
- The airway is kept open throughout CPR. Only use one hand for chest compressions. Keep the other hand on the forehead to maintain the head tilt. For children, use both hands for the head-tilt/chin-lift method when giving breaths.
- 20 breaths are given per minute.

## INFANT CPR—ONE RESCUER

### PROCEDURE

1 Check if the infant is responding. Shout at the infant. Gently tap an arm or leg.
2 Activate the EMS system or the agency's emergency response system if help is available.
3 Kneel at the infant's side near the head.
4 Logroll the infant onto his or her back. Keep the head, neck, and spine straight. Position the infant supine on a hard, flat surface.
5 Open the airway. Use the head-tilt/chin-lift method if injury is not suspected. Use the jaw-thrust method if you suspect injury.
6 Check for breathing. *Look* to see if the chest rises and falls. *Listen* for the escape of air. *Feel* for the flow of air on your cheek.
7 Cover the infant's nose and mouth with your mouth for rescue breathing (see Fig. 40-14).
8 Give 2 slow rescue breaths. Use enough force to make the chest rise. Take 1 to 1½ seconds for each breath. Let the chest deflate between breaths.
9 Check for circulation. Use the brachial pulse. Also check for breathing, coughing, and moving.
10 Locate hand position for chest compressions (Fig. 40-15). (Keep the airway open with one hand.)
  a Draw an imaginary line between the nipples. Find the sternum (breastbone).

  b Place 2 fingers on the sternum about 1 finger-width below the imaginary line.
11 Give 5 chest compressions followed by 1 slow breath. You will give 100 chest compressions per minute and 20 rescue breaths per minute.
  a Use the 2 fingers on the sternum for chest compressions. Press the sternum down about one-third to one-half the depth of the chest (about ½ to 1 inch).
  b Release pressure after each compression. Keep your fingers on the chest.
  c Count out loud in a rhythm. (Try: "1, 2, 3, 4, 5.")
  d Give 1 breath after every 5 chest compressions.
12 Check for circulation after 1 minute.
13 Do the following if there are no signs of circulation:
  a Activate the EMS system or emergency response system.
  b Continue CPR.
14 Give 1 rescue breath every 3 seconds if there are signs of circulation but breathing is absent or inadequate. You will give 20 rescue breaths per minute.

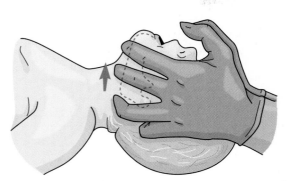

**FIG. 40-13** The jaw-thrust method. Fingers are on the lower jaw on each side. The jaw is lifted upward.

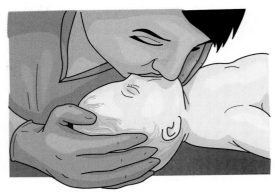

**FIG. 40-14** The infant's nose and mouth are covered during rescue breathing.

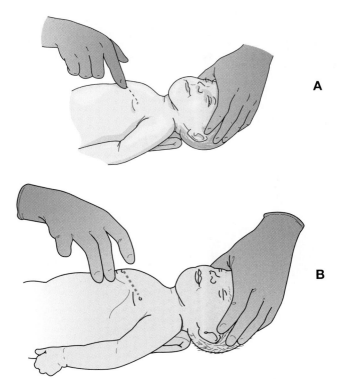

**A**

**B**

**FIG. 40-15** Locating hand position for infant chest compressions. **A,** Draw an imaginary line between the nipples. Find the sternum (breastbone). **B,** Place 2 fingers on the sternum about 1 finger-width below the imaginary line.

# CHILD CPR—ONE RESCUER

## PROCEDURE

1 Check if the child is responding. Shout at the child. Gently tap an arm or leg.
2 Activate the EMS system or the agency's emergency response system if help is available.
3 Kneel at the child's side near the head.
4 Logroll the child onto his or her back. Keep the head, neck, and spine straight. Position the child supine on a hard, flat surface.
5 Open the airway. Use the head-tilt/chin-lift method if injury is not suspected. Use the jaw-thrust method if you suspect injury.
6 Check for breathing. *Look* to see if the chest rises and falls. *Listen* for the escape of air. *Feel* for the flow of air on your cheek.
7 Cover the child's mouth with your mouth. Pinch the nostrils shut.
8 Give 2 slow rescue breaths. Use enough force to make the chest rise. Take 1 to 1½ seconds for each breath. Let the chest deflate between breaths.
9 Check for circulation. Use the carotid pulse. Check for breathing, coughing, or moving.
10 Locate hand position for chest compressions. (Keep the airway open with one hand.)
　a Find the middle of the sternum (breastbone).

　b Place the heel of one hand over the lower half of the sternum (Fig. 40-16). Keep your fingers off the chest.
11 Give 5 chest compressions followed by 1 slow breath. Give 100 chest compressions per minute and 20 rescue breaths per minute:
　a Use the heel of your hand on the sternum for chest compressions. Press the sternum down about one-third to one-half the depth of the chest (about 1 to 1½ inches).
　b Release pressure after each compression. Keep the heel of your hand on the chest.
　c Count out loud in a rhythm. (Try: "1, 2, 3, 4, 5.")
　d Give 1 breath after every 5 chest compressions.
12 Check for circulation after 1 minute.
13 Do the following if there are no signs of circulation:
　a Activate the EMS system or emergency response system.
　b Continue CPR.
14 Give 1 rescue breath every 3 seconds if there are signs of circulation but breathing is absent or inadequate. You will give 20 rescue breaths per minute.

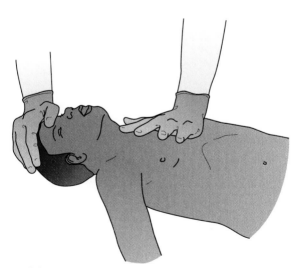

**FIG. 40-16** The heel of one hand is used for CPR on a child. The heel is placed over the lower end of the sternum. The fingers are off the chest.

## TWO-RESCUER INFANT OR CHILD CPR.

Sometimes two rescuers are available for infant or child CPR. One rescuer kneels by the victim's head. The rescuer checks for responsiveness and circulation and gives the rescue breaths. The other kneels at the infant's feet or the child's side to give chest compressions. For two-rescuer CPR on an infant, the American Heart Association prefers the 2 thumb encircling-hands technique for chest compressions (Fig. 40-17).

A rescue breath is given after every 5 compressions. The rescuer giving chest compressions will pause for the rescue breath. After 1 minute of CPR (100 chest compressions and 20 rescue breaths), the rescuer at the head will check for circulation.

Rescuers can switch positions when circulation is checked. The one giving rescue breaths will give chest compressions. The rescuer giving chest compressions will give the rescue breaths.

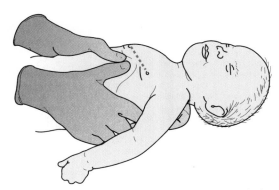

**FIG. 40-17** The 2 thumb encircling-hands technique. Both thumbs are used to give chest compressions on an infant. The thumbs are on the sternum about 1 finger-depth below the nipple line.

# FOREIGN-BODY AIRWAY OBSTRUCTION IN ADULTS

Foreign-body airway obstruction *(choking)* can lead to cardiac arrest. Air cannot pass through the air passages to the lungs. The body does not get oxygen.

Foreign bodies can cause airway obstruction. This often occurs during eating. A large, poorly chewed piece of meat is the most common cause. Laughing and talking while eating also are common causes. So is excessive alcohol intake. *See Focus on Older Persons: Foreign-Body Airway Obstruction (FBAO) in Adults.*

FBAO can occur in the unconscious person. Common causes are aspiration of vomitus and the tongue falling back into the airway. These occur during cardiac arrest.

Foreign bodies can cause partial or complete airway obstruction. With *partial obstruction,* some air moves in and out of the lungs. The person is conscious. Usually the person can speak. Often forceful coughing can remove the object.

With severe or *complete airway obstruction,* the conscious person clutches at the throat (Fig. 40-18). The person cannot breathe, speak, or cough. The person appears pale and cyanotic (bluish color). Air does not move in and out of the lungs. The conscious person is very frightened. If the obstruction is not removed, the person will die. FBAO is an emergency.

The Heimlich maneuver is used to relieve FBAO. It involves abdominal thrusts. The maneuver is performed with the person standing, sitting, or lying down. The finger sweep is used with the Heimlich maneuver when an adult becomes unconscious.

The Heimlich maneuver is not effective in very obese persons or pregnant women. Chest thrusts are used (Box 40-2).

Call for help when a person has an obstructed airway. Have someone activate the EMS system or the agency's emergency response system.

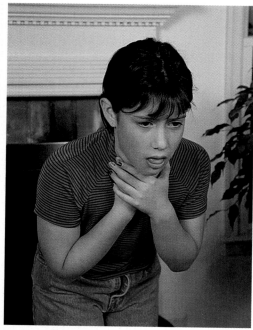

**FIG. 40-18** A choking person will clutch at the throat.

---

## FOCUS ON OLDER PERSONS

**FOREIGN-BODY AIRWAY OBSTRUCTION (FBAO) IN ADULTS**

Older persons are at risk for choking. Weakness, poorly fitting dentures, dysphagia, and chronic illnesses are common causes. They also can choke on hard candy, apples, or pieces of hot dog.

---

**BOX 40-2     OBSTRUCTED AIRWAY: CHEST THRUSTS FOR OBESE OR PREGNANT PERSONS**

**THE VICTIM IS SITTING OR STANDING**

1. Stand behind the person.
2. Place your arms under the person's underarms. Wrap your arms around the person's chest.
3. Make a fist. Place the thumb side of the fist on the middle of the sternum (breastbone).
4. Grasp the fist with your other hand.
5. Give backward chest thrusts until the object is expelled or the person becomes unconscious.

**THE VICTIM IS LYING DOWN OR UNCONSCIOUS**

1. Position the person supine.
2. Kneel next to the person.
3. Position your hands as for external chest compressions.
4. Give chest thrusts until the object is expelled or the person becomes unconscious.

## FBAO—THE RESPONSIVE ADULT

### PROCEDURE

1 Ask the person if he or she is choking.
2 Ask if the person can cough or speak.
3 Give abdominal thrusts (Fig. 40-19):
  a Stand behind the person.
  b Wrap your arms around the person's waist.
  c Make a fist with one hand.
  d Place the thumb side of the fist against the abdomen. The fist is in the middle above the navel and below the end of the sternum (breastbone).
  e Grasp your fist with your other hand.
  f Press your fist and hand into the person's abdomen with a quick, upward thrust.
  g Repeat thrusts until the object is expelled or the person loses consciousness.
4 Lower the unresponsive person to the floor or ground. Position the person supine.
5 Activate the EMS system or the agency's emergency response system.
6 Do a finger sweep to check for a foreign object.
  a Open the person's mouth. Use the tongue–jaw lift method (Fig. 40-20, *A*):
    —Grasp the tongue and lower jaw with your thumb and fingers.
    —Lift the lower jaw upward.
  b Insert your other index finger into the mouth along the side of the cheek and deep into the throat (Fig. 40-20, *B*). Your finger should be at the base of the tongue.
  c Form a hook with your index finger.
  d Try to dislodge and remove the object. Do not push it deeper into the throat.
  e Grasp and remove the object if it is within reach.
7 Open the airway with the head-tilt/chin-lift method.
8 Give 1 or 2 rescue breaths.
9 Reposition the person's head if the chest did not rise. Give 1 or 2 rescue breaths.
10 Give up to 5 abdominal thrusts (See procedure: *FBAO—The Unresponsive Adult*, p. 792.)
11 Repeat steps 6 through 10 (finger sweeps, rescue breathing, and abdominal thrusts) until rescue breathing is effective. Start CPR if necessary.

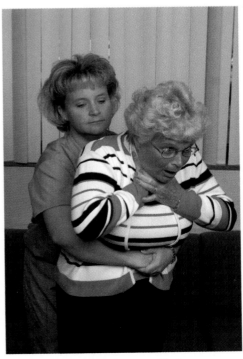

**FIG. 40-19** Abdominal thrusts with the person standing.

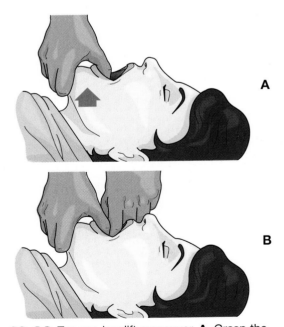

**FIG. 40-20** Tongue–jaw lift maneuver. **A,** Grasp the person's tongue and lift the jaw forward with one hand. **B,** Use the index finger of the other hand to check for a foreign object.

**THE UNRESPONSIVE ADULT.** You may find an adult who is unresponsive. You did not see the person lose consciousness, and you do not know the cause. Do not assume the cause is choking. Check for unresponsiveness, and start rescue breathing. Abdominal thrusts are done if you cannot ventilate the person. Then use the finger-sweep maneuver.

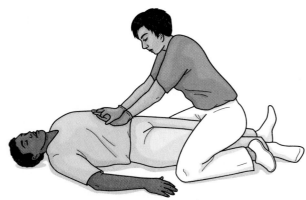

**FIG. 40-21** Abdominal thrusts with the person lying down. The rescuer straddles the thighs.

## FBAO—THE UNRESPONSIVE ADULT

### PROCEDURE

1 Check to see if the person is responding.
2 Call for help. Activate the EMS system or the agency's emergency response system.
3 Logroll the person to the supine position with his or her face up. Arms are at the sides.
4 Open the airway. Use the head-tilt/chin-lift method.
5 Check for breathing.
6 Give 1 or 2 slow rescue breaths. Reposition the person's head and open the airway if the chest does not rise. Give 1 or 2 rescue breaths.
7 Give 5 abdominal thrusts (Fig. 40-21) if you cannot ventilate the person.
   a Straddle the person's thighs.
   b Place the heel of one hand against the abdomen. It is in the middle above the navel and below the end of the sternum (breastbone).
   c Place your second hand on top of your first hand.
   d Press both hands into the abdomen with a quick, upward thrust. Give 5 thrusts.
8 Do a finger sweep to check for a foreign object. See step 6 in procedure: *FBAO—The Responsive Adult*, p. 791.
9 Repeat steps 6 through 8 until rescue breathing is effective. Start CPR if necessary.

# FBAO IN INFANTS AND CHILDREN

Children can choke on small objects such as pieces of hot dogs, marbles, hard candy, peanuts, and grapes. Peanut butter and popcorn also can cause choking. So can coins and small toys and toy parts.

Airway obstruction may be partial or complete. If the child has a strong cough, encourage the child to continue coughing. Try to relieve the obstruction if the cough weakens or when breathing problems increase. Activate the EMS system or the agency's emergency response system if efforts do not relieve the obstruction.

Signs of severe or complete airway obstruction occur *suddenly.* They include:

- Clutching at the throat (older child)
- Sudden onset of respiratory distress
- Cannot speak or cry
- Weak cough or cough with no sound
- High-pitched, noisy, or wheezing sounds with inspiration
- Increasing breathing problems
- Cyanosis (bluish color to the skin and lips)

**SAFETY ALERT:** *FBAO in Infants and Children*
Respiratory infections can cause airway obstruction in infants and children. Airway structures become swollen. The airway narrows or becomes completely obstructed. Air cannot enter the airway. The child needs immediate emergency care in a hospital.

The procedures that follow will not relieve airway obstruction caused by an infection. Do not try them if the child has a fever, rash, respiratory congestion, hoarseness, or other signs and symptoms of an infection. You will be wasting precious time. Activate the EMS system or the agency's emergency response system at once.

Also, abdominal thrusts are not given to infants. They can cause liver and other organ damage. Back blows and chest thrusts are used for infants.

## FBAO—THE RESPONSIVE INFANT

### PROCEDURE

1 See *Safety Alert: FBAO in Infants and Children.*
2 Hold the infant face down over your forearm. Kneel or sit to support your arm on your thigh. The infant's head is lower than the trunk. Hold the infant's jaw to support the head.
3 Give up to 5 back blows (Fig. 40-22, p. 794). Use the heel of your hand. Give the back blows between the shoulder blades. (Stop the back blows if the object is expelled.)
4 Turn the infant as a unit:
  a Support his or her head, neck, jaw, and chest with one hand.
  b Support the back with your other hand.
  c Turn the infant as a unit. The infant is in the back-lying position on your forearm.
5 Give up to 5 chest thrusts (Fig. 40-23, p. 794):
  a Locate hand position as for chest compressions.
  b Compress the chest upward toward the head. Use 2 or 3 fingers.
  c Stop chest thrusts if the object is expelled.
6 Give 5 back blows followed by 5 chest thrusts until the object is expelled or the child becomes unresponsive.

7 Do the following if the infant becomes unresponsive:
  a Activate the EMS system or the agency's emergency response system if you have help.
  b Open the airway with the tongue–jaw lift method. Give a rescue breath.
8 Look in the throat for an object. If you see an object, remove it with a finger sweep.
9 Repeat rescue breathing, back blows, chest thrusts, the tongue–jaw lift maneuver, and the finger sweep for a visible object until one of the following occurs:
  a The object is expelled.
  b The infant starts breathing.
  c You need to start CPR.
10 Activate the EMS system or the agency's emergency response system after following the procedure for 1 minute.
11 Continue the FBAO procedure or CPR until emergency personnel arrive.

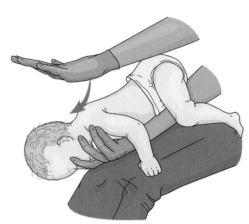

**FIG. 40-22** Back blows. The infant is held face down and supported with one hand. The rescuer's arm is supported on his or her thigh. Back blows are given between the shoulder blades with the heel of one hand.

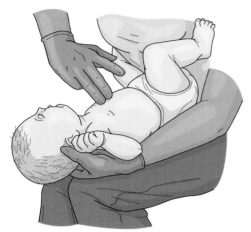

**FIG. 40-23** Chest thrusts. The infant is in the back-lying position. Hand position for chest thrusts is the same as for chest compressions.

# FBAO—THE RESPONSIVE CHILD

## PROCEDURE

1 See *Safety Alert: FBAO in Infants and Children,* p. 793.
2 Determine if the child is choking. Ask if the child is choking and if he or she can speak. Tell the child that you are going to help.
3 Stand behind the child.
4 Wrap your arms under the child's underarms and around the chest.
5 Make a fist with one hand. Place the thumb side of the fist on the child's abdomen. The fist is in the middle above the navel and below the sternum (breastbone).
6 Grab the fist with the other hand.
7 Give a quick inward and upward thrust.
8 Repeat abdominal thrusts until the object is expelled or the child becomes unresponsive.
9 Do the following if the child becomes unresponsive:
   a Activate the EMS system or the agency's emergency response system if you have help.

b Open the airway with the tongue–jaw lift method. Give a rescue breath.
10 Look in the throat for an object. If you see an object, remove it with a finger sweep.
11 Repeat rescue breathing, abdominal thrusts, the tongue–jaw lift maneuver, and the finger sweep for a visible object until one of the following occurs:
   a The object is expelled.
   b The child starts breathing.
   c You need to start CPR.
12 Activate the EMS system or the agency's emergency response system after following the procedure for 1 minute.
13 Continue the FBAO procedure or CPR until emergency personnel arrive.

**THE UNRESPONSIVE INFANT OR CHILD.** As with adults, you may find an infant or child unconscious. You cannot assume the cause is choking on a foreign object.

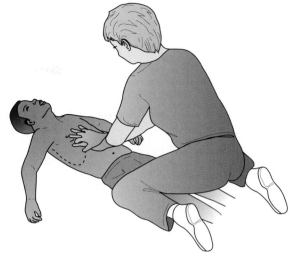

**FIG. 40-24** Abdominal thrusts for an unresponsive child.

## FBAO—THE UNRESPONSIVE INFANT OR CHILD

### PROCEDURE

1 See *Safety Alert: FBAO in Infants and Children*, p. 793.
2 Check if the infant or child is responding.
3 Activate the EMS system or the agency's emergency response system if you have help.
4 Open the airway.
5 Check for breathing. *Look* to see if the chest rises and falls. *Listen* for the escape of air. *Feel* for the flow of air on your cheek.
6 Give a rescue breath. Reposition the head if the chest does not rise. Open the airway, and give a rescue breath.
7 Do one of the following:
   a For an infant—give up to 5 back blows and 5 chest thrusts.
   b For a child—give up to 5 abdominal thrusts (Fig. 40-24).

8 Open the airway with the tongue–jaw lift maneuver. Give a rescue breath.
9 Look in the throat for an object. If you see an object, remove it with a finger sweep.
10 Repeat rescue breathing, abdominal thrusts (back blows and chest thrusts for an infant), the tongue–jaw lift maneuver, and the finger sweep for a visible object until one of the following occurs:
   a The object is expelled.
   b The infant or child starts breathing.
   c You need to start CPR.
11 Activate the EMS system or the agency's emergency response system after following the procedure for 1 minute.
12 Continue the FBAO procedure or CPR until emergency personnel arrive.

## RECOVERY POSITION

The recovery position is a side-lying position (Fig. 40-25). It is used when the person is breathing and has a pulse but is not responding. The position helps keep the airway open. Because the side-lying position allows fluids to drain from the mouth, it helps prevent aspiration of mucus and vomitus. It also prevents the tongue from falling toward the back of the throat.

Logroll the person into the recovery position. Keep the head, neck, and spine straight. Then keep the person in good alignment. A hand supports the head. *Do not use this position if the person might have neck injuries or other trauma.* Check the person's breathing and circulation often. If necessary, activate the EMS system or the agency's emergency response system. Start CPR if necessary.

*See Focus on Children: Recovery Position.*

## SELF-ADMINISTERED HEIMLICH MANEUVER

You yourself may choke. You can perform the Heimlich maneuver to relieve the obstructed airway. To do so:

1 Make a fist with one hand.
2 Place the thumb side of the fist above your navel and below the lower end of the sternum.
3 Grasp your fist with your other hand.
4 Press inward and upward quickly.
5 Press the upper abdomen against a hard surface if the thrust did not relieve the obstruction. Use the back of a chair, a table, or a railing.
6 Use as many thrusts as needed.

## AUTOMATED EXTERNAL DEFIBRILLATORS

Early defibrillation is part of the AHA's Chain of Survival. An abnormal heart rhythm called *ventricular fibrillation* (VF, V-fib) causes cardiac arrest. Rather than beating in a regular rhythm, the heart muscle shakes and quivers like a bowl of Jell-O. No blood is pumped out of the heart. Therefore the heart, brain, and other organs do not receive blood and oxygen.

VF must be stopped and a regular rhythm restored. If not, the person dies. A *defibrillator* is used to stop the VF. It delivers a shock to the heart. The shock stops the VF. This allows the return of a regular heart rhythm. Defibrillation as soon as possible after the onset of VF increases the person's chance of survival.

Automatic external defibrillators (AEDs) are computerized devices. They are found in hospitals, nursing centers, dental offices, and other health care agencies. They are on airplanes and in airports, health clubs, malls, office buildings, and many other public places. AHA basic life support courses teach health care providers and members of the public how to use them. Remember, the goal is early defibrillation.

You will learn to how to use an AED when you take a BLS course.

---

### ► FOCUS ON CHILDREN
#### RECOVERY POSITION

Remember, injuries are common causes of cardiac arrest in infants and children. If you suspect the child is injured, do not use the recovery position. Keep the child supine, and hold the airway open. Use the jaw-thrust method to keep the airway open.

---

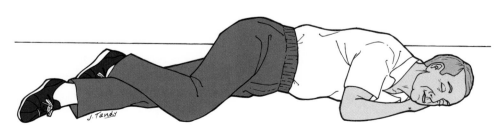

**FIG. 40-25** Recovery position.

# HEMORRHAGE

Life and body functions require an adequate blood supply. If a blood vessel is torn or cut, bleeding occurs. The larger the blood vessel, the greater the bleeding and blood loss. **Hemorrhage** is the excessive loss of blood in a short time. If the bleeding is not stopped, the person will die.

Hemorrhage may be internal or external. You cannot see internal hemorrhage. Bleeding occurs inside the body into tissues and body cavities. Pain, shock (p. 798), vomiting blood, coughing up blood, and loss of consciousness signal internal hemorrhage. There is little you can do for internal bleeding. Activate the EMS system. Then keep the person warm, flat, and quiet until medical help arrives. Do not give fluids.

If not hidden by clothing, external bleeding is usually seen. Bleeding from an artery occurs in spurts. There is a steady flow of blood from a vein. To control external bleeding:

- Follow the rules in Box 40-1, p. 779. This includes activating the EMS system.
- Have the person lie down.
- Do not remove any objects that have pierced or stabbed the person.
- Place a sterile dressing directly over the wound. Use any clean material (handkerchief, towel, cloth, sanitary napkin) if there is no sterile dressing.
- Apply pressure with your hand directly over the bleeding site (Fig. 40-26). Do not release the pressure until the bleeding stops.
- If direct pressure does not control bleeding, apply pressure over the artery above the bleeding site (Fig. 40-27). Use your first three fingers. For example, if bleeding is from the lower arm, apply pressure over the brachial artery. The brachial artery supplies blood to the lower arm. Continue to apply pressure to the wound with your other hand.
- Bind the wound when bleeding stops. Tape or tie the dressing in place. You can tie the dressing with such things as clothing, a scarf, a necktie, or a belt.

> **SAFETY ALERT:** *Hemorrhage*
> Contact with blood is likely with hemorrhage. Follow Standard Precautions and the Bloodborne Pathogen Standard to the extent possible. Wear gloves if possible. Practice hand hygiene as soon as you can.

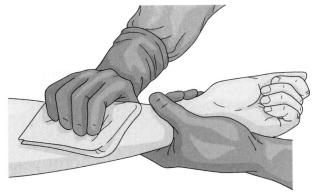

**FIG. 40-26** Direct pressure is applied to the wound to stop bleeding. The hand is placed over the wound.

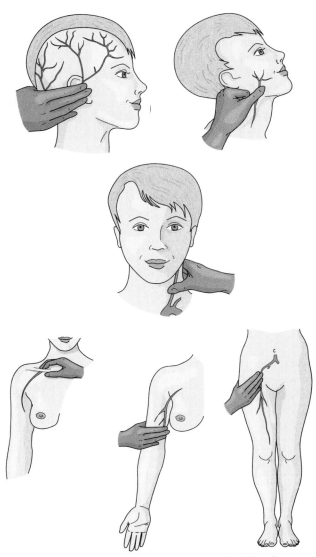

**FIG. 40-27** Pressure points to control bleeding.

# SHOCK

**Shock** results when organs and tissues do not get enough blood. Blood loss, heart attack (myocardial infarction), burns, and severe infection are causes. Signs and symptoms include:

- Low or falling blood pressure
- Rapid and weak pulse
- Rapid respirations
- Cold, moist, and pale skin
- Thirst
- Restlessness
- Confusion and loss of consciousness as shock worsens

Shock is possible in any person who is acutely ill or injured. Do the following to prevent and treat shock:

- Follow the rules in Box 40-1, p. 779. This includes activating the EMS system.
- Keep the person lying down.
- Maintain an open airway.
- Control hemorrhage.
- Keep the person warm. Place blankets over and under the person if possible.
- Reassure the person.
- Follow Standard Precautions and the Bloodborne Pathogen Standard.

## ANAPHYLACTIC SHOCK

Some people are allergic or sensitive to foods, insects, chemicals, and drugs. Many people are allergic to penicillin. An antigen is a substance that the body reacts to. The body releases chemicals to fight or attack the antigen. The person may react with an area of redness, swelling, or itching. Or the reaction can involve the entire body.

**Anaphylaxis** is life-threatening sensitivity to an antigen. (*Ana* means without. *Phylaxis* means protection.) It can occur within seconds. Signs and symptoms include:

- Sweating
- Shortness of breath
- Low blood pressure
- Irregular pulse
- Respiratory congestion
- Swelling of the larynx (laryngeal edema)
- Hoarseness
- Dyspnea

Anaphylactic shock is an emergency. The EMS system must be activated. The person needs special drugs to reverse the allergic reaction. Keep the person lying down and the airway open. Start CPR if cardiac arrest occurs.

# SEIZURES

**Seizures (convulsions)** are violent and sudden contractions or tremors of muscle groups. They are caused by an abnormality in the brain. Causes include head injury during birth or from trauma, high fever, brain tumors, poisoning, seizure disorders, and nervous system infections. Lack of blood flow to the brain can also cause seizures.

The major types of seizures are *partial seizures* and *generalized seizures*. Only a part of the brain is involved with a partial seizure. A body part may jerk. Or the person has hearing or vision problems or stomach discomfort. The person does not lose consciousness.

With generalized seizures, the whole brain is involved. The *generalized tonic-clonic seizure (grand mal seizure)* has two phases. In the tonic phase, the person loses consciousness. If standing or sitting, the person falls to the floor. The body is rigid because all muscles contract at once. The clonic phase follows. Muscle groups contract and relax. This causes jerking and twitching movements. Urinary and fecal incontinence may occur. A deep sleep is common after the seizure. Confusion and headache may occur on awakening.

The *generalized absence (petit mal) seizure* usually lasts a few seconds. There is loss of consciousness, twitching of the eyelids, and staring. No first aid is necessary. *See Focus on Children: Seizures.*

You cannot stop a seizure. However, you can protect the person from injury:

- Follow the rules in Box 40-1, p. 779. This includes activating the EMS system.
- Do not leave the person alone.
- Lower the person to the floor. This protects the person from falling.
- Place a folded blanket, towel, cushion, pillow, or other soft item under the person's head (Fig. 40-28). Or cradle the person's head in your lap. This prevents the person's head from striking the floor.
- Turn the person onto his or her side. Make sure the head is turned to the side.
- Loosen tight jewelry and clothing (ties, scarves, collars, necklaces) around the neck.
- Move furniture, equipment, and sharp objects away from the person. The person may strike these objects during uncontrolled body movements.
- Do not give the person food or fluids.
- Do not try to restrain body movements during the seizure.
- Do not put any object or your fingers between the person's teeth. The person can bite down on your fingers during the seizure.

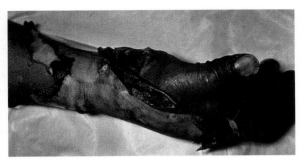

**FIG. 40-29** Full-thickness burn. (From Ignatavicius DD, Workman ML: *Medical-surgical nursing: critical thinking for collaborative care,* ed 4, Philadelphia, 2002, Saunders.)

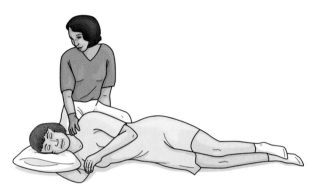

**FIG. 40-28** A pillow protects the person's head during a seizure.

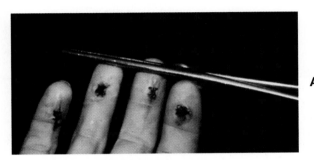

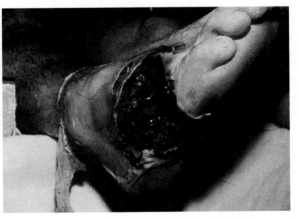

**FIG. 40-30** An electrical burn. **A,** The electrical current enters through the hand. **B,** The electrical current exits through the foot. (From Sanders M: *Mosby's paramedic textbook*, St Louis, 1994, Mosby.)

## BURNS

Burns can severely disable a person (Fig. 40-29). They can also cause death. Most burns occur in the home. Infants and children are at risk; so are older persons. Common causes of burns and fires are:

- Scalds from hot liquids
- Playing with matches and lighters
- Electrical injuries (Fig. 40-30)
- Cooking accidents (barbecues, microwaves, stoves, ovens)
- Falling asleep while smoking
- Fireplaces
- Space heaters
- No smoke detectors or nonfunctioning smoke detectors
- Sunburn
- Chemicals

The skin has two layers: the dermis and the epidermis. Burns are described as partial thickness or full thickness. *Partial-thickness burns* involve the dermis and part of the epidermis. They are very painful. Nerve endings are exposed. *Full-thickness burns* involve the dermis and the entire epidermis. Fat, muscle, and bone may be injured or destroyed. Full-thickness burns are not painful. Nerve endings are destroyed.

Some burns are minor; others are severe. Severity depends on burn size and depth, the body part involved, and the person's age. Burns to the face, eyes, ears, hands, and feet are more serious than burns to an arm or leg. Infants, young children, and older persons are at high risk for death.

Emergency care of burns includes the following:

- Follow the rules in Box 40-1, p. 779. This includes activating the EMS system.
- Do not touch the person if he or she is in contact with an electrical source. Have the power source turned off, or remove the electrical source. Use an object that does not conduct electricity (rope or wood) to remove the electrical source.

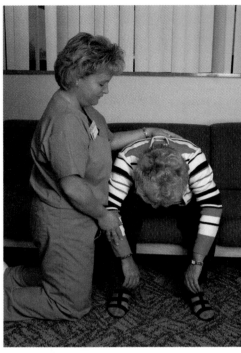

**FIG. 40-31** The person bends forward and lowers her head between her knees to prevent fainting.

- Remove the person from the fire or burn source.
- Stop the burning process. Put out flames with water, or roll the person in a blanket. Or smother flames with a coat, sheet, or towel.
- Do not remove burned clothing.
- Remove hot clothing that is not sticking to the skin. If you cannot remove hot clothing, cool the clothing with water.
- Remove jewelry and any tight clothing that is not sticking to the skin.
- Provide rescue breathing and CPR as needed.
- Cover burns with sterile, cool, moist coverings. Or use towels, sheets, or any other clean cloth. Keep the covering wet.
- Do not put oil, butter, salve, or ointments on the burns.
- Cover the person with a blanket or coat to prevent heat loss.
  *See Focus on Children: Burns. See Focus on Older Persons: Burns.*

# FAINTING

**Fainting** is the sudden loss of consciousness from an inadequate blood supply to the brain. Hunger, fatigue, fear, and pain are common causes. Some people faint at the sight of blood or injury. Standing in one position for a long time and being in a warm, crowded room are other causes. Dizziness, perspiration, and blackness before the eyes are warning signals. The person

looks pale. The pulse is weak. Respirations are shallow if consciousness is lost. Emergency care for fainting includes the following:
- Have the person sit or lie down before fainting occurs.
- If sitting, the person bends forward and places the head between the knees (Fig. 40-31).
- If the person is lying down, raise the legs.
- Loosen tight clothing (belts, ties, scarves, collars, and so on).
- Keep the person lying down if fainting has occurred. Raise the legs.
- Do not let the person get up until symptoms have subsided for about 5 minutes.
- Help the person to a sitting position after recovery from fainting. Observe for fainting.

# STROKE

Stroke (cerebrovascular accident) occurs when the brain is suddenly deprived of its blood supply (Chapter 33). Usually only part of the brain is affected. A stroke may be caused by a thrombus, an embolus, or hemorrhage if a blood vessel in the brain ruptures.

Signs of stroke vary. They depend on the size and location of brain injury. Loss of consciousness or semiconsciousness, rapid pulse, labored respirations, elevated blood pressure, and hemiplegia are signs of stroke. The person may have slurred speech or aphasia (the inability to speak). Loss of vision in one eye, unsteadiness, and falling also are signs. Seizures may occur.

Emergency care includes the following:

- Follow the rules in Box 40-1, p. 779. This includes activating the EMS system.
- Position the person in the recovery position on the affected side (see Fig. 40-25). The affected side is limp, and the cheek appears puffy.
- Elevate the head without flexing the neck.
- Loosen tight clothing (belts, ties, scarves, collars, and so on.)
- Keep the person quiet and warm.
- Reassure the person.
- Provide rescue breathing and CPR if necessary.
- Provide emergency care for seizures if necessary.

## QUALITY OF LIFE

Protect quality of life during emergencies. Treat the person with dignity and respect.

Protect the right to privacy and confidentiality. Do not expose the person unnecessarily. You may be in a place where you cannot close doors, shades, and curtains. The person may be in a lounge, dining area, or public place. Do what you can to provide privacy.

Onlookers can threaten privacy and confidentiality. During an emergency, your main concern is the person's illness or injuries. You cannot give care and manage onlookers at the same time. Ask someone else to deal with the onlookers. If someone else is giving care, keep onlookers away from the person.

People are curious. They want to know what happened, the extent of injuries or illness, and if the person will be okay. Do not discuss the situation. Information about the person's care, treatment, and condition is confidential. Only doctors diagnose. You can make observations about signs and symptoms. The doctor determines what is wrong with the person.

Protect the right to personal choice. Choices are few in emergencies. They are given when possible. Hospital care may be required. The person has the right to choose a hospital.

Protect personal items from loss and damage. Dentures and eyeglasses are often lost or broken in emergencies. Watches and jewelry are easily lost. Clothing may be torn or cut. Be very careful to protect the person's property. In public places, personal items are given to the family, police, or EMS personnel.

Physical and psychological safety are important. Protect the person from further injury. For example, protect the person from falls after a stroke. Protect the person having a seizure from head injuries. The person needs to feel safe and secure. Reassurance, explanations about care, and a calm approach are important. They help the person feel safe and secure.

# ■ REVIEW QUESTIONS ■

Circle the **BEST** answer.

1  The goals of first aid are to
   a  Call for help and keep the person warm
   b  Prevent death and prevent injuries from becoming worse
   c  Stay calm and give emergency care
   d  Calm the person and keep bystanders away

2  When giving first aid, you should
   a  Be aware of your own limits
   b  Move the person
   c  Give the person fluids
   d  Perform needed emergency measures

3  Cardiac arrest is
   a  The same as stroke
   b  The sudden stopping of heart action and breathing
   c  The sudden loss of consciousness
   d  When organs and tissues do not get enough blood

4  Which is *not* a sign of cardiac arrest?
   a  No pulse
   b  No breathing
   c  A sudden drop in blood pressure
   d  Unconsciousness

5  Mouth-to-mouth rescue breathing for an adult involves the following *except*
   a  Pinching the nostrils shut
   b  Placing your mouth tightly over the person's mouth
   c  Blowing air into the mouth as you exhale
   d  Covering the nose with your mouth

6  Chest compressions are performed on an adult. The chest is compressed
   a  $\frac{1}{2}$ to 1 inch with the index and middle fingers
   b  1 to $1\frac{1}{2}$ inches with the heel of one hand
   c  $1\frac{1}{2}$ to 2 inches with two hands
   d  With one hand in the middle of the sternum

7  Which does *not* determine adequate breathing?
   a  Looking to see if the chest rises and falls
   b  Counting respirations for 30 seconds
   c  Listening for the escape of air
   d  Feeling for the flow of air

8  Which pulse is used during adult CPR?
   a  The apical pulse
   b  The brachial pulse
   c  The carotid pulse
   d  The femoral pulse

9  How many breaths are given when CPR is started?
   a  1
   b  2
   c  3
   d  4

10  You are doing adult CPR alone. Which is *false*?
   a  Give 2 breaths after every 15 compressions
   b  Check for a pulse after 1 minute
   c  Give 1 breath after every fifth compression
   d  Count out loud

11  Adult CPR is being given by two people. Rescue breaths are given
   a  After every 5 compressions
   b  After every 15 compressions
   c  After every compression
   d  Only when the positions are changed

12  Chest compressions are given to an infant at a rate of
   a  60 per minute
   b  75 per minute
   c  80 per minute
   d  100 per minute

13  The most common cause of FBAO in adults is
   a  A loose denture
   b  Meat
   c  Marbles
   d  Candy

14  If airway obstruction occurs, the person usually
   a  Clutches at the throat
   b  Can speak, cough, and breathe
   c  Is calm
   d  Has a seizure

**15** Chest thrusts are used for FBOA in an adult. Which is *false?*
  **a** The person can be standing, sitting, or lying down.
  **b** A fist is made with one hand.
  **c** The thrusts are given inward and upward at the lower end of the sternum.
  **d** The hands are over the sternum.

**16** Poking motions are used with a finger sweep.
  **a** True
  **b** False

**17** Arterial bleeding
  **a** Cannot be seen
  **b** Occurs in spurts
  **c** Is dark red
  **d** Oozes from the wound

**18** A person is hemorrhaging from the left forearm. The first action is to
  **a** Lower the body part
  **b** Apply pressure to the brachial artery
  **c** Apply direct pressure to the wound
  **d** Cover the person

**19** A person is in shock. The signs of shock are
  **a** Rising blood pressure, rapid pulse, and slow respirations
  **b** Rapid pulse, rapid respirations, and warm skin
  **c** Falling blood pressure; rapid pulse and respirations; and cold, moist, and pale skin
  **d** Falling blood pressure; slow pulse and respirations; thirst; restlessness; and warm, flushed skin

**20** A person in shock needs
  **a** Rescue breathing
  **b** To be kept lying down
  **c** Clothes removed
  **d** The recovery position

**21** These statements relate to tonic-clonic seizures. Which is *false?*
  **a** There is contraction of all muscles at once.
  **b** Incontinence may occur.
  **c** The seizure usually lasts a few seconds.
  **d** There is loss of consciousness.

**22** A person was burned. There are no complaints or signs of pain. You know that
  **a** The burn is minor
  **b** The burn is partial thickness
  **c** The burn is full thickness
  **d** The dermis was destroyed

**23** Burns are covered with
  **a** A clean, moist cloth or dressing
  **b** Butter, oil, or salve
  **c** Water
  **d** Nothing

**24** A person is about to faint. Which is *false?*
  **a** Take the person outside for fresh air.
  **b** Have the person sit or lie down.
  **c** Loosen tight clothing.
  **d** Raise the legs if the person is lying down.

**25** A person is having a stroke. Emergency care includes the following *except*
  **a** Positioning the person on the affected side
  **b** Giving the person sips of water
  **c** Loosening tight clothing
  **d** Keeping the person quiet and warm

*Answers to these questions are on p. 820.*

# The Dying Person

41

# OBJECTIVES

- Define the key terms listed in this chapter
- Describe terminal illness
- Explain the factors that affect attitudes about death
- Describe how different age-groups view death
- Describe the five stages of dying
- Explain how to meet the needs of the dying person and family
- Describe hospice care
- Explain the importance of the Patient Self-Determination Act
- Explain what is meant by a "Do Not Resuscitate" order
- Identify the signs of approaching death and the signs of death
- Explain how to assist with postmortem care
- Perform the procedure described in this chapter

# KEY TERMS

**advance directive**  A document stating a person's wishes about health care when that person cannot make his or her own decisions

**postmortem**  After *(post)* death *(mortem)*

**reincarnation**  The belief that the spirit or soul is reborn in another human body or in another form of life

**rigor mortis**  The stiffness or rigidity *(rigor)* of skeletal muscles that occurs after death *(mortis)*

**terminal illness**  An illness or injury for which there is no reasonable expectation of recovery

Some deaths are sudden; others are expected. Health team members see death often. Many are unsure of their feelings about death. Dying persons and the subject of death cause them discomfort. Death and dying mean helplessness and failure to cure. They also remind us that our loved ones and we will die.

Your feelings about death affect the care you give. You will help meet the dying person's physical, psychological, social, and spiritual needs. Therefore you must understand the dying process. Then you can approach the dying person with caring, kindness, and respect.

# TERMINAL ILLNESS

Many illnesses and diseases have no cure. Some injuries are so serious that the body cannot function. Recovery is not expected. The disease or injury ends in death. An illness or injury for which there is no reasonable expectation of recovery is a **terminal illness.**

Doctors cannot predict the exact time of death. A person may have days, months, weeks, or years to live. People expected to live for a short time have lived for years. Others expected to live longer have died sooner than expected.

Modern medicine has found cures or has prolonged life in many cases. Future research will bring new cures. However, hope and the will to live strongly influence living and dying. Many people have died for no apparent reason when they have lost hope or the will to live.

# ATTITUDES ABOUT DEATH

Experiences, culture, religion, and age influence attitudes about death. Many people fear death. Others do not believe they will die. Some look forward to and accept death. Attitudes about death often change as a person grows older and with changing circumstances.

Dying people often need hospital, nursing center, hospice, or home care. The family is often involved in the person's care. They usually gather at the bedside to comfort the person and each other. When death occurs, the funeral director is called. He or she takes the body to the funeral home. There the body is prepared for funeral practices.

Many adults and children never have had contact with a dying person. Nor have they been present at the time of death. Some have not attended a visitation (wake) or funeral. They have not seen the process of dying and death. Therefore it is frightening, morbid, and a mystery.

## CULTURE AND RELIGION

Practices and attitudes about death differ among cultures. *See Caring About Culture: Death Rites.* In some cultures, dying people are cared for at home by the family. Some families prepare the body for burial.

Attitudes about death are closely related to religion. Some believe that life after death is free of suffering and hardship. They also believe in reunion with loved ones. Many believe sins and misdeeds are punished in the afterlife. Others believe there is no afterlife. To them, death is the end of life.

There also are religious beliefs about the body's form after death. Some believe the body keeps its physical form. Others believe that only the spirit or soul is present in the afterlife. **Reincarnation** is the belief that the spirit or soul is reborn in another human body or in another form of life.

Many people strengthen their religious beliefs when dying. Religion also provides comfort for the dying person and the family.

Many religions practice rites and rituals during the dying process and at the time of death. Prayers, blessings, and scripture readings are common in many religions.

---

### CARING ABOUT CULTURE
#### DEATH RITES

In *Vietnam*, quality of life is more important than length of life because of beliefs in reincarnation. Less suffering in the next life is expected. Therefore dying persons are helped to recall past good deeds and to achieve a fitting mental state. Death at home is preferred over death in the hospital. Upon death, the body is washed and wrapped in a clean, white sheet. In some areas a coin or jewels (a wealthy family) and rice (a poor family) are put in the dead person's mouth. This is from the belief that they will help the soul go through the encounters with gods and devils and the soul will be born rich in the next life. Relatives sew small pillows to place under the body's neck, feet, and wrists. The body is placed in a coffin for in-ground burial.

The *Chinese* have an aversion to anything concerning death. Autopsy and disposal of the body are not prescribed by religion. Donating body parts is encouraged. The eldest son makes all arrangements. The body is buried in a coffin. After 7 years, the body is exhumed and cremated. The urn is reburied in the tomb. White or yellow and black clothing is worn for mourning.

In *India*, Hindu persons are often accepting of God's will. The person's desire to be clearheaded as death nears must be assessed in planning medical treatment. A time and place for prayer are essential for the family and the person. Prayer helps them deal with anxiety and conflict. The Hindu priest reads from Holy Sanskrit books. Some priests tie strings (meaning a blessing) around the neck or wrist. After death, the son pours water into the mouth of the deceased. Blood transfusions, organ transplants, and autopsies are allowed. Cremation is preferred. Reincarnation is a Hindu belief.

From D'Avanzo CE, Geissler EM: *Pocket guide to cultural health assessment,* ed 3, St Louis, 2003, Mosby.

---

### FOCUS ON CHILDREN
#### ATTITUDES ABOUT DEATH

Infants and toddlers have no concept of death. Between the ages of 3 and 5 years, children are curious and have ideas about death. They know when family members or pets die. They notice dead birds or bugs. They think death is temporary. Children often blame themselves when someone or something dies. To them, death is punishment for being bad. Answers to questions about death often cause fear and confusion. Children who are told "He is sleeping" may be afraid to go to sleep.

Children between the ages of 5 and 7 years know death is final. They do not think that they will die. Death happens to other people. It can be avoided. Children relate death to punishment and body mutilation. It also involves witches, ghosts, goblins, and monsters. These ideas come from fairy tales, cartoons, movies, video games, and TV.

## AGE

Adults fear pain and suffering, dying alone, and the invasion of privacy. They also fear loneliness and separation from loved ones. They worry about the care and support of those left behind. Adults often resent death because it affects plans, hopes, dreams, and ambitions. *See Focus on Children: Attitudes About Death. See Focus on Older Persons: Attitudes About Death.*

## THE STAGES OF DYING

Dr. Elisabeth Kübler-Ross described five stages of dying. They are denial, anger, bargaining, depression, and acceptance:

- *Denial* is the first stage. Persons refuse to believe they are dying. "No, not me" is a common response. The person believes a mistake was made. Information about the illness or injury is not heard. The person cannot deal with any problem or decision about the matter. This stage can last for a few hours, days, or much longer. Some people are still in denial when they die.
- *Anger* is stage two. The person thinks "Why me?" There is anger and rage. Dying persons envy and resent those with life and health. Family, friends, and the health team are often targets of anger. The person blames others and finds fault with those who are loved and needed the most. It is hard to deal with the person during this stage. Anger is normal and healthy. Do not take the person's anger personally. Control any urge to attack back or avoid the person.
- *Bargaining* is the third stage. Anger has passed. The person now says "Yes, me, but. . . ." Often the person bargains with God for more time. Promises are made in exchange for more time. The person may want to see a child marry, see a grandchild, have one more Christmas, or live for some other event. Usually more promises are made as the person makes "just one more" request. You may not see this stage. Bargaining is usually private and on a spiritual level.

- *Depression* is the fourth stage. The person thinks "Yes, me" and is very sad. The person mourns things that were lost and the future loss of life. The person may cry or say little. Sometimes the person talks about people and things that will be left behind.
- *Acceptance* of death is the last stage. The person is calm and at peace. The person has said what needs to be said. Unfinished business is completed. The person accepts death. This stage may last for many months or years. Reaching acceptance stage does not mean death is near.

Dying persons do not always pass through all five stages. A person may never get beyond a certain stage. Some move back and forth between stages. For example, Mr. Jones reached acceptance but moves back to bargaining. Then he moves forward to acceptance. Some people stay in one stage until death.

## PSYCHOLOGICAL, SOCIAL, AND SPIRITUAL NEEDS

Dying people have psychological, social, and spiritual needs. They may want family and friends present. They may want to talk about their fears, worries, and anxieties. Some want to be alone. Often they need to talk during the night. Things are quiet. There are few distractions, and there is more time to think. You need to listen and use touch:

- *Listening.* The person needs to talk and share worries and concerns. Let the person express feelings and emotions in his or her own way. Do not worry about saying the wrong thing or finding comforting words. You do not need to say anything. Being there for the person is what counts.
- *Touch.* Touch shows caring and concern when words cannot. Sometimes the person does not want to talk but needs you nearby. Do not feel that you need to talk. Silence, along with touch, is a powerful and meaningful way to communicate.

Some people want to see a spiritual leader. Or they want to take part in religious practices. Provide privacy during prayer and spiritual moments. Be courteous to the spiritual leader. The person has the right to have religious objects nearby (medals, pictures, statues, or religious writings). Handle these valuables with care and respect.

# PHYSICAL NEEDS

Dying may take a few minutes, hours, days, or weeks. Body processes slow. The person is weak. Changes occur in levels of consciousness. To the extent possible, independence is allowed. As the person weakens, basic needs are met. The person may depend on others for basic needs and activities of daily living. Every effort is made to promote physical and psychological comfort. The person is allowed to die in peace and with dignity.

## VISION, HEARING, AND SPEECH

Vision blurs and gradually fails. The person naturally turns toward light. A darkened room may frighten the person. The eyes may be half-open. Secretions may collect in the corners of the eyes.

Because of failing vision, explain what you are doing to the person or in the room. The room should be well lit. However, avoid bright lights and glares.

Good eye care is essential (Chapter 16). If the eyes stay open, a nurse may apply a protective ointment. Then the eyes are covered with moist pads to prevent injury.

Hearing is one of the last functions lost. Many people hear until the moment of death. Even unconscious persons may hear. Always assume that the person can hear. Speak in a normal voice. Provide reassurance and explanations about care. Offer words of comfort. Avoid topics that could upset the person.

Speech becomes difficult. It may be hard to understand the person. Sometimes the person cannot speak. Anticipate the person's needs. Do not ask questions that need long answers. Ask "yes" or "no" questions. These should be few in number. Despite the person's speech problems, you must talk to him or her.

## MOUTH, NOSE, AND SKIN

Oral hygiene promotes comfort. Routine mouth care is given if the person can eat and drink. Frequent oral hygiene is given as death nears and when taking oral fluids is difficult. Oral hygiene is needed if mucus collects in the mouth and the person cannot swallow.

Crusting and irritation of the nostrils can occur. Nasal secretions, an oxygen cannula, or an NG tube is a common cause. Carefully clean the nose. Apply lubricant as directed by the nurse and the care plan.

Circulation fails and body temperature rises as death nears. The skin feels cool, pale, and mottled (blotchy). Perspiration increases. Skin care, bathing, and preventing pressure ulcers are necessary. Linens and gowns are changed whenever needed. Although the skin feels cool, only light bed coverings are needed. Blankets may make the person feel warm and cause restlessness.

## ELIMINATION

Urinary and fecal incontinence may occur. Use incontinence products or bed protectors as directed. Give perineal care as needed. Constipation and urinary retention are common. Enemas and catheters may be needed. The nurse may delegate enemas and catheter care to you (Chapters 18 and 19).

## COMFORT AND POSITIONING

Skin care, personal hygiene, back massages, oral hygiene, and good alignment promote comfort. Some persons have severe pain. The nurse gives pain relief drugs ordered by the doctor. Frequent position changes and supportive devices also promote comfort. You may need help to turn the person slowly and gently. Semi-Fowler's position is usually best for breathing problems.

## THE PERSON'S ROOM

The person's room should be comfortable and pleasant. It should be well lit and well ventilated. Unnecessary equipment is removed. Some equipment is upsetting to look at (suction machines, drainage containers). If possible, these items are kept out of the person's sight.

Mementos, pictures, cards, flowers, and religious items provide comfort. Arrange them within the person's view. The person and family arrange the room as they wish. This helps meet love, belonging, and self-esteem needs. The room should reflect the person's choices.

Often the person's room is by the nurse's station. The person can be watched carefully.

# THE FAMILY

This is a hard time for the family. It may be very hard to find comforting words. Show your feelings by being available, courteous, and considerate. Use touch to show your concern.

The family usually is allowed to stay as long as they wish. Sometimes family members stay during the night. The health team makes them as comfortable as possible.

You must respect the right to privacy. The person and family need time together. However, you cannot neglect care because the family is present. Most agencies let family members help give care. Or you can suggest that they take a break for a beverage or meal.

The family may be very tired, sad, and tearful. Watching a loved one die is very painful. So is dealing with the eventual loss of that person. The family goes through stages like the dying person. They need support, understanding, courtesy, and respect. A spiritual leader may provide comfort. Communicate this request to the nurse at once.

# HOSPICE CARE

Hospice care focuses on the physical, emotional, social, and spiritual needs of dying persons and their families (Chapter 1). It is not concerned with cure or life-saving measures. Pain relief and comfort are stressed. The goal is to improve the dying person's quality of life.

A hospice may be part of a hospital, nursing center, or home care agency. It may be a separate agency. Many hospices offer home care. Follow-up care and support groups for survivors are hospice services.

# LEGAL ISSUES

Much attention is given to the right to die. Many people do not want machines or other measures keeping them alive. Consent is needed for any treatment. When able, the person makes care decisions. Some people make end-of-life wishes known.

## THE PATIENT SELF-DETERMINATION ACT

The Patient Self-Determination Act and OBRA give persons the right to accept or refuse medical treatment. They also give the right to make advance directives. An **advance directive** is a document stating a person's wishes about health care when that person cannot make his or her own decisions. Advance directives usually forbid certain care if there is no hope of recovery. Living wills and durable power of attorney are common advance directives.

These laws protect quality of care. Quality of care cannot be less because of the person's advance directives.

Health care agencies must inform all persons of the right to advance directives on admission. This information is in writing. The medical record must document whether the person has made them.

**LIVING WILLS.** A living will is a document about measures that support or maintain life when death is likely. Tube feedings, ventilators, and CPR are examples. A living will may instruct doctors:
- Not to start measures that prolong dying
- To remove measures that prolong dying

**DURABLE POWER OF ATTORNEY.** Durable power of attorney for health care also is an advance directive. It gives the power to make health care decisions to another person. Usually this is a family member, friend, or lawyer. When a person cannot make health care decisions, the person with durable power of attorney can do so.

## "DO NOT RESUSCITATE" ORDERS

When death is sudden and unexpected, efforts are made to save the person's life. CPR is started (Chapter 40). The agency's emergency response system is activated. Nurses, doctors, and staff rush to the person's bedside. They bring emergency and life-saving equipment. CPR and other life-support measures are continued until the person is resuscitated or until the doctor declares the person dead.

Doctors often write "Do Not Resuscitate" (DNR) or "No Code" orders for terminally ill persons. This means that the person will not be resuscitated. The person is allowed to die with peace and dignity. The orders are often written after consulting with the person and family. The family and doctor make the decision if the person is not mentally able to. Some advance directives address resuscitation.

You may not agree with care and resuscitation decisions. However, you must follow the person's or family's wishes and the doctor's orders. These may be against your personal, religious, and cultural values. If so, discuss the matter with the nurse. An assignment change may be needed.

# QUALITY OF LIFE

A person has the right to die in peace and with dignity. Box 41-1, p. 810, contains the dying person's bill of rights. *See Focus on Long-Term Care: Quality of Life, p. 810.*

## BOX 41-1    THE DYING PERSON'S BILL OF RIGHTS

- I have the right to be treated as a living human being until I die.
- I have the right to maintain a sense of hopefulness, however changing its focus may be.
- I have the right to be cared for by those who can maintain a sense of hopefulness, however changing this might be.
- I have the right to express my feelings and emotions about my approaching death, in my own way.
- I have the right to participate in decisions concerning my care.
- I have the right to expect continuing medical and nursing attention even though "cure" goals must be changed to "comfort" goals.
- I have the right not to die alone.
- I have the right to be free from pain.
- I have the right to have my questions answered honestly.
- I have the right not to be deceived.
- I have the right to have help from and for my family accepting my death.
- I have the right to die in peace and dignity.
- I have the right to retain my individuality and not be judged for my decisions, which may be contrary to the beliefs of others.
- I have the right to discuss and enlarge my religious and/or spiritual experiences, regardless of what they may mean to others.
- I have the right to expect that the sanctity of the human body will be respected after death.
- I have the right to be cared for by caring, sensitive, knowledgeable people who will attempt to understand my needs and will be able to gain some satisfaction in helping me face my death.

Modified From Barbus AJ: *Am J Nurs* 75(1):99, 1975.

## FOCUS ON LONG-TERM CARE
### QUALITY OF LIFE

The dying person has rights under OBRA:

- *The right to privacy before and after death.* Do not expose the person unnecessarily. The person has the right not to have his or her body seen by others. Proper draping and screening are important.
- *The right to visit with others in private.* If the person is too weak to leave the room, the roommate may have to do so. The nurse and social worker develop a plan that satisfies everyone. Moving the dying person to a private room provides privacy. The family can also stay as long as they like.
- *The right to confidentiality before and after death.* Only those involved in care need to know the person's diagnosis and condition. The final moments and cause of death also are kept confidential. So are statements, conversations, and family reactions.
- *The right to be free from abuse, mistreatment, and neglect.* Some health team members avoid dying persons. They are uncomfortable with death and dying. Others have religious or cultural beliefs about being near dying people. Neglect is possible. So is abuse or mistreatment. Family, friends, or staff may be sources of such actions. The dying person may be too weak to report the abuse or mistreatment. Or the person may feel that punishment is deserved for needing so much care. The person has the right to receive kind and respectful care before and after death. Always report signs of abuse, mistreatment, or neglect to the nurse at once.
- *Freedom of restraint.* Restraints are used only if ordered by the doctor. Dying persons are often too weak to be dangerous to themselves or others.
- *The right to have personal possessions.* You must protect the person's property. The person may want photos and religious items nearby. Protect the person's property from loss or damage before and after death. They may be family treasures or mementos.
- *The right to a safe and home-like setting.* Dying persons depend on others for safety. Everyone must keep the setting safe and home-like. The center is the person's home. Try to keep equipment and supplies out of view. The room also should be free from unpleasant odors and noises. Do your best to keep the room neat and clean.
- *The right to personal choice.* The person has the right to be involved in treatment and care. The dying person may refuse treatment. Advance directives are common. Some persons cannot make treatment decisions. The family or legal representative does so. The decision may be to allow the person to die with peace and dignity. The health team must respect choices to refuse treatment or not prolong life.

# SIGNS OF DEATH

There are signs that death is near. These signs may occur rapidly or slowly:

- Movement, muscle tone, and sensation are lost. This usually starts in the feet and legs. It eventually spreads to other body parts. When mouth muscles relax, the jaw drops. The mouth may stay open. The facial expression is often peaceful.
- Peristalsis and other gastrointestinal functions slow down. Abdominal distention, fecal incontinence, impaction, nausea, and vomiting are common.
- Body temperature rises. The person feels cool or cold, looks pale, and perspires heavily.
- Circulation fails. The pulse is fast, weak, and irregular. Blood pressure starts to fall.
- The respiratory system fails. Cheyne-Stokes (Chapter 30), slow, or rapid and shallow respirations are observed. Mucus collects in the airway. This causes the *death rattle* that is heard.
- Pain decreases as the person loses consciousness. However, some people are conscious until the moment of death.

The signs of death include no pulse, respirations, or blood pressure. The pupils are fixed and dilated. A doctor determines that death has occurred and pronounces the person dead. *See Focus on Home Care: Signs of Death.*

# CARE OF THE BODY AFTER DEATH

Care of the body after *(post)* death *(mortem)* is called **postmortem** care. A nurse gives postmortem care. You may be asked to assist. Postmortem care begins when the doctor pronounces the person dead.

Postmortem care is done to maintain good appearance of the body. Discoloration and skin damage are prevented. Valuables and personal items are gathered for the family. The right to privacy and the right to be treated with dignity and respect apply after death.

Within 2 to 4 hours after death, rigor mortis develops. **Rigor mortis** is the stiffness or rigidity *(rigor)* of skeletal muscles that occurs after death *(mortis)*. The body is positioned in normal alignment before rigor mortis sets in. The family may want to see the body. The body should appear in a comfortable and natural position for this viewing.

In some agencies the body is prepared only for viewing. The funeral director completes postmortem care.

Postmortem care may involve repositioning the body. For example, soiled areas are bathed and the body placed in good alignment. Moving the body can cause remaining air in the lungs, stomach, and intestines to be expelled. When air is expelled, sounds are produced. Do not let these sounds alarm or frighten you. They are normal and expected.

---

## FOCUS ON HOME CARE
### SIGNS OF DEATH

Death often occurs in the home setting. Before the body is taken to the funeral home, the person must be pronounced dead. This is a legal requirement. So is contacting the coroner or medical examiner. State laws and agency policies vary. If a person dies at home, call the nurse. The nurse tells you what to do.

---

**DELEGATION GUIDELINES:** *Postmortem Care*

When assisting with postmortem care, you need this information from the nurse:

- If dentures will be inserted or placed in a denture container
- If tubes will be removed or left in place
- If the family wants to view the body
- Special agency policies and procedures

---

**SAFETY ALERT:** *Postmortem Care*

Standard Precautions and the Bloodborne Pathogen Standard are followed. You may have contact with infected blood, body fluids, secretions, or excretions.

# ASSISTING WITH POSTMORTEM CARE

## QUALITY OF LIFE

Remember to:
- Knock before entering the person's room
- Address the person by name
- Introduce yourself by name and title

## PRE-PROCEDURE

1 Follow *Delegation Guidelines: Postmortem Care.* See *Safety Alert: Postmortem Care*, p. 811.
2 Practice hand hygiene.
3 Collect the following:
   - Postmortem kit (shroud or body bag, gown, ID tags, gauze squares, safety pins)
   - Bed protectors
   - Wash basin
   - Bath towels and washcloths
   - Tape
   - Dressings
   - Gloves
   - Cotton balls
   - Gown
   - Valuables envelope
4 Provide for privacy.
5 Raise the bed for body mechanics.
6 Make sure the bed is flat.

## PROCEDURE

7 Put on the gloves.
8 Position the body supine. Arms and legs are straight. A pillow is under the head and shoulders.
9 Close the eyes. Gently pull the eyelids over the eyes. Apply moist cotton balls gently over the eyelids if the eyes will not stay closed.
10 Insert dentures if it is agency policy. If not, put them in a labeled denture container.
11 Close the mouth. If necessary, place a rolled towel under the chin to keep the mouth closed.
12 Follow agency policy about jewelry. Remove all jewelry, except for wedding rings if this is agency policy. List the jewelry that you removed. Place the jewelry and the list in a valuables envelope.
13 Place a cotton ball over the rings. Tape them in place.
14 Remove drainage containers. Leave tubes and catheters in place if there will be an autopsy. Ask the nurse about removing tubes.
15 Bathe soiled areas with plain water. Dry thoroughly.
16 Place a bed protector under the buttocks.
17 Remove soiled dressings. Replace them with clean ones.
18 Put a clean gown on the body. Position the body as in step 8.
19 Brush and comb the hair if necessary.
20 Cover the body to the shoulders with a sheet if the family will view the body.
21 Gather the person's belongings. Put them in a bag labeled with the person's name.
22 Remove supplies, equipment, and linens. Straighten the room. Provide soft lighting.
23 Remove the gloves. Decontaminate your hands.
24 Let the family view the body. Provide for privacy. Return to the room after they leave.
25 Decontaminate your hands. Put on gloves.
26 Fill out the ID tags. Tie one to the ankle or to the right big toe.
27 Place the body in the body bag, or cover it with a sheet. Or apply the shroud (Fig. 41-1).
   a Bring the top down over the head.
   b Fold the bottom up over the feet.
   c Fold the sides over the body.
   d Pin or tape the shroud in place.
28 Attach the second ID tag to the shroud, sheet, or body bag.
29 Leave the denture cup with the body.
30 Pull the privacy curtain around the bed. Or close the door.

## POST-PROCEDURE

31 Remove the gloves. Decontaminate your hands.
32 Strip the unit after the body has been removed. Wear gloves for this step.
33 Remove the gloves. Decontaminate your hands.
34 Report the following to the nurse:
   - The time the body was taken by the funeral director
   - What was done with jewelry and personal items
   - What was done with dentures

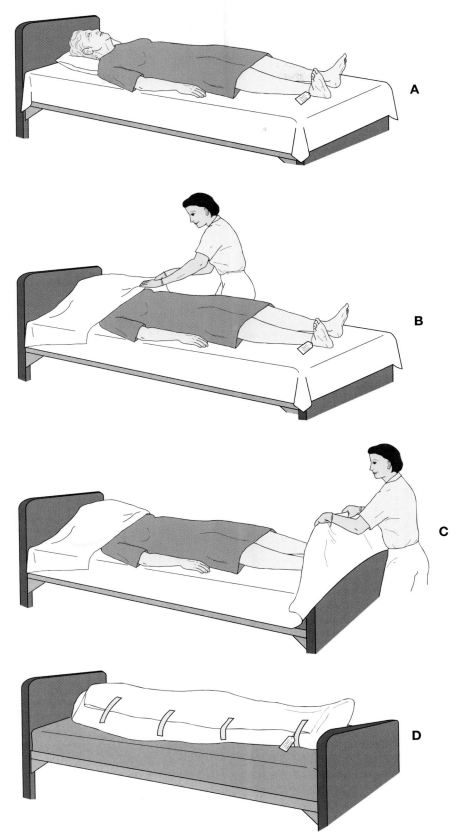

**FIG. 41-1** Applying a shroud. **A,** Place the body on the shroud. **B,** Bring the top of the shroud down over the head. **C,** Fold the bottom up over the feet. **D,** Fold the sides over the body. Tape or pin the sides together. Attach the ID tag.

# ■ REVIEW QUESTIONS ■

Circle the **BEST** answer.

1 Which is *true*?
  a Death from terminal illness is sudden and un-expected.
  b Doctors know when death will occur.
  c An illness is terminal when there is no reasonable hope of recovery.
  d All severe injuries result in death.

2 These statements relate to attitudes about death. Which is *false*?
  a Dying people are often cared for in health agencies.
  b Religion influences attitudes about death.
  c Infants and toddlers understand death.
  d Young children often blame themselves when someone dies.

3 Reincarnation is the belief that
  a There is no afterlife
  b The spirit or soul is reborn into another human body or another form of life
  c The body keeps its physical form in the afterlife
  d Only the spirit or soul is present in the afterlife

4 Children between the ages of 5 and 7 years view death as
  a Temporary
  b Final
  c Adults do
  d Going to sleep

5 Adults and older persons usually fear
  a Dying alone
  b Reincarnation
  c The five stages of dying
  d Advance directives

6 Persons in the stage of denial
  a Are angry
  b Make "deals" with God
  c Are sad and quiet
  d Refuse to believe they are dying

7 A dying person tries to gain more time during the stage of
  a Anger
  b Bargaining
  c Depression
  d Acceptance

8 When caring for a dying person, you should
  a Use touch and listen
  b Do most of the talking
  c Keep the room darkened
  d Speak in a loud voice

9 As death nears, the last sense lost is
  a Sight
  b Taste
  c Smell
  d Hearing

10 The dying person's care includes the following *except*
  a Eye care
  b Mouth care
  c Active range-of-motion exercises
  d Position changes

11 The dying person is positioned in
  a The supine position
  b The Fowler's position
  c Good body alignment
  d The dorsal recumbent position

12 A "Do Not Resuscitate" order was written. This means that
  a CPR will not be done
  b The person has a living will
  c Life-prolonging measures will be carried out
  d The person is kept alive as long as possible

13 Which are *not* signs of approaching death?
  a Increased body temperature and rapid pulse
  b Loss of movement and muscle tone
  c Increased pain and blood pressure
  d Cheyne-Stokes respirations and the death rattle

14 The signs of death are
  a Convulsions and incontinence
  b No pulse, respirations, or blood pressure
  c Loss of consciousness and convulsions
  d The eyes stay open, no muscle movements, and the body is rigid

15 Postmortem care is done
  a After rigor mortis sets in
  b After the doctor pronounces the person dead
  c When the funeral director arrives for the body
  d After the family has viewed the body

*Answers to these questions are on p. 820.*

# REVIEW QUESTION ANSWERS

## Chapter 1
## Introduction to Health Care Agencies

1  c
2  b
3  a
4  c
5  b
6  a
7  b
8  d
9  c
10  c
11  a
12  c

## Chapter 2
## The Nursing Assistant

1  d
2  c
3  a
4  b
5  a
6  a
7  a
8  b
9  a
10  c
11  b
12  c
13  a
14  a
15  d
16  a
17  d
18  c
19  a
20  b
21  a
22  a
23  a
24  c
25  c

## Chapter 3
## Work Ethics

1  c
2  d
3  c
4  d
5  b
6  d
7  c
8  b
9  c
10  d
11  c
12  b
13  a
14  a
15  b
16  c
17  d
18  c
19  b
20  a
21  d
22  c

## Chapter 4
## Communicating With the Health Team

1  a
2  c
3  d
4  b
5  d
6  c
7  d
8  d
9  c
10  d
11  b
12  a  Prefix
    b  Root
    c  Suffix
13  Prefix
14  Suffix
15  a  Right upper quadrant
    b  Right lower quadrant
    c  Left upper quadrant
    d  Left lower quadrant

16  d
17  a
18  c
19  f
20  e
21  b
22  Without or not
23  Bad, difficult, abnormal
24  Double, two, twice
25  Away from
26  Across, over
27  After, behind
28  Scant, small
29  Excessive, too much
30  By, through
31  Half
32  Decreased, less than normal
33  Toward
34  Pain
35  Inflammation
36  Creation of an opening
37  Removal of, excision
38  Blood condition
39  Condition
40  Excessive flow
41  Lack, deficiency
42  Disease
43  Incision, cutting into
44  Profuse flow, discharge
45  Surgical repair or reshaping
46  Skull
47  Heart
48  Breast
49  Vein
50  Urine
51  Breathing, respiration
52  Blue
53  Artery
54  Colon, large intestine
55  Joint
56  Stone
57  Stomach
58  Brain
59  Sugar, sweetness
60  Blood
61  Uterus
62  Liver
63  Muscle
64  Kidney

65 Vein
66 Eye
67 Bone
68 Nerve
69 Lung
70 Poison
71 Mind
72 Chest
73 j
74 f
75 d
76 h
77 a
78 g
79 i
80 b
81 e
82 c
83 BRP
84 ad lib
85 c/o
86 bid
87 HS; hs
88 I&O
89 NPO; npo
90 prn
91 postop; post op
92 q
93 w/c
94 stat

## Chapter 5
### Assisting With the Nursing Process

1 a
2 d
3 b
4 c
5 d
6 c
7 c
8 b
9 c
10 d

## Chapter 6
### Understanding the Person

1 c
2 d
3 c
4 b
5 a
6 d
7 a
8 d

9 b
10 d
11 c
12 a
13 c
14 a
15 d
16 d
17 c
18 d
19 d
20 b
21 b

## Chapter 7
### Body Structure and Function

1 a
2 b
3 d
4 c
5 c
6 a
7 b
8 c
9 d
10 d
11 b
12 a
13 b
14 b
15 b
16 c
17 d
18 a
19 d
20 a
21 b

## Chapter 8
### Growth and Development

1 b
2 c
3 b
4 a
5 b
6 c
7 b
8 a
9 c
10 c
11 c
12 c
13 a
14 b

15 c
16 a
17 d
18 c

## Chapter 9
### Care of the Older Person

1 a
2 d
3 c
4 b
5 c
6 a
7 b
8 c
9 a
10 c
11 d
12 c
13 a
14 d
15 a
16 c
17 a
18 a

## Chapter 10
### Safety

1 T
2 T
3 T
4 T
5 T
6 F
7 F
8 T
9 T
10 T
11 F
12 T
13 F
14 T
15 T
16 T
17 F
18 b
19 d
20 c
21 c
22 a
23 a
24 d
25 c
26 a
27 d

28 d
29 c
30 b
31 c
32 b
33 d
34 b
35 d
36 b
37 a
38 c
39 c
40 c
41 b
42 d

## Chapter 11
### Restraint Alternatives and Safe Restraint Use

1 F
2 F
3 F
4 T
5 T
6 T
7 T
8 T
9 F
10 F
11 F
12 T
13 F
14 T
15 T
16 F
17 d
18 a
19 c
20 b
21 c
22 a
23 d
24 a
25 c
26 c
27 d

## Chapter 12
### Preventing Infection

1 F
2 T
3 F
4 F
5 F
6 F

7 T
8 T
9 T
10 b
11 d
12 d
13 b
14 d
15 c
16 a
17 d
18 c
19 a
20 d
21 d
22 c
23 b
24 a

## Chapter 13
### Body Mechanics

1 d
2 b
3 a
4 c
5 c
6 b
7 a
8 a
9 b
10 a
11 b
12 a
13 a
14 a
15 a
16 b
17 b
18 a
19 d
20 b
21 c
22 c
23 c
24 b
25 a

## Chapter 14
### The Person's Unit

1 b
2 d
3 a
4 b
5 d
6 a

7 b
8 c
9 b
10 c
11 c
12 T
13 F
14 F
15 T
16 T
17 T
18 F

## Chapter 15
### Bedmaking

1 b
2 d
3 b
4 a
5 b
6 a
7 d
8 c

## Chapter 16
### Personal Hygiene

1 T
2 T
3 F
4 F
5 F
6 F
7 F
8 T
9 F
10 F
11 F
12 F
13 T
14 T
15 T
16 d
17 b
18 b
19 c
20 c
21 d

## Chapter 17
### Grooming

1 d
2 b
3 c
4 a

5  d
6  d
7  b
8  d
9  b
10  F
11  F
12  T
13  T
14  F

## Chapter 18
## Urinary Elimination

1  b
2  d
3  a
4  b
5  b
6  a
7  a
8  d
9  c
10  d

## Chapter 19
## Bowel Elimination

1  a
2  b
3  d
4  a
5  c
6  d
7  b
8  c
9  b
10  d

## Chapter 20
## Nutrition and Fluids

1  b
2  a
3  a
4  d
5  d
6  c
7  a
8  c
9  a
10  c
11  d
12  c
13  c
14  b
15  b

16  a
17  c
18  a
19  c
20  c

## Chapter 21
## Measuring Vital Signs

1  c
2  b
3  d
4  c
5  a
6  a
7  c
8  d
9  b
10  c
11  a
12  b

## Chapter 22
## Exercise and Activity

1  a
2  b
3  c
4  b
5  c
6  b
7  c
8  a
9  b
10  c
11  b
12  F
13  F
14  T
15  F
16  T

## Chapter 23
## Comfort, Rest, and Sleep

1  a
2  c
3  d
4  c
5  a
6  b
7  c
8  d
9  b
10  c
11  c
12  a

13  b
14  b

## Chapter 24
## Admissions, Transfers, and Discharges

1  F
2  T
3  T
4  T
5  F
6  T
7  T
8  F
9  T
10  T
11  T
12  F

## Chapter 25
## Assisting With the Physical Examination

1  b
2  d
3  c
4  b
5  c

## Chapter 26
## Collecting and Testing Specimens

1  d
2  b
3  a
4  c
5  d
6  b
7  a
8  c
9  a
10  b

## Chapter 27
## The Person Having Surgery

1  c
2  b
3  b
4  a
5  a
6  c
7  c
8  a

9  b
10  c
11  d
12  a
13  a
14  a
15  F
16  T
17  F
18  F
19  T
20  T
21  T
22  F
23  T
24  T

## Chapter 28
## Wound Care

1  b
2  c
3  a
4  c
5  b
6  c
7  a
8  d
9  a
10  a
11  b
12  a
13  d
14  c
15  c

## Chapter 29
## Heat and Cold
## Applications

1  d
2  b
3  d
4  b
5  c
6  b
7  d
8  a
9  d
10  c
11  a
12  b

## Chapter 30
## Oxygen Needs

1  a
2  c
3  c
4  b
5  d
6  c
7  d
8  a
9  b
10  d
11  b
12  d
13  d
14  c
15  b
16  c
17  d
18  b
19  c
20  d

## Chapter 31
## Rehabilitation and
## Restorative Care

1  c
2  b
3  a
4  d
5  a
6  a
7  c
8  c
9  T
10  T
11  T
12  F
13  T
14  T

## Chapter 32
## Hearing and Vision
## Problems

1  b
2  b
3  d
4  a
5  c
6  b
7  a
8  b
9  a
10  a

11  c
12  b
13  b
14  c

## Chapter 33
## Common Health Problems

1  a
2  c
3  a
4  d
5  c
6  a
7  a
8  d
9  c
10  b
11  a
12  a
13  a
14  d
15  b
16  c
17  d
18  a
19  d
20  a
21  b
22  b
23  c
24  a
25  c
26  a
27  d
28  c

## Chapter 34
## Mental Health Problems

1  b
2  b
3  a
4  c
5  d
6  d
7  c
8  c
9  b
10  c
11  d
12  d

## Chapter 35
## Confusion and Dementia

1  a
2  b
3  c
4  a
5  d
6  d
7  b
8  b
9  a
10  d
11  c
12  a

## Chapter 36
## Developmental Disabilities

1  d
2  b
3  d
4  b
5  a
6  d
7  c
8  c
9  d
10  b
11  a
12  c
13  b
14  d
15  c

## Chapter 37
## Sexuality

1  a
2  d
3  c
4  a
5  b
6  b
7  d
8  b
9  b
10  b

## Chapter 38
## Caring for Mothers and Newborns

1  c
2  d
3  b
4  d
5  d
6  b
7  c
8  c
9  c
10  c
11  d
12  d
13  d
14  a
15  c
16  c
17  T
18  T
19  F
20  T

## Chapter 39
## Assisted Living

1  a
2  a
3  b
4  d
5  b
6  b
7  d
8  b
9  a
10  b
11  c
12  d
13  d
14  c

## Chapter 40
## Basic Emergency Care

1  b
2  a
3  b
4  c
5  d
6  c
7  b
8  c
9  b
10  c
11  b
12  d
13  b
14  a
15  c
16  b
17  b
18  c
19  c
20  b
21  c
22  c
23  a
24  a
25  b

## Chapter 41
## The Dying Person

1  c
2  c
3  b
4  b
5  a
6  d
7  b
8  a
9  d
10  c
11  c
12  a
13  c
14  b
15  b

# APPENDIX A

# NATIONAL NURSE AIDE ASSESSMENT PROGRAM (NNAAP™) WRITTEN EXAMINATION CONTENT OUTLINE

The NNAAP Written Examination is comprised of seventy (70) multiple choice questions. Ten (10) of these questions are pre-test (non-scored) questions on which statistical information will be collected.

## I. PHYSICAL CARE SKILLS

A. Activities of Daily Living .... 7% of exam
  1. Hygiene
  2. Dressing and Grooming
  3. Nutrition and Hydration
  4. Elimination
  5. Rest/Sleep/Comfort
B. Basic Nursing Skills ....... 37% of exam
  1. Infection Control
  2. Safety/Emergency
  3. Therapeutic/Technical Procedures
  4. Data Collection and Reporting
C. Restorative Skills .......... 5% of exam
  1. Prevention
  2. Self Care/Independence

## II. PSYCHOSOCIAL CARE SKILLS

A. Emotional and Mental Health Needs .................... 10% of exam
B. Spiritual and Cultural Needs .................. 3% of exam

## III. ROLE OF THE NURSE AIDE

A. Communication .......... 10% of exam
B. Client Rights ............. 15% of exam
C. Legal and Ethical Behavior ... 5% of exam
D. Member of the Health Care Team ......................... 8% of exam

# NATIONAL NURSE AIDE ASSESSMENT PROGRAM (NNAAP™) SKILLS EVALUATION†

## LIST OF SKILLS

1. Washes hands
2. Measures and records weight of ambulatory client
3. Cleans entire mouth (including tongue and all surfaces of teeth), using gentle motions
4. Dresses client with affected right arm
5. Transfers client from bed to wheelchair
6. Assists client to ambulate
7. Cleans and stores dentures
8. Performs passive range-of-motion (ROM) on one shoulder
9. Performs passive range-of-motion (ROM) on one knee and one ankle
10. Measures and records urinary output
11. Assists clients with use of bedpan
12. Provides perineal care for incontinent client
13. Provides catheter care

14. Takes and records oral temperature
15. Takes and records radial pulse, and counts and records respirations
16. Takes and records client's blood pressure (one-step procedure)
17. Takes and records client's blood pressure (two-step procedure)
18. Puts one knee-high elastic stocking on client
19. Makes an occupied bed
20. Provides foot care
21. Provides fingernail care
22. Feeds client who cannot feed self
23. Positions client on side
24. Gives modified bed bath (face, and one arm, hand, and underarm)
25. Shampoos client's hair in bed

# APPENDIX B

## MINIMUM DATA SET (MDS) — *VERSION 2.0*
### FOR NURSING HOME RESIDENT ASSESSMENT AND CARE SCREENING

### *BASIC ASSESSMENT TRACKING FORM*

## SECTION AA. IDENTIFICATION INFORMATION

| 1. | RESIDENT NAME⊙ | |
|---|---|---|
| | | a. (First)　　　b. (Middle Initial)　　　c. (Last)　　　d. (Jr/Sr) |
| 2. | GENDER⊙ | 1. Male　　　　2. Female |
| 3. | BIRTHDATE⊙ | [ ][ ] — [ ][ ] — [ ][ ][ ][ ]  Month　Day　Year |
| 4. | RACE/⊙ ETHNICITY | 1. American Indian/Alaskan Native　4. Hispanic<br>2. Asian/Pacific Islander　5. White, not of<br>3. Black, not of Hispanic origin　　Hispanic origin |
| 5. | SOCIAL SECURITY⊙ AND MEDICARE NUMBERS⊙ [C in 1st box if non med. no.] | a. Social Security Number<br>[ ][ ][ ] — [ ][ ] — [ ][ ][ ][ ]<br>b. Medicare number (or comparable railroad insurance number) |
| 6. | FACILITY PROVIDER NO.⊙ | a. State No.<br>b. Federal No. |
| 7. | MEDICAID NO. ["+" if pending, "N" if not a Medicaid recipient]⊙ | |
| 8. | REASONS FOR ASSESS-MENT | [Note—Other codes do not apply to this form]<br>**a.** Primary reason for assessment<br>　1. Admission assessment (required by day 14)<br>　2. Annual assessment<br>　3. Significant change in status assessment<br>　4. Significant correction of prior full assessment<br>　5. Quarterly review assessment<br>　10. Significant correction of prior quarterly assessment<br>　0. *NONE OF ABOVE*<br><br>**b.** *Codes for assessments required for Medicare PPS or the State*<br>　*1. Medicare 5 day assessment*<br>　*2. Medicare 30 day assessment*<br>　*3. Medicare 60 day assessment*<br>　*4. Medicare 90 day assessment*<br>　*5. Medicare readmission/return assessment*<br>　*6. Other state required assessment*<br>　*7. Medicare 14 day assessment*<br>　*8. Other Medicare required assessment* |

**9. Signatures of Persons who Completed a Portion of the Accompanying Assessment or Tracking Form**

I certify that the accompanying information accurately reflects resident assessment or tracking information for this resident and that I collected or coordinated collection of this information on the dates specified. To the best of my knowledge, this information was collected in accordance with applicable Medicare and Medicaid requirements. I understand that this information is used as a basis for ensuring that residents receive appropriate and quality care, and as a basis for payment from federal funds. I further understand that payment of such federal funds and continued participation in the government-funded health care programs is conditioned on the accuracy and truthfulness of this information, and that I may be personally subject to or may subject my organization to substantial criminal, civil, and/or administrative penalties for submitting false information. I also certify that I am authorized to submit this information by this facility on its behalf.

| Signature and Title | Sections | Date |
|---|---|---|
| a. | | |
| b. | | |
| c. | | |
| d. | | |
| e. | | |
| f. | | |
| g. | | |
| h. | | |
| i. | | |
| j. | | |
| k. | | |
| l. | | |

---

**GENERAL INSTRUCTIONS**

*Complete this information for submission with all full and quarterly assessments (Admission, Annual, Significant Change, State or Medicare required assessments, or Quarterly Reviews, etc.)*

---

⊙ = Key items for computerized resident tracking

[ ] = When box blank, must enter number or letter　[a.] = When letter in box, check if condition applies

MDS 2.0 September, 2000

Resident _____    Numeric Identifier _____

# MINIMUM DATA SET (MDS) — *VERSION 2.0*
## FOR NURSING HOME RESIDENT ASSESSMENT AND CARE SCREENING
### *BACKGROUND (FACE SHEET) INFORMATION AT ADMISSION*

## SECTION AB. DEMOGRAPHIC INFORMATION

| 1. | DATE OF ENTRY | Date the stay began. Note — Does not include readmission if record was closed at time of temporary discharge to hospital, etc. In such cases, use prior admission date <br> ☐☐ — ☐☐ — ☐☐☐☐ <br> Month    Day    Year |
|---|---|---|
| 2. | ADMITTED FROM (AT ENTRY) | 1. Private home/apt. with no home health services <br> 2. Private home/apt. with home health services <br> 3. Board and care/assisted living/group home <br> 4. Nursing home <br> 5. Acute care hospital <br> 6. Psychiatric hospital, MR/DD facility <br> 7. Rehabilitation hospital <br> 8. Other |
| 3. | LIVED ALONE (PRIOR TO ENTRY) | 0. No <br> 1. Yes <br> 2. In other facility |
| 4. | ZIP CODE OF PRIOR PRIMARY RESIDENCE | ☐☐☐☐☐ |
| 5. | RESIDENTIAL HISTORY 5 YEARS PRIOR TO ENTRY | (*Check all settings* resident **lived in** during 5 years prior to date of entry given in item AB1 above) <br> Prior stay at this nursing home — a. <br> Stay in other nursing home — b. <br> Other residential facility—board and care home, assisted living, group home — c. <br> MH/psychiatric setting — d. <br> MR/DD setting — e. <br> *NONE OF ABOVE* — f. |
| 6. | LIFETIME OCCUPA-TION(S) [Put "/" between two occupations] | ☐☐☐☐☐☐☐☐☐☐☐☐☐☐☐☐ |
| 7. | EDUCATION (*Highest Level Completed*) | 1. No schooling    5. Technical or trade school <br> 2. 8th grade/less    6. Some college <br> 3. 9-11 grades    7. Bachelor's degree <br> 4. High school    8. Graduate degree |
| 8. | LANGUAGE | (*Code for correct response*) <br> **a. Primary Language** <br> 0. English    1. Spanish    2. French    3. Other <br> **b. If other, specify** |
| 9. | MENTAL HEALTH HISTORY | Does resident's RECORD indicate any history of mental retardation, mental illness, or developmental disability problem? <br> 0. No    1. Yes |
| 10. | CONDITIONS RELATED TO MR/DD STATUS | (*Check all conditions* that are related to MR/DD status that were manifested before age 22, and are likely to continue indefinitely) <br> Not applicable—no MR/DD (Skip to AB11) — a. <br> MR/DD with organic condition <br> Down's syndrome — b. <br> Autism — c. <br> Epilepsy — d. <br> Other organic condition related to MR/DD — e. <br> MR/DD with no organic condition — f. |
| 11. | DATE BACK-GROUND INFORMA-TION COMPLETED | ☐☐ — ☐☐ — ☐☐☐☐ <br> Month    Day    Year |

## SECTION AC. CUSTOMARY ROUTINE

| 1. | CUSTOMARY ROUTINE (*In year prior to DATE OF ENTRY to this nursing home, or year last in community if now being admitted from another nursing home*) | (*Check all that apply.* If all information UNKNOWN, check last box only.) |
|---|---|---|
| | | **CYCLE OF DAILY EVENTS** |
| | | Stays up late at night (e.g., after 9 pm) — a. |
| | | Naps regularly during day (at least 1 hour) — b. |
| | | Goes out 1+ days a week — c. |
| | | Stays busy with hobbies, reading, or fixed daily routine — d. |
| | | Spends most of time alone or watching TV — e. |
| | | Moves independently indoors (with appliances, if used) — f. |
| | | Use of tobacco products at least daily — g. |
| | | *NONE OF ABOVE* — h. |
| | | **EATING PATTERNS** |
| | | Distinct food preferences — i. |
| | | Eats between meals all or most days — j. |
| | | Use of alcoholic beverage(s) at least weekly — k. |
| | | *NONE OF ABOVE* — l. |
| | | **ADL PATTERNS** |
| | | In bedclothes much of day — m. |
| | | Wakens to toilet all or most nights — n. |
| | | Has irregular bowel movement pattern — o. |
| | | Showers for bathing — p. |
| | | Bathing in PM — q. |
| | | *NONE OF ABOVE* — r. |
| | | **INVOLVEMENT PATTERNS** |
| | | Daily contact with relatives/close friends — s. |
| | | Usually attends church, temple, synagogue (etc.) — t. |
| | | Finds strength in faith — u. |
| | | Daily animal companion/presence — v. |
| | | Involved in group activities — w. |
| | | *NONE OF ABOVE* — x. |
| | | **UNKNOWN**—Resident/family unable to provide information — y. |

## SECTION AD. FACE SHEET SIGNATURES

**SIGNATURES OF PERSONS COMPLETING FACE SHEET:**

**a.** Signature of RN Assessment Coordinator                Date

I certify that the accompanying information accurately reflects resident assessment or tracking information for this resident and that I collected or coordinated collection of this information on the dates specified. To the best of my knowledge, this information was collected in accordance with applicable Medicare and Medicaid requirements. I understand that this information is used as a basis for ensuring that residents receive appropriate and quality care, and as a basis for payment from federal funds. I further understand that payment of such federal funds and continued participation in the government-funded health care programs is conditioned on the accuracy and truthfulness of this information, and that I may be personally subject to or may subject my organization to substantial criminal, civil, and/or administrative penalties for submitting false information. I also certify that I am authorized to submit this information by this facility on its behalf.

| Signature and Title | Sections | Date |
|---|---|---|
| b. | | |
| c. | | |
| d. | | |
| e. | | |
| f. | | |
| g. | | |

MDS 2.0  September, 2000

☐ = When box blank, must enter number or letter    ☐ a. = When letter in box, check if condition applies

From Centers for Medicare and Medicaid Services, http://cms.hhs.gov/medicaid/mds20

Resident _____  Numeric Identifier _____

## MINIMUM DATA SET (MDS) — *VERSION 2.0*
## FOR NURSING HOME RESIDENT ASSESSMENT AND CARE SCREENING
### *FULL ASSESSMENT FORM*
(Status in last 7 days, unless other time frame indicated)

### SECTION A. IDENTIFICATION AND BACKGROUND INFORMATION

**1. RESIDENT NAME**

a. (First)   b. (Middle Initial)   c. (Last)   d. (Jr/Sr)

**2. ROOM NUMBER**

**3. ASSESSMENT REFERENCE DATE**

a. Last day of MDS observation period

Month — Day — Year

b. Original (0) or corrected copy of form (enter number of correction)

**4a. DATE OF REENTRY**

Date of reentry from most recent temporary discharge to a hospital in last 90 days (or since last assessment or admission if less than 90 days)

Month — Day — Year

**5. MARITAL STATUS**
1. Never married   3. Widowed   5. Divorced
2. Married   4. Separated

**6. MEDICAL RECORD NO.**

**7. CURRENT PAYMENT SOURCES FOR N.H. STAY**

(Billing Office to indicate; check all that apply in last 30 days)

| | | | |
|---|---|---|---|
| Medicaid per diem | a. | VA per diem | f. |
| Medicare per diem | b. | Self or family pays for full per diem | g. |
| Medicare ancillary part A | c. | Medicaid resident liability or Medicare co-payment | h. |
| Medicare ancillary part B | d. | Private insurance per diem (including co-payment) | i. |
| CHAMPUS per diem | e. | Other per diem | j. |

**8. REASONS FOR ASSESSMENT**

[Note—If this is a discharge or reentry assessment, only a limited subset of MDS items need be completed]

a. Primary reason for assessment
1. Admission assessment (required by day 14)
2. Annual assessment
3. Significant change in status assessment
4. Significant correction of prior full assessment
5. Quarterly review assessment
6. Discharged—return not anticipated
7. Discharged—return anticipated
8. Discharged prior to completing initial assessment
9. Reentry
10. Significant correction of prior quarterly assessment
0. NONE OF ABOVE

b. Codes for assessments required for Medicare PPS or the State
1. Medicare 5 day assessment
2. Medicare 30 day assessment
3. Medicare 60 day assessment
4. Medicare 90 day assessment
5. Medicare readmission/return assessment
6. Other state required assessment
7. Medicare 14 day assessment
8. Other Medicare required assessment

**9. RESPONSIBILITY/ LEGAL GUARDIAN**

(Check all that apply)

| | | | |
|---|---|---|---|
| Legal guardian | a. | Durable power attorney/financial | d. |
| Other legal oversight | b. | Family member responsible | e. |
| Durable power of attorney/health care | c. | Patient responsible for self | f. |
| | | NONE OF ABOVE | g. |

**10. ADVANCED DIRECTIVES**

(For those items with supporting documentation in the medical record, check all that apply)

| | | | |
|---|---|---|---|
| Living will | a. | Feeding restrictions | f. |
| Do not resuscitate | b. | Medication restrictions | g. |
| Do not hospitalize | c. | Other treatment restrictions | h. |
| Organ donation | d. | NONE OF ABOVE | i. |
| Autopsy request | e. | | |

### SECTION B. COGNITIVE PATTERNS

**1. COMATOSE**
(Persistent vegetative state/no discernible consciousness)
0. No   1. Yes   (If yes, skip to Section G)

**2. MEMORY**
(Recall of what was learned or known)

a. Short-term memory OK—seems/appears to recall after 5 minutes
0. Memory OK   1. Memory problem

b. Long-term memory OK—seems/appears to recall long past
0. Memory OK   1. Memory problem

**3. MEMORY/ RECALL ABILITY**

(Check all that resident was normally able to recall during last 7 days)

| | | | |
|---|---|---|---|
| Current season | a. | That he/she is in a nursing home | d. |
| Location of own room | b. | | |
| Staff names/faces | c. | NONE OF ABOVE are recalled | e. |

**4. COGNITIVE SKILLS FOR DAILY DECISION-MAKING**

(Made decisions regarding tasks of daily life)
0. INDEPENDENT—decisions consistent/reasonable
1. MODIFIED INDEPENDENCE—some difficulty in new situations only
2. MODERATELY IMPAIRED—decisions poor; cues/supervision required
3. SEVERELY IMPAIRED—never/rarely made decisions

**5. INDICATORS OF DELIRIUM— PERIODIC DISORDERED THINKING/ AWARENESS**

(Code for behavior in the last 7 days.) [Note: Accurate assessment requires conversations with staff and family who have direct knowledge of resident's behavior over this time].
0. Behavior not present
1. Behavior present, not of recent onset
2. Behavior present, over last 7 days appears different from resident's usual functioning (e.g., new onset or worsening)

a. EASILY DISTRACTED—(e.g., difficulty paying attention; gets sidetracked)

b. PERIODS OF ALTERED PERCEPTION OR AWARENESS OF SURROUNDINGS—(e.g., moves lips or talks to someone not present; believes he/she is somewhere else; confuses night and day)

c. EPISODES OF DISORGANIZED SPEECH—(e.g., speech is incoherent, nonsensical, irrelevant, or rambling from subject to subject; loses train of thought)

d. PERIODS OF RESTLESSNESS—(e.g., fidgeting or picking at skin, clothing, napkins, etc; frequent position changes; repetitive physical movements or calling out)

e. PERIODS OF LETHARGY—(e.g., sluggishness; staring into space; difficult to arouse; little body movement)

f. MENTAL FUNCTION VARIES OVER THE COURSE OF THE DAY—(e.g., sometimes better, sometimes worse; behaviors sometimes present, sometimes not)

**6. CHANGE IN COGNITIVE STATUS**

Resident's cognitive status, skills, or abilities have changed as compared to status of 90 days ago (or since last assessment if less than 90 days)
0. No change   1. Improved   2. Deteriorated

### SECTION C. COMMUNICATION/HEARING PATTERNS

**1. HEARING**

(With hearing appliance, if used)
0. HEARS ADEQUATELY—normal talk, TV, phone
1. MINIMAL DIFFICULTY when not in quiet setting
2. HEARS IN SPECIAL SITUATIONS ONLY—speaker has to adjust tonal quality and speak distinctly
3. HIGHLY IMPAIRED/absence of useful hearing

**2. COMMUNICATION DEVICES/ TECHNIQUES**

(Check all that apply during last 7 days)

| | |
|---|---|
| Hearing aid, present and used | a. |
| Hearing aid, present and not used regularly | b. |
| Other receptive comm. techniques used (e.g., lip reading) | c. |
| NONE OF ABOVE | d. |

**3. MODES OF EXPRESSION**

(Check all used by resident to make needs known)

| | | | |
|---|---|---|---|
| Speech | a. | Signs/gestures/sounds | d. |
| Writing messages to express or clarify needs | b. | Communication board | e. |
| American sign language or Braille | c. | Other | f. |
| | | NONE OF ABOVE | g. |

**4. MAKING SELF UNDERSTOOD**

(Expressing information content—however able)
0. UNDERSTOOD
1. USUALLY UNDERSTOOD—difficulty finding words or finishing thoughts
2. SOMETIMES UNDERSTOOD—ability is limited to making concrete requests
3. RARELY/NEVER UNDERSTOOD

**5. SPEECH CLARITY**

(Code for speech in the last 7 days)
0. CLEAR SPEECH—distinct, intelligible words
1. UNCLEAR SPEECH—slurred, mumbled words
2. NO SPEECH—absence of spoken words

**6. ABILITY TO UNDERSTAND OTHERS**

(Understanding verbal information content—however able)
0. UNDERSTANDS
1. USUALLY UNDERSTANDS—may miss some part/intent of message
2. SOMETIMES UNDERSTANDS—responds adequately to simple, direct communication
3. RARELY/NEVER UNDERSTANDS

**7. CHANGE IN COMMUNICATION/ HEARING**

Resident's ability to express, understand, or hear information has changed as compared to status of 90 days ago (or since last assessment if less than 90 days)
0. No change   1. Improved   2. Deteriorated

☐ = When box blank, must enter number or letter   a. = When letter in box, check if condition applies

MDS 2.0 September, 2000

Resident _____    Numeric Identifier _____

## SECTION D. VISION PATTERNS

| 1. | VISION | (Ability to see in adequate light and with glasses if used)<br>0. ADEQUATE—sees fine detail, including regular print in newspapers/books<br>1. IMPAIRED—sees large print, but not regular print in newspapers/books<br>2. MODERATELY IMPAIRED—limited vision; not able to see newspaper headlines, but can identify objects<br>3. HIGHLY IMPAIRED—object identification in question, but eyes appear to follow objects<br>4. SEVERELY IMPAIRED—no vision or sees only light, colors, or shapes; eyes do not appear to follow objects | |
|---|---|---|---|
| 2. | VISUAL LIMITATIONS/ DIFFICULTIES | Side vision problems—decreased peripheral vision (e.g., leaves food on one side of tray, difficulty traveling, bumps into people and objects, misjudges placement of chair when seating self) | a. |
| | | Experiences any of following: sees halos or rings around lights; sees flashes of light; sees "curtains" over eyes | b. |
| | | NONE OF ABOVE | c. |
| 3. | VISUAL APPLIANCES | Glasses; contact lenses; magnifying glass<br>0. No                        1. Yes | |

## SECTION E. MOOD AND BEHAVIOR PATTERNS

| 1. | INDICATORS OF DEPRES- SION, ANXIETY, SAD MOOD | (Code for indicators observed in last 30 days, irrespective of the assumed cause)<br>0. Indicator not exhibited in last 30 days<br>1. Indicator of this type exhibited up to five days a week<br>2. Indicator of this type exhibited daily or almost daily (6, 7 days a week) | |
|---|---|---|---|

| VERBAL EXPRESSIONS OF DISTRESS | | h. Repetitive health complaints—e.g., persistently seeks medical attention, obsessive concern with body functions | |
|---|---|---|---|
| a. Resident made negative statements—e.g., "Nothing matters; Would rather be dead; What's the use; Regrets having lived so long; Let me die" | | i. Repetitive anxious complaints/concerns (non-health related) e.g., persistently seeks attention/ reassurance regarding schedules, meals, laundry, clothing, relationship issues | |
| b. Repetitive questions—e.g., "Where do I go; What do I do?" | | SLEEP-CYCLE ISSUES | |
| c. Repetitive verbalizations— e.g., calling out for help, ("God help me") | | j. Unpleasant mood in morning | |
| | | k. Insomnia/change in usual sleep pattern | |
| d. Persistent anger with self or others—e.g., easily annoyed, anger at placement in nursing home; anger at care received | | SAD, APATHETIC, ANXIOUS APPEARANCE | |
| e. Self deprecation—e.g., "I am nothing; I am of no use to anyone" | | l. Sad, pained, worried facial expressions—e.g., furrowed brows | |
| | | m. Crying, tearfulness | |
| f. Expressions of what appear to be unrealistic fears—e.g., fear of being abandoned, left alone, being with others | | n. Repetitive physical movements—e.g., pacing, hand wringing, restlessness, fidgeting, picking | |
| | | LOSS OF INTEREST | |
| g. Recurrent statements that something terrible is about to happen—e.g., believes he or she is about to die, have a heart attack | | o. Withdrawal from activities of interest—e.g., no interest in long standing activities or being with family/friends | |
| | | p. Reduced social interaction | |

| 2. | MOOD PERSIS- TENCE | One or more indicators of depressed, sad or anxious mood were not easily altered by attempts to "cheer up", console, or reassure the resident over last 7 days<br>0. No mood            1. Indicators present,            2. Indicators present, indicators            easily altered            not easily altered | |
|---|---|---|---|
| 3. | CHANGE IN MOOD | Resident's mood status has changed as compared to status of 90 days ago (or since last assessment if less than 90 days)<br>0. No change            1. Improved            2. Deteriorated | |
| 4. | BEHAVIORAL SYMPTOMS | (A) Behavioral symptom frequency in last 7 days<br>0. Behavior not exhibited in last 7 days<br>1. Behavior of this type occurred 1 to 3 days in last 7 days<br>2. Behavior of this type occurred 4 to 6 days, but less than daily<br>3. Behavior of this type occurred daily | |

(B) Behavioral symptom alterability in last 7 days
0. Behavior not present OR behavior was easily altered
1. Behavior was not easily altered

| | | (A) | (B) |
|---|---|---|---|
| a. WANDERING (moved with no rational purpose, seemingly oblivious to needs or safety) | | | |
| b. VERBALLY ABUSIVE BEHAVIORAL SYMPTOMS (others were threatened, screamed at, cursed at) | | | |
| c. PHYSICALLY ABUSIVE BEHAVIORAL SYMPTOMS (others were hit, shoved, scratched, sexually abused) | | | |
| d. SOCIALLY INAPPROPRIATE/DISRUPTIVE BEHAVIORAL SYMPTOMS (made disruptive sounds, noisiness, screaming, self-abusive acts, sexual behavior or disrobing in public, smeared/threw food/feces, hoarding, rummaged through others' belongings) | | | |
| e. RESISTS CARE (resisted taking medications/ injections, ADL assistance, or eating) | | | |

| 5. | CHANGE IN BEHAVIORAL SYMPTOMS | Resident's behavior status has changed as compared to status of 90 days ago (or since last assessment if less than 90 days)<br>0. No change            1. Improved            2. Deteriorated | |
|---|---|---|---|

## SECTION F. PSYCHOSOCIAL WELL-BEING

| 1. | SENSE OF INITIATIVE/ INVOLVE- MENT | At ease interacting with others | a. |
|---|---|---|---|
| | | At ease doing planned or structured activities | b. |
| | | At ease doing self-initiated activities | c. |
| | | Establishes own goals | d. |
| | | Pursues involvement in life of facility (e.g., makes/keeps friends; involved in group activities; responds positively to new activities; assists at religious services) | e. |
| | | Accepts invitations into most group activities | f. |
| | | NONE OF ABOVE | g. |
| 2. | UNSETTLED RELATION- SHIPS | Covert/open conflict with or repeated criticism of staff | a. |
| | | Unhappy with roommate | b. |
| | | Unhappy with residents other than roommate | c. |
| | | Openly expresses conflict/anger with family/friends | d. |
| | | Absence of personal contact with family/friends | e. |
| | | Recent loss of close family member/friend | f. |
| | | Does not adjust easily to change in routines | g. |
| | | NONE OF ABOVE | h. |
| 3. | PAST ROLES | Strong identification with past roles and life status | a. |
| | | Expresses sadness/anger/empty feeling over lost roles/status | b. |
| | | Resident perceives that daily routine (customary routine, activities) is very different from prior pattern in the community | c. |
| | | NONE OF ABOVE | d. |

## SECTION G. PHYSICAL FUNCTIONING AND STRUCTURAL PROBLEMS

| 1. | (A) ADL SELF-PERFORMANCE—(Code for resident's PERFORMANCE OVER ALL SHIFTS during last 7 days—Not including setup)<br>0. INDEPENDENT—No help or oversight —OR— Help/oversight provided only 1 or 2 times during last 7 days<br>1. SUPERVISION—Oversight, encouragement or cueing provided 3 or more times during last 7 days —OR— Supervision (3 or more times) plus physical assistance provided only 1 or 2 times during last 7 days<br>2. LIMITED ASSISTANCE—Resident highly involved in activity; received physical help in guided maneuvering of limbs or other nonweight bearing assistance 3 or more times — OR—More help provided only 1 or 2 times during last 7 days<br>3. EXTENSIVE ASSISTANCE—While resident performed part of activity, over last 7-day period, help of following type(s) provided 3 or more times:<br>— Weight-bearing support<br>— Full staff performance during part (but not all) of last 7 days<br>4. TOTAL DEPENDENCE—Full staff performance of activity during entire 7 days<br>8. ACTIVITY DID NOT OCCUR during entire 7 days |
|---|---|

(B) ADL SUPPORT PROVIDED—(Code for MOST SUPPORT PROVIDED OVER ALL SHIFTS during last 7 days; code regardless of resident's self-performance classification)
0. No setup or physical help from staff
1. Setup help only
2. One person physical assist            8. ADL activity itself did not occur during entire 7 days
3. Two+ persons physical assist

| | | | (A) SELF-PERF | (B) SUPPORT |
|---|---|---|---|---|
| a. | BED MOBILITY | How resident moves to and from lying position, turns side to side, and positions body while in bed | | |
| b. | TRANSFER | How resident moves between surfaces—to/from: bed, chair, wheelchair, standing position (EXCLUDE to/from bath/toilet) | | |
| c. | WALK IN ROOM | How resident walks between locations in his/her room | | |
| d. | WALK IN CORRIDOR | How resident walks in corridor on unit | | |
| e. | LOCOMO- TION ON UNIT | How resident moves between locations in his/her room and adjacent corridor on same floor. If in wheelchair, self-sufficiency once in chair | | |
| f. | LOCOMO- TION OFF UNIT | How resident moves to and returns from off unit locations (e.g., areas set aside for dining, activities, or treatments). If facility has only one floor, how resident moves to and from distant areas on the floor. If in wheelchair, self-sufficiency once in chair | | |
| g. | DRESSING | How resident puts on, fastens, and takes off all items of street clothing, including donning/removing prosthesis | | |
| h. | EATING | How resident eats and drinks (regardless of skill). Includes intake of nourishment by other means (e.g., tube feeding, total parenteral nutrition) | | |
| i. | TOILET USE | How resident uses the toilet room (or commode, bedpan, urinal); transfer on/off toilet, cleanses, changes pad, manages ostomy or catheter, adjusts clothes | | |
| j. | PERSONAL HYGIENE | How resident maintains personal hygiene, including combing hair, brushing teeth, shaving, applying makeup, washing/drying face, hands, and perineum (EXCLUDE baths and showers) | | |

MDS 2.0 September, 2000

Resident_____  Numeric Identifier _____

| 2. | BATHING | How resident takes full-body bath/shower, sponge bath, and transfers in/out of tub/shower (EXCLUDE washing of back and hair.) *Code for most dependent* in self-performance and support.<br>**(A)** BATHING SELF-PERFORMANCE codes appear below | (A) | (B) |
|---|---|---|---|---|
| | | 0. Independent—No help provided | | |
| | | 1. Supervision—Oversight help only | | |
| | | 2. Physical help limited to transfer only | | |
| | | 3. Physical help in part of bathing activity | | |
| | | 4. Total dependence | | |
| | | 8. Activity itself did not occur during entire 7 days<br>*(Bathing support codes are as defined in Item 1, code B above)* | | |

| 3. | TEST FOR BALANCE<br>(see training manual) | *(Code for ability during test in the last 7 days)*<br>0. Maintained position as required in test<br>1. Unsteady, but able to rebalance self without physical support<br>2. Partial physical support during test;<br> or stands (sits) but does not follow directions for test<br>3. Not able to attempt test without physical help | |
|---|---|---|---|
| | | **a.** Balance while standing | |
| | | **b.** Balance while sitting—position, trunk control | |

| 4. | FUNCTIONAL LIMITATION IN RANGE OF MOTION<br><br>(see training manual) | *(Code for limitations during last 7 days that interfered with daily functions or placed resident at risk of injury)*<br>**(A)** RANGE OF MOTION     **(B)** VOLUNTARY MOVEMENT<br>0. No limitation       0. No loss<br>1. Limitation on one side   1. Partial loss<br>2. Limitation on both sides   2. Full loss | (A) | (B) |
|---|---|---|---|---|
| | | **a.** Neck | | |
| | | **b.** Arm—Including shoulder or elbow | | |
| | | **c.** Hand—Including wrist or fingers | | |
| | | **d.** Leg—Including hip or knee | | |
| | | **e.** Foot—Including ankle or toes | | |
| | | **f.** Other limitation or loss | | |

| 5. | MODES OF LOCOMO-TION | *(Check all that apply during last 7 days)* | | |
|---|---|---|---|---|
| | | Cane/walker/crutch | a. | |
| | | Wheeled self | b. | |
| | | Other person wheeled | c. | |
| | | Wheelchair primary mode of locomotion | d. | |
| | | NONE OF ABOVE | e. | |

| 6. | MODES OF TRANSFER | *(Check all that apply during last 7 days)* | | |
|---|---|---|---|---|
| | | Bedfast all or most of time | a. | |
| | | Bed rails used for bed mobility or transfer | b. | |
| | | Lifted manually | c. | |
| | | Lifted mechanically | d. | |
| | | Transfer aid (e.g., slide board, trapeze, cane, walker, brace) | e. | |
| | | NONE OF ABOVE | f. | |

| 7. | TASK SEGMENTA-TION | Some or all of ADL activities were broken into subtasks during **last 7 days** so that resident could perform them<br>0. No       1. Yes | |
|---|---|---|---|

| 8. | ADL FUNCTIONAL REHABILITA-TION POTENTIAL | Resident believes he/she is capable of increased independence in at least some ADLs | a. |
|---|---|---|---|
| | | Direct care staff believe resident is capable of increased independence in at least some ADLs | b. |
| | | Resident able to perform tasks/activity but is very slow | c. |
| | | Difference in ADL Self-Performance or ADL Support, comparing mornings to evenings | d. |
| | | NONE OF ABOVE | e. |

| 9. | CHANGE IN ADL FUNCTION | Resident's ADL self-performance status has changed as compared to status of **90 days ago** (or since last assessment if less than 90 days)<br>0. No change      1. Improved      2. Deteriorated | |
|---|---|---|---|

## SECTION H. CONTINENCE IN LAST 14 DAYS

| 1. | CONTINENCE SELF-CONTROL CATEGORIES<br>*(Code for resident's PERFORMANCE OVER ALL SHIFTS)* | | |
|---|---|---|---|
| | 0. CONTINENT—Complete control *[includes use of indwelling urinary catheter or ostomy device that does not leak urine or stool]* | | |
| | 1. USUALLY CONTINENT—BLADDER, incontinent episodes once a week or less; BOWEL, less than weekly | | |
| | 2. OCCASIONALLY INCONTINENT—BLADDER, 2 or more times a week but not daily; BOWEL, once a week | | |
| | 3. FREQUENTLY INCONTINENT—BLADDER, tended to be incontinent daily, but some control present (e.g., on day shift); BOWEL, 2-3 times a week | | |
| | 4. INCONTINENT—Had inadequate control BLADDER, multiple daily episodes; BOWEL, all (or almost all) of the time | | |

| a. | BOWEL CONTI-NENCE | Control of bowel movement, with appliance or bowel continence programs, if employed | |
|---|---|---|---|
| b. | BLADDER CONTI-NENCE | Control of urinary bladder function (if dribbles, volume insufficient to soak through underpants), with appliances (e.g., foley) or continence programs, if employed | |

| 2. | BOWEL ELIMINATION PATTERN | Bowel elimination pattern regular—at least one movement every three days | | |
|---|---|---|---|---|
| | | Constipation | b. | |
| | | Diarrhea | c. | |
| | | Fecal impaction | d. | |
| | | NONE OF ABOVE | e. | |

| 3. | APPLIANCES AND PROGRAMS | Any scheduled toileting plan | a. | | | |
|---|---|---|---|---|---|---|
| | | Bladder retraining program | | Did not use toilet room/commode/urinal | f. | |
| | | External (condom) catheter | b. | Pads/briefs used | g. | |
| | | Indwelling catheter | c. | Enemas/irrigation | h. | |
| | | Intermittent catheter | d. | Ostomy present | i. | |
| | | | e. | NONE OF ABOVE | j. | |

| 4. | CHANGE IN URINARY CONTI-NENCE | Resident's urinary continence has changed as compared to status of **90 days ago** (or since last assessment if less than 90 days)<br>0. No change     1. Improved     2. Deteriorated | |
|---|---|---|---|

## SECTION I. DISEASE DIAGNOSES

**Check only those diseases that have a relationship** to current ADL status, cognitive status, mood and behavior status, medical treatments, nursing monitoring, or risk of death. (Do not list inactive diagnoses.)

| 1. | DISEASES | *(If none apply, CHECK the NONE OF ABOVE box)* | | | | |
|---|---|---|---|---|---|---|
| | | **ENDOCRINE/METABOLIC/NUTRITIONAL** | | Hemiplegia/Hemiparesis | v. | |
| | | | | Multiple sclerosis | w. | |
| | | Diabetes mellitus | a. | Paraplegia | x. | |
| | | Hyperthyroidism | b. | Parkinson's disease | y. | |
| | | Hypothyroidism | c. | Quadriplegia | z. | |
| | | **HEART/CIRCULATION** | | Seizure disorder | aa. | |
| | | Arteriosclerotic heart disease (ASHD) | d. | Transient ischemic attack (TIA) | bb. | |
| | | Cardiac dysrhythmias | e. | Traumatic brain injury | cc. | |
| | | Congestive heart failure | f. | **PSYCHIATRIC/MOOD** | | |
| | | Deep vein thrombosis | g. | Anxiety disorder | dd. | |
| | | Hypertension | h. | Depression | ee. | |
| | | Hypotension | i. | Manic depression (bipolar disease) | ff. | |
| | | Peripheral vascular disease | j. | Schizophrenia | gg. | |
| | | Other cardiovascular disease | k. | **PULMONARY** | | |
| | | **MUSCULOSKELETAL** | | Asthma | hh. | |
| | | Arthritis | l. | Emphysema/COPD | ii. | |
| | | Hip fracture | m. | **SENSORY** | | |
| | | Missing limb (e.g., amputation) | n. | Cataracts | jj. | |
| | | Osteoporosis | o. | Diabetic retinopathy | kk. | |
| | | Pathological bone fracture | p. | Glaucoma | ll. | |
| | | **NEUROLOGICAL** | | Macular degeneration | mm. | |
| | | Alzheimer's disease | q. | **OTHER** | | |
| | | Aphasia | r. | Allergies | nn. | |
| | | Cerebral palsy | s. | Anemia | oo. | |
| | | Cerebrovascular accident (stroke) | t. | Cancer | pp. | |
| | | Dementia other than Alzheimer's disease | u. | Renal failure | qq. | |
| | | | | NONE OF ABOVE | rr. | |

| 2. | INFECTIONS | *(If none apply, CHECK the NONE OF ABOVE box)* | | | | |
|---|---|---|---|---|---|---|
| | | Antibiotic resistant infection (e.g., Methicillin resistant staph) | a. | Septicemia | g. | |
| | | | | Sexually transmitted diseases | h. | |
| | | Clostridium difficile (c. diff.) | b. | Tuberculosis | i. | |
| | | Conjunctivitis | c. | Urinary tract infection **in last 30 days** | j. | |
| | | HIV infection | d. | Viral hepatitis | k. | |
| | | Pneumonia | e. | Wound infection | l. | |
| | | Respiratory infection | f. | NONE OF ABOVE | m. | |

| 3. | OTHER CURRENT OR MORE DETAILED DIAGNOSES AND ICD-9 CODES | a. _____ | | | • | |
|---|---|---|---|---|---|---|
| | | b. _____ | | | • | |
| | | c. _____ | | | • | |
| | | d. _____ | | | • | |
| | | e. _____ | | | • | |

## SECTION J. HEALTH CONDITIONS

| 1. | PROBLEM CONDITIONS | *(Check all problems present in last 7 days unless other time frame is indicated)* | | | | |
|---|---|---|---|---|---|---|
| | | **INDICATORS OF FLUID STATUS** | | Dizziness/Vertigo | f. | |
| | | | | Edema | g. | |
| | | Weight gain or loss of 3 or more pounds within a 7 day period | a. | Fever | h. | |
| | | | | Hallucinations | i. | |
| | | Inability to lie flat due to shortness of breath | b. | Internal bleeding | j. | |
| | | | | Recurrent lung aspirations in **last 90 days** | k. | |
| | | Dehydrated; output exceeds input | c. | Shortness of breath | l. | |
| | | | | Syncope (fainting) | m. | |
| | | Insufficient fluid; did **NOT** consume all/almost all liquids provided during **last 3 days** | d. | Unsteady gait | n. | |
| | | | | Vomiting | o. | |
| | | **OTHER** | | NONE OF ABOVE | p. | |
| | | Delusions | e. | | | |

Resident _____

| 2. | PAIN SYMPTOMS | (Code the **highest level of pain** present in the **last 7 days**) | | |
|---|---|---|---|---|
| | | **a. FREQUENCY** with which resident complains or shows evidence of pain<br><br>0. No pain (**skip to J4**)<br>1. Pain less than daily<br>2. Pain daily | **b. INTENSITY** of pain<br>1. Mild pain<br>2. Moderate pain<br>3. Times when pain is horrible or excruciating | |

| 3. | PAIN SITE | (*If pain present, **check all sites** that apply in **last 7 days***) | | |
|---|---|---|---|---|
| | | Back pain | a. | |
| | | Bone pain | b. | |
| | | Chest pain while doing usual activities | c. | |
| | | Headache | d. | |
| | | Hip pain | e. | |
| | | Incisional pain | f. | |
| | | Joint pain (other than hip) | g. | |
| | | Soft tissue pain (e.g., lesion, muscle) | h. | |
| | | Stomach pain | i. | |
| | | Other | j. | |

| 4. | ACCIDENTS | (***Check all that apply***) | | |
|---|---|---|---|---|
| | | Fell in **past 30 days** | a. | |
| | | Fell in **past 31-180 days** | b. | |
| | | Hip fracture in **last 180 days** | c. | |
| | | Other fracture in **last 180 days** | d. | |
| | | NONE OF ABOVE | e. | |

| 5. | STABILITY OF CONDITIONS | Conditions/diseases make resident's cognitive, ADL, mood or behavior patterns unstable—(fluctuating, precarious, or deteriorating) | a. |
|---|---|---|---|
| | | Resident experiencing an acute episode or a flare-up of a recurrent or chronic problem | b. |
| | | End-stage disease, 6 or fewer months to live | c. |
| | | NONE OF ABOVE | d. |

## SECTION K. ORAL/NUTRITIONAL STATUS

| 1. | ORAL PROBLEMS | Chewing problem | a. |
|---|---|---|---|
| | | Swallowing problem | b. |
| | | Mouth pain | c. |
| | | NONE OF ABOVE | |

| 2. | HEIGHT AND WEIGHT | Record (**a.**) **height in inches** and (**b.**) **weight in pounds**. Base weight on most recent measure in **last 30 days**; measure weight consistently in accord with standard facility practice—e.g., in a.m. after voiding, before meal, with shoes off, and in nightclothes |
|---|---|---|
| | | **a.** HT (in.) [ ] [ ]   **b.** WT (lb.) [ ] [ ] |

| 3. | WEIGHT CHANGE | a. **Weight loss**—5 % or more in **last 30 days**; or 10 % or more in **last 180 days**<br>0. No          1. Yes |
|---|---|---|
| | | b. **Weight gain**—5 % or more in **last 30 days**; or 10 % or more in **last 180 days**<br>0. No          1. Yes |

| 4. | NUTRITIONAL PROBLEMS | Complains about the taste of many foods | a. |
|---|---|---|---|
| | | Regular or repetitive complaints of hunger | b. |
| | | Leaves 25% or more of food uneaten at most meals | c. |
| | | NONE OF ABOVE | d. |

| 5. | NUTRITIONAL APPROACHES | (**Check all that apply in last 7 days**) | | | |
|---|---|---|---|---|---|
| | | Parenteral/IV | a. | | |
| | | Feeding tube | b. | | |
| | | Mechanically altered diet | c. | | |
| | | Syringe (oral feeding) | d. | | |
| | | Therapeutic diet | e. | | |
| | | Dietary supplement between meals | f. | | |
| | | Plate guard, stabilized built-up utensil, etc. | g. | | |
| | | On a planned weight change program | h. | | |
| | | NONE OF ABOVE | i. | | |

| 6. | PARENTERAL OR ENTERAL INTAKE | (*Skip to Section L if neither 5a nor 5b is checked*) |
|---|---|---|
| | | a. Code the proportion of **total calories** the resident received through parenteral or tube feedings in the **last 7 days**<br>0. None                      3. 51% to 75%<br>1. 1% to 25%                4. 76% to 100%<br>2. 26% to 50% |
| | | b. Code the average **fluid intake** per day by IV or tube in **last 7 days**<br>0. None                      3. 1001 to 1500 cc/day<br>1. 1 to 500 cc/day       4. 1501 to 2000 cc/day<br>2. 501 to 1000 cc/day  5. 2001 or more cc/day |

## SECTION L. ORAL/DENTAL STATUS

| 1. | ORAL STATUS AND DISEASE PREVENTION | Debris (soft, easily movable substances) present in mouth prior to going to bed at night | a. |
|---|---|---|---|
| | | Has dentures or removable bridge | b. |
| | | Some/all natural teeth lost—does not have or does not use dentures (or partial plates) | c. |
| | | Broken, loose, or carious teeth | d. |
| | | Inflamed gums (gingiva); swollen or bleeding gums; oral abcesses; ulcers or rashes | e. |
| | | Daily cleaning of teeth/dentures or daily mouth care—by resident or staff | f. |
| | | NONE OF ABOVE | g. |

## SECTION M. SKIN CONDITION

| 1. | ULCERS<br><br>(Due to any cause) | (*Record the number of ulcers at each ulcer stage—regardless of cause. If none present at a stage, record "0" (zero). Code all that apply during **last 7 days**. Code 9 = 9 or more.*) [**Requires full body exam.**] | Number at Stage |
|---|---|---|---|
| | | **a.** Stage 1.   A persistent area of skin redness (without a break in the skin) that does not disappear when pressure is relieved. | |
| | | **b.** Stage 2.   A partial thickness loss of skin layers that presents clinically as an abrasion, blister, or shallow crater. | |
| | | **c.** Stage 3.   A full thickness of skin is lost, exposing the subcutaneous tissues - presents as a deep crater with or without undermining adjacent tissue. | |
| | | **d.** Stage 4.   A full thickness of skin and subcutaneous tissue is lost, exposing muscle or bone. | |

| 2. | TYPE OF ULCER | (*For each type of ulcer, **code for the highest stage in the last 7 days** using scale in item M1—i.e., 0=none; stages 1, 2, 3, 4*) | |
|---|---|---|---|
| | | **a.** Pressure ulcer—any lesion caused by pressure resulting in damage of underlying tissue | |
| | | **b.** Stasis ulcer—open lesion caused by poor circulation in the lower extremities | |

| 3. | HISTORY OF RESOLVED ULCERS | Resident had an ulcer that was resolved or cured **in LAST 90 DAYS**<br>0. No                      1. Yes | |
|---|---|---|---|

| 4. | OTHER SKIN PROBLEMS OR LESIONS PRESENT | (**Check all that apply** during **last 7 days**) | |
|---|---|---|---|
| | | Abrasions, bruises | a. |
| | | Burns (second or third degree) | b. |
| | | Open lesions other than ulcers, rashes, cuts (e.g., cancer lesions) | c. |
| | | Rashes—e.g., intertrigo, eczema, drug rash, heat rash, herpes zoster | d. |
| | | Skin desensitized to pain or pressure | e. |
| | | Skin tears or cuts (other than surgery) | f. |
| | | Surgical wounds | g. |
| | | NONE OF ABOVE | h. |

| 5. | SKIN TREATMENTS | (**Check all that apply** during **last 7 days**) | |
|---|---|---|---|
| | | Pressure relieving device(s) for chair | a. |
| | | Pressure relieving device(s) for bed | b. |
| | | Turning/repositioning program | c. |
| | | Nutrition or hydration intervention to manage skin problems | d. |
| | | Ulcer care | e. |
| | | Surgical wound care | f. |
| | | Application of dressings (with or without topical medications) other than to feet | g. |
| | | Application of ointments/medications (other than to feet) | h. |
| | | Other preventative or protective skin care (other than to feet) | i. |
| | | NONE OF ABOVE | j. |

| 6. | FOOT PROBLEMS AND CARE | (**Check all that apply** during **last 7 days**) | |
|---|---|---|---|
| | | Resident has one or more foot problems—e.g., corns, callouses, bunions, hammer toes, overlapping toes, pain, structural problems | a. |
| | | Infection of the foot—e.g., cellulitis, purulent drainage | b. |
| | | Open lesions on the foot | c. |
| | | Nails/calluses trimmed during **last 90 days** | d. |
| | | Received preventative or protective foot care (e.g., used special shoes, inserts, pads, toe separators) | e. |
| | | Application of dressings (with or without topical medications) | f. |
| | | NONE OF ABOVE | g. |

## SECTION N. ACTIVITY PURSUIT PATTERNS

| 1. | TIME AWAKE | (**Check appropriate time periods over last 7 days**)<br>Resident awake all or most of time (i.e., naps no more than one hour per time period) in the: | | |
|---|---|---|---|---|
| | | Morning | a. | |
| | | Afternoon | b. | |
| | | Evening | c. | |
| | | NONE OF ABOVE | d. | |

(If resident is comatose, skip to Section O)

| 2. | AVERAGE TIME INVOLVED IN ACTIVITIES | (**When awake and not receiving treatments or ADL care**)<br>0. Most—more than 2/3 of time        2. Little—less than 1/3 of time<br>1. Some—from 1/3 to 2/3 of time    3. None |
|---|---|---|

| 3. | PREFERRED ACTIVITY SETTINGS | (**Check all settings** in which activities are **preferred**) | | |
|---|---|---|---|---|
| | | Own room | a. | |
| | | Day/activity room | b. | |
| | | Inside NH/off unit | c. | |
| | | Outside facility | d. | |
| | | NONE OF ABOVE | e. | |

| 4. | GENERAL ACTIVITY PREFERENCES (adapted to resident's current abilities) | (**Check all PREFERENCES** whether or not activity is currently available to resident) | | | | |
|---|---|---|---|---|---|---|
| | | Cards/other games | a. | | Trips/shopping | g. |
| | | Crafts/arts | b. | | Walking/wheeling outdoors | h. |
| | | Exercise/sports | c. | | Watching TV | i. |
| | | Music | d. | | Gardening or plants | j. |
| | | Reading/writing | e. | | Talking or conversing | k. |
| | | Spiritual/religious activities | f. | | Helping others | l. |
| | | | | | NONE OF ABOVE | m. |

MDS 2.0 September, 2000

Resident _____     Numeric Identifier _____

| 5. | PREFERS CHANGE IN DAILY ROUTINE | Code for resident preferences in daily routines<br>0. No change     1. Slight change     2. Major change | |
|---|---|---|---|
| | | a. Type of activities in which resident is currently involved | |
| | | b. Extent of resident involvement in activities | |

## SECTION O. MEDICATIONS

| 1. | NUMBER OF MEDICA-TIONS | (*Record the number of different medications used in the last 7 days; enter "0" if none used*) | |
|---|---|---|---|
| 2. | NEW MEDICA-TIONS | (*Resident currently receiving medications that were initiated during the last 90 days*)<br>0. No         1. Yes | |
| 3. | INJECTIONS | (*Record the number of DAYS injections of any type received during the last 7 days; enter "0" if none used*) | |
| 4. | DAYS RECEIVED THE FOLLOWING MEDICATION | (*Record the number of DAYS during last 7 days; enter "0" if not used. Note—enter "1" for long-acting meds used less than weekly*) | |

| | | |
|---|---|---|
| a. Antipsychotic | | d. Hypnotic |
| b. Antianxiety | | e. Diuretic |
| c. Antidepressant | | |

## SECTION P. SPECIAL TREATMENTS AND PROCEDURES

| 1. | SPECIAL TREAT-MENTS, PROCE-DURES, AND PROGRAMS | a. SPECIAL CARE—*Check treatments or programs received during the last 14 days* |
|---|---|---|

**TREATMENTS**

| TREATMENTS | | | | PROGRAMS | |
|---|---|---|---|---|---|
| Chemotherapy | a. | | Ventilator or respirator | | l. |
| Dialysis | b. | | **PROGRAMS** | | |
| IV medication | c. | | Alcohol/drug treatment program | | m. |
| Intake/output | d. | | Alzheimer's/dementia special care unit | | n. |
| Monitoring acute medical condition | e. | | Hospice care | | o. |
| Ostomy care | f. | | Pediatric unit | | p. |
| Oxygen therapy | g. | | Respite care | | q. |
| Radiation | h. | | Training in skills required to return to the community (e.g., taking medications, house work, shopping, transportation, ADLs) | | r. |
| Suctioning | i. | | | | |
| Tracheostomy care | j. | | | | |
| Transfusions | k. | | NONE OF ABOVE | | s. |

b. THERAPIES - *Record the number of days and total minutes each of the following therapies was administered (for at least 15 minutes a day) in the last 7 calendar days (Enter 0 if none or less than 15 min. daily)*
[Note—count only post admission therapies]
(A) = # of days administered for **15 minutes or more**
(B) = total # of minutes provided in **last 7 days**

| | DAYS (A) | MIN (B) |
|---|---|---|
| a. Speech - language pathology and audiology services | | |
| b. Occupational therapy | | |
| c. Physical therapy | | |
| d. Respiratory therapy | | |
| e. Psychological therapy (by any licensed mental health professional) | | |

| 2. | INTERVEN-TION PROGRAMS FOR MOOD, BEHAVIOR, COGNITIVE LOSS | (*Check all interventions or strategies used in last 7 days—no matter where received*) | |
|---|---|---|---|
| | | Special behavior symptom evaluation program | a. |
| | | Evaluation by a licensed mental health specialist in **last 90 days** | b. |
| | | Group therapy | c. |
| | | Resident-specific deliberate changes in the environment to address mood/behavior patterns—e.g., providing bureau in which to rummage | d. |
| | | Reorientation—e.g., cueing | e. |
| | | NONE OF ABOVE | f. |

| 3. | NURSING REHABILITA-TION/ RESTOR-ATIVE CARE | Record the NUMBER OF DAYS each of the following rehabilitation or restorative techniques or practices was **provided to the resident for more than or equal to 15 minutes per day in the last 7 days** (*Enter 0 if none or less than 15 min. daily.*) |
|---|---|---|

| | | | |
|---|---|---|---|
| a. Range of motion (passive) | | f. Walking | |
| b. Range of motion (active) | | g. Dressing or grooming | |
| c. Splint or brace assistance | | h. Eating or swallowing | |
| TRAINING AND SKILL PRACTICE IN: | | i. Amputation/prosthesis care | |
| d. Bed mobility | | j. Communication | |
| e. Transfer | | k. Other | |

| 4. | DEVICES AND RESTRAINTS | (*Use the following codes for last 7 days:*)<br>0. Not used<br>1. Used less than daily<br>2. Used daily | |
|---|---|---|---|
| | | Bed rails | |
| | | a. — Full bed rails on all open sides of bed | |
| | | b. — Other types of side rails used (e.g., half rail, one side) | |
| | | c. Trunk restraint | |
| | | d. Limb restraint | |
| | | e. Chair prevents rising | |
| 5. | HOSPITAL STAY(S) | Record number of times resident was admitted to hospital with an overnight stay **in last 90 days** (or since last assessment if less than 90 days). (*Enter 0 if no hospital admissions*) | |
| 6. | EMERGENCY ROOM (ER) VISIT(S) | Record number of times resident visited ER without an overnight stay **in last 90 days** (or since last assessment if less than 90 days). (*Enter 0 if no ER visits*) | |
| 7. | PHYSICIAN VISITS | In the **LAST 14 DAYS** (or since admission if less than 14 days in facility) how many days has the physician (or authorized assistant or practitioner) examined the resident? (*Enter 0 if none*) | |
| 8. | PHYSICIAN ORDERS | In the **LAST 14 DAYS** (or since admission if less than 14 days in facility) how many days has the physician (or authorized assistant or practitioner) changed the resident's orders? *Do not include order renewals without change. (Enter 0 if none)* | |
| 9. | ABNORMAL LAB VALUES | Has the resident had any abnormal lab values during the **last 90 days** (or since admission)?<br>0. No       1. Yes | |

## SECTION Q. DISCHARGE POTENTIAL AND OVERALL STATUS

| 1. | DISCHARGE POTENTIAL | a. Resident expresses/indicates preference to return to the community | |
|---|---|---|---|
| | |     0. No        1. Yes | |
| | | b. Resident has a support person who is positive towards discharge | |
| | |     0. No        1. Yes | |
| | | c. Stay projected to be of a short duration— discharge projected **within 90 days** (do not include expected discharge due to death)<br>0. No       2. Within 31-90 days<br>1. Within 30 days    3. Discharge status uncertain | |
| 2. | OVERALL CHANGE IN CARE NEEDS | Resident's overall self sufficiency has changed significantly as compared to status of **90 days ago** (or since last assessment if less than 90 days)<br>0. No change   1. Improved—receives fewer   2. Deteriorated—receives<br>                     supports, needs less       more support<br>                     restrictive level of care | |

## SECTION R. ASSESSMENT INFORMATION

| 1. | PARTICIPA-TION IN ASSESS-MENT | a. Resident:       0. No    1. Yes | | |
|---|---|---|---|---|
| | | b. Family:        0. No    1. Yes    2. No family | | |
| | | c. Significant other:   0. No    1. Yes    2. None | | |

**2. SIGNATURE OF PERSON COORDINATING THE ASSESSMENT:**

a. Signature of RN Assessment Coordinator (sign on above line)

b. Date RN Assessment Coordinator signed as complete

| | | — | | | — | | | | |
|---|---|---|---|---|---|---|---|---|---|
| Month | | | Day | | | Year | | | |

MDS 2.0 September, 2000

Resident _____    Numeric Identifier _____

## SECTION T. THERAPY SUPPLEMENT FOR MEDICARE PPS

| 1. | SPECIAL TREAT- MENTS AND PROCE- DURES | **a. RECREATION THERAPY**—*Enter number of days and total minutes of recreation therapy administered (**for at least 15 minutes a day**) in the last 7 days (Enter 0 if none)* |
|----|---------|-------------------------------------------|

<table>
<tr><td></td><td></td><td colspan="2" align="right">DAYS    MIN</td></tr>
<tr><td></td><td></td><td>(A)</td><td>(B)</td></tr>
</table>

(A) = **# of days** administered for 15 minutes or more
(B) = **total # of minutes** provided in last 7 days

*Skip unless this is a Medicare 5 day or Medicare readmission/ return assessment.*

**b. ORDERED THERAPIES**—*Has physician ordered any of following therapies to begin in FIRST 14 days of stay—physical therapy, occupational therapy, or speech pathology service?*
0. No      1. Yes

*If not ordered, skip to item 2*

**c.** Through day 15, provide an estimate of the number of days when at least 1 therapy service can be expected to have been delivered.

**d.** Through day 15, provide an estimate of the number of therapy minutes (across the therapies) that can be expected to be delivered?

| 2. | WALKING WHEN MOST SELF SUFFICIENT | |
|----|---------|---|

*Complete item 2 if ADL self-performance score for TRANSFER (G.1.b.A) is 0,1,2, or 3 AND at least one of the following are present:*
¥ Resident received physical therapy involving gait training (P.1.b.c)
¥ Physical therapy was ordered for the resident involving gait training (T.1.b)
¥ Resident received nursing rehabilitation for walking (P.3.f)
¥ Physical therapy involving walking has been discontinued within the past 180 days

*Skip to item 3 if resident did not walk in last 7 days*

*(FOR FOLLOWING FIVE ITEMS, BASE CODING ON THE EPISODE WHEN THE RESIDENT WALKED THE FARTHEST WITHOUT SITTING DOWN. INCLUDE WALKING DURING REHABILITATION SESSIONS.)*

**a. Furthest distance walked** without sitting down during this episode.

0. 150+ feet      3. 10-25 feet
1. 51-149 feet     4. Less than 10 feet
2. 26-50 feet

**b. Time walked** without sitting down during this episode.

0. 1-2 minutes     3. 11-15 minutes
1. 3-4 minutes     4. 16-30 minutes
2. 5-10 minutes    5. 31+ minutes

**c. Self-Performance in walking** during this episode.

0. *INDEPENDENT*—No help or oversight
1. *SUPERVISION*—Oversight, encouragement or cueing provided
2. *LIMITED ASSISTANCE*—Resident highly involved in walking; received physical help in guided maneuvering of limbs or other nonweight bearing assistance
3. *EXTENSIVE ASSISTANCE*—Resident received weight bearing assistance while walking

**d. Walking support provided** associated with this episode (code regardless of resident's self-performance classification).

0. No setup or physical help from staff
1. Setup help only
2. One person physical assist
3. Two+ persons physical assist

**e. Parallel bars** used by resident in association with this episode.

0. No      1. Yes

| 3. | CASE MIX GROUP | Medicare | | | | | State | | | | |
|----|---------|----------|---|---|---|---|-------|---|---|---|---|

## RESIDENT ASSESSMENT PROTOCOL TRIGGER LEGEND FOR REVISED RAPS (FOR MDS VERSION 2.0)

**Key:**
● = One item required to trigger
❷ = Two items required to trigger
★ = One of these three items, plus at least one other item required to trigger
@ = When both ADL triggers present, maintenance takes precedence

> Proceed to RAP Review once triggered

| MDS ITEM | | CODE | Delirium | Cognitive Loss/Dementia | Visual Function | Communication | ADL-Rehabilitation Trigger A @ | ADL-Maintenance Trigger B @ | Urinary Incontinence and Indwelling Catheter | Psychosocial Well-Being | Mood State | Behavioral Symptoms | Activities Trigger A | Activities Trigger B | Falls | Nutritional Status | Feeding Tubes | Dehydration/Fluid Maintenance | Dental Care | Pressure Ulcers | Psychotropic Drug Use | Physical Restraints | |
|---|---|---|---|---|---|---|---|---|---|---|---|---|---|---|---|---|---|---|---|---|---|---|---|
| B2a | Short term memory | 1 | | ● | | | | | | | | | | | | | | | | | | | B2a |
| B2b | Long term memory | 1 | | ● | | | | | | | | | | | | | | | | | | | B2b |
| B4 | Decision making | 1,2,3 | | ● | | | | | | | | | | | | | | | | | | | B4 |
| B4 | Decision making | 3 | | | | | ● | | | | | | | | | | | | | | | | B4 |
| B5a to B5f | Indicators of delirium | 2 | ● | | | | | | | | | | | | | | | | | | ● | | B5a to B5f |
| B6 | Change in cognitive status | 2 | ● | | | | | | | | | | | | | | | | | | ● | | B6 |
| C1 | Hearing | 1,2,3 | | | | ● | | | | | | | | | | | | | | | | | C1 |
| C4 | Understood by others | 1,2,3 | | | | ● | | | | | | | | | | | | | | | | | C4 |
| C6 | Understand others | 1,2,3 | | ● | | ● | | | | | | | | | | | | | | | | | C6 |
| C7 | Change in communication | 2 | | | | | | | | | | | | | | | | | | | ● | | C7 |
| D1 | Vision | 1,2,3 | | | ● | | | | | | | | | | | | | | | | | | D1 |
| D2a | Side vision problem | √ | | | ● | | | | | | | | | | | | | | | | | | D2a |
| E1a to E1p | Indicators of depression, anxiety, sad mood | 1,2 | | | | | | | | | ● | | | | | | | | | | | | E1a to E1p |
| E1n | Repetitive movement | 1,2 | | | | | | | | | | | | | | | | | | | ● | | E1n |
| E1o | Withdrawal from activities | 1,2 | | | | | | | | ● | | | | | | | | | | | | | E1o |
| E2 | Mood persistence | 1,2 | | | | | | | | | ● | | | | | | | | | | | | E2 |
| E3 | Change in mood | 2 | ● | | | | | | | | | | | | | | | | | | ● | | E3 |
| E4aA | Wandering | 1,2,3 | | | | | | | | | | | ● | | | | | | | | | | E4aA |
| E4aA - E4eA | Behavioral symptoms | 1,2,3 | | | | | | | | | | ● | | | | | | | | | | | E4aA - E4eA |
| E5 | Change in behavioral symptoms | 1 | | | | | | | | | | ● | | | | | | | | | | | E5 |
| E5 | Change in behavioral symptoms | 2 | ● | | | | | | | | | | | | | | | | | | ● | | E5 |
| F1d | Establishes own goals | √ | | | | | | | | ● | | | | | | | | | | | | | F1d |
| F2a to F2d | Unsettled relationships | √ | | | | | | | | ● | | | | | | | | | | | | | F2a to F2d |
| F3a | Strong id, past roles | √ | | | | | | | | ● | | | | | | | | | | | | | F3a |
| F3b | Lost roles | √ | | | | | | | | ● | | | | | | | | | | | | | F3b |
| F3c | Daily routine different | √ | | | | | | | | ● | | | | | | | | | | | | | F3c |
| G1aA - G1jA | ADL self-performance | 1,2,3,4 | | | | | ● | | | | | | | | | | | | | | | | G1aA - G1jA |
| G1aA | Bed mobility | 2,3,4,8 | | | | | | | | | | | | | | | | | | ● | | | G1aA |
| G2A | Bathing | 1,2,3,4 | | | | | ● | | | | | | | | | | | | | | | | G2A |
| G3b | Balance while sitting | 1,2,3 | | | | | | | | | | | | | | | | | | ● | | | G3b |
| G6a | Bedfast | √ | | | | | | | | | | | | | | | | | | ● | | | G6a |
| G8a,b | Resident, staff believe capable | √ | | | | | ● | | | | | | | | | | | | | | | | G8a,b |
| H1a | Bowel incontinence | 1,2,3,4 | | | | | | | | | | | | | | | | | | ● | | | H1a |
| H1b | Bladder incontinence | 2,3,4 | | | | | | | ● | | | | | | | | | | | | | | H1b |
| H2b | Constipation | √ | | | | | | | | | | | | | | | | | | | ● | | H2b |
| H2d | Fecal impaction | √ | | | | | | | | | | | | | | | | | | | ● | | H2d |
| H3c,d,e | Catheter use | √ | | | | | | | ● | | | | | | | | | | | | | | H3c,d,e |
| H3g | Use of pads/briefs | √ | | | | | | | ● | | | | | | | | | | | | | | H3g |
| I1i | Hypotension | √ | | | | | | | | | | | | | | | | | | | ● | | I1i |
| I1j | Peripheral vascular disease | √ | | | | | | | | | | | | | | | | | | ● | | | I1j |
| I1ee | Depression | √ | | | | | | | | | | | | | | | | | | | ● | | I1ee |
| I1jj | Cataracts | √ | | | ● | | | | | | | | | | | | | | | | | | I1jj |
| I1ll | Glaucoma | √ | | | ● | | | | | | | | | | | | | | | | | | I1ll |
| I2j | UTI | √ | | | | | | | | | | | | | | | | ● | | | | | I2j |
| I3 | Dehydration diagnosis | 276.5 | | | | | | | | | | | | | | | | ● | | | | | I3 |
| J1a | Weight fluctuation | √ | | | | | | | | | | | | | | | | ● | | | | | J1a |
| J1c | Dehydrated | √ | | | | | | | | | | | | | | | | ● | | | | | J1c |
| J1d | Insufficient fluid | √ | | | | | | | | | | | | | | | | ● | | | | | J1d |
| J1f | Dizziness | √ | | | | | | | | | | | | | ● | | | | | | ● | | J1f |
| J1h | Fever | √ | | | | | | | | | | | | | | | | ● | | | | | J1h |
| J1i | Hallucinations | √ | | | | | | | | | | | | | | | | | | | ● | | J1i |
| J1j | Internal bleeding | √ | | | | | | | | | | | | | | | | ● | | | | | J1j |
| J1k | Lung aspirations | √ | | | | | | | | | | | | | | | | | | | ● | | J1k |
| J1m | Syncope | √ | | | | | | | | | | | | | | | | | | | ● | | J1m |

MDS 2.0 September, 2000

From Centers for Medicare and Medicaid Services, http://cms.hhs.gov/medicaid/mds20

## SECTION V. RESIDENT ASSESSMENT PROTOCOL SUMMARY

Numeric Identifier _____

| Resident's Name: | Medical Record No.: |
|---|---|

1. Check if RAP is triggered.

2. For each triggered RAP, use the RAP guidelines to identify areas needing further assessment. Document relevant assessment information regarding the resident's status.

- Describe:
  — Nature of the condition (may include presence or lack of objective data and subjective complaints).
  — Complications and risk factors that affect your decision to proceed to care planning.
  — Factors that must be considered in developing individualized care plan interventions.
  — Need for referrals/further evaluation by appropriate health professionals.

- Documentation should support your decision-making regarding whether to proceed with a care plan for a triggered RAP and the type(s) of care plan interventions that are appropriate for a particular resident.

- Documentation may appear anywhere in the clinical record (e.g., progress notes, consults, flowsheets, etc.).

3. Indicate under the Location of RAP Assessment Documentation column where information related to the RAP assessment can be found.

4. For each triggered RAP, indicate whether a new care plan, care plan revision, or continuation of current care plan is necessary to address the problem(s) identified in your assessment. The Care Planning Decision column must be completed within 7 days of completing the RAI (MDS and RAPs).

| A. RAP PROBLEM AREA | (a) Check if triggered | Location and Date of RAP Assessment Documentation | (b) Care Planning Decision—check if addressed in care plan |
|---|---|---|---|
| 1. DELIRIUM | | | |
| 2. COGNITIVE LOSS | | | |
| 3. VISUAL FUNCTION | | | |
| 4. COMMUNICATION | | | |
| 5. ADL FUNCTIONAL/ REHABILITATION POTENTIAL | | | |
| 6. URINARY INCONTINENCE AND INDWELLING CATHETER | | | |
| 7. PSYCHOSOCIAL WELL-BEING | | | |
| 8. MOOD STATE | | | |
| 9. BEHAVIORAL SYMPTOMS | | | |
| 10. ACTIVITIES | | | |
| 11. FALLS | | | |
| 12. NUTRITIONAL STATUS | | | |
| 13. FEEDING TUBES | | | |
| 14. DEHYDRATION/FLUID MAINTENANCE | | | |
| 15. DENTAL CARE | | | |
| 16. PRESSURE ULCERS | | | |
| 17. PSYCHOTROPIC DRUG USE | | | |
| 18. PHYSICAL RESTRAINTS | | | |

B. _____

1. Signature of RN Coordinator for RAP Assessment Process

2. ☐☐ — ☐☐ — ☐☐☐☐   Month  Day  Year

_____

3. Signature of Person Completing Care Planning Decision

4. ☐☐ — ☐☐ — ☐☐☐☐   Month  Day  Year

MDS 2.0 September, 2000

# RESIDENT ASSESSMENT PROTOCOL TRIGGER LEGEND FOR REVISED RAPS (FOR MDS VERSION 2.0)

Key:
- ● = One item required to trigger
- ❷ = Two items required to trigger
- ★ = One of these three items, plus at least one other item required to trigger
- @ = When both ADL triggers present, maintenance takes precedence

**Proceed to RAP Review once triggered**

| MDS ITEM | Description | CODE | Delirium | Cognitive Loss/Dementia | Visual Function | Communication | ADL-Rehabilitation Trigger A @ | ADL-Maintenance Trigger B @ | Urinary Incontinence and Indwelling Catheter | Psychosocial Well-Being | Mood State | Behavioral Symptoms | Activities Trigger A | Activities Trigger B | Falls | Nutritional Status | Feeding Tubes | Dehydration/Fluid Maintenance | Dental Care | Pressure Ulcers | Psychotropic Drug Use | Physical Restraints | |
|---|---|---|---|---|---|---|---|---|---|---|---|---|---|---|---|---|---|---|---|---|---|---|---|
| J1n | Unsteady gait | √ | | | | | | | | | | | | | | | | | | | ● | | J1n |
| J4a,b | Fell | √ | | | | | | | | | | | | | ● | | | | | | ● | | J4a,b |
| J4c | Hip fracture | √ | | | | | | | | | | | | | | | | | | | ● | | J4c |
| K1b | Swallowing problem | √ | | | | | | | | | | | | | | | | | | | ● | | K1b |
| K1c | Mouth pain | √ | | | | | | | | | | | | | | | | | ● | | | | K1c |
| K3a | Weight loss | 1 | | | | | | | | | | | | | | ● | | | | | | | K3a |
| K4a | Taste alteration | √ | | | | | | | | | | | | | | ● | | | | | | | K4a |
| K4c | Leave 25% food | √ | | | | | | | | | | | | | | ● | | | | | | | K4c |
| K5a | Parenteral/IV feeding | √ | | | | | | | | | | | | | | ● | ● | | | | | | K5a |
| K5b | Feeding tube | √ | | | | | | | | | | | | | | | ● | ● | | | | | K5b |
| K5c | Mechanically altered | √ | | | | | | | | | | | | | | ● | | | | | | | K5c |
| K5d | Syringe feeding | √ | | | | | | | | | | | | | | ● | | | | | | | K5d |
| K5e | Theraputic diet | √ | | | | | | | | | | | | | | ● | | | | | | | K5e |
| L1a,c,d,e | Dental | √ | | | | | | | | | | | | | | | | | ● | | | | L1a,c,d,e |
| L1f | Daily cleaning teeth | Not √ | | | | | | | | | | | | | | | | | ● | | | | L1f |
| M2a | Pressure ulcer | 2,3,4 | | | | | | | | | | | | | | ● | | | | | | | M2a |
| M2a | Pressure ulcer | 1,2,3,4 | | | | | | | | | | | | | | | | | | ● | | | M2a |
| M3 | Previous pressure ulcer | 1 | | | | | | | | | | | | | | | | | | ● | | | M3 |
| M4e | Impaired tactile sense | √ | | | | | | | | | | | | | | | | | | ● | | | M4e |
| N1a | Awake morning | √ | | | | | | | | | | | ❷ | | | | | | | | | | N1a |
| N2 | Involved in activities | 0 | | | | | | | | | | | ❷ | | | | | | | | | | N2 |
| N2 | Involved in activities | 2,3 | | | | | | | | | | | | ● | | | | | | | | | N2 |
| N5a,b | Prefers change in daily routine | 1,2 | | | | | | | | | | | | ● | | | | | | | | | N5a,b |
| O4a | Antipsychotics | 1-7 | | | | | | | | | | | | | | | | | | | ★ | | O4a |
| O4b | Antianxiety | 1-7 | | | | | | | | | | | | | ● | | | | | | ★ | | O4b |
| O4c | Antidepressants | 1-7 | | | | | | | | | | | | | ● | | | | | | ★ | | O4c |
| O4e | Diuretic | 1-7 | | | | | | | | | | | | | | | | ● | | | | | O4e |
| P4c | Trunk restraint | 1,2 | | | | | | | | | | | | | ● | | | | | | | ● | P4c |
| P4c | Trunk restraint | 2 | | | | | | | | | | | | | | | | | | ● | | ● | P4c |
| P4d | Limb restraint | 1,2 | | | | | | | | | | | | | | | | | | | | ● | P4d |
| P4e | Chair prevents rising | 1,2 | | | | | | | | | | | | | | | | | | | | ● | P4e |

MDS 2.0 September, 2000

From Centers for Medicare and Medicaid Services, http://cms.hhs.gov/medicaid/mds20

# APPENDIX C

# USEFUL SPANISH VOCABULARY AND PHRASES*

## CHAPTER 2: THE NURSING ASSISTANT

| | |
|---|---|
| Miss | señorita (seh-nyoh-ree-tah) |
| Mrs. | señora (seh-nyoh-rah) |
| Mr. | señor (seh-nyohr) |
| Hello! | ¡Hola! (Oh-lah) |
| I am going to cover you. | Lo voy acubrir. (Loh boy ah-koo-breer) |

## CHAPTER 3: WORK ETHICS

| | |
|---|---|
| Excuse me. | Con permiso. (kohn pehr-mee-soh) |
| Good morning, sir. | Buenos días, señor. (Boo-eh-nohs dee-ahs, seh-nyohr) |
| Good afternoon! | ¡Buenas tardes! (Boo-eh-nahs tahr-dehs) |
| How may I help you? | ¿En qué puedo servirle? (Ehn keh poo-eh-doh sehr-beer-leh) |
| Thank you for talking to me! | ¡Gracias por hablar conmigo! (Grah-see-ahs pohr ah-blahr kohn-mee-goh) |
| Good morning, Mrs. Ortiz! | !Buenos días, señora Ortiz! (Boo-eh-nohs dee-ahs, seh-nyo-rah ohr-tees) |
| Good morning, doctor! | !Buenos días, doctor! (Boo-eh-nohs dee-ahs, dohk-tohr) |
| You are welcome. | De nada. (Deh nah-dah) |
| Good afternoon! | !Buenas tardes! (Boo-eh-nahs tahr-dehs) |
| employ | emplear (ehm-pleh-ahr) |
| My name is... | Mi nobres es.../Me llamo... (Mee nohm-breh ehs/ Meh yah-moh) |
| Please! | ¡Por favor! (Pohr fah-bohr) |
| Thank you! | ¡Gracias! (Grah-see-ahs) |
| Thank you very much! | ¡Muchas gracias! (Moo-chahs grah-see-ahs) |
| What can I help you with? | ¿En qué puedo ayudarlo? (Ehn keh poo-eh-doh ah-yoo-dahr-loh) |
| Yes, sir. | Sí, señor. (See, seh-nyohr) |

*This appendix is presented for your convenience. Please note: This listing does not include all chapters; only those for which vocabulary and phrases directly relate to the content in this textbook.

Translations taken from Joyce EV, Villanueva ME: *Say it in Spanish: A Guide for Health Care Professionals*, ed 2, Philadelphia, 2000, WB Saunders.

# CHAPTER 4: COMMUNICATING WITH THE HEALTH TEAM

| Number | English | Spanish | Pronunciation |
|---|---|---|---|
| 1 | one | uno | (oo-noh) |
| 2 | two | dos | (dohs) |
| 3 | three | tres | (trehs) |
| 4 | four | cuatro | (koo-ah-troh) |
| 5 | five | cinco | (seen-koh) |
| 6 | six | seis | (seh-ees) |
| 7 | seven | siete | (see-eh-teh) |
| 8 | eight | ocho | (oh-choh) |
| 9 | nine | nueve | (noo-eh-beh) |
| 10 | ten | diez | (dee-ehs) |
| 11 | eleven | once | (ohn-seh) |
| 12 | twelve | doce | (doh-seh) |
| 13 | thirteen | trece | (treh-seh) |
| 14 | fourteen | catorce | (kah-tohr-seh) |
| 15 | fifteen | quince | (keen-seh) |
| 16 | sixteen | dieciséis | (dee-ehs-ee-seh-ees) |
| 17 | seventeen | diecisiete | (dee-ehs-ee-see-eh-teh) |
| 18 | eighteen | dieciocho | (dee-ehs-ee-oh-choh) |
| 19 | nineteen | diecinueve | (dee-ehs-ee-noo-eh-beh) |
| 20 | twenty | veinte | (beh-een-teh) |
| 30 | thirty | treinta | (treh-een-tah) |
| 40 | forty | cuarenta | (koo-ah-rehn-tah) |
| 50 | fifty | cincuenta | (seen-koo-ehn-tah) |
| 60 | sixty | sesenta | (seh-sehn-tah) |
| 70 | seventy | setenta | (seh-tehn-tah) |
| 80 | eighty | ochenta | (oh-chehn-tah) |
| 90 | ninety | noventa | (noh-behn-tah) |
| 100 | one hundred | cien | (see-ehn) |

| Time | Standard | Military (hours P.M.) |
|---|---|---|
| one o'clock | la una<br>(la oo-nah) | las trece horas<br>(lahs treh-seh oh-rahs) |
| two o'clock | las dos<br>(lahs dohs) | las catorce horas<br>(lahs kah-tohr-seh oh-rahs) |
| three o'clock | las tres<br>(lahs trehs) | las quince horas<br>(lahs keen-seh oh-rahs) |
| four o'clock | las cuatro<br>(lahs koo-ah-troh) | las dieciséis horas<br>(lahs dee-ehs-ee-seh-ees oh-rahs) |
| five o'clock | las cinco<br>(lahs seen-koh) | las diecisiete horas<br>(lahs dee-ehs-ee-see-eh-teh oh-rahs) |
| six o'clock | las seis<br>(lahs seh-ees) | las dieciocho horas<br>(lahs dee-ehs-ee-oh-choh oh-rahs) |
| seven o'clock | las siete<br>(lahs see-eh-teh) | las diecinueve horas<br>(lahs dee-ehs-ee-noo-eh-beh oh-rahs) |
| eight o'clock | las ocho<br>(lahs oh-choh) | las veinte horas<br>(lahs beh-een-teh oh-rahs) |
| nine o'clock | las nueve<br>(lahs noo-eh-beh) | las veintiuna horas<br>(lahs beh-een-tee-oo-nah oh-rahs) |

| Time | Standard | Military (hours P.M.) |
|------|----------|----------------------|
| ten o'clock | las diez (lahs dee-ehs) | las veintidós horas (lahs beh-een-tee-dohs oh-rahs) |
| eleven o'clock | las once (lahs ohn-seh) | las veintitrés horas (lahs beh-een-tee-trehs oh-rahs) |
| twelve o'clock/ midnight | las doce/la media noche (lahs doh-seh/lah meh-dee-ah non-cheh) | las cero horas (lahs seh-roh-oh-rahs) las veinticuatro horas (lahs beh-een-tee-koo-ah-troh oh-rahs) |

---

| | | | |
|---|---|---|---|
| abdomen | abdomen (ahb-doh-mehn) | which? | ¿cuál? (koo-ahl) |
| communication | comunicación (koh-moo-nee-kah-see-ohn) | who? | ¿quién? (kee-ehn) |
| black | negro (neh-groh) | how many? | ¿cuántos? (koo-ahn-tohs) |
| blue | azul (ah-sool) | how much? | ¿cuánto? (koo-ahn-toh) |
| clear | claro (klah-roh) | no, not | no (noh) |
| green | verde (behr-deh) | no one, nobody | nadie (nah-dee-eh) |
| red | rojo (roh-hoh) | nothing | nada (nah-dah) |
| yellow | amarillo (ah-mah-ree-yoh) | never, not ever | nunca, jamás (noon-kah, hah-mahs) |
| white | blanco (blahn-koh) | neither | tampoco (tahm-poh-koh) |
| Monday | lunes (loo-nehs) | neither....nor | ni....ni (nee....nee) |
| Tuesday | martes (mahr-tehs) | not one, not any | ninguno (neen-goo-noh) |
| Wednesday | miércoles (mee-ehr-koh-lehs) | without | sin (seen) |
| Thursday | jueves (hoo-eh-behs) | Every two hours. | Cada dos horas. (Kah-dah dohs oh-rahs) |
| Friday | viernes (bee-ehr-nehs) | Hello, I'm John Goodguy. | Hola, soy John Goodguy. (Oh-lah, soh-ee John Goodguy) |
| Saturday | sábado (sah-bah-doh) | Hello, Mrs. Mora. | Hola, señora Mora. (Oh-lah, seh-nyoh-rah Moh-rah) |
| Sunday | domingo (doh-meen-goh) | | |
| what? | ¿qué?/¿qué tal? (keh/keh tahl) | How are you? | ¿Cómo está? (Koh-moh ehs-tah) |
| when? | ¿cuándo? (koo-ahn-doh) | How do you feel? | ¿Cómo te sientes? (Koh-moh teh see-ehn-tehs) |
| where? | ¿dónde? (dohn-deh) | How do you feel now? | ¿Cómo se siente ahora? (Koh-moh seh see-ehn-teh ah-oh-rah) |
| why? | ¿por qué? (pohr keh) | | |
| for whom? | ¿para quién? (pah-rah kee-ehn) | | |
| for what? | ¿para qué? (pah-rah keh) | | |

# CHAPTER 5: ASSISTING WITH THE NURSING PROCESS

|  |  |
|---|---|
| Do you know where we are? | ¿Sabe dónde está? (Sah-beh dohn-deh ehs-tah) |
| Do you know the day? | ¿Qué día es hoy? (Keh dee-ah ehs oh-ee) |
| Where does it hurt? | ¿Dónde le duele? (Don-deh leh doo-eh-leh) |
| Point. | Apunte./Señale. (Ah-poon-teh/Seh-nyah-leh) |
| Did you fall? | ¿Se cayó? (Seh kah-yoh) |
| Do you have any symptoms: nausea, dizziness, other unusual feelings? | ¿Tiene algún síntoma como náuseas, vértigo, otra sensación rara? (Tee-eh-neh ahl-goon seen-toh-mah koh-moh nah-oo-seh-ahs, behr-tee-goh, oh-trah sehn-sah-see-ohn rah-rah) |
| Does the pain move from one place to another? | ¿El dolor se mueve de un lugar a otro? (Ehl doh-lohr seh moo-eh-beh deh oon loo-gahr ah oh-trah) |
| Does the pain get better if you stop and rest? | ¿Se mejora el dolor si se detiene y descansa? (Seh meh-hoh-rah ehl doh-lohr see seh deh-tee-eh-neh ee dehs-kahn-sah) |
| Has the pain gotten worse or gotten better? | ¿Se ha puesto el dolor peor o mejor? (Seh ah poo-ehs-toh ehl doh-lohr peh-ohr oh meh-hohr) |
| How often do you have the pain? | ¿Qué tan seguido tiene el dolor? (Keh tahn seh-gee-doh tee-eh-neh ehl doh-lohr) |
| How severe is the pain? | ¿Qué tan severo es el dolor? (Keh tahn seh-beh-roh ehs ehl doh-lohr) |
| On a scale from 1 [insignificant] to 10 [unbearable] | En una escala del 1 [insignificante] al 10 [intolerable]: (Ehn oo-nah ehs-kah-lah dehl oo-noh [een-seeg-nee-fee-kahn-teh] ahl deeehs [een-toh-leh-rah-bleh]) |
| Is the pain there all the time, or does it come and go? | ¿Está el dolor allí todo el tiempo, o va y viene? (Ehs-tah ehl doh-lohr ah-yee toh-doh ehl tee-ehm-poh, oh bah ee bee-ehn-eh?) |
| What caused the pain? | ¿Qué causó el dolor? (Keh kah-oo-soh ehl doh-lohr) |
| What did you do that caused the pain? | ¿Qué hacía cuando apareció el dolor? (Keh ah-see-ah koo-ahn-doh ah-pah-reh-see-oh ehl doh-lohr) |
| What makes the pain better? | ¿Qué hace mejorar el dolor? (Keh ah-seh meh-hoh-rahr ehl doh-lohr) |
| What is wrong? | ¿Qué pasa? (Keh pah-sah) |
| Is there any pain? | ¿Tiene algún dolor? (Tee-eh-neh ahl-goon doh-lohr) |
| What is hurting you? | ¿Qué le duele? (Keh leh doo-eh-leh) |
| How are you? | ¿Cómo está? (Koh-moh ehs-tah) |
| Do you have vision problems? | ¿Tienes problemas con la visión? (Tee-eh-nehs proh-bleh-mahs kohn lah bee-see-ohn) |
| Do you wear glasses? | ¿Usas anteojos/lentes? (Oo-sahs ahn-teh-ohhohs/lehn-tehs) |
| Do you have problems with your teeth? | ¿Tienes promblemas con los dientes? (Tee-eh-nehs prog-bleh-mahs kohn lohs dee-ehn-tehs) |
| At what time do you go to sleep? | ¿A qué hora te acuestas a dormir? (Ah keh oh-rah teh ah-koo-ehs-tahs ah dohr-meer) |
| How many hours do you sleep? | ¿Cuantás horas duermes? (Koo-ahn-tahs oh-rahs doo-ehr-mehs) |
| Do you wake up at night? | ¿Te despiertas en la noche? (Teh dehs-pee-ehr-tahs ehn lah noh-che) |
| Have you had headaches? | ¿Ha tenido dolor de cabeza? (Ah teh-nee-doh doh-lohr deh kah-beh-sah) |
| Do you have dizzy spells? | ¿Tiene mareos? (Tee-eh-neh mah-reh-ohs) |
| Swelling of the ankles? | ¿Hinchazón en los tobillos? (Een-chah-sohn ehn lohs toh-bee-yohs) |
| nausea | náusea (nah-oo-seh-ah) |
| normal | normal (nohr-mahl) |
| Are you nauseated? | ¿Está nauseado?/ ¿Tiene náuseas? (Ehs-tah nah-oo-seh-ah-doh/ Tee-eh-neh nah-oo-seh-ahs) |

Are you okay? | ¿Está bien?/¿Se siente bien?
| | (Ehs-tah bee-ehn/
| |   Seh see-ehn-teh bee-ehn)

Do you feel | ¿Se siente nauseado?
nauseated? | (Seh see-ehn-teh nah-oo-
| |   seh-ah-doh)

Do you feel weak? | ¿Se siente débril?
| | (Seh see-ehn-teh deh-beel)

Do you have | ¿Tiene dolor?
pain? | (Tee-eh-neh doh-lohr)
Is there any pain? | ¿Tiene algún dolor?
| | (Tee-eh-neh ahl-goon
| |   doh-lohr)

Is there anything that | ¿Hay algo que le preocupa?
worries you? | (Ah-ee ahl-goh keh leh
| |   preh-oh-koo-pah)

Is there anything else | ¿Hay otra cosa que le
bothering you? | moleste?
| | (Ah-ee oh-trah koh-sah
| |   keh-leh moh-lehs-teh)

Is there numbness/a | ¿Está entumecido/
tingling sensation/ | adormecido/tiene ardor
burning in your | en su pierna/brazo/
leg/arm/foot/ | pie/mano?
hand? | (Ehs-tah ehn-too-meh-see-
| |   doh/ah-dohr-meh-see-do/
| |   tee-eh-neh ahr-dohr ehn
| |   soo pee-ehr-nah/brah-soh/
| |   pee-eh/mah-noh)

Tell me if there is | Dime si duele.
pain. | (Dee-meh see doo-eh-leh)
Tell me if it hurts. | Dime si esto te duele.
| | (Dee-meh see ehs-toh teh
| |   doo-eh-leh)

The pain is in one | ¿El dolor es fijo?
place? | (Ehl doh-lohr ehs fee-hoh)
The pain is localized, | El dolor está fijo, agudo.
sharp. | (Ehl doh-lohr ehs-tah ehn ehl
| |   lah-dohl kohs-tah-doh)

The pain is on the | El dolor está en el
side. | lado/costado.
| | (Ehl doh-lohr ehs-tah ehn ehl
| |   lah-dohl kohs-tah-doh)

The pain is sharp? | ¿El dolor es agudo?
| | (Ehl doh-lohr ehs
| |   ah-goo-doh)

What brought you | ¿Qué lo trajo al hospital?
to the hospital? | (Keh loh trah-hoh ahl
| |   ohs-pee-tahl)

What is the matter? | ¿Qué le pasa/sucede?
| | (Keh leh pah-sah/
| |   soo-seh-deh)

What is the pain | ¿Qué tipo de dolor tiene?
like? | (Keh tee-oh deh doh-lohr
| |   tee-eh-neh)

What other | ¿Qué otra molestia tiene?
discomfort | (Keh oh-trah moh-lehs-tee-ah
do you have? | tee-eh-neh)
What symptoms | ¿Qué síntomas tiene?
do you have? | (Keh seen-toh-mahs
| |   tee-eh-neh)

When you have pain, | Cuando tiene dolor, ¿le dan
do you get | náuseas?
nauseated? | (Koo-ahn-doh tee-eh-neh
| |   doh-lohr, leh dahn
| |   nah-oo-seh-ahs)

## CHAPTER 6: UNDERSTANDING THE PERSON

Let me know how | Dígame cómo se siente.
you feel. | (Dee-gah-meh koh-moh seh
| |   see-ehn-teh)

My name is... | Mi nombre es.../Me llamo...
| | (Mee nohm-breh ehs/
| |   Meh yah-moh)

Good-bye! | ¡Hasta luego!
| | (Ahs-tah loo-eh-goh)

Hi! | !Hola!
| | (Oh-lah)

Good morning. | Buenos días.
| | (Boo-eh-nohs dee-ahs)

Good afternoon. | Buenas tardes.
| | (Boo-eh-nahs tahr-dehs)

Good evening. | Buenas noches.
| | (Boo-eh-nahs noh-chehs)

Do you speak | ¿Habla inglés?
English? | (Ah-blah een-glehs)
Thank you! | ¡Gracias!
| | (Grah-see-ahs)

Thank you very | ¡Muchas gracias!
much! | (Moo-chahs grah-see-ahs)
You are welcome. | De nada.
| | (Deh nah-dah)

respect | respeto
| | (rehs-peh-toh)

the family | la familia
| | (lah fah-mee-lee-ah)

father | padre
| | (pah-dreh)

dad | papá
| | (pah-pah)

mother | madre
| | (mah-dreh)

mom | mamá
| | (mah-mah)

husband | esposo
| | (ehs-poh-soh)

wife | esposa
| | (ehs-poh-sah)

| | |
|---|---|
| sister | hermana (ehr-mah-nah) |
| brother | hermano (ehr-mah-noh) |
| son | hijo (ee-hoh) |
| daughter | hija (ee-hah) |
| niece | sobrina (soh-bree-nah) |
| nephew | sobrino (soh-bree-noh) |
| grandmother | abuela (ah-boo-eh-lah) |
| grandfather | abuelo (ah-boo-eh-loh) |
| grandparents | abuelos (ah-boo-eh-lohs) |
| aunt | tía (tee-ah) |
| uncle | tío (tee-oh) |
| stepfather | padrastro (pah-drahs-troh) |
| stepmother | madrastra (mah-drahs-trah) |
| stepson | hijastro (ee-hahs-troh) |
| stepdaughter | hijastra (ee-hahs-trah) |
| children | hijos (eeh-hohs) |
| great-grandparents | bisabuelos (bee-sah-boo-eh-lohs) |
| mother-in-law | suegra (soo-eh-grah) |
| father-in-law | suegro (soo-eh-grah) |
| sister-in-law | cuñada (koo-nyah-dah) |
| brother-in-law | cuñado (koo-nyah-doh) |
| cousins | primos (pree-mohs) |
| cousin (female) | prima (pree-mah) |
| cousin (male) | primo (pree-moh) |
| grandchildren | nietos (nee-eh-tohs) |
| godparents | padrinos (pah-dree-nohs) |
| godfather | padrino (pah-dree-noh) |
| godmother | madrina (mah-dree-nah) |

| | |
|---|---|
| Do you understand? | ¿Comprende?/¿Entiende? (Kohm-prehn-deh/ Ehn-tee-ehn-deh) |
| Are you cold? | ¿Tiene frío? (Tee-eh-neh free-oh) |
| Are you hot? | ¿Tiene calor? (tee-eh-neh kah-lohr) |
| Are you hungry? | ¿Tiene hambre? (Tee-eh-neh ahm-breh) |
| Are you sleepy? | ¿Tiene sueño? (Tee-eh-neh soo-eh-nyoh) |
| Are you thirsty? | ¿Tiene sed? (Tee-eh-neh sehd) |
| Is that enough? | ¿Es suficiente? (Ehs soo-fee-see-ehn-teh) |
| Is that a lot? | ¿Es mucho? (Ehs moo-choh) |
| Is that too much? | ¿Es demasiado? (Ehs deh-mah-see-ah-doh) |
| Are you comfortable? | ¿Está cómoda? (Ehs tah koh-moh-dah) |
| A nurse will see you. | Una enfermera la atenderá. (Ooh-nah ehn-fehr-meh-rah lah ah-tehn-deh-rah) |
| Good! | ¡Bueno! (Boo-eh-noh) |
| Good afternoon, Miss González. | Buenas tardes, señorita González. (Boo-eh-nahs tahr-dehs, seh-nyoh-ree-tah Gohn-sah-lehs) |
| Good luck! | ¡Buena suerte! (Boo-eh-nah soo-ehr-teh) |
| Have a good day! | ¡Pase un buen día! (Pah-seh oon boo-ehn dee-ah) |
| Hello. | Hola (Oh-lah) |
| I am through. | Ya terminé. (Yah tehr-mee-neh) |
| I will see you tomorrow. | Le veré mañana. (Lah beh-reh mah-nyah-nah) |
| I will return shortly. | Regresaré en seguida. (Reh-greh-sah-reh ehn seh-ghee-dah) |
| If you don't understand, please let me know. | Si no entiende, dígame por favor. (See noh ehn-tee-ehn-deh, dee-gah-meh pohr fah-bohr) |
| Visiting hours are from nine in the morning to nine at night. | Las horas de visita son de las nueve de la mañana a las nueve de la noche. (Lahs oh-rahs deh bee-see-tah shon deh lahs noo-eh-beh deh lah mah-nyah-nah ah lahs noo-eh-beh deh lah noh-cheh) |

| | |
|---|---|
| Visiting hours are from two to eight P.M. | Las horas de visita son de las dos a las ocho de la noche. (Lahs oh-rahs deh bee-see-tah sohn deh lahs dohs ah loahs oh-choh deh lah noh-cheh) |

## CHAPTER 7: BODY STRUCTURE AND FUNCTION

| | |
|---|---|
| ligament | ligamento (lee-gah-mehn-toh) |
| organ | órgano (ohr-gah-noh) |
| pancreas | páncreas (pahn-kreh-ahs) |
| saliva | saliva (sah-lee-bah) |

## CHAPTER 8: GROWTH AND DEVELOPMENT

| | |
|---|---|
| infancy | infancia (een-fahn-see-ah) |

## CHAPTER 10: SAFETY

| | |
|---|---|
| What can I help you with? | ¿En qué puedo ayudarlo? (Ehn keh poo-eh-doh ah-yoo-dahr-loh) |
| This is the call bell. | Este es el timbre. (Ehs-teh ehs ehl teem-breh) |
| coma | coma (koh-mah) |
| comatose | comatoso (koh-mah-toh-soh) |
| Call if you need help. | Llame si necesita ayuda. (Yah-meh see neh-seh-see-tah ah-yoo-dah) |
| No smoking. | No se permite fumar. (Noh seh pehr-mee-teh foo-mahr) |
| Wear this bracelet all the time. | Use esta pulsera todo el tiempo. (Oo-seh ehs-tah pool-seh-rah toh-doh ehl tee-ehm-poh) |
| You cannot smoke here. | No puede fumar aquí. (Noh poo-eh-deh foo-mahr ah-kee) |
| You cannot smoke in your room. | No puede fumar en el cuatro. (Noh poo-eh-deh foo-mahr ehn ehl koo-ahr-toh) |

## CHAPTER 12: PREVENTING INFECTION

| | |
|---|---|
| Wash well all fruits and vegetables. | Lave bien frutas y verduras. (Lah-beh bee-ehn froo-tahs ee behr-doo-rahs) |
| Wash hands before eating. | Lave las manos antes de comer. (Lah-beh lahs mah-nohs ahn-tehs deh koh-mehr) |
| bacteria | bacteria (bahk-teh-ree-ah) |
| inflammation | inflamación (een-flah-mah-see-ohn) |
| pathogen | patogénico (pah-toh-heh-nee-koh) |

## CHAPTER 13: BODY MECHANICS

| | |
|---|---|
| I will put you on the stretcher. | Voy a ponerlo en la camilla. (Boy ah poh-nher-loh ehn lah kah-mee-yah) |
| Sit in the chair. | Siéntese en la silla. (See-ehn-teh-seh ehn lah see-yah) |
| spinal | espinal (ehs-pee-nahl) |
| Do you need the headboard up? | ¿Necesita levantar más la cabecera? (Neh-seh-see-tah leh-bahn-tahr mahs lah kah-beh-seh-rah) |
| I am going to help you lie down. | Voy a ayudarlo a acostarse. (Boy ah ah-yoo-dahr-loh ah ah-kohs-tahr-seh) |
| I am going to help you lie on the stretcher. | Voy a ayudarlo a acostarse en la camilla. (Boy ah ah-yoo-dahr-loh ah ah-kohs-tahr-seh ehn lah kah-mee-yah) |
| I will help you sit. | Le ayudaré a sentarse. (Leh ah-yoo-dah-reh ah sehn-tahr-seh) |
| Turn on your side. | Voltéese de lado. (Bhol-teh-eh-seh deh lah-doh) |
| Turn to your side. | Voltéate de lado. (Bhol-teh-ah-teh deh lah-doh) |

## CHAPTER 14: THE PERSON'S UNIT

| | |
|---|---|
| These buttons move the bed up/down. | Estos botones mueven la cama arriba/abajo. (Ehs-tohs boh-tah-nehs moo-eh-behn lah kay-mah ah-ree-bah/ah-bah-hoh) |
| You can raise the head. | Puede levantar la cabeza. (Poo-eh-deh leh-bahn-tahr lah kah-beh-sah) |
| You can raise the feet. | Puede levantar los pies. (Poo-eh-deh leh-bahn-tahr lohs pee-ehs) |
| The rails lower down. | El barandal se baja. (Ehl bah-rahn-dahl seh bah-hah) |
| Your towels are in the bathroom. | Sus toallas están en el baño. (Soos too-ahyahs ehs-tahn ehn ehl bah-nyoh) |
| There is an emergency light. | Hay una luz para emergencias. (Ah-ee oo-nah loos pah-rah eh-mehr-hehn-see-ahs) |
| Pull the cord in the bathroom. | Jale el cordón en el baño. (Hah-leh ehl kohr-dohn ehn ehl bah-nyoh) |
| The bell will sound. | La campana sonará. (Lah kahm-pah-nah soh-nah-rah) |
| This button lowers (raises) the headboard. | Este botón baha (sube) la cabecera de la cama. (Ehs-teh boh-tohn bah-hah (soo-beh) lah kah-beh-seh-rah deh lah kah-mah) |
| The chair turns into a bed. | Esta silla se hace cama. (Ehs-tah see-yah seh ah-seh kah-mah) |
| This is the radio. | Este es el radio. (Ehs-teh ehs ehl rah-dee-oh) |
| This is the call bell/buzzer. | Este es la campana/el timbre. (Ehs-teh ehs lah kahm-pah-nah/ehl teem-breh) |
| You have a private bathroom. | Tiene un baño/inodoro privado. (Tee-eh-neh oon bah-nyoh/ ee-noh-doh-roh pree-bah-doh) |

## CHAPTER 15: BEDMAKING

| | |
|---|---|
| linen | lino (lee-noh) |
| Do you need more pillows? | ¿Necesita más almohadas? (Neh-seh-see-tah mahs ahl-moh-ah-dahs) |

## CHAPTER 16: PERSONAL HYGIENE

| | |
|---|---|
| I am going to clean your teeth. | Voy a limpairle los dientes. (Boy ah leem-pee-ahr-leh lohs dee-ehn-tehs) |
| Rinse your mouth. | Enjuague su boca. (Ehn-hoo ah-geh soo boh-kah) |
| Here is a glass of water to rinse with. | Aquí está un vaso de agua para que se enjuague. (Ah-kee-ehs-tah oon bah-soh deh ah-goo-ah pah-rah keh seh ehn-hoo-ah-geh) |
| Open your mouth, please. | Abra la boca, por favor. (Ah-brah lah boh-kah, pohr fah-bohr) |
| There is a shower. | Hay una ducha/regadera. (Ah-ee oo-nah doo-chah/ reh-gah-deh-rah) |
| There is also a bathtub/tub. | También hay una bañera/ tina. (Tahm-bee-ehn ah-ee oo-nah bah-nyeh-rah/tee-nah) |
| Use dental floss. | Use hilo dental. (Oo-seh ee-loh dehn-tahl) |

## CHAPTER 17: GROOMING

| | |
|---|---|
| Mrs. . . ., I need to help you change clothes. | Señora . . ., necesito ayudarle a cambiar su ropa. (Señora . . ., neh-seh-see-toh ah-yoo-dahr-leh ah kahm-bee-ahr soo roh-pah) |

## CHAPTER 18: URINARY ELIMINATION

| | |
|---|---|
| When was the last time you used the toilet? | ¿Cuándo fue la última vez gue hizo del baño/que obró? (Koo-ahn doh foo-eh lah ool-tee-mah behs keh ee-soh dehl bah-nyoh/ keh oh-broh) |
| How often do you urinate? | ¿Cuántas veces ornia? (Koo-ahn-tahs beh-sehs oh-ree-nah) |
| Do you want the bedpan? | ¿Quiere el pato/el bacín? (Kee-eh-reh ehl pah-toh/ ehl bah-seen) |
| Do you have problems with starting to urinate? | ¿Tiene dificultad para empezar a orinar? (Tee-eh-neh dee-fee-kool-tahd pah-rah ehm-peh-sahr ah oh-ree-nahr) |
| Do you want to pass urine? | ¿Quiere orinar? (Kee-eh-reh oh-ree-nahr) |
| Everytime you go to the bathroom to void, you must place the urine in the container. | Cada vez que vaya al baño a orinar, debe poner la orina en el recipiente. (Kah-dah behs keh bah-yah ahl bah-nyoh ah oh-ree-nahr, deh-beh poh-nehr lah oh-ree-nah ehn ehl reh-see-pee-ehn-teh) |
| I will ask you to void. | Le diré que orine. (Leh dee-reh keh oh-ree-neh) |

## CHAPTER 19: BOWEL ELIMINATION

| | |
|---|---|
| Are you constipated? | ¿Está esterñido? (Ehs-tah ehs-treh-nyee-doh) |
| Do you have diarrhea? | ¿Tiene diarrea? (Tee-eh-neh dee-ah-reh-ah) |
| Do you wish to have a bowel movement? | ¿Quiere evacuar/hacer del baño? (Kee-eh-reh eh-bah-koo-ahr/ ah-sehr dehl bah-nyoh) |
| A bowel movement. | Hacer del baño. (Ah-sehr dehl bah-nyoh) |
| Do you want to have a bowel movement? | ¿Quiere evacuar?¿Quiere obrar? (Kee-eh-reh eh-bah-koo-ahr/Kee-eh-reh oh-brahr) |
| I will collect a sample of feces. | Voy a recoger una muestra de excremento. (Boy ah reh-koh-hehr oo-nah moo-ehs-trah deh ehx-kreh-mehn-toh) |

## CHAPTER 20: NUTRITION AND FLUIDS

| | |
|---|---|
| Have you eaten? | ¿Ha comido? (Ah koh-mee-doh) |
| What did you eat? | ¿Qué comido? (Keh koh-mee-doh) |
| Do you take a special diet? | ¿Toma dieta especial? (Toh-mah dee-eh-tah ehs-peh-see-ah-lehs) |
| What foods do you like? | ¿Qué alimentos le gustan? (Keh ah-lee-mehn-tohs leh goos-tahn) |
| What foods do you dislike? | ¿Qué alimentos le disgustan? (Keh ah-lee-mehn-tohs leh dees-goos-tahn) |
| How many times do you eat per day? | ¿Cuántas veces come por día? (Koo-ahn-tahs beh-sehs koh-meh pohr dee-ah) |
| What did you eat for breakfast? | ¿Qué comió en el desayuno? (Keh koh-mee-oh ehn ehl deh-sah-yoo-noh) |
| I am going to give you a list. | Voy a darle una lista. (Boy ah dahr-leh oo-nah lees-tah) |

For breakfast:
Para el desayuno:
(Pah-rah ehl deh-sah-yoo-noh)

eggs
huevos
(oo-eh-bohs)

toast
pan tostado
(pahn tohs-tah-doh)

coffee
café
(kah-feh)

milk
leche
(leh-cheh)

juice
jugo
(joo-goh)

fruit
fruta
(froo-tah)

How do you like your coffee?
¿Comó le gusta el café?
(Koh-moh leh goos-tah ehl kah-feh)

black
negro
(neh-groh)

with cream
con crema
(kohn kreh-mah)

with sugar
con azúcar
(kohn ah-soo-kahr)

What kind of coffee?
¿Qué clase de café?
(Keh klah-seh deh kah-feh)

regular
regular
(reh-goo-lahr)

decaffeinated
descafeinado
(dehs-kah-feh-ee-nah-doh)

instant
instantáneo
(eens-tahn-tah-neh-oh)

What kind of juices?
¿Qué clase de jugos?
(Keh klah-seh deh joo-gohs)

orange
naranja
(nah-rah-hah)

grape
uva
(oo-bah)

apple
manzana
(mahn-sah-nah)

grapefruit
toronja
(toh-rohn-hah)

prune
ciruela
(see-roo-eh-lah)

tomato
tomate
(toh-mah-teh)

How do you like the eggs fixed?
¿Cómo le gustan los huevos?
(Koh-moh leh goos-tahn lohs oo-eh-bohs)

scrambled
revueltos
(reh-boo-ehl-tohs)

over-easy
volteados
(bohl-teh-ah-dohs)

fried
fritos
(free-tohs)

hard-boiled
duros
(doo-rohs)

with ham
con jamón
(kohn hah-mahn)

We have cereals.
Tenemos cereales.
(Teh-neh-mohs seh-reh-ah-lehs)

oatmeal
avena
(ah-beh-nah)

cream of wheat
crema de trigo
(kreh-mah deh tree-goh)

corn flakes
hojitas de maíz/corn flakes
(oh-hee-tahs de mah-ees/hohrn fleh-ee-ks)

Do you like them hot/cold?
¿Le gustan calientes/fríos?
(Leh goos-tahn kah-lee-ehn-tehs/free-ohs)

We have meats:
Tenemos carnes:
(Teh-nehmohs kahr-nehs)

beef
res
(rehs)

hamburger
hamburguesa
(ahm-boor-geh-sah)

steak
bistec
(bees-tehk)

roast
rostizado
(rohs-tee-sah-doh)

pork
puerco
(poo-ehr-koh)

chops
chuletas
(choo-leh-tahs)

ribs
costillas
(kohs-tee-yahs)

chicken
pollo
(poh-yoh)

fried chicken
pollo frito
(poh-yoh free-toh)

baked chicken
pollo asado
(poh-yoh ah-sah-doh)

breast
pechuga
(peh-choo-gah)

leg
pierna
(pee-ehr-nah)

wings
alas
(ah-lahs)

fish
pescado
(pehs-kah-doh)

breaded
empanizado
(ehm-pah-nee-sah-doh)

broiled fish
pescado al horno
(pehs-kah-doh ahl ohr-noh)

Among the vegetables that we serve are:
Entre los vegetales que servimos hay:
(Ehn-treh lohs beh-heh-tah-lehs keh sehr-bee-mohs ah-ee)

| | |
|---|---|
| potatoes | papas (pah-pahs) |
| baked potatoes | papas asadas (pah-pahs ah-sah-dahs) |
| french fries | papas fritas (pah-pahs free-tahs) |
| mashed potatoes | puré de papas (poo-reh deh pah-pahs) |
| green beans | ejotes/habichuelas eh-hoh-tehs/ah-bee-choo-eh-lahs) |
| peas | chícharos (chee-chah-rohs) |
| corn | maíz/elote (mah-ees/eh-loh-teh) |
| beans | frijoles/habas (free-hoh-lehs/ah-bahs) |
| pinto beans | frijol pinto (free-hohl peen-toh) |
| refried | refritos (reh-free-tohs) |
| salad | ensalada (ehn-sah-lah-dah) |
| lettuce | lechuga (leh-choo-gah) |
| We also have desserts: | También tenemos postres: (Tahm-bee-ehn teh-neh-mohs pohs-trehs) |
| ice cream | nieve/helado (nee-eh-beh/eh-lah-doh) |
| vanilla | vainilla (bah-ee-nee-yah) |
| chocolate | chocolate (choh-koh-lah-teh) |
| strawberry | fresa (freh-sah) |
| pies | pasteles (pahs-teh-lehs) |
| pecan | nuez (noo-ehs) |
| apple | manzana (mahn-sah-nah) |
| cookies | galletas (gah-yeh-tahs) |
| candy | dulces (dool-sehs) |
| The water is in the glass/pitcher. | El aqua están en el vaso/ la jarra. (Ehl ah-goo-ah ehs-tah ehn ehl bah-soh/lah hah-rah) |
| Do you want water? | ¿Quere agua? (Kee-eh-reh ah-goo-ah) |
| Do you need ice? | ¿Necesita hielo? (Neh-seh-see-tah ee-eh-loh) |

| | |
|---|---|
| The fork, spoon, and knife are wrapped in the napkin. | El tenedor, cuchara y cuchillo están envueltos en la servilleta. (Ehl teh-neh-dohr, koo-chah-rah ee koo-chee-yoh ehs-tahn ehn-boo-ehl-tohs ehn lah sehr-bee-yeh-tah) |
| There is a straw. | Hay un popote. (Ah-ee oon poh-poh-teh) |
| The salt and pepper are in these packets. | La sal y pimienta están en estos paquetes. (Lah sahl ee pee-mee-ehn-tah ehs-tahn ehn ehs-tohn pah-keh-tehs) |
| The cover is hot. | La cubeirta está caliente. (Lah koo-bee-ehr-tah ehs-tah kah-lee-ehn-teh) |
| It keeps the food warm. | Guarda la comida tibia. (Goo-ahr-dah lah koh-mee-dah tee-bee-ah) |
| Select your foods from the menu after breakfast. | Seleccione las comidas del menú después del desayuno. (Seh-lehk-see-oh-neh lahs koh-mee-dahs dehl meh-noo dehs-poo-ehs dehl deh-sah-yoo-noh) |
| dehydration | deshidratación (deh-see-drah-tah-see-ohn) |
| nutrition | nutrición (noo-tree-see-ohn) |
| salt | sal (sahl) |
| Do you want: | ¿Quiere: (Kee-eh-reh) |
| a glass of water? | un vaso de agua? (oon bah-soh deh ah-goo-ah) |
| a glass of juice? | un vaso de jugo? (oon bah-soh deh hoo-goh) |
| Do you want: | ¿Quiere: (Kee-eh-reh) |
| something to eat? | algo de comer? (ahl-goh deh koh-mehr) |
| something to drink? | algo de tomar/beber? (ahl-goh deh toh-mahr/ beh-behr) |
| something to read? | algo de leer? (ahl-goh deh leh-ehr) |
| After meals. | Después de las comidas. (Dehs-poo-ehs deh lahs koh-mee-dahs) |
| Are you hungry? | ¿Tiene hambre? (Tee-eh-neh ahm-breh) |
| Difficulty in swallowing . . . | Diffcultad al tragar . . . (Dee-fee-kool-tahd ahl-tra-gahr) |

| | |
|---|---|
| Do you want a cup of coffee? | ¿Quiere una taza de café? (Kee-eh-reh oo-nah tah-sah deh-kah-feh) |
| Do you want a glass of juice? | ¿Quiere un vaso con jugo? (Kee-eh-reh oon bah-soh kohn hoo-goh) |
| Do you want a glass of water? | ¿Quiere un vaso con agua? (Kee-eh-reh oon bah-soh kohn ah-goo-ah) |
| Do you want something to drink? | ¿Quiere algo de tomar/beber? (Kee-eh-reh ahl-goh deh toh-mahr/beh-behr) |
| How do you like your eggs fixed? | ¿Comó le gustan los huevos? (Koh-moh leh goos-tahn lohs oo-eh-bohs) |
| How do you like your coffee? | ¿Cómo le gusta el café? (Koh-moh leh goos-tah ehl kah-feh) |
| How many glasses of water do you drink? | ¿Cuántos vasos de agua toma? (Koo-ahn-tohs bah-sohs de ah-goo-ah toh-mah) |
| The meals are served at. . . . | Los alimentos se sirven a. . . (Lohs ah-lee-mehn-tohs seh seer-behn ah) |
| When was the last time you ate? | ¿Cuándo fue la última vez que comió? (Koo-ahn-doh foo-eh lah ool-tee-mah behs keh koh-mee-oh) |
| You have to choose three meals a day. | Tiene que escoger tres comidas diarias. (Tee-eh-neh keh ehs-koh-hehr trehs koh-mee-dahs dee-ah-ree-ahs) |

## CHAPTER 21: MEASURING VITAL SIGNS

| | |
|---|---|
| I will start by taking vital signs. | Voy a empezar por tomar los signos vitales. (Boy ah ehm-peh-sahr pohr toh-mahr lohs seeg-nohs bee-tah-lehs) |
| Take the temperature rectally. | Tome la temperatura por el recto. (Toh-meh lah tehm-peh-rah-too-rah pohr ehl rehk-toh) |
| bradycardia | bradicardia (brah-dee-kahr-dee-ah) |
| fever | fatal (fah-tahl) |
| pulse | pulso (pool-soh) |

| | |
|---|---|
| rectal | rectal (rehk-tahl) |
| stethoscope | estetoscopio (ehs-teh-tohs-koh-pee-oh) |
| systole | sístole (sees-toh-leh) |
| thermometer | termómetro (tehr-moh-meh-troh) |
| I will take the radial pulse. | Voy a tomar su pulso radial. (Boy ah toh-mahr soo pool-soh rah-dee-ahl) |
| I will take your blood pressure. | Voy a tomar tu presión de sangre. (Boy ah toh-mahr too preh-see-ohn deh sahn-greh) |

## CHAPTER 22: EXERCISE AND ACTIVITY

| | |
|---|---|
| Please stay/remain in bed. | Por favor, quédeses en la cama. (Pohr fah-bohr, keh-deh-seh ehn lah kan-mah) |
| Lift your arm. | Levanta tu brazo. (leh-bahn-tah too brah-soh) |
| Extend it. | Extiéndelo. (Ehx-tee-ehn-deh-loh) |
| Flex it. | Dóblalo. (Doh-blah-loh) |
| Rotate it. | Gíralo./Dale vuelta. (Hee-rah-loh/Dah-leh boo-ehl-tah) |
| Bend your elbow. | Dobla el codo. (doh-blah ehl koh-doh) |
| Turn your forearm. | Voltea el antebrazo. (Bohl-teh-ah ehl ahn-teh brah-soh) |
| Open your hand. | Abre tu mano. (Ah-breh too mah-noh) |
| Close it. | Ciérrala. (See-eh-rah-lah) |
| Open the fingers wide. | Separa bien los dedos. (Seh-pah-rah bee-ehn lohs deh-dohs) |
| Bend the wrist. | Dobla la muñeca. (Doh-blah lah moo-nyeh-kah) |
| Extend your wrist. | Extiende tu muñeca. (Ehx-tee-ehn-deh too moo-nyeh-kay) |
| Lift your leg. | Levanta la pierna. (Leh-bahn-tah lah pee-ehr-nah) |

Bend it. — Dóblala. (Doh-blah-lah)

Bend your hip. — Dobla tu Cadera. (Doh-blah too kah-deh-rah)

Straighten your knee. — Endereza la rodilla. (Ehn-deh-reh-sah lah roh-dee-yah)

Move your leg. — Mueve tu pierna. (Moo-eh-beh too pee-ehr-nah)

Forward. — Adelante. (Ah-deh-lahn-teh)

Backward. — Atrás. (Ah-trahs)

Turn it to the left. — Voltéalo hacia la izquierda. (Bohl-teh-ah-loh ah-see-ah lah ees-kee-ehr-dah)

Turn it to the right. — Voltéalo hacia la derecha. (Bohl-teh-ah-loh ah-see-ah lah deh-reh-chah)

Lift your foot. — Levanta tu pie. (Leh-bahn-tah too pee-eh)

Bend your toes. — Dobla tus dedos (del pie). (Doh-blah toos deh-dohs (dehl pee-eh)

Lower your foot. — Baja el pie. (Bah-hah ehl pee-eh)

Flex the foot upward. — Dobla el pie hacia arriba. (Doh-blah ehl pee-eh ah-see-ah ah-ree-bah)

Straighten your leg. — Endereza tu pierna. (Ehn-deh-reh-sah too pee-ehr-nah)

Please walk. — Camina, por favor. (Kah-mee-nah, pohr fah-bohr)

exercise — ejercicio (eh-hehr-see-see-oh)

syncope — síncope (seen-koh-peh)

Activities are part of the plan. — Las actividades son parte del plan. (Lahs ahk-tee-bee-dah-dehs sohn pahr-teh dehl plahn)

Are you dizzy? — ¿Tiene mareos? (Tee-eh-neh mah-reh-ohs)

Do you feel dizzy? — ¿Se siente mareado? (Seh see-ehn-teh mah-reh-ah-doh)

Extend your arm. — Extiende tu brazo. (Ehx-tee-ehn-deh too brah-soh)

Extend your leg and foot. — Extiende tu pierna y pie. (Ehx-tee-ehn-deh too pee-ehr-nah ee pee-eh)

Flex your foot upward. — Dobla el pie para arriba. (Doh-blah ehl pee-eh pah-rah ah-ree-bah)

Flex your arm. — Dobla tu brazo. (Doh-blah too brah-soh)

Now raise the left arm. — Ahora levante el brazo izquierdo. (Ah-oh-rah leh-bahn-teh ehl brah-soh ees-kee-ehr-doh)

Turn the forearm. — Voltea el antebrazo. (Bhol-teh-ah ehl ahn-teh-brah-soh)

# CHAPTER 23: COMFORT, REST, AND SLEEP

At what time do you get up? — ¿A qué hora se levanta? (Ah keh oh-rah seh leh-bahn-tah)

At what time do you go to bed? — ¿A qué hora se acuesta? (Ah keh oh-rah seh ah-koo-ehs-tah)

How many hours do you sleep? — ¿Cuántas horas duerme? (Koo-ahn-tahs oh–rahs doo-ehr-meh)

Do you sleep during the day? — ¿Duerme durante el día? (Doo-ehr-meh doo-rahn-teh ehl dee-ah)

How long? — ¿Cuánto tiempo? (Koo-ahn-toh tee-ehm-poh)

Rest now. — Descanse ahora. (Dehs-kahn-seh ah-oh-rah)

At what time do you go to sleep? — ¿A qué hora se acuesta a dormir? (Ah keh oh-rah seh ah-koo-ehs-tah ah dohr-meer)

Do you wake up at night? — ¿Se despierta en la noche? (Seh dehs-pee-ehr-tah ehn lah noh-chen)

Are you cold? — ¿Tiene frío? (Tee-eh-neh free-oh)

Are you comfortable? — ¿Está cómoda? (Ehs-tah koh-moh-dah)

Are you hurting? — ¿Tiene dolor? (Tee-eh-neh doh-lohr)

| English | Spanish (pronunciation) |
|---|---|
| Are you sleepy? | ¿Tiene sueño? (Tee-eh-neh soo-eh-nyoh) |
| Do you have chest pain? | ¿Tiene dolor en el pecho? (Tee-eh-neh doh-lohr ehn ehl peh-choh) |
| Does it still hurt? | ¿Todavía le duele? (Toh-dah-bee-ah leh doo-eh-leh) |
| Does the pain move from one place to another? | ¿El dolor se mueve de un lugar a otro? (Ehl doh-lohr seh moo-eh-beh deh oon loo-gahr ah oh-troh) |
| Has the pain gotten worse or gotten better? | ¿Se ha puesto el dolor peor o mejor? (Seh ah poo-ehs-toh ehl doh-lohr peh-ohr oh meh-hohr) |
| How often do you have the pain? | ¿Qué tan seguido tiene el dolor? (Keh tahn seh-gee-doh tee-eh-neh ehl doh-lohr) |
| I am going to let you rest. | Voy a dejarlo descansar. (Boy ah deh-hahr-loh dehs-kahn-sahr) |
| If it hurts, tell me. | Si duele, avísame. (See doo-eh-leh, ah-bee-sah-meh) |
| On a scale from 1 [insignificant] to 10 [unbearable]. . . | En una escala del 1 [insignificante] al 10 [intolerable]. . . (Ehn oo-nah ehs-kah-lah dehl oo-noh [een-seeg-nee-gee-kahn-teh] ahl dee-ehs [een-toh-leh-rah-bleh]) |
| Pain? | ¿Dolor? (Doh-lohr) |
| Point when it hurts. | Señale cuando duela. (Seh-nyah-leh koo-ahn-doh doo-eh-lah) |
| Rest. | Descanse (Des-kahn-seh) |

# CHAPTER 24: ADMISSIONS, TRANSFERS, AND DISCHARGES

| English | Spanish (pronunciation) |
|---|---|
| I am going to ask many questions! | ¡Voy a hacerle muchas preguntas! (Boy ah ah-sehr-leh moo-chahs preh-goon-tahs) |
| The meals are served | Los alimentos se sirven (Lohs ah-lee-mehn-tohs seh seer-behn) |
| at seven A.M. | a las siete de la mañana. (ah lahs see-eh-teh deh lah mah-nyah-nah) |
| at eleven thirty. | a las once y media. (ah lahs ohn-seh ee meh-dee-ah) |
| at five P.M. | a las cinco de la tarde. (ah lahs seen-koh deh lah tahr-deh) |
| Phone for local calls. | Teléfono para llamadas locales. (Teh-leh-foh-noh pah-rah yah-mah-dahs loh-kah-lehs) |
| This is the radio. | Este es el radio. (Ehs-teh ehs ehl rah-dee-oh) |
| The television has four channels. | El televisor tiene cuatro canales. (Ehl teh-leh-bee-sohr tee-eh-neh koo-ah-troh kay-nah-lehs) |
| Change into the gown. | Póngase esta bata. (Phn-gah-seh ehs-tah bah-tah) |
| I need to ask you some questions. | Necesito hacerle unas preguntas. (Neh-seh-see-toh ah-sehr-leh oo-nahs preh-goon-tahs) |
| I am going to give you a tour of the floor. | Voy a darle un recorrido por el piso. (Boy ah dahr-leh oon reh-koh-ree-doh pohr ehl pee-soh) |
| This is the lobby. | Esta es la sala de espera. (Ehs-tah ehs lah sah-lah deh ehs-peh-rah) |
| The elevators work twenty-four hours. | Los elevadores funcionan las veinticuatro horas. (Lohs eh-leh-bah-dohrehs foon-see-oh-nahn lahs beh-een-tee-koo-ah-troh oh-rahs) |
| In case of fire, take the stairs. | En caso de fuego, use la escalera. (Ehn kah-soh deh foo-eh-goh, oo-seh lah ehs-kah-leh-rah) |
| There are bathrooms for guests in the corner. | Hay baños para las visitas en la esquina. (Hay bah-nyohs pah-rah lahs bee-see-tahs ehn lah ehs-kee-nah) |
| This is your room. | Este es su cuarto. (Ehs-teh ehs soo koo-ahr-toh) |
| You can tape pictures to the wall. | Puede pegar retratos en la pared. (Poo-eh-deh peh-gahr reh-trah-tohs ehn lah pah-rehd) |

| | | | |
|---|---|---|---|
| You can put cards on the shelf. | Puede poner trajetas en el estante. (Poo-eh-deh poh-nehr tahr-hehtahs ehn ehl ehs-tahn-teh) | Did you bring an artificial eye? | ¿Trajo un ojo artificial? (Trah-hoh oon prohs-teh tee-koh) |
| You can have flowers. | Puede tener flores. (Poo-eh-deh teh-nehr floh-rehs) | Did you bring an artificial limb? | ¿Trajo un prostético? (Trah-hoh oon oh-hoh ahr-tee-fee-see-ahl) |
| This is the call bell/ buzzer. | Esta es la campana/el timbre. (Ehs-tah ehs lah kahm-pah-nah/ehl teem-breh) | Did you bring contact lenses? | ¿Trajo lentes de contacto? (Trah-hoh lehn-tehs deh kohn-tahk-toh) |
| This button lowers (raises) the headboard. | Este botón baja (sube) la cabecera de la cama. (Ehs-teh boh-tohn bah-hah (soo-beh) lah kah-behseh-rah deh lah kah-mah) | Did you bring dentures? | ¿Trajo una dentadura postiza? (Trah-hoh oon-ah dehn-tah-doo-rah pohs-tee-sah) |
| Do you need more pillows? | ¿Necesita más almohadas? (Neh-seh–see-tah mahs ahl-moh-ah-dahs) | Did you bring glasses? | ¿Trajo anteojos/lentes? (Trah-hoh ahn-teh-oh-hohs/lehn-tehs) |
| You have a private bathroom. | Tiene un baño/inodoro privado. (Tee-eh-neh oon bah-nyoh/ee-noh-doh-roh pree-bah-doh) | Did you bring jewelry?/cash? | ¿Trajo joyas?/diner? (Trah-hoh hoh-yahs/dee-neh-roh) |
| There is a shower. | Hay una ducha/regadera. (Ahee oo-nah doo-chah/reh-gah-deh-rah) | I will show you your room. | Le mostraré su cuarto. (Leh mohs-trah-reh soo koo-ahr-tah) |
| There is also a bathtub/tub. | También hay una bañera/tina. (Tahm-bee-ehn ah-ee oo-nah bah-nyeh-rah/tee-nah) | | |

## CHAPTER 26: COLLECTING AND TESTING SPECIMENS

| | | | |
|---|---|---|---|
| Your clothes go in the closet. | Su ropa va en el closet/ropero. (Soo roh-pah bah ehn ehl kloh-seht/roh-peh-roh) | I am going to explain how to collect the urine. | Le voy a explicar cómo juntar la orina. (Leh boy ah ehx-plee-kahr koh-moh hoon-tahr lah oh-ree-nah) |
| You can make local phone calls. | Puede hacer llamadas locales. (Poo-eh-deh ah sehr-yah-mah-dahs loh-kah-lehs) | Every time you urinate, put it in the container. | Cada vez que orine, póngala en el frasco. (Kah-dah behs keh oh-ree-neh, pohn-gah-lah ehn ehl frahs-koh) |
| Dial 9, wait for the tone, then dial the number you want to call. | Marque el nueve, espere el tono, luego marque el número que quiera llamar. (mahr-keh ehl noo-eh-beh, ehs-peh-reh ehl toh-noh, loo-eh-doh mahr-key ehl noo-meh roh keh kee-eh-rah yah-mahr) | The container will be kept in the bucket with ice. | El frasco se mantendrá en una tina con hielo. (Ehl frahs-koh seh mahn-tehn-drah ehn oo-nah tee-nah kohn ee-eh-loh) |
| You can call collect. | Puede llamar por cobrar. (poo-eh-deh yah-mahr pohr koh-brahr) | Remember that you will do this for 24 hours. | Recuerde que hará esto por veinticuatro horas. (Reh-koo-ehr-deh keh ah-rah ehs-toh pohr beh-een-tee-koo-ah-troh oh-rahs) |
| You cannot smoke in your room. | No puede fumar en el cuarto. (Noh poo-eh-deh foo-mahr ehn ehl koo-ahr-toh) | If there is no ice in the bucket, call me. | Si no hay hielo en la tina, llámeme. (See noh ah-ee ee-eh-loh ehn lah tee-nah, yah-meh-meh) |
| Did you bring a hearing aid? | ¿Trajo un aparato para oír? (Trah-hoh oon ah-pah-rah-toh pah-rah oo-eer) | I also need a urine sample. | También necesito una muestra de orina. (Tahm-bee-ehn neh-seh-see-toh oo-nah moo-ehs-trah deh oh-ree-nah) |

| I am going to explain the collection of the urine. | Le voy a explicar la colección de orina. (Leh boy ah ehx-plee-kahr lah koh-lehk-see-ohn de oh-ree-nah) |
|---|---|

## CHAPTER 27: THE PERSON HAVING SURGERY

| anesthesia | anestesia (ah-nehs-teh-see-ah) |
|---|---|
| embolism | embolismo (ehm-boh-lees-moh) |

## CHAPTER 28: WOUND CARE

| hematoma | hematoma (eh-mah-toh-mah) |
|---|---|
| ulcer | úlcera (ool-seh-rah) |

## CHAPTER 30: OXYGEN NEEDS

| Breathe in. | Respire. (Rehs-pee-reh) |
|---|---|
| Breathe out. | Saque el aire. (Sah-keh ehl ah-ee-reh) |
| Now, take a deep breath. | Ahora, respira hondo. (Ah-oh-rah, rehs-pee-rah ohn-doh) |
| Cough! | ¡Tose! (Toh-seh) |
| Cough harder! | ¡Tose más fuerte! (Toh-seh mahs foo-ehr-teh) |
| Let it out. | Exhala. (Ehx-ah-lah) |
| oxygen | oxígen (ohx-ee-heh-noh) |
| Are you having problems breathing? | ¿Tiene problemas al respirar? (Tee-eh-neh proh-bleh-mahs ahl rehs-pee-rahr) |
| Cough deeply. | Tosa más fuerte. (Toh-sah mahs foo-ehr-teh) |
| Does it hurt to breathe? | ¿Te duele al respirar? (Teh doo-eh-leh ahl toh-sehr) |
| Does it hurt to cough? | ¿Te duele al toser? (Teh doo-eh-leh ahl toh-sehr) |

## CHAPTER 31: REHABILITATION AND RESTORATIVE CARE

| independence | independencia (een-deh-pehn-dehn-see-ah) |
|---|---|

## CHAPTER 32: HEARING AND VISION PROBLEMS

| glaucoma | glaucoma (glah-oo-koh-mah) |
|---|---|
| vertigo | vértigo (behr-tee-goh) |
| vision | visión (bee-see-ohn) |

## CHAPTER 33: COMMON HEALTH PROBLEMS

| What causes AIDS? | ¿Qué causa el SIDA? (Keh kah-oo-sah ehl see-dah) |
|---|---|
| A virus known as HIV . . . | El virus causal del SIDA se conoce como VIH . . . (Ehl bee-roos kah-oo-sahl dehl see-dah seh koh-noh-seh koh-moh beh-ee-ah-cheh[VIH]) |
| Who is at risk of getting AIDS? | ¿Quién está en riesgo de contraer el SIDA? (Kee-ehn ehs-tah ehn ree-ehs-goh deh kohn-trah-ehr ehl see-dah) |
| sexually active homosexual and bisexual males or females | homosexuales activos y hombres o mujeres bisexuales (oh-moh-sehx-oo-ah-lehs ahk-tee-bohs ee ohm-brehs oh moo-heh-rehs bee-sehx-oo-ah-lehs) |
| intravenous drug abusers | los que abusan de las drogas intravenosas (lohs keh ah-boo-sah deh lahs droh-gahs een-trah-beh-noh-sahs) |
| hemophiliacs and recipients of blood/blood components | hemofílicos, donadores de sangre o transfusión con sangre contaminada (eh-moh-fee-lee-kohs, doh-nah-doh-rehs deh sahn-greh oh trahns-foo-see-ohn kohn sahn-greh kohn-tah-mee-nah-dah) |

fetus of infected mothers

fetos de madres contamnadas
(feh-tohs deh mah-drehs kohn-tah-mee-nah-dahs)

Infected persons can transmit the virus.

Las personas infectadas pueden transmitir el virus
(Lahs pehr-soh-nahs een fehk-tah-dahs poo-ehdehn-trahns-mee-teer ehl bee-roos)

Can casual contact cause AIDS?

¿Los contactos eventaules puden causar SIDA?
(Lohs kohn-tahk-tohs eh-behn-too-ah-lehs poo-ehdehn kah-oo-sahr see-dah)

HIV is not transmissible by casual contact, nor . . .

El VIH no es transmitido en forma casual, ni por . . .
(Ehl VIH noh ehs trahns-mee-tee-doh ehn fohr-mah kah-soo-ahl, nee pohr:)

living in the same house as infected persons

vivir en la misma casa con personas infectadas
(bee-beer ehn lah mees-mah kah-sah kohn pehr-soh-nahs een-fehk-tah-dahs)

eating food handled by persons with AIDS

comer comida preparada por personas infectadas con SIDA
(koh-mehr koh-mee-dah preh-pah-rah-dah pohr pehr-soh-nahs een-fehk-tah-dahs kohn see-dah)

coughing, sneezing, kissing, or swimming with infected persons

tos, estornudo, besar, o nadar con personas infectadas
(tohs, ehs-tohr-noo-doh, beh-sahr oh nah-dahr kohn pehr-soh-nahs een-fehk-tah-dahs)

How serious is AIDS?

¿Qué tan serio es el SIDA?
(Keh tahn seh-ree-oh ehs-ehl see-dah)

AIDS has a high fatality rate approaching 100%.

El SIDA tiene una tasa cercana al 100 por ciento de mortalidad.
(Ehl see-dah tee-eh-neh oo-nah tah-sah sehr-kah-nah ahl see-ehn pohr see-ehn-toh deh mohr-tah-lee-dahd)

Is there a danger from donated blood?

¿Qué peligro hay por sangre donada?
(Keh peh-lee-groh ah-ee pohr sahn-greh doh-nah-dah)

The risk of contracting HIV is not high. Blood banks and other centers use sterile equipment and disposable needles.

El riesgo de contraer VIH no es alto. Los bancos de sangre y otros centros usan equipos estériles y agujas desechables.
(Ehl ree-ehs-goh deh kohn-trah-ehr VIH noh ehs ahl-toh. Lohs bahn-kohs deh sahn-greh ee oh-trohs sehn-trohs oo-sahn eh-kee-pohs ehs-teh-ree-lehs ee ah-goo-hahs deh-seh-chah-blehs)

The U.S. Public Health Service recommends:

El Departamento de Salud Pública de los Estados Unidos recomienda:
(Ehl Deh-pahr-tah-mehn-toh deh Sah-lood Poo-blee-kah deh lohs Ehs-tah-dohs Oo-nee-dohs reh-koh-mee-ehn-dah)

1. Know sexual background/ habits of partners.

1. Conozca los hábitos sexuales de su pareja.
(Koh-nohs-kah lohs ah-bee-tohs sex-oo-ah-lehs deh soo pah-reh-hah)

2. Use a condom or prophylactic.

2. Use un condón o profiláctico.
(Oo-seh oon kohn-dohn oh proh-fee-lahk-tee-koh)

3. If your partner is in a high risk group, cease sexual relations.

3. Si su compañera está en el grupo de alto riesgo, suspenda las relaciones sexuales.
(See soo kohm-pah-nyeh-rah ehs-tah ehn ehl groo-pah deh ahl-toh ree-ehs-goh, soos-pehn-dah lahs reh-lah-see-ohn-ehs sehx-oo-ahl-ehs)

4. Eliminate multiple sexual partners.

4. Elimine múltiples compañeros sexuales.
(Eh-lee-mee-neh mool-tee-plehs kohm-pha-nyeh-rohs sehx-oo-ah-lehs)

5. Don't use intra-venous drugs with contami-nated needles; don't share needles or syringes.

5. No use drogas intravenosas con agujas contaminadas; no comparta aguijas o jeringas.
(Noh oos-eh droh-gahs een-trah-veh-noh-sahs kohn ah-goo-hahs kohn-tah-mee-nah-dahs; noh kohm-pahr-tah ah-goo-hahs oh hehr-een-gahs)

asthma — asma
(ahs-mah)

cancer — cáncer
(kahn-sehr)

cardiac — cardíaco
(kahr-dee-ah-koh)

chemotherapy — quimioterapia
(kee-mee-oh-teh-rah-pee-ah)

hepatitis — hepatits
(eh-pah-tee-tees)

insulin — insulina
(een-soo-lee-nah)

venereal — venéreo
(beh-neh-reh-oh)

vomit — vómito
(boh-mee-toh)

Does the pain get better if you stop and rest? — ¿Se mejora el dolor si se detiene y descansa?
(Seh meh-hoh-rah ehl doh-lohr see-seh deh-tee-eh-neh ee dehs-kahn-sah)

## CHAPTER 34: MENTAL HEALTH PROBLEMS

claustrophobia — claustrofobia
(klah-oos-troh-foh-bee-ah)

obsession — obsesión
(ohb-seh-see-ohn)

panic — pánico
(pah-nee-koh)

## CHAPTER 35: CONFUSION AND DEMENTIA

delirious — delirio
(deh-lee-ree-oh)

## CHAPTER 36: DEVELOPMENTAL DISABILITIES

epilepsy — epilepsia
(eh-peel-ehp-see-ah)

## CHAPTER 37: SEXUALITY

sex — sexo
(sehx-oh)

sexual — sexual
(sehx-oo-ahl)

## CHAPTER 38: CARING FOR MOTHERS AND NEWBORNS

Is he/she . . . — ¿Está . . .
(Ehs-tah...)

breast-feeding? — tomando pecho?
(toh-mahn-doh peh-choh)

taking formula? — tomando fórmula?
(toh-mahn-doh fohr-moo-lah)

What formula does he take? — ¿Qué fórmula toma?
(Keh fohr-moo-lah toh-mah)

How many ounces does he take? — ¿Cuántas onzas toma?
(Koo-ahn-tahs ohn sahs-toh-mah)

How often do you feed the baby? — ¿Qué tan a menudo alimenta al bebé?
(keh tahn ah meh-noo-doh ah-lee-mehn-tah ahl beh-beh)

Does he/she have: fever/diarrhea/colic? — ¿Tiene: fiebre/diarrea/cólico?
(Tee-eh-neh: fee-eh-breh/dee-ah-rreh-ah/koh-lee-koh)

Does the baby sleep all night? — ¿Dureme el bebé toda la noche?
(Doo-ehr-meh ehl beh-beh toh-dah lah noh-cheh)

How many times does he wake up? — ¿Cuántas veces se despierta?
(Koo-ahn-tahs beh-sehs seh dehs-pee-ehr-tah)

Does he cry a lot? — ?Llora mucho?
(Yoh-rah moo-choh)

When was the last time he had a bowel movement? — ¿Cuándo fue la última vez que evacuó/hizo del baño?
(Koo-ahn-doh foo-eh lah ool-tee-mah behs keh eh-bah-koo-oh/ee-soh dehl bah-nyoh)

Is he urinating well? — ¿Orina bien?
(Oh-ree-nah bee-ehn)

Have you seen blood in the urine? — ¿Ha visto sangre en la orina?
(Ah bees-toh sahn-greh ehn lah oh-ree-nah)

| | |
|---|---|
| How many diapers have you changed since yesterday? | ¿Cuántos pañales le ha cambiado desde ayer? (Koo-ahn-tohs pah-nyah-lehs leh ah kahm-bee-ah-doh dehs-deh ah-yehr) |
| When did you notice the skin rash? | ¿Cuándo se díco cuenta de la piel rosada? (Koo-ahn-doh seh dee-oh koo-ehn-tah deh lah pee-ehl roh-sah-dah) |
| How many times has he vomited? | ¿Cuántas veces ha vomitado? (Koo-ahn-tahs beh-sehs ah boh-mee-tah-doh) |
| Is it a lot? | ¿Es mucho? (Ehs moo-choh) |
| Does the vomit have blood? | ¿Tiene sangre el vómito? (Tee-eh-neh sahn-greh ehl boh-mee-toh) |
| What color? | ¿De qué color? (Deh keh koh-lohr) |
| Does it have undigested food? | ¿Tiene restos de comida? (Tee-eh-neh rehs-tohs deh koh-mee-dah) |
| Does it smell bad? | ¿Huele mal? (Oo-eh-leh mahl) |
| Is he coughing? | ¿Está tosiendo? (Ehs-tah toh-see-ehn-doh) |
| Do not put on plastic pants! | No le ponga clzones de plástico! (Noh leh pohn-gah kahl-sohn-ehs deh plahs-tee-koh) |
| Sterilize the bottles. | Esterilice las botellas/ los biberones. (Ehs-teh-ree-lee-seh lahs boh-teh-yahs/lohs bee-beh-roh-nehs) |
| Help him to burp. | Póngalo a repetir/eructar. (Pohn-gah-loh ah reh-peh-teer/eh-rook-tahr) |
| Pat his back gently. | Dé palmaditas en la espalda. (Deh pahl-mah-dee-tahs ehn lah ehs-pahl-dah) |
| sanitary | sanitario (sah-nee-tah-ree-oh) |

## CHAPTER 39: ASSISTED LIVING

| | |
|---|---|
| Take the medicine with juice. | Tome la medicina con jugo. (Toh-meh lah meh-dee-see-nah kohn joo-goh) |
| Take it with a full glass of water. | Tómela con un vaso lleno de agua. (Toh-meh-lah kohn oon bah-soh yeh-noh deh ah-goo-a) |
| Do not drink alcohol with this medicine. | No tome alcohol con esta medicina. (Noh toh-meh ahl-kohl kohn ehs-tah meh-dee-see-nah) |
| It can cause drowsiness. | Le puede causar sueño. (Leh poo-eh-deh kah-oo-sahr soo-eh-nyoh) |
| Do not drive! | ¡No maneje/conduzca! (Noh mah-neh-heh/ kohn-doos-kah) |
| Do not operate machinery! | ¡No maneje/opere una máquina/maquinaria! (Noh mah-neh-heh/oh-peh-reh oo-nah mah-kee-nah/ah-kee-nah-ree-ah) |
| Take on an empty stomach. | Tómela con el estómago vacío. (Toh-meh-lah kohn ehl ehs-toh-mah-goh bah-see-oh) |
| Take one hour before eating. | Tómela una hora antes de comer. (Toh-meh-lah oo-nah oh-rah ahn-tehs de koh-mehr) |
| Take the medicine with food. | Tome la medicina con comida. (Toh-meh lah mehdee-see-nah kohn koh-mee-dah) |
| medication | medicamento (meh-dee-kah-mehn-toh) |
| medicine | medicina (meh-dee-see-nah) |

## CHAPTER 40: BASIC EMERGENCY CARE

| | |
|---|---|
| We are going to the hospital. | Vamos al hospital. (Bah-mohs ahl ohs-pee-tahl) |
| We are going in the ambulance. | Vamos en la ambulancia. (Bah-mohs ehn lah ahm-boo-lahn-see-ah) |

# GLOSSARY

**abbreviation** A shortened form of a word or phrase

**abduction** Moving a body part away from the midline of the body

**abrasion** A partial-thickness wound caused by the scraping away or rubbing of the skin

**abuse** The intentional mistreatment or harm of another person

**accountable** Being responsible for one's actions and the actions of others who perform delegated tasks; answering questions about and explaining one's actions and the actions of others

**acetone** A substance that appears in urine from the rapid breakdown of fat for energy; ketone body or ketone

**active physical restraint** A restraint attached to the person's body and to a fixed (immovable) object; it restricts movement or body access

**activities of daily living (ADL)** The activities usually done during a normal day in a person's life

**acute illness** A sudden illness from which a person is expected to recover

**acute pain** Pain that is felt suddenly from injury, disease, trauma, or surgery

**adduction** Moving a body part toward the midline of the body

**admission** Official entry of a person into an agency

**adolescence** The time between puberty and adulthood; a time of rapid growth and physical and social maturity

**advance directive** A document stating a person's wishes about health care when that person cannot make his or her own decisions

**affect** Feelings and emotions

**allergy** A sensitivity to a substance that causes the body to react with signs and symptoms

**alopecia** Hair loss

**ambulation** The act of walking

**AM care** Routine care before breakfast; early morning care

**amputation** The removal of all or part of an extremity

**anaphylaxis** A life-threatening sensitivity to an antigen

**anesthesia** The loss of feeling or sensation produced by a drug

**anorexia** The loss of appetite

**anterior** At or toward the front of the body or body part; ventral

**anxiety** A vague, uneasy feeling in response to stress

**aphasia** The inability *(a)* to speak *(phasia)*

**apical-radial pulse** Taking the apical and radial pulses at the same time

**apnea** The lack or absence *(a)* of breathing *(pnea)*

**arterial ulcer** An open wound on the lower legs and feet caused by poor arterial blood flow

**artery** A blood vessel that carries blood away from the heart

**arthritis** Joint *(arthr)* inflammation *(itis)*

**arthroplasty** The surgical replacement *(plasty)* of a joint *(arthro)*

**asepsis** Being free of disease-producing microbes

**aspiration** Breathing fluid or an object into the lungs

**assault** Intentionally attempting or threatening to touch a person's body without the person's consent

**assessment** Collecting information about the person; a step in the nursing process

**assisted living facility** Provides housing, personal care, support services, health care, and social activities in a homelike setting

**atrophy** The decrease in size or a wasting away of tissue

**base of support** The area on which an object rests

**battery** Touching a person's body without his or her consent

**bedsore** A pressure ulcer, pressure sore, or decubitus ulcer

**benign tumor** A tumor that grows slowly and within a local area

**biohazardous waste** Items contaminated with blood, body fluids, secretions, or excretions; *bio* means life, and *hazardous* means dangerous or harmful

**Biot's respirations** Rapid and deep respirations followed by 10 to 30 seconds of apnea

**bisexual** A person who is attracted to both sexes

**blood pressure** The amount of force exerted against the walls of an artery by the blood

**body alignment** The way the head, trunk, arms, and legs are aligned with one another; posture

**body language** Messages sent through facial expressions, gestures, posture, hand and body movements, gait, eye contact, and appearance

**body mechanics** Using the body in an efficient and careful way

**body temperature** The amount of heat in the body that is a balance between the amount of heat produced and the amount lost by the body

**bradycardia** A slow *(brady)* heart rate *(cardia);* less than 60 beats per minute

**bradypnea** Slow *(brady)* breathing *(pnea);* respirations are fewer than 12 per minute

**braille** A writing system that uses raised dots for each letter of the alphabet; the first 10 letters also represent 0 through 9

**calorie** The amount of energy produced when the body burns food

**cancer** Malignant tumor

**capillary** A tiny blood vessel; food, oxygen, and other substances pass from the capillaries to the cells

**cardiac arrest** The heart and breathing stop suddenly and without warning

**carrier** A human or animal that is a reservoir for microbes but does not have signs and symptoms of infection

**case management** A nursing care pattern; a case manager (an RN) coordinates a person's care from admission through discharge and into the home setting

**catheter** A tube used to drain or inject fluid through a body opening

**catheterization** The process of inserting a catheter

**cell** The basic unit of body structure

**cerumen** Earwax

**chart** The medical record

**Cheyne-Stokes respirations** Respirations gradually increase in rate and depth and then become shallow and slow; breathing may stop *(apnea)* for 10 to 20 seconds

**chronic illness** An ongoing illness, slow or gradual in onset, for which there is no known cure; the illness can be controlled and complications prevented

**chronic pain** Pain lasting longer than 6 months; it is constant or occurs off and on

**chronic wound** A wound that does not heal easily

**circadian rhythm** Daily rhythm based on a 24-hour cycle; the day-night cycle or body rhythm

**circulatory ulcer** An open wound on the lower legs and feet caused by decreased blood flow through the arteries or veins; vascular ulcer

**circumcision** The surgical removal of foreskin from the penis

**civil law** Laws concerned with relationships between people

**clean-contaminated wound** Occurs from the surgical entry of the reproductive, urinary, respiratory, or gastrointestinal system

**clean technique** Medical asepsis

**clean wound** A wound that is not infected; microbes have not entered the wound

**closed fracture** The bone is broken but the skin is intact; simple fracture

**closed wound** Tissues are injured but the skin is not broken

**colostomy** A surgically created opening *(stomy)* between the colon *(colo)* and abdominal wall

**coma** A state of being unaware of one's surroundings and being unable to react or respond to people, places, or things

**combining vowel** A vowel added between two roots or between a root and a suffix to make pronunciation easier

**comfort** A state of well-being; the person has no physical or emotional pain and is calm and at peace

**communicable disease** A disease caused by pathogens that spread easily; a contagious disease

**communication** The exchange of information—a message sent is received and interpreted by the intended person

**compound fracture** Open fracture

**compress** A soft pad applied over a body area

**compulsion** Repeating an act over and over again

**confidentiality** Trusting others with personal and private information

**conflict** A clash between opposing interests or ideas

**conscious** Awareness of the environment and experiences; the person knows what is happening and can control thoughts and behaviors

**constipation** The passage of a hard, dry stool

**constrict** To narrow

**contagious disease** Communicable disease

**contaminated wound** A wound with a high risk of infection

**contamination** The process of becoming unclean

**contracture** The lack of joint mobility caused by abnormal shortening of a muscle

**contusion** A closed wound caused by a blow to the body; a bruise

**convulsion** A seizure

**courtesy** A polite, considerate, or helpful comment or act

**crime** An act that violates a criminal law

**criminal law** Laws concerned with offenses against the public and society in general

**culture** The characteristics of a group of people—language, values, beliefs, habits, likes, dislikes, customs—passed from one generation to the next

**cyanosis** Bluish skin color

**Daily Reference Values (DRVs)** The maximum daily intake values for total fat, saturated fat, cholesterol, sodium, carbohydrate, and dietary fiber

**Daily Value (DV)** How a serving fits into the daily diet; expressed in a percent (%) based on a daily diet of 2000 calories

**dandruff** The excessive amount of dry, white flakes from the scalp

**deafness** Hearing loss in which it is impossible for the person to understand speech through hearing alone

**decubitus ulcer** A pressure ulcer, pressure sore, or bedsore

**defamation** Injuring a person's name and reputation by making false statements to a third person

**defecation** The process of excreting feces from the rectum through the anus; a bowel movement

**defense mechanism** An unconscious reaction that blocks unpleasant or threatening feelings

**dehiscence** The separation of wound layers

**dehydration** The excessive loss of water from tissues; a decrease in the amount of water in body tissues

**delegate** To authorize another person to perform a task

**delirium** A state of temporary but acute mental confusion

**delusion** A false belief

**delusion of grandeur** An exaggerated belief about one's importance, wealth, power, or talents

**delusion of persecution** A false belief that one is being mistreated, abused, or harassed

**dementia** The loss of cognitive and social function caused by changes in the brain

**development** Changes in mental, emotional, and social function

**developmental disability** A disability occurring before 22 years of age

**developmental task** A skill that must be completed during a stage of development

**diarrhea** The frequent passage of liquid stools

**diastole** The period of heart muscle relaxation; the period when the heart is at rest

**diastolic pressure** The pressure in the arteries when the heart is at rest

**digestion** The process of physically and chemically breaking down food so that it can be absorbed for use by the cells

**dilate** To expand or open wider

**diplegia** Similar body parts are affected on both sides of the body

**dirty wound** An infected wound

**disability** A lost, absent, or impaired physical or mental function

**disaster** A sudden catastrophic event in which many people are injured and killed and property is destroyed

**discharge** Official departure of a person from an agency

**discomfort** Pain

**disinfection** The process of destroying pathogens

**distal** The part farthest from the center or from the point of attachment

**distraction** To change the person's center of attention

**dorsal** At or toward the back of the body or body part; posterior

**dorsal recumbent position** The back-lying or supine position; the supine position with the legs together; horizontal recumbent position

**dorsiflexion** Bending the toes and foot up at the ankle

**douche** The introduction of a fluid into the vagina and the immediate return of the fluid

**drawsheet** A small sheet placed over the middle of the bottom sheet; it helps keep the mattress and bottom linens clean and dry; the cotton drawsheet

**dysphagia** Difficulty *(dys)* swallowing *(phagia)*

**dyspnea** Difficult, labored, or painful *(dys)* breathing *(pnea)*

**dysuria** Painful or difficult *(dys)* urination *(uria)*

**early morning care** AM care

**edema** The swelling of body tissues with water

**ego** The part of the personality dealing with reality; deals with thoughts, feelings, good sense, and problem solving

**ejaculation** The release of semen

**elective surgery** Surgery done by choice to improve the person's life or well-being

**electrical shock** When electrical current passes through the body

**embolus** A blood clot *(thrombus)* that travels through the vascular system until it lodges in a distant blood vessel

**emergency surgery** Surgery done immediately to save life or function

**emotional illness** Mental illness, mental disorder, psychiatric disorder

**enema** The introduction of fluid into the rectum and lower colon

**enteral nutrition** Giving nutrients through the gastrointestinal tract *(enteral)*

**enuresis** Urinary incontinence in bed at night

**epidermal stripping** Removing the epidermis (outer skin layer) as tape is removed from the skin

**episiotomy** An incision *(otomy)* into the perineum

**erectile dysfunction** Impotence

**ergonomics** The science of designing a job to fit the worker

**esteem** The worth, value, or opinion one has of a person

**ethics** Knowledge of what is right conduct and wrong conduct

**evaluation** To measure if goals in the planning step were met; a step in the nursing process

**evening care** HS care or PM care

**evisceration** The separation of the wound along with the protrusion of abdominal organs

**expressive aphasia** Difficulty expressing or sending out thoughts

**expressive-receptive aphasia** Difficulty expressing or sending out thoughts and difficulty receiving information

**extension** Straightening a body part

**external rotation** Turning the joint outward

**fainting** The sudden loss of consciousness from an inadequate blood supply to the brain

**false imprisonment** Unlawful restraint or restriction of a person's freedom of movement

**fecal impaction** The prolonged retention and buildup of feces in the rectum

**fecal incontinence** The inability to control the passage of feces and gas through the anus

**feces** The semi-solid mass of waste products in the colon

**first aid** Emergency care given to an ill or injured person before medical help arrives

**flatulence** The excessive formation of gas in the stomach and intestines

**flatus** Gas or air passed through the anus

**flexion** Bending a body part

**flow rate** The number of drops per minute *(gtt/min)*

**Foley catheter** An indwelling or retention catheter

**footdrop** The foot falls down at the ankle; permanent plantar flexion

**Fowler's position** A semi-sitting position; the head of the bed is raised between 45 and 90 degrees

**fracture** A broken bone

**fraud** Saying or doing something to trick, fool, or deceive a person

**friction** The rubbing of one surface against another

**full-thickness wound** The dermis, epidermis, and subcutaneous tissue are penetrated; muscle and bone may be involved

**full visual privacy** Having the means to be completely free from public view while in bed

**functional incontinence** The person has bladder control but cannot use the toilet in time

**functional nursing** A nursing care pattern focusing on tasks and jobs; each nursing team member has certain tasks and jobs to do

**gait belt** A transfer belt

**gangrene** A condition in which there is death of tissue

**gastrostomy tube** A tube inserted through a surgically created opening *(stomy)* into the stomach *(gastro)*; stomach tube

**gavage** Tube feeding

**general anesthesia** The loss of consciousness and all feeling or sensation

**geriatrics** The branch of medicine concerned with the problems and diseases of old age and older persons; the care of aging people

**germicide** A disinfectant applied to the skin, tissues, or non-living objects

**gerontology** The study of the aging process

**glucosuria** Sugar *(glucos)* in the urine *(uria)*; glycosuria

**glycosuria** Sugar *(glycos)* in the urine *(uria)*; glucosuria

**goal** That which is desired in or by the person as a result of nursing care

**gossip** To spread rumors or talk about the private matters of others

**graduate** A measuring container for fluid

**ground** That which carries leaking electricity to the earth and away from an electrical item

**growth** The physical changes that are measured and that occur in a steady, orderly manner

**guided imagery** Creating and focusing on an image

**hallucination** Seeing, hearing, or feeling something that is not real

**harassment** To trouble, torment, offend, or worry a person by one's behavior or comments

**hazardous substance** Any chemical in the workplace that can cause harm

**health team** Staff members who work together to provide health care

**hearing loss** Difficulty hearing normal conversations

**hematoma** A collection of blood under the skin and tissues

**hematuria** Blood *(hemat)* in the urine *(uria)*

**hemiplegia** Paralysis on one side of the body

**hemoglobin** The substance in red blood cells that carries oxygen and gives blood its color

**hemoptysis** Bloody *(hemo)* sputum *(ptysis* means "to spit")

**hemorrhage** The excessive loss of blood in a short time

**hemothorax** Blood *(hemo)* in the pleural space *(thorax)*

**heterosexual** A person who is attracted to members of the other sex

**hirsutism** Excessive body hair in women and children

**holism** A concept that considers the whole person; the whole person has physical, social, psychological, and spiritual parts that are woven together and cannot be separated

**homosexual** A person who is attracted to members of the same sex

**horizontal recumbent position** The dorsal recumbent position

**hormone** A chemical substance secreted by the glands into the bloodstream

**hospice** A health care agency or program for persons who are dying

**HS care** Care given at bedtime (hour of sleep [HS]); evening care or PM care

**hyperextension** Excessive straightening of a body part

**hyperglycemia** High *(hyper)* sugar *(glyc)* in the blood *(emia)*

**hypertension** Blood pressure measurements that remain above *(hyper)* a systolic pressure of 140 mm Hg or diastolic pressure of 90 mm Hg

**hyperthermia** A body temperature *(thermia)* that is much higher *(hyper)* than the person's normal range

**hyperventilation** Respirations are rapid *(hyper)* and deeper than normal

**hypoglycemia** Low *(hypo)* sugar *(glyc)* in the blood *(emia)*

**hypotension** When the systolic blood pressure is below *(hypo)* 90 mm Hg and the diastolic pressure is below 60 mm Hg

**hypothermia** A very low *(hypo)* body temperature *(thermia)*

**hypoventilation** Respirations are slow *(hypo)*, shallow, and sometimes irregular

**hypoxemia** A reduced amount *(hypo)* of oxygen *(ox)* in the blood *(emia)*

**hypoxia** Cells do not have enough *(hypo)* oxygen *(oxia)*

**id** The part of the personality at the unconscious level; concerned with pleasure

**ileostomy** A surgically created opening *(stomy)* between the ileum (small intestine [*ileo*]) and the abdominal wall

**immunity** Protection against a disease or condition; the person will not get or be affected by the disease

**implementation** To perform or carry out measures in the care plan; a step in the nursing process

**impotence** The inability of the male to have an erection; erectile dysfunction

**incision** An open wound with clean, straight edges; usually intentionally made with a sharp instrument

**indwelling catheter** A catheter left in the bladder so urine drains constantly into a drainage bag; retention or Foley catheter

**infancy** The first year of life

**infected wound** A wound containing large amounts of microbes and that shows signs of infection; a dirty wound

**infection** A disease resulting from the invasion and growth of microbes in the body

**insomnia** A chronic condition in which the person cannot sleep or stay asleep all night

**intake** The amount of fluid taken in

**intentional wound** A wound created for therapy

**internal rotation** Turning the joint inward

**intravenous (IV) therapy** Giving fluids through a needle or catheter inserted into a vein; IV, IV therapy, and IV infusion

**intubation** Inserting an artificial airway

**invasion of privacy** Violating a person's right not to have his or her name, picture, or private affairs exposed or made public without giving consent

**involuntary seclusion** Separating a person from others against his or her will; keeping the person confined to a certain area or away from his or her room without consent

**jejunostomy tube** A tube inserted into the intestines through a surgically created opening *(stomy)* into the middle part of the small intestine *(jejunum)*

**job description** A list of responsibilities and functions the agency expects you to perform

**Kardex** A type of card file that summarizes information found in the medical record—drugs, treatments, diagnosis, routine care measures, equipment, and special needs

**ketone** Acetone; ketone body

**ketone body** Acetone; ketone

**knee-chest position** The person kneels and rests the body on the knees and chest; head is turned to one side, arms are above the head or flexed at the elbows, back is straight, and body is flexed about 90 degrees at the hips

**Kussmaul respirations** Very deep and rapid respirations

**laceration** An open wound with torn tissues and jagged edges

**laryngeal mirror** An instrument used to examine the mouth, teeth, and throat

**lateral** At the side of the body or body part

**lateral position** The side-lying position

**law** A rule of conduct made by a government body

**libel** Making false statements in print, writing, or through pictures or drawings

**licensed practical nurse (LPN)** A nurse who has completed a 1-year nursing program and has passed a licensing test; called *licensed vocational nurse (LVN)* in some states

**licensed vocational nurse (LVN)** Licensed practical nurse

**lithotomy position** The person lies on the back with the hips at the edge of the exam table, knees are flexed, hips are externally rotated, and feet are in stirrups

**local anesthesia** The loss of feeling or sensation in a small area

**lochia** The vaginal discharge that occurs after childbirth

**logrolling** Turning the person as a unit, in alignment, with one motion

**malignant tumor** A tumor that grows fast and invades other tissues; cancer

**malpractice** Negligence by a professional person

**mechanical ventilation** Using a machine to move air into and out of the lungs

**medial** At or near the middle or midline of the body or body part

**medical asepsis** Practices used to remove or destroy pathogens and to prevent their spread from one person or place to another person or place; clean technique

**medical diagnosis** The identification of a disease or condition by a doctor

**medical record** A written account of a person's condition and response to treatment and care; chart

**medication reminder** Reminding the person to take drugs, observing them being taken as prescribed, and charting that they were taken

**melena** A black, tarry stool

**menarche** The first menstruation and the start of menstrual cycles

**menopause** The time when menstruation stops and menstrual cycles end

**menstruation** The process in which the lining of the uterus breaks up and is discharged from the body through the vagina

**mental** Relating to the mind; something that exists in the mind or is done by the mind

**mental disorder** Mental illness, emotional illness, psychiatric disorder

**mental health** The person copes with and adjusts to everyday stresses in ways accepted by society

**mental illness** A disturbance in the ability to cope or adjust to stress; behavior and function are impaired; mental disorder, emotional illness, psychiatric disorder

**metabolism** The burning of food for heat and energy by the cells

**metastasis** The spread of cancer to other body parts

**microbe** A microorganism

**microorganism** A small *(micro)* living plant or animal *(organism)* seen only with a microscope; a microbe

**micturition** Urination or voiding

**morning care** Care given after breakfast; hygiene measures are more thorough at this time

**nasal speculum** An instrument used to examine the inside of the nose

**nasogastric (NG) tube** A tube inserted through the nose *(naso)* into the stomach *(gastro)*

**nasointestinal tube** A tube inserted through the nose *(naso)* into the small intestine *(intestinal)*

**need** Something necessary or desired for maintaining life and mental well-being

**negligence** An unintentional wrong in which a person fails to act in a reasonable and careful manner and causes harm to a person or to the person's property

**nocturia** Frequent urination *(uria)* at night *(noct)*

**non-pathogen** A microbe that does not usually cause an infection

**nonverbal communication** Communication that does not use words

**normal flora** Microbes that live and grow in a certain area

**nosocomial infection** An infection acquired during a stay in a health agency

**NREM sleep** The phase of sleep when there is *no rapid eye movement;* non-REM sleep

**nursing assistant** A person who gives basic nursing care under the supervision of an RN or LPN/LVN

**nursing care plan** A written guide about the person's care

**nursing diagnosis** Describes a health problem that can be treated by nursing measures; a step in the nursing process

**nursing intervention** An action or measure taken by the nursing team to help the person reach a goal

**nursing process** The method RNs use to plan and deliver nursing care; its five steps are assessment, nursing diagnosis, planning, implementation, and evaluation

**nursing team** The individuals who provide nursing care—RNs, LPNs/LVNs, and nursing assistants

**nutrient** A substance that is ingested, digested, absorbed, and used by the body

**nutrition** The processes involved in the ingestion, digestion, absorption, and use of foods and fluids by the body

**objective data** Information that is seen, heard, felt, or smelled; signs

**observation** Using the senses of sight, hearing, touch, and smell to collect information

**obsession** A recurrent, unwanted thought or idea

**obstetrics** The branch of medicine concerned with the care of women during pregnancy, labor, and childbirth and for the 6 to 8 weeks after birth

**old** Persons between 75 and 84 years of age

**old-old** Persons 85 years of age and older

**oliguria** Scant amount (olig) of urine (uria); less than 500 ml in 24 hours

**ombudsman** Someone who supports or promotes the needs and interests of another person

**open fracture** The broken bone has come through the skin; compound fracture

**open wound** The skin or mucous membrane is broken

**ophthalmoscope** A lighted instrument used to examine the internal structures of the eye

**oral hygiene** Mouth care

**organ** Groups of tissues with the same function

**orthopnea** Breathing (pnea) deeply and comfortably only when sitting (ortho)

**orthopneic position** Sitting up (ortho) and leaning over a table to breathe

**orthostatic hypotension** Abnormally low (hypo) blood pressure when the person suddenly stands up (ortho and static); postural hypotension

**ostomy** A surgically created artificial opening

**otoscope** A lighted instrument used to examine the external ear and the eardrum (tympanic membrane)

**output** The amount of fluid lost

**overflow incontinence** Urine leaks when the bladder is too full

**oxygen concentration** The amount (percent) of hemoglobin containing oxygen

**pack** A treatment that involves wrapping a body part with a wet or dry application

**pain** To ache, hurt, or be sore; discomfort

**panic** An intense and sudden feeling of fear, anxiety, terror or dread

**paranoia** A disorder (para) of the mind (noia); false beliefs (delusions) and suspicion about a person or situation

**paraphrasing** Restating the person's message in your own words

**paraplegia** Paralysis from the waist down

**partial-thickness wound** The dermis and epidermis of the skin are broken

**passive physical restraint** A restraint near but not directly attached to the person's body; it does not totally restrict freedom of movement and allows access to certain body parts

**pathogen** A microbe that is harmful and can cause an infection

**patient-focused care** A nursing care pattern; services are moved from departments to the bedside

**pediatrics** The branch of medicine concerned with the growth, development, and care of children; they range in age from the newborn to teenagers

**pediculosis (lice)** Infestation with lice

**pediculosis capitis** Infestation of the scalp (capitis) with lice

**pediculosis corporis** Infestation of the body (corporis) with lice

**pediculosis pubis** Infestation of the pubic (pubis) hair with lice

**penetrating wound** An open wound in which the skin and underlying tissues are pierced

**percussion hammer** An instrument used to tap body parts to test reflexes; reflex hammer

**percutaneous endoscopic gastrostomy (PEG) tube** A tube inserted into the stomach *(gastro)* through a stab or puncture wound *(stomy)* made through *(per)* the skin *(cutaneous)*; a lighted instrument *(scope)* allows the doctor to see inside a body cavity or organ *(endo)*

**pericare** Perineal care

**perineal care** Cleaning the genital and anal areas; pericare

**peristalsis** Involuntary muscle contractions in the digestive system that move food through the alimentary canal; the alternating contraction and relaxation of intestinal muscles

**personality** The set of attitudes, values, behaviors, and traits of a person

**phantom pain** Pain felt in a body part that is no longer there

**phobia** Fear, panic, or dread

**planning** Setting priorities and goals; a step in the nursing process

**plantar flexion** The foot *(plantar)* is bent *(flexion)*; bending the foot down at the ankle

**plaque** A thin film that sticks to the teeth; it contains saliva, microbes, and other substances

**plastic drawsheet** A drawsheet placed between the bottom sheet and the cotton drawsheet to protect the mattress and bottom linens from dampness and soiling; waterproof drawsheet

**pleural effusion** The escape and collection of fluid *(effusion)* in the pleural space

**PM care** HS care or evening care

**pneumothorax** Air *(pneumo)* in the pleural space *(thorax)*

**pollutant** A harmful chemical or substance in the air or water

**polyuria** Abnormally large amounts *(poly)* of urine *(uria)*

**posterior** Dorsal

**postmortem** After *(post)* death *(mortem)*

**postoperative** After surgery

**postpartum** After *(post)* childbirth *(partum)*

**postural hypotension** Orthostatic hypotension

**posture** Body alignment

**preceptor** A staff member who guides another staff member

**prefix** A word element placed before a root; it changes the meaning of the word

**preoperative** Before surgery

**pressure sore** A bedsore, decubitus ulcer, or pressure ulcer

**pressure ulcer** Any injury caused by unrelieved pressure; decubitus ulcer, bedsore, or pressure sore

**primary caregiver** The person mainly responsible for providing or assisting with the child's basic needs

**primary nursing** A nursing care pattern; an RN is responsible for the person's total care

**pronation** Turning the joint downward

**prone position** Lying on the abdomen with the head turned to one side

**prosthesis** An artificial replacement for a missing body part

**proximal** The part nearest to the center or to the point of origin

**pseudodementia** False *(pseudo)* dementia

**psychiatric disorder** Mental illness, mental disorder, emotional illness

**psychiatry** The branch of medicine concerned with mental health problems

**psychosis** A state of severe mental impairment

**puberty** The period when reproductive organs begin to function and secondary sex characteristics appear

**pulse** The beat of the heart felt at an artery as a wave of blood passes through the artery

**pulse deficit** The difference between the apical and radial pulse rates

**pulse rate** The number of heartbeats or pulses felt in 1 minute

**puncture wound** An open wound made by a sharp object; entry of the skin and underlying tissues may be intentional or unintentional

**purulent drainage** Thick green, yellow, or brown drainage

**quadriplegia** Paralysis from the neck down

**radiating pain** Pain felt at the site of tissue damage and in nearby areas

**range of motion (ROM)** The movement of a joint to the extent possible without causing pain

**receptive aphasia** Difficulty receiving information

**recording** The written account of care and observations

**reflex** An involuntary movement

**reflex incontinence** The loss of urine at predictable intervals when the bladder is full

**regional anesthesia** The loss of feeling or sensation in a large area of the body

**registered nurse (RN)** A nurse who has completed a 2-, 3-, or 4-year nursing program and has passed a licensing test

**regurgitation** The backward flow of food from the stomach into the mouth

**rehabilitation** The process of restoring the person to the highest possible level of physical, psychological, social, and economic function

**reincarnation** The belief that the spirit or soul is reborn in another human body or in another form of life

**relaxation** To be free from mental and physical stress

**religion** Spiritual beliefs, needs, and practices

**REM sleep** The phase of sleep when there is *rapid eye movement*

**reporting** The oral account of care and observations

**reservoir** The environment in which a microbe lives and grows

**respiration** The process of supplying the cells with oxygen and removing carbon dioxide from them; breathing air into (inhalation) and out of (exhalation) the lungs

**respiratory arrest** When breathing stops; breathing stops but heart action continues for several minutes

**respiratory depression** Slow, weak respirations at a rate of fewer than 12 per minute

**responsibility** The duty or obligation to perform some act or function

**rest** To be calm, at ease, and relaxed; no anxiety and stress

**restorative aide** A nursing assistant with special training in restorative nursing and rehabilitation skills

**restorative nursing care** Care that helps persons regain their health, strength, and independence

**restraint** Any item, object, device, garment, material, or drug that limits or restricts a person's freedom of movement or access to one's body

**retention catheter** A Foley or indwelling catheter

**reverse Trendelenburg's position** The head of the bed is raised, and the foot of the bed is lowered

**rigor mortis** The stiffness or rigidity (*rigor*) of skeletal muscles that occurs after death (*mortis*)

**root** A word element containing the basic meaning of the word

**rotation** Turning the joint

**sanguineous drainage** Bloody drainage (*sanguis*)

**seizure** The violent and sudden contractions or tremors of muscle groups; convulsion

**self-actualization** Experiencing one's potential

**self-esteem** Thinking well of oneself and seeing oneself as useful and having value

**semi-Fowler's position** The head of the bed is raised 30 degrees; or the head of the bed is raised 30 degrees, and the knee portion is raised 15 degrees

**serosanguineous drainage** Thin, watery drainage (*sero*) that is blood-tinged (*sanguineous*)

**serous drainage** Clear, watery fluid (*serum*)

**service plan** A written plan listing the services needed by the person and who provides them

**sex** Physical activities involving the reproductive organs; done for pleasure or to have children

**sexuality** The physical, psychological, social, cultural, and spiritual factors that affect a person's feelings and attitudes about his or her sex

**shearing** When skin sticks to a surface while muscles slide in the direction the body is moving

**shock** Results when organs and tissues do not get enough blood

**side-lying position** The lateral position

**signs** Objective data

**simple fracture** Closed fracture

**Sims' position** A left side-lying position in which the upper leg is sharply flexed so it is not on the lower leg and the lower arm is behind the person

**skin tear** A break or rip in the skin; the epidermis separates from the underlying tissues

**slander** Making false statements orally

**sleep** A state of unconsciousness, reduced voluntary muscle activity, and lowered metabolism

**spastic** Uncontrolled contractions of skeletal muscles

**sphygmomanometer** A cuff and measuring device used to measure blood pressure

**spore** A bacterium protected by a hard shell

**sputum** Mucus from the respiratory system that is expectorated (expelled) through the mouth

**standard of care** The skills, care, and judgment required by the health team member under similar conditions

**stasis ulcer** An open wound on the lower legs and feet cause by poor blood return through the veins; venous ulcer

**sterile** The absence of *all* microbes

**sterile field** A work area free of *all* pathogens and non-pathogens (including spores)

**sterile technique** Surgical asepsis

**sterilization** The process of destroying *all* microbes

**stethoscope** An instrument used to listen to the sounds produced by the heart, lungs, and other body organs

**stoma** An opening; see *colostomy* and *ileostomy*

**stomatitis** Inflammation *(itis)* of the mouth *(stomat)*

**stool** Excreted feces

**straight catheter** A catheter that drains the bladder and then is removed

**stress** The response or change in the body caused by any emotional, physical, social, or economic factor

**stress incontinence** When urine leaks during exercise and certain movements

**stressor** The event or factor that causes stress

**subconscious** Memory, past experiences, and thoughts of which the person is not aware; they are easily recalled

**subjective data** Things a person tells you about that you cannot observe through your senses; symptoms

**suction** The process of withdrawing or sucking up fluid *(secretions)*

**suffix** A word element placed after a root; it changes the meaning of the word

**suffocation** When breathing stops from the lack of oxygen

**sundowning** Signs, symptoms, and behaviors of AD increase during hours of darkness

**superego** The part of the personality concerned with right and wrong

**supination** Turning the joint upward

**supine position** The back-lying or dorsal recumbent position

**suppository** A cone-shaped, solid drug that is inserted into a body opening; it melts at body temperature

**surgical asepsis** The practices that keep items free of *all* microbes; sterile technique

**symptoms** Subjective data

**syncope** A brief loss of consciousness; fainting

**system** Organs that work together to perform special functions

**systole** The period of heart muscle contraction; the period when the heart is pumping

**systolic pressure** The amount of force needed to pump blood out of the heart into the arterial circulation

**tachycardia** A rapid *(tachy)* heart rate *(cardia);* more than 100 beats per minute

**tachypnea** Rapid *(tachy)* breathing *(pnea);* respirations are 24 or more per minute

**tartar** Hardened plaque

**task** A function, procedure, activity, or work that does not require an RN's professional knowledge or judgment

**team nursing** A nursing care pattern; a team of nursing staff is led by an RN who decides the amount and kind of care each person needs

**terminal illness** An illness or injury for which there is no reasonable expectation of recovery

**thrombus** A blood clot

**tinnitus** Ringing in the ears

**tissue** A group of cells with similar functions

**tort** A wrong committed against a person or the person's property

**transfer** Moving a person from one room or nursing unit to another

**transfer belt** A belt used to support persons who are unsteady or disabled; a gait belt

**transsexual** A person who believes that he or she is a member of the other sex

**transvestite** A person who becomes sexually excited by dressing in the clothes of the other sex

**trauma** An accident or violent act that injures the skin, mucous membranes, bones, and internal organs

**Trendelenburg's position** The head of the bed is lowered, and the foot of the bed is raised

**tumor** A new growth of abnormal cells; tumors are benign or malignant

**tuning fork** An instrument vibrated to test hearing

**umbilical cord** The structure that carries blood, oxygen, and nutrients from the mother to the fetus

**unconscious** Experiences and feelings that cannot be recalled

**unintentional wound** A wound resulting from trauma

**ureterostomy** The surgical creation of an artificial opening *(stomy)* between the ureter *(uretero)* and the abdomen

**urge incontinence** The loss of urine in response to a sudden, urgent need to void; the person cannot get to a toilet in time

**urgent surgery** Surgery needed for the person's health; it is done soon to prevent further damage or disease

**urinary frequency** Voiding at frequent intervals

**urinary incontinence** The loss of bladder control

**urinary urgency** The need to void at once

**urination** The process of emptying urine from the bladder; micturition or voiding

**vaccination** The administration of a vaccine to produce immunity against an infectious disease

**vaccine** A preparation containing dead or weakened microbes

**vaginal speculum** An instrument used to open the vagina so it and the cervix can be examined

**vascular ulcer** A circulatory ulcer

**vein** A blood vessel that carries blood back to the heart

**venous ulcer** A stasis ulcer

**ventral** Anterior

**verbal communication** Communication that uses written or spoken words

**vertigo** Dizziness

**vital signs** Temperature, pulse, respirations, and blood pressure

**voiding** Urination or micturition

**will** A legal statement of how a person wants property distributed after death

**word element** A part of a word

**work ethics** Behavior in the workplace

**workplace violence** Violent acts (including assault or threat of assault) directed toward persons at work or while on duty

**wound** A break in the skin or mucous membrane

**young-old** Persons between 65 and 74 years of age

# INDEX